PATHOPHYSIOLOGY
Clinical Concepts of Disease Processes

PATHOPHYSIOLOGY
Clinical Concepts of Disease Processes

Sylvia Anderson Price, R.N., B.S., M.P.H.
Lorraine McCarty Wilson, R.N., B.S., M.S.

Assistant Professors of Nursing
University of Michigan–Ann Arbor

McGraw-Hill Book Company
New York   St. Louis   San Francisco   Auckland   Bogotá   Düsseldorf
Johannesburg   London   Madrid   Mexico   Montreal   New Delhi
Panama   Paris   São Paulo   Singapore   Sydney   Tokyo   Toronto

NOTICE

Medicine is an ever-changing science. As new research and clinical experience broaden our knowledge, changes in treatment and drug therapy are required. The editors and the publisher of this work have made every effort to ensure that the drug dosage schedules herein are accurate and in accord with the standards accepted at the time of publication. Readers are advised, however, to check the product information sheet included in the package of each drug they plan to administer to be certain that changes have not been made in the recommended dose or in the contraindications for administration. This recommendation is of particular importance in regard to new or infrequently used drugs.

Library of Congress Cataloging in Publication Data
Main entry under title:

Pathophysiology.

  Includes index.
  1. Physiology, Pathological.   2.   Nursing.
I.   Price, Sylvia Anderson.   II.   Wilson, Lorraine McCarty.
RB113.P363   616.07   77-13124
ISBN 0-07-050857-7

PATHOPHYSIOLOGY
Clinical Concepts of Disease Processes

2 3 4 5 6 7 8 9 0   HDHD   7 8 3 2 1 0 9 8

This book was set in Optima by Monotype Composition Company, Inc.
The editors were Orville W. Haberman, Jr., and Henry C. De Leo;
the designer was Barbara Ellwood;
the production supervisor was Robert C. Pedersen.
Photographs were taken by Edward Sherman and Wendell Rideout.
The illustrations were done by Margaret Croup Brudon.
Halliday Lithograph Corporation was printer and binder.

CONTENTS

LIST OF CONTRIBUTORS

Gerald D. Abrams, M.D.
Professor of Pathology
Department of Pathology
University of Michigan
Medical School

Daniel J. Fall, M.D.
Clinical Assistant Professor
of Internal Medicine
University of Michigan

Penny J. Ford, R.N., M.S.
Cardiovascular Clinical
Nurse Specialist
Doctoral Candidate at
Teacher's College
Columbia University

Cathy M. Idema, R.N., M.P.H.
Head Nurse, Community Health Nursing
University of Michigan

Marie Trava King, R.N., B.S.N., M.S.N.
St. Joseph's School of Nursing
Baltimore, Maryland

Mary Carter Lombardo, R.N., M.S.N.
Neurology Clinical
Nurse Specialist
Baltimore, Maryland

Larry S. Matthews, M.D.
Associate Professor of Surgery
Section of Orthopaedic Surgery
University of Michigan
Medical School

Sylvia Anderson Price, R.N., B.S., M.P.H.
Assistant Professor of Nursing
Former Coordinator of Pathophysiology Course
University of Michigan

David E. Schteingart, M.D.
Professor of Internal Medicine
University of Michigan
Medical School

William R. Solomon, M.D.
Associate Professor of Internal Medicine
University of Michigan
Medical School

Kenneth A. Stoutenborough, M.D.
Clinical Assistant Professor
Department of Internal Medicine
Michigan State University
College of Human Medicine
Blodgett and St. Mary Hospitals
Grand Rapids, Michigan

Lorraine McCarty Wilson, R.N., B.S., M.S.
Assistant Professor of Nursing
Coordinator of Pathophysiology Course
University of Michigan

PREFACE

Human pathophysiology is the science that focuses on the illnesses of humans. It is the study of disease, or "lack of ease." *Disease* refers to a state characterized by certain alterations in the body; alterations that presumably involve structure even though that structure may be microscopic. However, disease should not be regarded as a static state. Disease itself is a dynamic process. It is an abnormal form of life. Disease may be acute or insidious in its onset, variable in its duration, and it results in either the recovery (partial or complete) or death of the person.

Pathophysiology emphasizes the *dynamic* aspects of disease. It is concerned with the disruption of normal physiology; with the alterations, derangements, and mechanisms involved in disruption and how they manifest themselves as signs, symptoms, physical, and laboratory findings. Pathophysiology provides the basic link between the sciences of anatomy, physiology, and biochemistry and its application to clinical practice. The study of pathophysiology is essential to understanding the rationale for medical and surgical therapy.

In preparing this text on pathophysiology for health professionals, we are aware that the rapid accumulation of knowledge in the biomedical sciences poses a problem not only for the student but for the practitioner as well. The student must master clinically significant facts and must be prepared to continue learning as a practitioner. The role of the practitioner in the health care delivery system is also changing. Nurses and other health professionals are working more independently and they are assuming a more collaborative role with other practitioners. It is important for these practitioners to understand why certain manifestations of disease occur and why specific therapeutic regimens are prescribed. Therefore, we designed this book to meet the above objectives.

The uniqueness of this book is that the subject is presented in a self-instructional format. Objectives have been given for each part and chapter. These objectives focus the student's attention on the important concepts in the subject. Conceptual material is followed by questions and answers on the content presented. The answers give the student additional insight. This self-instructional method enables the student to actively participate in the learning process through reading, reasoning, and demonstrating in writing his or her mastery of the concepts. Active participation in the learning process is enhanced by this approach which also requires the student to apply concepts and not to merely memorize factual material. The authors believe that this method enables one to achieve maximum understanding of the subject material. In addition, the pace may be one that the student finds most comfortable.

Since numerous subject areas are involved, we have incorporated selected areas into what is referred to as "core" content. Our selection is based on areas where we feel in-depth coverage of the subject is deficient.

The subject is presented in the following fashion. First, the general concepts of disease are discussed. Additional parts examine the various disorders of an organ or organ system. Emphasis is placed on understanding the roots of a given disorder, which is an essential factor in the development of insight. For example, consider diseases of the kidney. The student who thoroughly understands the nephron, which is the fundamental work unit of the kidney, is better able to predict what diseases will occur when certain pathophysiological processes involve the kidney. That student will understand the basis for such diseases as pyelonephritis, glomerulonephritis, and the nephroses. Also, the student will understand the symptomatology and the rationale for the treatment.

In attempting to provide a text for the sophisticated learning needs of today's health professionals, the material is discussed in greater depth than is found in similar pathophysiology texts. In order to reduce the subject matter to manageable dimensions, the authors have focused on relevant concepts that are applicable to optimum practices of modern health care delivery.

ACKNOWLEDGMENTS

Our sincere appreciation:

To Margaret Croup Brudon, an outstanding medical illustrator whose work was consistently excellent and creative and was most gracious in making accommodations when necessary.

To Cathy Dilworth Somer, former Nursing Editor at McGraw-Hill Book Company, who encouraged and gave us support for the initial project.

To Orville W. Haberman Jr., Nursing Editor and Mary Ann Linder, Assistant to the Editor at McGraw-Hill Book Company, for their support, encouragement and dedication to the completion of this tremendous undertaking.

To Gary A. Snyder, Field Representative, McGraw-Hill Book Company, College Division, for his suggestion of the title which captures the essence of this book.

To Anne Marie Pizzuti and Paula Wilson Saari, formerly our teaching assistants in Pathophysiology who conscientiously reviewed the manuscript and made many valuable suggestions.

To David and Ann Wilson for their assistance in the translation of ideas into sketches.

To the Community-Based BSN Program Special Project Grant, School of Nursing, The University of Michigan for granting permission to use portions of the pathophysiology materials prepared through that grant in the preparation of this text.

To The University of Michigan Independent Study Unit for granting permission to use the histology slides from the program by Lorraine Wilson and Sylvia Price, *Normal Renal Function and Renal Pathophysiology* (35-mm slide program), Ann Arbor, 1975.

To Myrna K. Hendricks, Mary Plummer, and Virginia Hinderer for the excellent quality of their work in typing the manuscript.

We also appreciate the review and suggestions on selected portions of the manuscript offered by the following: Giles Bole, Nancy F. Creason, Shirley Duggan, Nancy M. Janz, Martin J. Nemiroff, Phyllis Coindreau Patterson, Roseann Rich, Jacquelyn Smith, Joanne F. Timm, and Nina H. Williams.

Sylvia Anderson Price
Lorraine McCarty Wilson

PATHOPHYSIOLOGY
Clinical Concepts of Disease Processes

PART I Introduction to General Pathology: Mechanisms of Disease

GERALD D. ABRAMS

The intent of Part I of the text is to provide the reader with the background necessary for the understanding of the many different diseases to which human beings fall victim. The number of specific human diseases is immense, and the variety is great, given the fact that no organ or organ system within the body is exempt from disease. However, the basic ways in which an organ can become diseased are quite limited, and the large and bewildering array of diseases actually represents different combinations and permutations of a smaller number of basic biological processes leading to the alterations of structure and function that are recognized clinically. It is on these basic biological processes that this first section will be focused.

The study of such basic disease processes is usually called *general pathology*. Pathology is the science or study of disease. In its broadest sense, pathology is literally abnormal biology, the study of sick or disordered life. As a basic biological science, the study of pathology includes such fields as plant pathology, insect pathology, and veterinary and comparative pathology, as well as human pathology, which is the major focus of this text.

Pathology, in the context of human medicine, is not only a basic or theoretical science but also a clinical medical specialty. Pathologists are specialists in laboratory medicine, providing a consultative service to other physicians, thereby assisting in the diagnosis and treatment of disease. The scope of laboratory medicine is such as to include all of the many types of studies performed on samples derived from patients, including samples of tissue, blood, and other body fluids. Some laboratory studies which fall under the general heading of "anatomic pathology" involve the study and assessment of morphologic alterations in cells and tissues. Surgical pathology, exfoliative cytology, and autopsy pathology are included in this division. Many types of studies are done by other than morphologic means, and these areas of "clinical pathology" include such things as clinical chemistry, microbiology, hematology, immunology, and immunohematology.

In this part the specifics of individual diseases will not be discussed. However, fundamental disease processes, such as inflammation, neoplasia, and immunologic injury, will be described. Following the elucidation of these fundamental processes, the details of specific illnesses will be addressed in later parts of the text.

OBJECTIVES

At the end of Part I you will be able to:

1 Describe the essential features of basic disease processes including the body's reactions to injury and infection, the immune response, disturbances of circulation, and abnormalities of cellular growth.

2 Interpret the natural history and clinical manifestations of specific illnesses in terms of their etiology and pathogenesis.

CHAPTER 1 General Concepts of Disease— Health vs. Disease

OBJECTIVES   **At the completion of Chap. 1 you should be able to:**

1 Define *pathology*.

2 Distinguish between anatomic and clinical pathology.

3 Explain the concept of normalcy.

4 Describe the essential components involved in the disease process.

5 Differentiate between etiology and pathogenesis in relation to disease.

6 Identify and use the following terms when describing the manifestations of a disease: symptom, sign, lesion, sequel, complication.

CONCEPT OF NORMALCY

In terms of their personal experiences, most people have some notion of what it is to be "normal" and would define disease or illness in terms of deviation from or absence of that normal state. However, on closer scrutiny, the concept of normalcy turns out to be a complex one which cannot be defined succinctly; and correspondingly, the concept of disease is far from simple.

Selecting any parameter of measurement which might be applied to an individual or group of individuals, we define *normal* as some sort of average value for that parameter. Thus, average values for parameters such as height, weight, and blood pressure are derived from observations on many individuals. Implicitly, a certain amount of variation from the average is accepted as being permissible or normal. Thus, the usual concept of normalcy involves both an average value and some range of variation either above or below that value.

Variation in normal values actually stems from several different sources. First, it is recognized that individuals differ from one another because of differences in their genetic makeup. Thus, no two individuals in the world, except for those derived from the same fertilized ovum, have exactly the same genes. Then, there is variation related to the fact that individuals differ in their life experiences and in their interaction with the environment. Third, even in a single individual, many physiologic parameters vary because of the way in which the control mechanisms of the body function. For instance, measurement of blood glucose concentrations in a healthy person would reveal significant variations at different times during the day, depending upon food intake, activities of the individual, and so forth. These variations would generally occur within a certain range. The situation is somewhat analogous to a room with thermostatically controlled temperature which may dip slightly below the desired or ideal level before such a drop is sensed by the thermostat. The corrective action then triggered by the thermostat may, in turn, overshoot the ideal slightly before the heat input is halted. Indeed such variations in body temperature, even in the normal state, do occur in all individuals. Finally, for those physiologic parameters that must be measured by fairly intricate means, a significant amount of variation in observed values may be derived from error or imprecision inherent in the measurement process itself.

Because of the above considerations, establishing limits on this "normal" range of variation from an average value is a matter of some complexity. This complexity relates to such things as knowing the degree of physiologic oscillation of a particular measurement, accounting for the degree of variation among normal individuals even under baseline conditions, and figuring the precision of the measurement method. Then, finally, the biological significance of the measurement must be estimated. It is thus evident that single measurements, observations, or laboratory results which seem to be indicative of abnormality must always be judged in the context of the entire individual. A single reading of elevated blood pressure does not make an individual hypertensive; a single slightly elevated blood glucose level does not relegate an individual to the category of diabetics; and a single hemoglobin value lower than average does not necessarily indicate anemia.

Finally, to place all of the above considerations in perspective, it should be noted that concepts of normalcy and even disease are, to an extent, arbitrary and are influenced by cultural values as well as by biological realities. For example, in our culture, a defect of central nervous system function manifesting itself as a significant reading disability would be labeled as an abnormality, whereas the same defect might never be noted in a primitive culture. Furthermore, a trait which might be average and thus normal in one population might be considered distinctly abnormal in another. Consider, for instance, how a "normal" person from our population would be viewed by a group of central African pygmies; or conversely, how an infant from a primitive culture, with the "normal" chronic diarrhea and poor weight gain might be viewed in one of our well-baby clinics!

CONCEPT OF DISEASE

Bearing in mind these nuances in the concept of normalcy, disease can be defined as a form of life beyond the limits of normal. The most useful yardstick of these limits of normal relates to the ability of the individual to meet the demands placed on the body, to adapt to these demands or changes in the external environment in order to maintain reasonable constancy of the internal environment. All cells in the body need a certain amount of oxygen and nutrients for their continuing survival and function and also require an environment which affords such things as narrow ranges of temperature, water content, acidity, and salt concentration. Thus, the maintenance of internal constancy is an essential feature of the normal body. When some of the structures and functions of the body deviate from the norm to the point that this constancy is destroyed or threatened or that the individual can no longer meet environmental challenges, disease is said to exist.

Another important element in the concept of disease is the recognition that disease does not involve the development of a completely new form of life but rather is an extension or distortion of the normal life processes that are present in the individual. Even in the case of an obviously infectious disease, where the body is literally invaded, the infectious agent itself does not constitute the disease but only serves to evoke the changes in the subject that ultimately are manifested as disease. Thus, disease is actually the sum of the physiological processes which have been distorted. In order to understand and adequately treat the disease one must take into account the identity of the normal processes interfered with, the character of the disturbances, and the secondary effects of such disturbances on other vital processes.

An alternative view of disease, certainly not unknown in history, holds that disease is actually a new form of life, a sort of possession of the body by an outside agent. From this notion it would follow that some form of exorcism, which is directed at driving out that agent, is proper therapy of disease. However, even in the instance of an invasive infectious agent, attempted treatment with antibiotics alone may not be sufficient to cure the patient if proper attention is not directed toward the intrinsic bodily processes.

A theme that will recur, with variations, throughout this volume is that disease above all is part and parcel of the patient. *Normal and abnormal processes represent different points on the same continuous spectrum.* In other words, the seeds of disease actually lie within the adaptive machinery of the body itself. The very same machinery which allows us to become immune to certain infections evokes reactions such as hay fever and asthma when some of us are challenged by certain environmental agents. Similarly, the machinery of cellular proliferation that allows us to repair wounds and constantly to renew cell populations in various tissues may run amok, giving rise to cancer.

THE DEVELOPMENT OF DISEASE

Etiology

Etiology, in its most general definition, is the assignment of causes or reasons for phenomena. A description of the etiology of a disease includes the identification of those causal factors that acting in concert provoke the particular disease. Thus, the tubercle bacillus is designated as the etiologic agent of tuberculosis. Other etiologic factors in the development of tuberculosis which influence the course of the infection include the age, nutritional status, and even the occupation of the individual. It is important enough to repeat that even in the case of an infectious disease such as tuberculosis the agent itself does not constitute the disease. Rather, the resultant of all of the responses to that agent, all of the perversions of biological processes, constitutes the disease. In the etiology of a particular disease, physical, chemical, infectious, or nutritional factors in the environment as well as a variety of intrinsic characteristics of the host may be important.

Pathogenesis

Pathogenesis of a disease refers to the development or evolution of the disease. To continue with the above example, a description of the pathogenesis of tuberculosis would indicate the mechanisms whereby the invasion of the body by the tubercle bacillus ultimately leads to the observed abnormalities.

When considering the totality of human disease, the number of etiologic factors and the number of separately named diseases seem to be endless. However, even though there are many different diseases, the situation is not as difficult as indicated by sheer numbers. The response mechanisms of the body are finite. Therefore, disease A differs from disease B because it varies somewhat in terms of this or that pathogenetic mechanism being exaggerated. Thus, the understanding of a manageable number of pathogenetic mechanisms permits understanding of a very large number of seemingly different diseases.

Manifestations of disease

Early in the development of a disease, the etiologic agent or agents may provoke a number of changes in biological processes which can be detected by laboratory analysis even though there is no recognition by the patient that these changes have occurred. Thus, many diseases have a *subclinical stage* during which the patient functions normally even though the disease processes are well established. It is important to understand that the structure and function of many organs provide a large reserve or safety margin, so that functional impairment may become evident only when disease has become quite advanced anatomically. For example, chronic renal disease could completely destroy one kidney and partly destroy the other before any symptoms related to decreased renal function would be perceived.

As certain biological processes are encroached upon, the patient begins to feel subjectively that something is wrong. These subjective feelings are termed *symptoms* of disease. By definition, symptoms are subjective and can only be reported by the patient to an observer. When, however, the manifestations of the disease involve objectively identifiable aberrations, these are termed *signs* of the disease. Nausea, malaise, and pain are symptoms, while fever, reddening of the skin, and a palpable mass are signs of disease. A demonstrable structural change produced in the course of a disease is referred to as a *lesion*. Lesions may be evident at a gross and/or a microscopic level. The outcome of a disease is sometimes referred to as a *sequel* (plural, *sequelae*). For example, the sequel to an inflammatory process in a given tissue might be a scar in that tissue. The sequel to acute rheumatic inflammation of the heart might be scarred, deformed cardiac valves. A *complication* of disease is a new or separate process that may arise secondarily because of some change produced by

the original entity. For example, bacterial pneumonia may be a complication of viral infection of the respiratory tract.

Finally, it is essential to emphasize that disease is dynamic rather than static. The manifestations of disease in a given patient may change from day to day as biologic equilibriums shift and as compensatory mechanisms are brought into play. Environmental influences that are brought to bear upon the patient will also affect the disease. Every disease has a *range* of manifestations, a *natural history* which varies from patient to patient.

QUESTIONS

General concepts of disease—health vs. disease—Chap. 1

Directions: Answer the following questions on a separate sheet of paper.

1 Define pathology.

2 What is the difference between anatomic and clinical pathology? List at least three examples of types of studies included under each of these divisions.

3 What is the difference between etiology and pathogenesis?

4 Explain the concept of normalcy.

Directions: Circle the letter preceding each item below that correctly answers each question. More than one answer may be correct.

5 In the course of a disease process, an objective clinical finding is termed a:
a Symptom b Sign c Lesion d Sequel
e Complication

6 Which of the following would be considered symptoms?
a Edema b Pallor c Cyanosis d Headaches

CHAPTER 2 Heredity, Environment, and Disease; Interaction of Heredity and Environment

OBJECTIVES   **At the completion of Chap. 2 you should be able to:**

1 Differentiate between extrinsic and intrinsic factors in relation to the disease process.

2 Describe the importance of hereditary factors in disease.

3 Describe how DNA is involved in programming the function of cells.

4 Explain what occurs with regard to DNA during the process of cell division.

5 Describe the process of differentiation.

6 Explain the process by which genes control the development of a particular trait.

7 Define *mutation*.

8 Differentiate between dominant and recessive characters.

9 Explain the ways in which chromosomal abnormalities can develop.

10 Describe the importance of karyotypic anomalies.

11 Identify the way in which genetic abnormalities may be expressed as disease.

12 Discuss the purposes of genetic counseling.

EXTRINSIC FACTORS IN DISEASE

If one were asked to list some of the important causes of human disease, such things as infectious agents, mechanical trauma, toxic chemicals, radiation, extremes of temperature, nutritional problems, and even psychological stress would likely be mentioned. All of these, along with many others usually placed on such a list, actually represent variations in the environment which can produce disease when brought to bear upon the subject. Certainly it is true that such *extrinsic factors* are exceedingly important causes of human misery, and attention is directed to them in an attempt to prevent and alleviate disease. However, since disease is actually part of the life of the afflicted individual—the sum of the physiological processes which have been distorted—a view of disease causation that takes into account only extrinsic factors is necessarily incomplete. The intrinsic

biological processes must also be taken into consideration.

INTRINSIC FACTORS IN DISEASE

Many characteristics of the individual host must be considered as *intrinsic factors* in disease, inasmuch as they will have significant impact on the evolution of various conditions. Age, sex, and even abnormalities acquired in the course of previous illnesses are factors that need to be considered in the pathogenesis of a disease. Above all, the genetic constitution or genome of the individual is an essential part of the "equation." This is true because the anatomic characteristics of the host, the myriad of physiological mechanisms of everyday life, and the modes of responding to injury are all determined by the genetic information assembled at the moment of conception of the individual. A more familiar way of stating this principle is that in studying the biology of disease one must always take into account both heredity and environment.

Interaction of extrinsic and intrinsic factors—a spectrum

One often hears the question, Is this disease hereditary? In a sense, that question is improper and, recognizing that heredity is almost always vitally important, should be phrased, To what extent is heredity important in this disease? The exceptions to this principle are relatively few and quite extreme. Admittedly, heredity plays no real role in determining the outcome when one is involved in an explosion or struck by a speeding truck; but, such instances aside, it is always a factor. Even in an exogenous infectious disease, it is clear that genetic factors can influence susceptibility to the infectious agent and also the pattern of disease produced by that agent.

With regard to the relative balance of heredity and environment in the causation of disease there exists a broad spectrum. At one end of the spectrum are those diseases which are largely determined by some environmental agent irrespective of the individual's hereditary background, while at the other end are those diseases which represent faulty heredity, that is, faulty genetic programming of the body's machinery. These latter diseases include those usually identified as *hereditary diseases*, diseases which are expressed in almost any bearer of the faulty genetic information regardless of extrinsic influences. Between these two ends of the spectrum most human diseases occur and involve a significant interplay between genetic and extrinsic factors. A brief commentary on heredity and an exploration of some of the ways that inherited abnormality can be expressed would be instructive at this point.

THE NATURE OF THE GENOME

The "stuff" of heredity

Deoxyribonucleic acid, or DNA, is the chemical material which is responsible for storing, duplicating, and transmitting literally all of the information needed for programming the function of a given single cell and even of an entire individual. There is an endless variety of ways that the chemical building blocks of DNA can be assembled, so that there are virtually limitless numbers of different kinds of DNA. A given particle of DNA may "instruct" a cell to produce a specific chemical product. To do this, the DNA "tells" the cell what raw materials to select from the passing circulatory stream and how to assemble them into the desired product. Similarly, other kinds of DNA can instruct cells to develop certain kinds of structures. Ultimately it is the DNA that determines exactly how the billions of cells which make up the body are assembled, and, in fact, whether the indi-

vidual will be a dog, a cat, or a human. Portions of the DNA also determine the limits of the individual's stature, the facial features, and a multitude of traits and processes that characterize the individual. Some DNA is even used to control other DNA, by instructing the cell when to "switch on" and use some portion of the DNA information stored in it. Finally, DNA molecules can instruct the cell to make exact duplicates of themselves when the cell is about to divide, ensuring that the genetic information is passed on appropriately to the two daughter cells.

In a nondividing cell, the DNA is found almost entirely within the nucleus. Even with the microscope, individual DNA molecules cannot be seen as distinct structures but only as part of ill-defined, deeply staining material within the nucleus (Fig. 2-1). As the cell begins to divide, the material in the nucleus arranges itself into strands called *chromosomes* (Fig. 2-2). The cells of the human body generally contain 46 chromosomes, or 23 pairs each (22 pairs of autosomes plus 1 pair of sex chromosomes). During the process of cell division the DNA is duplicated, and there is splitting of each chromosome and then a separation of the newly formed structures, so that identically endowed daughter cells are formed. In this fashion, beginning with the fertilized ovum at the moment of conception, identical genetic information is passed to every cell of the developing

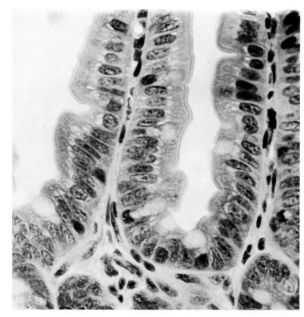

FIGURE 2-1 Nuclei of nondividing cells. The ovoid nuclei of these intestinal lining cells are arranged in regular rows. The DNA that controls the cells is within these nuclei, forming part of the deeply stained material called chromatin. (Photomicrograph, ×800.)

body. As a result of this process in a given individual, a cell of the epidermis will have exactly the same genetic information as a cell within the liver. The reason that a skin cell differs from a liver cell is that in the course of development different portions of the "program" encoded in the DNA have actually been *expressed*. The process by which cells having within them the same genetic information begin to diverge in their structure and function is referred to as *differentiation*.

Within the body there occurs a special kind of cell division which does not involve an even distribution of genetic material to the two daughter cells. This special type of division is involved in the formation of sperm and ova. In these instances, before the finished product is formed, a type of reduction division occurs such that only 23 chromosomes, that is *one* member of each pair, end up in each sperm or ovum. Then, at the moment of conception, the union of the two half-sets of chromosomes produces a fertilized ovum having the proper number of chromosomes, one of each pair from each parent.

The genetic shuffle

The unit of heredity is the *gene,* a portion of DNA that controls the development of a particular trait, ultimately by specifying the production of some chemical product within the cells of the body. Any given chromosome contains a tremendous number of genes which are arranged so that genes controlling a particular trait are located on a specific position (locus) on a definite chromosome pair. Of a given pair of chromosomes in the somatic cells of an individual, one is derived from

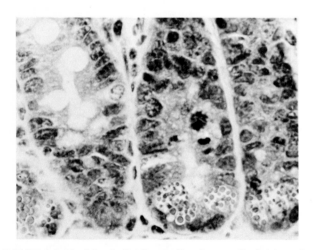

FIGURE 2-2 Nuclei of dividing cells. As a cell divides, the nuclear material is arranged in strands called chromosomes. The starlike figure to the right of center is a cluster of chromosomes in a dividing cell. Just below this is a pair of horizontally oriented dark masses which actually represent masses of chromosomes dividing into two daughter cells. (Photomicrograph, ×800.)

each parent, and, correspondingly, at a specified position on the chromosomes is a pair of genes, one gene from each parent. Tremendous genetic variability from individual to individual is due to the fact that there is a random sorting of chromosomes in each germ cell during reduction division which is coupled with random union of sperm and ovum. Thus, although relatives are more likely to share portions of their DNA than are nonrelated individuals, the only individuals possessing identical genomes are twins derived from the same fertilized ovum, i.e., identical twins. Another source of genetic variation is a change occurring in some portion of the DNA of a germ cell. Such a chemical change in the DNA is termed a *mutation,* the result being that the trait programmed by that particular gene may be altered in the individual receiving it.

The presence of individual genes cannot be detected with a microscope, but their presence can be inferred merely from the appearance of a demonstrable trait, a *phenotypic* trait, in the bearer. At a given genetic locus, if the paternal and maternal genes differ, one may be *dominant* so that the trait determined by that gene is phenotypically evident in the individual even if the second gene is different. The effect of the second gene is thus not expressed, and the trait determined by that gene is termed *recessive*. A recessive gene will not express itself phenotypically unless it is matched by a similar recessive gene from the other parent. Thus a particular trait, seemingly absent in both parents, may appear in the child if one recessive gene of the pair is supplied by each parent. Inheritance of a particular trait governed by a single gene pair as described is sometimes called *Mendelian* inheritance. However, many phenotypic traits are not so simply determined but are the result of the additive effect of multiple genes.

Abnormality of the hereditary material in an individual may thus arise and be expressed in a variety of ways. A particular abnormality may appear in a child without being a total surprise if the phenotypic expression of that trait is evident in the parents or immediate family. On the other hand, an abnormality may appear without previous evidence of the trait in a family either by the combination of two preexisting recessive genes, by the process of mutation in the germ cell of one of the parents, or by a complex polygenic combination not present in either parent. In addition, abnormalities of entire chromosomes, or major portions of a chromosome, may arise during the development of germ cells and then be transmitted to the individual created by that germ cell.

PHENOTYPIC EXPRESSION OF GENETIC ABNORMALITY

Chromosomal anomalies

The coarsest sort of abnormality of genetic material is that which is associated with a visible morphologic peculiarity of chromosomes. Chromosomal abnormalities can develop in a variety of ways as cells divide. If such accidents occur during the production of germ cells, the individual formed from such abnormal ova or sperm will carry the chromosomal abnormality in all cells of the body, because as the original fertilized egg (with its abnormal chromosome) divides, subsequent generations of daughter cells receive the chromosomal abnormality which has been reproduced in the process of cell division. One common way for a chromosomal abnormality to develop is for one or more chromosomes to break and have their broken ends "stick" inappropriately to other chromosomes, with the formation of a fused, abnormal chromosome. Another type of abnormality involves faulty separation of the two chromosomes of a given pair during the special reduction division which normally leads to a chromosome number of 23 in sperm or ova. If such faulty separation occurs, a germ cell would be formed with a *pair* of chromosomes in a particular location instead of a single chromosome, which results in 24 chromosomes instead of 23. Fertilization of such a cell, for instance, an ovum, by a normal sperm with 23 chromosomes would yield a cell with 47 chromosomes—with a *triplet* instead of a *pair* of chromosomes in a given location.

The presence of a chromosomal abnormality in an individual patient can be detected by sampling some living cells, usually white blood cells, encouraging them to divide in an artificial culture, and then studying the details of microscopic anatomy of the chromosomes formed during cell division. The array of chromosomes observed in this fashion is referred to as a *karyotype*.

The results of karyotypic anomalies can be extremely serious, presumably because of the large quantity of DNA and the many genes involved, and the fact that genes on other chromosomes will be operating in a situation of abnormal imbalance. It has been found that many spontaneously aborted embryos or fetuses have abnormal chromosomes, which indicates that the abortion occurred because the chromosomal abnormality

present at the moment of conception was lethal to the developing individual. However, some chromosomal abnormalities do permit birth of a live baby, though they produce severe defects in that individual. Because of the grossness of the genetic defect in such instances, multiple organ systems are often involved.

An example of a chromosomal abnormality, which unfortunately is not rare, is the common form of Down's syndrome, or mongolism, in which there is an extra chromosome in one pair, yielding a total chromosome number of 47. As shown in Fig. 2-3 the typical karyotype of a mongol shows three chromosomes in the so-called 21 position, the condition being referred to as *trisomy 21*. Affected individuals have a number of familiar and distinctive physical traits. They are generally mentally retarded and have a variety of internal anatomic abnormalities. The basic problem in this form of mongolism stems from a failure of separation of one chromosome pair that occurs in the development of the maternal germ cell, the ovum. Evidence indicates that advanced maternal age carries an increased risk of this sort of accident. Given the high risk of such pregnancies, it may be desirable to make or to rule out the diagnosis of mongolism before the fetus becomes independently viable. This is accomplished by studying the chromosomes of fetal cells obtained by puncturing the amniotic sac around the fetus and aspirating a bit of amniotic fluid which contains some of the cells of the fetus. This procedure, which is called *amniocentesis*, does not generally harm the developing fetus.

Many other chromosomal anomalies have been described in individuals who have multiple defects. It is estimated that 10 to 15 percent of infants born with

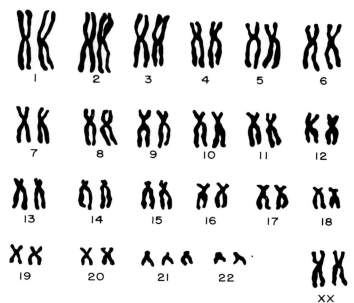

FIGURE 2-3 *Karotype of a female with Down's syndrome (mongolism). In the position conventionally designated as 21 are three chromosomes instead of two. This trisomy 21 is present in all of the cells of the affected individual and is expressed in terms of abnormalities in several organ systems.*

multiple malformations and mental retardation have abnormal karyotypes. Approximately 5 percent of still-borns have abnormal chromosomes, as do approximately one-half of spontaneous abortuses. Fortunately, however, genetic abnormalities so gross as to involve karyotypic abnormality constitute but a small fraction of hereditary abnormality.

Single gene abnormalities

Abnormalities of a single gene are more prevalent than the defects described above. These genetic abnormalities cannot be identified by microscopic examination of cells since the karyotype of the affected individual is normal. The presence of the abnormal gene is inferred by the detection of an abnormal phenotypic trait in the individual and in the family tree. Single gene abnormalities, both dominant and recessive, can be expressed in a variety of ways, ranging from simple localized anatomic defects to subtle and complex disturbances of bodily chemistry.

Localized malformations are perhaps the most readily observed effects of single gene abnormalities. When, for instance, a dozen individuals in three generations of a family have identically deformed hands and the pattern of incidence follows the laws of Mendelian inheritance, there is no difficulty in recognizing what is involved. However, it should be noted that the bulk of birth defects do not fit into this single gene category but are more often the result of several, separate gene abnormalities, possibly along with some environmental effects, or are the result of an intrauterine accident such as drug exposure or rubella. *Congenital* and *hereditary* are not synonymous terms. An abnormality may be congenital, i.e., present at birth, and not be genetically determined. Conversely, a genetically determined abnormality may manifest itself for the first time in some instances only when the patient is middle-aged.

Single gene abnormalities may be expressed as *inborn errors of metabolism*. This designation refers to a situation in which an abnormal gene leads to the production of a faulty product or to an absence of production of that product. If the product is an enzyme, the result of the genetic abnormality is the loss of services of that enzyme, a situation sometimes referred to as *enzymopathy*. Enzymopathies have three general sorts of consequences. First, if the lack of enzyme prevents some metabolic reaction from occurring, the subject may exhibit the lack of the result of that reaction. The albino illustrates this in the lack of melanin, the brown pigment of the body, because of a genetically determined deficiency of an enzyme essential to its production.

A second sort of consequence of enzymopathy involves the accumulation of some substance in the body when, with an essential enzyme missing, the substance cannot be properly eliminated from the body. The precise results of such a *storage disease* depend on where in the body the substance accumulates. For example, in the adult-type Gaucher's disease a complex lipid accumulates within cells scattered in the liver, spleen, lymph nodes, and bone marrow of affected individuals (Fig. 2-4). Signs and symptoms of this storage disease may be quite mild and may not appear until adult life, when normal cells of the bone marrow begin to be crowded out by the Gaucher cells or when the spleen becomes enlarged and results in the formation of an abdominal mass. Tay-Sachs disease is an even more serious example. In this condition, due to a missing enzyme, the affected subject progressively accumulates a certain lipid within the neurons of the brain. Resulting degeneration of these cells leads to blindness, paralysis, and death, usually before 4 years of age.

The third type of consequence of enzymopathy is

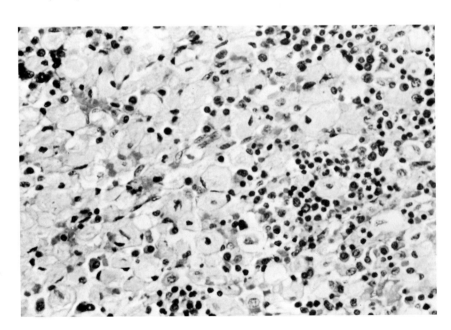

FIGURE 2-4 Gaucher cells in the bone marrow. Much of this field, especially on the left, is occupied by large, pale cells stuffed with stored lipid. These Gaucher cells crowd out the normal blood-forming elements, seen relatively concentrated at the right. Similar changes occur in many other organs. (Photomicrograph, ×500.)

typified by the disease phenylketonuria, or PKU, in which the genetic defect leads to accumulation of improperly metabolized substances which have a toxic effect on certain bodily functions, especially those of the growing, developing brain. The result in the untreated case is severe mental retardation. Fortunately, in this disease early diagnosis, with dietary restriction of the substances which are not properly metabolized, can circumvent the disastrous effects on the growing infant.

In yet another category of single gene abnormality, aberrant DNA may lead to the production of an abnormal protein molecule such as the hemoglobin molecule. A slight deviation in the structure of the hemoglobin may give it unusual physical properties which can be magnified into a serious disease. For example, in sickle-cell anemia the abnormal recessive gene "instructs" the red blood cells to produce hemoglobin molecules which are prone to deform when the oxygen concentration in the blood is reduced. These sickled red cells form tangled masses and are rapidly destroyed, producing a variety of severe signs and symptoms characteristic of anemia.

Other single gene abnormalities cover a broad spectrum of phenotypic expression. Thus, there are genetically determined defects in the growth of bones, hereditary disorders in the chemistry of connective tissue, and genetically determined diseases such as cystic fibrosis in which there is an abnormality of many exocrine secretions, such as sweat and pancreatic and bronchial secretions. (Because of the last abnormality, affected individuals frequently die prematurely of pulmonary infection.) There have also been recognized a number of genetically determined conditions in which the individual is normal in all respects except for an unusual response to some environmental agent such as a drug. This latter sort of phenomenon has resulted in the recent development of the field of *pharmacogenetics*, the study of hereditary variations in response to drugs. The list of abnormal phenotypes determined by Mendelian inheritance includes many hundreds of diverse conditions.

However, even more prevalent than any of the situations outlined above are the many things that "run in families" but do not follow the usual patterns of Mendelian or single gene inheritance. Analysis of many of these diseases reveals that the interaction of several separate genes and several environmental factors determines the outcome. An excellent example of this type of pattern is observed in atherosclerotic coronary artery disease (refer to Part V). Evidence indicates that the incidence of coronary artery disease is more prevalent in members of the immediate family of patients with the disease than in the general population. However, it is equally clear that environmental factors such as cigarette smoking, diet, and perhaps psychological stress make a significant contribution to the incidence and severity of the disease, along with associated conditions such as diabetes and high blood pressure. In such polygenic or *multifactorial* disease, the approach to prevention can clearly proceed along nongenetic lines with the expectation that environmental manipulation such as dietary limitations or alternatives in life-style and smok-

ing habits will be beneficial regardless of genetic constitution.

To recapitulate, some human diseases arise as a direct result of abnormality of DNA, the "stuff" of heredity. The basic problem may be one involving a single gene, multiple genes, or even an entire chromosome; and the expression of the abnormality may range from a localized anatomic malformation, to a complex chemical and metabolic problem, to an increased susceptibility to something in the environment.

PREVENTIVE MEDICINE AND GENETIC COUNSELING

Very often the pronouncement to a patient that some condition is "hereditary" is met with feelings of hopelessness and despair and a sense of the irreversibility of what one has been dealt by nature. These feelings are, to an extent, a realistic expression of the fact that the era of genetic engineering has not yet arrived, that it is not yet possible to reverse such things as Tay-Sachs disease in a dying infant. Nonetheless, the total perspective of genetics and disease is far different than what is conjured up by the grim situations that first come to mind.

Many conditions that are inherited are not inevitably *expressed* in the bearer of the abnormal DNA despite the presence of a single or even several abnormal genes. As previously discussed, the ravages of phenylketonuria can be prevented, even in an infant with a hereditary lack of critical enzymes, by careful dietary manipulation. The progression of coronary artery disease can be influenced by manipulations ranging from drug treatment to changes in personal habits. The task of human genetics in such instances is not simply one of noting and cataloging the inevitable, but is one of identifying subjects at unusual risk on a genetic basis and minimizing that risk by some environmental manipulation. Modifying the expression of genetic abnormality is an advancing frontier of biomedicine.

In those conditions that have not yielded even partly to such an approach, the outlook is necessarily somewhat different and is based ultimately on prevention of the disease, that is, through prevention of the birth of individuals afflicted with the disorder in question. This process, in turn, has two operational levels, both of which involve decisions on the part of the concerned individuals. At the first level, a pregnancy likely to yield an abnormal individual can be electively avoided by the couple. At the second level, a pregnancy can be terminated by elective abortion prior to independent viability of a fetus determined to be affected with the condition in question. In the first example it is essential that the parents are accurately informed of the risk of conceiving an individual with an abnormality. The subject of risk often arises when an earlier pregnancy has already yielded an affected infant or when there is a strong family history of some particular condition. Also, there is a general risk in belonging to a population group where there is an increased incidence of some condition such as the group of Eastern European Jews where there is an increased incidence of Tay-Sachs disease. For some conditions it is now possible by means of specific tests applied to normal parents to detect the presence of a recessive gene which in a *double dose* would yield an afflicted infant. This is the case, for instance, with both Tay-Sachs disease and sickle-cell disease. In these situations if both parents are found to be carriers of the gene, then the couple can be informed that the likelihood of producing an affected infant would be one pregnancy in four. Based on this knowledge the parents could decide, in keeping with their own particular religious or ethical systems, whether to avoid pregnancy entirely, whether to take the calculated risk, or whether to proceed with the pregnancy and seek prenatal diagnosis of the anticipated condition with possible termination of the pregnancy. For example, in Tay-Sachs disease it is now possible to secure fetal cells by amniocentesis and determine their content of the particular enzyme involved in the disease. This type of approach has allowed couples to produce families when the risk of pregnancy would previously not have been considered by them.

Extremely difficult and sensitive decisions in this area must ultimately be made by the prospective parents. This requires that accurate and understandable information related to the nature and prognosis of the particular disease, the mode of its inheritance, and the probability of the disease appearing in the offspring be made available. In many instances this is the task of a person who has special skills in genetic counseling.

Identifying a condition as hereditary is not without pitfalls for the inexperienced. As emphasized above, many congenital conditions may be essentially nonhereditary, while nearly identical conditions may in fact be hereditary. Even conditions that are definitely *familial*, in terms of their greater frequency in a given family, may be nonhereditary but due to some environmental influence exposing the entire family. Even more important, a given individual may appear to be afflicted with disease A associated with a gene but actually may have disease B which closely mimics disease A but is associated with a different gene and with a different pattern of inheritance. The subject might even be afflicted with disease C, which could be a nonhereditary look-alike. The counselor must be aware of such mimicry and be able to interpret appropriate studies which range from chromosomal and chemical analyses of cells secured from patient and or family, to careful evaluation of the family tree for evidence of disease.

In summary, the medical counselor must have the skill and perception to render as accurate a diagnosis as currently possible. The counselor must possess the ability to explain to the parents humanely but understandably the nature and prognosis of the disease and its impact on affected individuals, the mode of available treatment, and the means of preventing the occurrence of the disease. The ultimate decision as to any action is made by the parents or patients in the light of available options, and therapeutic measures are administered by the members of the health team in accordance with that decision. While the issues are perhaps more obvious in the case of so-called hereditary disease, the sequence just outlined is not unique. It describes the essence of medical practice.

QUESTIONS

Heredity, environment, and disease, interaction of heredity and environment—Chap. 2

Directions: Answer the following questions on a separate sheet of paper.

1 List the ways in which DNA is responsible for storing, duplicating, and transmitting all of the information needed for programming the functions of a cell.

2 What occurs in relation to DNA during the process of cell division?

3 List the ways in which chromosomal abnormalities can develop.

4 Discuss the purposes of genetic counseling.

Directions: Circle the letter preceding each item below that correctly answers the question. More than one answer may be correct.

5 Which of the following are extrinsic factors in relationship to the disease process?
a Microorganisms *b* Race *c* Sex *d* Nutrition

6 Which of the following best describes a *hereditary* disease?
a Largely determined by an environmental agent. *b* Faulty genetic "programming" of the body's machinery results only from external influences. *c* Expressed in nearly every bearer of faulty genetic information regardless of external influences. *d* An infectious agent is the usual causal agent.

7 Differentiation refers to the process by which:
a There is a decrease in the number of cells in a given population. *b* Cells having within them the same genetic information begin to diverge in their structure and function. *c* There is a chemical change in the DNA. *d* The nucleus arranges itself into strands.

8 Which of the following are characteristic features of autosomal *dominant* disorders?
a Not expressed as disease if dominant gene is

present. *b* Manifest as disease when only one abnormal gene is present and the partner on the homologous chromosome is normal. *c* The trait will be altered when an individual has a mutation of a single dominant gene. *d* Individuals who are homozygous for dominant genes are usually less severely affected than those who are heterozygous for recessive genes.

9 Which of the following genetic diseases are inherited as autosomal *recessive* disorders?
a Sickle-cell anemia *b* Down's syndrome
c Phenylketonuria (PKU) *d* Tay-Sachs disease

10 Which of the following diseases is an example of a genetic disease due to an abnormal karyotype?
a Phenylketonuria (PKU) *b* Albinism
c Down's syndrome *d* Sickle-cell anemia

Directions: Circle T if the statement is true and F if it is false. Correct the false statements.

11 T F The presence of individual abnormal genes can be detected with a microscope.

12 T F The term *genetic trait* means that the trait is inherited because of the DNA which is passed from generation to generation.

13 T F An arrangement of the chromosomes present in a cell is called a karyotype.

14 T F An inborn error of metabolism results from a genetically determined enzymatic defect that may involve the body's handling of protein, carbohydrates, lipids, etc.

CHAPTER 3 Cellular Injury and Death

OBJECTIVES   **At the completion of Chap. 3 you should be able to:**

1 Describe the organization of a hypothetical "typical" cell.

2 List the modalities by which cells may be injured or killed.

3 Describe the sequential stages of cell damage.

4 Describe the relationship of these stages to functional abnormalities of a cell.

5 Distinguish between the several forms of degenerative changes that occur in injured cells.

6 State at least one example of each of these degenerative cell changes.

7 Differentiate between atrophy and hypertrophy.

8 Explain the concept "point of no return" in relation to cell injury.

9 Explain the concept of necrosis.

10 Identify the types and causes of necrosis.

11 State at least one example of each type of necrosis.

12 Describe the effects of necrosis.

13 Explain what happens to necrotic tissue in the body.

14 Identify and distinguish the various types of pathological calcification.

15 Define *somatic death*.

16 Describe the typical postmortem changes.

CELLULAR ORGANIZATION

Although within the body there are many different kinds of cells with highly specialized functions, all cells, to a large extent, have similar life-styles and similar structural elements. They have parallel requirements for such things as oxygen and nutrient supplies, for constancy of temperature, for water supply, and for means of waste disposal. The cell is literally the unit of life, the smallest entity that manifests the various phenomena which are associated with living. Therefore, the cell is also the basic unit of disease.

The organization of a hypothetical "typical" cell is diagrammed in Fig. 3-1. The cell is bounded by a *cell membrane*, which not only gives the cell its shape but also attaches it to other cells. Even more importantly, the cell membrane serves as the gateway to and from the cell, allowing only certain things to pass in either direction, and even actively transporting some things in a selective fashion. It is also the cell membrane that must receive

many of the control signals from around the body and transmit these signals to the interior of the cell.

Within the cell is the *nucleus*, which serves as the control center by virtue of the fact that the DNA is concentrated within it. The instructions coded within the nuclear DNA are actually executed within the *cytoplasm*, which is a watery medium containing many structures so small that they can be seen only with the electron microscope. These ultramicroscopic organs are termed *organelles*, and they are highly specialized as to function even within the confines of a single cell.

The *mitochondria* are organelles devoted to energy production within the cell. They are the power plant of the cell, for within them various foodstuffs are oxidized to produce the driving force for other cellular activities. The *endoplasmic reticulum* and *Golgi apparatus* constitute a sort of manufacturing, processing, and plumbing system within the cytoplasm. These structures are actually composed of a network of connecting tubules in which various degradative and synthetic activities occur. In particular, protein synthesis is carried out in relation to the endoplasmic reticulum under control of RNA (ribonucleic acid) in the *ribosomes*. The cytoplasmic RNA is actually produced and directed by nuclear DNA to act as a sort of assembly team in relation to the executive role of DNA. The ribosomes are responsible for assembly of raw materials into specific structures according to the directions supplied by DNA. The Golgi apparatus is a packaging device, wrapping the cell products for export (secretion) or for storage within the cell. The *lysosomes* are membrane-bound packages of digestive enzymes prepared by the cell and held inactive until needed. Yet other organelles not shown in Fig. 3-1 account for additional special functions within the cell, such as providing rigidity and/or movement in the manner of a musculoskeletal system. The various organelles represent a total organism in microcosm, and their activity must be closely coordinated and controlled to preserve cellular intregity.

MODALITIES OF CELLULAR INJURY

There are many ways in which cells can be injured or killed, but important modalities of injury tend to fall into several categories. One of the most common factors in cellular injury is a *deficiency of oxygen or other critical nutrient material*. Cells are particularly dependent upon a continuous supply of oxygen, because it is the energy of oxidative chemical reactions which drives the machinery of the cell and maintains the integrity of the various components of the cell. Therefore, without oxygen the

various maintenance and synthetic activities of cells quickly come to a halt. A second important type of injury is *physical*, which involves actual disruption of cells, or at least disturbance of the usual spatial relationships between the various organelles or of the structural integrity of one or more types of organelles. Thus, mechanical and thermal means of injury are significant in the causation of human disease. *Living infectious agents* constitute a third category of injurious modalities, and there is a wide variety of means by which particular organisms injure cells. *Chemical agents* constitute a final common means of cellular injury. Not only do toxic substances find their way into cells from the environment, but accumulation of endogenous substances (as with genetically determined metabolic "errors") may likewise injure cells.

THE CELL UNDER ATTACK

When an injurious stimulus is applied to a cell, the first important effect is what has been called a *biochemical lesion*. This involves a change in the chemistry of one or more metabolic reactions within the cell. It is interesting to note that very few types of injury are actually understood at this level. Although biochemical changes can be

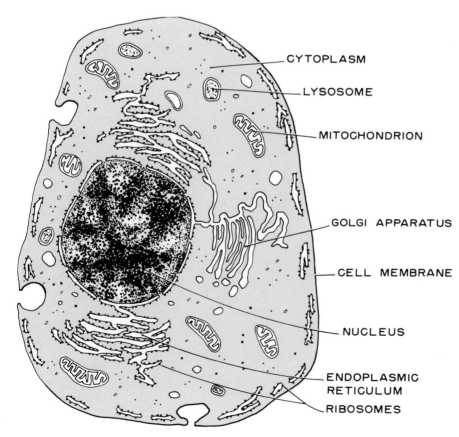

CYTOPLASM

LYSOSOME

MITOCHONDRION

GOLGI APPARATUS

CELL MEMBRANE

NUCLEUS

ENDOPLASMIC RETICULUM

RIBOSOMES

FIGURE 3-1 Diagram of a hypothetical typical cell. The structural basis for division of labor within the cell is shown diagrammatically. It should be noted that in the living body the cell membrane not only bounds the cell and controls access to the interior but also joins the cell with others to form tissues.

noted in injured cells, very often the abnormalities noted are second- or third-order effects rather than evidence of the primary biochemical lesion. When a biochemical lesion is established, the cell may or may not manifest a functional abnormality. In the case of many injuries, the cell possesses sufficient reserve to perform without significant functional impairment; in other instances there can be a failure of contraction, secretion, or other activities of the cell. Finally, accompanying these biochemical and functional abnormalities there may *or may not* be a detectable morphological change in the affected cell. The limitation here is one of technique. Changes that are evident upon routine microscopic examination are generally late changes, since many biochemical and functional abnormalities may have occurred before the anatomic abnormality becomes evident. With the advent of electron microscopy it is becoming possible to detect earlier and earlier microscopic lesions, but with presently available techniques it is still true that many functionally impaired cells may not yield evidence of their impairment in morphological terms.

The result of an attack upon a cell is not always impairment of function. In fact, there are cellular mechanisms of *adaptation* to various kinds of adversity. For example, a common reaction of a muscle cell placed under abnormal stress is to gain strength by enlargement, a process called *hypertrophy.* Thus, the heart muscle cells of an individual with high blood pressure will enlarge in order to cope with the strain of pumping against increased resistance. A similar type of adaptation occurs in regard to certain chemical challenges. Barbiturates and certain other substances are ordinarily metabolized in liver cells, under the influence of enzyme systems found within these cells in association with the endoplasmic reticulum. In an individual taking barbiturates, there is often a striking increase in the amount of endoplasmic reticulum within liver cells, and this is associated with an increased enzyme content in these cells and an increased ability to metabolize the drug.

MORPHOLOGICAL CHANGES IN SUBLETHALLY INJURED CELLS

Often when cells are injured but not killed, they manifest easily identifiable morphological changes. These sublethal changes are at least potentially reversible. That is, if the injurious stimulus can be withdrawn, the cells return to their previous state of health. On the other hand, these changes may be a step toward cell death if the noxious influence cannot be corrected. Sublethal changes in cells are traditionally called *degenerations* or *degenerative changes.* Although any cells of the body may manifest such changes, metabolically active cells such as liver, kidney, and heart cells are commonly in-

volved. Degenerative changes tend to involve the cytoplasm of cells, while nuclei maintain their integrity as long as the cell is not lethally injured. Although there are infinite numbers of injurious agents or specific ways of attacking cells, the repertory of morphological expression of injury is actually quite limited.

The commonest form of cellular degenerative change involves the accumulation of water within the affected cells. The injury in effect causes loss of volume control on the part of the cells. Ordinarily, in order to maintain constancy of its internal environment, a cell must expend metabolic energy to pump sodium ion out of the cell. This occurs at the level of the cell membrane. Anything which disturbs energy metabolism in the cell or slightly injures the cell membrane may render the cell unable to pump out sufficient sodium ion. The natural osmotic result of increased intracellular concentration of sodium is an influx of water into the cell. The result is a morphological change termed *cellular swelling.* An older name for this change was *cloudy swelling,* reflecting the fact that an organ whose cells suffered this change acquired a peculiar parboiled appearance grossly and the affected cells acquired an unusual granular appearance of the cytoplasm microscopically. These changes reflect the fact that when water accumulates within the cytoplasm, the cytoplasmic organelles also absorb it, causing mitochondrial swelling, dilatation of the endoplasmic reticulum, and so forth. Microscopically the changes of cellular swelling are quite subtle and involve simply an enlargement of the cell and a slight change in its texture. The gross counterpart of this is the enlargement of the affected tissue or organ usually detectable by a moderate increase in weight. If the noxious influence which has produced cellular swelling can be removed, after a period of time the cells usually begin to extrude sodium, and along with it water, and the volume returns to normal. This change is but a slight perturbation of the normal state of affairs.

If there is a severe influx of water, some of the cytoplasmic organelles such as the endoplasmic reticulum may be converted into water-filled sacs. Upon microscopic examination, the cytoplasm of the cell is seen to be vacuolated (Fig. 3-2). This is termed *hydropic change* or sometimes *vacuolar change.* The gross appearance of affected organs and the significance of the change is identical to that of cellular swelling.

A more striking and significant change than simple cellular swelling involves the intracellular *accumulation of lipid* within affected cells. This type of change commonly involves the kidneys, heart muscle, and liver, particularly the latter. Microscopically, the cytoplasm of the affected cells appears vacuolated in a fashion quite similar to that seen in hydropic change, but the content of the vacuoles is lipid instead of water. In the case of the liver, the amount of lipid accumulating within a cell is often immense, so that the nucleus of the cell is pushed to one side and the cytoplasm of the cell is occupied by one huge lipid-containing vacuole (Fig. 3-3). The counterpart of such changes with respect to the gross appearance of affected tissues involves swelling of the tissues, increase in weight of the affected organ, and very often a distinct yellowish cast to the tissue due to contained lipid. Severely affected livers are in fact often bright yellow and greasy to touch. This type of change is termed *fatty change* or sometimes *fatty degeneration*, or *fatty infiltration*.

Fatty change occurs commonly because it can be produced by so many different mechanisms, particularly in the liver. Hepatocytes (and other types of cells), normally are involved in an active metabolic exchange of lipids. These substances are constantly mobilized from adipose tissue into the bloodstream from which they are extracted by the liver cells. Some of the lipid which is absorbed by the cell is oxidized, while some of it is combined with protein synthesized by the cell and then exported from the cell (i.e., into the bloodstream) in the form of lipoprotein. Accumulation of fat within the cell can be produced by interfering with the usual

exchange processes at any of several points. For example, if an excess of lipid is presented to the liver cell, the metabolic and synthetic capabilities of the cell may be exceeded, whereupon the lipid will accumulate intracellularly. If, on the other hand, even normal amounts of lipid reach the cell and oxidation is impaired by some cellular injury, lipid will accumulate. Finally, if the process of lipoprotein synthesis and export is interfered with at any of several points, lipid will also accumulate. For these reasons one may encounter a fatty liver in diverse situations ranging from malnutrition, which will impair protein synthesis, to overfeeding, which will

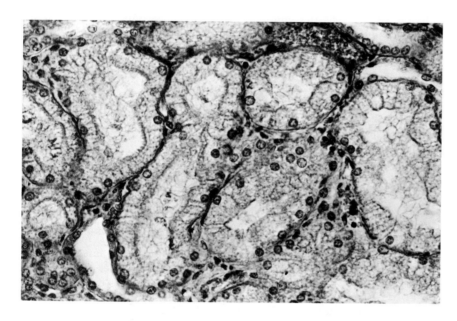

FIGURE 3-2 Hydropic change in renal tubular epithelium. The epithelial cells lining these convoluted tubules are enlarged and have vacuolated, lacy-appearing cytoplasm due to intracellular accumulation of water. (Photomicrograph, ×500.)

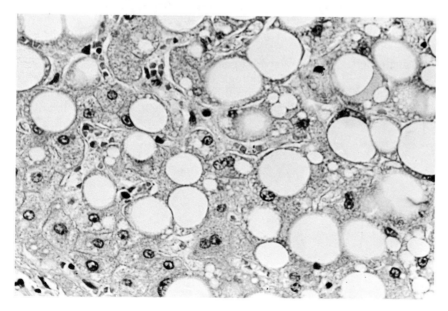

FIGURE 3-3 Fatty change in liver. Many liver cells have several small "holes" in their cytoplasm or a single huge vacuole which distorts the entire cell. These apparently empty spaces contained abundant lipid which was dissolved during histologic preparation. The liver cells at the lower left are virtually normal. (Photomicrograph, ×500.)

in effect swamp the liver with lipids. Hypoxia will sufficiently impair cellular metabolism to produce fatty accumulation, and numerous toxic substances from the environment will affect the cells in such a manner as to promote lipid accumulation. One of the most potent and widespread toxins in our environment to produce fatty livers is alcohol. This substance is directly toxic to the liver cells as well as indirectly injurious to individuals whose alcohol intake is extreme, because this often leads to malnutrition. Fatty change is potentially reversible but frequently reflects a severe injury to the cell and thus constitutes a step on the way to cell death.

Another response of cells under attack is to undergo a reduction in mass, quite literally a shrinkage. Such an acquired reduction in the size of a cell, a tissue, or an organ is referred to as *atrophy*. Seemingly the atrophic cell or tissue is able to achieve an equilibrium under the adverse conditions imposed upon it by virtue of reducing the total demand it must meet. Grossly, of course, atrophic tissues or organs are smaller than normal.

In the course of becoming atrophic the cell must absorb some of its constituents. This involves what is sometimes called *autophagocytosis*, literally a self-eating process. This involves the enzymatic digestion of portions of the cell contained within cytoplasmic vacuoles. This same process occurs not only in the cell undergoing atrophy but also in the wear and tear of everyday cellular existence. That is to say, cytoplasmic organelles are damaged from time to time and are sequestered within a cytoplasmic vacuole and digested enzymatically. The digestion process tends to leave traces of residual indigestible material which gradually accumulate within the cells. This material is derived for the most part from membranous structures within the cells and generally has a dark-brown color. As cells age, they accumulate more and more of this intracytoplasmic pigment, which is referred to as *lipofuscin, aging pigment,* or *wear-and-tear pigment*. As cells become atrophic, lipofuscin may become even more concentrated because of increased autophagocytic activity. Sometimes the atrophic tissue is pigmented even grossly; the process responsible is referred to as *brown atrophy*.

If the noxious influence on a cell is severe enough or long enough continued, the cell will reach a point at which it can no longer compensate and cannot carry on metabolically. At some hypothetical point of no return, the processes become irreversible, and the cell is in effect dead. At this hypothetical instant of death, when the cell just reaches the *point of no return,* it may not be possible to recognize morphologically that the cell is irreversibly dead. However, if a group of cells that has reached this state remains in the living host for even a few hours, additional things occur which permit the recognition of the cells or the tissue as being dead. All cells have within them a variety of enzymes, many of them lytic. While the cell is alive, these enzymes do no damage to the cell, but they are released upon cell death and begin to dissolve various cellular constituents. In addition, as the dead cells change chemically, the living tissues immediately adjacent respond to the changes and mount an acute inflammatory reaction (see Chap. 4). Part of this latter reaction is the delivery of many leukocytes or white blood cells to the area, and these assist in the digestion of the dead cells. Thus, from their own digestive enzymes or as a result of the inflammatory process, the cells that have reached the point of no return begin to undergo discernible morphological changes.

When a cell or group of cells or tissue in a living host are recognizably dead, they are referred to as *necrotic. Necrosis,* then, represents local cell death. If the whole subject dies, the dead body is not referred to as necrotic.

In general, although the lytic changes which occur in necrotic tissue may involve the cytoplasm of cells, it is the nuclei which manifest the changes most clearly indicative of cell death. Commonly, the nucleus of the dead cell shrinks, develops an irregular outline, and stains densely with the usual dyes used by pathologists. This process is referred to as *pyknosis,* and the nuclei are termed *pyknotic*. Alternatively, nuclei may crumble, leaving scattered fragments of chromatin material within the cell. This process is referred to as *karyorrhexis*. Finally, in some instances, the nuclei of dead cells lose their staining ability and simply disappear, the process being referred to as *karyolysis* (see Fig. 3-4).

The morphologic appearance of necrotic tissue varies depending upon the results of lytic activities within the dead tissue. If the activity of lytic enzymes is inhibited

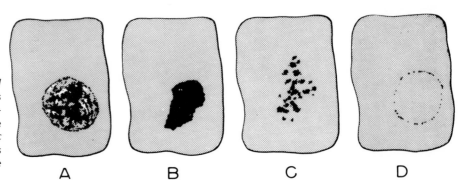

FIGURE 3-4 Nuclear changes in cell death. The morphological changes most clearly indicative of cell death involve the nucleus. Diagrammed above are a normal nucleus (A), a pyknotic nucleus (B), a karyorrhectic nucleus (C), and one which has undergone karyolysis (D).

A   B   C   D

somewhat by local conditions, the necrotic cells will maintain their outline, and the tissue will maintain its architectural features for some period of time. This type of necrosis is called *coagulative necrosis* and is particularly common when necrosis has been caused by deprivation of blood supply (Fig. 3-5). In some instances the necrotic tissue gradually liquefies by enzymatic action, the process being called *liquefactive necrosis*. This is particularly likely to occur in an area of necrotic brain, and the result is literally a hole in the brain filled with fluid (Fig. 3-6). In yet other instances the necrotic cells disintegrate, but the finely divided cellular fragments remain in the area for months or even years, virtually undigested. This type of necrosis is referred to as *caseous necrosis* because of the fact that the area so affected has the appearance of crumbly cheese when viewed grossly (see Fig. 3-7). The prototype situation

giving rise to caseous necrosis is tuberculosis, although this type of necrosis can arise in many other situations.

Certain special local conditions can give rise to yet other variants of necrosis. *Gangrene* is defined as coagulative necrosis, usually due to deprivation of blood supply, with superimposed growth of saprophytic bacteria. Gangrene thus occurs in necrotic tissues that are exposed to living bacteria. This is especially common in the extremities (Fig. 3-8) or in a segment of bowel which becomes necrotic (Fig. 3-9). Sometimes the shriveled, blackened tissue of a gangrenous area on an extremity is described as being the seat of *dry gangrene*,

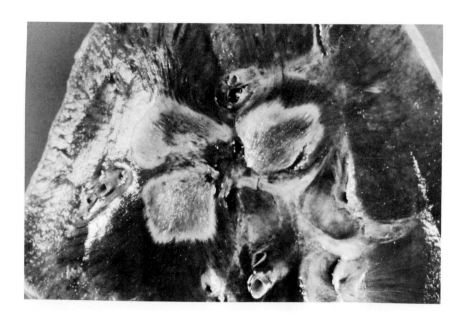

FIGURE 3-5 Coagulative necrosis. In this close-up of the cut surface of a kidney, three pale areas of necrosis can be seen. The architectural outlines are obviously maintained in the dead tissue, hence the designation as coagulative necrosis. (Since the renal papillae are involved, this condition is specifically termed renal papillary necrosis.)

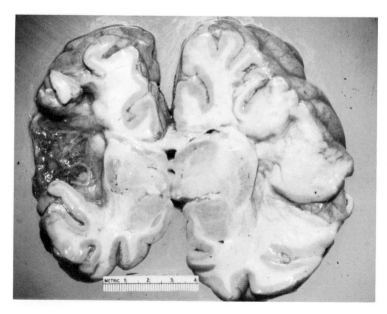

FIGURE 3-6 Liquefactive necrosis. A large defect is seen at the left in this section of brain. The brain substance in this area became necrotic due to deprivation of blood supply. As is generally true in this organ, the necrotic tissue gradually softened, then liquefied, leaving a permanent defect.

while an internal area which cannot become desiccated is designated as *moist gangrene*. In either situation the process involves the growth of saprophytic bacteria superimposed upon necrotic tissue.

Necrotic adipose tissue constitutes another special case. If the duct system of the pancreas is ruptured, either by trauma or in the course of spontaneous disease of the pancreas, the pancreatic enzymes ordinarily carried within the ducts may be spilled into the surroundings. The secretions of the pancreas contain many powerful hydrolytic enzymes, including lipases which cleave the lipids of adipose tissue. When this cleavage occurs, free fatty acids are formed by enzymatic action,

and these are rapidly combined with metallic ions (such as calcium) in the area producing deposits of soaps. This phenomenon, referred to as *enzymatic fat necrosis* or *pancreatic fat necrosis*, is largely restricted to the abdominal cavity since that represents the area exposed to leaking pancreatic enzymes. If adipose tissue elsewhere becomes necrotic, spillage of lipid from the dead cells may evoke an inflammatory response, but there is no formation of the yellow, chalky deposits characteristic of enzymatic fat necrosis.

Effects of necrosis

The most obvious effect of necrosis, of course, is *loss of function* of the dead area. If the necrotic tissue represents a small fraction of an organ with a large reserve (e.g., the kidney), there may be no functional impact on the host. On the other hand, if the area of necrosis

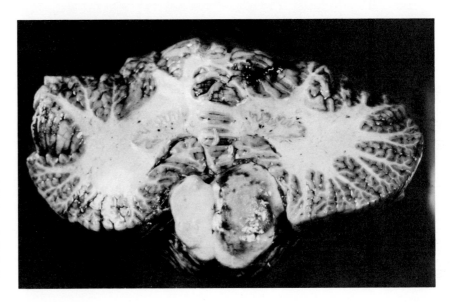

FIGURE 3-7 Caseous necrosis. A large necrotic area is evident in the brainstem at the right of center. In this instance, the dead tissue crumbled but did not liquefy. Because of a fancied gross resemblance to cheese, this type of necrosis is termed caseous. (This particular lesion was the result of tuberculosis, one of many causes of caseation.)

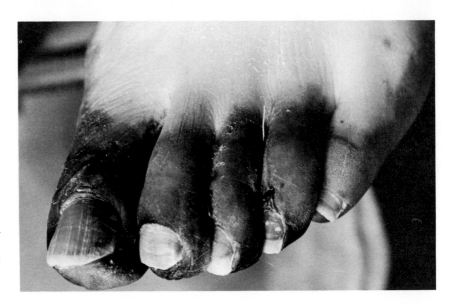

FIGURE 3-8 Gangrene. The toes of this foot have become necrotic because of poor blood supply. Saprophytic microorganisms are growing in the blackened dead tissue. On the extremities gangrene of this sort is frequently termed "dry."

is in a portion of brain, severe neurologic deficit or even death might be the result. In addition, the necrotic area in some instances can become a *focus of infection*, representing an excellent culture medium for the growth of certain organisms which might then spread elsewhere in the body. Even without becoming infected, the presence of necrotic tissue within the body may evoke certain *systemic changes*, such as fever, increased numbers of leukocytes within the circulating blood, and a variety of subjective symptoms. Finally, the necrotic tissue often *leaks its constituent enzymes* into the bloodstream as the cells die and the permeability of cell membranes increases. It is possible to analyze a specimen of blood and determine the level of various enzymes such as creatine phosphokinase (CPK), lactic dehydrogenase (LDH), or glutamic-oxaloacetic transaminase (GOT). Then an increased level of one or another enzyme may indicate that the patient does in fact have an area of necrosis hidden deep in some tissue. This principle has given rise to an important diagnostic field, clinical enzymology.

FATE OF NECROTIC TISSUE

Most often when an area of tissue becomes necrotic, the event evokes an inflammatory response on the part of the adjacent tissues (see Chap. 4). As a result of this inflammatory response, the dead tissue is ultimately demolished and removed, making way for the reparative process which replaces the necrotic area with regenerating cells of the sort lost or, in many instances, with scar tissue. If the necrotic tissue is located on a body surface, e.g., along the lining of the gastrointestinal tract, it may simply slough off, leaving a gap in the continuity of the surface which is referred to as an *ulcer*. Finally if the necrotic area is neither demolished nor cast off, it commonly will be encapsulated by fibrous connective tissue and will ultimately be impregnated with calcium salts

precipitated from the circulating blood in the area of necrosis. This process of calcification may lead to the necrotic area becoming stony hard and remaining so for the life of the individual.

PATHOLOGICAL CALCIFICATION

The deposition of insoluble calcium salts from the bloodstream which renders tissues rigid and hard is of course perfectly normal in the formation of bones and teeth. Elsewhere when such a phenomenon occurs, it is abnormal and is referred to as *pathological calcification* or *heterotopic calcification*. This may occur in several situations. Most commonly, as described above, injured tissue or necrotic tissue which is not quickly demolished may become the site of calcification. This particular form of calcification is referred to as *dystrophic*. Since an area of caseous necrosis by its very nature remains undigested for long periods of time, it commonly becomes calcified. Thus, because tiny foci of tuberculosis or other infections occur in lung and in the lymph nodes draining the lung, small foci of dystrophic calcification commonly appear in these areas. They are not particularly important biologically but often appear on x-rays because of the opacity of the dense deposits of calcium salts. Another common site of dystrophic calcification is in the walls of arteries which have become atherosclerotic (see Chap. 7). In fact, the texture of this "hardening of the arteries" is due to the calcium deposition.

In certain other circumstances calcium salts may be deposited in the soft tissues of the body in the absence

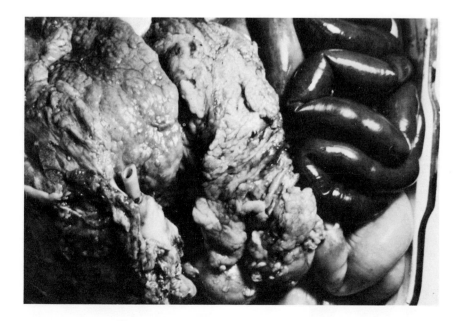

FIGURE 3-9 Gangrene. In this instance, a major portion of small intestine has been deprived of its blood supply. The gangrenous loops of intestine at the upper right contrast with the viable ones at the lower right. Saprophytes flourish in the necrotic tissue. Internal gangrene of this sort is inevitably "moist" as contrasted to that on the extremities.

of prior tissue damage or necrosis. This type of calcification is referred to as *metastatic calcification*. This process occurs not because of an abnormality of tissues but because there is an abnormal concentration of calcium and phosphorus salts within the circulating blood. Specifically, if the concentration of these substances rises beyond a certain critical level, their solubility product is exceeded, and precipitation occurs in a variety of tissues, especially lung, kidney, stomach, and the walls of blood vessels. The concentrations of calcium and phosphates in the blood are in turn affected by activity of the parathyroid glands, renal function, intake of calcium and vitamin D in the diet, and the integrity of the skeleton. Thus, metastatic calcification may be

seen with hyperparathyroidism, decreased renal function, abnormal diet, and destructive lesions of the skeletal system which liberate large quantities of calcium salts from the bones.

Calcium salts may also be deposited in the form of stones or *calculi* within the duct systems of a variety of organs. Calculi are formed from a variety of locally available materials, i.e., materials within the secretions of the particular organ. Thus, although they frequently contain calcium as one constituent, many calculi are not primarily calcific. Some calculi form as a result of encrustation of necrotic debris within a duct, while others form because of an imbalance in the constituents of a particular secretion such that there is precipitation from what is ordinarily a dissolved state. For a variety of reasons, then, calculi are commonly encountered in the biliary tract (Fig. 3-10), the pancreas, the salivary glands, the prostate, and the urinary system.

While calculi are often silent and discovered inciden-

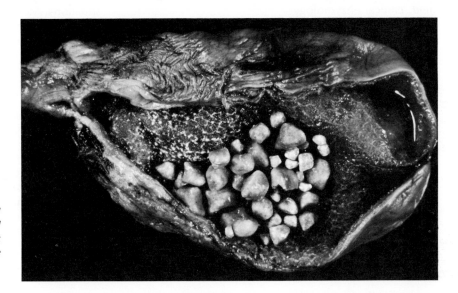

FIGURE 3-10 Gallstones within the gall bladder. Calculi of this sort are composed largely of bile pigments and cholesterol. It is apparent that stones of this size may be propelled into the common bile duct, where they can obstruct the flow of bile.

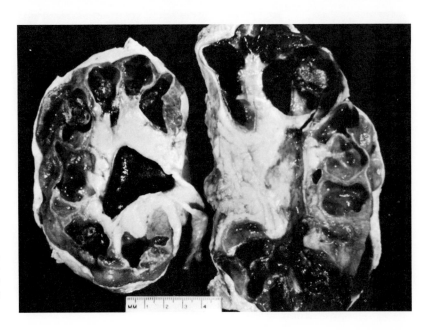

FIGURE 3-11 Renal calculi. Numerous large stones are present within the calyces and pelvis of these hemisected kidneys. The associated obstruction of urine flow and infection have led to marked loss of renal parenchyma.

tally if at all, many move along the duct system of the particular organ and cause pain and bleeding. Frequently calculi will move until they lodge in the narrow part of the duct system and produce obstruction of the outflow of the particular secretion. When this occurs, there is often infection of the obstructed organ and atrophy of the parenchyma (Fig. 3-11).

SOMATIC DEATH

Death of the entire individual, as contrasted to localized death or necrosis, is referred to as *somatic death*. In past years the definition of somatic death was a relatively simple matter. An individual was declared dead when "vital functions" ceased beyond any chance of reversal. Thus, if an individual stopped breathing and could not be resuscitated, the heart rather quickly stopped beating as a result of anoxia, and the individual was indisputably dead. Today, with technological advances, a patient can be attached to a mechanical respirator if breathing stops. If the patient's heart begins to falter, an electrical pacemaker may be put in place. With such "life-sustaining" machinery available, the definition of death becomes an exceedingly difficult one. In fact, it should be pointed out that not all cells of the body die at once. Living tissue cultures have been established from tissues removed from corpses. In hospitals today a common definition of somatic death concerns the activity of the central nervous system, specifically the brain. When the brain is dead, electrical activity ceases and the electro-encephalogram becomes "flat." When the absence of electrical activity has been demonstrated for a predetermined period of time under rigidly defined circumstances, medical authorities will consider the patient dead despite the fact that heart and lungs could be kept going artificially for some time.

Following death certain so-called postmortem changes ensue. Because of a chemical reaction in the muscles of the dead subject, a stiffness called *rigor mortis* develops. The phrase *algor mortis* refers to the inevitable cooling of a dead subject as the body temperature approaches environmental temperature. Another set of changes is referred to as *livor mortis* or postmortem lividity. Generally, such lividity is due to the fact that when the circulation stops, the blood within the vessels settles according to the pull of gravity, and the tissues lowermost in the body develop a purple discoloration due to their increased content of blood. At a microscopic level, as the individual tissues within the corpse die, their enzymes are released locally, and lytic reactions begin. These reactions, termed *postmortem autolysis* (literally self-dissolution), are very similar to the changes seen in necrotic tissue but, of course, are not accompanied by an inflammatory reaction. The speed of onset of various postmortem changes is extremely variable, depending on individual as well as on associated environmental characteristics. Thus the amazingly accurate pinpointing of the time of death by medical authorities in detective fiction is largely just that, fiction.

QUESTIONS

Cellular injury and death—Chap. 3

Directions: Circle the letter preceding each item below that correctly answers the question. More than one answer may be correct.

1 The part of the cell which serves as the control center because DNA is concentrated within it is the:
a Cell membrane b Cytoplasm c Mitochondria d Nucleus

2 Within the cytoplasm of the cell, protein synthesis is carried out in association with:
a Lysosomes b Endoplasmic reticulum c Mitochondria d Lipofuscin granules

3 Structural alterations in cells which are REVERSIBLE include all of the following EXCEPT:
a Cloudy swelling or cellular swelling b Hydropic change c Fatty infiltration d Karyolysis

4 Accumulation of lipid within liver cells may be related to:
a Starvation of the patient b Excessive alcohol intake by the patient c Obesity d Toxic injury to liver cells e All of the above

5 An increase in the size of a tissue or an organ due to an increase in the size of the individual cells without an increase in the number of component cells would be termed:
a Atrophy b Hypertrophy c Autophagocytosis d Karyolysis

6 The death of cells or tissue within a living host is:
a Somatic death b Putrefaction c Necrosis d Inflammation

7 Necrosis that results in a cheeselike appearance of affected tissue due to disintegration of the dead cells and that is frequently caused by tuberculosis is termed:
a Liquefactive b Caseous c Coagulative d Enzymatic fat

8 Gangrene is most likely to develop in a large area of ischemic necrosis in the:
a Heart b Pancreas c Brain d Intestine

9 A type of calcification which occurs when damaged or dead cells cannot be eliminated from the body is:
a Dystrophic b Metastatic c Calcinosis d Hypertrophic

10 Which of the following would probably *not* be associated with the presence of a calculus (stone) in the excretory duct of an organ?
a Colic b Bleeding into the duct system of the organ c Infection d Proliferation of the secretory cells of the organ e Obstruction to the flow of the particular secretion

causing them to stiffen produces _____

_____.

Directions: Fill in the blanks with the correct words.

11 The sequence of events involved in cellular degenera-

tion includes _____,

_____, and finally

_____ alterations.

12 Three major categories of pathological calcification

are _____, _____

_____, and _____.

13 Following death, a chemical reaction in the muscles

Directions: Match the type of necrosis in col. A with its characteristic manifestation or description in col. B.

Column A

14 ____ Coagulative
         necrosis
15 ____ Liquefactive
         necrosis
16 ____ Caseation
17 ____ Enzymatic fat
         necrosis
18 ____ Gangrene

Column B

a Massive necrosis with
  superimposed bacterial
  growth
b Characteristic of tuberculosis or fungal infections
c Characteristic of brain
d Characteristic necrosis of
  heart and kidney due to
  ischemia
e Related to rupture of the
  pancreatic duct system

CHAPTER 4 Response of the Body to Injury

OBJECTIVES

At the completion of Chap. 4 you will be able to:

1 Define *inflammation* and identify some possible causes.

2 Explain why inflammation is considered a major defense mechanism of the body.

3 Explain why inflammation can originate only within viable tissue and in a living host.

4 Distinguish inflammation from infection.

5 Identify the cardinal signs of acute inflammation and the mechanism responsible for each.

6 Identify the forces which normally govern the transport of fluid between the intravascular and interstitial spaces.

7 Describe the major events (vascular and cellular response) of acute inflammation and their order of occurrence.

8 Name several local chemical mediators of the inflammatory response and describe their role.

9 Describe the margination, adhesion, and emigration of blood leukocytes.

10 Define and contrast *exudate* and *transudate*.

11 Define *lymphadenitis* and describe the mechanism causing it in inflammation.

12 Define *chemotaxis* and *chemotactic substances*.

13 Describe the defensive or adaptive role of phagocytosis.

14 Define *opsonin* and *lysosome*.

15 Describe the morphological and functional characteristics of the five types of blood leukocytes.

16 Differentiate between monocytes, macrophages, and histiocytes.

17 Describe the role of mast cells in acute inflammation.

18 Contrast the characteristics of neutrophils and macrophages.

19 Identify the major locations, components, and function of the reticuloendothelial system (RES) or macrophage system.

20 Differentiate between acute, subacute, and chronic inflammation on the basis of duration and predominant cell types.

21 Describe the characteristics of a granuloma, the mechanism responsible for its formation, and the causative agents involved.

22 Differentiate between these patterns of inflammation on the basis of variations in their exudate and give examples of each: serous, fibrinous, catarrhal, purulent, pseudomembranous, phlegmonous (cellulitis).

23 Identify the components of pus.

24 Define *suppuration, abscess, empyema, sinus, fistula, ulcer.*

25 Describe the possible fate of inflamed areas.

26 Define and differentiate between *healing by first intention* and *healing by second intention* in terms of time, sequence of events, outcome, and factors determining which course will be followed.

27 Identify the local and systemic factors affecting healing.

28 List several complications of wound healing.

29 Describe the systemic effects of inflammation.

AN OVERVIEW OF THE INFLAMMATORY REACTION

Whenever cells or tissues of the body are injured or killed, so long as the host survives, there is a striking response on the part of the surviving adjacent tissues. This response to injury is called *inflammation.* More specifically, inflammation is a vascular reaction whose net result is the delivery of fluid, dissolved substances, and cells from the circulating blood into the interstitial tissues in an area of injury or necrosis.

There is a natural tendency to view inflammation as something undesirable since, under ordinary circumstances, one would rather not have an inflamed throat, skin, soft tissue, or the like. However it cannot be emphasized too strongly that inflammation is actually a beneficial and defensive phenomenon, the net result of which is the neutralization and elimination of an offending agent, the demolition of necrotic tissue, and the establishment of conditions necessary for repair and restitution. The beneficial character of the inflammatory reaction is dramatically demonstrated in our hospitals by what happens when patients cannot produce a needed inflammatory reaction, e.g., when it has become necessary to administer high doses of drugs which have the side effect of suppressing such reactions. Under these conditions there is a high incidence of extremely severe, rapidly spreading, or even lethal infections caused by ordinarily harmless microorganisms.

The inflammatory reaction is actually a dynamic and continuous succession of well-coordinated events. In order to manifest an inflammatory reaction a tissue must be alive and in particular must possess a functional microcirculation. One corollary to this requirement is that if an area of tissue necrosis is extensive, the inflammatory reaction will not be found in its midst, but rather at its edges, i.e., at the interface between the dead tissue and living tissue with an intact circulation. Another corollary is that if a particular injury kills the host instantly, there will be no evidence of an associated inflammatory reaction, since this would take time to develop.

The causes of inflammation are numerous and varied. There is no profit in attempting to list these causes, but it is essential to understand that *inflammation and infection are not synonymous.* Thus, *infection* (the presence of living microorganisms within the tissue) is but one cause of inflammation, and in many instances inflammation occurs under conditions of perfect sterility, such as when a portion of tissue dies because of deprivation of blood supply. Because of the broad range of situations which result in inflammation, an understanding of the process is basic to much of biology and medicine. Without an understanding of the process one cannot begin to comprehend the principles of infectious disease, the principles of surgery, wound healing, and the response to a variety of kinds of trauma, or the principles of how the body copes with catastrophes of tissue death such as strokes, "heart attacks," and the like.

Despite the large number of causes of inflammation and the varieties of situations in which it appears, the train of events set in motion tends to be the same in general outline, with various types of examples of inflammation differing largely in quantitative detail. Happily, therefore, one can study the inflammatory reaction as a general phenomenon and deal with the quantitative variations secondarily.

GROSS FEATURES OF ACUTE INFLAMMATION

Acute inflammation is the *immediate* response of the body to injury or cell death. The gross features are familiar to all of us, as a moment's reflection on past scrapes, cuts, and minor infections will recall. In fact, these obvious features of inflammation were described some 2000 years ago and are still known as *cardinal signs of inflammation.* These include pain, redness, warmth, swelling, and altered function, or, in the classical Latin, *dolor, rubor, calor, tumor,* and *functio laesa.*

Redness

Redness, or rubor, is usually the first thing to be noted in an area that is in the process of becoming inflamed. As the inflammatory reaction begins, the arterioles supplying the area become dilated, thus allowing more blood into the local microcirculation. Capillaries previously empty or perhaps only partly distended quickly become packed with blood (Fig. 4-1). This condition, termed *hyperemia* or *congestion,* accounts for the local blush of acute inflammation. The production of hyperemia at the start of an inflammatory reaction is controlled by the body both neurogenically and chemically, via the release of substances like histamine.

Heat

Heat, or calor, parallels the redness of an acute inflammatory reaction. Actually, heat is a characteristic only of the inflammatory reactions at the body surface, which is normally cooler than the 37°C temperature of the interior of the body. An area of cutaneous inflammation becomes warmer than the surroundings because there is more blood (at 37°C) being conducted from the inside of the body to the surface in the affected area than in a normal area. This phenomenon of local warmth is not observed in inflamed areas deep within the body, since such tissues will already be at the core temperature of 37°C, and local hyperemia would make no difference.

Pain

The pain, or dolor, of an inflammatory reaction is probably produced in a variety of ways. Change in local pH

or in the local concentration of certain ions can stimulate nerve endings. Similarly, the release of certain chemicals such as histamine or other bioactive chemicals can stimulate the nerves. In addition, swelling of the inflamed tissues leading to increased local pressure can undoubtedly produce pain.

Swelling

Perhaps the most striking aspect of acute inflammation is the local swelling (tumor). This is produced by the transfer of fluid and cells from the bloodstream to the interstitial tissues. This mixture of fluid and cells that accumulates in an area of inflammation is termed an *exudate.* Early in the course of inflammatory reactions most of the exudate is fluid. A classic example of such exudate fluid is that which appears quickly within a blister following a minor burn of the skin. Somewhat later, white blood cells, or leukocytes, leave the bloodstream and accumulate as part of the exudate.

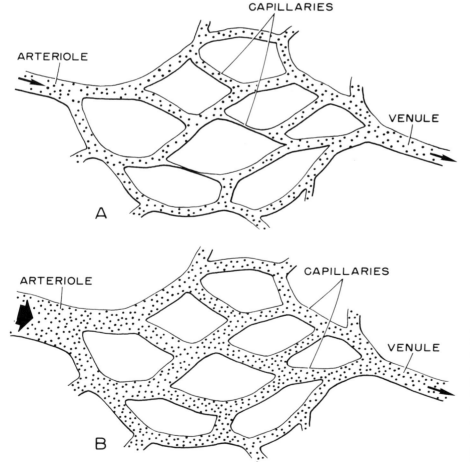

FIGURE 4-1 Mechanism of hyperemia in acute inflammation. The caliber of the arteriole controls the volume flow of blood into a capillary bed. In the normal state (A), the flow is such that some capillaries appear collapsed and others extremely narrow. With arteriolar dilatation (B), the increased volume of blood flowing into the capillaries distends them and produces the gross red-purple discoloration of tissue due to increased blood content.

Altered function

The fact of altered function, *functio laesa,* is a familiar one. In a superficial way, it is easy to understand why a swollen, painful part with an abnormal circulation and abnormal local chemical environment should function abnormally. In truth, however, we do not understand in detail the means whereby function of an inflamed tissue is impaired.

FLUID ASPECTS OF INFLAMMATION

Exudation

In order to understand the very rapid flux of fluid across vessel walls into the tissue in an area of inflammation it is necessary to recall the principles governing fluid transport under more normal conditions. Ordinarily, the walls of the smallest vascular channels (such as capillaries and venules) will allow small molecules to pass but will retain large molecules such as plasma proteins within the vascular lumen. The result of this semipermeable character of the vessels is that there is an

osmotic force tending to keep fluid within the vasculature. This is counterbalanced by the outward thrust of hydrostatic pressure within the vessels. A simplified diagram of the balance of forces is shown in Fig. 4-2. It can be seen that the lymphatics function to siphon off fluid which has reached the interstices of the tissue, and an equilibrium is thus normally maintained.

Shifts of fluid in the evolving inflammatory reaction are exceedingly rapid, as illustrated by the previously cited example of a blister following thermal injury. When such inflammatory exudates are analyzed, it is found that they contain significant amounts of plasma protein. Thus, a key event in acute inflammation is the alteration of permeability of the tiny vessels in the area leading to protein leakage. This is followed by a shift in osmotic balance and, in effect, water follows protein, producing swelling of the tissues. The arteriolar dilatation which produces local hyperemia and redness also results in an increase in intravascular pressure locally as vessels become engorged. This, too, augments the fluid shift (Fig. 4-2). The major factor, however, is the increase in vascular permeability to protein.

It is the endothelial cells which line the small vessels that are responsible for the usual semipermeable character of the vessels, and it is these same cells which change their relationship to one another in acute inflammation, producing the leakage of protein and fluid. Figure 4-3 shows the situation diagrammatically. In the normal small vessel at the left, the endothelial lining cells are

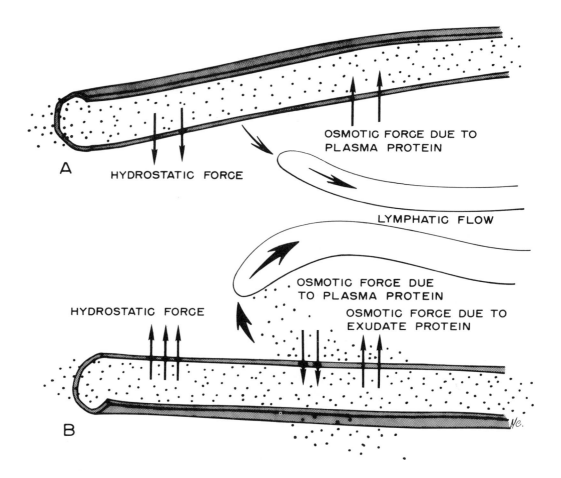

joined tightly to one another. The dots in the lumen represent large molecules such as those of serum proteins or of large marker particles injected experimentally to simulate protein molecules. Ordinarily these large molecules or particles cannot penetrate the intercellular junctions. However, if one induces an inflammatory reaction locally, there develops an actual separation between contiguous endothelial cells in the area, and the marker particles (and presumably the protein molecules) exit from the lumen as shown at the right of Fig. 4-3. If one uses a pigmented marker particle for such an experiment, entire vessels become discolored, and it becomes possible to see which part of the microcirculation is actually leaking in the course of inflammation. In most instances studied in this fashion, the leak seems to occur chiefly at the venular end of the microcirculation rather than within the true capillaries (Fig. 4-3).

The regularity of this response, even with diverse stimuli, the frequent presence of a latent period between application of the inflammatory stimulus and the beginning of leakage, and the ability to frustrate the reaction with certain chemical agents all indicate that chemically active *mediators* must be released locally to account for the separation of endothelial cells and the permeability changes. A variety of substances including histamine, plasma kinins, and prostaglandins, to mention but a few, have been identified as probable mediators of acute inflammation. Probably different combinations of mediators are important in different circumstances associated with inflammation. In addition, independently of mediators, it is likely that some injurious modalities lead to direct damage of vascular endothelium with associated leakage of protein and fluid through openings thus created.

Lymphatics and flow of lymph

The lymphatic system participates in the acute inflammatory reaction in parallel with the blood vascular system. Ordinarily there is a slow percolation of interstitial fluid into lymphatic channels in the tissue, and the lymph thus formed is carried centrally in the body ultimately to rejoin venous blood. As an area becomes inflamed, there is usually a striking increase in the flow of lymph draining from the area. It is known that in the course of acute inflammation, the contiguous lining cells of the smallest lymphatics separate somewhat, just as

FIGURE 4-2 *Factors involved in fluid exchange between blood vessels and tissues. In the normal or resting state (A), hydrostatic forces tend to push fluid into the interstitial spaces. This is largely balanced by the osmotic force exerted by plasma protein (dots) which ordinarily do not pass through vessel walls. The fluid which does pass into the interstices drains via the lymphatics. In acute inflammation (B), protein escapes from the vessels as permeability increases. This, along with a smaller contribution from the increased hydrostatic pressure related to hyperemia, accounts for a significant fluid flux. Lymphatic flow is correspondingly increased.*

they do within the venules, thus allowing more ready access of material from the interstices of tissues into the lymphatics. There is even evidence that lymphatic channels are maintained in an open position as a tissue swells by a system of connective tissue fibers anchored to the walls of the lymphatics. In any event, not only does the flow of lymph increase but the protein and cell content of the lymph likewise increase during acute inflammation. On the one hand, this increased flow of material through lymphatics is beneficial since it tends to minimize the swelling of the inflamed tissue by draining off a portion of the exudate. On the other hand, the price we pay is that potentially injurious agents can be carried by the lymphatics from a primary site of inflammation to a distant point in the body. By such means, for instance, infectious agents may spread. The spread is often limited by the filtering action of regional lymph nodes through which the lymph flows as it moves centralward in the body; but agents or materials carried within the lymph may pass through the nodes and reach the bloodstream. For these reasons one must always be aware of the possible involvement of the lymphatic system in inflammation of any cause. When a lymphatic vessel itself becomes inflamed, this is termed *lymphangitis*. If a lymph node becomes inflamed, the phenomenon is termed *lymphadenitis*. Regional lymphadenitis is an exceedingly common accompaniment of inflammation. One familiar example is the enlarged, tender cervical lymph nodes seen with tonsillitis. (The more general term *lymphadenopathy* is used to describe virtually any abnormality of lymph nodes. In practice the term refers not only to lymphadenitis, but to any *enlargement* of lymph nodes, most nodal reactions being accompanied by enlargement.)

CELLULAR ASPECTS OF INFLAMMATION

Margination and emigration

Early in acute inflammation as arterioles dilate, the flow of blood into the inflamed area increases. Soon, however, the character of the blood flow changes. As fluid leaks out of the microcirculation with its increased permeability, large numbers of the so-called formed elements (red blood cells, platelets, and white blood cells), are left behind, and the viscosity of the blood increases. The circulation within the affected area then slows, leading to some important consequences. In a normal situation (Fig. 4-4A), the flow of blood is more or less streamlined, and the formed elements do not bump up against the sides of the vessel appreciably. As the viscosity of the blood increases and the flow slows, the leukocytes begin to *marginate*, that is, they move to the periphery of the stream, along the lining of the vessel

(Fig. 4-4B). With progression of the phenomenon, the marginated leukocytes begin to adhere to the endothelium. The result is an appearance reminiscent of a cobblestone street, leading to the designation of this event as *pavementing*. Actually margination and pavementing are but preludes to emigration of the leukocytes from the blood vessels to the surrounding tissue.

Figure 4-4C is a diagrammatic representation of leukocytic emigration. Leukocytes move in an ameoboid fashion. They seem able to protrude a pseudopod into the potential space between two endothelial cells and then push gradually through to appear on the other side, a process requiring a matter of minutes. The net result, given the fact that this event is repeated in innumerable venules and that more and more leukocytes are delivered into the area via the circulating blood, is that tremendous numbers of cells are delivered into the area of inflammation in a relatively short time. Literally millions of cells emigrate into even a small area of inflammation within a period of several hours.

Chemotaxis

The active motility of the leukocytes in the interstices of inflamed tissues once they emigrate is apparently not random but directionally oriented. This is accomplished by a variety of chemical "signals." The phenomenon of

directional orientation of movement is referred to as *chemotaxis*. Many different things may provide a chemotactic signal to attract leukocytes, ranging from infectious agents, to damaged tissues, to substances activated within the protein fraction of plasma leaking from the bloodstream. Thus, a smooth combination of increased delivery of leukocytes to the area (hyperemia), changes in blood flow resulting in margination and pavementing, and chemotactic orientation of leukocyte motion results in the rapid accumulation of a significant leukocytic component in the exudate.

Types of leukocytes and their functions

The leukocytes which circulate in the bloodstream and emigrate into inflammatory exudates originate in the bone marrow, where not only leukocytes, but also red blood cells and platelets are continuously produced (see Part III). Normally, within the bone marrow there can be found large numbers of immature leukocytes of various kinds and a "pool" of mature leukocytes being held in reserve for release into the circulating blood. The numbers of each type of leukocyte circulating in the peripherial blood are closely controlled within certain limits (see Part III) but are altered "on demand" when an inflammatory process arises. That is to say, with the instigation of an inflammatory response, feedback signals to the bone marrow alter the rate of production and release of one or more kinds of leukocytes into the bloodstream.

Granulocytes constitute a class of leukocytes which includes neutrophils, eosinophils, and basophils. These

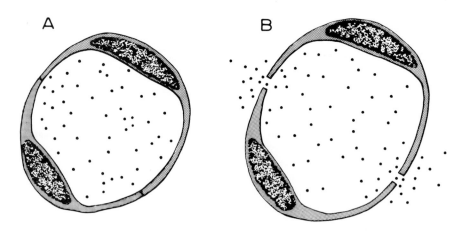

FIGURE 4-3 Mechanism of increased vascular permeability in acute inflammation. In normal vessels (A), the junctions between endothelial lining cells are sufficiently tight to keep large molecules (dots) within the lumen. In acute inflammation (B), contraction of endothelial cells creates gaps allowing leakage of macromolecules. As shown in (C), the permeability change is at the venular side of the microcirculatory bed.

three types of cells are named by virtue of the granules within their cytoplasm visible after the application of certain dyes. Two additional types of leukocytes, monocytes and lymphocytes, do not contain the numerous cytoplasmic granules that characterize the above-named cells. Although each of the types of cells listed is available in the circulating blood, the appearance of leukocytes within exudates is not a random affair but probably represents the result of specific chemotactic signals arising in the evolution of the inflammatory process.

The first cells to appear in large numbers within exudates in the early hours of inflammation are neutrophils. The nuclei of these cells are irregularly lobed or polymorphous (Fig. 4-5). These cells are therefore called *polymorphonuclear neutrophils, PMNs* or *"polys."* These cells have a developmental sequence within the bone marrow which requires approximately 2 weeks for completion. When they are released into the circulating blood, their circulatory half-life is 6 hours or so. There are approximately 5000 neutrophils per cubic millimeter of blood in circulation at any given time, with approximately 100 times this number being held in reserve as mature cells within the bone marrow ready to be released on signal. Amazingly, although literally billions of neutrophils per day are replaced by the bone marrow, their production and release is quite rigidly controlled. When released into the bloodstream, polymorphonuclear neutrophils are ordinarily incapable of further cell division or significant synthesis of cellular products. The numerous granules visible within the cytoplasm of the neutrophils, however, actually represent membrane-bound packets of enzymes, i.e., *lysosomes*, produced during maturation of the cells. These enzymes include a wide variety of hydrolases, including proteases, lipases, phosphatases, etc. In addition, associated with the granules are a variety of antimicrobial substances. Thus, in effect, the mature polymorphonuclear neutrophil is a traveling bag of enzyme-loaded and antimicrobial particles.

Polymorphonuclear neutrophils are capable of active ameboid motion and are able to engulf a variety of materials by a process termed *phagocytosis*. As illustrated in Fig. 4-6, the neutrophil approaches the particle (for instance, a bacterium) to be phagocytized, flows its cytoplasm around the particle, and eventually takes the particle into the cytoplasm enveloped in a membrane-bound vesicle which pinches off from the cell membrane of the neutrophil. This phagocytic process is aided by certain substances which coat the object to be ingested and render it more easily internalized by the leukocyte. These kinds of leukocytosis-promoting substances, called *opsonins*, include immunoglobulin antibodies and components of the so-called complement system (see Chap. 5). Having ingested a particle and incorporated it into the cytoplasm in a *phagocytic vacuole* or *phagosome*, the next task of the leukocyte is to kill the particle, if it is a living microbial agent, and to digest it. Killing of living agents is accomplished in a variety of ways including alteration in intracellular pH following phagocytosis, release of antibacterial substances into the phagocytic vacuole, and production of antibacterial sub-

stances such as hydrogen peroxide as a result of cellular metabolic processes initiated following the phagocytic event. The digestion of phagocytized particles is generally accomplished within the vacuoles by fusion of lysosomes with the phagosome. The previously inactive digestive enzymes are now activated within the so-called *phagolysosome*, resulting in the enzymatic digestion of the object.

Under certain other circumstances, these same potent digestive enzymes of the neutrophils may be released into the host tissues rather than into intracellular phagolysosomes. When this occurs, the neutrophilic enzymes become potent agents of tissue injury. This extracellular release occurs with death and disintegration of neutrophils; it occurs following phagocytosis of certain crystals such as urates by neutrophils (because phagocytosis of these crystals is followed by rupture of phagolysosomes); and it also occurs when neutrophils attempt to ingest immune complexes under certain circumstances. These kinds of situations will be described more fully below.

The *eosinophil* is another type of granulocyte which may appear in inflammatory exudates, although usually in relatively small numbers. Eosinophils have irregular nuclei much like neutrophils, but the cytoplasmic granules stain a bright red with the dye eosin and are much more prominent than the lavender-colored granules of neutrophils. The granules of eosinophils are actually packets of enzymes quite similar to those of neutrophils. In fact, functionally eosinophils do many of the same things: responding to chemotactic stimuli, phagocytizing various kinds of particles, and even killing certain microorganisms. What appears to be distinctive about eosinophils, however, is that they respond to certain unique chemotactic stimuli generated in the course of allergic reactions and that they contain enzymes which are capable of counteracting the effects of certain inflammatory mediators released in such reactions. Apparently correlated with these features is the fact that eosinophils tend to accumulate in significant concentrations at the site of allergic reactions, where they may be acting as "firemen."

The third type of granulocyte is the *basophil*, whose cytoplasm is crowded with large granules which stain a deep blue with basic dyes. Although these cells come from the bone marrow like other granulocytes, they have many features in common with certain cells of the connective tissues called *mast cells* or *tissue basophils*. The granules of both of these kinds of cells contain a variety of enzymes, heparin, and histamine. Blood basophils seem to respond to chemotactic signals released in the course of certain immunologic reactions. Ordinarily they are present in very small numbers in exudates. Blood basophils and tissue mast cells are stimulated to release the contents of their granules into the surroundings in a variety of injurious circumstances including both immunologic and nonspecific reactions. In fact, the mast cells are a major source of histamine early in any acute inflammatory reaction. The immunologic means of stimulating granule release by mast cells or basophils will be discussed in Chap. 5.

The *monocyte* is an important form of leukocyte which differs from the granulocytes by virtue of its nuclear morphology and the relatively agranular character of its cytoplasm (Fig. 4-5). The monocyte originates within the bone marrow just as do the granulocytes, but its circulatory life is 3 to 4 times longer than that of granulocytes. In the course of acute inflammatory reactions monocytes begin to emigrate approximately at the same time as do neutrophils, but they do so in much smaller numbers and at a slower rate. Consequently in the early hours of inflammation there are relatively few such cells within exudate. However, as exudates age, the

percentage of these cells frequently increases. The same cell which is called a monocyte in the circulating blood is called a *macrophage* when it appears within exudates. In fact, the same type of cell is found wandering in small numbers through the connective tissues of the body even in the absence of overt inflammation. These wandering macrophages in the connective tissues are frequently referred to as *histiocytes*.

In many ways the functions of macrophages most closely parallel those of polymorphonuclear neutrophils in that macrophages are actively motile cells which respond to chemotactic stimuli, are actively phagocytic, and are able to kill and digest a variety of agents. A number of important differences between macrophages and neutrophils exists. For one thing, the life cycle of macrophages is very different in that these cells may survive weeks or even possibly months within the tissues as compared to the short-lived neutrophils. In addition, when the monocyte enters the bloodstream from the bone marrow and when it enters the tissues from the bloodstream, it is not a fully mature cell in the sense that the neutrophil is. This latter cell is incapable of further

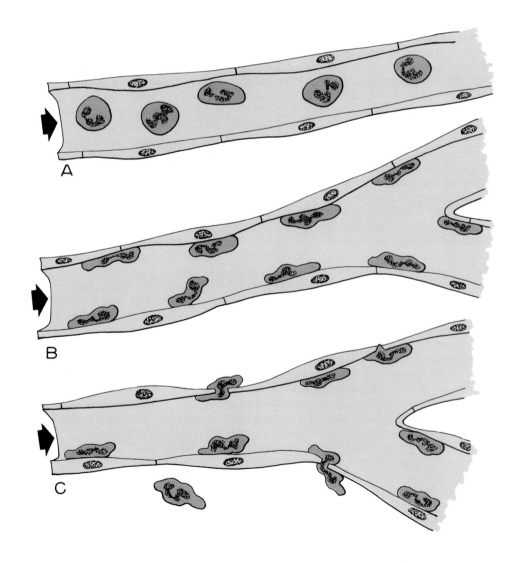

A

B

C

division and is also incapable of active synthesis of digestive enzymes. Monocytes, on the other hand, can be stimulated under some circumstances to divide within the tissues, and they are capable of responding to local conditions by synthesizing a variety of intracellular enzymes. This ability to undergo "on-the-job training" is a vital property of macrophages, particularly in certain immunologic reactions where they are literally trained by lymphocytes. In such circumstances macrophages are known to increase their metabolic activities, become more effective in phagocytosis, and become more efficient in killing and digesting certain microbes. In addition, macrophages may alter their form as they undergo such changes, giving rise to cells which have been traditionally referred to as *epithelioid cells*. Macrophages are also able to fuse together to form *multinucleated giant cells*. These forms will be illustrated below.

Although macrophages are significant components of various exudates, they are widely distributed in the body under normal baseline conditions. This was recognized many years ago and the term *reticuloendothelial system* (RES) was coined in recognition of the existence of a population of mononuclear cells sharing the same property, namely, phagocytosis. The RES is gradually coming to be called the *macrophage system*, because this name is actually more descriptive. As ordinarily conceived, the RES, or macrophage system, includes not only the blood monocytes and tissue histiocytes or wandering macrophages but a large population of more or less fixed mononuclear phagocytic cells closely related to the more mobile members of the system. This population of less mobile cells includes lining cells along blood channels within the spleen, the liver (where the cells are known as Kupffer cells), and the bone marrow. Similar fixed macrophages are present along many of the lymphatic channels within the lymph nodes of the body. There are, in addition, many macrophages within the serosal cavities of the body, within the lungs, and even within the central nervous system.

The important functions of this system involve, of course, the vigorous phagocytic activities of the component cells. These cells are responsible literally for cleaning the blood, the lymph, and the interstitial spaces of foreign material, thus performing a vital defensive function. Experimentally if one injects even millions of microorganisms into the circulating blood, they are removed within a matter of a few hours by the many millions of macrophages located strategically around the body. This is exceedingly important in everyday life inasmuch as the release of at least a few microorganisms into the circulating fluids of the body is a fairly frequent event.

It is known, for instance, that with vigorous brushing of the teeth, defecation, or, in fact, with certain medical or dental manipulations, organisms frequently enter the bloodstream. Because of the phagocytic activities of the macrophage system such episodes of *bacteremia* are transient and trivial. The macrophages in the body cavities and connective tissues perform a similar police function. In addition, the uptake of foreign material by macrophages is an essential first step in the chain of events which leads to the induction of an immune response (see Chap. 5). Finally, an important everyday function of the RES involves the processing of the hemoglobin of red blood cells which have reached the end of their life span. It is the function of macrophages to trap and recycle the components of this essential substance. These cells are capable of splitting hemoglobin into an iron-containing moiety and a non-iron-containing moiety. The iron is recycled in the body for the building of other red blood cells in the bone marrow and the non-iron-containing moiety, which is known as *bilirubin,* is carried in the bloodstream to the liver, where the hepatocytes extract the bilirubin from the bloodstream and secrete it as part of the bile.

One type of leukocyte, the *lymphocyte,* has not yet been mentioned. Lymphocytes generally are present in exudates only in very small numbers until the exudates are quite old, that is, until the inflammatory reactions have become chronic. Since the known functions of lymphocytes are all within the immunologic realm, these cells will be more fully described in Chap. 5.

Having described the essential features of the acute inflammatory response, it might be well to reflect at this point on the beneficial or adaptive nature of the response, each component of which has a unique importance. The function of the vasodilatation early in acute inflammation is to bring to the area the "raw materials" for the reaction. It is known that if the arteriolar dilatation and increased blood flow are frustrated by local conditions or by the administration of certain drugs, later aspects of the inflammatory reaction are significantly frustrated. The increased vascular permeability accomplishes not only the outpouring of fluid which may act to dilute noxious agents but also accomplishes the transfer of some important protein substances such as opsonins or other antibodies to the "battleground." Furthermore, one of the proteins which leaks into the area of inflammation is *fibrinogen,* which quickly precipitates to form *fibrin* which may act as kind of a sealer or "glue" in wounds, and because of its fibrillar character may act as a scaffold for migration of phagocytic leukocytes and ultimately for repair. The mobilization of leukocytes is of obvious defensive value not only in terms of the apprehension of invading microbes but also because leukocytes are responsible for demolition of tissue debris so that repair processes can begin.

FIGURE 4-4 Blood flow and cellular phenomena in acute inflammation. Normally (A), formed elements of the blood, especially the leukocytes shown in the diagram, are carried in the mainstream. As the circulation slows (B), margination of leukocytes occurs. This is a prelude to emigration of leukocytes between endothelial cells (C).

PATTERNS OF INFLAMMATION

Although the inflammatory reaction tends to evolve by the mechanisms described above, a number of different patterns of inflammation can emerge based on the type of exudate that is formed, the particular organ or tissue involved, and the duration of the inflammatory process. The nomenclature of inflammatory processes takes into account each of these variables. Different sorts of exudates are given descriptive names. The duration of the inflammatory response is designated as *acute* during the phase of active exudation; as *chronic* when there is evidence of advanced repair along with the exudation; and as *subacute* when there is but early evidence of repair along with the exudation. The location of the inflammatory reaction is designated by the suffix *-itis* appended to organ name (e.g., appendicitis, tonsillitis, arthritis, etc.).

Noncellular exudates

In some instances of inflammation, the exudate consists almost entirely of fluid and dissolved substances with very few leukocytes. The simplest sort of noncellular exudate is a *serous* exudate, which consists basically of the protein which leaks from permeable blood vessels in an area of inflammation along with the accompanying fluid. The most familiar example of serous exudate is blister fluid. Similar accumulations of serous exudate are frequent within body cavities such as the pleural cavity or the peritoneal cavity and, although not as strik-ing, serous exudates frequently spread through connective tissues.

Sometimes collections of fluid occur in body cavities for reasons other than inflammation, usually increased hydrostatic pressure or depletion of plasma protein. Such noninflammatory collections are termed *transudates,* and are protein-poor and cell-poor compared to exudates. A related type of noncellular exudate is *fibrinous* exudate. Such an exudate forms when the protein which is extravasated in an area of inflammation contains abundant fibrinogen. This fibrinogen precipitates to form fibrin, which is a sort of sticky, elastic meshwork (perhaps more familiar as the backbone of blood clot). Fibrinous exudates are frequently encountered on inflamed serosal surfaces such as the pleura and the pericardium, where the precipitated fibrin is compacted into a shaggy layer on the involved membrane (Fig. 4-7). When such a shaggy layer of fibrin has accumulated on serosal surfaces, it is frequently accompanied by the symptom of pain when one surface rubs on another. Thus, for instance, the patient with pleuritis feels pain upon respiration when the roughened surfaces rub together during inspiration. This rubbing of shaggy surfaces also produces a sign called *friction rub,* which is audible through the stethoscope over the affected area, be it pleura, pericardium, or the like.

Yet another noncellular exudate is the *mucinous* or *catarrhal* exudate. This type of exudate can form only on the surface of a mucous membrane, where there are cells capable of secreting mucin. This type of exudate differs from others in that it represents a cellular secretion rather than something which escapes from the bloodstream. Mucin secretion is obviously a normal property of mucous membranes, and mucinous exudate represents nothing more than an acceleration of a basic physiological process. The most familiar and homely example of a mucinous exudate is the runny nose which accompanies many upper respiratory infections.

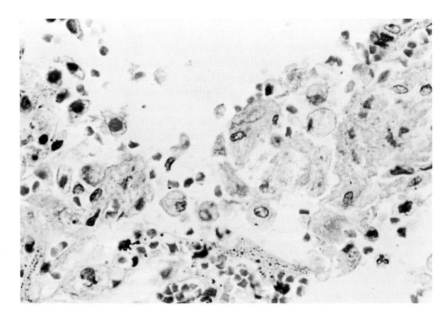

FIGURE 4-5 Macrophages and neutrophils in lung. In this instance relatively small numbers of leukocytes have emigrated from the bloodstream, and the field has been chosen to show these cells in relative isolation. In the space to the lower right corner are a few neutrophils, one of which has a distinctly trilobed nucleus (in sections such as this, granules are not as apparent as in blood films). Coursing horizontally across the field at bottom center is a distended capillary containing many red blood cells. In the space just above this are several macrophages with ovoid or indented nuclei and abundant cytoplasm. (Photomicrograph ×500.)

Probably the most common exudates are those which consist predominantly of polymorphonuclear neutrophils, in such numbers as to overshadow the fluid and proteinaceous parts of exudate. Such neutrophilic exudates are referred to as *purulent*. Purulent exudates (Fig. 4-8) are very commonly formed in response to bacterial infection. They are also seen in response to many aseptic injuries and are prominent in situations where tissues have become necrotic almost anywhere in the body.

Not infrequently (most often with bacterial infection) extremely high concentrations of neutrophils accumulate in a tissue, and many of these cells die and liberate their powerful hydrolytic enzymes into the surroundings. Under such circumstances the enzymes of the neutrophils literally digest the underlying tissue and liquefy it. This combination of neutrophil aggregation and liquefaction of underlying tissues is referred to as *suppuration,* and the exudate thus formed is referred to as *suppurative exudate*, or, more commonly, *pus*. Thus, pus consists of polymorphonuclear neutrophils, living, dying, and disintegrated, liquefied digestion products of underlying tissue, fluid exudate of the inflammatory process, and, very often, the inciting bacteria. The significant difference between suppurative and purulent inflammation is that with suppuration, there is liquefactive necrosis of underlying tissue. Figure 4-9 illustrates the significant difference between purulent and suppurative inflammation.

When localized suppuration occurs within a solid tissue, the resulting lesion is termed an *abscess*. As seen in Fig. 4-9, an abscess is quite literally a hole in the involved tissue filled with pus. Abscesses are difficult lesions for the body to handle because of their tendency to expand with the liquefaction of more tissue, their tendency to burrow, and their resistance to healing. In fact when an abscess has formed, it is difficult to deliver therapeutic agents such as antibiotics into the abscess via the bloodstream. In general the handling of abscesses by the body is greatly aided by draining them surgically, thus allowing the closed space previously filled with pus to collapse and heal. If abscesses are not surgically drained by pathways chosen by the surgeon, they tend to expand, destroying additional structures in their path. An abscess in lung might burrow until it communicates with the pleural cavity, and if the contents are discharged into the pleural cavity and infection spreads, the result might be *empyema,* which is a purulent inflammatory process involving the entire pleural cavity. Occasionally an abscess will rupture onto a surface and produce a draining tract which ends blindly in the space of the abscess. Any such blind tract communicating with a surface is referred to as a *sinus*. If, on the other hand, an abscess extended to two separate surfaces, it might result in an abnormal tract communicating between two

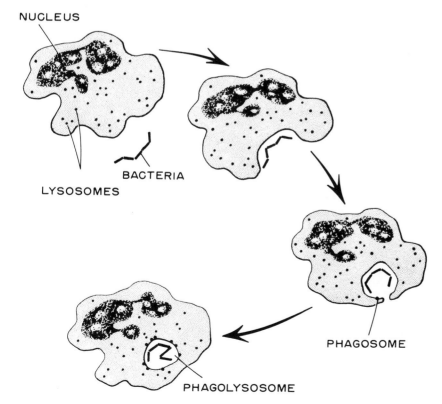

NUCLEUS

BACTERIA

LYSOSOMES

PHAGOSOME

PHAGOLYSOSOME

FIGURE 4-6 Diagram of phagocytosis. Neutrophils and monocytes ingest particles by flowing their cytoplasm around the objects and internalizing them in an envelope of cell membrane, the phagosome. The digestive enzymes of the lysosomes are then released into the phagolysosome.

organs or between the lumen of a hollow organ and the body surface. Such an abnormal communication is referred to as a *fistula*. (Fistulas are named according to their communications, e.g., gastrocolic, bronchopleural, colocutaneous.)

When purulent inflammation extends diffusely through a tissue, the process is referred to as *phlegmonous*. Perhaps more commonly the term *cellulitis* is used clinically to describe an area of phlegmonous inflammation. Such a spreading purulent process is seen usually as a result of bacterial infection when the particular agent is capable of spreading rapidly through the loose connective tissue of the body.

As one would expect, there are frequently mixtures of noncellular and cellular exudates, and these are named accordingly. Thus there are *fibrinopurulent* exudates which consist of fibrin and polymorphonuclear

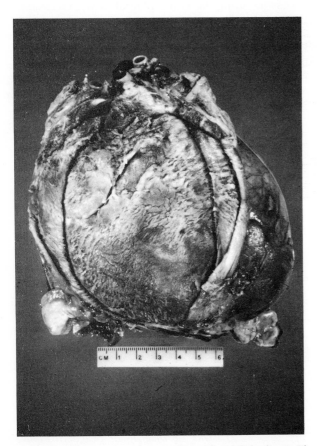

FIGURE 4-7 Fibrinous exudate on the surface of the heart. The pericardium has been opened and instead of the normally smooth epicardial surface, a shaggy layer of fibrin is evident. This has formed from fibrinogen that has exuded from underlying vessels. Classically this condition has been termed "bread-and-butter heart."

neutrophils, *mucopurulent* exudates consisting of mucin and neutrophils, *serofibrinous* exudates, etc. Certain of these exudates such as mucinous and mucopurulent are, of course, unique to mucous membranes.

Frequently in association with damage to mucous membranes, a necrotic area may actually slough off, leaving a gap in the continuity of the mucosal surface. Such a defect is termed an *ulcer*. Most often the bed of an ulcer will be surfaced by fibrinopurulent exudate emanating from the underlying blood vessels (Fig. 4-10). Sometimes broad areas of mucous membrane will become necrotic, and the dead cells may become enmeshed in a web of fibrinopurulent exudate which coats the mucosal surface. Such an area grossly resembles a ragged mucous membrane and hence this type of process is referred to as *pseudomembranous* or simply *membranous* inflammation (Fig. 4-11). The classical example of pseudomembranous inflammation in bygone days was the pseudomembrane of diphtheria within the respiratory tract. Thus such membranes are occasionally referred to as *diptheritic*. Pseudomembranous inflammation is now more commonly observed within the gastrointestinal tract, particularly the colon, as the result of an upset in the microbial ecology of the tract usually brought about by the administration of antibiotics.

A unique and distinctive pattern of inflammation which can occur virtually anywhere is *granulomatous* inflammation. This type of inflammation is characterized by the massing of large numbers of macrophages and their aggregation into nodular clumps referred to as *granulomas*. Although many inflammatory exudates contain appreciable numbers of macrophages, in granulomatous inflammation the field is dominated literally by sheets of these cells or their derivatives such as epithelioid cells or multinucleated giant cells. Granulomas take time to evolve and generally pass through rather nondescript acute stages where there is exudation of fluid, neutrophils, and protein. It is the continued emigration of monocytes and also the local proliferation of these cells which leads to their massing as a granuloma. Granulomas usually form because of the persistence within the tissues of some offensive agent resistant to the efforts of the body to dispose of it. Such agents can include insoluble but sterile materials or particularly resistant microorganisms. The prototypical microorganism which evokes the formation of granulomas is the *Mycobacterium tuberculosis*, or tubercle bacillus. The response to this organism is characteristically granulomatous, and usually the macrophages mass in nodular aggregates of epithelioid cells and giant cells. This sort of a nodular mass of epithelioid cells is referred to as a *tubercle* (Fig. 4-12). Granulomas also form in response to foreign bodies such as suture materials (Fig. 4-13). In general the presence of a granuloma is the hallmark of "tissue indigestion." As the granuloma evolves in some instances, the macrophages acquire increasing ability to handle the offensive agent, in which case it is eliminated. In other instances the agent remains refractory, and the net effect of the granuloma formation is to wall off that agent from the remainder of the body.

Given the presence of an inflammatory reaction, the happiest result that can be obtained occurs when there actually has been little or no destruction of underlying tissue. In such instances when the offending agent has been neutralized and removed, the stimulus for continuing exudation of fluid and cells gradually disappears. The small blood vessels in the area regain their usual semipermeability, fluid flux ceases, and emigration of leukocytes likewise stops. The fluid which has been previously exuded is gradually absorbed by the lymphatics, and the cells of the exudate disintegrate, wander off via the lymphatics, or are actually eliminated from the body (as, for instance, by being coughed up in the case of exudates within the lung). The net result of this process is that the previously inflamed tissue is left precisely as it was before the reaction started. This phenomenon is referred to as *resolution*.

In contrast, when significant amounts of tissue have been destroyed, resolution cannot occur. There must be *repair* of the destroyed tissue by proliferation of adjacent

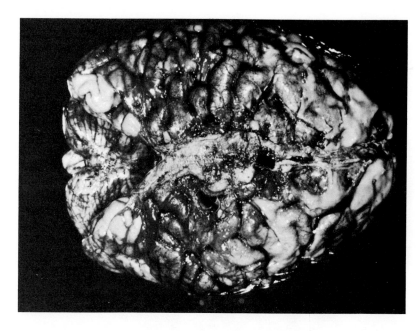

FIGURE 4-8 Purulent exudate within the cerebral meninges. The membranes covering the brain contain literally millions of neutrophils forming a purulent exudate. The creamy patches of exudate are especially prominent at the right. The gyri in the center of the photo are dark because of intense vascular congestion, part of the inflammatory response. (This is pneumococcal meningitis.)

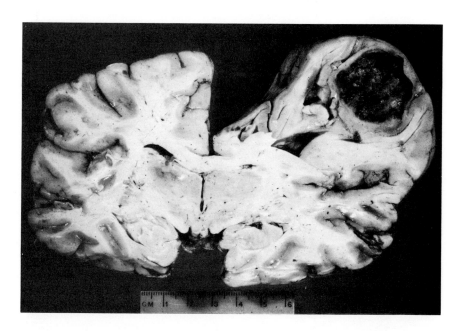

FIGURE 4-9 Brain abscess. As a result of bacterial infection in the cerebral hemisphere on the right, large numbers of neutrophils emigrated into the region. Liquefaction of the regional tissue by lysosomal enzymes of the neutrophils produced the defect illustrated.

surviving host cells. Repair actually involves two separate but coordinated components. One, referred to as *regeneration,* actually involves proliferation of parenchymal elements identical to those lost, the net result being replacement of those lost elements by the same kind of cells. The second component of repair involves the proliferation of connective tissue elements leading to the formation of *scar.* In most tissues there is a combination of these two activities.

The abilities of different kinds of cells and tissues to regenerate differs widely. Most epithelial tissues, such as the covering of the skin, the lining of the mouth, pharynx, and gastrointestinal tract, regenerate beautifully following loss of a portion of the tissue. Other epithelial cells, such as those of the liver parenchyma, renal tubules, or the secretory elements of certain glands, regenerate well providing that the outlines of the tissue are maintained without extensive collapse during the inflammatory process. Unfortunately some tissues regenerate very poorly or not at all. Useful regeneration is extremely limited in involuntary and voluntary muscle if it is present at all, and there is absolutely no regeneration in heart muscle, which is unfortunate given the frequency of necrosis of portions of myocardium in our population. Finally it should be pointed out that there is

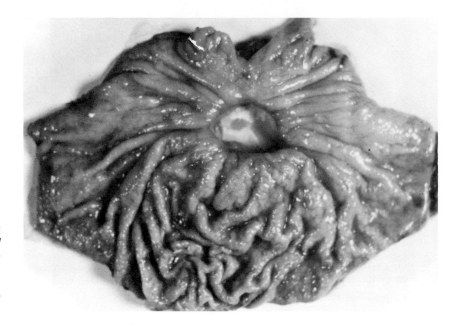

FIGURE 4-10 *Gastric ulcer. A gap such as this in the continuity of a surface is termed an ulcer. An inflammatory reaction is invariably present in the base. Blood vessels may be eroded, giving rise to hemorrhage, or the full thickness of wall may be perforated.*

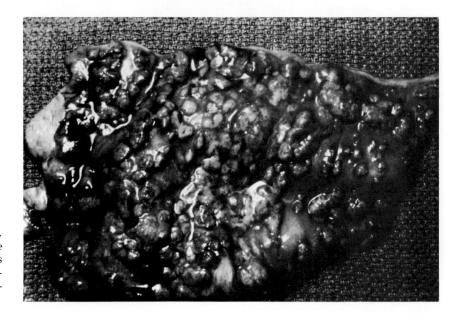

FIGURE 4-11 *Pseudomembranous colitis. The many plaquelike lesions on the colonic mucosal surface represent patches of "pseudomembrane" consisting of fibrinopurulent exudate and necrotic epithelial debris.*

no regeneration of neurons or nerve cells within the central nervous system. When such cells are lost, the loss is permanent.

Repair by formation of scar is an efficient process in virtually any tissue of the body. Formation of scar involves proliferating connective tissue from areas adjoining the necrotic tissue extending into the area as it is demolished by the inflammatory reaction. Such ingrowth of a proliferating young connective tissue into an area of inflammation is referred to as *organization*, and the connective tissue itself is referred to as *granulation tissue*. The components of granulation tissue actually include proliferating fibroblasts, proliferating capillary sprouts (the endothelial cells are sometimes referred to as *angioblasts*), various leukocytes of the inflammatory process, fluid portions of the exudate, and a loose semi-

fluid connective tissue ground substance. Organization occurs in situations where abundant tissue has become necrotic, it occurs when inflammatory exudates persist and do not resolve, and it occurs where masses of blood (hematomas) or blood clots do not resolve quickly. The fibroblasts and angioblasts of granulation tissue originate from preexisting fibroblasts and capillaries in the surroundings, and their migration is somehow oriented so there is gradual extension of this tissue into the appropriate area (Fig. 4-14).

The earliest evidence of organization usually occurs

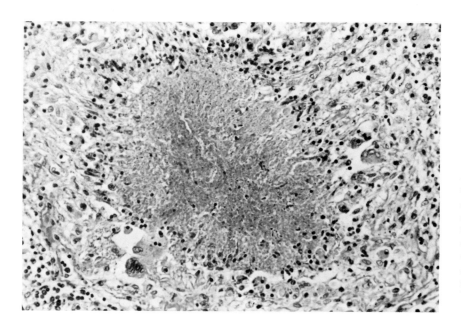

FIGURE 4-12 Epithelioid tubercle. A tubercle is a mass of macrophages which have acquired an "epithelioid" appearance. The zone of ill-defined light-staining cells at the periphery of the field (outer one-third) consists of epithelioid macrophages and multinucleated giant cells (three o'clock and seven o'clock). The center of the tubercle has undergone caseous necrosis. The small dark cells are lymphocytes. (Photomicrograph, ×315.)

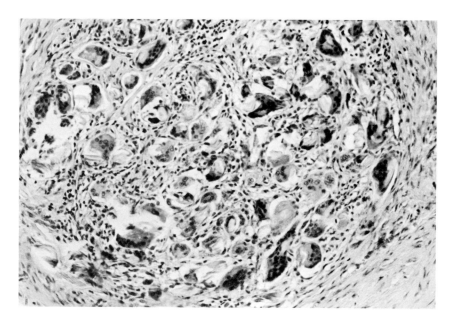

FIGURE 4-13 Foreign body granuloma. In this instance the granuloma is a mass of macrophages which have fused to form many giant cells. Many of these have engulfed fibrils, which represent fragments of suture material. (Photomicrograph, ×200.)

several days after the start of the inflammatory reaction. By the end of a week or so, the granulation tissue is still very loose and cellular. At this point the fibroblasts of the granulation tissue gradually begin to secrete the soluble precursors of the protein *collagen*, which gradually precipitates as fibrils in the interstices of the granulation tissue. With the passage of time, more and more collagen is deposited in the granulation tissue, which is now gradually maturing to a rather dense collagenous connective tissue or scar (Fig. 4-15). While the scar achieves much of its strength by the end of 2 weeks

or so, there is a continuing remodeling process and a continuing increase in the density and strength of the scar over the ensuing weeks. The granulation tissue which at first was quite cellular and vascular gradually becomes less cellular and less vascular and more densely collagenous. The gross counterpart of this evolution is familiar in the appearance of healing incisions, where the resulting scar is at first somewhat loose and quite pink because of the vascularity, ultimately becoming denser and paler as the blood vessels regress.

The coordination of scar formation and regeneration is perhaps most easily illustrated in the case of the healing of cutaneous wounds. The simplest type of healing is that seen in the body's handling of wounds such as surgical incisions where the wound edges can be brought together for the healing process to begin.

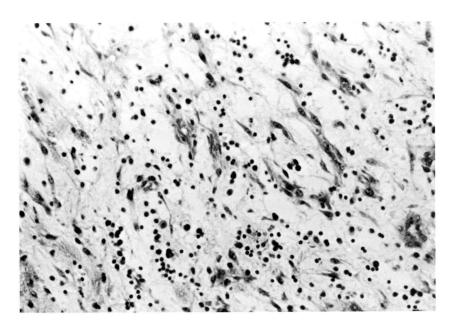

FIGURE 4-14 Early organization. The field depicts granulation tissue growing into an area of repair. The elongated, spindle-shaped cells are fibroblasts. Capillary sprouts are recognized as tubular structures, round in cross section (as at the lower right). The small dark cells are leukocytes, and the interstitial spaces contain exudate fluid and connective tissue ground substance. Compare with Fig. 4-15. (Photomicrograph, ×315.)

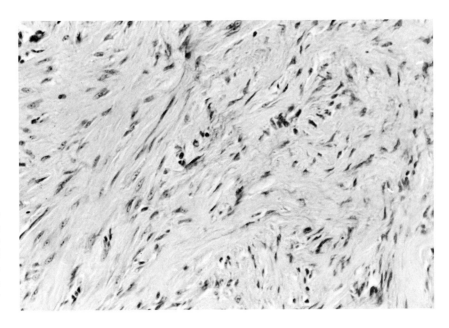

FIGURE 4-15 Maturing scar. As granulation tissue matures, the fibroblasts synthesize collagen which comes to form the tough scar. In this field, the interstitial material has a "stringy" appearance due to abundant collagen in fibrillar form. As scar ages, it becomes less cellular, more densely collagenous. (Photomicrograph, ×315.)

Such healing is referred to as *primary healing* or *healing by first intention*. As seen in Fig. 4-16, immediately after wounding the wound edges are bound together by a bit of blood clot, the fibrin of which acts somewhat like a glue. Immediately thereafter an acute inflammatory reaction develops at the edges of the wound, and the inflammatory cells, particularly macrophages, enter the blood clot and begin to demolish it. On the heels of this exudative inflammatory reaction, the ingrowth of granulation tissue into the area formerly occupied by the clot begins. Thus in a period of several days the wound is bridged by granulation tissue which is destined to mature to a scar. While this is going on (Fig. 4-16), the surface epithelium at the edges begins to regenerate, and within a period of a few days a thin layer of epithelium migrates across the wound surface. As the scar beneath matures, this epithelium also thickens and matures so that it comes to resemble the adjacent skin. The net result (Fig. 4-16) is a reconstituted skin surface and an underlying scar which may be virtually invisible or barely visible as a thickened line. Many skin wounds heal in just this fashion with no medical attention. In others, sutures are placed to hold the wound edges in apposition until healing can occur. Sutures can be removed when organization and epithelial regeneration have progressed to the point where the edges will not gape when the sutures are removed. Thus, in an area of skin where there is relatively little tension, sutures can be removed in several days, long before maximal strength of the scar has been achieved, and in fact

before appreciable amounts of collagen have been laid down. In other areas under stress, sutures must be left in place longer to hold the tissue together until a tough scar can form.

A second pattern of healing occurs when the wounding of skin is such that the edges cannot be brought together during the healing process. This is referred to as *healing by second intention* or sometimes *healing by granulation* (Fig. 4-17). This type of healing is qualitatively identical to that described above. The difference lies only in the fact that much more granulation tissue is formed, much more epithelial regeneration is necessary, and usually a larger scar is formed. The entire process, of course, takes longer than healing by primary intention. Very often in such large open wounds, granulation tissue can be observed covering the floor of the wound as a delicate nappy carpet which bleeds easily on touch. In other situations the granulation tissue actually grows beneath a scab, and epithelial regeneration likewise occurs beneath the scab. Ultimately in such circumstances the scab is cast off when healing is complete. Most of us can recall having impatiently removed a scab approximately in the stage shown in Fig. 4-17B to reveal a central pinpoint of bleeding granulation tissue where epithelial regeneration is not yet total. Although

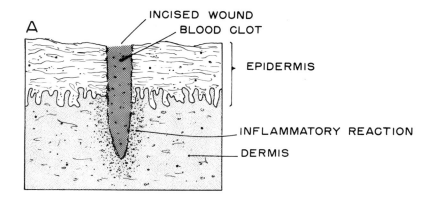

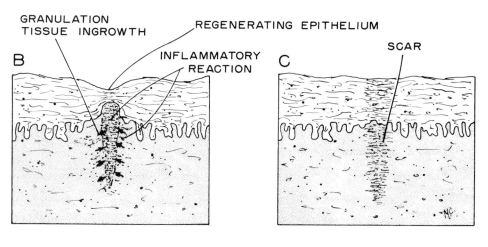

FIGURE 4-16 Healing of an incised, primarily closed wound. The wound edges are initially held together by blood clot (A) and perhaps also by sutures. An acute inflammatory response is mounted in the adjacent tissue, and leads to ingrowth of granulation tissue after several days (B). At this stage epidermal regeneration is under way. The usual result is complete epidermal regeneration and a compact dermal scar, which forms as the granulation tissue matures.

there is evidence of advanced repair side by side with continuing exudation. Evidence of advanced repair includes extensive regenerative proliferation and extensive formation of scar with abundant collagen.

identical in many ways to healing by primary intention, secondary healing is less desirable (not that there is often a choice!) because of the time involved and the termination in a much larger and potentially disfiguring scar.

Healing in virtually any tissue of the body occurs by a process paralleling that described for the skin, with local variations depending upon the ability of the tissues to regenerate, etc.

The designation of an inflammatory process as acute, subacute, or chronic reflects the duration in terms of the extent of repair. Acute inflammation by definition has no reparative aspects, consisting only of the exudative phenomena of inflammation. In subacute inflammation there is beginning granulation tissue ingrowth and perhaps beginning regeneration. In chronic inflammation

FACTORS AFFECTING INFLAMMATION AND HEALING

In some situations the inflammatory process may be impaired from the beginning, i.e., in its exudative stages. The entire inflammatory process is dependent upon an intact circulation to the affected area. Thus, when there is a deficiency of blood supply to an area, the result may be very sluggish inflammatory processes, persistent infections, and poor healing. Another requisite for efficient exudative inflammation is a liberal supply of leukocytes in the circulating blood. Patients whose marrow is destroyed or depressed, as, for instance, by malignant disease or as the result of adverse reaction to drugs, are unable to produce cellular exudates with normal function and as a result are liable to severe infections. More

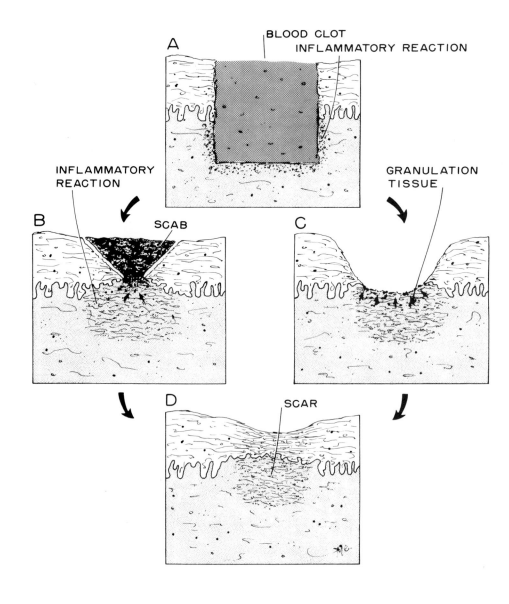

rarely the functions of leukocytes may be impaired (e.g., abnormal chemotaxis, abnormal phagocytosis, or abnormal intracellular killing and digestion), and the patient is rendered similarly liable to aggressive infections.

Many factors can affect the healing of wounds or other areas of tissue injury and inflammation. The healing process, dependent as it is on cellular proliferation and synthetic activity, is particularly sensitive to local deficiencies of blood supply (with attendant impairment of raw material delivery), and is also sensitive to the nutritional state of the host. Patients who are markedly malnourished do not heal wounds optimally. The healing of wounds is also adversely affected by the presence of foreign material or necrotic tissue in the wound, by the presence of wound infection, and by incomplete immobilization and apposition of wound edges.

Even if healing proceeds adequately on a cellular level, there are occasionally complications as an end result. It is in the nature of scar tissue to shorten and to become more dense and compact with the passage of time. The result of this is sometimes *contracture*, which may disfigure an area, limit motion at a joint, etc. If the scar tissue encircles a tubular structure, e.g., the urethra, the result may be a *stricture*, which narrows the structure in question and may produce serious difficulty. When serosal surfaces are inflamed and the exudate does not resolve, granulation tissue and eventually scar may come to bind serosal surfaces together forming what are called *adhesions*. In many areas such as the pleura or the pericardium, adhesions are generally trivial as far as organ function is concerned. Within the peritoneal cavity, however, adhesions, whether between loops of bowel or between abdominal viscera and the body wall, may produce webs which can constrict portions of the gastrointestinal tract or can actually entrap them, forming internal hernias which may strangulate and become gangrenous. Another complication seen occasionally in healing wounds of the body wall is the so-called *incisional hernia*. In this situation the granulation tissue and scar which bridge the surgical defect in the body wall gradually yield to intraperitoneal pressure forming a bulging sac in the incision. Another minor local complication of healing is the protrusion of a bit of granulation tissue above the surface of the healing wound forming what is sometimes called "proud flesh" or a *pyogenic granuloma*. Healing generally proceeds well when such excrescences are cauterized or nipped off. A complication of healing occasionally encountered is the so-called *amputation* or *traumatic neuroma* which simply represents regenerative prolifera-

tion of nerve fibers into the area of healing where they become entrapped in dense scar. Such a neuroma may constitute an unsightly or even painful lump within a scar. Finally some individuals, apparently on a genetic basis, handle the production and/or remodeling of collagen in a healing wound abnormally, so that an excess of collagen is formed, leading to a protrusion called a *keloid*. These are somewhat commoner in blacks and Orientals and in younger patients. Keloids are biologically trivial but cosmetically may assume great importance.

SYSTEMIC ASPECTS OF INFLAMMATION

The emphasis of all of the foregoing description has been on strictly local aspects of the response to injury. It must be pointed out that systemic accompaniments of the local reaction are frequently present. *Fever* is a familiar phenomenon occurring in parallel with many local inflammatory processes, noninfectious as well as infectious. While many causes of fever exist, a final pathway of mediation seems to be the release of so-called *endogenous pyrogens* from neutrophils and macrophages. These substances affect the temperature-regulating centers in the hypothalamus, in effect resetting the body's "thermostat" and producing fever. Another striking accompaniment of local inflammation is the set of hematologic changes commonly observed. Stimuli emanating from the locus of inflammation influence the process of maturation and the release of leukocytes from the bone marrow leading to an increase in the circulating numbers of one or another type of leukocyte, the increase being referred to as *leukocytosis*. Changes in certain blood proteins also occur along with alterations in the so-called sedimentation rate of the blood. With severe injuries, striking metabolic and endocrinologic changes occur. Finally local inflammatory reactions are often accompanied by a variety of ill-defined "constitutional" symptoms including malaise, anorexia or loss of appetite, and varying degrees of disability or even prostration. The causes and mediation of most of these systemic changes are poorly understood or unknown.

QUESTIONS

Response of the body to injury—Chap. 4

Directions: Circle the letter preceding each item below that correctly answers the question. More than one answer may be correct.

1 The best definition of inflammation is:
   a Accumulation of water in the cells due to failure of the sodium pump *b* Invasion of tissue by living

FIGURE 4-17 Healing of an open wound by second intention. The process is qualitatively similar to that shown in Fig. 4-16, but involves more extensive epithelial regeneration and formation of more abundant scar. Diagram A indicates the situation shortly after wounding. Diagram B represents healing under a scab, while Diagram C shows an open wound with visible granulation tissue. The end result D involves a large scar and often a thin area of "new" epidermis devoid of hair and other appendages.

pathogenic organisms c Margination of leukocytes along the vascular lining d Local reaction of the tissues to an injury

2 The *ultimate* purpose of the inflammatory response is to:
a Increase fatty infiltration in the affected tissue in preparation for the process of healing b Release lysosomes which promote the synthesis of cellular proteins to promote healing c Localize, destroy, neutralize, and remove injurious agents in preparation for the process of healing d Restore function by promoting hydropic changes in cells

3 An acute inflammatory reaction in the host can be expected:
a Following cell injury by pathogenic bacteria b Following introduction of a *sterile* but irritating foreign material c Around an area of necrosis in a sterile area d In the center of a necrotic area e Shortly following death

4 Which of the following are cardinal signs of acute inflammation?
a Calor b Rigor c Functio laesa d Algor
e Rubor

5 Which of the cardinal signs of inflammation result from increased blood flow in the affected area?
a Swelling b Heat c Pain d Redness

6 Manifestations of inflammation resulting from increased vascular permeability include:
a Swelling b Heat c Pain d Redness

7 Which of the following are believed to be causes of pain in an inflamed area?
a Pressure of the exudate b Changes in the pH due to acidic breakdown products c Release of chemical mediators which stimulate nerve endings d Increased flow of lymph

8 The two *major* forces which normally govern the transport of fluid between the intravascular and interstitial spaces are:
a The hydrostatic pressure of the blood b The contractility of endothelial cells c The osmotic pressure of the plasma proteins d The permeability of connective tissue

9 Which one of the following reactions occurs in an acute inflammatory response?
a Lymph flow decreases producing edema. b Arterioles in the area dilate to produce active congestion. c Protein follows water into the interstitial spaces. d The permeability of the venules decrease due to the release of local chemical mediators.

10 An exudate differs from a transudate in that:
a Exudates contain more cells derived from the blood. b Transudates are much smaller in quantity. c A transudate is a result of a noninflammatory situation. d Exudates have a higher protein content than transudates.

11 The rapid shift of fluid into the interstitial tissue during inflammation is a result of:
a Increased hydrostatic pressure within the vessel b Increased osmotic pressure within the vessel c Increase in the lymphatic flow d Increase in the permeability of the vessel walls to protein

12 Local chemical substances accounting for increases in blood vessel diameter and/or permeability include:
a Histamine b Plasma kinins c Corticosteroids
d Prostaglandins

13 In an acute inflammatory reaction, the first cells to appear at the site of injury are generally the:
a Monocytes b Lymphocytes c Plasma cells
d Polymorphonuclear neutrophils (PMNs)

14 The cells least likely to be found in large numbers (dominant in the exudate) in chronic inflammation are:
a Lymphocytes b Plasma cells c Macrophages
d Fibroblasts e Neutrophils (PMNs)

15 Opsonization refers to:
a Removal of extracellular debris by specific digestive enzymes b Enzymatic destruction of large particles of foreign material over a long period of time c Destruction of the fibrin barrier formed around some bacterial infection sites d A process by which bacteria are rendered more susceptible to phagocytosis

16 The polymorphonuclear neutrophil is associated with:
a Phagocytosis of bacteria in acute inflammation b Cytoplasmic granules (lysosomes) which stain bright red with eosin dye c Heparin production d Synthesis of antibody in allergic reactions

17 Basophils:
a Have many features in common with mast cells in connective tissue b Have cytoplasmic granules which stain deep blue with basic dyes c Are generally present in large numbers in exudates d Are granulocytes which contain histamine and heparin in their cytoplasmic granules

18 The mechanisms of leukocytosis in the course of an inflammatory reaction include:
a Increased production of leukocytes by the bone marrow b Increased life span of leukocytes during inflammation c Increased release of leukocytes from the bone marrow reserves into the blood d Stimulation of the vascular endothelium by pyrogens

19 The reticuloendothelial system:
a Has also been called the macrophage system b Provides major defense against the spread of infection in the body c Removes foreign material from circulating blood, lymph, and tissue spaces d Includes as components blood monocytes, wandering macrophages, and fixed mononuclear phagocytic

cells *e* Is present in the bone marrow, spleen, lymph nodes, and liver

20 Epithelioid cells:
a Are altered epithelial cells *b* Are common components of granulomatous inflammation *c* Serve to wall off an agent which cannot be destroyed or eliminated from the body *d* Are the primary cells of epithelial tumors *e* Are altered macrophages

21 Pus contains:
a Dead and dying neutrophils *b* Microorganisms *c* Tissue debris *d* Water and solutes

22 Which of the following cells are capable of regeneration (provided the basic framework of the cells are preserved) following necrosis?
a Myocardial cells *b* Epithelial cells of the gastrointestinal tract *c* Neurons *d* Hepatocytes *e* Lymphoid cells

23 What *two* cell types play the primary role in organization?
a Fibroblasts producing collagen *b* Osteoblasts producing mature scar tissue *c* Endothelial cells producing new blood vessels *d* Parenchymal cells producing new connective tissue

24 Which of the following may organize?
a Unresolved exudate *b* Necrotic tissue *c* Persistent blood clots *d* Collagen fibers

25 In comparison to healing by first intention, one would expect healing by secondary intention to involve:
a Good apposition of wound edges *b* A longer time for the process to be completed *c* Less scarring *d* Formation of more granulation tissue *e* A greater amount of exudate

26 The outcome of inflammation is affected by:
a Vascularity of the tissue *b* Nutritional status of the host *c* Presence of debris *d* Immunologic capability

27 Systemic manifestations associated with inflammation include:
a Leukocytosis *b* Malaise (vague feeling of discomfort) *c* Fever *d* Agranulocytosis

Directions: Circle T if the statement is true and F if it is false. Correct false statements.

28 T F When a specific area of the body is infected, the regional lymph nodes may act as filters preventing further spread of the bacteria in the body.

29 T F A chemotactic effect can be exerted only by the injurious agent.

30 T F Monocytes and neutrophils both respond to chemotactic signals.

31 T F Mast cells are the primary source of histamine.

32 T F Lysosomes are packets of digestive enzymes within the cytoplasm of neutrophils and other cells.

33 T F Monocytes differ from neutrophils in that they are capable of synthesizing intracellular enzymes and dividing after migration to the tissues while neutrophils are not.

34 T F When a circulating monocyte appears in an exudate, it is called a mast cell.

35 T F Granulation tissue consists primarily of proliferating young connective tissue.

36 T F Healing by secondary intention requires a longer time period and leaves a larger scar than healing by primary intention.

37 T F Granulomas may result from a foreign material such as a nonabsorbable suture left in the body or from certain bacteria such as the tubercle bacillus which are resistant to phagocytosis or enzymatic digestion.

38 T F Granuloma formation indicates that the body cannot easily overcome or eliminate the agent responsible.

39 T F Giant cells are formed by the fusion of neutrophils in chronic granulomatous inflammation.

40 T F Subacute inflammations show evidence of advanced repair along with exudation.

41 T F A keloid represents disordered wound healing and is caused by the proliferation of nerve fibers and their entrapment in dense scar tissue.

Directions: Match the following types of exudates in col. A to the statements in col. B.

Column A
42 ____ Catarrhal
43 ____ Suppurative
44 ____ Phlegmonous (cellulitis)
45 ____ Serous
46 ____ Pseudomembranous

Column B
a Poorly limited spreading or diffuse inflammation
b Occurs only on mucous membranes and contains mucin
c Includes a web of fibrinopurulent exudate coating the necrotic mucosal surface
d Contains very few cells (e.g., blister fluid)
e Contains many living and dead neutrophils and debris liquefied by enzymes released from the dead neutrophils

Directions: Fill in the blanks with the correct words.

47 A(n) _____ is a lesion within solid tissue containing dead cells, liquefied tissue, neutrophils, and often bacteria.

48 A(n) _____ is a local gap in the body surface or the lining of a mucuous membrane.

49 The accumulation of pus in the pleural cavity is called _____ .

50 A blind tract opening to the body surface is called a _____ tract.

51 An abnormal communication tract between two organs or the lumen of a hollow organ and the body surface is called a _____ .

52 The suffix for inflammation is _____ .

53 _____ is the term describing the movement of leukocytes from the axial stream to the periphery of the blood vessel lumen.

54 _____ is the term used to describe leukocytes inserting pseudopodia in intercellular junctions and sliding and wriggling through to the extravascular spaces.

55 The resorption of exudate with return of the area to normal is called _____ .

56 _____ is the replacement of dead or injured tissues by new cells of parenchymal or stromal origin.

57 Inflammation of the lymph nodes is termed _____ .

58 Place the following events in the correct sequence as they occur in an inflammatory reaction.
a Tissue injury *b* Increased local blood flow leading to heat and redness *c* Emigration of leukocytes *d* Slowing of blood flow; margination of leukocytes *e* Increased vascular permeability

CHAPTER 5 Response of the Body to Immunological Challenge

OBJECTIVES   **At the completion of Chap. 5 you should be able to:**

1 Describe in general terms the biological significance of immune responses.

2 Describe the nature of antigens.

3 Describe the two basic modes of immunologic response which may be elicited when lymphoid tissue is exposed to antigens.

4 State the general properties associated with immunologic reactions.

5 Identify three sorts of phenomena manifested by antigen-stimulated lymphocytes.

6 Describe the components of the lymphoid system including their location, structure, interconnections, and functions.

7 Trace the development of lymphocytes.

8 Describe the steps in the process of immunoglobulin synthesis.

9 Contrast the sequence of events that occurs when an antigen is first introduced into the body and when that material is reintroduced into the same individual.

10 Compare active and passive immunization.

11 Characterize the several different classes of immunoglobulins as to occurrence and function.

12 Identify characteristics that are common to the several different types of immunoglobulins.

13 Describe the means of histamine release in the course of immuno-logic reactions.

14 Describe the means by which the complement system may be acti-vated and the consequences of such activation.

15 Describe the cellular phenomena which may occur when lymphocytes interact with antigen in the effector phase of a cellular immune response.

16 Differentiate between the mechanisms of antibody-mediated (imme-diate) and cell-mediated (delayed) hypersensitivity according to the type of response, cell changes, and reactions.

17 Describe the four basic types of immunologic injuries as classified by Gell and Coombs.

18 List three types of allergic reactions due to humoral immunity and three types due to cellular immunity.

THE NATURE OF IMMUNOLOGICAL REACTIONS

Antigens

When a foreign material is introduced into the tissues of a living host, there is generally a response mounted to the presence of that material. That response has the general characteristics of the inflammatory reaction described in Chap. 4. Many foreign materials, if introduced into the host body on multiple occasions, elicit precisely the same response on each occasion. Certain foreign materials, however, are capable of inducing a change in the host such that reactions to subsequent exposures are different than the reaction to the first introduction of the material. Such altered responses on the part of the host are referred to as immunologic responses, and the materials eliciting them are termed *antigens* or *immunogens. The essence of an immune response is that the offending material is neutralized, destroyed, or eliminated from the host body more rapidly than would otherwise be the case.*

As indicated above, not all foreign materials are antigenic. Those materials which do function as antigens are generally of relatively high molecular weight, usually in excess of 10,000. Most antigens are proteins, but certain polysaccharides, polypeptides, and nucleic acids of large size may also function antigenically. Antigens may be chemically pure substances, or, as is often the case, might be incorporated in complex form as part of the structure of a bacterium, a virus, or even of a living tissue. In provoking a response the entire molecule of antigen does not necessarily play a vital role. In fact it appears that only certain active portions of the molecule, called *determinant groups,* are specifically essential to the reactions. From the standpoint of general biology as well as of human medicine it is important to note that certain small molecules which are unable in and of themselves to act as antigens are able to join chemically with larger molecules such as proteins within the host body, creating a sort of complex which may then behave as an antigen. In such an instance, the specificity of the reactions provoked is related in large part to determinant groups of the small molecule. Such molecules are called *haptens,* and the larger molecules are referred to as *carriers.*

Properties of the immune response

The "business" of the immune response, i.e., the expeditious elimination of antigenic material, is accomplished by the host body in two sorts of ways. The first type of response, the *humoral immune response,* is effected by *immunoglobulins,* which are proteins synthesized by the host in response to introduction of the antigenic material. These immunoglobulins are capable of reacting specifically with the antigens which provoke their pro-duction and in so reacting, sometimes with the aid of one or another "amplification systems," lead to elimination of the antigen. The second sort of immunologic reaction, the *cell-mediated reaction,* is mediated directly by lymphocytes which have proliferated in response to introduction of the antigen and which react specifically with the antigen (without the intervention of ordinary immunoglobulins).

Immunologic reactions, whether mediated by immunoglobulin antibodies or directly by cells, display the property of *self-recognition.* That is to say, these reactions will be mounted only against materials which are sensed as being foreign and will not ordinarily be mounted against constituents of the host's own body. A second property of immunologic response is *memory,* by virtue of which the production of immunoglobulin antibodies or the expansion of a clone of specifically reactive cells proceeds more rapidly with repeated introduction of the antigen. The cellular mechanisms of the body, in effect, remember the antigen. Last but not least, *specificity* is an extremely important property of immunologic reactions. That is to say, the antibodies whose formation is elicited by a particular antigen react uniquely with that antigen (or with molecules bearing virtually identical determinant groups).

Immunoreactive tissues

The part of the immune response which leads to the production of immunoglobulin antibodies or to the proliferation of antigen-reactive cells is sometimes referred to as the *afferent limb* or *induction phase* of the immune response. Lymphocytes and macrophages are the cells chiefly responsible for this portion of the response. More specifically, it is the so-called lymphoid tissues of the body which are involved. Once antibody has been synthesized or antigen-reactive cells have proliferated, they become widely disseminated in various tissues of the body so that when antigens are re-introduced in almost any location, an efficient immunologic reaction may ensue. In other words, the effector cells or immunoglobulin molecules, although produced in the lymphoid tissues, may participate in the *efferent limb* or *effector phase* of the immunologic response virtually anywhere in the body.

BIOLOGY OF LYMPHOCYTES AND LYMPHOID TISSUES

Properties of lymphocytes

Lymphocytes are, morphologically speaking, among the most nondescript cells of the body (see Figs. 5-2 to 5-5). Lymphocytes, in general, have large, roughly spherical, rather deeply staining nuclei and relatively little cytoplasm. Even under scrutiny with the electron microscope lymphocytes tend to be rather uninspiring in appearance, with relatively little in the way of intracytoplasmic organelles. As seen with the ordinary microscope, lymphocytes tend to differ from one another largely in respect to their size and amount of cytoplasm.

Although lymphocytes certainly give no such hint from their drab morphology, they are in point of fact extremely dynamic cells and are remarkably heterogeneous in a variety of respects. Probably the variation in size is the most trivial aspect of lymphocyte heterogeneity. Lymphocytes actually differ in terms of how they differentiate in the course of development; they differ in their life cycles; they stream along different pathways in the body; they have different surface characteristics; and most importantly, they serve different functions. Some lymphocytes, when properly stimulated, are capable of secreting soluble substances termed *lymphokines,* which have exceedingly important effects on other cells within the body. Other types of lymphocytes, when properly stimulated, actually modulate their structure, acquire the cytoplasmic "machinery" of protein synthesis, and become producers of immunoglobulin antibody. When lymphocytes have undergone this type of modulation, they are referred to as *plasma cells* (Fig. 5-1). When viewed with the electron microscope, the abundant basophilic cytoplasm which develops as a lymphocyte becomes a plasma cell is seen to contain an extensive rough endoplasmic reticulum which is the locus of immunoglobulin synthesis. Some lymphocytes are also capable, when properly stimulated, of undergoing what is termed *blast transformation.* That is, they become dividing lymphoblasts and give rise to expanding numbers of cells having the same properties. These various reactions of different kinds of lymphocytes are triggered by reactions which occur at the level of the cell membrane.

Components of the lymphoid system

Lymphocytes are virtually ubiquitous in the body but tend to be concentrated in certain tissues (the lymphoid tissues) which together constitute a coordinated system. The components of this system include lymph nodes, spleen, thymus, lymphoid tissues associated with mucosal surfaces, and bone marrow.

Lymph nodes (Fig. 5-2) are the most numerous components of this system. These encapsulated masses of lymphoid tissues are present in virtually every area of the body, perhaps the most familiar being the nodes palpable in the neck or groin. They are interposed in the course of lymphatic channels in the manner of filters. The entering or afferent lymphatics pierce the capsule of the node, and the lymph immediately enters an anastomosing system of sinusoids lined by reticuloendothelial macrophages. The node is, in effect, a meshwork of sinusoids with nodules of lymphoid tissue called *follicles* arranged in the meshwork at the periphery of the node (the cortex). In the inner part, or medulla of the node, cords of lymphoid tissue are formed between the sinusoids. In both cortex and medulla of lymph nodes, myriads of lymphocytes are able to interact with one another and with macrophages, often in the presence of antigenic materials percolating through the node after having entered by the afferent lymphatics. Efferent lymphatics exit from the node from the region of the medulla. An important detail of lymph node structure is the fact that lymph nodes also have a rich blood supply, which is important to the traffic of lymphocytes within the body.

The *spleen* is, in effect, a large mass of lymphoid and reticuloendothelial cells interposed in the course of the bloodstream. Instead of being filled with lymph, the sinusoids of the spleen are filled with blood. Interspersed in this meshwork of blood sinusoids with their reticuloendothelial cell lining are nodules of lymphoid tissue similar to those in the cortex of lymph nodes

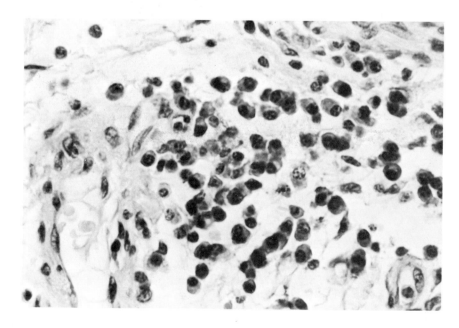

FIGURE 5-1 *Plasma cells in tissue. These cells represent lymphocytes which have been modulated into immunoglobulin-synthesizing cells. They differ from "ordinary" lymphocytes by virtue of their relatively abundant, deeply staining cytoplasm. (Photomicrograph, ×800.)*

(Fig. 5-3). As in the case of the lymph nodes, the structure of the spleen allows close interaction between lymphocytes, macrophages, and materials carried in the bloodstream.

The *thymus* is a somewhat less familiar lymphoid tissue which is located in the thorax anterior to the upper part of the heart and great vessels. This organ consists of a reticular framework densely infiltrated with lymphocytes arranged in the pattern of cortex and medulla (Fig. 5-4). The lymphoid tissue of the thymus has a rich blood supply.

An extremely important component of the lymphoid system is the lymphoid tissue associated with *mucosal surfaces* in the body such as in the gastrointestinal tract and the respiratory tract. Although in any one area this type of lymphoid tissue does not form particularly large nodules, the diffuseness of its distribution renders this tissue highly important. It is also strategically placed in terms of antigen reactivity and defensive function by virtue of being at the interface between the host and the environment. This type of lymphoid tissue is particularly prominent within the gastrointestinal tract, distributed diffusely in the so-called lamina propria of the mucosa (see Fig. 5-5) and in nodular aggregates referred to as Peyer's patches.

Finally, the *bone marrow* should be designated as an important part of the lymphoid system. Although atten-

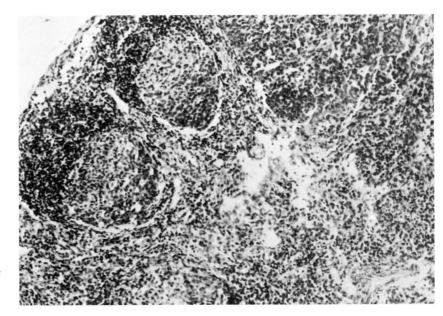

FIGURE 5-2 Lymph node. The capsule and the underlying sinusoid are seen at the upper left. Two prominent lymphoid follicles are evident in the subjacent cortex. The open spaces (center and right) are sinusoids, while the intervening clusters of cells are cords of lymphocytes comprising the medulla. (Photomicrograph, ×200.)

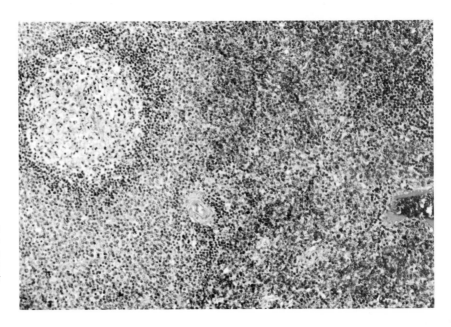

FIGURE 5-3 Spleen. At the upper left is a lymphoid follicle in the so-called white pulp. This is similar to the cortical follicles of lymph nodes. The right half of the field is occupied by "red pulp," a meshwork of blood sinusoids and intervening cells. (Photomicrograph, ×200.)

tion is usually focused on hematopoietic elements in the marrow which are responsible for producing granulocytes, platelets, and red blood cells, many millions of lymphocytes are scattered within the bone marrow.

Lymphocytic traffic within the body

The various components of the lymphoid system are joined together by a sort of double plumbing system, the blood vascular system and the lymphatic system. At any given time millions of lymphocytes are moving within both the blood and the lymph. The various lymphatic channels in the body drain fluid from the interstices of organs and tissues and conduct it centralward, where ultimately the various channels join together and enter the bloodstream via a large vein in the thorax. Thus, there is a constant flow of lymph back into the blood and a constant formation of lymph by movement of fluid from the blood out into the tissues. In a similar fashion there is a constant recirculation of lymphocytes themselves. If one were to sample the lymph within the large central lymphatic channel (the thoracic duct) many lymphocytes would be found. In fact sufficient numbers of lymphocytes flow through the thoracic duct to replace the total number in circulation in the bloodstream several times per day.

Most of the lymphocytes flowing in the thoracic duct are actually being "recycled." In recent years it has been recognized that lymphocytes leave the bloodstream by specialized venules within lymphoid tissues; they spend variable lengths of time within the lymphoid tissues and then circulate via the stream of lymph to rejoin the lymphocytes in circulating blood. Lymphocytes differ quite strikingly from one another with respect to their movements around the body. Some lymphocytes are remarkably long-lived (many months or even years) and travel and recycle extensively. Other lymphocytes are relatively short-lived and do not move around quite as

freely. It also appears that certain groups of lymphocytes may have preferential "homing" patterns with respect to various parts of the lymphoid system. The key point here is that there exists within the lymphoid system provision for moving lymphocytes from one area to another. The biological importance of this lies in the fact that members of a particular clone of lymphocytes which initially proliferate in one given location may circulate around the body and be available for interaction with antigen at many locations.

Ontogeny of lymphocytes

The body's supply of lymphocytes begins embryologically in the yolk sac and liver, and the supply function is ultimately taken over by the lymphocyte population of the bone marrow. Lymphocytes are continually exported from the bone marrow, and some of them migrate to the thymus, where their development is conditioned. That is to say, by virtue of their exposure to certain substances within the thymus, these lymphocytes acquire certain reactive properties. Such cells are known as *thymus-dependent* lymphocytes or *T-lymphocytes*. These lymphocytes are subsequently exported from the thymus, and they populate the various other lymphoid tissues of the body. Other lymphocytes are apparently independent of the thymic influence and thus have properties which differ from the T-lymphocytes. The thymus-independent cells are referred to as B-lymphocytes. It is these sorts of lymphocytes which modulate under appropriate conditions to become plasma cells. The populating of so-called peripheral lymphoid tissues by B- and T-lymphocytes is not a random affair, and these tissues

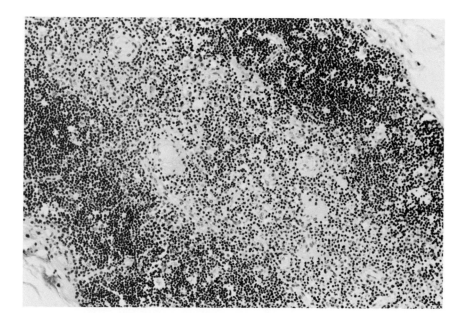

FIGURE 5-4 Thymus. The framework of this organ is infiltrated by myriads of lymphocytes, more densely in the cortex (periphery), less so in the medulla. The thymic tissue tends to atrophy with age. (Photomicrograph, ×200.)

have actually been mapped in terms of preferential concentration of one or another type of cell. Although these specific localizations are not important for purposes of the present discussion, it is vital to reemphasize that the design of lymphoid tissue is such as to allow the interaction of T-lymphocytes, B-lymphocytes, macrophages, and antigenic materials carried in blood or lymph or entering via a mucosal surface.

ANTIBODY-MEDIATED IMMUNITY

Induction of immunoglobulin synthesis

The requisites for synthesis of immunoglobulins or antibodies are such that no one organ has a monopoly on antibody production. Generally speaking, when antigen can be brought into the presence of macrophages, B-lymphocytes, and T-lymphocytes, immunoglobulin production may result. Conditions are right within the lymph nodes, the spleen, and certain of the nodular lymphoid tissues along mucosal surfaces. Thus if antigen enters the subcutaneous tissues, such as commonly is the case with injections, the material drains via the lymphatics to the regional lymph nodes where antibody production subsequently takes place. If antigen enters the bloodstream directly, the spleen is a major locus of antibody production. In either situation there may be "spillover," so that, for instance, following subcutaneous injection, antigen may actually pass through the regional lymph nodes to get into the blood circulation to the spleen. In a similar fashion, antigenic material entering by mucosal surfaces may stimulate the associ-ated lymphoid tissues or may drain to regional lymph nodes.

When an antigen enters a lymphoid tissue, the initial step involves uptake of the antigenic material by macrophages. These cells are responsible either for presenting the antigen in the proper form to the lymphocytes or possibly for processing the antigen to produce a highly immunogenic molecule of some sort. The antigen then functions to "select" certain lymphocytes and react with them. That is to say, there are within the lymphoid tissues at least a small number of lymphocytes whose surface receptors are such as to react with the determinant groups of the antigen. The net result of such interaction is an increase in the number of lymphocytes of that particular type, and a modulation of the B-lymphocytes into antibody-producing plasma cells. In the case of most antigens, a population of T-lymphocytes functions as "helper cells," somehow influencing B-lymphocyte activities. The net result of this interaction that is appreciated both grossly and microscopically is an enlargement of the reacting lymph node, a marked increase in the number of lymphocytes within it, and an expansion of the follicles within the cortex and the cords of cells within the medulla. As the plasma cells synthesize immunoglobulin antibody, it is secreted into the lymph and thence circulates widely in the body. Part of the result of the induction in an immune reaction is the production of "memory lymphocytes." Presumably such cells circulate widely in the body so that cellular memory of the antigen does not remain a localized affair.

When an antigen is first introduced into the body, there is a latent period usually amounting to several days before significant amounts of antibody appear in the circulating fluids. This time is required for the various cellular interactions, proliferation, and modulation to occur. In this so-called *primary response* the level of antibody rises somewhat slowly and then gradually diminishes as the immunoglobulin is catabolized. The

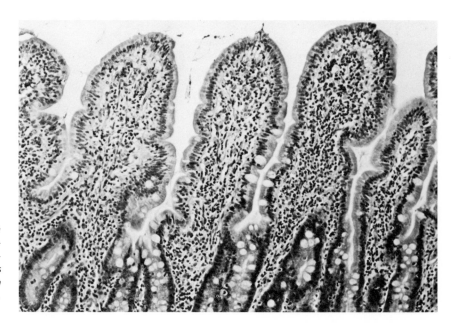

FIGURE 5-5 Mucosal lymphoid tissue. In this section of small intestine, large numbers of lymphocytes are present in the connective tissue beneath the epithelium. This is of obvious importance given the antigen load impinging on a mucosal surface. (Photomicrograph, ×200.)

nature of immunologic memory is such that when
antigen is introduced the second time, even in another
location, and even after immunoglobulin levels have
dwindled, the machinery of antibody production is put
into motion much more rapidly, so that immunoglobulin
appears after a shorter latent period and usually reaches
higher levels in the circulating fluids.

These principles provide the rationale for immunization against many diseases. Immunization is referred to
as *active* when the antigen is introduced into the host,
who subsequently activates the machinery of immunoglobulin synthesis. *Passive immunization* is accomplished by injecting preformed immunoglobulin directly
into a host, i.e., with another individual or animal having
done the immunologic "work." With passive immunization, once the immunoglobulin has been catabolized by
the recipient, there is no memory, so the host is protected only during the circulatory life of the administered antibody. With active immunization, however,
memory is induced (stimulated by an occasional
"booster" injection), so that if the host is even challenged by the agent of the corresponding disease, antibody production will be prompt and efficient, thus
protecting the individual.

The nature of immunoglobulin molecules

Immunoglobulins, or antibodies, are protein molecules
which possess as part of their structure unique sequences of amino acids permitting highly specific interactions with the corresponding antigens. Each molecule
of immunoglobulin (Ig) consists of four peptide chains,
2 heavy (H) chains and 2 light (L) chains, chemically
bonded together. Immunoglobulins belong to several
different classes, each one of which is characterized by
a certain constancy of structure (in the H chains) in
addition to the variable, antigen-reactive portion of the
molecule. These classes are named with the letters G,
M, A, E, D, and are usually designated as IgG, IgM,
IgA, IgE, and IgD. The constant portions of these various
immunoglobulin molecules determine the general biological effects of the particular kind of antibody, while
the variable regions determine specifically which antigens will be reacted with. The antibodies most commonly found in circulating fluids and in many tissues
belong to the IgG group. These antibodies are important
in resistance to infection and are able to cross the
placenta from mother to child, passively immunizing the
latter. IgM antibodies are found largely within circulating
fluids and are generally the first sort to be synthesized
early in the antibody response. IgA antibodies are produced in the lymphoid tissues along mucosal surfaces,
and these molecules are actually combined with a protein in the mucosa and secreted onto the mucosal
surfaces as so-called secretory antibody. This type of
antibody protects the exposed surface against certain
agents in the lumen. IgE antibodies are produced within
lymphoid tissues (usually near boundary surfaces in the
body) and secreted into the circulating fluids, but they
rapidly attach to the myriads of mast cells or tissue basophils around the body. These cells have specific recep-

tors on their surfaces for a portion of the IgE molecule.
Via their effects on the release of chemical mediator
substances from the mast cells, IgE molecules are involved in the regulation of vascular permeability and
mucosal secretion. Relatively little is known of the function of IgD.

Functions of immunoglobulin molecules

The basic function of any immunoglobulin molecule is,
of course, to react with the corresponding antigen. This
particular interaction involves the variable portion of the
immunoglobulin molecule. The biological effects of the
interaction, i.e., those which lead to antigen neutralization or elimination, are mediated by other portions of
the immunoglobulin molecule. The results of these
latter kinds of reactions take a number of forms. If the
antigen is a soluble protein molecule, for instance, one
result of the interaction with antibody (usually of the IgG
or IgM class) is the linking together of numerous antigen
and antibody molecules to form a large latticework
which results in the formation of a precipitate. Such
precipitation reactions can be demonstrated in vitro and
presumably may be important in vivo where insoluble
precipitates would be more rapidly cleared by phagocytic cells than soluble molecules would be. If the
antigen is on the surface of a large structure such as a
bacterial cell, the interaction with immunoglobulin may
again form a complexly linked structure, but this time the
result will be agglutination of numerous bacteria bearing
the antigen on their surfaces. Another function of immunoglobulin may be to coat an antigenic particle and,
by interacting with receptors on the surface of phagocytic cells such as neutrophils or macrophages, render
that particle more easily phagocytized (opsonization).
Immunoglobulin may also interact with the pharmacologically important part of toxin molecules, thus
neutralizing the toxin. Secretory immunoglobulin of the
IgA class appears to function by preventing adherence of
antigen (e.g., antigen on the surface of a microorganism)
to the mucosa. These sorts of direct effects of antigen-
antibody interaction can be visualized as having the net
effect of eliminating the offensive material with dispatch.
Certain kinds of immunoglobulin molecules, in addition,
serve as effectors of immune responses in conjunction
with certain "amplification systems."

Antibodies of the IgE class act in conjunction with
mast cells when responding to antigen. These particular
immunoglobulin molecules have such a high affinity for
receptors on the surface of mast cells that they are
rapidly fixed to a variety of tissues in the body and do not
circulate in both fluids in high concentrations. The fixation of IgE antibody to the surface of mast cells does
not in and of itself alter the function of these cells or
injure them. It does, however, prepare them for action.
The mode of attachment of IgE molecules to mast cells

is such that, in effect, their antigen-reactive portions remain free. When antigen molecules contact the corresponding IgE fixed to the surface of mast cells, the antigen-antibody interaction (apparently by changing molecular configurations at the level of the cell membrane) is such as to trigger release of the contents of the mast cells. Three particularly important pharmacologically active mediator substances are released from mast cells by this interaction. One of these mediators is histamine, which is capable of altering vascular permeability, causing contraction of certain smooth muscle, and increasing the rate of secretion of certain mucosal cells. A second mediator is referred to as SRS-A, slow-reacting substance of anaphylaxis. This material is also capable of increasing vascular permeability, causing contraction of certain smooth muscle, and altering pulmonary physiology. Interestingly, a third substance released from mast cells under these circumstances is ECF-A, the eosinophil chemotactic factor of anaphylaxis. As the name suggests, this substance is responsible for

the accumulation of eosinophils at the locus of this type of antigen-antibody interaction. The net effect of antigen-antibody interaction, then, is the explosive release of substances which alter the physiology of the microcirculation locally. Some evidence indicates that this sort of reaction may be important in the defense of mucosal surfaces against certain agents in the environment. Unfortunately, as will be described below, the same sort of reaction is responsible for certain allergic responses.

Another means whereby the interaction of immunoglobulin and antigen is biologically amplified is via the *complement system*. This system is actually a set of nine functional components. These interacting components of the complement system are proteins which circulate in the blood in an inactive form. So-called complement-fixing antibodies, immunoglobulins of the IgG and IgM type, are capable of activating the various proteins of the sequence. As shown in Table 5-1, the interaction of antigen and antibody results in the activation of the first component of the system. Activated C_1 in turn interacts with the second and fourth components of the system, yielding a product C_{142} which then activates the so-called third component. Portions of the activated third component go on to interact with the later components of the system. The activation of the entire sys-

TABLE 5-1
The complement system

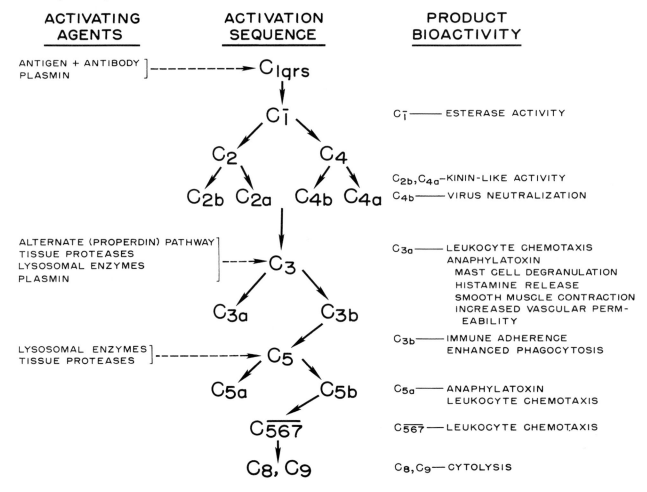

tem through C_8 and C_9, when it occurs on a cell surface, radically alters the cell membrane, leading to lysis. If the original antigen-antibody interaction occurred on the surface of a bacterial cell, the activation of this system would lead to lysis of that bacterium, clearly an event of some significance. Reference to Table 5-1 will also reveal that fragments of various of the activated components earlier in the sequence have exceedingly important biological activities. Thus portions of C_3 and C_5 are capable of releasing histamine from mast cells, leading to contraction of smooth muscle and alteration of vascular permeability. These fragments are sometimes referred to as anaphylatoxins. Portions of the third component are also important in opsonization. Finally fragments of the third and the fifth components and a complex of the fifth, sixth, and seventh components are strongly chemotactic for leukocytes. Clearly, activation of the various parts of the complement system provides an immense biological leverage to the original antigen-antibody interaction. It should be noted here that although the complement system is an important amplifier of immunologic reactions, it also serves importantly in nonimmunologic settings. There are ways of activating the third component and subsequent components in the system directly without the intervention of antigen-antibody interactions; and it appears on the basis of current evidence that a number of components of the complement system are important mediators of any nonspecific inflammatory response. Although this discussion has emphasized the adaptive or beneficial aspects of the complement system, it should be pointed out once again that we usually pay a price for having various response mechanisms within the body. The complement system is, in fact, involved in a number of potentially harmful reactions, as described later in this chapter.

CELL-MEDIATED IMMUNITY

The nature of the response

This second of the two modes of immunologic response of the body does not involve circulating immunoglobulin molecules as effectors of the response. Instead, the various interactions with antigens are directly mediated by T-lymphocytes which are specifically reactive with a particular antigen. The reason why some antigens should stimulate immunoglobulin production and others should induce the development of cell-mediated immunity is not entirely clear. The difference seems to lie in the mode of presentation of the antigen to the host. Simple proteins when injected almost always evoke humoral-type responses, i.e., those mediated by immunoglobulin. It seems that when the antigen is complex, especially part of something like a bacterial body or part of some other living cell, cellular immunity is effectively evoked. The two types of immunity are not necessarily mutually exclusive; and in the course of an infectious disease, elements of both kinds of immunologic reactions are demonstrable.

Induction of the cell-mediated response

The afferent or inductive limb of the cellular immune response takes place within the lymphoid tissues of the body just as it does in the case of humoral immunity. The end point of the process, however, is proliferation of a clone of T-lymphocytes specifically reactive with a particular antigen, but no synthesis of immunoglobulin. The specifically reactive lymphocytes enter the circulating fluids of the body, migrate widely, and are available virtually anywhere to react with the antigen when it is reintroduced.

Cellular immune functions

The specifically reactive T-lymphocytes which proliferate during the inductive phase of the response ultimately function as effectors of the immune reaction without the assistance of circulating immunoglobulin molecules. (Since the immune function actually resides in the lymphocytes themselves, a state of cell-mediated immunity cannot be transferred passively by means of serum the way humoral immunity can be.) The rapid destruction or elimination of the antigen is accomplished either by the lymphocytes themselves or by means of the actions of other cells influenced by the lymphocytes.

In cell-mediated reactions biological amplification is provided by various lymphokines, the soluble substances released by T-lymphocytes when stimulated by the appropriate antigen. A number of different lymphokine activities have been described, and these have different cellular targets. Some lymphokines are able to induce blast transformation and proliferation of other lymphocytes, in effect recruiting the services of such cells. Among the substances secreted by lymphocytes which influence other lymphocytes is *transfer factor*, which is capable of transferring the specific reactivity from one set of lymphocytes to another. Other substances, termed *lymphotoxins*, seem able to cause necrosis of the living cells which bear the corresponding antigens on their surfaces. Appropriately sensitized lymphocytes appear to be capable of killing target cells not only by use of lymphotoxins but by some mechanism involving direct contact of the "killer lymphocytes" with the target cells, or by less direct effects involving the recruitment of macrophages. Still other lymphokines exert their major effects on macrophages. One such lymphokine, macrophage migration inhibiting factor (MIF), is able to suppress the migration of macrophages in vitro. Such an effect in vivo might well serve to keep macrophages in an area where lymphocytes had come into contact with the antigens with which they were reactive. Lymphocytes are also capable of secreting substances which are chemotactic for macrophages. The in vivo counterpart of this activity would be the efficient formation of macrophage-rich exudates in areas of challenge. Finally, certain lymphokines have the effect of activating or "arming" macrophages, rendering them more effective as phagocytic and microbicidal cells. Thus, the activities of various lymphokines are such as to alter cellular events in an area of antigen introduction in a way admirably designed to accelerate handling and disposal of that antigenic material.

The classic example of cellular immune function is encountered in the development and evolution of tuberculosis. It has long been known that previous experience of tuberculous infection results in some measure of resistance to the disease upon later challenge. It has been known for many years that this protection is not mediated by any demonstrable immunoglobulin antibody but seems to reside within host cells. More specifically, it is possible to demonstrate by appropriate experiments that macrophages derived from individuals who have had a tuberculous infection at some time in the past are better able to deal with tubercle bacilli than macrophages derived from naïve hosts. In the latter, intracellular killing of phagocytized living organisms proceeds very slowly if at all; whereas in the macrophages from the experienced individual, the rate of intracellular killing is enhanced. Furthermore, it can be shown that when tubercle bacilli are introduced into experienced hosts, the inflammatory reaction in response to the bacilli evolves much more rapidly and efficiently than in inexperienced hosts. Although in the expression of protection against tubercle bacilli the macrophages are the essential cells, it is now known that the accumulation and function of these cells is actually enhanced by T-lymphocytes which are specifically reactive with antigens of the tubercle bacilli. In short, what happens is that the initial exposure to tubercle bacilli leads to proliferation of specifically reactive lymphocytes (usually 2 weeks or so after the infection) and dissemination of these cells around the body. The result of subsequent contact between these lymphocytes and additional tubercle bacilli is the release of lymphokines leading to the critical effects on macrophages. Interestingly, the interaction between lymphocytes and antigens of tubercle bacilli is highly specific, but once these cells activate the macrophages, the superior properties of the macrophages seem to function equally well against a variety of agents regardless of antigenic specificity. It should be emphasized that a state of cellular immunity evolves even during the first infection with the tubercle bacilli and is, in fact, responsible for assisting the host in arresting that infection. During the first 2 weeks or so following introduction of tubercle bacilli, bacillary multiplication proceeds relatively unhindered by the host's inflammatory response. During this time the macrophages that appear within the exudate around the organisms seem incapable of coping with them. When specifically reactive lymphocytes appear on the scene at the end of the induction phase, the inter-

action of these cells with antigen leads to the progressive increase in the microbicidal efficiency of macrophages, and the host eventually (in most instances) arrests the spread of the infection.

These same sorts of cellular reactions form the basis for skin testing to detect the cellular immune state. If a bit of protein derived from tubercle bacilli is injected into the skin of an individual who has never been infected with the tubercle bacillus, there ensues a very mild, nonspecific acute inflammatory reaction as would occur in response to any minimally irritating foreign material. This inflammatory response is transient, and by 24 hours after the injection the site usually appears completely normal. This is considered a negative test. On the other hand, if antigen is injected into the skin of an individual who has been infected with the tubercle bacillus at some time in the past, a pronounced local inflammatory response evolves slowly, so that by 24 hours after injection the local area is indurated (that is, thickened and swollen). Microscopic examination (Fig. 5-6) reveals that the induration is due to dense infiltration of the area by mixture of lymphocytes and macrophages. This constitutes a positive reaction. Actually, only a few of the many lymphocytes at the site of the reaction are specifically antigen-reactive cells. The remaining lymphocytes and macrophages have been "recruited" into the area as a result of substances released by the antigen-reactive cells. It should be noted that a positive test does *not* mean that the subject has the clinical disease, tuberculosis. A positive reaction indicates that the subject has contacted the organism at some time, with the resulting development of a clone of reactive T-lymphocytes. A person with a positive skin test could have the disease but most often does not. The test is clinically useful in differential diagnosis and in screening. In the former instance, if the subject has evidence of a disease which could be tuberculosis but might not be, a negative skin test (i.e., evidence of the subject not having previous contact with the tubercle bacillus) would be evidence in favor of some other etiologic diagnosis. In the latter instance, skin testing is useful in screening populations such as medical and nursing personnel who are exposed occupationally to tuberculosis. Continuing negativity on tests repeated at regular intervals affords reasonable assurance that no infection has been acquired. If a previously negative individual converts to positive, this indicates infection since the previous test. With such a finding, appropriate tests can be undertaken to make certain that clinically significant disease does not exist, and a program of prophylactic administration of antituberculous drugs might be undertaken to eliminate the very slight possibility that infection might progress. Once an individual has been found to be positive on skin test there is usually no point in repeating the test at later intervals since such positivity is most often permanent.

A measure of protection against tuberculosis can be afforded skin test–negative individuals by means of vaccination designed to induce a cellular immune state. The material generally used is referred to as BCG (bacillus of Calmette and Guérin), which is a live but attenuated strain of tubercle bacillus. These organisms are incapable of producing a progressive infection in normal individuals, but will result in the development of a clone of T-lymphocytes specifically reactive against tuberculoproteins. The protection afforded by such a procedure is not total and is usually not deemed desirable in relatively low-risk situations. Persons in such situations are more efficiently handled by serial skin testing and chemoprophylaxis as indicated.* More recently, BCG vaccination has been employed in the attempted immunotherapy of malignant disease. The rationale for this approach is that once activated by the BCG, the cellular immune defenses of the host may also operate against the cancer cells.

IMMUNITY AND HYPERSENSITIVITY

Relationship between the two

The several humoral and cell-mediated reactions outlined above are clearly of adaptive value to the host. When one speaks of immunity, one generally refers to such beneficial phenomena mediated by the immunologic apparatus of the body. However, the price we pay for having this adaptive machinery is that occasionally the interaction of antibodies or T-lymphocytes with antigen may result in injury to the host. These injurious reactions are frequently referred to as *hypersensitivity* reactions. The term *allergy* is also used to describe certain clinically observed hypersensitivity reactions in humans.

According to terminology evolved many years ago, hypersensitivity reactions mediated by immunoglobulins are sometimes referred to as *immediate-type hyper-*

*This is more efficient since tuberculin-negative subjects do not require frequent chest x-rays to rule out acute tuberculosis, while tuberculin-positive subjects (including those positive due to BCG) do.

sensitivity reactions while those mediated by cellular immune mechanisms are called *delayed hypersensitivity* reactions. (Sometimes the latter reactions are also referred to as tuberculin-type hypersensitivity reactions or bacterial hypersensitivity reactions, because of prototypical examples.) While this terminology is occasionally employed currently, it is less than completely precise because of considerable overlapping in the velocity of the various kinds of reactions. A more useful classification of immunologic injuries is that proposed by Gell and Coombs. This scheme recognizes four types of mechanisms: Type I reactions are mediated by IgE antibodies fixed to the surface of mast cells. Type II reactions are mediated by IgG- or IgM-type antibodies reacting with antigens on the surface of the target cell. Type III reactions are mediated through the formation of antigen-antibody complexes, largely with IgG antibodies. Type IV reactions are mediated by sensitized T-lymphocytes.

Modes of tissue injury

In Type I reactions, also referred to as *anaphylactic-type* reactions, the subject must be sensitized by prior exposure to a particular antigen. During the inductive phase of the response IgE antibodies are made, circulated, and fixed to the surface of mast cells widely scattered about the body. When antigen is then reintroduced into the subject, interaction of antigen with mast-cell-fixed antibody results in explosive release of substances contained within the cells. If the amount of antigen introduced is small and of local extent, mediator release is local, and the result is nothing more than an area of vasodilatation and increased permeability leading to a bit of local

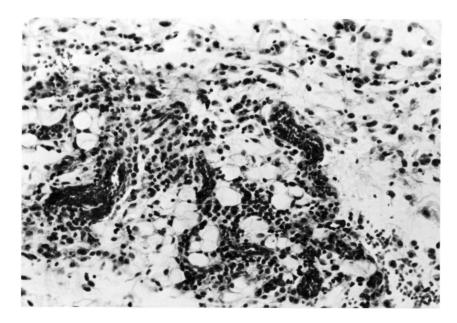

FIGURE 5-6 Positive tuberculin skin test. The area of antigen injection becomes densely packed with lymphocytes and macrophages, especially perivascularly. This gives us the gross induration which constitutes the positive reaction. (Photomicrograph, ×315.)

swelling. (This mechanism of reaction forms the basis for skin testing by the allergist.) If, however, a larger amount of antigen is introduced intravenously into the sensitized subject, release of mediators may be massive and widespread. A classic example of this type of *generalized anaphylactic reaction* can be relatively easily produced experimentally in the guinea pig. The animal is initially sensitized by injection of some foreign antigen by a variety of routes. When that same antigen is subsequently introduced by intravenous injection, signs of distress appear within a few moments, and the animal may die quickly after a period of agitation or even convulsions. Autopsy of such an animal reveals that the lungs are markedly hyperinflated. This phenomenon is due to bronchiolar obstruction which leads to trapping of inspired air within the lungs, ventilatory failure, and rapid suffocation. This chain of events is due to the release of mediator substances from mast cells, the chief target then being the bronchiolar smooth muscle, which is thrown into a state of continuous spastic contraction. The precise pattern of response to widespread mediator release from mast cells varies from species to species but can be equally dramatic in humans in a number of different situations (see Part II).

Type II reactions are basically *cytotoxic.* In these sorts of reactions, the circulating IgG or IgM antibody unites with the corresponding antigen on the surface of a cell (i.e., the antigen is either attached to or a part of the cell's surface). The net result of the interaction might be accelerated phagocytosis of the target cell or might be actual lysis of the target cell following activation of the eighth and ninth components of the complement sequence. If the target cell is a foreign one such as a bacterium, the outcome of this type of reaction is beneficial. However, as is sometimes the case, the target cell may be a host erythrocyte, in which case the result may be a form of hemolytic anemia.

Type III reactions take a number of forms, but they are mediated ultimately by immune complexes, that is, complexes of antigen with antibody, usually of the IgG type. The prototype of this sort of reaction is the so-called *Arthus reaction.* Classically, this type of reaction is elicited by first sensitizing an experimental animal to some foreign protein and subsequently challenging the subject by an intracutaneous injection of the same antigen. The reaction typically evolves over a period of several hours, passing through a phase of swelling and redness and ultimately becoming necrotic and hemorrhagic in severe examples. The microscopic appearance of a typical Arthus reaction is shown in Fig. 5-7. The essence of the lesion is severe vascular damage brought about by large numbers of neutrophils which infiltrate vessel walls in the region of the challenge. In this phenomenon, the basic mechanism involves the formation of antigen-antibody complexes in vascular walls as injected antigen diffuses into the walls and combines with antibody diffusing out of the circulation. A key element in the reaction is activation of the complement cascade by the immune complexes within vascular walls. This activation results in the formation of chemotactic factor (C_{567}) which attracts neutrophils from the circulation. The final effectors of vascular damage are the powerful lytic enzymes released from lysosomes of the leukocytes which are attracted. It is important to note that the reaction triggered by the immune complexes bears no immunologic relationship to the vascular walls. The presence of the immune complexes within vascular walls and the subsequent damage to those walls represent a sort of mechanical outcome of the circumstances of challenge. Similar immune complexes could be formed in other situations and produce parallel reactions.

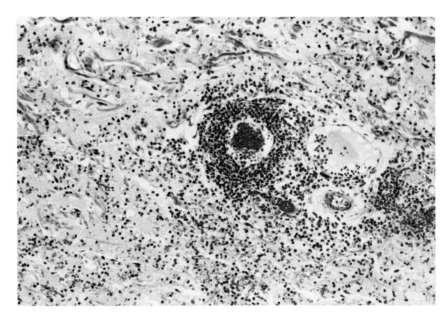

FIGURE 5-7 Arthus reaction. In the center of the field is a blood vessel densely infiltrated by neutrophils which are attracted to the site by the Type III reaction. Severe damage is inflicted on the vessel by the leukocytic enzymes. (Photomicrograph, ×200.)

This, in fact, is what occurs in so-called *serum sickness,* which is another classical sort of immune complex disease. The basic mechanism of production of serum sickness involves the formation of immune complexes within the circulatory system, with subsequent deposition of these complexes in a number of locations. The entire chain of events can be initiated by a *single* injection of foreign protein provided that the amount injected is relatively massive. If the amount of the foreign material is sufficient, abundant antigen will still be in circulation when immunoglobulin production and release begin several days after the original injection. As antibody is formed, it enters the circulation and combines with the still-circulating antigen, forming circulating immune complexes. These complexes are deposited in many points of the vascular system, and at each of those points complement is activated, leukocytes are attracted, and a vasculitis similar to that of the Arthus phenomenon is produced (Fig. 5-8). Another important component of serum sickness is the characteristic renal lesion. The circulating immune complexes are filtered out as the blood passes through renal glomeruli, and the glomeruli are injured by the complexes, producing the characteristic *glomerulonephritis* of serum sickness. Again it should be noted that tissue damage is initiated by the deposition of immune complexes which in themselves are not immunologically related to the tissues injured. Thus, in a real sense, the numerous vessels and glomeruli involved in serum sickness are "innocent bystanders."

Immune complex, or Type III, reactions precisely analogous to those described above can be elicited in humans, as will be described in Part II. Thus, serum sickness is a potential clinical problem and immune complex glomerulonephritis develops in a number of settings, including certain infections.

Type IV reactions mediated by the contact of sensitized T-lymphocytes with the corresponding antigen can be seen in a number of settings. Tuberculosis affords a classic example. The protective or beneficial effects of T-lymphocyte-mediated reactions in tuberculosis have been described above. Accompanying these sorts of reactions there is often extensive necrosis of tissue, which, in fact, is quite characteristic of the disease. Such necrosis is now recognized to be a result of cell-mediated immunity rather than being directly caused by any toxic moiety of the tubercle bacillus. It appears that necrosis is the result of lymphocytotoxicity, i.e., the effect of lymphocytes activated by the tuberculoprotein of the bacilli.

Type IV reactions are also exemplified by so-called *allergic contact dermatitis,* which can be induced experimentally as well as having a spontaneous human counterpart. In this type of situation a simple chemical material is applied to the skin of the subject, and the material acts as a *hapten,* combining with proteins in the skin. The complex molecules thus formed induce the proliferation of a clone of sensitized lymphocytes which subsequently interact with the antigen in the skin. The cells of the skin then bear the brunt of lymphocytotoxicity and of the secondary effects triggered by lymphokines released in the reaction. The clinical counterparts of this are described in Part II.

This type of reaction is also mounted in the rejection of foreign grafts. When a living tissue from one individual is grafted into another, whether a patch of skin or an entire organ such as a kidney, unless the donor and recipient are genetically identical, the graft tissue is sensed by the recipient's immune system as being foreign and antigenic. After a brief induction phase, lymphocytes specifically sensitized to so-called *histocompatibility* or *transplant antigens* of the graft invade

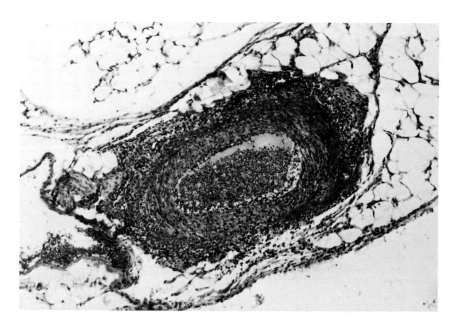

FIGURE 5-8 Serum sickness. This mesenteric artery is being damaged by leukocytes in a mechanism analogous to that depicted in Fig. 5-7. The circumstances of immune complex formation differ. (Photomicrograph, ×125.)

the graft and lead to its destruction or rejection by a number of mechanisms involving either direct lymphocytotoxicity or the involvement of macrophages. While T-lymphocytes play a major role in graft rejection, under some circumstances immunoglobulins play a significant parallel role. It is these sorts of rejection reactions which limit our ability to replace defective organs in one individual with those taken from another.

QUESTIONS

Response of the body to immunologic challenge—Chap. 5

Directions: Answer the following questions on a separate sheet of paper.

1 What is the essential biological significance of an immune response?

2 Describe the nature of antigens in terms of their structure and their effects on the host.

3 Describe two different modes of immunologic responses which may be evoked when lymphoid tissue is exposed to antigens.

4 List three properties generally associated with immunologic reactions.

5 What are the possible reactions of lymphocytes stimulated by antigen?

6 Describe the mechanism by which antibodies appear to be formed.

Directions: Circle the T for true and the F for false. Correct any false statements.

7	T	F	The sinusoids of the spleen are filled with lymph.
8	T	F	Lymphocytes are widely distributed within the bone marrow.
9	T	F	If antigen enters the bloodstream directly, the regional lymph nodes are a major locus of antibody production.
10	T	F	Passive immunization refers to the situation wherein an antigen is introduced into the host and the process of immunoglobulin synthesis is activated.
11	T	F	People normally have only minute amounts of IgE present in their blood serum.
12	T	F	Immediate hypersensitivity is a cell-mediated response.

13   T   F   Mediators of cellular immunity are sensitized T-lymphocytes and are elaborated when the cell encounters its antigen.

Directions: Circle the letter preceding each item below that correctly answers each answer. More than one answer may be correct.

14 All of the following are components of the lymphoid system EXCEPT:
a Lymph nodes   *b* Spleen   *c* Liver   *d* Thymus
e Bone marrow

15 The thymus converts stem cells from the bone marrow to:
a T-lymphocytes   *b* B-lymphocytes   *c* Both *a* and *b*
d Neither *a* nor *b*

16 When an antibody reacts with its corresponding antigen:
a A precipitate may be produced from a previously soluble antigen   *b* A biologically "toxic" complex may be formed   *c* The elimination of the antigen (in the intact host) may be accelerated   *d* A particulate antigen may be caused to agglutinate   *e* All of the above

17 An antibody which can coat the surface of bacteria so that phagocytosis by PMNs and macrophages is enhanced is called a(n):
a Hapten   *b* Agglutinin   *c* Opsonin   *d* Precipitin

18 When stimulated by antigen, sensitive T-lymphocytes release:
a SRS-A   *b* ECF-A   *c* Secretory IgA
d Macrophage inhibiting factor

19 IgE antibody has a special affinity for:
a Mast cells   *b* Eosinophils   *c* Basophils
d Histiocytes

20 The principal role of IgE in allergic reactions is to:
a Form a precipitating complex with allergens
b Fix the complement with tissue-damaging effects
c Generate eosinophilic chemotactic factor   *d* Combine with allergen on the mast cell surface and induce secretion of contained materials

21 Which of the following is an important function of IgG?
a Protection of mucosal surfaces   *b* Mediation of the tuberculin skin test   *c* Defense against pyogenic infections   *d* Participation in anaphylactic reactions

22 Complement activation would be anticipated with:
a Reactions of antigens with cell-bound IgE   *b* Reactions of antigens with sensitized T-lymphocytes   *c* Reactions of antigens with IgG   *d* Addition of antigens alone to complement-rich serum

23 Biological effects of activation of complement components include all of the following EXCEPT:
a Production of lesions in target cell membranes
b Release of histamine with resulting vascular permeability changes   *c* Attraction of white blood cells

d Development of "transfer factor" in sensitized lymphocytes   *e* Facilitation of phagocytosis by white blood cells

24 Mast cell granules contain substances that are involved in hypersensitivity reactions. Which of the following statements is/are true regarding these substances?
a Histamine effects are never evident before 1 hour. *b* SRS-A causes increased vessel permeability. *c* ECF-A causes constriction of bronchial smooth muscle.   *d* Histamine causes lymphokine generation.

25 Reactions due to delayed hypersensitivity may have any of the following features EXCEPT:
a Involvement of nonsensitive macrophages recruited by specifically sensitive lymphoid cells *b* Mediation by circulating IgM antibody   *c* Passive transfer by means of specifically sensitized lymphocytes   *d* Responsibility for immunity to some bacterial and fungal infections

26 All of the following statements about anaphylaxis are true EXCEPT:
a A condition caused by an immunological reaction *b* Potentially fatal condition   *c* May occur in minutes or even seconds of exposure to causative agent *d* Patient possibly not previously exposed to the causative agent or a closely related one   *e* Thought to be mediated by IgE

27 Which of the following are characteristic of serum sickness?
a It is a delayed hypersensitivity reaction.   *b* It requires many periods of exposure to a particular antigen.   *c* It is IgE-mediated.   *d* Circulating antibody-antigen complexes are present as the disease evolves.   *e* It may occur following administration of animal serums to an individual not previously sensitized to the antigen.

28 Delayed hypersensitivity reactions such as the positive tuberculin response reflect a recruitment of cells by factors released by:
a IgE   *b* Neutrophils   *c* Lymphocytes *d* The complement system   *e* Macrophages

29 An example of a Type III hypersensitivity reaction is:
a An Arthus reaction   *b* A delayed hypersensitivity reaction   *c* Cell surface antigen combining with antibody   *d* An anaphylactic reaction

Directions: Match the characteristics in col. A with the type of immune mechanism generally involved in col. B.

Column A	Column B
30 _____ Antibody-mediated	*a* Humoral
31 _____ Mediated by sensitized T-lymphocytes	immunity
32 _____ B-lymphocytes involved	*b* Cellular immunity
33 _____ Can be induced by simple protein molecules	
34 _____ Response more likely to be immediate	
35 _____ Anaphylactic shock following penicillin injection	
36 _____ Positive tuberculin skin test	

CHAPTER 6 The Response of the Body to Infectious Agents

OBJECTIVES At the completion of Chap. 6 you should be able to:

1 State the general requirements for the establishment of an infection.

2 Distinguish an infection from an infectious disease.

3 Identify the modes of entry of an infectious agent into the host.

4 Describe the local and systemic means of dissemination in the host body once an infectious agent is established.

5 Describe the normal body defenses against penetration and spread of infectious agents in the following and give examples of each:
  a Skin and mucosal surface
  b Inflammatory reaction
  c Reticuloendothelial system

6 Define *bacteremia, septicemia, septicopyemia.*

7 List the direct and indirect means of transmission of organisms from the source to a susceptible host.

8 Describe the characteristics of an organism which affect its transmissibility, invasiveness, and pathogenicity.

9 Identify several mechanisms by which microorganisms cause injury.

10 Define *commensalism, mutualism.*

11 Describe the concept of an opportunistic infection.

12 Identify the host and environmental factors which determine resistance, susceptibility, and outcome of an infection.

13 Explain why the normal microbial flora of the body is essential for the health of the human host.

Infection is a universal aspect of life. Plants and animals of all sizes and descriptions are infested with a variety of living microbes, and human beings are certainly no exception. The purpose of the following discussion is not to catalog the many specific infections to which human beings fall victim but rather to discuss in a most general way the biological principles which govern the interaction between host and infectious agents. In particular, a goal of this chapter is to provide a proper perspective of the universe of infection, i.e., to establish firmly the view that infectious *disease* is but an occasional outcome of the interaction between host and microbe.

HOST DETERMINANTS OF INFECTION

A requirement for the production of any infection is that the infectious organism must be able to *adhere to, colonize,* or *invade* the host and proliferate at least to some extent. It is not surprising, therefore, that in the course of evolution, animal species, including human beings, have evolved certain elaborate defense mechanisms at the various interfaces with the environment.

Skin and oropharyngeal mucosa

A major interface between the environment and the human body is, of course, the skin. Figure 6-1 shows the structure of a typical area of human skin. Clearly the intact skin with its keratinized or horny layer at the outer surface and multilayered epithelium beneath constitutes an excellent *mechanical* barrier to infection. Ordinarily it is exceedingly difficult for any microorganism to breach this mechanical barrier. However, cuts, abrasions, or areas of maceration (such as in folds of the body which are kept constantly moist) may allow infectious agents to enter. In addition to being a simple mechanical barrier, the skin also has a certain ability to *decontaminate* itself. Thus, organisms which adhere to the outer layers of skin (assuming they do not simply die as they dry out) will be shed as the outer flakes of skin fall off. In addition to this physical sort of decontamination there is a chemical decontamination attributable to the properties of sweat and sebaceous secretions which bathe the surface of the skin. Finally, associated with the skin is a so-called *normal flora* (described more fully later in this chapter), which may exert a sort of *biological* decontaminative effect by inhibiting the multiplication of organisms which land on the cutaneous surface.

The lining of the mouth and much of the pharynx is similar to the skin in that it is surfaced by a multilayered epithelium which constitutes a formidable mechanical barrier to microbial invasion. This mechanical barrier, however, may actually be breached along gingival margins and in the region of the tonsils. The oropharyngeal mucosa is also decontaminated by the flow of saliva, which simply washes many particles away mechanically. In addition, there are substances in the saliva that are inhibitory to certain microorganisms. Finally, there is a rich microbial flora within the mouth and pharynx that may also act to impair the growth of some potential invaders.

The gastrointestinal tract

The gastric mucosa is of a glandular sort and is not a particularly impressive mechanical barrier. Frequently there are small defects or erosions of the gastric lining, but these are of no consequence in relation to infection, because the gastric environment is extremely hostile to many microorganisms. This is due largely to the pronounced acidity of gastric secretions. Also, the stomach tends to empty its contents relatively rapidly into the small intestine. The lining of the small intestine (Fig. 6-2) is likewise not particularly tough mechanically, and it is potentially easily penetrated by many bacteria. However, peristaltic propulsion of intestinal contents is extremely rapid in the small intestine, and bacterial populations are thereby kept quite sparse within the lumen. When intestinal motility is impaired, microbial

counts are sharply elevated within the small intestine, and invasion of the mucosa may then occur. Several other features of the small intestine assist in the rapid propulsion of organisms through the tract. Abundant mucus is constantly secreted by intestinal lining cells, forming a viscous blanket over the intestinal surface, trapping bacteria and propelling them distally by peristalsis. In addition, adhesion of bacteria to the mucosal surface is inhibited by the presence of antibodies within the intestinal secretions. In the large intestine (Fig. 6-3) the lining is likewise not particularly tough mechanically. In this location propulsion is not especially rapid, and in fact there is relative stagnation of intestinal contents. Here, the major defense against establishment of invading microbes is the presence of astronomical numbers of "normal" microbial inhabitants which coexist peacefully with the host. This mass of normal bacteria has many ecological ways of discouraging invaders either by competition for foodstuffs or by actually secreting antibacterial (antibiotic) substances.

Respiratory tract

Represented in Fig. 6-4 is a microscopic view of the mucosal surface typical of conducting portions of the respiratory tract (e.g., the lining of the nose, the nasopharynx, the trachea, and the bronchi). The epithelium consists of tall cells, some of which are mucus-secreting, but most of which are equipped with cilia at their lumenal surfaces. These tiny projections beat like whips with the action stroke directed upward towards the mouth, nose, and exterior of the body. The mucus-secreting cells produce a sticky blanket which rides on top of the cilia and glides continuously upward. If microbes are inhaled, they tend to impinge on the

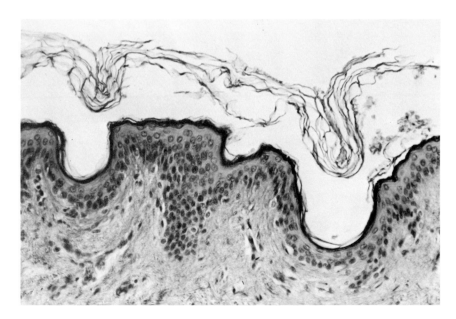

FIGURE 6-1 Skin. The epidermis consists of multiple layers of cells, the most superficial of which are flattened and keratinized. (The apparent looseness of this keratinized zone is an artifact of tissue handling.) In toto, these layers constitute a formidable mechanical barrier. (Photomicrograph, ×315.)

mucus blanket, to be moved outward and either expectorated or swallowed. This action is enhanced by the presence of antibodies within the secretions. If some agents elude these defenses and reach the air spaces in the lung itself, the macrophages always present there provide another line of defense.

OTHER DEFENSIVE BARRIERS

Other surfaces in the body are similarly equipped with defensive mechanisms. Within the urinary tract the lining is a multilayered epithelium which provides a mechanical barrier, but one of the main antimicrobial defenses is the flushing action of urine flow. Anything which interferes with the normal flow of urine, whether it be obstruction of a ureter or simply bad habits of long-delayed micturition, will promote infection. The ocular conjunctiva is likewise defended in part mechanically and in part by the flow of tears. The vaginal mucosa is a tough, multilayered epithelium whose mechanical properties are augmented by a rich resident flora and by mucous secretions.

Inflammation as a defense

If an infectious agent manages to penetrate one or another of the barriers of the body and enter the tissues, the *next line of defense* is the *acute inflammatory reaction*. From the discussion in Chap. 4, the value of the inflammatory reaction in this regard should be

evident. It might be reemphasized at this point that the inflammatory reaction is an arena in which humoral (antibody) and cellular aspects of bodily defense converge. The antimicrobial activities of the phagocytes, for instance, are augmented by the opsonizing effects of antibodies and complement components. The defensive properties of macrophages, as another example, may be enhanced by so-called *cellular immune mechanisms* (see Chap. 5).

In the event that the acute inflammatory reaction is not sufficient to handle the invader, the infection may spread elsewhere in the body. The usual means of spread is largely passive as regards microbial action, and usually involves currents of body fluid carrying the organisms. Locally, even the outpouring of exudate fluid may move the organisms about, and a phagocyte may actually be an agent of spread if it does not kill the ingested organism but wanders to another location. Spread tends to occur across natural spaces. For instance, if something perforates part of the gastrointestinal tract and the contained microorganisms enter the peritoneal cavity, they can spread along the entire peritoneal surface. If some agent reaches a connective tissue plane, such as along a muscle, it may spread rapidly along that plane. When infectious organisms gain access to the meninges (the coverings around the central nervous system), there is frequently rapid spread along the entire cerebrospinal axis.

Lymphatics in infection

For reasons outlined in Chap. 4, the flow of lymph is accelerated in acute inflammation. This means, unfortunately, that infectious agents on occasion may also spread quite rapidly along the course of lymphatics with the flowing lymph. Sometimes lymphangitis is the result, but more often the infectious agents are carried directly

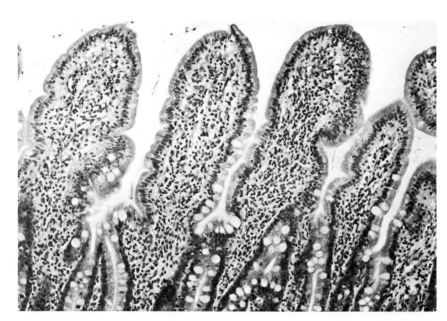

FIGURE 6-2 Small intestine. The epithelium separating bowel contents from underlying tissue is actually quite delicate and is not a particularly good mechanical barrier. The surface is protected by mucus secreted by the light-staining "goblet cells," by antibody produced by the underlying lymphoid tissues, and by peristaltic emptying. (Photomicrograph, ×200.)

to the lymph nodes, where they are rapidly phagocytized by reticuloendothelial macrophages. In such instances the effluent lymph moving centrally beyond a lymph node may be freed of living organisms.

The final defenses

If spreading infectious agents are not arrested within lymph nodes or if such agents directly invade venous channels at the primary site, there may be actual infection of the bloodstream. Bursts of bacteria in the bloodstream are actually not uncommon, and the episodes of so-called *bacteremia* are usually handled quickly and effectively by the macrophages of the reticuloendothelial system. If large numbers of organisms are fed into the bloodstream, however, and if these organisms are sufficiently resistant, the macrophage system may be overwhelmed. This will result in persistence of organisms in circulation, with associated symptoms of malaise, prostration, and signs of fever, chills, etc. This condition is called *septicemia*, often referred to by the laity as "blood poisoning." Finally in some instances organisms reach such high numbers that they are circulating in clumps, lodging in many organs, and producing myriads of microabscesses (Fig. 6-5). This overwhelming situation is called *septicoyemia*, or simply *pyemia*.

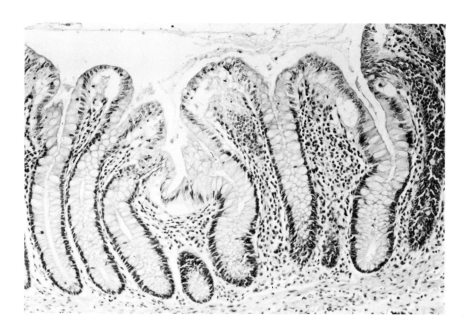

FIGURE 6-3 Colon. This epithelium contains many mucus-secreting cells. A sheet of mucus is visible over the mucosal surface. The rich microbial flora which "defends" the colon is not visible in this preparation. (Photomicrograph, ×200.)

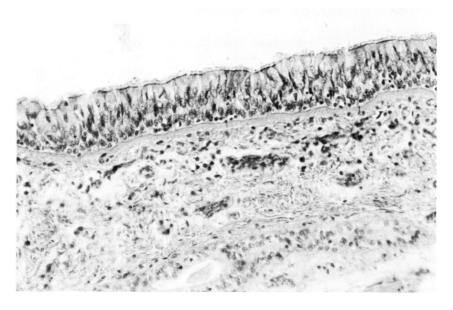

FIGURE 6-4 Trachea. This type of epithelium is equipped with cilia, visible as a fringe along the upper surface. These are responsible for propelling a protective mucous blanket over the exposed surface of the air passages. (Photomicrograph, ×315.)

MICROBIAL DETERMINANTS OF INFECTION

Transmissibility

An obviously essential feature in the production of infection is the transport of the living infectious agent to the host. Perhaps the most obvious means of transmission of infection is *directly* from person to person, e.g., by coughing, sneezing, kissing, etc.

Organisms are transmitted *indirectly* in a variety of ways. Infected individuals shed organisms into the environment, and these are deposited on various surfaces and can be resuspended in air at a later time, thus spreading indirectly to other hosts. Similarly, organisms can get into the soil, the water, the food, or other chains of indirect transmission. Around hospitals, infection can also be spread via exudates and excreta. Blood transfusions may also be a means of spreading infection, as in the case of viral hepatitis. More complex types of indirect transmission involve vectors such as insects. These may act in a strictly mechanical fashion, carrying the microbial agents from one place to another, or may act in a biological fashion, i.e., by serving as intermediate hosts in some essential part of a life cycle of the infectious agent.

Certain intrinsic characteristics of microorganisms sharply influence their transmissibility or communicability. Organisms which are very resistant to drying, e.g., spore-forming organisms, are readily transmissible through the environment. On the other hand, some organisms, e.g., the spirochetes of syphilis, are extremely sensitive to drying and temperature change, factors which sharply limit the mode of this transmission. In hospitals a sort of natural selective factor which influences the communicability of microbial agents is their resistance to antibiotics. It is distressingly common to find antibiotic-resistant strains of microorganisms emerging and then being communicated relatively freely in the hospital environment.

Invasiveness

Once communicated to a new host, the microbial agent must establish itself on or in the host in order to produce infection. There is great variability in the means adopted by various infectious agents for becoming established on or in the host individual. *Cholera,* for instance, is caused by an organism that never invades the tissues but only colonizes the lining of the intestine, apparently by being able to adhere to some component of the surface and thus avoid being washed away. There are some other organisms, e.g., those which produce bacillary dysentery, which invade only the superficial lining of the bowel but never go any farther into the body. Then there are organisms such as the causative agent of typhoid, which not only invades the superficial lining of the bowel

but eventually reaches the bloodstream and disseminates around the body. Another efficient spreader is the spirochete of syphilis, which penetrates mucous membrane or skin at the portal of entry and is disseminated via the bloodstream with great rapidity.

Some organisms, even after gaining access to the tissues and becoming established, never spread to any extent. The organisms which produces tetanus, for instance, do not actually spread around the body. When they grow locally, they secrete a toxin which is carried via the bloodstream to produce the widespread effects that characterize the disease. The reasons for these differences in invasiveness of various organisms are not clearly understood but undoubtedly are related to specific chemical requirements of the organism and the extent to which these requirements can be met in various locales.

Microorganisms have evolved certain ways of breaching host barriers or eluding defense mechanisms. For example, some organisms develop a slimy capsule such that the phagocytic cells of the host cannot ingest them efficiently. In the course of evolution other organisms have developed the enzymatic means of spreading through the ground substance of connective tissue by a sort of chemical digestive process. Yet other organisms are able to secrete toxins which kill leukocytes, thus eluding capture. Some organisms have even evolved a resistance to the intracellular environment within phagocytes, and these organisms (for instance, the tubercle bacillus) tend to persist as intracellular parasites.

Ability to produce disease

At the level of explaining in a chemical or molecular way the mechanism whereby the presence of an infectious agent produces disease, our knowledge has been relatively meager and is only now growing. Best understood are those situations in which the infectious agent actually secretes a soluble *exotoxin* which then circulates and produces well-defined physiologic changes by acting on specific cells. Thus the chemical mechanisms of disease production in tetanus and in diphtheria, for instance, are relatively well understood.

Many other microorganisms, such as the gram-negative bacteria, contain as part of their structure a complex *endotoxin* which is released with lysis of the microorganism. Although the biological role of such endotoxins is far from completely understood, it is known that the release of endotoxin can be associated with the production of fever and under more extreme circumstances, such as gram-negative speticemias, with the production of a shock syndrome.

Some organisms actually injure the host, largely by immunologic means. The tubercle bacillus, for instance, appears to have no direct toxin of its own. Rather, the patient becomes allergic to the tubercle bacillus (cell-mediated immune mechanism), and the caseous necrosis typical of the disease is produced on an immunologic basis. In a similar vein, some organisms affect the host by contributing to the formation of antigen-antibody complexes which may subsequently be injurious, e.g., via the development of immune complex glomerulonephritis.

At the far end of the spectrum are viruses which are obligate intracellular parasites. In effect, viruses are simply chunks of genetic material (DNA, RNA) equipped to insert themselves into host cells. The cells are subsequently injured (if at all) by the new genetic information being expressed in altered cell function. One expression of such added genetic information is the replication of additional infectious virus, which may be accompanied by lysis of the affected cell. The cell may also be altered without actually becoming necrotic. In fact, the cell may even be stimulated to proliferate, as in the case of virally induced tumors. Viruses may also injure the host by evoking a variety of immunologic reactions in which some moiety of the virus behaves as an antigen.

MODES OF INTERACTION OF HOST AND MICROBE

It is common to view the interaction between a host and an infectious agent in terms of all out war or a "fight to the death." There is a great tendency to view infectious agents as intrinsically "bad" things, designed to produce disease. However, the real business, biologically speaking, of any living agent is not to produce disease but to produce more of the same kind of agents. In effect, a given microbial agent "could not care less" about producing disease in the host individual. In fact an ideal infectious agent would simply reproduce within a given host (who constitutes a food supply) and not harm the host or otherwise "rock the boat."

Thinking in evolutionary terms, if a particular infectious agent were to be so effective in producing disease that it would be lethal to each host it entered, the organism would rapidly run out of a food supply and quickly become extinct. The other side of the coin is that if a particular host species is to survive in the course of evolution, one of the things that it must face successfully is infectious agents within the environment. Natural selection obviously would favor the hardier hosts. So, in the course of evolution, more resistant hosts and less

lethal infectious agents tend to be developed. Thus, the dictates of evolution are such that most interactions between host and infectious agent should turn out eventually to be rather happy ones, producing significant harm to neither party. When a relationship between host and infectious agent is inoffensive to either species, that type of interaction is referred to as *commensalism*. When the interaction affords both parties some benefit, the interaction is referred to as *mutualism*. Commensalism and mutualism are the most frequent outcomes of infectious interactions in nature, and the production of *infectious disease* is in an evolutionary sense (and in fact numerically) an aberrant circumstance.

By this line of reasoning one would predict that most infectious diseases should be mild, or even that most infections should be unaccompanied by disease. As a matter of fact, it does turn out, even for most microbial "pathogens," that the presence of the organism on or in the host is most commonly trivial or inapparent and only as the exception is significant disease produced. Thus, for every individual suffering from an infectious disease of a particular sort there are probably several individuals in the population who are *infected* with the same organism and are *not at all sick*. Pneumococcus, staphylococcus, meningococcus, and many other pathogens can be recovered easily from perfectly healthy individuals in the population.

There are certainly exceptions to the principle that infection is most often mild or even inapparent. Interestingly these exceptions can usually be explained on evolutionary grounds. Rabies, for instance, is almost 100 percent fatal to human beings. Our species has not evolved with the virus but is only accidentally inserted into the chain of infection which usually involves other mammalian species better adapted to the infection. The same is true of many other animal diseases in which human beings "get in the way," becoming much more ill than the particular animal species adapted to that infection. Another sort of evolutionary exception is seen

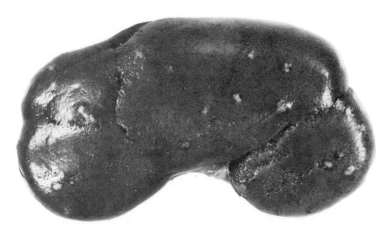

FIGURE 6-5 *Kidney in septicopyemia. The light-colored lesions scattered over the cortical surface are actually microabscesses formed as a result of lodgement of blood-borne bacteria.*

when "new" organisms are introduced into previously isolated human populations. Thus, when primitive tribes are suddenly invaded by individuals from the outside world or when island populations are exposed to agents that are commonplace in our experience (e.g., measles), the attack and fatality rates may be striking. This same evolutionary principle is involved in the spread of certain strains of influenza virus around the world. In this latter instance the virus behaves as if it were "new" because of the development of antigenic traits which are unknown to the population at risk.

For these reasons it has become obvious that simply knowing the line of transmission of an infectious agent from host to host does not explain fully the incidence of an infectious *disease*. To understand the epidemiology of such a disease completely, we must understand those aspects of the interaction between host and microbe which convert an ordinarily innocuous or inapparent infection into a clinically significant infectious disease.

Opportunistic infection

The concept of *opportunistic infection* reflects our recognition of the fact that there are many organisms which we do not think of as doing much to a healthy individual but which, given the wrong circumstances, will take over and produce an infectious disease. Such organisms are referred to as opportunists because they seemingly take advantage of the special circumstances of the host. Many opportunists are organisms which reside constantly within the host, and these are sometimes referred to as *endogenous* infectious agents. Some *exogenous* agents are likewise opportunistic in their behavior.

Opportunistic infections emerge when some factor or set of factors has compromised intrinsic defense mechanisms of the host or has in some way altered the ecology of the normal resident microbes (see later). Many opportunistic infections are seen in our hospitals in patients who have been significantly debilitated by diseases which impair their nutrition, their immunologic reactions, or their ability to produce effectively functioning leukocytes. Leukemias and other forms of cancer are high on the list of such diseases associated with opportunistic infections. Similarly, pharmacological agents which must be administered in the treatment of certain diseases may have as an undesirable side effect, the suppression of immunologic or inflammatory reactions, thus paving the way for opportunistic infections. Adrenal cortical steroids, which behave in many ways as anti-inflammatory agents, are high on this list, as are cytotoxic agents given in the course of cancer chemotherapy or immunosuppressive therapy. Antimicrobial therapy sometimes also leads to opportunistic infection apparently via suppression of part of the normal microbial flora, altering the critical ecological balance such that another member of the flora may emerge and grow out of all proportion, thus, producing disease. Antimicrobial therapy may also render a host more susceptible to some agent which ordinarily could not get a foothold because of the normal microbial flora.

Many other things happen to hospitalized patients that tend to tip the scales in favor of an infectious organism rather than the patient. These include certain phenomena associated with anesthesia, shock, and burns, to mention but a few instances. Finally there are many examples of diseases that predispose individuals to the occurrence of infectious diseases. For example, certain cancers which involve the lymphoid tissues of the body result in *defective cellular immune reactions*. Individuals with these deficiencies develop infectious diseases due to agents ordinarily controlled by the lymphocyte-macrophage system. Finally, one infectious disease may predispose to another. For example, an individual may develop a viral "cold" and thereby become likely to develop bacterial pneumonia as a complication.

There are numerous environmental factors in the community at large that tip the scales in favor of a particular organism rather than the host. An example of such an environmental factor involving a single individual would be occupational exposure such as to silica dust predisposing to tuberculosis. Entire populations of individuals may be involved at one time, such as in famine conditions where depression of host response results in virtual epidemics of diseases such as tuberculosis. Finally, in deference to our grandmothers who seemed to know about such things, it should be pointed out that meteorologic changes may also influence the incidence of *infectious disease* as compared to infection. A variety of studies has indicated in this regard that certain infectious agents can be found within human populations the year round, but *symptomatic* infections with those agents have a seasonal incidence, perhaps related to the weather.

None of the above discussion is intended to belittle the importance of germs in disease or to discourage attempts at interrupting the cycle of transmission of infectious agents between individuals. What should be emphasized, though, is that a given organism may be a necessary condition for the production of a particular disease without in itself being a sufficient condition. It is the complex interaction of many host and environmental factors that ultimately determines the precise outcome in a given instance of infection. For these reasons when one considers the "virulence" or the "pathogenicity" of a particular microorganism, it must be done in relation to the status of the given host at that time.

NORMAL MICROBIAL FLORA

In the above discussion, in several places, the *normal or indigenous microbial flora* was mentioned. It should be emphasized that the host together with this microbial flora constitutes a sort of ecosystem whose equilibriums are an essential part of what we consider health.

Quantitatively, the normal microbial flora of animal hosts (including the human species) represents a staggering sort of load. For example, a significant fraction of the dry weight of feces actually consists of bacterial carcasses. We all excrete trillions of organisms each day from the gastrointestinal tract. The skin likewise has a large resident flora, estimated to be in concentration of greater than 10,000 organisms per square centimeter of skin. It should be pointed out that these are not simply organisms adhering to dirty skin but organisms which live deep within the various epithelial structures of the skin (and in fact are shed in larger numbers with scrubbing). Astronomical numbers of organisms also live within the mouth. Scrapings taken from the surfaces of teeth or gums may contain millions of organisms per milligram of material, and saliva may contain as many as 100 million organisms per milliliter.

Another point to be emphasized is that this impressive microbial flora is not a random population. Of the many species of microbes encountered within the environment as we move about each day, only relatively few have become adapted in the course of their own evolution to the particular environments that we afford in various tissues. Therefore, within certain limits the flora of a given animal species is predictable, and within a given species such as our own the flora of particular tissues is quite predictable. An interesting point about the flora is that in most tissues that have been studied carefully the anaerobic bacteria seem to outnumber the aerobic bacteria. This is especially true in the bowel, where the ratio is as high as 1000:1.

Biologists have known of the existence of the normal microbial flora for many decades, but opinions concerning the significance of the flora have varied tremendously through the years. In the early years of this century some authorities had a very dim view of the flora, judging it at best to be a neutral mass, and at worst to be a cause of the degenerative diseases of aging. Gradually this view has been replaced, with the increasing recognition that no animal species would evolve with a particular flora in a disadvantageous relationship. To the contrary, one would predict that a mutually advantageous relationship should evolve.

Clearly, indigenous microbes do many good things for us. Many chemical reactions within the lumen of the bowel, for instance, are actually carried out by the resident microbes. The ecologic functions of such microbes in repelling potential invaders has already been alluded to. In fact, however, carrying this argument on evolutionary grounds even further, one would predict that many traits of our species have evolved as they did partly as a result of the presence of the microbial associates. In everyday terms this means that a number of anatomic and physiologic traits of the host that we consider normal and innate actually develop as a response to the presence of the flora. Putting this in another way, the host depends for normalcy to a significant extent upon the microbial flora. It is known, for instance, that the structure and function of the lining of the gastrointestinal tract are influenced by the presence of the flora, that the motility of the tract is influenced by the

flora, and that many of the reactions of the tract to challenge are similarly conditioned by the flora.

Although such considerations are perhaps more obvious within the gastrointestinal tract, the direct and indirect effects of the indigenous flora are not limited to that area. There is reason to believe that even immunologic function and leukocyte function are influenced by the flora.

The actual means by which the microbial flora acts upon the host are not well understood. In fact, even the identity of some components of the flora in human beings is far from clear. We are only now beginning to learn what it is that controls the usual ecologic balance of the flora itself; a combination of factors involving microbe-to-microbe and host-to-microbe interactions. What is evident at this point, however, is that when one disrupts the normal ecology of the microbal flora, it is done at significant risk to the host.

QUESTIONS

The response of the body to infectious agents—Chap. 6

Directions: Answer the following questions on a separate sheet of paper.

1 What are the criteria used to determine that a host is infected? Does a host who is infected necessarily have an infectious disease?

2 Name at least five portals of entry of infectious agents into the host. Describe the characteristics of the defenses at each of these portals.

3 Briefly describe what can occur if an acute inflammatory reaction is unable to contain an invading microorganism locally?

4 What is the final line of defense against widespread dissemination of an infectious agent throughout the body?

5 What is meant by an opportunistic infection?

6 What are some situations which can change an inapparent infection into an infectious disease?

7 Briefly discuss the interaction of the human host and the bacteria forming the normal flora on body surfaces. What value does this relationship provide for the host?

8 List several known mechanisms causing tissue injury by infectious agents.

Directions: Circle the letter preceding each item below that correctly answers each question. More than one answer may be correct.

9 All of the following may directly deter or prevent the invasion and spread of infectious agents EXCEPT:
a Inflammatory response   b Intact skin
c Alveolar macrophages   d Fibroblasts
e Reticuloendothelial system

10 When microorganisms reach such a high number in the circulation that they lodge in tissues and form abcesses, the condition is termed:
a Septicemia   b Bacteremia   c Septicopyemia
d Polycythemia

11 In relationships between hosts and infectious agents evolution has favored:
a Weak, nonresistant hosts   b Hardier, resistant hosts   c Very lethal infectious agents
d Less lethal infectious agents

Match the organisms listed in col. A with their specific invasive characteristic in col. B.

Column A

12 _____ Cholera vibrio
13 _____ Typhoid bacillus
14 _____ Syphilis spirochete
15 _____ Tetanus bacillus

Column B

a Penetrates the mucous membrane or skin and enters the bloodstream; disseminated widely in body
b Invades the lining of the bowel and enters the bloodstream
c Colonizes bowel lumen, never invades
d Remains local but secretes a toxin which is carried in the bloodstream

Match the terms in col. A which indicate the type of relationship between two dissimilar organisms living in close association (e.g., human being and microorganism) to their correct interpretation in col. B.

Column A

16 _____ Commensalism
17 _____ Parasitism
18 _____ Mutualism

Column B

a The association is beneficial to one but detrimental to the other.
b The association is beneficial to one without injury to the other.
c The association is beneficial to both.

CHAPTER 7 Disturbances of Circulation

At the completion of Chap. 7 you should be able to:

1 Describe the two mechanisms by which congestion (hyperemia) may be produced.

2 State at least one example of each type of congestion.

3 Identify the systemic causes of passive congestion.

4 Describe the effects of chronic passive congestion in areas such as the lungs, liver, and veins.

5 Differentiate between acute passive congestion and chronic passive congestion in terms of their effects on the involved tissue.

6 Define *edema*.

7 Discuss the pathogenesis of edema in terms of factors governing fluid flux across vascular membranes.

8 Compare an exudate to a transudate as to pathogenesis and give an example of each type.

9 Describe the significance of generalized edema.

10 Define the following terms associated with hemorrhage: *hematoma, petechiae, ecchymoses*.

11 Describe the various causes of hemorrhage.

12 Describe the body's mechanisms for stopping hemorrhage.

13 Describe the local and systemic effects of hemorrhage.

14 Discuss the etiology, pathogenesis, and morphology of thrombi.

15 Distinguish between factors predisposing to the development of thrombi in arteries and veins.

16 Contrast the consequences of arterial and venous thrombi.

17 Describe the process of embolism.

18 Trace the route when fragments of venous thrombi from deep veins of the leg or pelvis break off and are dislodged into the circulation.

19 Describe the potential consequences of pulmonary arterial emboli, caisson disease, air emboli, and traumatic fat emboli.

20 Define *arteriosclerosis*.

21 Differentiate between Monckeberg's sclerosis, arteriolosclerosis, and atherosclerosis in terms of morphology and clinical significance.

22 Identify for atherosclerosis the area(s) of involvement, unit lesion, etiology, incidence, and consequences.

23 Discuss the possible causes of ischemia and the effects on affected tissue.

24 Describe the possible outcome of occlusion of major blood vessels.

25 Define an *infarct*.

26 Discuss the factors which determine whether an ischemic area actually undergoes infarction.

27 Describe the morphologic features of an infarct.

28 Cite examples of infarcts commonly encountered clinically.

CONGESTION

Simply stated, *congestion* is an overabundance of blood *within* the vessels in a given region. Another word for congestion is *hyperemia*. When observed grossly, an area of tissue or an organ which is congested has a deeper red (or purplish) color than usual because of the increase in blood within the tissue. Microscopically the capillaries in a hyperemic tissue are dilated and engorged with blood. Basically there are two mechanisms by which congestion may be produced: (1) by an actual increase in the amount of blood flowing into an area or (2) by a decrease in the amount of blood draining from an area.

Active congestion

When the flow of blood into an area is increased and produces congestion, the phenomenon is referred to as *active congestion,* in the sense that more blood than usual is actively flowing into the area. This increase in local blood flow is accomplished by dilatation of arterioles which behave as valves governing the flow into the local microcirculation. One common example of active congestion is the hyperemia accompanying acute inflammation which accounts for the redness described in Chap. 4 (see Fig. 4-1). Another example of active congestion is a blush, which is basically a matter of vasodilatation produced in response to a neurogenic stimulus. A physiological example of active congestion is the delivery of more blood upon "demand" of a working tissue such as an actively contracting muscle. By its very nature, active congestion is often short-lived. As the stimulus to arteriolar dilatation is withdrawn, the flow of blood to the affected area is decreased, and the situation returns to normal.

Passive congestion

As the name suggests, *passive congestion* does not involve an increase in the amount of blood flowing into an area but rather some impairment in drainage of blood from the area. Anything which compresses the venules and veins draining a tissue may produce passive congestion. When one places an elastic tourniquet about the arm prior to drawing blood from a vein, one is actually inducing an artificial form of passive congestion. A similar and more significant change could be produced, for instance, by a tumor compressing the local venous drainage to an area. In addition to such local causes of passive congestion there are central or systemic reasons for impaired venous drainage. Not infrequently the heart fails in its pumping action (see Part V), and this leads to impaired venous drainage. For instance, if the left side of the heart fails in its pumping action, the flow of blood returning to the heart from the lung will be somewhat impaired. Under such circumstances blood will be dammed back into the lung, producing passive congestion of the pulmonary vasculature. Similarly if the right side of the heart fails, the damming up of blood affects systemic venous return, and many tissues throughout the body become passively congested. In point of fact, very often patients suffer simultaneously from right- and left-sided cardiac failure.

Passive congestion may be relatively short-lived, in which case it is termed *acute passive congestion,* or it may be of long standing, in which case it is termed *chronic passive congestion.* If the passive congestion is short-lived, there are no effects on the involved tissue. In chronic passive congestion, however, there may be permanent changes in the tissues. These changes are due in large part to the fact that in a passively congested area if the change in blood flow is marked enough, there is an element of tissue hypoxia which may lead to shrinkage or even loss of cells of the involved tissue. In certain organs this also leads to an increase in the amount of fibrous connective tissue. In many areas there is also evidence of local breakdown of red blood cells, which results in the deposition of hemoglobin-derived pigments within the tissues.

The effects of chronic passive congestion are particularly notable in lungs and liver. In the case of the lungs (Fig. 7-1), the walls of air spaces tend to become thickened, and numerous macrophages containing *hemosiderin* pigment are formed as a product of the breakdown of hemoglobin from red blood cells which escape the congested vessels into the air spaces. Such hemosiderin-containing macrophages are sometimes termed *heart failure cells* and can be found in the sputum of patients in chronic left-sided cardiac failure. In the case of the liver, chronic passive congestion leads to marked dilatation of the blood channels in the center of each hepatic lobule, with shrinkage of liver cells in this area. The result of this is a striking gross appearance of the liver (Fig. 7-2) produced by the hyperemic centrilobular zone alternating with the less affected peripheral areas of each lobule. This gross appearance is sometimes referred to as "nutmeg liver" because of the fancied resemblance of the cut surface of such a liver to the cut surface of a nutmeg.

Another effect of chronic passive congestion is dilatation of the veins in the affected area. As the walls of affected veins are chronically stretched, they become somewhat fibrotic, and the veins also tend to lengthen. Because veins are fixed at various points along their length they necessarily become tortuous as they lengthen, i.e., they twist back and forth between points of fixation. Dilated, somewhat tortuous, thick-walled veins are referred as *varicose veins* or *varices*. Varicose veins in the legs are a familiar sight. Also common are *hemorrhoids*, which are actually varicose veins of the anus (in the hemorrhoidal plexus of veins). More importantly, venous varices sometimes form in the lower esophagus in cases of chronic liver disease (see Part IV), and rupture of such congested varices may lead to fatal hemorrhage.

EDEMA

Edema is an accumulation of excess fluid between the cells of the body or within the various body cavities. When edema accumulates in a cavity, it is usually called an *effusion*, e.g., pericardial effusion, pleural effusion. An accumulation of fluid in the peritoneal cavity is usually termed *ascites*. Massive generalized edema is frequently referred to as *anasarca*. *Hydrops* and *dropsy* are older terms also referring to edema.

Etiology and pathogenesis

The development of edema can be explained by considering the various forces normally controlling fluid exchange across vessel walls (see Fig. 4-2 and Chap. 4). Local factors include the hydrostatic pressure within the microcirculation and the permeability of vessel walls.

Increases in hydrostatic pressure will tend to force fluid into the interstitial spaces of the body. For this simple reason, congestion and edema tend to go together. As was explained in the discussion of inflammation, a local increase in the permeability of vessel walls to protein will allow these large molecules to escape the vessels, and fluid will follow osmotically. Therefore, edema is a prominent part of the acute inflammatory reaction. Another local cause of edema formation is obstruction of lymphatic channels, which are normally responsible for drainage of the interstitial fluid. When these channels become obstructed for any reason, an important pathway of egress of fluid is lost, leading to accumulation of edema, referred to as *lymphedema*. Lymphedema is seen in a variety of inflammatory conditions affecting the lymphatics but is perhaps most commonly encountered in hospitals following either excision or irradiation of local lymphatics as part of cancer therapy. A specific example of this type of edema is swelling of the upper extremity sometimes seen following radical mastectomy.

Systemic factors may also favor edema formation. Since fluid balance is dependent on osmotic properties of serum protein, conditions accompanied by a lower concentration of this protein may lead to edema. In the so-called *nephrotic syndrome*, massive amounts of protein are lost in the urine, and the patient becomes hypoproteinemic and edematous. The hypoproteinemia of advanced liver disease may also favor the formation of edema. In famine situations massive edema may likewise accompany the nutritional hypoproteinemia.

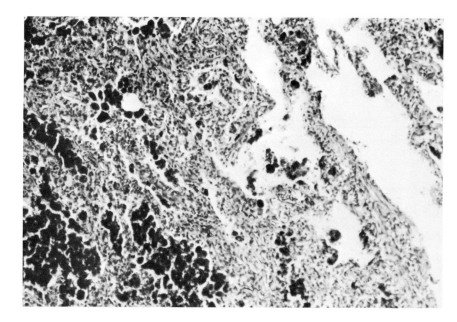

FIGURE 7-1 *Chronic passive congestion of lung. Alveolar septa are thickened (evident at the right), and many air spaces contain deeply pigmented macrophages containing hemosiderin. (Photomicrograph, ×200.)*

Transudates vs. exudates

When fluid accumulates in a tissue or space because of increased vascular permeability to protein, this accumulation is referred to as an *exudate*. Thus, inflammatory edema represents an exudate. When fluid accumulates in the tissues or spaces because of reasons other than change in vascular permeability, the accumulation is referred to as a *transudate*. In hospital situations probably cardiac failure is the leading cause of transudate formation. Sometimes it becomes important clinically to determine whether a particular fluid accumulation represents a transudate or an exudate. Exudates by their very nature tend to contain more protein than transudates and tend, therefore, to have higher specific gravities. In addition, the protein of exudates often includes fibrinogen, which will precipitate as fibrin, causing clotting of the exudate fluid. Transudates do not clot generally. Finally, exudates will frequently contain leukocytes as part of the inflammatory process, while transudates tend to be cell-poor.

Morphology of edema

The morphology of edema involves simply a swelling of the affected part because of too much fluid contained within the interstices. The swelling is generally of a soft sort, and the fluid actually can be moved about. This latter feature is utilized clinically in diagnosing subtle degrees of edema. While a massively swollen ankle is easily diagnosed on sight, a slight degree of edema may be present without being particularly visible. In this instance gentle pressure of a thumb against the side of the ankle will tend to displace some of the edema fluid temporarily, and when the thumb is removed after a few moments, a depression is left in the tissues. This is referred to as *pitting edema*. This same mobility of edema fluid within the interstices of tissues accounts for certain postural effects. Sometimes, when first admitted to the hospital, a patient will have demonstrably edematous ankles, because in the ambulatory situation the edema moves with gravity towards the lower extremities. However, when the patient has been in bed for a time with the lower extremities not in a dependent position, the ankles may become slimmer, and edema may become demonstrable over the sacrum instead.

Effects of edema

Edema is important primarily as an indicator of something being amiss. In other words, the swollen ankles per se do not harm the patient other than, perhaps, in a cosmetic sense but do serve as an indicator of protein loss, congestive heart failure, etc. In certain locations edema in and of itself is extremely important. Edema of the lungs, as, for instance, in left-sided heart failure, is an acute medical emergency if extensive. If a sufficient number of air spaces in the lungs fill with edema fluid, the patient may literally drown. Massive pulmonary edema can be lethal within a matter of minutes. Lesser degrees of pulmonary edema which can be tolerated in a ventilatory sense may be dangerous to bedridden patients. In such instances the fluid may collect posteriorly at the lung bases and serve as a focus for the development of bacterial pneumonia, sometimes referred to as *hypostatic pneumonia*. Edema is also life-threatening when it affects the brain. This is so because the skull represents a closed space with no room to spare. As the brain becomes edematous, it swells and is compressed against the bony confines of the skull. At some point, in severe cases, increased intracranial pressure will compromise blood flow within the brain, leading to death.

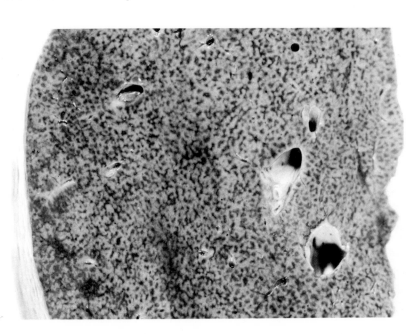

FIGURE 7-2 Chronic passive congestion of liver. Dark areas are hyperemic centrilobular zones, while light areas are less affected peripheral zones. The result is this typical "nutmeg" pattern.

Hemorrhage is the escape of blood from confines of the cardiovascular system, with accumulation in the tissues or spaces of the body, or with actual escape from the body. Special descriptive terms are used to designate various circumstances of hemorrhage. An accumulation of blood with tissues is referred to as a *hematoma*. When the blood escapes into various spaces in the body, it is named according to the space, e.g., *hemopericardium*, *hemothorax* (hemorrhage into the pleural space), *hemoperitoneum*, *hematosalpinx* (hemorrhage into the fallopian tube). Pinpoint hemorrhages visible on cutaneous or mucosal surfaces or on cut surfaces of organs are referred to as *petechiae*. Larger, blotchy areas of hemorrhage are referred to as *ecchymoses*, and a condition characterized by widespread blotchy hemorrhages is sometimes referred to as *purpura*.

Etiology of hemorrhage

The commonest cause of hemorrhage is loss of integrity of vascular walls, which permits the escape of blood. This is most often due to external trauma such as we all experience from time to time with injuries accompanied by bruising. (The discoloration of a bruise is due to the blood accumulated in the interstices of the traumatized tissue.) Vascular walls may be disrupted as a result of disease as well as trauma.

A number of mechanisms exist within the body to counteract hemorrhage (see Part III). One mechanism of hemostasis involves the *blood platelets,* which are made in the bone marrow and circulate in the blood in large numbers. Platelets act directly to plug small leaks in vessels by aggregating in the area and blocking the flow. Platelets also lead to hemostasis by triggering the *clotting mechanism* of the blood. The "backbone" of a blood clot is fibrin, which is precipitated from its circulating precursor, fibrinogen. The precipitation of fibrin is controlled by a number of clotting factors which are activated under certain circumstances (see Chap. 18).

Hemorrhage may be caused by an abnormality of these hemostatic mechanisms. For instance, hemorrhage accompanies a state of *thrombocytopenia*, a deficiency in the number of circulating platelets. Thrombocytopenia can arise because of destruction or suppression of the bone marrow, e.g., by malignancy or by some drug, with consequent failure of platelet production. Thrombocytopenia may also occur if circulating platelets are rapidly destroyed, as occurs in certain diseases. When the platelet count in the peripheral blood drops beyond a certain point, the patient begins to bleed "spontaneously," meaning that the trauma of normal motion leads to widespread hemorrhages. A deficiency of any of the various clotting factors may likewise lead to hemorrhage. Such deficiency can be hereditary (e.g., hemophilia), but can also be acquired. Certain of the blood clotting factors are synthesized in the liver, and with advanced hepatic disease the level of such factors available in the blood may drop precipitously. Paradoxically, in certain situations excessive clotting of the blood may lead to an acquired deficiency of platelets and/or clotting factors. Usually this involves the formation of myriads of tiny clots around the body, so-called *disseminated intravascular coagulation* (DIC), and the acquired deficiency state is sometimes referred to under the general heading, *consumptive coagulopathy*.

Effects of hemorrhage

The *local effects* of hemorrhage are related to the presence of extravasated blood in the tissues and can range from trivial to lethal. Perhaps the most trivial local effect is a bruise, which may be of only cosmetic importance. The initial bluish discoloration of the bruise is related directly to the presence of spilled red blood cells accumulated in the tissue. These extravasated erythrocytes break down fairly rapidly and are phagocytized by macrophages arriving as part of the associated inflammatory response. These macrophages process the hemoglobin in the same manner used in the normal recycling of old red cells but in a much more accelerated, concentrated fashion. As the hemoglobin is metabolized within these cells, it is split into an iron-containing moiety called *hemosiderin* and a non-iron-containing moiety which, in tissues, is termed *hematoidin* (although it is chemically identical with *bilirubin*). Hemosiderin has a rusty-brown color, and hematoidin a light-yellow color. It is the play of these pigments in a resolving bruise that produces the familiar range of colors as the "black-and-blue mark" fades through varying shades of brown and yellow, ultimately to disappear as the macrophages wander off, and restitution of the tissue is complete. Sometimes, when a hematoma is of considerable volume, it may actually organize rather than resolve completely, leaving some degree of local scarring.

At the other extreme, strictly local hemorrhage may be fatal, even if of small volume, if it is in the wrong place. Thus, as seen in Fig. 7-3, a relatively small volume of hemorrhage in a vital area of the brain can produce death. Similarly if a few hundred milliliters of blood are aspirated into the tracheobronchial tree, the patient may be suffocated. Another area wherein a relatively small volume of hemorrhage may produce death is the pericardial sac. If hemopericardium develops quickly and the tough fibrous pericardial sac does not have the opportunity to stretch, pressure within the sac builds up rapidly as blood accumulates. Sometimes the pressure is sufficient with accumulation of only a few hundred milliliters, that diastolic filling of the heart is impaired, leading to death by *cardiac tamponade*.

The systemic effects of blood loss are related directly to the volume of blood extravasated. Obviously, if a major portion of the circulatory volume is lost, as with massive trauma, the patient may die of *exsanguination* very quickly. It should be noted that a patient may exsanguinate with absolutely no external evidence of hemorrhage. This occurs when the extravasated blood accumulates within a large body cavity such as the pleural cavity or peritoneal cavity. This type of lethal internal hemorrhage is seen all too often in crushing injuries associated with motor vehicle accidents, when broken ribs lacerate a lung or abdominal trauma results in rupture of the spleen or liver. (In emergency room practice such internal hemorrhage is identified by needle aspiration of the cavity in question.) The effects of a given volume of hemorrhage are also related to the rate at which the loss occurs, a larger volume loss being better tolerated if it occurs gradually rather than instantaneously.

Short of death, the rapid loss of a sufficient volume of blood may lead to a condition of *shock*. A detailed consideration of the various shock syndromes is beyond the scope of this discussion, but it should be pointed out that shock can be produced not only by loss of blood volume but because of neurogenic causes, cardiac causes, or even accompanying systemic sepsis. Although the various shock syndromes differ in detail, they are all basically accompanied by a decrease in blood pressure and by an element of loss of control over the regulation of blood flow, leading ultimately to inadequate perfusion and oxygenation of the vital tissues of the body.

If a patient survives the acute loss of a given volume of blood, the circulatory volume is quickly regained by an influx of fluid into the cardiovascular system. This leads to a relative dilution of the red blood cell mass remaining, and the patient at that point would be found to be somewhat anemic. Under such conditions the marrow is stimulated to produce red blood cells in an accelerated fashion, and the anemia would gradually be corrected. Under conditions of chronic loss of even relatively small volumes of blood, the compensatory abilities of the marrow may be exceeded, and the patient may become progressively more anemic. Not infrequently, patients with chronic loss of blood present themselves with signs and symptoms of the anemia rather than of the blood loss itself. Thus, many a patient with a cancer of the colon which oozes blood for many months unnoticed into the feces, may ultimately seek medical attention because of fatigue, pallor, lack of energy, etc. Thus, occult loss of blood is a consideration in the investigation of many anemias.

THROMBOSIS

The process of formation of a blood clot or coagulum within the vascular system (i.e., the blood vessels or the heart) during life is referred to as *thrombosis*. The coagulum of blood is called a *thrombus*. The accumulation of blood which clots outside of the vascular system, e.g., a hematoma, is *not* referred to as a thrombus. Furthermore, the clots that form within the cardiovascular system after death are not called thrombi. They are called *postmortem clots*.

Thrombosis is obviously of great adaptive value in case of hemorrhage. That is to say, a thrombus acts as a very effective hemostatic plug. However, thrombosis may also occur inappropriately when the normal control mechanisms are defective and, under these circumstances, prove to be harmful to the host.

Etiology and pathogenesis of thrombosis

Three sets of factors ordinarily guard against inappropriate thrombus formation. First of all, the normal vascular system has a smooth, slick lining of endothelial cells to which platelets and fibrin do not readily adhere.

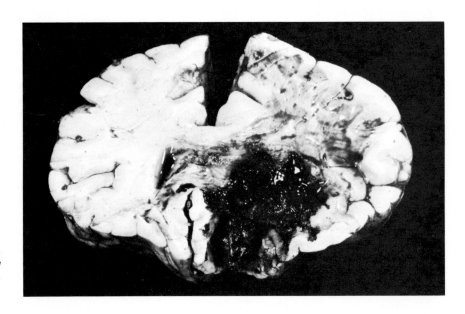

FIGURE 7-3 Cerebral hemorrhage. In an instance such as this, a relatively small volume of hemorrhage may lead to death because of local destructive effects.

Secondly the normal flow of blood within the vascular system is a fairly streamlined one so that platelets are not hurled against lining surfaces. Finally, the clotting mechanism (see Chap. 18) has built into it a number of chemical checks and balances to control clot formation. Correspondingly, there are three basic kinds of situations in which clots form inappropriately: those in which there is abnormality of the vessel wall and lining, those in which blood flow is abnormal, and those in which the coagulability of the blood itself is increased.

The flow of blood on the arterial side of the circulation is a high-pressure flow of rapid velocity, and the arteries themselves are rather thick-walled and not easily deformed. For these reasons the usual cause of arterial thrombosis is disease in the lining and wall of the artery, particularly atherosclerosis (see discussion later). On the venous side of the circulation the blood flow is one of low pressure and relatively lower velocity, and the veins are sufficiently thin-walled that they can be deformed readily by external pressures. For these reasons, the usual causes of thrombosis on the venous side of the circulation relate to diminished flow of blood. Finally, chemical changes occur in the blood of patients with a variety of diseases, leading to a hypercoagulable state which may further complicate any of the above situations.

Morphology and fate of thrombi

Thrombi consist of varying combinations of aggregated platelets, participated fibrin, and enmeshed red blood cells and leukocytes. The precise configuration of a thrombus depends on the conditions under which it was formed. If the thrombus begins to form in flowing blood, very often the first element is a clump of platelets adhering to the endothelium. This could occur because of abnormal flow allowing platelets to settle against or

to be hurled against the endothelium; or could occur because of a roughening of the endothelial lining, which would produce a nidus for platelet aggregation. As platelets aggregate, they release substances which encourage the precipitation of fibrin, so that soon the platelet aggregates come to be surrounded by fibrin and trapped blood cells. Successive waves of events of this sort can lead to a complex, ribbed structure of a thrombus. On the other hand, if a thrombus forms in a vessel in which the flow has virtually stopped, the clot may simply consist of a diffuse meshwork of fibrin trapping the formed elements of the blood more or less homogeneously. It should be noted here that, in contrast to the processes just described, postmortem clotting occurs quite slowly so that the formed elements of the blood layer out before the clot solidifies, giving rise to a stratified structure in which red blood cells, white blood cells, and fibrin may be quite separate. Such postmortem clots tend to be more elastic than true thrombi and are much less likely to be adherent to vascular walls.

Thrombi may occur literally in any part of the cardiovascular system for a variety of causes. Figure 7-4 illustrates a thrombus from a large deep vein of the leg. Such thrombi are all too common in our hospitalized, bedridden patients. Their occurrence is generally related to the decreased rate of flow through these veins, in turn secondary to the loss of pumping action of muscular activity. The situation is aggravated in many instances by sluggish peripheral circulation related to chronic cardiac failure. It cannot be emphasized too strongly that *phlebothrombosis*, the formation of thrombi in veins, is an ever-present danger stalking hospitalized patients.

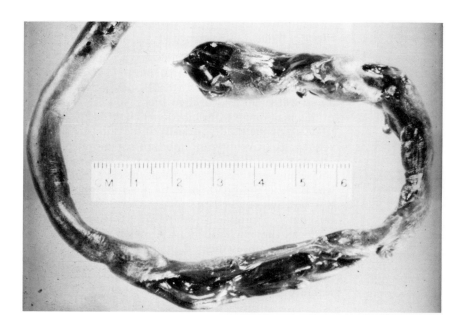

FIGURE 7-4 Venous thrombus. This thrombus was extracted from a leg vein at autopsy. Such a finding is unfortunately quite common and is associated with many dire consequences. Reference to the scale emphasizes the magnitude of the clot.

Such thrombi may develop relatively silently or may be accompanied by signs and symptoms of inflammation of the vein wall, which are presumably secondary to the presence of the thrombus. (When inflammatory signs dominate, the condition is sometimes referred to as *thrombophlebitis*.) The most feared consequences of such venous thrombi is the breaking off of a portion which is then transported in the bloodstream and lodges at a distant site.

Figure 7-5 illustrates a thrombus within the left atrium of the heart. In this instance the thrombus formed because of an abnormal flow and pattern of circulation through the atrium related to stenosis of the mitral valve. Occasionally such atrial thrombi may behave as "ball valves," suddenly occluding the atrioventricular orifice and producing instant death. More often such thrombi act as the source of fragments which are propelled distally in the bloodstream.

Figure 7-6 illustrates a thrombus on a cardiac valve.

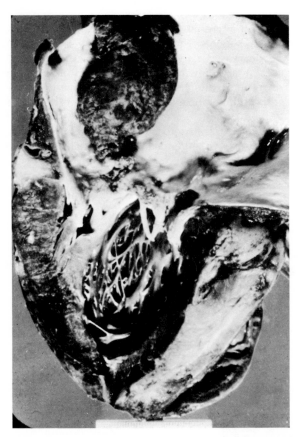

FIGURE 7-5 Atrial thrombus. A huge thrombus has formed in the left atrium because of malfunction of the scarred mitral valve. The position of this clot renders it of great potential danger.

In this instance the cause is bacterial infection of the valve, and the thrombus is frequently referred to as a *vegetation*. Vegetations of infective endocarditis are exceedingly dangerous because of local damage to the valve, and because fragments may be propelled to other sites in the body where additional vessels may become occluded and infected.

Figure 7-7 illustrates a thrombus within the left ventricle of the heart. When a thrombus such as this one is adherent to the wall of the cardiovascular system but does not totally occlude the area, it is referred to as a *mural thrombus*. The reason for the formation of a ventricular mural thrombus is usually the death of the underlying myocardium with an associated inflammatory reaction reaching the lining of the heart.

Figure 7-8 illustrates a thrombus within an artery. Clearly evident in the picture is the thickening of the wall of the artery which has given rise to the thrombus. The roughening in this instance is due to a disease (atherosclerosis) and is a precipitating cause of thrombosis.

Very often, when the subject survives the formation of a thrombus, the fate of the thrombus is to undergo resolution. The body possesses fibrinolytic mechanisms which, along with the action of leukocytes, may lead to the dissolution of clots. Probably all of us form tiny thrombi now and then, and these are resolved without ever reaching the clinical horizon. On the other hand, the fate of some large thrombi is to undergo organization, with granulation tissue growing in from an adjacent vascular lining. In such instances, the involved vessel may become permanently plugged by scar. Sometimes the vascular channels within the young granulation tissue organizing a thrombus may anastomose in a manner as to provide new channels through the area occupied by thrombus. This phenomenon is referred to as *recanalization*. Unfortunately, in many instances, before the thrombus either organizes or resolves, portions of it break off and are propelled in the bloodstream, ultimately lodging elsewhere and occluding additional vessels.

Effects of thrombi

The consequences of thrombosis are perhaps most obvious in the case of arterial thrombi. If an artery is occluded by a thrombus, the tissues served by that artery will suffer loss of their blood supply. The results of this may range from functional abnormality of tissue to death of the tissue or death of the subject. The consequences of venous thrombi are somewhat different. The anatomy of the venous system is such that if one vein is plugged, chances are that the blood will find its way back to the heart via some anastomosing channel. It is only when very large veins are occluded by thrombus that local problems with passive congestion become evident. The most ominous problem associated with venous thrombi is their fragmentation and transport to distant points in the body. Similarly, the effects of cardiac thrombi are largely related to their moving elsewhere within the cardiovascular system.

Definition and types

The carriage of a physical mass in the bloodstream from one place to another with lodgement in the new location is termed *embolism*. The physical mass itself is called an *embolus*. The commonest emboli in human subjects are derived from thrombi and are termed *thromboemboli*. Many other things, however, can become embolic. Bits of tissue can embolize if they enter the vascular system, usually with trauma. Cancer cells may embolize, constituting a devastating means of spread of the disease (see Chap. 8). Foreign materials injected into the cardiovascular system may embolize. Droplets of liquid which form in the circulation under a variety of circumstances or are injected into the circulation may embolize, and even gas bubbles may become embolic.

Pathogenesis, routes, and effects of embolism

The commonest sources of emboli within the body are venous thrombi, most often in the deep veins of the legs or the pelvis. When fragments of such venous thrombi break off and float with the flow of blood, they enter

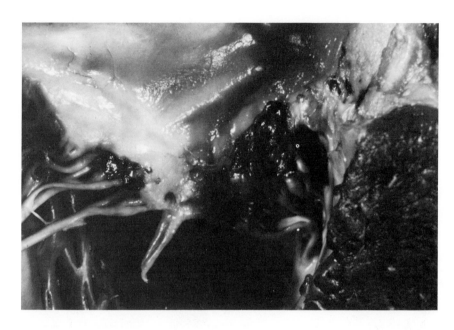

FIGURE 7-6 Infective endocarditis. The dark vegetations on this mitral valve are actually thrombotic masses formed around foci of bacterial infection of the valve. The valve was previously scarred (note thickening of leaflets and chordae) and therefore was susceptible to infection during a burst of bacteremia.

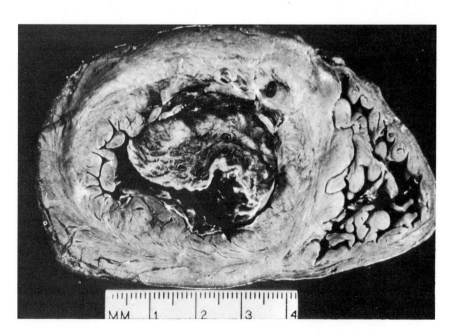

FIGURE 7-7 Mural thrombus in heart. In this transverse section of left ventricle a large mural thrombus overlies an area of previous myocardial necrosis.

the vena cava and then the right side of the heart. Such fragments do not lodge along this path because of the large size of the vessels and cardiac chambers involved. The blood leaving the right ventricle, however, flows into the main pulmonary artery, which branches into right and left pulmonary arteries, which in turn branch to smaller vessels. For these reasons of anatomy, emboli originating in venous thrombi usually terminate as *pulmonary arterial emboli.* When a very large fragment of thrombus becomes an embolus, a major portion of the pulmonary arterial supply may suddenly be occluded (Fig. 7-9). This can produce virtually instantaneous death of the subject. On the other hand, smaller pulmonary arterial emboli may be silent, may lead to pulmonary hemorrhage secondary to the vascular damage, or may actually result in necrosis of a portion of lung. Pulmonary emboli of various sizes can be found in a significant fraction of patients dying within hospitals, sometimes contributing to the death of the subject, sometimes being only of incidental importance. Showers of tiny pulmonary emboli over a long period of time may produce sufficient occlusion of the pulmonary vascular bed as to cause the right side of the heart to become overloaded and to fail.

Emboli which lodge on the arterial side of the circu-

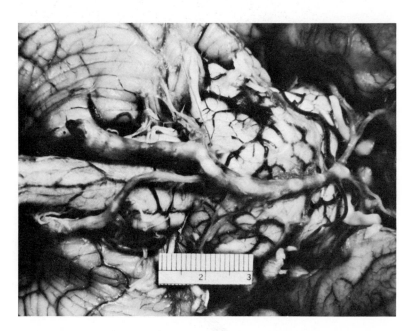

FIGURE 7-8 Thrombus in a sclerotic artery. The artery above the brainstem (left of center) is athero-sclerotic and gnarled. The lumen is occluded by a thrombus which protrudes from the cut end at the left.

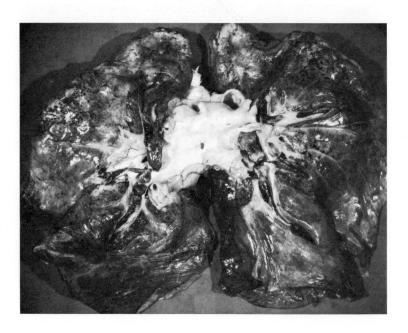

FIGURE 7-9 Massive pulmonary emboli. The opened pulmonary arteries supplying these lungs are seen in the center of the photo. The several dark cylindrical masses are emboli which originated from venous thrombus in a leg, similar to that shown in Fig. 7-4. The patient died within moments of lodgement of the emboli.

lation take their origin on the "left side" of the circulatory system either in the left cardiac chambers or in the large arteries. The only way that an embolus originating on the venous side of the circulation could lodge on the arterial side is to bypass the lungs via a defect in the interatrial or interventricular septum of the heart. This situation, termed *paradoxical embolism*, is exceedingly rare. Most often an arterial embolus is found to have originated from an intracardiac thrombus or, more rarely, from a mural thrombus in the aorta or one of its large branches.

Gas bubbles may become embolic in a variety of circumstances. One such circumstance has been termed *caisson disease*, more popularly known as "the bends." This situation arises when a subject has been living under markedly increased atmospheric pressure such as within a pressurized caisson or in underwater diving gear. In such circumstances increased amounts of atmospheric gases are dissolved within the bloodstream. If decompression is sufficiently abrupt, the result is analogous to what is seen when a warm bottle of soda pop is suddenly opened. The myriads of tiny gas bubbles appearing within the circulation are carried to a variety of places in the body where they lodge in the microcirculation and occlude the blood flow to those tissues. In hospitals an analogous circumstance sometimes arises when atmospheric air enters venous channels due to faulty handling of an intravenous infusion or indwelling vascular catheter; or sometimes in the course of a surgical procedure when large vascular channels must be traversed. With massive air embolism a large "bolus" of air may enter the right side of the heart, and at autopsy a large foamy mass of air and blood is seen distending the heart and pulmonary vessels.

An example of embolism of liquid droplets is so-called *traumatic fat embolism*. As the name suggests, these emboli, composed of fat globules, tend to form within the circulation following trauma. The usual point of lodgement is the microcirculation of the lung. Minor degrees of fat embolism probably follow most surgical procedures where fatty tissue is incised, allowing lipidic material to enter vascular channels. In such circumstances the few scattered emboli which lodge in the lung are completely silent and trivial. A similar circumstance arises when bones are fractured, apparently with liberation of lipid into the sinusoids of the bone marrow. Again, such scattered pulmonary fat emboli as result in this circumstance are trivial and clinically inapparent. Occasionally, however, following traumatic injury, fat embolism may be massive. It is not clear that all of the fat droplets in such a circumstance originate from trauma to adipose cells. Some evidence suggests that in this type of circumstance there is actually coalescence of lipid normally carried within the bloodstream. In any event, with sufficiently massive fat embolism, symptoms of respiratory distress may appear, usually in the first day or two after trauma. In severe instances the emboli lodge in a variety of places in the body beyond the lungs, including the skin and, more importantly, the central nervous system. In both of these latter areas each microscopic fat embolus is associated with a petechial

hemorrhage. In the case of the brain, a tiny focus of necrosis surrounds each occluded vessel. In these rare instances, fat embolism can be fatal, usually because of cerebral damage.

ATHEROSCLEROSIS

Arteriosclerosis, or "hardening of the arteries," is an exceedingly important disease phenomenon in most developed countries. The term arteriosclerosis actually encompasses any condition of arterial vessels that result in a thickening and/or hardening of the walls. Three conditions are generally included under this heading: *Monckeberg's sclerosis, arteriolosclerosis*, and *atherosclerosis*. Monckeberg's sclerosis involves deposition of calcium salts in the muscular wall of medium-sized arteries. Although this can be detected grossly and even seen on x-rays, this form of arteriosclerosis is not clinically significant since the lining of the involved vessel is not roughened and the lumen is not narrowed. Arteriolosclerosis refers to a thickening of arterioles, seen frequently in patients with elevated blood pressure and to some extent in association with aging. The most important type of arteriosclerosis is atherosclerosis, and generally when the term arteriosclerosis is used, it is used synonymously with atherosclerosis.

Atherosclerosis is a disease which involves the aorta, its large branches, and medium-sized arteries such as those supplying portions of the extremities, the brain, the heart, and the major internal viscera. Atherosclerosis does not involve arterioles, and it does not involve the venous side of the circulation. The disease is a multifocal one, and the unit lesion, or *atheroma* (also termed *atherosclerotic plaque*), consists of an elevated mass of fatty material associated with fibrous connective tissue, very often with secondary deposits of calcium salts and blood products. The plaques of atherosclerosis begin in the intima or inner layer of the vessel wall but with growth may extend to encroach upon the media or musculoelastic portion of the vessel wall.

Morphology of atherosclerosis

The typical gross appearance of moderately severe atherosclerosis is shown in Fig. 7-10. Recalling that a smooth endothelial lining of vessels is an important protection against thrombus formation, it is not at all difficult to realize why atherosclerosis should involve considerable liability to arterial thrombosis. The microscopic appearance of an atheroma is illustrated in Fig. 7-11. The dominance of both fibrous and fatty material in the lesion is evident (in fact, the term athero and sclerosis refers to the *mushy* and to the *hard* character of the lesions, respectively). In large vessels such as the aorta even numerous and severe atheromas do not generally lead to occlusion of the lumen but only to roughening of the lining surface. In smaller vessels, the atheromas may actually become circumferential, leading to marked narrowing of the lumen (Fig. 7-12).

Etiology and incidence of atherosclerosis

Atherosclerosis is truly a multifactorial disease, and it is therefore not possible to cite a single or dominant etiologic factor. The various factors which contribute to the development of atherosclerosis are so widespread in the populations of more affluent countries that none but the youngest individuals in the population are spared from the disease. In fact, autopsies performed on young adults dying "in their prime" as a result of

trauma always reveal lesions of atherosclerosis, sometimes surprisingly severe. In general, the earliest fatty deposits can be seen in young children, and these tend to increase with age (speaking of the population as a whole). The rate at which atheromas increase in size and number is influenced by a wide variety of factors. Certainly genetic factors are important here, and atherosclerosis and its complications often tend to run in families. Subjects with abnormalities of their blood lipids are often susceptible to accelerated atherosclerosis, as are individuals with diabetes mellitus. Blood pressure is an important factor in the incidence and severity of atherosclerosis. Patients with hypertension are much likelier to have earlier and more severe atherosclerosis; and the severity of the disease is correlated with the blood pressure even in the so-called normal range. In this regard it is interesting to note that atherosclerosis is not seen within the pulmonary arteries (usually a low-pressure circuit) unless the pressure is abnormally elevated, a state termed *pulmonary hypertension*. Without unduly lengthening the listing of "risk factors" in the

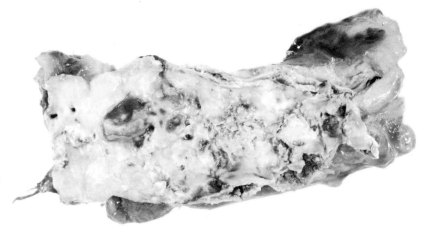

FIGURE 7-10 Atherosclerosis of aorta. This photo depicts the intimal (lining) surface of the abdominal aorta. Instead of being pearly and smooth, the surface is a roughened mass of atherosclerotic plaques.

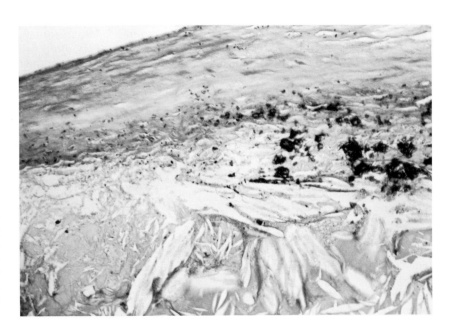

FIGURE 7-11 Atherosclerotic plaque. The clefts in the depths of the plaque represent large deposits of cholesterol. The dark material at the right is a dystrophic calcific deposit, and the horizontal band across the top is a fibrous "cap" of the lesion. The elevated rough lesions in Fig. 7-10 have this microscopic appearance.

development of atherosclerosis, it should be empha- sized that *cigarette smoking* is a major environmental factor leading to increased severity of atherosclerosis. The precise way in which these various factors contribute to the pathogenesis of the lesions of atherosclerosis has not been completely elucidated.

Consequences of atherosclerosis

The consequences of atherosclerosis depend in part on the size of the artery involved. If the artery is a medium-sized one such as a major branch of the coronary artery with a lumen perhaps a few millimeters in diameter, atherosclerosis may lead gradually to narrowing or even total obstruction of the lumen. In contrast to this slowly developing occlusion, complications of atherosclerosis may lead to an abruptly developing occlusion. One such circumstance is thrombus formation superimposed upon the intimal roughening produced by atherosclerotic plaques. Thrombosis tends to be occlusive in a small or medium-sized artery but may be in the form of a rela- tively thin mural deposit in a large vessel like the aorta. Another complication of atherosclerosis is hemorrhage into the soft center of the plaque. In a vessel the size of the coronary artery this may result in swelling of the plaque with sudden occlusion of the lumen. Another complication which may lead to acute arterial occlusion is a rupture of the plaque with swelling up of the soft lipidic contents into the lumen and lodgement in a nar- rower "downstream" segment of the vessel. Finally, if extensive and severe enough, lesions of atherosclerosis may encroach upon the muscular and elastic wall (the media) of an artery, thus weakening it. In the abdom- inal aorta, a frequent site of severe artherosclerosis, the result of such medial damage may be the formation of an atherosclerotic *aneurysm* which is a ballooning of the weakened arterial wall (Fig. 7-13). Although a thrombus

may form within such an aneurysm because of the abnormal swirling of the blood and because of the roughened intima, the feared complication of an aneu- rysm is rupture with exsanguination.

ISCHEMIA AND INFARCTION

Ischemia is simply inadequacy of blood supply in an area. When tissues are rendered ischemic, they suffer by virtue of being deprived of necessary oxygen and nu- trients. It is also possible that the accumulation of meta- bolic wastes within the poorly perfused tissue may also contribute to tissue damage. Literally anything which affects the flow of blood may produce tissue ischemia. One tends to think first of local arterial obstruction in the production of ischemia, related to atherosclerosis, thrombosis, or embolism. In less usual circumstances, venous obstruction may lead to ischemia when the flow of blood through the tissue virtually reaches a standstill. There are even systemic causes of tissue ischemia. For instance, if heart failure is sufficiently severe, a tissue might become ischemic simply because of the low level of perfusion. Similarly, prolonged shock may lead to significant tissue ischemia.

The effects of ischemia are conditioned by a number of variables such as the intensity of the ischemia, the rate of onset, and the metabolic demands of the partic- ular tissue. In some instances of ischemia, usually in- volving muscular tissues, pain may be a symptom of diminished blood supply. For example, an elderly person

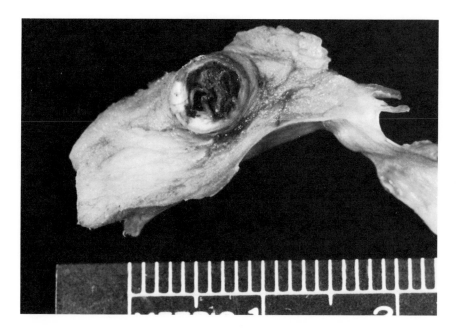

FIGURE 7-12 Atherosclerotic ar- tery. The circumferential atheroma has left only a tiny lumen (at eight o'clock) in this cross section of coronary artery. Conse- quences in terms of blood flow are ob- vious.

with atherosclerosis of the leg arteries and consequent decrease in blood flow, may have sufficient blood supply when at rest but not during activity. When such an individual walks briskly, increasing the metabolic demand of the leg muscles, the onset of relative ischemia may cause pain and limping. The same type of thing happens in the heart muscle with narrowing of the coronary arterial circulation. In such an instance, a patient may, with activity, develop a feeling of oppression or squeezing pain within the chest, this phenomenon being referred to as *angina pectoris*. By definition, anginal pain recedes with rest, when the metabolic demand of the heart muscle diminishes to the point where the narrowed coronary arterial circulation is adequate.

Another effect of ischemia, if it is of gradual onset and prolonged duration, is that the involved tissue may atrophy, that is, shrink. A common example of this is readily observed in a patient who has atherosclerosis which diminishes the circulation to the lower extremities. Often the legs exhibit loss of muscle mass, and the skin becomes smooth, thin, and hairless, all the result of chronic ischemia.

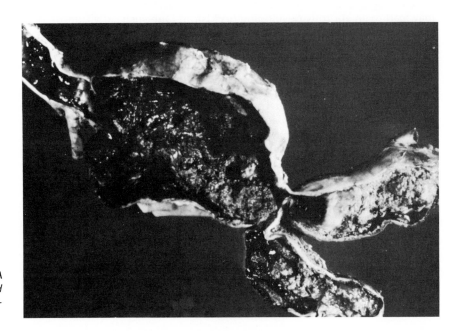

FIGURE 7-13 Atherosclerotic aneurysms. A large aneurysm distorts the distal aorta and each iliac artery. The walls of such aneurysms are prone to rupture.

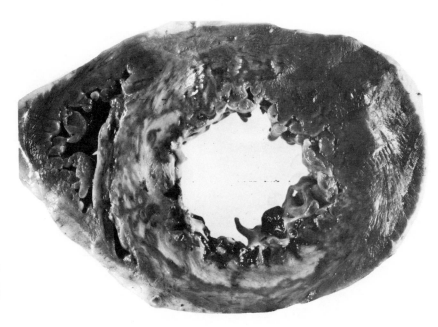

FIGURE 7-14 Myocardial infarct. Myocardial ischemia has resulted in coagulative necrosis (light area) of much of the septum and ventricular wall.

The most extreme effect of ischemia is the death of the ischemic tissue. An area of ischemic necrosis is termed an *infarct,* and the process of forming an infarct is termed *infarction.* Whether or not an ischemic area actually undergoes infarction is conditioned by a variety of local and systemic factors. For instance, a degree of arterial occlusion will be better tolerated if it occurs slowly, if the metabolic demand of the tissue is low, and if there is development of collateral circulation (that is, auxiliary supply of the involved area by branches of neighboring arteries). In addition, the effects of a given degree of ischemia will be worsened if the oxygen carriage within the blood is diminished for any reason.

The morphological features of infarcts vary from organ to organ, but in general the tissue necrosis produced by ischemia is accompanied by an element of hemorrhage from damaged vessels at the edges of the infarcted area. In loose tissues such as the lung, this hemorrhage is extensive, and the infarcted area literally becomes stuffed with blood producing a *hemorrhagic* or *red infarct.* In other organs, e.g., the kidney or the heart, the hemorrhage accompanying infarction is minimal, and the infarct tends to be *pale.* It should be borne in mind that in hemorrhagic as well as in pale infarcts the basic cause of the damage is ischemia of the tissues. In most infarcts the necrosis produced by ischemia is of coagulative type, and the outlines of the tissue are maintained (Fig. 7-14). In the lung, hemorrhage dominates the picture, while in the brain an area of infarction gradually softens and undergoes liquefactive change so that the result is a hole in the tissue.

The presence of infarcted tissue excites an inflammatory reaction at the margins interfacing with viable tissue. Soon neutrophils and macrophages invade the dead area to begin the job of demolition. Subsequently, the area is gradually organized as demolition proceeds, and the usual outcome is scarring of the infarcted area. In many organs an infarct is not particularly important in and of itself, given the amount of reserve of that organ. Thus even a moderately large renal infarct will not endanger the life of the subject because of the ability of one kidney or even part of one kidney to maintain homeostasis. The presence of a pulmonary infarct likewise is not particularly threatening in terms of ventilatory function. In this latter instance, however, the occurrence of pulmonary infarction is somewhat ominous, because it is usually the result of pulmonary embolism. Therefore, there is always concern that larger and more threatening emboli may originate from the source of the first embolus. In the case of the brain and of the myocardium, the results of infarction are much more significant because there is less reserve in these organs, each area being important; and in particular because in these two areas there is no possibility of regeneration of infarcted elements. Finally, in some areas exposed to bacterial populations, the infarcted tissue will serve as a focus of growth of saprophytic microorganisms. Thus, infarcts of bowel quickly become gangrenous, and infarcts of portions of the extremity are initially recognized as areas of gangrene.

QUESTIONS

Disturbances of circulation—Chap. 7

Directions: Answer the following questions on a separate sheet of paper.

1 Describe how the mechanisms involved in active congestion differ from those in passive congestion?

2 Explain how congestion could be produced by a cardiac problem.

3 What are the effects on the involved tissue of acute passive congestion and chronic passive congestion?

4 Define *edema.*

Directions: Circle the letter next to each item which correctly answers the following questions. More than one answer may be correct.

5 Which of the following is the best example of *active* congestion?
a The lung in acute left ventricular failure b The tissues of the leg in femoral vein thrombosis c The red "halo" around an area of cutaneous inflammation

6 The individual with chronic right-sided heart failure who develops persistent hyperemia of the liver has which type of congestion?
a Active b Chronic active c Chronic passive d Acute passive

7 Chronic passive congestion may lead to which of the following changes in the liver?
a Dilatation of the blood channels in the centrilobular zone of each hepatic lobule b Enlargement of liver cells of each hepatic lobule c Constriction of blood channels in the peripheral zone of each hepatic lobule d Shrinkage of liver cells in the centrilobular zone of each hepatic lobule

8 The accumulation of fluid in the peritoneal cavity is called:
a Pericardial effusion b Peritonitis c Ascites d Pleural effusion

9 Which of the following would likely contribute to the formation of edema?
a Elevation of venous pressure in a tissue b Dehydration c Marked decrease in serum protein d Arterial obstruction in a tissue e Increased phagocytosis in lymph nodes draining the area

10 In acute inflammatory states the following statements apply:
a Protein molecules move from inside the vessels of the area to the interstitial spaces b Arterioles in the area dilate to produce active congestion c Water

"follows" protein into the interstitial spaces *d* Edema develops because of diminution of lymphatic drainage

11 Which of the following edematous conditions is potentionally the *most* serious?
a Pleural effusion *b* Ascites *c* Cerebral edema
d Facial edema

12 Exudates differ from transudates in that:
a Exudates tend to contain more leukocytes.
b Transudates have a higher specific gravity than exudates. *c* Exudates have a higher protein content than transudates. *d* Exudates contain large numbers of basophils.

13 Pinpoint hemorrhages visible on cutaneous or mucosal surfaces are referred to as:
a Ecchymoses *b* Petechiae *c* Hematomas

Directions: Answer the following questions on a separate sheet of paper.

14 What is the commonest cause of a hemorrhage?

15 What are two basic mechanisms for stopping hemorrhage?

16 Describe the local and systemic effects of hemorrhage.

17 Describe two clinical implications of thrombosis.

18 List some local causes of ischemia.

19 Describe possible effects of ischemia.

Directions: Circle the letter next to each item which correctly answers the following questions. More than one answer may be correct.

20 Thrombi consist of all of the following EXCEPT:
a Aggregate platelets *b* Precipitated fibin
c Basophils *d* Enmeshed erythrocytes and leukocytes

21 In the formation of a thrombus which event usually occurs first?
a Platelet aggregation *b* Precipitation of fibrin
c Vascular dilatation *d* Hemolysis

22 Thrombosis is favored by all of the following EXCEPT:
a Decreased viscosity of the blood *b* Venous stasis
c Increase in blood platelets *d* Rough vessel lining

23 The carriage of a physical mass in the bloodstream from one place to another with lodgement in the new location is:
a Ischemia *b* Infarction *c* Embolism
d Thrombosis

24 Emboli which lodge on the arterial side of the circulation generally originate from a(n):

a Mural thrombus in the aorta *b* Right atrium
c Intracardiac thrombus *d* Femoral vein

25 If decompression is sufficiently abrupt or when atmospheric air enters venous channels, gas bubbles may appear within the circulation, where they lodge in the microcirculation and occlude the blood flow to the area. Examples of this condition would include:
a A diver who has been living under increased atmospheric pressure *b* A surgical procedure when large vascular channels were traversed *c* A patient with a fractured femur *d* Generalized traumatic injury involving adipose tissue

26 All of the following conditions contribute to atherosclerosis EXCEPT:
a Certain genetic factors *b* Increased serum cholesterol levels *c* Diabetes mellitus *d* Hypotension
e Cigarette smoking

27 The atherosclerotic plaque usually initially involves the:
a Arterioles *b* Intima of an artery
c Media of an artery *d* Intima of a vein

28 All of the following generally cause ischemia EXCEPT:
a Diminished clotting factors *b* Local arterial obstruction *c* Thrombosis *d* Atherosclerosis

29 Which of the following describes an infarcted area located in the lung?
a The hemorrhage accompanying infarction is minimal, and the infarction tends to be pale. *b* The hemorrhage is extensive, and the infarcted area tends to be red. *c* The infarction gradually softens and undergoes liquefactive change.

Directions: Circle T if true, F if false. Correct the false statement in the space provided below each item.

30 T F Monckeberg's sclerosis is a clinically significant form of arteriosclerosis since the lining of the involved vessel is roughened and the lumen is narrowed.

31 T F Atherosclerosis is the most important form of arteriosclerosis.

32 T F An atheroma is an elevated mass of fatty material and associated fibrous connective tissue.

33 T F Atherosclerosis can usually be ascribed to a single etiologic factor.

34 T F Complications of atherosclerosis may lead to an abruptly developing occlusion.

35 T F The results of infarction in the brain and myocardium are very significant particularly because there is no possibility of regeneration of infarcted elements.

36 T F Infarct is a term used to denote a type of circulatory abnormality.

CHAPTER 8 Disturbances of Growth, Cellular Proliferation, and Differentiation

OBJECTIVES   **At the completion of Chap. 8 you should be able to:**

1 Distinguish between agenesis, hypoplasia, and atrophy as to etiology and possible consequences.

2 List at least two common causes of atrophy.

3 Contrast hypertrophy and hyperplasia.

4 Identify an example of physiological and of nonphysiological hyperplasia.

5 Describe the phenomenon referred to as metaplasia.

6 Explain the significance of dysplasia.

7 Define a neoplasm.

8 Differentiate between benign and malignant neoplasms according to architecture, rate of growth, and pattern of enlargement and spread.

9 State two dangerous properties of malignant neoplasms which distinguish them from benign neoplasms.

10 Trace the pathways by which malignant neoplasms disseminate through the body.

11 Describe the effects of benign and malignant neoplasms on the host.

12 Explain the pattern of organization of tumor cells and stroma.

13 Identify the terms used to describe the microscopic resemblance of tumor cells to their normal ancestors.

14 Explain the basis of exfoliative cytology.

15 State the criteria used in the classification of neoplasms.

16 Identify with an example the following terms used to describe neoplasms: adeno-, -oma, polyp, papilloma, carcinoma, fibroma, osteoma, chondroma, sarcoma, lymphoma.

17 Describe the possible cellular basis of malignant behavior.

18 Describe the environmental and genetic factors that seem to be involved in the causation of neoplasia.

19 Describe the rationale used in determining the treatment modalities for neoplasia.

ORGANS AND TISSUES SMALLER THAN NORMAL

Not infrequently one encounters a tissue, or organ, or part of the body that is smaller than normal. This situation can arise in two ways: as a result of a developmental defect or as an acquired abnormality. Stated in a slightly different way, the organ or tissue may never have grown to a definitive size, or, alternatively, it may have reached definitive size and then secondarily have shrunk.

In the course of development it may come to pass that the embryonic rudiment of an organ never forms. This phenomenon is referred to as *agenesis,* and the result is the absence of the particular organ. Thus, for instance, as a result of agenesis some individuals are born with but a single kidney. A related situation is *aplasia,* which involves the embryonic rudiment of an organ failing to grow at all once it has formed (some use the terms agenesis and aplasia interchangeably and, indeed, there is little practical difference). Yet another abnormal developmental situation is that in which the embryonic rudiment forms and grows but never quite reaches definitive or adult size, yielding a dwarfed organ. This phenomenon is called *hypoplasia.* Hypoplasia might, like agenesis and aplasia, involve any portion of the body, might involve one of a pair of organs, or might even involve both organs of a pair. Minor degrees of hypoplasia of some organ might be well tolerated for long periods of time, the net effect being some encroachment on the usual degree of reserve of that organ.

Organs which reach definitive size in the course of development and then secondarily shrink are referred to as *atrophic.* Atrophy has a variety of causes, and some instances of atrophy are actually normal or physiological, as, for instance, the atrophy of certain parts of the embryo or fetus in the course of development. Some forms of atrophy are inevitable with advancing age, such as the endocrine atrophy which occurs when hormonal support is withdrawn from a tissue like the mammary gland. An extremely common cause of atrophy is chronic ischemia. Another common cause of atrophy, primarily involving skeletal muscle, is so-called disuse atrophy. When, for instance, a broken leg is placed in an immobilizing cast for a period of weeks or months, the mass of the extremity is significantly reduced due to atrophy of the unused muscle. In this situation the individual muscle cells are of reduced size, but the state is a reversible one. In other instances of atrophy there is actually a loss of cellular elements.

ORGANS AND TISSUES LARGER THAN NORMAL

Hypertrophy

Hypertrophy is defined as an enlargement of a tissue or organ because of enlargement of individual cells. Hypertrophy can be seen in a variety of tissues but is particularly prominent in various types of muscle. An increased workload on a muscle is a very strong stimulus to hypertrophy. The bulging biceps of the weight lifter is an obvious example of muscular hypertrophy. The same type of thing happens as an important adaptive response in the case of the myocardium. If a subject has an abnormal cardiac valve which imposes an unusual mechanical load, say, on the left ventricle, or if the ventricle is pumping against an elevated systemic blood pressure, the result is hypertrophy of the myocardium with thickening of the ventricular wall. A similar phenomenon can occur in smooth muscle which is forced to work against an increased load. Thus the wall of the urinary bladder may become hypertrophic when there is obstruction to the free overflow of urine. In each of these instances hypertrophic enlargement of cells is actually accompanied by an increase in the contractile elements of the tissue and thus the response is an adaptive one. Hypertrophy is stimulus-related so that it tends to regress at least to some extent if the abnormal workload is withdrawn.

Hyperplasia

Hyperplasia is an increase in the absolute number of cells within a tissue leading to an increase in the size of that tissue or organ. This obviously can occur only in a tissue capable of cell division. (In such tissues hyperplasia may also be accompanied by hypertrophy of individual cells.) Hyperplasia occurs in a wide variety of tissues under many different circumstances, some of them completely physiological. For instance, with the hormonal stimulus of pregnancy and lactation there is extensive proliferation of epithelial elements within the breast with an increase in the size of breast tissue due to this hyperplasia. An example of nonphysiological hyperplasia is a callus, which is a thickening of skin developing in response to a mechanical stimulus. Microscopic examination of a callus reveals a marked increase in the number of epidermal cells and in the number of layers of cells in the epidermis, clearly an adaptive response.

Although certainly an abnormal stimulus (e.g., associated with endocrine inbalance) may give rise to hyperplasia which is nonadaptive, many examples of hyperplasia represent "rational" responses on the part of the body to some imposed demand. As with hypertrophy, if the abnormal circumstance is reversed, the signal to cellular proliferation is withdrawn, and there is regression of the hyperplasia and return to more normal conditions. In the above example, the enlarged breast shrinks to a more normal size following lactation, and the callus gradually disappears when the mechanical stimulus to the skin is no longer applied.

ABNORMAL DIFFERENTIATION

Metaplasia

The character of cellular *differentiation* in a given tissue may also change under abnormal circumstances. Differentiation is the process by which the progeny of dividing *stem cells* become specialized to perform a particular task. For instance dividing cells in the deepest layer of the epidermis gradually migrate upward, and as they do so, they acquire the specialized protective characteristics of outer epidermal cells and produce a proteinaceous substance known as keratin. Similarly within the lining of the respiratory tract some of the dividing cells in the epithelium develop into tall columnar cells with cilia on their luminal surfaces.

When differentiating cell systems of this type are placed under adverse circumstances, the pattern of differentiation may change so that the dividing cells begin to differentiate into types of cells not ordinarily found in the area but that would be perfectly reasonable elsewhere in the body. This phenomenon is referred to as *metaplasia*. For instance, when the lining of the uterine cervix is chronically irritated, portions of the columnar epithelium are replaced by an epidermislike squamous epithelium (Fig. 8-1). Presumably, this "squamous metaplasia" is adaptive, i.e., the squamous epithelium is more resistant to irritation than the original epithelium. The process of metaplasia seems to be under tight control, that is, the "new" type of differentiation is perfectly regular as well as being adaptive. Metaplasia is potentially reversible, so that if the cause of the original change can be eliminated, the stem cells in the population once again differentiate to form the specialized types of cells usually found in that locale.

DYSPLASIA

Dysplasia is an abnormality in the differentiation of proliferating cells such that there occurs an abnormal degree of variation in the size, shape, and appearance of the cells with a disturbance in the usual arrangement of those cells (Fig. 8-2). In essence, dysplasia represents a degree of loss of control over the affected cell population. Minor degrees of dysplasia are frequently en-

countered in association with areas of inflammation, and these are potentially reversible if the irritant stimulus can be reversed. However, in some instances the stimulus leading to dysplasia cannot be identified, and the changes may become progressively more severe, terminating eventually in the development of malignant disease.

NEOPLASIA

A *neoplasm*, literally a "new growth," is an abnormal mass of proliferating cells. The cells of a neoplasm are derived from previously normal cells, but in undergoing neoplastic change they acquire a certain degree of autonomy. Neoplastic cells are autonomous in the sense of growing at a rate which is uncoordinated with the needs of the host and functioning quite independently of the usual homeostatic controls over most other cells of the body. The growth of neoplasic cells is usually progressive, i.e., it does not reach equilibrium, but results rather in an ever increasing mass of cells having the same properties. A neoplasm serves no adaptive purpose as far as benefiting the host and, in fact, is frequently harmful. Finally, in keeping with the autonomous character of neoplastic cells, even if the stimulus that caused the neoplasm is withdrawn, the neoplasm continues to grow progressively.

The word *tumor* is used more or less synonymously with the word neoplasm. Originally the word tumor meant simply swelling or lump, so that occasionally the phrase "true tumor" is used to denote a neoplasm as contrasted with some other sort of lump. Two basic types of neoplasms are distinguished on the basis of their

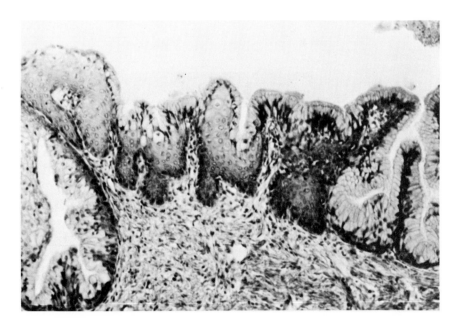

FIGURE 8-1 Squamous metaplasia. In this lining epithelium of uterine cervix, the usual cell type is columnar, as at the right. Most of the epithelium has altered its differentiation to form an epidermislike squamous epithelium. (Photomicrograph, ×200.)

behavior. Some are referred to as *benign*, while others are termed *malignant*. *Cancer* is a general term referring to any malignant neoplasm. Thus, there are many tumors or neoplasms which are noncancerous.

Characteristics of benign neoplasms

A benign (i.e., noncancerous) neoplasm is a strictly local affair. The proliferating cells which constitute the neoplasm tend to be quite cohesive so that as the mass of neoplastic cells grows, there is centrifugal expansion of the mass with a fairly well-defined border. Since the proliferating cells do not fall away from each other, the edges of the neoplasm tend to move outward more or less smoothly, pushing adjacent tissue away in the process. In so doing, benign neoplasms frequently acquire a capsule of compressed connective tissue separating them from their surroundings. Above all, as indicated in Fig. 8-3A, the benign neoplasm remains a strictly local affair. The rate of growth of benign neoplasms is often rather leisurely, and some seem to plateau and remain at a more or less stable size for many months or years.

Characteristics of malignant neoplasms

Many of the characteristics of malignant neoplasms contrast sharply with those of their benign counterparts. Malignant neoplasms generally grow more rapidly than benign ones and almost always grow in a relentlessly progressive manner if not removed. The cells of a malignant neoplasm are not as cohesive as benign cells, and consequently the pattern of expansion of a malignant neoplasm is often quite irregular (Fig. 8-3B). Malignant neoplasms tend not to be encapsulated, and they are usually not easily separable from their surroundings in the way that benign neoplasms are. In fact malignant neoplasms characteristically *invade* their surroundings rather than simply pushing them aside. Malignant cells, whether in clusters, cords, or singly, seem to cut their way through adjacent tissue in a destructive fashion. The gross features of benign and malignant neoplasms are contrasted in Figs. 8-4 and 8-5.

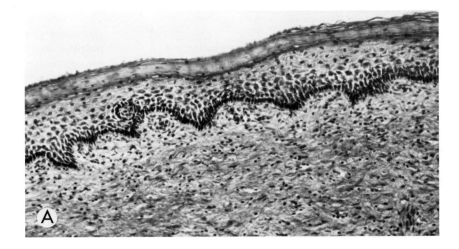

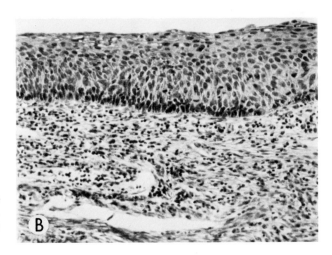

FIGURE 8-2 *Dysplasia vs. normal. In the normal epithelium* (A) *the cells are very regular in a given zone and the layering is orderly. In dysplasia* (B) *there is marked morphological variation in the cells and layering is disordered. (Photomicrograph, ×200.)*

An additional property of malignant neoplasms, the most devastating of all, is related to the ability of proliferating cancer cells to break away from the parent tumor (the so-called *primary* tumor) and enter the circulation to float elsewhere. When such embolic cancer cells lodge, they are able to extravasate, continue their proliferation, and form a *secondary* focus of tumor. Actually a single primary focus of cancer can give rise to numerous embolic fragments which in turn may form dozens or even hundreds of secondary nodules at considerable distance from the primary. The process of discontinuous spread of malignant neoplasms is referred to as *metastasis*, and the daughter foci or areas of secondary growth are referred to as *metastases* (singular, *metastasis*). Thus, the two dangerous properties of malignant neoplasms which distinguish them from noncancerous neoplasms are the ability to invade normal tissue and the ability to form metastases. A benign neoplasm has neither one of these abilities.

Metastasis can occur by a variety of routes. Invasion of blood vascular channels gives rise to hematogenous metastasis in a pattern which at first may be quite predictable. That is to say, for instance, if cancer cells originating from a primary location in the wall of the gastrointestinal tract enter the venous drainage of the tract, they very likely will lodge in the liver, since portal venous blood must flow through that organ before returning to the heart. On the other hand, hematogenously borne cells originating from, say, a malignant neoplasm in the leg, will flow via the vena cava to the right side of the heart and then to the lungs, where the secondary foci may grow. In an analogous fashion malignant cells may invade lymphatic channels and float centralward with the streaming of lymph. In such instances metastasis would be expected to appear in the regional lymph node group filtering the lymph emanating from a particular organ. Thus, for instance, lymphogenous metastases from a primary cancer of the breast may be anticipated in the axillary lymph nodes, and lymphogenous metastases from a primary cancer in the oral cavity would be sought in cervical lymph node groups. In addition to metastasizing via blood vessels and lymphatics, cancer cells may metastasize directly by being transported across a body cavity (e.g., the peritoneal cavity) and implanting on a distant surface of that cavity. In this fashion a malignant neoplasm which invades through the entire thickness of the wall of an abdominal organ may "seed" the entire peritoneal cavity, producing literally hundreds of metastases by the direct route. Similarly, if malignant cells are picked up on surgical instruments in the course of an operation they may be implanted elsewhere in the incision, ultimately to grow into metastatic foci. Figures 8-6 to 8-8 illustrate metastases encountered at autopsy.

In all likelihood, most cancer cells which enter the blood or lymphatic circulation or various body cavities fail to form progressively growing metastases. This is due in part to the fact that the growth of such cells is inhibited by various bodily defenses (e.g., immunologic) and is also related to the fact that growth conditions in an organ of secondary lodgement may not be adequate for the particular cells. Presumably on this basis many cancers have characteristic patterns of metastasis which become important in diagnosis and treatment.

Effects of neoplasms on the host

Neoplasms affect the host in a variety of ways. Since benign neoplasms do not invade or metastasize, the problems they cause are generally local. These can range from trivial to lethal. For example, a small, strictly benign

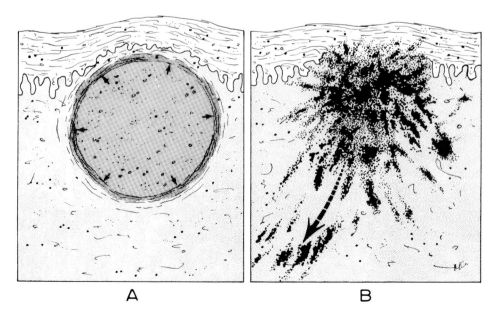

A   B

FIGURE 8-3 Diagram of benign vs. malignant growth. A "typical" benign neoplasm (A) is cohesive, centrifugally expanding, smooth-bordered, and often encapsulated. Adjacent tissue is compressed. A malignant neoplasm (B) is less cohesive, has an irregular border, and invades adjacent tissue. Malignant cells are also capable of metastasis (dotted arrow).

tumor in the loose subcutaneous tissue of the arm might constitute a cosmetic problem but little else. At the opposite end of the spectrum, a perfectly benign tumor (in the sense defined above) growing in a vital area such as the cranial cavity might actually kill the patient by virtue of exerting pressure on some vital part of the brain as the neoplasm expanded locally. For such reasons "benign" does not necessarily mean inconsequential.

Local problems caused by benign neoplasms might involve plugging of various body passages. A vein or a part of the gastrointestinal tract might become obstructed by a perfectly benign neoplasm impinging upon it. Benign neoplasms can also become ulcerated and infected, and they may give rise to significant hemorrhage. Finally, benign tumors are capable of producing striking effects which are not mechanical, but related rather to the metabolic properties of the tumor cells. For instance, the cells of the islets of Langerhans of the pancreas may give rise to a benign neoplasm only a few millimeters in diameter that would never produce mechanical problems. Sometimes, however, such neoplastic cells retain the function of parent cells and produce insulin. Because neoplasms do not respond appropriately to homoestatic signals, such a neoplasm of islet cells might produce insulin inappropriately and in great

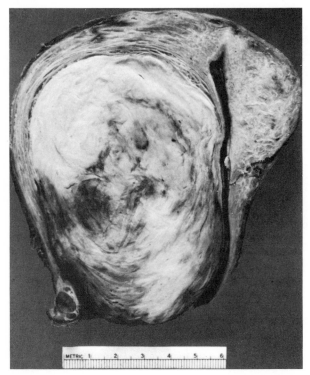

FIGURE 8-4 Benign neoplasm. In this section of uterus, the right half is normal. On the left is a large benign neoplasm (a leiomyoma).

excess, causing abnormally low blood sugar levels. Patients with such neoplasms might thus suffer a variety of systemic signs and symptoms of hypoglycemia.

Malignant neoplasms are capable of doing everything that benign tumors do, but usually in a much more aggressive, destructive fashion related to the generally faster growth rate of malignant neoplasms and to their ability to invade, destroy local tissues, and spread to form distant metastases. Many advanced malignant neoplasms even appear to compete nutritionally with the patient, literally trapping nutrient materials to the detriment of the host. Thus, all too frequently patients with advanced cancers have the appearance of severe malnutrition, a state referred to as *tumor cachexia*. Commonly the life of such a debilitated patient with an advanced cancer is finally terminated by an episode of pneumonia or systemic sepsis.

Host impact on neoplasms

Although a key event in the life history of any neoplasm is the development of a "runaway" clone of proliferating cells which are unresponsive to homeostatic signals within the body, even highly malignant neoplasms are not completely autonomous. Obviously, neoplasms are in need of a supply of oxygen and nutrients for the proliferating neoplastic cells, and these must be supplied by the host. In fact, neoplastic cells are able to evoke from the neighboring nonneoplastic tissues the formation of a vascular supply to nourish the tumor cells. Thus, the supporting framework or *stroma* of neoplasms includes not only a fibrous connective framework but also numerous finely branching, thin-walled blood vessels (Fig. 8-9). The connective tissue cells and blood vessels are actually not part of the neoplastic clone of cells but represent nonneoplastic host cells whose proliferation has been stimulated by substances related from the tumor cells.

On the other hand, it has become evident that various processes within the host body may modulate the growth of neoplastic cells and in effect constitute antineoplastic defenses. It has been demonstrated that many neoplastic cells are sufficiently different antigenically from the corresponding normal host cells that the body may mount an immunologic reaction against the neoplasm. Although there is no doubt of the existence of such immunologic defenses, the current state of knowledge about them does not permit the routine widespread use of immunotherapeutic measures at present. There have been promising demonstrations of beneficial immunologic effects in the treatment of certain neoplasms; and efforts are now made to consider the immunologic status of the host when planning and conducting various modes of antineoplastic therapy.

Structure of neoplasms

As indicated above, neoplasms consist of the proliferating neoplastic cells associated with a logisitical support system referred to as a *stroma*. The pattern of organization of tumor cells and stroma varies widely between neoplasms, and, in fact, the relative balance of stromal elements may lend the neoplasm distinctive characteristics. A tumor which contains an extremely dense fibrous stroma is very hard grossly and is sometimes referred to as *scirrhous*. A tumor which consists predominantly of neoplastic cells with relatively little stroma is much softer and is sometimes referred to as *medullary*.

Since neoplastic cells are derived from previously normal cell populations, they have many of the characteristics of that normal cell population metabolically and microscopically. Tumors vary in the degree of this resemblance. If the microscopic resemblance of tumor cells to their normal ancestors is close the neoplasm is frequently referred to as *well-differentiated* (Fig. 8-10). If the resemblance of neoplastic cells to their forebears is very slight, so that the tumor consists largely of unspecialized proliferating elements, the neoplasm is frequently termed *poorly differentiated, undifferentiated, or anaplastic.* The neoplasm in Fig. 8-9 is rather poorly differentiated. The level of differentiation may be expressed in terms of the structure of individual cells, in terms of the production of some cell products such as mucin or keratin, or in the arrangement of neoplastic cells in relation to one another. Thus, for instance, a well-differentiated neoplasm arising from a mucin-producing glandular epithelium may be composed of tumor cells which individually resemble the nonneoplastic glandular tissue, are arranged in a pattern of tubules or glands like the parent tissue, and may manifest mucin secretion. An anaplastic tumor arising from such a tissue might lack individual cellular resemblance, might lack glandular arrangement, and might manifest no evidence of mucin secretion. In general, benign neoplasms are very well differentiated, i.e., they resemble parent tissues very closely. Malignant neoplasms occupy a rather broad spectrum with regard to differentiation. Many highly aggressive destructive cancers are poorly differentiated or anaplastic microscopically, but in some instances even well-differentiated neoplasms may behave in a malignant fashion.

In the case of many malignant neoplasms, individual cells manifest morphological abnormalities which seem to mirror the malignant behavioral potential of the cells. Many cancer cells have an altered ratio of nuclear volume to cytoplasmic volume, irregular contour of nuclei, and irregular chromatin patterns. These individual cytologic manifestations of malignancy form the basis of exfoliative cytology, that is, the examination of individual cells which have exfoliated or dropped from the surface of tissues into the secretion bathing those tissues. The familiar pap smear named after the originator of the method, George Papanicolau, is a smear of this sort made of any of a variety of body fluids including such things as pleural fluid, gastric aspirate, sputum specimens, bronchial washings, and uterine cervical scrapings. Specimens for cytologic examination can frequently be obtained with minimal inconvenience to the patient and provide exceedingly valuable diagnostic information should morphologically malignant cells be found on the smear. Figure 8-11 illustrates benign and malignant cells seen in a cytologic smear.

Classification and nomenclature of neoplasms

A classification of neoplasms is important in terms of predicting the possible or probable course of disease in a particular patient and thereby planning rational modes of therapy. The usual contemporary scheme of classification of neoplasms utilizes several different sets of criteria. The most important of these is the distinction between benign and malignant biological behavior. If a

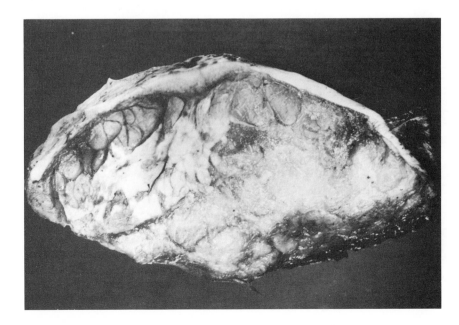

FIGURE 8-5 Malignant neoplasm. In this section of breast, a whitish tissue infiltrates the breast to the left of center. This is a malignant neoplasm; specifically, a carcinoma. Contrast the gross features of this with the benign neoplasm in Fig. 8-4.

particular neoplasm had invaded neighboring nonneoplastic tissue or has produced metastases, it is obviously malignant. In the absence of these obvious manifestations of malignant potential, the classification depends on the microscopic characteristics of the particular neoplasm. The appearance of individual cells, their level of differentiation, their arrangement, and the presence or absence of certain cell products may mirror in a predictive way the behavioral potential of the particular tumor. Other parts of the classification scheme take into account the cell type of origin of the neoplasm and the organ of origin of the neoplasm. Classification of neoplasms on the basis of these several kinds of criteria is useful in that years of accumulated experience have shown that a tumor with a particular appearance of cells, of a certain level of differentiation, arranged in a certain way, originating in a certain organ will behave with a degree of predictability. This allows the medical team to plan therapy based on knowing what has happened to many patients with similar neoplasms in the past.

This kind of classification of neoplasms is expressed in a system of naming that serves as a sort of shorthand, condensing abundant information into a relatively few terms. An attempt to display the entire system of tumor nomenclature at this point would prove tedious. Abundant specific information is contained in subsequent chapters. However, a few generalizations here might be in order. Many neoplasms encountered in our species arise from epithelium which includes cells covering surfaces, lining organs, and forming glands of various kinds. The root *adeno-* is used to denote something of glandular origin. The suffix *-oma* refers to a neoplasm (with some exceptions). Thus in the usual system of nomenclature an *adenoma* is a benign neoplasm of glandular epithelial origin. Examples of such neoplasms would include adenomas of thyroid gland, adrenal gland, or the lining glandular epithelium within the gastrointestinal tract. In the instance of neoplasms arising and projecting from lining epithelia, topographic terms are sometimes used. Thus an adenoma of the colonic lining epithelium which projects into the lumen either as a broad-based mass or hangs into the lumen on a "stem" is frequently referred to as a *polyp*. Such a growth projecting into the lumen of an organ in fingerlike projections is often referred to as a *papilloma*. These topographic terms are not restricted in their usage, however, so that the usual nasal polyp, for instance, is not a neoplasm at all but a

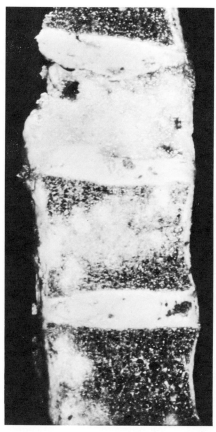

FIGURE 8-6 *Vertebral metastases. The whitish nodules of metastatic carcinoma within the bone grew from cells originating in lung and spreading hematogenously.*

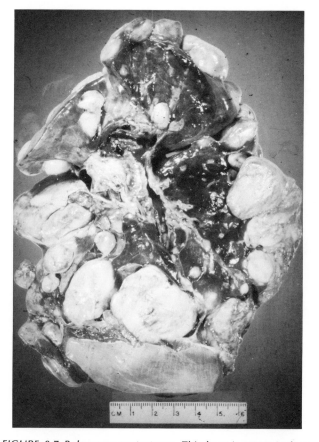

FIGURE 8-7 *Pulmonary metastases. This lung is extensively replaced (as was the contralateral lung) by malignant neoplasm originating in kidney.*

polypoid fold of swollen nasal mucosa. A malignant neoplasm arising from epithelium is referred to as *carcinoma*. Various qualifying prefixes and adjectives can then be added to the name. A malignancy of glandular epithelium would be referred to as an *adenocarcinoma*, while a malignant neoplasm arising from a squamous epithelium would be referred to as a *squamous cell carcinoma*. The designation of a neoplasm might also include some comment about the level of differentiation, so that one encounters such phrases as "well-differentiated, mucin-forming adenocarcinoma" or "well-differentiated, keratinizing squamous cell carcinoma." In addition, topographic descriptors may be used such as "papillary adenocarcinoma" or "fungating (literally mushrooming) carcinoma" for a projecting lesion, etc.

Neoplasms derived from the supporting tissues of the body are named according to the specific tissue of origin. Thus a benign neoplasm of a fibrous tissue would be termed a *fibroma*, a benign neoplasm of bone would be referred to as an *osteoma*, a benign neoplasm of cartilage would be referred to as a *chondroma*, etc. A

malignant neoplasm derived from supporting tissue is referred to as a *sarcoma*. The specific tissue of origin is prefixed to this term. Thus a malignant neoplasm arising from fibrous tissue is a *fibrosarcoma*, one arising from bone is an *osteosarcoma*, and one arising from cartilage is a *chondrosarcoma*.

Neoplasms arising from lymphoid tissue are referred to as *lymphomas*. Such neoplasms generally behave in a malignant fashion, so that the term lymphoma generally is used synonymously with *malignant lymphoma*. Lymphomas may arise from lymphoid tissue anywhere in the body, i.e., not only from lymph nodes and spleen, but from lymphoid cells in virtually any organ. Lymphomas may come to involve the bone marrow extensively, and in many patients the lymphoma cells circulate in the blood in large numbers, giving rise

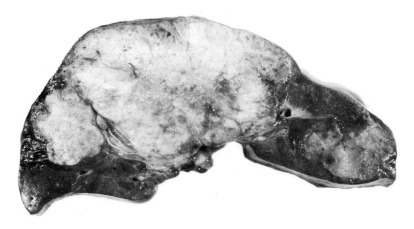

FIGURE 8-8 *Hepatic metastases. Many neoplasms spread to liver, particularly, as in this case, those arising in gastrointestinal tract. The whitish tissue is metastatic carcinoma.*

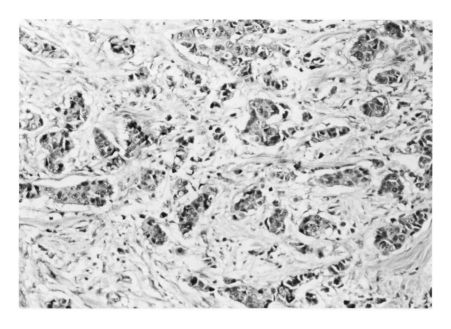

FIGURE 8-9 *Microscopic structure of a neoplasm. The dark clumps of cells are the actual carcinoma cells (i.e., of the malignant clone) while the remaining tissue is a fibrovascular stroma supplied by the host tissue.*

to *leukemia*. The term leukemia literally means "white blood" and pertains not only to lymphoid malignancy but also to malignancy of bone marrow cells with circulating malignant elements. The nomenclature of leukemias and lymphomas is quite complicated and will be discussed more fully in Part III.

Many special names are used for neoplasms arising in specific sites and from particular specialized tissues. Thus, gliomas arise from the glial supportive cells in the central nervous system, mesotheliomas arise from the lining cells of body cavities, retinoblastoma arises within the eye, etc.

Biology of cancer

As indicated above, cancer cells are derived from previously normal cell populations within the body. What is not yet understood completely is what is actually happening at a cellular level during the "transformation" or cancerigenic event, i.e., what is actually happening to a cell when it becomes a cancer cell. In the last analysis, the behavior of cancer cells is "antisocial" with regard to normal cells of the body. Malignant cells disobey the usual territorial rules and grow in inappropriate locations. They do not respond to the usual restraints on the size of cell populations or on the rate of growth of those populations. Evidence is beginning to accumulate which indicates that the important abnormalities of cancer cells seem to lie within the membranes of the cell. It is obviously on the cell membrane that homeostatic signals are received from other cells and from other points in the body and transmitted to the interior of the cell. Abnormalities in this important membrane

may thus result in abnormal reception of control signals or abnormal responses to them. There is also evidence that events at the cell membrane are important in controlling cellular proliferation. The antigenic structure of cell membranes is certainly important with regard to the immunologic interactions of the cell with its surroundings.

Several explanations in terms of cellular genetics and control mechanisms can be invoked to explain the "phenotypic" expression of malignancy in cells. A classical notion is that of *somatic mutation,* which suggests that the basic cancerigenic event involves a chemical change in the DNA of a cell, that is a mutation. This type of event would be similar to a mutation occurring in a germ cell but would instead involve a nongerm cell or somatic cell. This notion of mutation would explain the fact that once a cell is transformed into a neoplastic cell, its characteristics breed true, giving rise to an expanding clone of cells with similar properties. Another way of explaining a change in cells is the addition of genetic information to the genome of the cells. This, of course, is precisely what happens when a cell is infected by a virus. More recently, evidence has been found that the transformational or cancerigenic event may involve neither mutation nor addition to the total genetic information of the cell but may instead involve a change in the *expression* of genetic information present normally. According to this notion, there is within the total genome of any somatic cell the information necessary for the expression of malignant behavior, but this information is normally not expressed during adult life. Accordingly, the transformation of the normal cell to a tumor cell may involve inappropriate derepression of genes normally present. By this mechanism, cancer may be a disease of abnormal differentiation.

It is not possible to speak of a single etiology of cancer. There are obviously many different types of cancer with different epidemiologic patterns of occur-

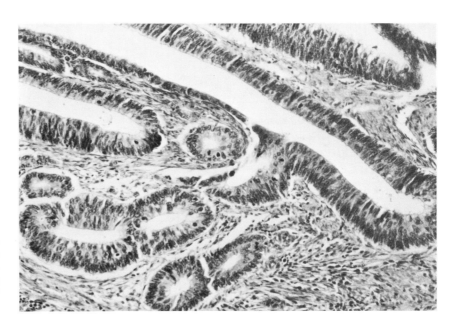

FIGURE 8-10 Well-differentiated adeno-carcinoma. This carcinoma of colon resembles the parent tissue to the extent of forming glands that are easily recognizable (see Fig. 6-3); thus it is "well-differentiated." (Photomicrograph, ×200.)

rence and different etiologic factors. In most instances of human neoplasia the causes are yet unknown. The weight of circumstantial and experimental evidence, however, seems to indicate that the environment is the source of most tumorigenic agents. There is certainly no doubt that many chemical substances within the environment are carcinogenic. This is evident from animal experimentation, from the incidence of certain tumors in industrial workers, and above all from the devastating incidence of lung cancer in cigarette smokers. The role of viruses in tumorigenesis has been elucidated in many species of animals; and while total proof is yet lacking in our species, there is little reason to believe we differ from other animals in this regard. Physical agents within the environment are also known to be potentially tu-

morigenic. Such agents would include ionizing radiations such as x-radiation and even ultraviolet radiation such as encountered in exposure to the sun.

Needless to say, genetic factors are also important in the causation of neoplasms. Again, animal experimentation has shown that it is possible to develop strains of individuals that are highly susceptible to one or another type of neoplasm on a genetic basis. It should be pointed out, however, that even in a strain of mice with a very high incidence of breast cancer, not all individuals are

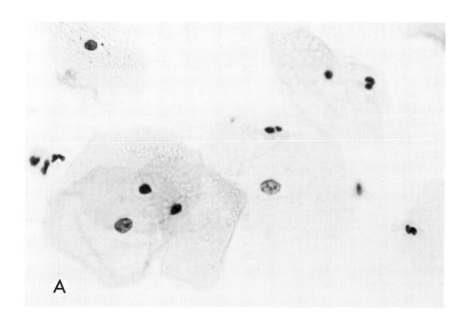

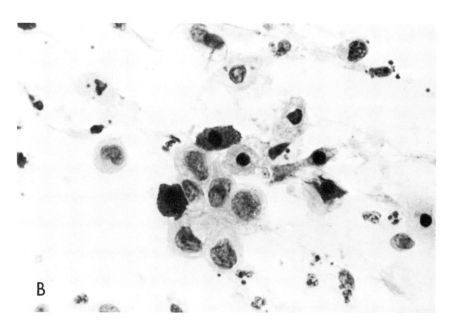

FIGURE 8-11 Benign and malignant cells in vaginal cytologic smears. In (A) the cells are benign. The ratio of nucleus to cytoplasm is small and nuclei are regular. In (B), taken from a patient with carcinoma of the uterine cervix, the ratio of the nucleus to cytoplasm is increased, and the nuclei are irregular. These features allow the diagnosis of malignancy. (Photomicrograph, ×800.)

affected, indicating the operation of certain environmental factors in addition to the genetic factors. The breeding habits of our species being what they are, there tends to be a dilution of this sort of genetic effect, and certainly in human beings there is nothing approaching the situation of inbred strains of rodents. Nonetheless genetic factors do seem to be important in human neoplasia. Generally there is not inheritance of an *overall susceptibility* to cancer of various kinds, but rather an inherited increased likelihood of developing one particular type of tumor or another. Thus, females in a family where several related women have developed breast cancer, particularly at an early age, are more likely than the general population to develop a breast cancer but probably no more likely to develop a bladder cancer. In most instances we do not know what is actually being inherited in those individuals who are genetically more susceptible to the development of a particular neoplasm. Even in such individuals there must be a significant interaction between genetic and environmental factors; and an exciting avenue of research is the attempt to identify individuals at a genetic risk and separate them somehow from the precipitating environmental factors. Finally it must be emphasized that neoplasms are sufficiently common in our species that several persons within a family group may develop a neoplasm for other than genetic reasons. That is to say, the occurrence of multiple neoplasms within a family may be totally unrelated to significant hereditary factors. Even when there appears to be a genuine *familial* incidence of a particular neoplasm, this may be related to some environmental factor within the family rather than a strictly genetic affair.

Clinical aspects of neoplasia

From the foregoing brief introduction to concepts of neoplasia, it should be evident that the variety of signs and symptoms that can be produced by neoplasms is virtually endless. Therefore, the astute clinician is constantly aware of the possible presence of a neoplasm with many modes of patient presentation. However, since there is nothing unique about the signs and symptoms produced by neoplasms, the diagnosis even when apparently "obvious" must be confirmed morphologically by the pathologist, i.e., on biopsy. Cytologic examination may yield presumptive diagnostic information, but this is usually confirmed by biopsy prior to treatment.

In the instance of a small, benign neoplasm, the biopsy itself might well be curative as well as diagnostic. If the total neoplasm was excised by the biopsy procedure and if the neoplasm is histologically benign, the disease has been eliminated. In other instances, not only must the diagnosis be ascertained microscopically, but the *extent* of the neoplasm must be determined before definitive therapy is undertaken. In other words, different stages in the growth of a cancer might require different therapeutic modalities. The extent of invasion of a neoplasm, the presence or absence of metastases, etc., are determined by combinations of radiologic, pathologic, and endoscopic means. In the case of malignant neoplasms, curative therapy involves eradication or removal of the neoplasm by means of surgery, irradiation, chemotherapy, or combinations thereof. More recently, in some centers, immunotherapy is being undertaken on a trial basis. It should be emphasized that even when a particular neoplasm is deemed "incurable" when discovered, the above modes of therapy may produce significant palliation. The details of the clinical approach to significant neoplasms will be outlined in subsequent chapters.

QUESTIONS

Disturbances of growth, cellular proliferation, and differentiation—Chap. 8

Directions: Match the term in col. A related to disturbances of cellular growth and proliferation to its proper description in col. B.

Column A	Column B
1 ____ Aplasia	a Abnormal degree of variation in size, shape, and appearance of the cells with an abnormal arrangement of cells
2 ____ Hyperplasia	
3 ____ Hypertrophy	
4 ____ Metaplasia	b Lack of differentiation or specialization in a group of neoplastic cells; representation as a mass of pleomorphic primitive cells
5 ____ Dysplasia	
6 ____ Neoplasia	
7 ____ Anaplasia	
	c Structure fails to grow in the course of organogenesis
	d Increase in the absolute number of cells leading to an increase in the size of that tissue or organ
	e Dividing cells differentiate into types of cells not ordinarily found in the area, but types of cells that would be perfectly reasonable elsewhere
	f Increase in size of existing cells without an increase in their number
	g An abnormal mass of proliferating cells, possessing a significant degree of autonomy
	h Increase in the size of existing cells of a tissue without an increase in the number

Directions: Circle the letter preceding each item below that correctly answers each question. More than one answer may be correct.

8 Which of the following are types of abnormal development?
  a Hyperplasia *b* Agenesis *c* Aplasia *d* Atrophy

9 Failure to reach definitive or adult size is:
  a Atrophy *b* Hypoplasia *c* Both *a* and *b*
  d Neither *a* nor *b*

10 The pressure of an enlarged prostate causes urethal obstruction. The resultant thickening of the bladder wall muscle is referred to as:
  a Hypertrophy *b* Hypoplasia *c* Atrophy
  d Neoplasia

11 A callus formed on the hand of a gardener from handling a hoe is an example of:
  a Dysplasia *b* Hyperplasia *c* Metaplasia
  d Neoplasia

12 Neoplasia differs from all other pathological processes in that it:
  a Involves proliferation of the cells of affected tissues
  b Is relatively autonomous of the body's controls
  c Is detrimental to the host *d* May affect the host's nutritional state adversely

13 Malignant neoplasms differ from benign neoplasms in that malignant neoplasms:
  a Have an infiltrative pattern of growth *b* Are encapsulated *c* Give rise to metastases *d* Compress adjacent tissue

14 A carcinoma of the stomach would be most likely to produce its earliest metastases in:
  a Bone *b* Lung *c* Liver *d* Kidney

15 An osteosarcoma of the femur would be most likely to produce its earliest metastases in the:
  a Kidney *b* Liver *c* Brain *d* Lung

16 A benign neoplasm of glandular epithelial origin would be termed:
  a Carcinoma *b* Myoma *c* Adenoma
  d Chondroma

17 A malignant neoplasm arising in fibrous tissue (mesenchymal origin) would be termed as:
  a Fibroma *b* Carcinoma *c* Fibrocarcinoma
  d Fibrosarcoma

Directions: Circle the T for true and the F for false. Correct the false statements.

18 T F Neoplastic cells are sufficiently different antigenically from the normal host cells that the body may mount an immunologic reaction against the neoplasm.

19 T F At present, there is widespread routine use of immunotherapeutic measures in the treatment of neoplasms.

20 T F A tumor which contains dense fibrous stroma and very hard growth is referred to as a medullary tumor.

21 T F Benign neoplasms tend to be very well differentiated, i.e., they resemble parent tissues very closely.

22 T F A Papanicolau smear is a cytologic diagnostic examination used only for uterine cervical scrapings or secretions.

Directions: Complete the following statements by filling in the blanks.

23 Some causes of atrophy are _____, _____, and _____.

24 Two dangerous properties of malignant neoplasms which distinguish them from benign neoplasms are (a) _____ and (b) _____ _____.

Directions: Answer the following questions on a separate sheet of paper.

25 List at least three pathways by which malignant neoplasms disseminate through the body.

26 How do neoplasms (benign and malignant) affect the host?

27 What are the criteria used in the classification of neoplasms?

28 What is actually happening at a cellular level during the "transformation" or cancerigenic event?

29 In terms of cellular control mechanisms explain the "phenotypic" expression of malignancy in cells.

30 What are the environmental and genetic factors that seem to be related to the causation of neoplasia?

31 What are the criteria used to determine the therapeutic modalities for treatment of neoplasia?

BIBLIOGRAPHY

AMBROSE, E. J. and F. J. C. ROE: *Biology of Cancer*, 2d ed., Halstead Press, New York, 1975.

BELLANTI, J. A.: *Immunology*, Saunders, Philadelphia, 1971.

COCKBURN, A.: *The Evolution and Eradication of Infectious Diseases*, Johns Hopkins, Baltimore, 1963.

GOOD, R. A. and D. W. FISHER: *Immunobiology*, Sinauer Associates, Stamford, Conn., 1971.

GOULD, S. E.: *Pathology of the Heart and Blood Vessels*, 3d ed., Charles C Thomas, Springfield, 1968.

JAWETZ, E., J. MELNICK, and E. ADELBERG: *Review of Medical Microbiology,* 11th ed., Lange, Palo Alto, 1974.

KENT, T. H.: *General Pathology,* Little, Brown, Boston, 1974.

LA VIA, M. and R. B. HILL, JR.: *Principles of Pathobiology,* Oxford, New York, 1975.

McKUSICK, V. A.: *Human Genetics,* 2d ed., Prentice-Hall, Englewood Cliffs, N.J., 1969.

PEACOCK, E. E. and W. VAN WINKLE: *Surgery and Biology of Wound Repair,* Saunders, Philadelphia, 1970.

PREHN, R. T. and L. M. PREHN: "Pathobiology of Neo-plasia," *American Journal of Pathology,* **80**: 529–550, 1975.

ROBBINS, S. and M. ANGELL: *Basic Pathology,* 2d ed., Saunders, Philadelphia, 1976.

ROSS, R. and J. A. GLOMSET: "Pathogenesis of Athero-sclerosis," *New England Journal of Medicine,* **295**: 369–377, 420–425, 1976.

SIMON, H. J.: *Attenuated Infection,* Lippincott, Philadel-phia, 1960.

SODEMAN, W. A., and W. A. SODEMAN, JR.: *Pathologic Physiology, Mechanisms of Disease,* 5th ed., Saun-ders, Philadelphia, 1974.

WEISMANN, G.: *Mediators of Inflammation,* Plenum, New York, 1974.

ZWEIFACH, B. W., L. GRANT, and R. T. McCLUSKEY: *The Inflammatory Process,* 2d ed., Academic Press, New York, 1973.

PART II Disturbances of Immune Mechanisms

WILLIAM R. SOLOMON

Unfavorable effects of immune processes underlie much human disease and may impair the function of any major organ system. In addition, characteristic changes in immune reactants that provide essential diagnostic clues *accompany* many conditions as effects or secondary causes. It is now clear that normal antibody and cell-mediated responses involve serial steps, each of which is modulated by groups of specific cells. Defects in these control processes may be the source of excessive or inappropriate immune reactions. Less commonly, disease results when normally protective immediate and delayed hypersensitivity mechanisms become impaired or fail to develop normally.

It is often difficult to confront the fact that protective immunity and allergic diseases share common processes of tissue response to substances recognized as "foreign" by the host. Immune mechanisms provide essential defense against invasion by injurious organisms and the emergence of malignant tumors, functions which have ensured their retention throughout vertebrate evolution. However, these same processes may be called forth by relatively innocuous extrinsic agents and occasionally may focus the reaction on host tissue components. In these circumstances the *net* effects of exposure and specific host response are unfavorable; patterns of overt illness that result are recognized as immunological diseases. These conditions are diverse in type and range in severity from trivial, chronic disorders of the skin or mucous membranes to catastrophic events that may be fatal within seconds. Furthermore, since immunological diseases are determined by host reactivity as well as by the type and strength of antigenic exposure, regional differences in their prevalence are prominent. Overall, however, these disorders are remarkably common, and their impact on human comfort and productivity is evident universally.

OBJECTIVES

At the completion of Part II you should be able to:

1 Describe the relationship between the immune processes and immediate and delayed hypersensitivity mechanisms.

2 Identify the etiology, pathogenesis, diagnosis, and treatment of selected immunologic diseases.

CHAPTER 9 Familiar Allergic Disorders: Anaphylaxis and the Atopic Diseases

OBJECTIVES

At the completion of Chap. 9 you should be able to:

1 Identify the immunological processes which are most clearly recognized as immunologic disease.

2 Define *hypersensitivity* and *sensitization*.

3 Identify the characteristics of allergy as an immunologic response.

4 Describe the tissue changes elicited by the reaction of immunoglobulin G (IgG) with antigen.

5 Describe immunoglobulin E–mediated (Type I) allergic problems as to type of cells involved, location, and reactions that occur.

6 Identify the characteristics of an acute systemic (anaphylactic) reaction in terms of etiology, onset, signs and symptoms, and tissue response.

7 Explain the treatment modalities for anaphylaxis.

8 List the usual requirements necessary to elicit anaphylactic sensitization in human beings.

9 Describe the characteristics of the atopic state in terms of familial predisposition, tissues most often affected, involved allergens, type of antibody necessary to mediate the reaction, and circumstances in which immune responses occur.

10 Identify for seasonal and perennial allergic rhinitis the common etiologies, signs and symptoms, distinctive features, complications, diagnostic procedures, and treatment.

11 Explain, for wheal-and-flare–eliciting skin tests, the techniques utilized and significance of a positive reaction in evaluating respiratory allergy.

12 Explain for the radioallergosorbent test (RAST) the purpose of the procedure and compare its clinical value to direct testing.

13 List three principal considerations which dominate the management of respiratory allergy as exemplified by allergic rhinitis.

14 State at least two examples of the treatment modalities used in the management of respiratory allergy.

15 Identify the classes, actions, side effects, and mode of administration of medications used in treating respiratory allergy as exemplified by allergic rhinitis.

16 Appreciate, for hyposensitization, the indications, practical characteristics, and efficacy of the procedure as well as its possible modes of action.

Immunological processes are most evident as clinically perceived reactions of immediate or delayed hypersensitivity. In this context, *hypersensitivity* denotes the capacity, acquired through prior contact with a specific, chemically characterizable agent, to hyperreact to that agent. The cellular events that follow exposure and establish a capacity for responses of hypersensitivity are termed *sensitization*. Reexposure to defined antigens may reveal that sensitized cells, as well as one or more types of immunoglobulins, have been produced in the course of this specific "defensive" response. Not surprisingly, clinical hypersensitivity reactions in human beings often show evidence of more than one immunological process, each with its specific amplification system(s). Such complexity is easy to accept where the "invader" is itself antigenically complex, (e.g., a microorganism) but can be elicited also by *single, defined* proteins.

Just as one antigen can elicit a varied (or diversified) specific immune response, so also can a single antigen-antibody interaction provoke different effects depending on the circumstances (or test system) in which it is observed. This implies, for example, that human IgG molecules specific for an antigen may precipitate the antigen from solution, agglutinate insoluble particles coated with the antigen, or activate complement proteins after interacting with the antigen in either form. The effects observed depend largely on antigen-antibody concentrations, the relative proportions of these reactants, and the presence of additional components which often serve as "indicators" in laboratory test systems. When such interactions occur in vivo, their effects depend upon similar factors as well as local tissue re-

sponses to the primary antigen-antibody reaction and to activation of secondary amplification mechanisms (see also Chap. 5).

Studies of antibody structure and function have shown that antigen *specificity* is directed by the (two) combining sites present on the Fab (antibody fragment) portions of immunoglobulin molecules. These antigen-reactive sequences of amino acids give *direction* to antibody-mediated processes. The biological consequences of the reaction generally are identified with the Fc fragment (crystallizable fragment) of antibodies. The Fc portion determines the tissue localization of immunoglobulins, and receptors on phagocytic cells may recognize this region, facilitating the uptake of antigen-antibody complexes and of particles bearing surface-bound immunoglobulins. Activation of the "classical" complement pathway also appears to involve the Fc region; as a result, activities including target cell lysis, leukocyte attraction, and release of permeability-enhancing factors may be generated. In addition, the class-specific properties of immunoglobulins, which allow these molecules to serve as *antibodies* are expressed on the Fc region.

Although it is the least plentiful of the five recognized antibody classes, immunoglobulin E (IgE) plays a disproportionately major role in human allergic* responses. IgE molecules bind readily to surface receptors of tissue mast cells and blood basophils. As a result, *bound* IgE is *concentrated* in the respiratory and gastrointestinal tracts as well as in the intravascular compartment (i.e., circulating blood) although it is readily demonstrated at other sites, including skin. When adjacent IgE molecules combine with groupings of a multiple reactive antigen, a series of events can occur, shown in Fig. 9-1, with liberation from the cell of tissue-reactive "mediator"

*The term *allergy* was proposed by von Pirquet in 1906 to denote all instances of acquired, altered reactivity that promote "supersensitivity." Current usage equates allergy with clinically evident responses of immediate or delayed hypersensitivity.

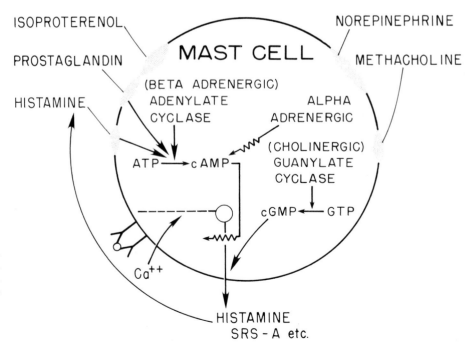

FIGURE 9-1 Factors that affect the release of mediator substances by mast cells. Smooth lines indicate potentiation of an effect; wavy lines signify inhibitory influences. Many agents act on cell surface receptors to modify secondarily the intracellular levels of cyclic AMP and GMP which, respectively, diminish and facilitate mediator release.

substances including histamine, slow-reacting substance of anaphylaxis (SRS-A), and an eosinophil chemotactic factor of anaphylaxis (ECF-A); additional substances that attract neutrophils and lead to the formation of kinins also have been described. Individual characteristics of some of these agents are summarized in Table 9-1; however, their combined effects promote dilatation and hyperpermeability of small blood vessels (principally venules), spasm of the walls of hollow viscera, and increased secretion by mucous membranes. Heightened venule permeability should promote diminished circulating blood volume and arterial pressure as well as collections of fluid outside of vessels. In fact, these effects are all more or less easily observed in clinically significant human responses involving IgE.

ANAPHYLAXIS—A TYPE I DISORDER

Acute systemic reactions—often resulting in death—first were recognized in several species almost 100 years ago during immunization experiments with foreign toxins. In many animals, sensitization did not confer protection; rather, on readministration of the toxin, there was prompt development of shock, airway obstruction, and/or visceral congestion in species-specific patterns. The term *anaphylaxis* (*ana* = back or reverse; *phylaxis* = protection) was derived from this paradoxical outcome. Similar human reactions were noted early in this century and remain the most rapidly developing and dangerous form of allergic response. Acute systemic reactions generally follow the *injection* of a potent antigen (*allergen*) into a highly sensitive subject, although, rarely, exposure occurs by ingesting the offending agent. In the past, antiserums (especially equine) derived from other species were most often responsible for these reactions; more recently, injected penicillins have become the principal offenders, with serums, ACTH, insulin, and other drugs less often implicated. Comparable reactions also may follow insect stings and the less frequent attacks of other venomous creatures upon *sensitive* subjects.

Acute systemic reactions generally begin within minutes after introduction of an allergen; a delay longer than 1 hour is distinctly rare. In extreme sensitivity, injection of an allergen may cause death or a sublethal reaction almost instantly, the most severe responses often appearing the most promptly. Affected pèrsons report a sense of uneasiness, rapidly followed by light-headedness, which may lead to syncope (loss of consciousness). Itching of the palms and scalp is often felt and may herald hives (urticaria) that cover much of the skin surface. Localized tissue swellings (angioedema*) may appear within minutes and distort especially the eyelids, lips, tongue, hands, feet, and genitalia. Swelling (edema) of the uvula and larynx are less evident to inspection but are especially prominent in human anaphylaxis, and may cause death by respiratory obstruction. Laryngeal edema causes prominent air hunger, impaired phonation, noisy breathing, and a "barking" or high-pitched cough. Respiratory difficulty also may arise due to bronchial narrowing, with audible wheezes mimicking spontaneous asthma (see Chap. 10). Less often, spasm of the gut, bladder, or uterus is prominent, with cramping pain, loss of visceral contents, or vaginal spotting. Figure 9-2 summarizes the most prominent manifestations of human anaphylaxis.

All current evidence suggests that clinical anaphylaxis in both animals and humans involves a sudden multifocal reaction of allergen with mast cell–bound, specific IgE, followed by widespread tissue response to the mediator substances (e.g., histamine, SRS-A) released; other factors appear to be of secondary importance at

Angioedema denotes a discrete swelling involving tissues deep to skin or mucous membranes and produced by a localized increase in vascular permeability.

TABLE 9-1
Mediators of inflammation released by human mast cells*

MEDIATOR	CHEMICAL CHARACTERISTICS	BIOLOGICAL ACTIVITY
Histamine	Simple amine mol wt 111	Contracts visceral smooth muscle; increases permeability of capillaries and venules; increases respiratory mucous gland activity; produces sensation of itching
Slow-reacting substance of anaphylaxis (SRS-A)	Acid lipid or lipoprotein mol wt ~500	Causes *prolonged* visceral smooth-muscle spasm; dilates and increases permeability of venules
Eosinophil chemotactic factor of anaphylaxis (ECF-A)	Pair of acidic tetrapeptides	Attracts eosinophils selectively
Platelet-activating factor (PAF)	Phospholipid(s?) mol wt < 500	Aggregates and degranulates platelets
Neutrophil chemotactic factor (NCF-A)	Not defined mol wt > 10,000	Causes directed migration of neutrophils
Basophil kallikrein†	Not defined	Causes formation of bradykinin

*Serotonin is present in human *platelets* and in the mast cells of other species. Additional materials released by human mast cells probably remain to be discovered.
†Released from basophils but not as yet described from mast cells.

best. Many features of these responses—including urticaria—can be induced by injection of agents that directly release mediators from mast cells in vivo, although *not* by parenteral histamine alone. Differences among species in patterns of anaphylactic response seem to reflect differences both in the distribution of mast cells and in relative responsiveness of tissues to mediator substances.

Effective treatment of anaphylaxis, requires, first, assurance of a patent airway. Careful and continuous observation is essential since oropharyngeal intubation, or, more commonly, tracheostomy may become necessary to prevent asphyxia. Hypotension, which, if severe and/or prolonged, may lead to brain, kidney, or heart damage, poses a threat only slightly less grim. Since this problem reflects primarily loss of intravascular fluid due to leaky vessels, it may be corrected most specifically by replacing plasma volume with normal saline, half-normal saline, or plasma. Several thousand milliliters of fluid often are required to restore normal blood pressure. Vasoconstrictor drugs (e.g., norepinephrine) can be of further value but offer limited benefit without adequate volume replacement. Epinephrine remains the preferred drug to limit or reverse the anaphylactic process and should be the first agent administered. A dose of 0.3 ml of 1:1000 epinephrine may be injected subcutaneously (see Chap. 10) and repeated several times, if needed, at intervals of 15 minutes; small children may receive 0.022 ml/kg to a maximum of 0.3 ml per dose. The absorption of epinephrine from subcutaneous depots is slow with severe hypotension; when shock is present, the drug may be diluted to 1:10,000 and infused slowly intravenously to provide comparable total doses. Injected antihistaminics (e.g., diphenhydramine or chlorpheniramine) may speed the resolution of urticaria and relieve cramps originating in hollow viscera. Adrenocortical steroids are often given for their favorable effects

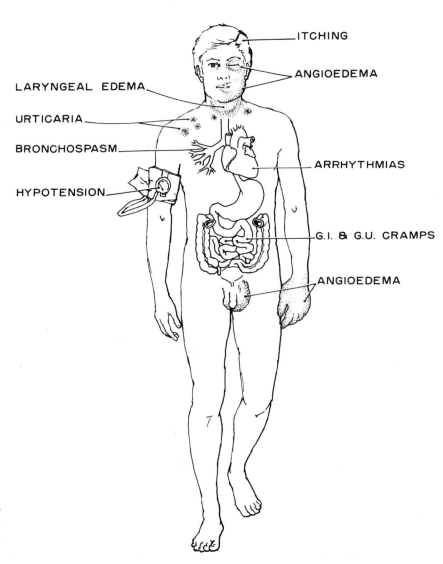

FIGURE 9-2 Prominent manifestations of human anaphylaxis. Laryngeal edema and profound hypotension usually pose the greatest dangers for affected persons.

on inflammation and abnormal vascular permeability; however, any benefit derived from such agents is *not* realized immediately. While the steroids rarely may be lifesaving in *prolonged* shock, they should be considered only after the airway is secure, volume repletion has been begun, and epinephrine administered.

Systemic reactions, comparable to those induced by drugs and serums, follow insect stings (bee, wasp, hornet, yellow jacket) and, rarely, bites (e.g., deerfly) in some persons. These responses, too, appear to be IgE-mediated and, without treatment mentioned above, may terminate fatally. Besides avoiding situations favored by stinging insects, susceptible persons are urged to carry commercially prepared, preloaded syringes of epinephrine whenever feasible. Such persons must be prepared to self-administer the drug in 0.3-ml subcutaneous doses and to apply a tourniquet if an extremity has been attacked. "Immunotherapy," or "hyposensitization," with incremental injected doses of sterile, aqueous, whole-body extracts of the responsible insect(s) is a time-honored approach which may decrease reactivity after many months (see "Allergic Rhinitis" later in this chapter); however, some treatment failures *do* occur. Current evidence suggests that immunotherapy with pure venoms will offer important advantages if these materials can be made available in the necessary amounts.

THE ATOPIC DISEASES

Anaphylactic sensitization in human beings generally requires the *injection* of potent allergens, although certain gastrointestinal and respiratory parasites also elicit prominent IgE responses. In addition, many persons make specific IgE responses to *mucosal* contact, (viz., by inhalation or ingestion) with quite innocuous materials including foods, pollens, and animal emanations (danders). The presence of allergen-specific IgE fixed to tissue may be demonstrated conveniently by performing skin tests and observing the development in 5 to 15 minutes of local redness (erythema)—often with a central hive (wheal). A *proportion* of persons, easily sensitized for such Type I (IgE-mediated) responses by mucosal exposure, also manifest one or more related illnesses, of which the most common types—allergic rhinitis, allergic (extrinsic) asthma, and atopic dermatitis —will be described subsequently. In addition, gastrointestinal allergy, allergic conjunctivitis, and instances of acute urticaria and angioedema (see earlier footnote) may coexist. Those with gastrointestinal allergy may show, in response to specific foods, perioral pruritus (itching), tongue and mucous-membrane swelling, difficulty in swallowing (dysphagia), nausea, vomiting, abdominal cramps, diarrhea, and perianal itching— singly or in combination. *Food allergy* may also affect distant organs including the skin and bronchi and rarely may underlie generalized reactions. These familiar conditions often are grouped as "atopic diseases," and the predisposition that favors their occurrence is termed *atopy.** The pathophysiological basis of atopy still is not entirely clear; however, prominent IgE production from mucosal exposure to (benign) allergens appears to be a principal marker. The tissue-fixing, IgE antibodies formed in this manner are often termed atopic *reagins.* In addition, health histories of affected subjects commonly include *more than one* of the atopic conditions. Furthermore, familial clustering of these conditions is very prominent, although it seems to be the atopic constitution, rather than any specific form of illness, that is hereditable. In most North American reports, more than one-half of overtly affected subjects have close relatives with atopic conditions, while in subjects free of atopic disease, a positive family history is definable only in circa 10 percent.

Allergic rhinitis

Nasal allergy is the most commonly encountered atopic condition, affecting as many as 20 percent of certain pediatric and young-adult populations in North America and western Europe. Elsewhere, rates of this and other atopic illnesses appear to be lower, although prevalence data often are incomplete. Persons with allergic rhinitis experience prominent nasal stuffiness, excessive nasal secretion (rhinorrhea), and sneezes that often occur in rapid succession. Pruritus (Fig. 9-3) of the nasal

*Atopy is derived from the Greek ατοπια, meaning strange or out-of-place. The term probably was chosen to express the inappropriateness of an immune response to entirely innocuous environment agents.

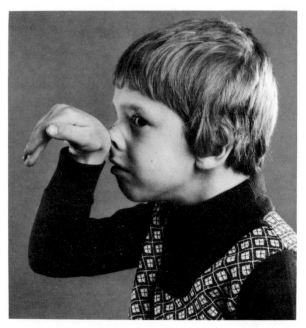

FIGURE 9-3 Upward deflection of the nasal tip is a common mannerism among children with allergic rhinitis. This "allergic salute" serves briefly to allay pruritus and open the nasal airway.

mucosa, throat, and ears often is distressing and is accompanied by conjunctival redness, ocular pruritus, and lacrimation. The involved mucous membranes show dilatation of blood vessels (especially venules) and extensive edema with prominent accumulation of eosinophils in both tissue and secretions. Many of these features, including the pruritus, can be duplicated by applying histamine alone to the normal mucosa, and allergic rhinitis may reflect, quite simply, the tissue effects of recognized, mast cell-derived mediator substances (see earlier in this chapter).

Although no *absolute* distinction is implied, allergic rhinitis is often divided into "seasonal" and "perennial" forms. Seasonal allergic rhinitis, or "hay fever," usually involves a specific period of symptoms in successive years, reflecting sensitivity principally to airborne pollens and/or fungus spores (Fig. 9-4) with defined schedules of prevalence. Seasonal rhinitis is mild in many persons who do not seek medical care but can be an exhausting illness for some because of continual sneezing, copious rhinorrhea, and unremitting pruritus. Intense pallor and swelling of mucous membranes usually accompany these dramatic symptoms, and eosinophils abound in nasal secretions (Fig. 9-5). By contrast, perennial rhinitis seldom shows major annual variations in severity, and symptoms are often dominated by unremitting nasal obstruction; prominent offenders include foods, house dust, and animal emanations to which daily exposure is commonplace. Not surprisingly, persons with multiple clinical sensitivities often experience perennial rhinitis with one or more predictable seasonal flares annually.

Although perennial allergic rhinitis rarely is a source of dramatic symptoms, persistent partial nasal obstruction can promote distressing complications. In most instances, the chronic rhinitic person resorts to mouth breathing with resulting complaints of snoring and oropharyngeal dryness. Dark circles and redundant tissue often develop beneath the eyes; while popularly termed "allergic shiners," these changes may reflect long-standing nasal obstruction of any cause. The swollen mucosa readily sustains bacterial infection and obstruction of paranasal sinus openings is common, leading to recurrent or chronic sinusitis. Drainage from foci of nasal infection promotes sore throat and can foster bronchial soiling and infection. Especially with recurrent infection, the swollen nasal mucosa is prone to form local projections, or *polyps*, that further obstruct the airway. In addition, especially in children, the pharyngeal openings of the eustachian tubes may become blocked by swollen mucosa, enlarged lymphoid tissue, or exudate. Without access to air, the middle ears fill with fluid, creating a *chronic serous otitis* marked by hearing loss and, often, recurrent middle ear infection.

Although it is acknowledged that allergic rhinitis sufferers tend to develop bronchial asthma with above-normal frequency, the extent of this increased risk remains unclear. In one population of rhinitic persons, *unselected for symptom severity*, less than 10 percent were observed to develop asthma as a new manifestation. However, this sequence has been recorded far more often in persons whose problems eventually prompted evaluation by an allergist. In general, the risk of subsequent asthma appears to rise with increasing severity of rhinitis, with prominent sinobronchial infection, and when asthma has been present in the past.

Although the pruritus, repetitive sneezing, and watery, profuse rhinorrhea of hay fever are distinctive, they are not unique to this disorder, and the symptoms of perennial rhinitis readily mimic those of other conditions. The *distinctive* feature of allergic rhinitis is that *compatible symptoms* appear or worsen predictably in response to *specific allergen exposures*. Therefore, in diagnosis, careful analysis of the factors precipitating rhinitis is of overriding importance. Many persons with

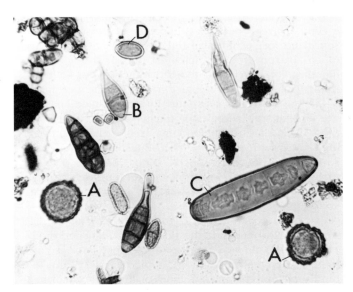

FIGURE 9-4 Particles recovered during atmospheric sampling in late summer. Prominent sources of hay fever including ragweed pollen grains (A), and fungus spores of Alternaria *(B) and* Helminthosporium *(C) species are evident. Many spores, such as those of mushrooms (D), remain to be evaluated as allergens.*

nonallergic vasomotor rhinitis experience similar nasal stuffiness and rhinorrhea without response to identifiable allergens. Instead, their complaints relate alone to airborne irritants, extremes of temperature and humidity, pregnancy, the menstrual cycle, and emotional factors. Long-standing nasal complaints due to recurrent or chronic infection, nasal polyps, marked deviation of the nasal septum, hypothyroidism, and antihypertensive or ovulatory suppressant drugs also must be distinguished from perennial allergic rhinitis.

A clinical history of symptoms on exposure provides the clearest indication of offenders in respiratory allergy. Symptom variations during and after travel deserve special attention, and the effects of overt exposure to agents including house dust, animals and fur products, feathers, seed derivatives, silk, and kapok fibers may be sought directly. Where casual observations are insufficient, history may be "created" by markedly increasing and/or reducing specific exposures, such as to foods or house pets, for brief periods to observe the results. In addition, the time or place of symptom occurrence may furnish etiological clues not readily evident to the sufferer. Specific pollen sensitivities, for example, may be deduced if the resulting symptoms can be dated precisely and "seasons" of prevalence for local airborne pollens are known (Fig. 9-6). Similarly, recognition of the heavy fungus exposures associated with leaf collection, lawn care, and gardening as well as with hiking in tall vegetation helps to explain associated symptoms.

Wheal-and-flare–eliciting skin tests provide useful *correlates* for a detailed clinical evaluation and are widely performed. However, even strongly positive reactions indicate only the immunological "apparatus" for response and provide no assurance that symptoms arise from exposure to the allergens in question. The ultimate value of skin tests is to support or contradict impressions formed during clinical fact-finding. In common clinical practice, aqueous extracts are used, and testing is performed initially by pricking the skin through

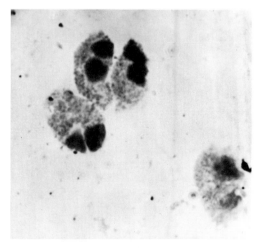

FIGURE 9-5 *Eosinophils from nasal secretions of a child with florid ragweed hay fever. Bilobed nuclei and discrete, round granules are familiar features of these cells.*

applied drops of these materials to produce epidermal or "prick" tests or by injecting small quantities (usually 0.02 ml) intracutaneously (Figs. 9-7 and 9-8). Since even this volume of extract may be hazardous in highly sensitive persons, prick tests are usually done first and negative reactors are considered for intracutaneous (IC) testing; where IC tests are done exclusively, very dilute materials must be used. Since occasional persons manifest whealing with minimal skin trauma (i.e., "dermographism"), all reactions must be compared with those at control sites tested with the sterile diluent alone. Wheal and erythema reactions may be reduced factitiously by oral antihistaminic drugs (see later in this section), and of these hydroxyzine (Atarax, Vistaril) may cause suppression lasting 2 to 3 days. Cortisonelike drugs, by contrast, have little effect on immediate skin reactivity, while suppression due to theophylline and sympathomimetic amines is minor, at best.

Few additional test procedures furnish help in evaluating respiratory allergy. Initial hopes that levels of total serum IgE could distinguish between symptomatic atopics and others have not been sustained. Recently, however, measurement of allergen-specific IgE has become possible in vitro using venous blood. This procedure, the radioallergosorbent test (RAST), diagrammed in Fig. 9-9, offers certain logistic advantages over direct testing and eliminates rare adverse reactions that accompany that procedure; however, neither the sensitivity nor the specificity of RAST exceeds that of conventional skin tests.

The demonstration of eosinophils as the predominating cell in nasal or lacrimal secretions strongly suggests an associated (Type I) allergic inflammatory process. In suitably stained material, the bilobed nuclei and abundant, discrete, red, refractile granules of eosinophils are evident by oil-immersion microscopy (Fig. 9-5).

Three principal considerations dominate the management of respiratory allergy as exemplified by allergic rhinitis: (1) efforts to reduce allergen (and irritant) exposure, (2) suppressive medications to mitigate symptom severity *nonspecifically*, and (3) *specific* hyposensitization to reduce responsiveness to *unavoidable* allergen challenge. Avoidance measures are most feasible for allergens associated with home and work situations, such as house dust, animal emanations, and agricultural products. However, even pollen exposure can be reduced significantly by remaining indoors with windows closed—a strategy that often requires air conditioning for success. House dust avoidance is fostered by providing smooth, simple surfaces that facilitate cleaning (e.g., bare floors, uncluttered table and dresser tops) as well as by elimination or plastic encasing of bedding and upholstered furnishings (Fig. 9-10). Filters or electrostatic particle precipitators are helpful where central forced air heating is used but do not replace a careful antidust program at room level. Recent recognition that mites in house dust often contribute to its allergenic potency provides a new rationale for these traditional measures.

Where sensitivity to animal emanations (dander) is confirmed, total avoidance of the source usually is justified. Although danders are popularly equated with hair, far more potent allergen sources include epidermal scales, saliva, and lacrimal secretions. House pets are the most persistently troublesome dander sources. However, occupational exposures also may plague laboratory workers, veterinarians, and livestock handlers. In addition, products derived from animal sources may retain sensitizing properties for prolonged periods; these include feather- and down-filled mate-

rials, fur-trimmed clothing and toys, furniture and rug pads (cattle and horse hair), and raw silk. Mohair and camel's hair fabrics are occasionally implicated as allergen sources, although commercially processed sheep wool appears not to be an offender.

Tobacco smoke is an acknowledged respiratory irritant, containing a remarkable assortment of toxic agents, but without proven activity as an allergen. By contrast, plant products such as cottonseed, flaxseed and castor bean meals are among the most potent sensitizers and are major-symptom sources in industry.

For several decades, antihistaminic drugs have been the most useful agents in the symptomatic (i.e., nonspecific) treatment of allergic nasal disease. While many antihistaminics share anticholinergic, antiserotonin, and/or tranquilizing properties, their capacity to compete with histamine for tissue receptors seems to underlie their effectiveness in hay fever, etc. These drugs are

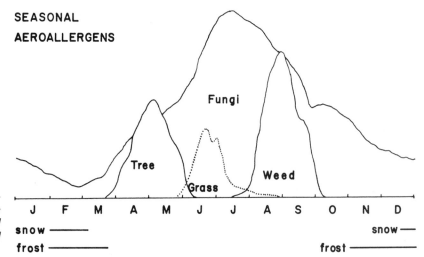

FIGURE 9-6 Patterns or airborne-allergen prevalence typical of central North America. The relationship of symptoms to tree, grass, and weed pollen sensitivity can often be deduced from their periods of occurrence.

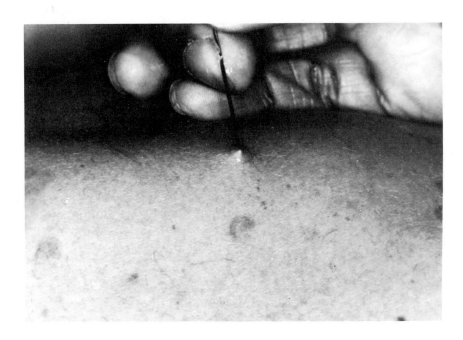

FIGURE 9-7 Technique of epidermal (prick) testing.

generally effective orally and may be administered in several doses daily for prolonged periods, if necessary. Side effects are common though seldom severe in normal persons and generally include drowsiness, lethargy, mucous membrane dryness, and occasionally, nausea, cramps, or lightheadedness. However, because of these symptoms and a frequent impairment of depth perception, activities involving moving vehicles, dangerous machinery, or fine hand-eye coordination in general must be undertaken with care by those receiving antihistaminics. In practice, several antihistaminic agents often must be tried before an optimal (or even a satisfactory) one is identified, and the results of such trials defy prediction from the outset. In choosing drugs for comparison by individuals, it must be recalled that many marketed preparations are merely different *forms* of a few agents (e.g., chlorpheniramine) and that efficacy trials should compare *different* chemical species. Patients often report a waning of previous antihistaminic effectiveness, requiring substitution (or addition) of different agents.

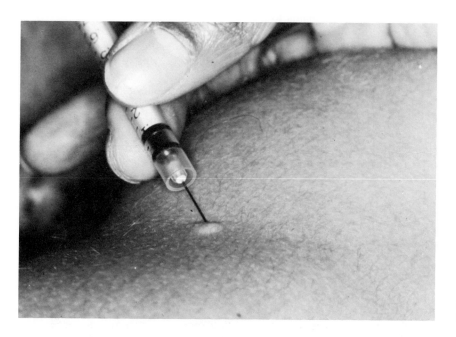

FIGURE 9-8 Technique of intradermal (intracutaneous) skin testing.

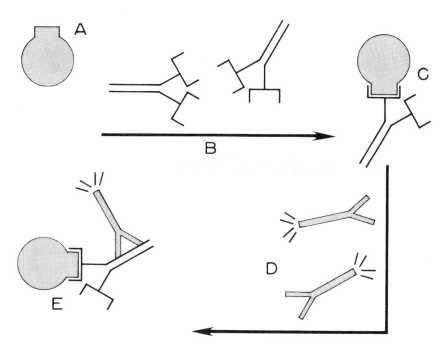

FIGURE 9-9 The radioallergosorbent test (RAST), a technique for quantitating allergen-specific immunoglobulin E. In this procedure allergens are linked chemically to carrier particles (A), and the resulting conjugate reacted (B) with serum presumably containing specific IgE. If IgE is bound (C), it will react with and bind radiolabeled antihuman IgE (D) to form a radioactive complex (E). By counting bound radioactivity, the original specific IgE present may be calculated.

Sympathomimetic amines offer additional benefit in allergic rhinitis and are often marketed in combinations with antihistaminics. Drugs including ephedrine and isoephedrine act as mucosal decongestants and, by causing more or less psychomotor stimulation, offset the sedative effects of histamine antagonists. Whether orally administered sympathomimetic drugs *significantly* affect the release of mediator substances from tissue mast cells is unclear, although (opposing) beta- and alpha-type adrenergic effects (see Chap. 10) both are possible. In addition, these agents produce side effects that may impair ocular, cardiac, gastrointestinal, and genitourinary function (see Chap. 10). The *topical* use of sympathomimetic agents as drops, sprays, and vapors is widespread and provides prompt mucosal shrinkage, which is helpful in acute illness (e.g., bacterial sinusitis). Unfortunately, these preparations are easily obtained and frequently overused. With prolonged abuse, an irritant effect often supervenes so that each dose gives transient decongestion followed by a prolonged obstructive response, prompting further medication. In habituated persons, the resulting mucosal inflammation, or *rhinitis medicamentosa,* produces obdurate nasal stuffiness and a congested, often violaceous, appearance. In approaching this problem, complete withdrawal of topical nasal medication is mandatory and, where possible, oral agents are substituted. At times several weeks of topical nasal dexamethasone spray must be given to make this change tolerable.

Intranasal steroids are useful also in suppressing the primary symptoms of allergic rhinitis but are reserved for brief, seasonal periods of exquisite severity. In addition, systemic corticosteroids will suppress hay fever manifes-

tations when other remedies have failed. However, the widespread side effects of these agents makes their chronic administration for nasal allergy unacceptable. Current efforts to develop poorly absorbed or rapidly metabolized steroids with largely local effects may provide additional useful medications.

Except for antibiotics when indicated, very few additional drugs offer benefit to rhinitis sufferers. Aspirin in conventional oral doses may have limited value for occasional persons with allergic and nonallergic vasomotor rhinitis. Evidence is accumulating that cromolyn sodium (see Chap. 10) may attenuate manifestations of allergic rhinitis and conjunctivitis by appropriate topical application. However, the place of this drug and certain oral congeners in managing upper airway disease remains to be defined.

Immunotherapy (hyposensitization) continues to provide an important *allergen-specific* approach to the treatment of respiratory allergy. This procedure typically entails the subcutaneous injection of incremental doses of extracts of a recognized allergen over prolonged periods in an attempt to somehow modify clinical reactivity. After reaching an empirically indicated "maximum" level, this dose is maintained pending evaluation of symptoms, and adjustments in the program are carried out accordingly. Valid indications for immunotherapy may include allergic rhinitis and/or conjunctivitis inadequately controlled despite optimal avoidance measures and antihistaminic treatment, as well as allergic asthma. In each instance, sensitivity to *specific, inhalant* allergens must be confirmed, since any nonspecific benefits of injection treatment are unpredictable; food factors are approached by diet modification exclusively. A typical treatment schedule is illustrated in Fig. 9-11. Properly controlled clinical trials have confirmed the value of hyposensitization for grass and ragweed pollen and have suggested that tree pollen and house dust immunotherapy *may* be beneficial. Other materials have

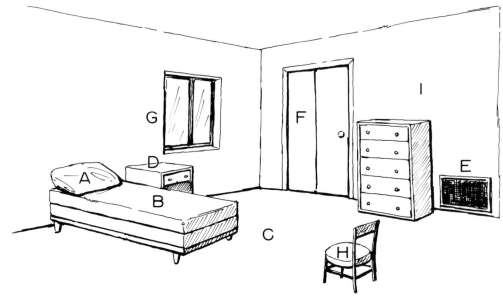

FIGURE 9-10 Measures designed to minimize exposure to house dust (and other inhalant allergens) as applied to a bedroom. Objectives include covering pillows (A), mattresses, and box springs (B) with plastic casings; maintaining a bare floor (C) and uncluttered surfaces (D); applying final filters to warm air ducts (E); keeping closet doors closed (F); and minimizing window coverings (G), wall decorations (I), and upholstered furnishings (H).

been shown to be valueless (e.g., respiratory bacterial vaccines) or remain unstudied (e.g., fungus extracts). Trials of pollen extracts have indicated also that (1) optimal symptom suppression is seen when the largest well-tolerated, extract doses are given, (2) symptom suppression due to treatment may carry over to a subsequent year when injections are withheld, and (3) a "placebo," or inert, material by injection may decrease symptoms in one-third to one-half of subjects in control groups.

The basis of the efficacy of immunotherapy remains unclear although several tissue effects that might promote benefit are known. It was initially assumed that the procedure effected active immunization against a pollen toxin, although this rationale has been entirely discredited. Subsequently, it has been postulated that immunotherapy might "turn off" specific IgE production. However, RAST values and skin test positivity do not substantially decrease during extended successful treatment, and specific IgE values usually rise early in the injection sequence. The appearance in serum of IgG antibodies specific for the injected allergen is well documented, and these factors can compete with IgE for allergen, giving them "blocking" capabilities. Although a general correlation between blocking antibody titer and clinical improvement is seen, the relationship is far from perfect, and exceptions (e.g., with high titers and unabated rhinitis) imply that other factors must also contribute. Recently described elevations, with immunotherapy, of IgG and IgA (blocking) antibodies in respiratory tract secretions suggest an alternative mechanism of tissue effect. In addition, blood basophils from persons receiving high-dose immunotherapy have been noted to release progressively less histamine on allergen challenge in vitro and, in some cases, to become wholly

ALLERGY TREATMENT

TENTATIVE DOSAGE SCHEDULE

To Doctor (referring) Date

Address

Suggestions for hyposensitization to appropriate inhalant allergens

In case of

In administering allergy extracts extreme care must be observed to prevent allergic reaction. Fresh aqueous epinephrine (adrenalin) 1/1000 and a tourniquet should always be available for instant use. One cc. tuberculin luer syringe and 26 or 27 gauge needles length are best to give the extract. Doses are given subcutaneously and slowly in an extremity. Frequent retraction of the luer plunger will detect any evidence of blood. If this occurs do not give dose at that location; try again at another site. All patients should be observed for a period of at least 20 minutes following each dose of extract. In the event of allergic reaction (such as syncope, generalized itching of the skin, nausea, tightness of the chest or hay fever) 0.3cc of epinephrine 1/1000 is given in the opposite arm and 0.1 epinephrine given at the site of the injection. In more severe reactions, also apply tourniquet above injection site and use antihistamines. If a reaction occurs, the next dose must be at least 0.1cc less than the amount which produced the reaction. Hold at this sub-symptom dose for at least 3 successive times before attempting again to increase.

Treatment should be given 1-2 x /wk until 0.5ml. of 1:50 or maintenance dose is reached; then once every 1 — 4 weeks, depending upon symptoms.

Begin

Date — 1:50,000 Extract conc.	Date — 1:5000 Extract conc.	Date — 1:500 Extract conc.	Date — 1:50 Extract conc.
0.05cc	0.05cc	0.05cc	0.05cc
0.1 cc	0.07cc	0.07cc	0.07cc
0.2 cc	0.1 cc	0.1 cc	0.1 cc
0.4 cc	0.15cc	0.15cc	0.15cc
0.5	0.20cc	0.2 cc	0.2 cc
	0.3 cc	0.25cc	0.25cc
	0.4 cc	0.3 cc	0.3 cc
	0.55	0.4 cc	0.4 cc
		0.5 cc	0.5 cc

Probable maintenance dose

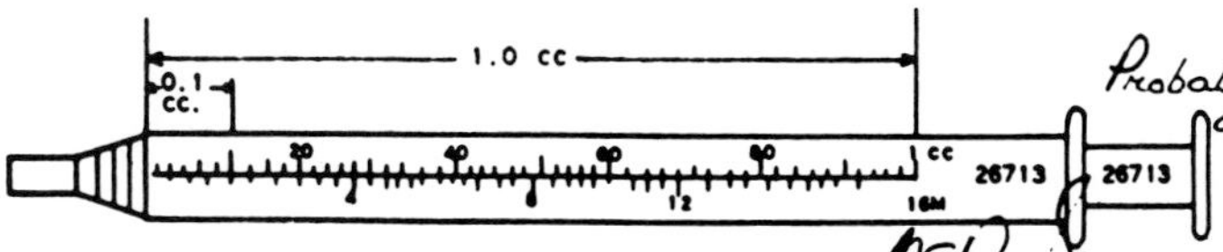

N.K. Solomon, M.D.

Phone: Area Code 313
764-6142

The University Hospital
Ann Arbor, Michigan

H2068678

FIGURE 9-11 Dosage schedule form used at the Allergy Clinic of the University Hospital, Ann Arbor, for patients whose injection treatment will be administered by their personal physicians. The steps shown form a commonly useful sequence, although additional dilutions or dosage volumes may be desirable for specific persons.

unresponsive. The importance of this effect is not clear, and some workers have alleged that its allergen-specificity is questionable. At present, therefore, although the clinical value of hyposensitization for selected allergens is established, the responsible mechanisms are not; current evidence justifies major interest in the role of blocking factors, however.

Although serious, *long-term* adverse effects of immunotherapy are nowhere evident, significant, transient, local or systemic reactions can occur. Locally, redness, whealing, and tender swelling lasting up to 36 hours may develop if dosage is excessive. These reactions usually mandate a reduction in the amount of allergen next injected. However, their severity also may be decreased by wiping the needle with a sterile swab before injection to remove adhering extract and applying firm pressure to the site following injection to prevent retrograde dissection of fluid along the needle track. Acute systemic reactions often are preceded by increasingly prominent local swellings but may occur in their absence. Generalized reactions exemplify human anaphylaxis but also may be accompanied by or confined to rhinitis and/or asthma symptoms; management has been described previously. Since extract should be given into a site sufficiently distal to allow placement of a proximal tourniquet, this opportunity also should be exploited. In addition, 0.1 to 0.2 ml of epinephrine is commonly introduced at the point of previous injection to slow allergen absorption. Although adverse reactions may occur capriciously, their risk increases with conditions that elevate cutaneous blood flow, including high environmental temperature, fever, physical exertion, hyperthyroidism, and pregnancy. Human error also is a factor frequently due to misreading of previously recorded doses or of vial labels; confusion of persons with similar names commonly is implicated. In general, reactions that will require treatment have onset within 20 minutes following injection; therefore most clinics require their patients to remain quietly seated in a well-ventilated room for 15 to 20 minutes after receiving injections. The low but inescapable risk of systemic reactions and a corresponding need for rapid, complex treatment measures leaves little justification for self-administration of extract by any patient.

At present, skin testing and most injection treatment are carried out with sterile, aqueous extracts containing, usually, an antimicrobial agent (e.g., phenol or Merthiolate) and occasionally a protein stabilizer such as human serum albumin. Attempts to establish standards of biological potency for these materials have not succeeded, and they commonly are rated on a "weight-by-volume" basis. In this system, a 1:500 ragweed pollen extract is the solution resulting when one gram of defatted ragweed pollen is extracted under defined conditions in five hundred milliliters of fluid. Alternative approaches based on assays of total protein or total nitrogen are no more instructive. Comparisons of extract potency based upon their ability to inhibit RAST carried out with standard reaginic serums appear feasible in the future. In addition, interest has become increasingly focused on therapeutic materials suitable for infrequent administration and combining low skin reactivity with prominent immunizing potency. Currently, alum-precipitated aqueous extracts are available with modest long-acting properties, although local and systemic adverse reactions can occur. Future directions emphasize the use of allergens aggregated by or absorbed to carriers as well as those chemically modified by agents such as formalin or glutaraldehyde.

QUESTIONS

Familiar allergic disorders: anaphylaxis and the atopic diseases—Chap. 9

Directions: Circle the letter preceding each item below that correctly answers each question. More than one answer may be correct.

1 Immunologic processes which are most clearly recognized as immunologic disease are reactions of:
  a Delayed hypersensitivity *b* Immediate hypersensitivity *c* Both *a* and *b* *d* Neither *a* nor *b*

2 All of the following are important characteristics of clinical hypersensitivity (allergy) as an immunologic response EXCEPT:
  a Specificity—reaction is to a specific, exogenous antigen. *b* Response usually involves immunologic mechanisms. *c* Reaction is abnormal (inappropriate or damaging). *d* Prior contact with a specific substance (allergen) is not necessary to elicit a response.

3 Reactions of immunoglobulin G (IgG) may include which of the following?
  a Forms a precipitating complex with allergens
  b Readily binds to surface receptors of blood eosinophils *c* Directly liberates mediator substances from the cell *d* Activates complement proteins after interacting with the antigen

4 IgE antibody has specific affinity for:
  a Mast cells *b* Eosinophils *c* Basophils
  d Histiocytes

5 Which of the following characteristics may be associated with IgE?
  a A tissue-fixing antibody associated with allergic rhinitis *b* Participates in reactions leading to release of histamine *c* Is involved in immunologically induced wheal-and-flare reactions *d* All of the above

6 Manifestations of acute systemic (anaphylactic) reaction include all of the following EXCEPT:
  a Pruritus of the scalp and palms of the hands
  b Eczema *c* Severe laryngeal edema and bronchial obstruction *d* Hypovolemic shock caused by exudation of fluid from the vascular compartment

7 All of the following statements about anaphylaxis are true EXCEPT:
a It is a condition caused by an immunologic reaction. b It is a potentially fatal condition c It is thought to be mediated by IgG. d Acute systemic reactions generally begin within minutes after introduction of an allergen.

8 Important considerations to be made in treating acute systemic (anaphylactic) reactions include which of the following?
a Maintaining a patent airway b Improving vascular or blood vessel integrity or intactness c Supporting the blood pressure d Promoting rapid absorption of the allergen e Administration of antipruritic lotions to the skin

9 A 30-year-old male has collapsed following an IM penicillin injection; he is unconscious with generalized hives and his blood pressure is 60/20. *Initial* treatment should be:
a IM penicillinase b Subcutaneous adrenalin and IM Benadryl (diphenhydramine) c IV corticosteroids in normal saline d Subcutaneous adrenalin and IV saline e IV corticosteroids and IM Benadryl

10 Characteristics of the atopic state include:
a A strong family history of chronic bronchitis and emphysema b The occurrence of typical infantile eczema without evident precipitating allergens c The genetically inherited predisposition to become hypersensitive d Presence of numerous wheal-and-flare reactions on testing the skin with food and pollen extracts

11 Atopic diseases include all of the following conditions EXCEPT:
a Bronchial asthma b Hay fever c Allergic eczematous contact dermatitis d Allergic rhinitis

12 Which of the following are typical signs and/or symptoms of perennial allergic rhinitis?
a Nasal stuffiness b Bouts of cough and wheezing c Rhinorrhea d Allergic shiners

13 Persons with seasonal allergic rhinitis or hay fever:
a Are less likely than normal to have had asthma or atopic dermatitis b Usually have other members in their family with atopic conditions c Develop sensitivity to penicillin in over 70 percent of cases d Typically wheeze with exposure to offending allergens

14 A 20-year-old male has a large wheal-and-flare reaction on skin testing with ragweed pollen extract; a comparable test with the diluent is nonreactive. He may be told, with confidence, that:
a He has large amounts of IgG blocking antibody specific for ragweed pollen allergens in his blood. b He has ragweed hay fever. c He is immune to ragweed pollen and will never have difficulty related to it in the future. d He has IgE antibodies specific for ragweed pollen allergens fixed at skin sites.

15 Antihistaminic drugs:
a Prevent the release of histamine from mast cells

b Prevent the release of histamine from macrophages c Are highly beneficial in treatment of severe asthma d At least partially control symptoms in a majority of patients with hay fever

16 Which of the following drugs should be immediately available when intracutaneous skin tests are being performed with atopic allergens?
a Epinephrine b Cortisone tablets c Horse serum d Antihistamine tablets

17 All of the following are recognized effects of hyposensitization (immunotherapy) EXCEPT:
a This will cause an immediate decrease in IgE in the blood. b This causes an increase in IgG which may compete with IgE for antigens. c Decreased histamine release from sensitized mast cells occurs with specific amounts of allergen. d Treated persons are able to tolerate progressively larger amounts of *injected* allergen.

18 Injection treatment (hyposensitization) would be most appropriate for:
a A 30-year-old mother of three with severe wheezing due to a guinea pig present in the home for 3 months b A 60-year-old vice-president of IBM with angioedema following ingestion of abalone (and other snails) c A 30-year-old veterinarian with well-identified asthma due to dog dander d A 9-month-old infant with severe eczema known to be worsened by egg e A 20-year-old nursing student with grass and ragweed pollen hay fever, readily controlled with an antihistamine-decongestant drug preparation

Directions: Answer the following questions on a separate sheet of paper.

19 Describe the pathogenesis of an acute systemic (anaphylactic) reaction.

20 What accounts for differences among species in patterns of an anaphylactic response?

21 What are the necessary conditions for anaphylactic sensitization in human beings?

22 List three principal considerations which dominate the management of respiratory allergy as exemplified by allergic rhinitis.

Directions: Circle the T for true and the F for false. Correct the false statements.

23 T F In North America and western Europe the most commonly encountered atopic condition is allergic rhinitis.

24 T F The distinctive feature of allergic rhinitis is that compatible symptoms appear

or worsen predictably in response to specific exposures.

25   T   F   Strongly positive wheal-and-flare–eliciting skin tests provide assurance that symptoms of allergic respiratory conditions do arise from exposure to the allergens in question.

26   T   F   The preferred method of skin testing for clinical evaluation of respiratory allergy is to inject highly concentrated aqueous extracts of allergenic material intracutaneously.

27   T   F   The radioallergosorbent test (RAST) is used to measure allergen-specific IgE using venous blood in vitro.

CHAPTER 10 Bronchial Asthma—Allergic and Otherwise

OBJECTIVES   **At the completion of Chap. 10 you should be able to:**

1 Define *bronchial asthma.*

2 Describe the tissue changes associated with *uncomplicated* asthma.

3 Explain the pattern of ventilatory dysfunction in asthma.

4 Identify for distressed asthmatic patients the signs and symptoms related to their condition.

5 Describe the relationship of atopy to bronchial asthma.

6 Relate autonomic innervation to the abnormal bronchial lability that is characteristic of asthmatic persons.

7 Describe the relationship of viral and respiratory infection with asthma in both children and adults.

8 Explain the significance of exercise in provoking an asthma attack.

9 List the signs and symptoms that differentiate asthma from other obstructive airway problems.

10 Identify for allergic aspergillosis the pathogenesis, signs and symptoms, treatment, and prognosis.

11 Compare chronic bronchitis, pulmonary emphysema, and bronchial asthma (unassociated with atopic factors) in terms of pathologic anatomy, symptoms, and diagnosis.

12 Explain the rationale for long-term treatment considerations in bronchial asthma.

13 Identify the drugs, mode of administration, dosages, side effects, and range of serum levels used in both acute and long-term management of asthma.

14 Identify the problems related to self-administration of adrenergic agents.

15 Describe the appropriate urgent treatment of asthma.

16 Identify for severe asthma or status asthmaticus the signs and symptoms, complications, treatment, and prognosis.

Asthma is a clinically defined condition marked by recurrent, discrete episodes of *reversible* bronchial narrowing, separated by periods in which ventilation approaches normal. Tissue changes in uncomplicated asthma (Fig. 10-1) are confined to bronchial airways and consist of smooth-muscle spasm, mucosal edema, and hypersecretion of viscid mucus. Mobilization of luminal secretions is compromised by airway narrowing and by the shedding of ciliated bronchial epithelial cells that normally subserve the clearance of mucus. A fundamental inability to achieve normal rates of flow (Fig. 10-2) during respiration (especially expiration) results in uneven lung aeration and a loss of the normal spatial matching of ventilation and pulmonary blood flow (Fig. 10-3). Depending on their severity, these defects may produce no symptoms or merely a sense of tracheal irritation; alternatively, respiratory distress may be intolerable. Airstream turbulence and the vibrations of bronchial mucus lead to audible wheezing during asthmatic attacks; however, this physical sign also is prominent in other obstructive airway problems. Distressed asthmatic people commonly breathe more rapidly than normal (even though this tends to increase resistance to air flow) and avoid unnecessary activity. In addition, the chest assumes a position of maximum inspiration, which is voluntarily achieved at first and serves to dilate the airways. Later this appearance is sustained due to incomplete emptying of alveoli resulting in progressive hyperinflation of the thorax (Fig. 10-4). In *uncomplicated* asthma, cough is prominent only as attacks resolve, when it serves to clear accumulated secretions. Between bouts of asthma the patient is typically free of wheezes and symptoms, although heightened bronchial reactivity and defects in ventilation remain demonstrable by special techniques. However, with chronicity, symptomless interludes may disappear, leading to a state of continuous asthma—often with secondary infection.

Although atopy is readily implicated in many instances

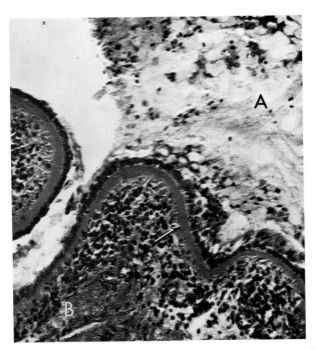

FIGURE 10-1 *Bronchial changes in chronic asthma. This small bronchus shows increased width of the epithelial basement membrane (arrow) and partial loss of mucosal cells. The lumen (A) is filled with mucus and cellular debris while the submucosa (B) is densely infiltrated with inflammatory cells including many eosinophils. (From J. M. Sheldon, R. G. Lovell, and K. P. Mathews, A Manual of Clinical Allergy, 2d ed., Saunders, Philadelphia, 1967.)*

of bronchial asthma, a substantial number of asthmatics lack demonstrable allergic factors even after exhaustive study. Such persons, including many infants as well as middle-aged and older adults, are often said to have "intrinsic" asthma, although their problem is more properly idiopathic (i.e., unexplained).

A subset of adults with idiopathic asthma also manifest nasal polyps, recurrent sinusitis, and severe airway obstructive responses to *aspirin*. Less frequently, other nonsteroidal anti-inflammatory drugs (e.g., indomethacin) or the FDA approved food coloring tartrazine (Yellow No. 5) also precipitate severe attacks in these patients. Moderate asthma is usually persistent in these patients even when recognized offenders are avoided, however, and prominent vasomotor rhinitis frequently ushers in the disease. A willingness to accept the patient's report of respiratory distress after aspirin is essential, since *no* safe confirmatory test is available.

Asthmatic people as a group, both those with and without allergic mechanisms, share an abnormal bronchial lability which promotes airway narrowing by many factors which have no effect on normals. The basis of this tendency remains unclear; however, asthmatic airways behave as if their beta-adrenergic innervation (which most effectively defends airway patency) were incompetent, and much evidence suggests that, at least functionally, partial "beta blockage" exists in typical asthma. Without adequate bronchodilator tone, bronchoconstrictor influences, known to be mediated normally by parasympathetic (cholinergic) and alpha-adrenergic pathways, would tend to predominate. In clinical practice, the bronchial lability of asthmatics may be confirmed by demonstrating their brisk airway obstructive responses to extremely *low* concentrations of inhaled histamine and methacholine; (the latter is a substance with activity resembling acetylcholine). Similar mechanisms probably contribute to bouts of asthma that often follow inhalation of cold air as well as exposure to myriad mists, dusts, and volatile irritants. Poorly understood nervous pathways are available also to mediate airway closure in response to psychic stimuli, which commonly worsen symptoms in both adults and children. (Asthma due *solely* to emotional factors is exceptionally rare, however.) Reflex pathways promoting bronchospasm with forced chest deflation are also especially effective in asthmatics and are activated by maneuvers such as laughing, blowing up a balloon, or providing a full expiration for ventilatory testing.

Flares of asthma commonly accompany viral or bacterial respiratory infections and may progress in severity, ultimately requiring inpatient care. Where responsible pathogens have been sought in childhood asthmatic patients, rhinovirus and parainfluenza virus infections have been especially implicated. The presence of significant secondary infection may be manifested by fever, purulent expectoration, elevated white blood cell count, or recovery of pathogens from sputum; however, often persistent asthma provides the *only* signal. Many children with infection-triggered asthma in preschool years go on to develop classical nasal allergy or allergic (atopic) asthma in later life. However, there are few indications that microbial sensitivity is responsible for asthma accompanying infection. Rather, since invading organisms frequently destroy already compromised ciliated epithelium and localize agents of inflammation in labile bronchi, their adverse effect on asthma is predictable. In addition, animal studies have suggested that microbial substances may further weaken beta-adrenergic activity.

Many severe asthmatics experience increased wheezing and dyspnea (abnormal shortness of breath) promptly with exertion of any intensity. In addition, a specific form of exercise-induced asthma (EIA) is often noted in which, following several minutes of brisk activity and often well after its termination, significant bronchospasm occurs. EIA is most commonly evident in children and characteristically appears in subjects symptomless before beginning exertion. Although a *minimum* total energy expenditure is necessary, above this critical level the risk of symptoms varies with the type of activity; generally, at comparable work levels, sprint running is most and swimming least conducive to EIA.

Since bronchial asthma is an abnormal *pattern* of response rather than a discrete disease, differential diagnosis requires attention to the clinical form and major determinants of this syndrome,* as well as to its distinction from other obstructive airway problems. Rarely, persons who overbreathe with psychic stress or children with noisy respiration due to large adenoids, a short neck, or a "floppy" epiglottis are suspected of having asthma. In adults, at least, this possibility often may be excluded by demonstrating a normal test response to inhalation of methacholine, while the childhood problems usually are clarified by careful examination and resolve, in time, with developmental changes. However, at any age, the impaction of a foreign body or growth of a localized tumor in the bronchi (or larynx) may lead to *diffuse* wheezing, simulating asthma. More

*A syndrome is a set of signs and symptoms that occur together and characterize a specific illness.

typical recurrent symptoms may be encountered in certain forms of diffuse vascular inflammation (vasculitis) and with secreting carcinoid tumors when these are metastatic to the liver.

Severe airway obstruction, capable of producing respiratory failure and associated with fever, is characteristic of the bronchiolitis of small children. This illness is often recurrent and appears frequently due to infection with respiratory syncytial virus. Severe local inflammation promotes closure of the small, distal airways involved, although humoral immune mechanisms may also contribute to this process.

A striking picture occurs in occasional allergic asthmatic people due to carriage of the fungus *Aspergillus fumigatus* in their bronchial lumina. Although there is little or no tissue invasion, this organism excites an intense, apparently immunologically directed, inflammatory response with fever, pulmonary infiltrates on chest x-ray, and prominent tissue and peripheral blood eosinophilia. Affected persons experience fatigue, weight loss, severe asthma, and expectoration of bronchial mucus plugs that may show the fungus as minute, dark growth points. Immediate (wheal-and-flare) skin reactivity to the organism is striking, and total serum IgE levels are extremely high. IgG precipitating antibodies with specificity for this fungus also are demonstrable in over 70 percent of this group. Suppression of the disease with adequate doses of adrenal cortical steroids (see later in this chapter) is feasible and also essential if irreversible bronchial damage (bronchiectasis) is to be averted (Fig. 10-5).

Especially in older adults, chronic bronchitis and pulmonary emphysema often require distinction from bronchial asthma when the latter is unassociated with atopic

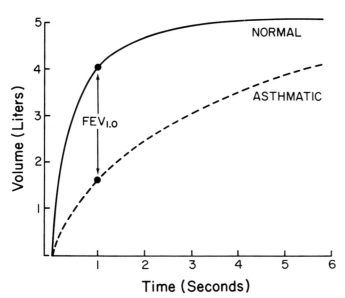

FIGURE 10-2 Forced expiratory curves produced by two 20-year-old males—one normal and one with moderately severe asthma. The slope of these curves at any point is equivalent to flow rate. An inability to move air quickly is the major ventilatory defect in asthma.

factors. *Chronic bronchitis* denotes a prolonged and often slowly progressive condition of bronchial inflammation and hypersecretion manifested by cough and sputum production extending over months and years. In addition, a proportion of chronic bronchitic people also experience episodic bouts of airway obstruction—in effect, a form of idiopathic asthma—late in the disease. *Pulmonary emphysema,* by contrast, presents prominent, *irreversible* anatomic changes with diffuse loss of the alveolar walls that normally exert outward traction on the bronchi that they surround. Deprived of this source of support, the airways tend to close in expiration wherever pressure outside their walls exceeds that in their lumina. Affected persons develop predictable periods of dyspnea and wheezing with any increase (usually exertional) in respiratory effort rather than experiencing *spontaneous attacks,* typical of asthma, which tend to begin at rest or, often, during sleep. Because the prognosis of emphysema is quite unfavorable, with variably increasing disability the rule, this diagnosis cannot be proposed lightly. However, since, with recurrent infection, asthmatic individuals also may acquire chronic bronchitis, and severely bronchitic patients ultimately may show emphysema as well, a sharp distinction between these disorders may be impossible at times. On the other hand, when chest hyperinflation, evident on x-ray or physical evaluation, is casually (and erroneously) designated "emphysema," a grave stigma may be implied without basis. In fact, the hyperinflation and resulting thoracic deformity of young asthmatics may be totally reversed with successful treatment, leaving them anatomically and functionally normal.

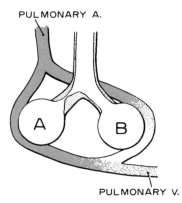

FIGURE 10-3 *Mismatching of ventilation and perfusion in asthma. Due to narrowing of its bronchus, alveolus A does not properly oxygenate its share of pulmonary artery blood; B functions normally. As a result of O_2 saturation of pulmonary venous blood is abnormally low. In asthma, a shift of blood flow from A- to B-type alveoli occurs but is usually inadequate. Furthermore, hyperventilation of B with room air cannot compensate for the "shunting" at A.*

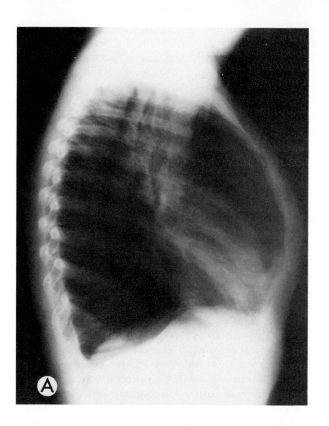

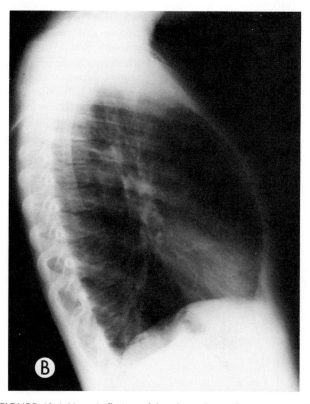

FIGURE 10-4 *Hyperinflation of the chest shown by an 8-year-old boy with asthma. X-ray (A) was taken during severe status asthmaticus which later required mechanical ventilation. (Note especially the broad space between the heart and sternum.) Film (B) was taken during a symptom-free interlude 4 months later and shows far less severe changes.*

The protracted course typical of asthma and its associated state of bronchial hyperreactivity determine a chronic need for treatment measures. Where atopic factors are evident, efforts to reduce exposure to and immunotherapy for selected inhalant allergens (see Chap. 9) have established value and, again, deserve attention. Avoidance of irritants—especially tobacco smoke—and prompt treatment of unresolved bacterial respiratory infections are frequently overlooked, although of major benefit to asthmatic people generally.

Perfumes, aerosol cleaners and cosmetics, strong cooking odors, solvents, and paint fumes also pose potentially avoidable risks that must be appreciated. Cold air is an additional bronchoconstrictor influence that may be mitigated by wearing a scarf or gauze mask over the nose and mouth as a heat exchanger. Adding moisture to dry indoor air (to maintain a relative humidity of at least 30 percent) is desirable, although poorly maintained humidifiers can become sources of microbial aerosols. In addition, programs of regular medication can effectively reduce bronchial lability and thereby raise the threshold for obstructive airway responses.

At present, the maintenance of adequate blood levels of theophylline is a first objective in the drug treatment of bronchial asthma (Fig. 10-6). The desired effect of theophylline is exerted by its inhibition of intracellular enzymes (viz., phosphodiesterases) which degrade the nucleotide, 3'5'-cyclic adenosine monophosphate (cyclic AMP). This substance mediates beta-adrenergic effects in many tissues, and, as intracellular levels of cyclic AMP rise in bronchial smooth muscle, relaxation (a beta effect) is notably increased. Cyclic AMP levels also strongly modify the allergen-induced release of inflammatory mediators (e.g., histamine, SRS-A, and ECF-A) from IgE-sensitized mast cells or blood basophils (Fig. 10-6). In these systems, increasing cyclic AMP levels serve to reduce mediator liberation and thereby provide an additional mode of effectiveness for both theophylline and direct beta-adrenergic agonists in bronchial asthma.* Serum levels of theophylline correlate closely with the occurrence of favorable or of toxic effects. Toxicity is uncommon below a concentration of 20 μg/ml, but its risk rises progressively above this point; similarly, favorable effects generally are absent below 10 μg/ml. Serum levels in the desired range of 10 to 20 μg/ml are usually achieved by administering doses of 5 to 6 mg of anhydrous theophylline per kilogram of body weight every 6 hours. However, individuals may differ as much as fivefold in their rates of hepatic metabolism of this drug. As a result, regular doses well above or below 5 to 6 mg/kg may be essential for a *safe* therapeutic effect. Theophylline administration must be approached cautiously—especially where liver function is impaired—since convulsions, cardiac rhythm disturbance, or hypotension may be the first sign(s) of serious overdosage. More commonly, headache, nausea, vomiting, diarrhea (which is rarely bloody), or muscle tremor are the principal manifestations of toxicity. Direct assay of the serum theophylline level has become increasingly available recently and affords a rational guide for dosage determination. This drug is well absorbed when given orally although administration every 6 hours is required. Elixirs of theophylline offer more rapid absorption, facilitating the acute treatment of asthmatic attacks, although adequate blood levels are maintained only briefly. Theophylline salts such as aminophylline (theophylline ethylenediamine) also may be given rectally as aqueous solutions or in cocoa butter suppositories; however, absorption is erratic, and this route is rarely preferred. In addition, sterile solutions of aminophylline are widely used for intravenous treatment of serious asthma (see later) but cause grave pain and tissue injury if injected by other routes.

Drugs with intrinsic beta-adrenergic effects continue to be useful for both acute and long-term management of asthma (although most also manifest a measure of alpha activity). The effectiveness of these agents is thought to reflect *direct* stimulation of an enzyme, adenyl cyclase, which promotes the synthesis of 3'5'-

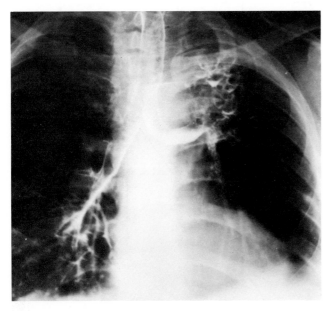

FIGURE 10-5 Left upper lobe saccular bronchiectasis demonstrated by bronchography in an adult with long-standing allergic bronchopulmonary aspergillosis. Bronchi in lower lung fields are essentially uninvolved. (Film courtesy of Dr. Terry Silver.)

*Considering the central importance of beta-adrenergic activity for bronchial patency, it is not surprising that beta-blocking drugs (e.g., propranolol) commonly worsen asthma. Present evidence suggests that alpha-adrenergic and cholinergic effects directly oppose those of beta stimulation; that is to say, they foster bronchial smooth-muscle spasm and augment mediator release from challenged mast cells.

cyclic AMP (Fig. 10-6). Cyclic AMP–induced effects (i.e., relaxation of bronchial smooth muscle and inhibition of mediator release from mast cells and basophils) are, therefore, shared by beta-adrenergic agents with theophylline, and additive effects of these two groups of drugs often result. Epinephrine, by subcutaneous injection, remains the most widely useful agent for relief of brief, acute asthmatic attacks. A dose of 0.3 ml of a 1:1000 solution is appropriate for most adults, while 0.022 ml/kg may be used (up to 0.3 ml) for small children. The therapeutic effect of aqueous epinephrine is maximum 10 to 15 minutes after injection and essentially gone after 1 hour. Therefore successive injections at 20-minute intervals are often employed to obtain a gradual, incremental effect.*

Beta-adrenergic drugs are available for inhalation as well as for oral administration. Unlike epinephrine, these

*Efforts to obtain an epinephrine product with prolonged activity have been only partially successful. Sus-phrine is widely used for this purpose and has superceded intramuscular epinephrine in oil. Recently interest has shifted to the sustained effects of newer injected agents such as terbutaline.

agents are commonly self-administered by patients, creating a potential for voluntary overdosage. Unwanted side effects do vary among these drugs; however, all tend to produce sleeplessness, psychomotor stimulation, and muscle tremor. In addition, loss of appetite, constipation, and difficulty in urination can result—especially in the elderly—although patients rarely associate these difficulties with their medications. The beta-adrenergic agents tend to raise the force of cardiac contraction, elevate heart rate, and increase the activity of abnormal foci of electrical activity in the myocardium and conducting system. These effects are potentially harmful in many types of cardiovascular disease and may increase blood flow to poorly ventilated areas of lung, resulting in a lowering of arterial oxygen tension. Recently introduced agents (metaproterenol, terbutaline, salbutamol) appear to impose lower cardiovascular side effects than longer established remedies such as ephedrine and isoproterenol.

Problems related to self-administration of adrenergic agents have arisen, especially with aerosol preparations administered either from pressurized cannisters or hand bulb–driven nebulizers. Several agents are available by this route for rapid relief of established asthma attacks, and at times aerosol use virtually becomes a conditioned reflex. Such behavior rapidly leads to overdosage—especially when asthma is severe and only barely respon-

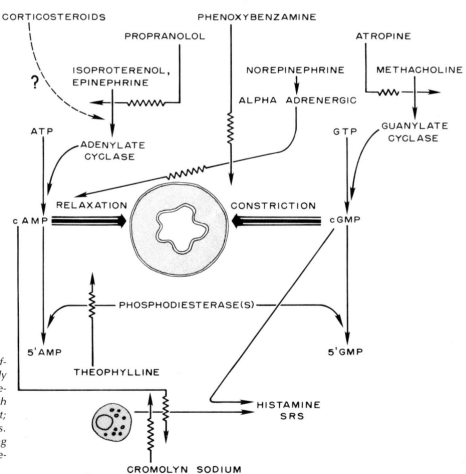

FIGURE 10-6 Actions of drugs that affect bronchial patency either directly or by modifying mediator substance release from mast cells (below). Smooth lines indicate potentiation of an effect; wavy lines signify inhibitory influences. The central importance and opposing effects of cyclic AMP and GMP deserve special attention.

sive to physiologic and therapeutic actions of adrenergic agents. Aerosol users commonly experience side effects as described above and may be predisposed to dangerous disturbances of cardiac rhythm by associated hypoxia and toxicity of fluorinated hydrocarbons (viz., freons) used as gaseous propellants. In addition (Fig. 10-7) protracted overuse of nebulizers often leads to temporarily altered bronchial reactivity in which inhalation of the drug induces brief (about 5 to 10 minute) improvement followed by a sustained obstructive response. In such responders, severe, sustained asthma may improve promptly when aerosols are *stopped*. These concerns mandate careful patient selection and close professional control of nebulizers used in all instances.

Especially in controlling *allergic* (extrinsic, atopic) asthma, regular use of disodium cromoglycate (cromolyn sodium) may provide a valuable supplement or, rarely, an alternative to conventional bronchodilator drugs. Both the structure and tissue effects of cromolyn are unique among antiasthmatic agents; indeed, inhibition of mediator release from allergen-challenged, sensitized mast cells remains its only established effect. Oral absorption of cromolyn is poor, and it is administered, in 20-mg doses, by inhalation of the dry powder in a lactose carrier. The drug substantially blocks obstructive airway responses to aerosolized allergen extracts inhaled under test conditions by sensitive subjects and, remark-

ably, also prevents anticipated exercise-induced asthma in many persons. Regular treatment with cromolyn often reduces the overall asthma burden, benefiting, especially, young allergic persons; however, improvement has been observed even in some with adult-onset, idiopathic disease. Having no intrinsic bronchodilator effect, cromolyn is without value in treating attacks of asthma and often must be withheld until acute symptom flares have been resolved. As with other inhaled medications, the delivery unit must be directed toward the pharynx and the patient instructed to take a deep breath, pausing briefly at peak inspiration before exhaling slowly.

Adrenal cortical steroids have proven to be extremely effective antiasthmatic drugs. However, in view of their potential side effects, these agents are reserved for symptoms not otherwise controllable by a combination of safer measures. The anti-inflammatory properties of steroids and their ability to increase the tissue effects of beta-adrenergic agents are well documented; however, additional effects may contribute to their antiasthmatic potency. These drugs are especially helpful when given in high-dose "bursts" for brief periods to terminate sustained, epinephrine-resistant asthma but also may be required in long-term, outpatient programs. When used chronically, the *minimum* steroid dose required to maintain tolerable function and comfort is the one appropriate. In many persons, corticosteroid control of asthma may be maintained at a lower cost in side effects by administering medication on alternate days. For this purpose, relatively short-acting agents (e.g., prednisone) are especially appropriate in single early morning doses. Although *several* times the daily drug requirement may be necessary on alternate days (qod), there usually is a lessening of somatic side effects including growth retardation in children. In addition, comparable control of symptoms is possible, potentially using qod steroids, with *less* suppression of the patient's adrenal cortical function as reflected by levels of serum cortisol measured 48 hours after medication. However, in a small number of steroid-dependent asthmatic people, qod drugs, in any reasonable dose, will not suffice.

Corticosteroids also may be given by inhalation to achieve a predominantly local bronchial effect; currently, beclomethasone dipropionate is the preferred preparation in doses of 100 mg 4 times a day. The addition of beclomethasone may confer success on an otherwise inadequate program lacking oral corticosteroids, or reduce the daily or qod steroid dose required for control of asthma. Overly aggressive treatment with beclomethasone by aerosol has led to pharyngeal irritation and a predisposition to oropharyngeal *Candida* infections. In addition, excessively rapid withdrawal of systemic steroids may precipitate adrenal cortical insufficiency and permit a sudden flare of previous sup-

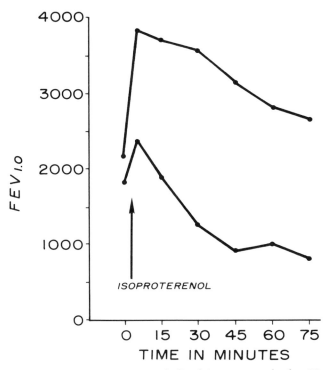

FIGURE 10-7 Responses to nebulized isoproterenol of a 23-year-old chronic asthmatic person. The lower curve was obtained after 5 months of isoproterenol overuse with up to 30 inhalations per day; a brief rise in $FEV_{1.0}$ followed by a sustained fall is shown. The upper curve is a response to isoproterenol after 6 months of abstinence from the drug showing a normal $FEV_{1.0}$ rise.

pressed inflammatory problems (e.g., allergic rhinitis, rheumatoid arthritis, etc.).

Few additional medications have proven merit in managing long-term asthma. Antihistaminic drugs rarely are beneficial—even in allergic asthma—and, by their drying effect on secretions, may compound the problem of sputum mobilization when airway obstruction is severe. The expectorant properties of iodides and glyceryl guaiacolate remain controversial at doses that do not produce gastrointestinal irritation uniformly. In addition, unpredictable adverse responses to iodides may include painful parotid swelling ("iodide mumps"), prolonged fever, worsening of acne, and the appearance of other skin rashes. Benefits of simple systemic hydration should not be overlooked when sputum mobilization is a problem, and many mild asthma attacks may be curtailed if the patient sits calmly, breathes slowly, and drinks small portions of a warm liquid. Theoretical considerations also have focused interest upon alpha-adrenergic and cholinergic antagonists as possible bronchodilators; however, the antiasthmatic potential of these drugs remains to be established.

The treatment approach to severe asthma

Although proper management can assure a good prognosis for most asthmatics, flares of the disease *do* occur requiring hospitalization and rarely resulting in fatalities. A sustained increase in symptoms often follows respiratory infection or the sudden withdrawal of a necessary suppressive medication; nebulizer abuse is sometimes crucial. However, allergen exposure *alone* rarely precipitates hospitalization.

Medical aid is often sought only after many days of increasing symptoms. During this period, poor fluid and calorie intake coupled with increased respiratory work and fluid loss may produce significant dehydration and metabolic acidosis as well as augmenting bronchial mucus plugging. As previously emphasized, the extent of airway obstruction is not uniform and, despite vascular compensation, leads to an imperfect matching of ventilation and blood flow in local areas of lung. As a result of these disparities, portions of the pulmonary blood flow escape aeration producing hypoxia and tending to impede CO_2 clearance. The deficit for CO_2 is overcome readily by the asthmatic person's respiratory effort, which can clear this readily diffusible gas by hyperventilating a *minority* of adequately perfused alveoli. As a result, the partial pressure of CO_2 (pCO_2) in arterial blood is often *below* the normal value (40 mmHg) with asthma of mild or moderate severity. A rise to normal or elevated pCO_2 levels, therefore, signifies that an advanced and perilous stage of obstruction (and ventilation-perfusion mismatching) has been reached. Similar compensation is not possible even transiently for deficient oxygen uptake; as a result, arterial pO_2 values fall progressively as asthma worsens. Substantial increases in respiratory work compound these defects by markedly raising the O_2 cost of breathing and its penalty in CO_2 production. Ultimately, ventilation may not suffice even for the metabolic needs of the respiratory system. Figure 10-8 summarizes changes observed in several parameters during increasingly severe asthma.

Epinephrine administration remains an appropriate first step in the urgent treatment of asthma. Standard

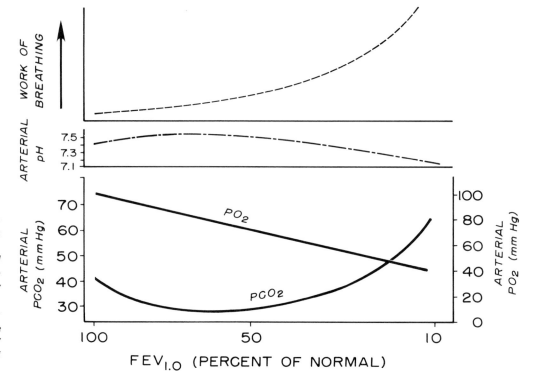

FIGURE 10-8 Changes in the work of breathing as well as in arterial pH, pO_2, and pCO_2 observed in asthmatic patients with increasingly severe airway obstruction (left to right). Hyperventilation is adequate to decrease pCO_2 and raise pH until airway narrowing and plugging are severe.

amounts may be given subcutaneously at 20-minute intervals for a gradual incremental effect; however if three or, at most, four such sequential doses fail, other measures must be substituted. Epinephrine-fast asthma often yields to intravenous aminophylline, although oral theophyllines (including hydroethanolic preparations) rarely suffice. Since many hours of self-medication with ephedrinelike drugs or with theophylline as tablets, elixirs, and suppositories may have occurred, an estimate of *residual* drug effects is mandatory. Where possible, rapid determination of theophylline serum levels can be used to predict dosage requirements initially. Persons without theophylline "on board" may receive 5 to 6 mg/kg of the drug intravenously by manual injection over at least 10 minutes, or by a "drip" infusion. Care will minimize instances of vomiting, hypotension, and seizures; however a treatment facility must be prepared to handle these side effects promptly. Severe asthma, persistent for at least 24 hours, which is not substantially benefited by optimal doses of epinephrine and theophylline is often termed *status asthmaticus*. This condition presents a serious threat to life and should prompt intensive *inpatient* care.

Most hospitalized asthmatics require supplementary hydration to replace water deficits which may amount to several liters. The oral route rarely is adequate to achieve this, and a significant risk of aspiration must be faced unless fluids and medication are given parenterally to patients with air hunger. Hypoxemia is present almost uniformly in status asthmaticus and should be corrected to a level of at least 70 mmHg following initial arterial blood gas determinations. Supplementary humidified oxygen is best provided by 24 percent or 28 percent Venti-mask or (Fig. 10-9) lacking these units, by nasal prongs.

Where bronchial unresponsiveness to epinephrine has been confirmed, this agent is withheld initially, although some patients may benefit from regular doses of inhaled adrenergic agents. However, aminophylline remains the mainstay of bronchodilator therapy, and after an initial "priming" dose of 5 to 6 mg/kg, this amount is given by continuous drip during each succeeding 6- to 8-hour period. Appropriate dosage adjustments are facilitated by determining serum theophylline levels. In addition, the need for antibiotic drugs must be decided after appropriate cultures are obtained.

Adrenal cortical steroids may be lifesaving in status asthmaticus and are usually begun if significant improvement is not evident within several hours of admission. High doses are given promptly, as well, to those who have *required* steroids either to terminate previous bouts of severe asthma or, within the previous 6 to 9 months, as a regular outpatient medication. Preparations of hydrocortisone or methylprednisolone for intravenous infusion are preferred, although even with these, several hours often are required for manifestation of initial effects.

A favorable outcome in status asthmaticus often hinges on the willingness of responsible personnel to monitor the patient's condition closely, to recognize deterioration promptly, and to anticipate problems. Prominent complications can include pneumothorax, pneumomediastinum, aspiration, drug toxicity or idio-

syncrasy, and cardiac failure or rhythm disturbance. Widespread plugging of airways may develop rapidly, manifested by a *decrease* in wheezing—but also by distant breath sounds over affected areas, (an ominous combination). Obvious deterioration often is heralded by drowsiness, confusion, and decreased muscle tone, as well as by a flagging of respiratory effort signalling general physical exhaustion. This situation readily leads to inadequate alveolar ventilation with mounting hypoxia and rising arterial levels of CO_2. The clinical state and arterial pCO_2 correlate closely, and an *upward trend* is disquieting even though the absolute value may be normal (i.e., 40 mmHg) or only minimally elevated. When pCO_2 levels exceeding 55 mmHg are encountered, despite a period of optimal treatment, they commonly signify a need for mechanical ventilation to reestablish adequate gas transfer. A volume-cycled respirator is usually chosen for this purpose after placement of a *soft,* cuffed endotracheal tube; tracheostomy rarely is required. Details of respirator care are beyond the scope of this discussion. Ventilatory assistance in status asthmaticus usually is needed for only 24 to 60 hours, when improvement engendered by bronchodilators, steroids, antibiotics, etc., usually has become evident.

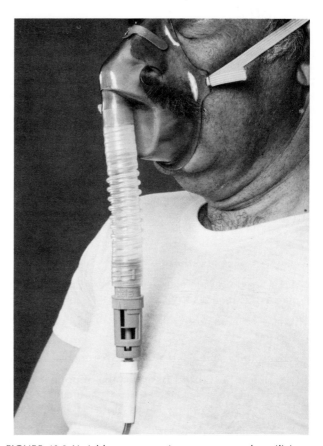

FIGURE 10-9 Variable concentration oxygen mask, utilizing a Venturi effect, is a useful device for controlled O_2 administration. With this particular device, inspired O_2 concentrations between 30 and 55 percent may be chosen.

For gravely ill asthmatic children, prolonged, carefully controlled, intravenous (IV) infusion of isoproterenol has been proposed as an alternative to conventional measures and, in skilled hands, this approach often can obviate mechanical ventilation. However, IV isoproterenol (Isuprel) carries a prohibitive risk of cardiovascular complications, including arrhythmias in those beyond adolescence, and its place in treating children remains to be defined.

For many inpatients with severe asthma, attaining an audibly clear chest is a realistic and useful predischarge goal, even though ventilatory test results (expiratory time, 1-second forced expiratory volume, maximum mid-expiratory flow rate, etc.) may remain somewhat abnormal; in others, irreversible bronchopulmonary changes may preclude a wheeze-free state. In either case, intensive treatment is continued until the anticipated maximum benefit is manifest, and then preparations are made for an outpatient program. During recovery bronchial responsiveness to epinephrine generally reappears and adrenergic agents (e.g., injected Sus-phrine or terbutaline every 8 hours) may be re-utilized. Sputum production often increases during recovery; however clearance of secretions may remain difficult despite optimal hydration and use of iodides or glyceryl guaiacolate (which have equivocal expectorant properties.) Chest physiotherapy (viz., repetitive manual percussion of the chest with postural drainage) is available now in most hospitals. This approach appears to promote sputum mobilization and can, at times, dislodge obstinate bronchial plugs, permitting reexpansion of atelectatic areas.

QUESTIONS

Bronchial asthma—allergic and otherwise—Chap. 10

Directions: Answer the following questions on a separate sheet of paper.

1 Define *bronchial asthma.*

2 What are the tissue changes associated with uncomplicated asthma?

3 What is the pattern of ventilatory dysfunction in asthma?

4 What is the relationship of atopy to bronchial asthma?

5 Describe a postulated basis for the abnormal bronchial lability that is characteristic of asthmatic people. In clinical practice, how is this bronchial lability confirmed?

6 Why do flares of asthma commonly accompany viral or bacterial respiratory infections?

7 Explain why drugs with intrinsic beta-adrenergic effects continue to be useful for acute and long-term management of asthma.

8 What are the measures used in the long-term treatment of bronchial asthma?

Directions: Circle the letter preceding each item below that correctly answers each question. More than one answer may be correct.

9 Which of the following manifestations are typical of distressed asthmatic people?
a "Allergic salute" due to pruritus of nasal mucosa
b Hyperinflation of the thorax c Rhinorrhea
d Dyspnea e Prolonged expiration and wheezing

10 All of the following substances may be responsible for severe airway obstructive responses in a subset of adults with idiopathic asthma EXCEPT:
a Aspirin b Corticosteroid anti-inflammatory drugs
c Indomethacin d Tartrazine (yellow no. 5) food coloring

11 Which of the following may precipitate individual attacks of asthma?
a Volatile irritants from organic solvents b Exposure to mists and dusts in industrial plants c Inhalation of cold air d Psychic stimuli e All of the above

12 In bronchial asthma:
a Bronchial smooth muscle is atrophic. b Medium- and small-sized bronchi are plugged with viscid mucus. c The lungs show diffuse destruction of alveolar walls. d The patient is usually free of symptoms between attacks.

13 Theophylline blood serum levels should be maintained in the range of _____ to _____ μg/ml for optimal therapeutic effect in asthma:
a 5 to 10 b 10 to 15 c 10 to 20 d 20 to 30

14 Serum levels of theophylline in the desired range are usually achieved by administering doses of _____ _____ mg/kg of body weight every 6 hours.
a 1 to 3 b 4 to 6 c 7 to 9 d 10 to 12

15 Which of the following are side effects of theophylline?
a Headache b Nausea c Bloody diarrhea
d Vomiting e All of the above

16 Aminophylline may be given appropriately to treat asthma:
a Orally as a liquid or tablet b Intravenously
c Rectally as a suppository d By inhalation

17 Jane S. was 6 when she suffered her first asthmatic attack. She was admitted to the hospital emergency room in acute respiratory distress. Jane was very anxious and had shortness of breath. Her temperature was 99.2°F rectally, her pulse was 100 per minute, and her respirations were 30 per minute. Chest examination revealed expiratory wheezing and normal resonance. She was felt to be experiencing an

acute attack of asthma. Appropriate initial treatment would include:
a Phenobarbital 25 mg orally *b* 0.2 ml of 1:1000 epinephrine subcutaneously *c* Aminophylline 50 mg rectally *d* Potassium iodide 2 g orally

18 Prominent manifestations of status asthmaticus include all of the following EXCEPT:
a Wheezing evident only on exertion *b* Widespread plugging of airways *c* Hypoxemia *d* Confusion

19 In status asthmaticus, when arterial $p\mathrm{CO_2}$ levels exceeding 55 mmHg are encountered despite a prolonged period of optimal treatment there is usually need for:
a Mechanical ventilation (a volume-cycled respirator is usually chosen after placement of a soft, cuffed endotracheal tube) *b* A tracheostomy *c* Both *a* and *b* *d* Neither *a* nor *b*

Directions: Match the T for true and the F for false. Correct the false statements.

20   T   F   Exercise-induced asthma is most commonly evident in older adults with idiopathic asthma and characteristically appears in subjects who are symptomless before beginning exertion.

21   T   F   Diffuse wheezing is a manifestation characteristic only of asthma.

22   T   F   In over 70 percent of asthmatic people with allergic aspergillosis, serum pre-

cipitins are demonstrable, and almost all have elevated IgE levels.

Directions: Match the disease condition in col. A with the appropriate description in col. B. More than one letter may be used in Col. A.

Column A	Column B
23 ____ Chronic bronchitis	*a* Irreversible anatomic changes with diffuse loss of alveolar walls.
24 ____ Pulmonary emphysema	*b* A prolonged and slowly progressive condition of bronchial inflammation and hypersecretion.
25 ____ Bronchial asthma	*c* Predictable periods of dyspnea and wheezing with any increase in respiratory effort.
	d Daily cough and increased sputum production extending over months and years.
	e Spontaneous attacks of wheezing and dyspnea often occurring at rest; between attacks the patient is typically wheeze- and symptom-free.

CHAPTER 11 Atopic Dermatitis—Urticaria

ATOPIC DERMATITIS

Atopic dermatitis is a common, chronic skin disorder (or group of related disorders) found with particular frequency among persons manifesting allergic rhinitis and asthma of their family members. In addition, high total serum IgE levels and multiple positive immediate skin test reactions are commonly noted with this condition. These associations appear to justify regarding atopic dermatitis as a de facto "atopic disease." However, the lesions of atopic dermatitis are not readily explained in terms of the transient wheal-and-flare response typical of IgE-mediated reactions. Rather, established skin lesions of atopic dermatitis show edema and variable infiltration with mononuclear cells and eosinophils as

well as fluid collections (forming clinically evident vesicles). Rupture of numerous tiny blisters leads to crusting and scaling. These changes and severe pruritus, which precedes and accompanies the eruption, are associated with an excessively dry skin. Sweating also is impaired in this condition, and sweat retention often leads to prominent, heat-induced itching. In addition, sebaceous secretions are deficient, and the skin shows both a low threshold for pruritus-inducing stimuli and an abnormal tendency to lichenification (viz., thickening of the skin with accentuation of normal markings).

Atopic dermatitis most commonly appears in the first year of life (as "infantile eczema") with red, raised, pruritic, scaling areas involving the cheeks, scalp, and diaper area. In a majority of children, the condition remits by age 5 but often only after the neck, antecubital and popliteal fossae, wrists, ankles, and waist have also become affected. The latter areas are prominently involved when this problem still is present in late childhood or when, following onset in infancy or adolescence, it persists into adult life (Fig. 11-1).

Intractable itching and painful cracks in the skin are major sources of discomfort for eczematous persons. In addition, the abraded, fissured epidermis is readily infected by bacteria—especially staphylococci—and by viruses which localize in skin. As a result, contact with herpes simplex virus, the "cold sore" agent, may produce a generalized eruption (Fig. 11-2), fever, and toxicity. An even more severe illness,* *eczema vaccinatum,* may follow exposure to vaccinia virus, and eczematous persons must scrupulously avoid receiving smallpox vaccination as well as exposure to unhealed vaccination sites.

As many as one-half of eczematous children may manifest overt respiratory allergy prior to puberty. Despite this strong association, it is rare to identify one or more allergens that substantially determine the activity of any case of atopic dermatitis. In persons with strong skin reactivity, factors such as house dust, animals, etc., may worsen the rash but appear to act by direct contact with an abraded epidermis rather than through dissemination after inhalant exposure. Foods—especially egg white—can be shown to flare skin lesions in a minority of children and deserve careful attention. Although the importance of ingestant allergens appears to decline sharply with increasing age, prolonged avoidance of food offenders, identified by challenge, clearly is justified.

Without a basis for allergen-specific measures in most

*Recently the high mortality rate associated with eczema vaccinatum has been substantially reduced by administration of vaccinia immune globulin and by improved supportive care.

cases, the approach to treatment of atopic dermatitis remains largely symptomatic (i.e., nonspecific symptom suppression). Locally applied agents are quite useful, but care to avoid potential irritants and topical sensitizers is essential. Prolonged use of bland, inexpensive lubricants is the foundation of most treatment programs and often suffices to keep the disorder quiescent. Oil-in-water emulsions (e.g., water washable base USP and Dermabase) may be adequate and act as minimally greasy vanishing creams. More effective lubrication can be obtained with water-in-oil emulsions (ointments) including hydrophilic ointment USP, Eucerine, and Aquaphor. Inert oils such as yellow and white petrolatum provide maximum greasiness and protection from dry air, etc., but their occlusive properties often promote retention of debris and troublesome pruritus.

Topical corticosteroids are widely useful in atopic dermatitis, but these costly preparations should be employed for their anti-inflammatory properties alone rather than general lubrication. Where indicated, topically applied steroids may be covered with an occluding layer of polyethylene to promote absorption of the drug, a strategy especially feasible at night. Steroids have largely replaced the once-popular coal tar preparation as anti-inflammatory agents. Tars are still used rarely to reduce lichenification and cracking, although urea-containing ointments are more cosmetically acceptable agents to promote healing and restoration of skin texture.

In managing atopic dermatitis, reduction of pruritus is both an end in itself and a means of interrupting the harmful "scratch-itch" cycle. Oral antipruritic agents

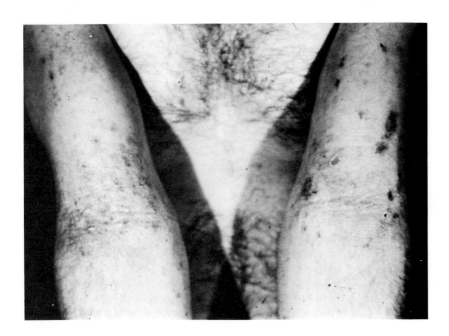

FIGURE 11-1 Chronic lesions of atopic dermatitis on the flexor surfaces of the arms of a young male; erosions, pigmentary changes, and a deepening of skin creases (lichenification) are evident. (From J. M. Sheldon, R. G. Lovell, and K. P. Mathews, A Manual of Clinical Allergy, 2d ed., Saunders, Philadelphia, 1967.)

such as diphenhydramine (Benadryl) and hydroxyzine (Atarax, Vistaril) are especially useful at night when subconscious scratch responses can do serious damage. Finger and toenails also should be kept as short as possible (consistent with comfort) to minimize trauma, and, for young children, soft, padded mittens or frank restraint of the extremities may be essential to sustain improvement. Well-washed cotton clothing is generally preferred, and, as a rule, fibers such as wool and synthetics that "snag" the skin must be avoided because of palpable irritant effects. Chapping due to cold dry air is quite harmful to eczematous persons, and well-maintained sources of humidification can offset the tendency of this condition to worsen in winter; organic solvents that defat even normal skin also must be scrupulously avoided. A more subtle drying effect is inflicted by the regular use of soap and water or by contact with water alone. This problem may be approached, in part, by using skin cleaners with low emulsifying activity. In addition, regular use of topical lubricants after washing or of emulsified oils in bath water is often helpful. However, frequent bathing by eczematous per-

sons is desirable only rarely, and water temperature should be maintained in a "tepid" range since body heating commonly will increase pruritus.

Acute flares of atopic dermatitis are especially frequent in children and present prominent redness, vesicle formation, and oozing, which may require inpatient care. Brief periods of high-dose systemic corticosteroids will usually speed resolution, and the need for antimicrobial agents requires careful consideration. In addition, cool soaks will reduce itching and remove cutaneous debris. Where involvement is general, cool tap-water baths, with or without agents such as colloidal oatmeal, may provide an antipruritic effect more efficiently. As acute lesions begin to resolve, shake lotions are often useful, followed by progressively greasier applications more typical of chronic care programs.

URTICARIA

Hives (urticaria) are familiar skin lesions and, at some time, probably affect at least 25 percent of the population. Many clinical forms of urticaria exist, and it appears that a variety of determinants ultimately will be recognized. At present, it seems clear that *some* types of urticaria reflect immunologic processes (especially those involving IgE) while others remain totally unexplained. This practical reality must be faced, since the resemblance of urticarial wheals to IgE-mediated skin reactions often has prompted the false inference that hives per se indicate allergy. Microscopically, most urticarial lesions present only edema, variable dilatation of vessels, and occasional neutrophils and eosinophils; in some patients, however, *grossly* identical lesions also show a definite vasculitis. The discrete, raised, pruritic, nontender lesions of urticaria appear most often on the trunk and proximal extremities, individual wheals rarely lasting over 36 hours; angioedema (see Chap. 9) manifested by painless, minimally pruritic, swelling of subcutaneous and submucosal tissues is occasionally associated.

Most episodes of urticaria are brief and self-limited, especially in childhood when hives commonly are related to preceding respiratory infections. In a minority of adults and, rarely, children, however, unexplained hives may persist for many months or years. The evaluation of such persons requires, first, exclusion of a serious underlying disease as the factor promoting urticaria; prominent among these are lymphomas, systemic lupus erythematosus, hyperthyroidism, and nonlymphoid neoplasms. While chronic foci of bacterial infection and intestinal parasites are often sought in these patients, they are rarely shown to cause the chronic hives.

Like anaphylactic reactions, urticaria can result from IgE-mediated responses to protein allergens. In both situations, the implicated agents usually are ingestants—especially such foods as egg, fish, diverse shellfish, and nuts, including the peanut. In addition, drugs and drug metabolites capable of stable bonding to proteins (e.g., penicillin derivatives), or themselves com-

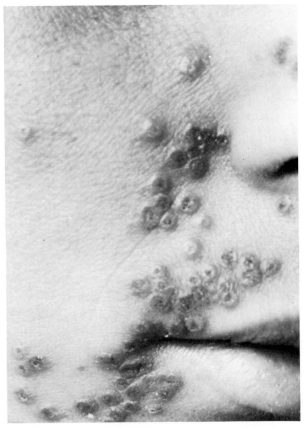

FIGURE 11-2 Facial lesions of eczema herpeticum in a young adult with life-long atopic dermatitis.

plete antigens, are prominent factors in systemic or urticarial Type I reactions (see Chap. 9). However, many drugs also appear to cause urticaria by mechanisms exclusive of IgE. Aspirin is probably the most frequent offender in this group and has been said to worsen nonspecifically 25 percent of chronic urticaria cases.

Physical factors are the major determinants in a proportion of patients with chronic urticaria, and of these environmental influences cold is probably most frequently implicated. Cold urticaria especially affects young adults and may appear with the most minor degrees of chilling. Hives develop in some as skin temperature falls but generally require rewarming for their appearance. Cold urticaria can be associated with large rises in plasma histamine levels (e.g., in venous blood from a chilled extremity), and headache as well as hypotension may result. This effect has led to disaster occasionally when affected persons have developed syncope while swimming, and drowned as a result. Urticaria also may be elicited specifically by local heating, the lesions being immediate in some subjects and delayed as long as several hours in others. Total-body heating (e.g., a warm bath) also can worsen pruritus and whealing of diverse additional causes. In addition, *cholinergic urticaria* is a clinically distinct syndrome in which physical exertion, emotional stress, and environmental warmth elicit crops of tiny wheals, each surrounded by a broad border of redness. Affected persons commonly show abnormally large whealing or erythematous responses to intradermal methacholine, although the pathogenetic significance of this reactivity remains unclear. A period of sustained running usually elicits typical wheals permitting confirmation of the diagnosis. Local urtication (hive formation) or angioedema also may follow exposure to sustained pressure, various wavelengths of light, or vibratory stimuli. Some of these rare conditions appear to be familial. Furthermore, in certain examples of heat-, light-, or cold-induced urticaria, local specific reactivity can be conferred on normal subjects by transfer of IgE in serum of affected persons. At present, it is not clear whether these "passive transfer" phenomena involve classical antigen-antibody reactions or alternative mechanisms.

Urticaria due to pressure most commonly occurs in those with dermographism (Fig. 11-3) in whom firm stroking will produce definite whealing responses. Dermographism is long-standing in a small proportion of normal persons but also may be acquired, appearing after adverse drug reactions or in disease states promoting infiltration of skin by mast cells. Dermographic persons typically develop wheals at pressure points including the buttocks and soles of the feet as well as beneath watch straps, belts, and tight underclothing.

Instances of angioedema accompanying acute urticaria are occasionally confused with hereditary angioedema (HANE), a familial defect in the control of inflammation. HANE manifests recurrent bouts of edema involving peripheral structures as well as the larynx and bowel, the last producing intense abdominal pain and often leading to exploratory laparotomies. These episodes rarely appear before age 10 and may recur indefinitely although their frequency often decreases after the sixth decade. Physical trauma (often quite subtle) may precede the edema, but many bouts are unexplained. Laryngeal edema poses a serious threat to life in these patients, and pedigree analysis usually reveals one or more instances in each family where this complication has caused death by asphyxiation. Swelling in this condition usually develops over many hours, regresses equally slowly, and is *not* accompanied by urticaria. HANE patients are known to share low activity levels of the factor that normally inhibits the acti-

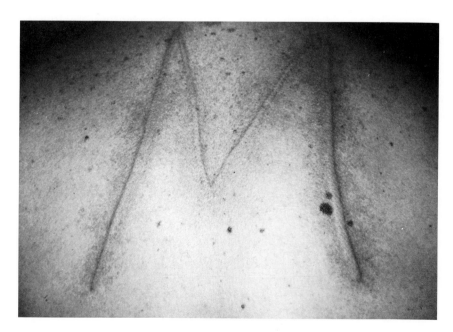

FIGURE 11-3 Dermographism evident 2 minutes after stroking the back lightly with a fingernail. The subject had occasional urticarial wheals at the beltline and on his buttocks.

vated first component of the complement system C1 as well as additional components concerned with clotting, inflammation, and fibrinolysis. As a result of this deficiency, C1 effects are unopposed, and C1 proceeds to activate and consume the early sequence components C4 and C2, which on assay are demonstrably low in this condition. A kininlike peptide has been described as a by-product of C2 activation, and its excessive generation in HANE may underlie this condition. Treatment measures are properly focused on preservation of the airway, avoidance of needless laparotomy, and general support. Currently available drugs contribute little to acute care; however, regular use of either methyltestosterone or epsilon-aminocaproic acid and its congeners may reduce the frequency of attacks.

Few additional conditions lend confusion to the evaluation of ordinary urticaria and angioedema. Occasionally, penetrants such as stinging plant hairs or insects produce troublesome whealing reactions, and the possibility of dermographism should not be overlooked. Chronic, pruritic, raised papules, termed *papular urticaria*, often follow insect bites, especially on the legs in childhood, but the persistence and induration (viz., firm consistency) of these lesions usually sets them apart. Typical urticaria may accompany serious primary disease or may follow trivial viral syndromes; however, frequently no cause is evident initially. Drugs or chemical additives in foods and beverages are often identified as sources of urticaria and should be evaluated carefully, although confirmatory in vitro tests rarely are available. Similarly, a painstaking review of historical details may provide evidence implicating foods, physical agents, or psychogenic factors.

Since bouts of hives generally are self-limited and vary in duration as well as in severity, the value of treatment measures for affected individuals often is difficult to discern. However, epinephrine has demonstrated effectiveness in speeding the resolution of acute urticaria and angioedema. Agents such as diphenhydramine and hydroxyzine also are acknowledged to have value in this condition, although both cause prominent sedation. Adrenal cortical steroids have been beneficial in severe acute hives but often fail to influence the course of longer established disease. In chronic urticaria, justifiable reassurance and use of optimal antihistaminic-sympathomimetic medications are of paramount importance; of these, hydroxyzine often is the single most valuable agent. Although repeated study of such patients rarely is fruitful, all concerned should remain receptive to clues that may implicate a responsible factor.

QUESTIONS

Atopic dermatitis—urticaria—Chap. 11

Directions: Circle the letter preceding each item below that correctly answers each question. More than one answer may be correct.

1 Patients with atopic dermatitis usually have increased serum levels of:
 a IgE b IgM c IgG d IgA

2 All of the following descriptions are typical of the skin lesions of atopic dermatitis EXCEPT:
 a Edematous b Typical wheal-and-flare response c Crusting and scaling d Infiltrated with mononuclear cells and eosinophils

3 Atopic dermatitis occurs with particular frequency among persons manifesting:
 a Hay fever b Allergic rhinitis c Allergic eczematous contact dermatitis d Bronchial asthma

4 Which of the following are characteristics of infantile eczema?
 a Usually appears in the first year of life b Is associated with a great increase in sebaceous activity producing an excessively oily skin c In all cases resolves permanently by 3 years of age d Is associated with red, raised, pruritic, scaling areas involving the cheeks, scalp, and diaper area

5 All of the following are potential complications of infantile eczema EXCEPT:
 a Infection with pyogenic (pus-forming) bacteria b Massive hemorrhage into affected skin c Sweat retention and severe itching d Thickening and lichenification of skin

6 In children acute flares of atopic dermatitis which are characterized by prominent redness, vesicle formation, and oozing may be treated by all of the following EXCEPT:
 a Systemic corticosteroids b Antipruritic agents c Oral cold tar preparations d Antimicrobial agents

7 Most urticarial lesions show microscopically:
 a Edema b Variable dilatation of vessels c Neutrophils and eosinophils d Severe destructive vasculitis

8 Which of the following characteristics are true of urticaria?
 a There are pruritic, nontender lesions. b There is inflammatory swelling of subcutaneous tissue. c Lesions appear most often on the face, palms, and soles. d Angioedema is always present.

9 The evaluation of persons with unexplained hives which persist for months or years requires exclusion of which of the following diseases?
 a Hay fever b Lymphomas c Bronchial asthma d Systemic lupus erythematosus

10 In the causation of chronic urticaria, which of the following physical factors is probably the most frequently responsible?
 a Cold b Light c Heat d Vibration

11 All of the following factors may elicit *generalized* cholinergic urticaria EXCEPT:
 a Physical exertion b Emotional stress c Environmental cold d Intradermal methacholine

12 Hereditary angioedema (HANE):
 a Involves the same mechanism as angioedema ac-

companying acute urticaria *b* Manifests recurrent bouts of edema involving peripheral structures as well as the larynx and bowel *c* Produces laryngeal edema which usually develops in a matter of minutes and is accompanied by urticaria *d* Implies low activity levels of the factor that normally inhibits the activated first component of the complement system

Directions: Circle the T for true and the F for false. Correct the false statements.

13   T   F   In persons with atopic dermatitis, factors such as house dust, animal danders, etc., commonly worsen the rash through inhalant exposure.

14   T   F   The approach to the treatment of atopic dermatitis remains largely symptomatic.

15   T   F   Topical corticosteroids are used properly in atopic dermatitis for their general lubricating properties.

16   T   F   Oral antipruritic agents such as diphenhydramine and hydroxyzine are especially useful in atopic dermatitis at night when subconscious scratch responses can do serious damage.

17   T   F   Coal tar preparations are, at present, the most widely used preparations to reduce lichenification and cracking.

18   T   F   In order to prevent chapping due to cold dry air in eczematous persons organic solvents should be used.

19   T   F   Both anaphylactic reactions and urticaria can result from IgE-mediated response to protein allergens.

20   T   F   Hives per se indicate allergy.

21   T   F   Local urtication (hive formation) may follow exposure to local body heating.

22   T   F   Dermographism in normal persons may appear after adverse drug reactions or in disease states promoting infiltration of skin by mast cells.

Directions: Answer the following questions on a separate sheet of paper.

23 List the usually implicated agents in both anaphylactic reactions and urticaria.

24 Discuss the treatment measures used for acute urticaria and angioedema.

CHAPTER 12 Autoimmune and Immune Complex-Induced Diseases

OBJECTIVES   **At the completion of Chap. 12 you should be able to:**

1 Define *autoantibodies*.

2 Illustrate with an example the way in which immune responses to autologous (i.e., host-derived) tissue components could arise.

3 Explain the way in which autoaggressive immune reactions may originate.

4 Describe Goodpasture's syndrome as an apparent example of antibody-mediated human autoimmunity.

5 Identify the characteristics of idiopathic thrombocytopenic purpura (ITP), its relationship to antiplatelet antibodies, and its treatment.

6 Illustrate, with examples, immunohemolytic (IH) processes.

7 Explain the Coombs' test and the significance of a positive reaction.

8 For hemolytic reactions to transfused blood, describe the signs and symptoms, population at risk, complications, feasibility of prevention, and desirable precautions.

9 In addition to manifestations of hemolysis, list the forms of adverse reactions that may accompany transfusions of blood or blood products.

10 Describe the effects of infusing serums containing potent leuko-agglutinins.

11 Describe the nature and origin of adverse reactions to transfusion in persons deficient in IgA.

12 State how the reactions described in objective no. 11 may be averted.

13 Explain for spontaneously developing immunohemolytic (IH) phenomena (viz., "warm" red blood cell autoantibodies and "cold" autoantibodies to red blood cells) the hypersensitivity reaction, age group affected, disease entities, signs and symptoms, and treatment.

14 Describe the clinical manifestations of serum sickness following a first exposure to horse serum.

15 Describe the pathogenesis of serum sickness.

16 Identify the etiology, onset, signs and symptoms, type of hypersensitivity reaction, laboratory findings, and associated clinical conditions of serum sickness.

17 Describe the reactions that occur with prolonged antigen exposure in individuals making only modest antibody responses.

18 Describe the characteristics of allergic eczematous contact dermatitis by identifying the type of hypersensitivity it connotes, abnormality produced, areas involved, examples of topical irritants and sensitizers, treatment, and characteristics of the diagnostic tests used.

Although injury to the host often is *incidental* to immune processes, host tissues, understandably, are rarely the target of antibody or cell-mediated attack. In many conditions, autoantibodies (i.e., antibodies reactive with autologous tissue components) arise, providing valuable diagnostic markers. However, only rarely do these serum factors appear to be responsible for direct tissue injury.

Although the appearance of autoantibodies denotes a failure of safeguards which normally prevent their emergence, responsible factors are rarely identifiable. In some instances (e.g., ocular pigment and endocrine gland cell components) the inciting antigens are normally sequestered and may remain "foreign" even to mature lymphoid tissues. If injury releases these heretofore locally confined materials into the general circulation, an immune response might readily occur with secondary damage to the injured organ and related structures. This mechanism does, in fact, appear to operate in certain eye conditions (e.g., sympathetic ophthalmia) and in several endocrine deficiency states. Immune responses to host tissue components could arise also following more subtle injury incident to microbial invasion. The possibility that infecting bacteria and viruses may produce *limited* changes in host tissue components rendering them "foreign" to immune surveillance has also been proposed. Antibodies (or sensitized lymphocytes) resulting from this process might have specificities broad enough to permit reaction with *native* as well as modified tissue determinants. In addition, autoimmune phenomena could result if an invading organism (or other introduced agent) and host tissues shared an antigen or closely similar antigenic groups as a result of parallel evolution. Although invoked especially with regard to the pathogenesis of poststreptococcal glomerulonephritis and rheumatic fever, this mechanism remains unsupported. Finally, it is reasonable to speculate that autoaggressive immune reactions may originate with mutant ("forbidden") clones of lymphoid cells programmed to recognize normal host components as "foreign."

Although the disorder is rare, Goodpasture's syndrome has attracted considerable attention as an apparent example of antibody-mediated human autoimmunity causing major damage to internal organs. The typical clinical picture of recurrent pulmonary hemorrhage (Fig. 12-1) and anemia coupled with progressive kidney failure has been described in Part VII; however, the relative severity of these features varies among patients. Most Goodpasture's cases present no evident cause, although the disease *has* followed viral and chemical insults to the lungs. Circulating antibodies, reactive with glomerular (kidney) and alveolar (lung) basement membranes, are usually present and, along with complement components, form linear deposits at these sites in vivo. The associated tissue damage is thought to reflect complement-mediated cytotoxicity and local effects of recruited neutrophils.

Human antibody-dependent, autoimmune disorders most often affect formed elements of the blood, with platelets and red blood cells attacked predominantly. Increasing evidence has linked the disease idiopathic thrombocytopenic purpura (ITP) with circulating IgG molecules reactive with host platelets. Even when fixed to platelet surfaces, these antibodies do not cause localization of complement proteins or lysis of platelets in the free circulation. However, platelets bearing Ig molecules are more readily removed and destroyed by macrophages in the spleen and liver. Evidence support-

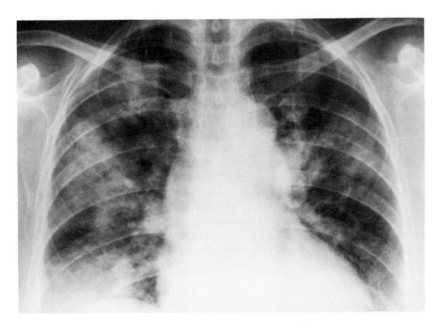

FIGURE 12-1 *Frontal chext x-ray during active pulmonary involvement in Goodpasture's syndrome. (Film courtesy of Dr. Terry Solver.)*

ing this mechanism for thrombocytopenia has come from studies of ITP patients and experimental subjects who have shown severe but brief platelet deficits after receiving ITP serums; transient thrombocytopenia, noted in infants delivered by mothers with ITP, also is consistent. ITP may follow infections—especially in childhood—but often appears without prior event and commonly resolves after days or weeks. Persistent ITP usually may be suppressed by corticosteroids which are thought to act largely by reducing platelet removal by spleen and liver. However, when the disease has lasted 6 or more months, the prospect of prolonged high-dose steroid treatment with its inherent side effects generally prompts a splenectomy. Platelet counts usually rise and may become normal after this procedure despite continued sequestration by the liver; in either case, lower steroid requirements result in most patients.

Red blood cell membranes carry literally hundreds of described antigens, and immunoglobulins reacting with one or more of these are found in ill as well as otherwise normal persons. Depending upon the type, specificity, and number of antibody molecules involved, their fixation to membrane sites may have no effect or may shorten cell life by extravascular removal or intravascular lysis. Where decreased survival results, stigmata of increased turnover of heme pigments (see Part III) usually can be demonstrated, and frank anemia will develop if the host's erythropoietic capacity cannot fully compensate. Generically, these conditions often are described as immunohemolytic (IH) processes. Hemolytic transfusion reactions are a distinctive form of IH process occurring usually when a recipient already sensitized to "foreign" human red blood cell antigens by pregnancy or prior transfusion receives blood containing these antigens. Far less often, transfused blood contains antibodies reactive with the recipient's erythrocytes. However, most IH processes arise through production by the host of antibodies reactive with his or her own red blood cells.

The Coombs' test provides information central to the description of IH disorders. In this procedure antibodies derived from other species (e.g., goat) and directed toward human immunoglobulins and/or complement are mixed with washed human erythrocytes. If these cells have, bound to their surfaces, the appropriate human serum components, then the foreign antiserum, by reacting with molecules on adjacent cells, will tend to link the cells and cause them to clump visibly (Fig. 12-2). In practice, the foreign (Coombs') serum is usually mixed directly with cells from drawn blood. A positive (clumping) reaction in this "direct Coombs' test" indicates that circulating cells with significant numbers of bound immunoreactive molecules are present. At times, the direct test is negative despite the presence in serum of antibodies reactive with human erythrocytes other than those of the host. These may be detected by in-

cubating the serums with human red blood cells of compatible ABO and Rh types and then performing a direct Coombs' test. Red blood cell agglutination in this "indirect Coombs' test" serves as an indicator of unsuspected serum antibody and as an important warning of danger prior to an intended blood transfusion. Direct Coombs' reactions are often performed with antiserums specific for human IgG or the third component of serum complement (C3).

Hemolytic reactions to transfused blood provide the most dramatic and dangerous IH phenomena observed clinically. These responses almost always appear *during* infusion of the offending blood and are marked by rapid intravascular lysis of red blood cells due to the circulating antibodies. Those at risk largely comprise persons sensitized to red blood cells antigens by prior pregnancy, transfusion, or unknown factors that may include bacterial or viral infection. Victims of transfusion reactions tend to manifest chills, fever, and low back pain—occasionally preceded by urticaria or flushing and often by uneasiness and mild air hunger. In addition, when cell lysis is massive, the resulting debris may trigger widespread *intravascular* clotting with consumptive depletion of coagulation factors and bleeding from wounds and venipuncture sites. Survivors of severe acute reactions also share a high risk of acute kidney failure promoted by shock and massive hemoglobinuria.

Considering these dire consequences, every reasonable measure to prevent or mitigate hemolytic transfusion reactions is justified. Basic to this effort are care in identifying the source and proper recipient of blood products as well as continual surveillance of persons receiving blood—especially of those whose mobility or awareness is impaired. Any serious question of an incipient reaction should prompt discontinuance of the questioned infusion, maintenance of intravenous access, and close clinical observation. A carefully drawn venous sample from the recipient should be checked for serum hemoglobin and the compatibility of donor and recipient reconfirmed. Without exception, *all* materials used for transfusion should be saved to facilitate serological and microbiological testing. Special precautions to monitor urine output are essential, and examination of serial centrifuged specimens for hemoglobin may be instructive. Maintenance of adequate hydration and urine flow are important considerations in all survivors, and osmotic diuresis with cautiously administered IV mannitol (beginning with an adult dose of 25 g) may help in achieving this goal. Safe fluid therapy demands precise and regular evaluation of cardiopulmonary and renal function. Measures to combat shock, pulmonary edema, acute renal failure, and/or defibrination may be required.

In addition to manifestations of hemolysis, several forms of adverse reaction may accompany transfusion of blood or blood products. Urticaria alone occurs rarely in recipients and, especially in atopic persons, may reflect trace amounts of food or other allergens in transfused

FIGURE 12-2 Reaction sequences in the direct (A) and indirect (B) Coombs' tests.

serum. In those requiring blood repeatedly or following multiple pregnancies, antibodies directed to human leukocyte membrane antigens often develop. With subsequent transfusion of "foreign" whole blood, these factors are available to agglutinate leukocytes and, at times, platelets. These reactions are the most common source of transfusion-associated fever, although vital organs are little affected. Suitable blood for those with leukoagglutinins may be obtained by filtration through nylon fibers or reconstitution from the frozen state, both preparations being essentially leukocyte-free. Where *serums* containing potent leukoagglutinins have been infused, recipients have developed fever, cough, shortness of breath, and lung shadows on chest x-ray; several days have been required for full resolution. Persons deficient in IgA also may suffer severe reactions from transfused IgA in plasma as a result of antibodies formed

to this immunoglobulin. Clinically, these episodes often resemble anaphylaxis with dyspnea, flushing, abdominal cramps, and diarrhea as well as fever and chills. These reactions may be averted by using IgA-deficient donors or thoroughly washed red blood cells. In addition to these problems, personnel supervising transfusion therapy must be alert for possible air embolism, volume overload, septicemia from microbial contamination, chilling from excessively cold blood, and calcium or platelet deficiency following massive blood replacement.

Spontaneously developing IH phenomena are divisible into three general categories: (1) types associated

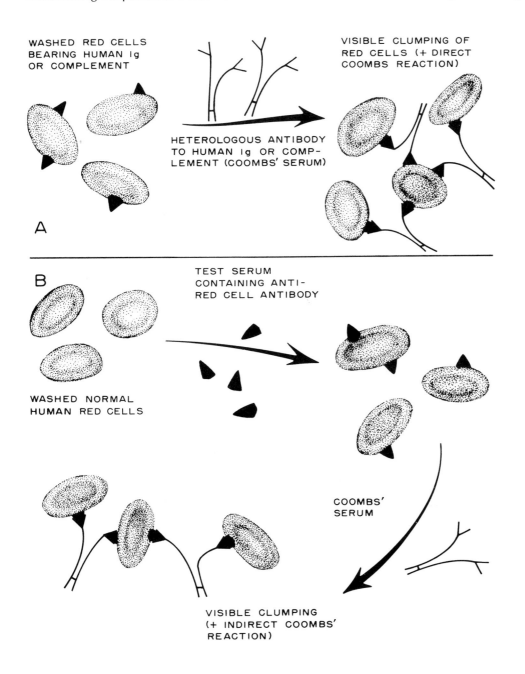

WASHED RED CELLS
BEARING HUMAN Ig
OR COMPLEMENT

HETEROLOGOUS ANTIBODY
TO HUMAN Ig OR COMP-
LEMENT (COOMBS' SERUM)

VISIBLE CLUMPING OF
RED CELLS (+ DIRECT
COOMBS REACTION)

A

B

TEST SERUM
CONTAINING ANTI-
RED CELL ANTIBODY

WASHED NORMAL
HUMAN RED CELLS

COOMBS'
SERUM

VISIBLE CLUMPING
(+ INDIRECT COOMBS'
REACTION)

with medications (see Chap. 13); (2) types with "warm" red blood cell autoantibodies reacting at 37°C; and (3) a group of conditions with "cold" antibodies that bind at lower temperatures and often only in a range of 4 to 15°C. Warm autoantibodies are usually of the IgG class and are recognized primarily in middle-aged adults. In more than one-half of these, a serious primary disease such as chronic lymphocytic leukemia, lymphoid (and rarely nonlymphoid) tumors, or systemic lupus erythematosus will become evident, and these conditions substantially determine the prognosis for affected individuals. The IH disorder may be evident only as a positive Coombs' test (with antihuman IgG) or rarely may lead to fulminant, fatal hemolysis. Most commonly, however, chronic morbidity results with pallor, fatigue, and weakness as well as recurrent fever and jaundice; dyspnea arising from heart failure, angina pectoris, and vascular thrombosis are also common. Splenic enlargement is a frequent finding, and this organ also is the main site of red blood cell destruction. Splenic trapping of erythrocytes is most marked when both IgG autoantibody and C3 are present on their surfaces. Where treatment is necessary, adrenocortical steroids are a proper first consideration, inducing remissions in over two-thirds of patients although relapses are common when these drugs are withdrawn. Splenectomy is undertaken where steroids, in acceptable doses, have proven inadequate alone. In addition immunosuppressive (cytotoxic) agents (e.g., cyclophosphamide and azathioprine) may provide additional value in highly selected patients. Since warm hemolysins commonly react with cells of essentially all potential normal donors, transfusions pose extreme difficulties and are avoided if possible. Where no other choice remains, addition of Coombs' serum following incubation of the patient's serum and panels of cells permit the least incompatible ones to be chosen.

Cold autoantibodies to red blood cells generally bind at temperatures well below 32°C; however, these molecules become dissociated at warmer levels required for the "fixation" (i.e., cell-surface localization) of complement. Because of this, hemolysis may be absent and red blood cell agglutination minor despite extremely high levels of autoantibody. IgM class cold agglutinins are demonstrable often in infectious mononucleosis and *Mycoplasma pneumoniae* infections, although decreased red blood cell survival rarely results. Chronic cold-dependent hemolysis is evident, however, in certain elderly persons, many of whom have lymphoid neoplasms and IgM autoantibodies. Besides stigmata of chronic hemolysis, these patients display signs of red blood cell agglutination (e.g., pain, cyanosis) in the peripheral circulation on exposure to cold. High titers of cold agglutinins in serum are prominent, and complement components are usually demonstrable on the red blood cells. Treatment considerations usually focus on the associated malignancy (where present), although

corticosteroids or immunosuppressive drugs have seemed beneficial in individual cases. A quite different situation involving IgG hemolysins has been seen with syphilis as well as viral infections and in some apparently normal persons. Termed *paroxysmal cold hemoglobinuria*, this condition presents short bouts of back and extremity pain, fever, chills, and hemoglobinuria precipitated by cold exposure. Sensitization of red blood cells usually occurs below 15°C, and, on rewarming, complement factors are fixed to membrane sites permitting brisk hemolysis.

Antibodies apparently reactive with normal tissue components are associated with diverse additional human disease states. However, in the majority of these conditions, antibody-induced *damage* has not been demonstrated, although, in some instances (e.g., systemic lupus erythematosus), pathogenic immune complexes are recognized. Since these various serum factors currently are associated more with diagnostic than pathogenetic considerations, they are discussed briefly in chapters treating diseases of major organ systems.

SERUM SICKNESS AND OTHER (TYPE III) CONDITIONS INDUCED BY CIRCULATING IMMUNE COMPLEXES

Serum sickness was among the earliest recognized hypersensitivity diseases and is considered the prototypic immune complex–induced illness. Originally observed following large volumes of unfractionated equine antiserums administered for prophylaxis of diphtheria, tetanus, etc., this condition is most prevalent today after drugs (e.g., penicillin and sulfonamides). The development of serum sickness requires administration (usually by injection) of an antigenic material that will remain in the circulation until a specific antibody response occurs, as shown in Fig. 12-3. At that time, the slowly diminishing blood levels of antigen drop sharply, denoting the formation of immune (antigen-antibody) complexes which are cleared from circulation rapidly by macrophage-monocyte scavenging and other mechanisms (viz., "immune elimination"). Complexes are formed initially in considerable antigen excess with small aggregates comprising one antibody molecule and two antigen molecules (or determinate groups) predominating. As antibody synthesis and immune elimination proceed following a single antigen dose, a state of antibody excess develops progressively. Between these extremes is a (usually brief) period when modest antigen excess occurs and somewhat larger complexes with molecular proportions approaching three antigen to two antibody predominate. Such complexes are capable of activating complement components and probably other amplification systems that mediate inflammation. Furthermore these complexes, due to their physical properties, are readily deposited in the walls of small vessels in many organs including the kidneys; inflammatory changes follow at these sites.

After initial exposure to an appropriate sensitizer, manifestations of serum sickness classically appear in 10 to 14 days; shorter latent periods precede second or subsequent attacks if exposure is repeated. Frequently the most prominent manifestation (Fig. 12-4) is urticaria—often severe and confluent—and angioedema, although skin lesions rarely may resemble bruises or the rash of measles. In addition, many persons develop fever, muscle soreness, and malaise. Lymphadenopathy, with enlarged and tender nodes, is often generalized and may be especially striking in those groups draining the site of introduction of the causative agent. Joint pain (arthralgia) may occur alone, or frank arthritis may affect several large joints together or sequentially. Although genitourinary symptoms are rare, urinalysis may reveal excessive excretion of albumin and, occasionally, of erythrocytes and white blood cells. Gastrointestinal complaints of nausea, vomiting, and abdominal pain infrequently dominate the picture, and, rarely, cardiac or peripheral nerve dysfunction is seen. In view of these diverse manifestations it is often difficult to distinguish serum sickness from certain infectious (especially viral) processes as well as conditions including rheumatic fever, sickle-cell crisis, glomerulonephritis, and bacterial endocarditis. Laboratory findings offer limited guidance in this differential process, although a modest leukocytosis, elevated red blood cell sedimentation rate, and *transient* depression of serum complement activity are characteristic of serum sickness.

As indicated above, complement-fixing immune complexes, presumably containing specific IgG and/or IgM, are implicated strongly in the causation of serum sickness. In addition, a majority of affected persons show tissue-fixing antibodies that mediate wheal-and-flare skin reactivity to the implicated antigen and may contribute

to clinical urticaria and angioedema.* There is growing evidence that the reactions of these factors with antigen promote release of mast cell–derived mediator substances which increase the permeability of small-vessel walls and thereby favor the deposition of complement-fixing complexes. In support of this mechanism are data *suggesting* that prophylactic use of antihistaminic agents may reduce the incidence of clinical serum sickness in high risk human populations—an effect also clearly shown in animal models.

Serum sickness typically is a brief illness and may require substantially no medication in many cases. However, considerable relief of discomfort may be achieved with regular doses of aspirin for fever and rheumatic complaints, as well as antihistaminic drugs and, if needed, epinephrine, to suppress urticaria and angioedema. Where these measures do not suffice, especially if urinary tract or neurological changes are pronounced, a brief course of corticosteroid treatment is justifiable. Careful prospective avoidance of the implicated antigen is essential, since acute systemic reactions as well as a more prompt reappearance of serum sickness may develop if exposure reoccurs.

Prolonged antigen exposure occurring in individuals making only *modest* antibody responses can promote a

*A majority of these factors probably are IgE; however, in a few cases studied, this activity also seemed to reside in other immunoglobulin classes.

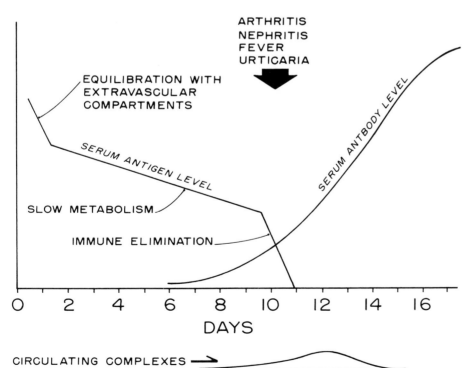

FIGURE 12-3 *Trends in immune reactants during the course of serum sickness.*

chronic condition in which complexes, formed in relative antigen excess, circulate. This situation may be produced readily in laboratory animals and, in human beings, occurs with systemic lupus erythematosus, bacterial endocarditis, and prolonged infections including malaria, syphilis, and leprosy. Deposition of immune complexes affects especially the kidney, where antigen as well as host antibody and complement (singly or in combination) may be demonstrated along the glomerular basement membrane or between adjacent capillaries (Fig. 12-5). As an apparent result of these deposits, inflammatory cells accumulate, the basement membranes thicken, and glomerular cells swell and proliferate, obliterating normal nephron structure. Changes in other organs also are recognized due largely to accumulation of complexes in vascular walls.

A syndrome of fever, arthritis, urticaria, and low serum complement levels has been observed early in the course of hepatitis B infection associated with circulating complexes of viral surface antigen (HbsAg) and host antibody. As liver involvement becomes manifest, this syndrome clears; its subsidence correlates, in time, with rising antibody titers and, usually, disappearance of HbsAg from serum. It seems probable that additional examples of immune complex–induced systemic vascular damage will be appreciated in the future. In addition, effects of locally formed complexes have been implicated increasingly in conditions including extrinsic allergic alveolitis (hypersensitivity pneumonitis) and rheumatoid synovitis. While offending antigens remain speculative in many cases, long-standing viral infections and pollutant chemicals deserve special consideration.

CONTACT DERMATITIS—A TYPE IV RESPONSE

Delayed-type hypersensitivity (DTH), mediated by specifically sensitized lymphocytes, provides a major defensive resource opposing attack by fungi, viruses, and bacteria adapted to intracellular growth as well as a deterrent to growth of malignant cells. Inflammation,

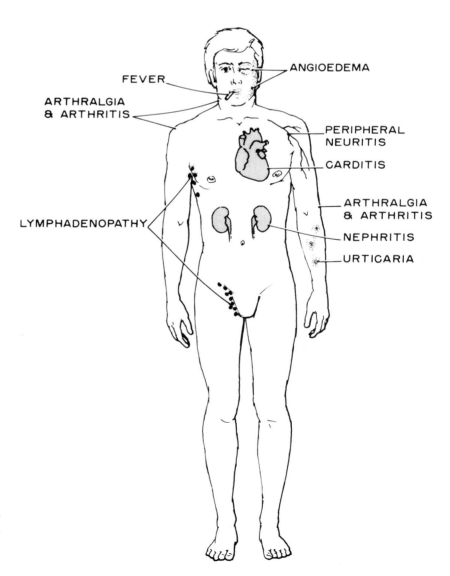

FIGURE 12-4 Manifestations that may occur during serum sickness. Despite these diverse possibilities, many patients experience only fever with skin and/or joint problems.

incident to these necessary responses, often injures normal host tissues. However, there are relatively few situations in which DTH underlies a response which is not substantially protective; of these, the most familiar is allergic eczematous contact dermatitis (AECD). Indeed, in the North American population as a whole, AECD (especially that due to poison ivy and its relatives) is the most frequently encountered *allergic* disorder.

AECD typically presents a pruritic, reddened, thickened area of skin which often shows relatively fragile vesicles (Fig. 12-6). Edema of the involved area often is intense at the outset and, if the face, genitalia, or a distal extremity is involved, may simulate angioedema. With chronicity, although pruritus remains, the rash comes to resemble "eczema" of any cause, with prominent lichenification and scaling. Involved skin shows an influx of mononuclear cells, especially about minute blood vessels, and separation, by edema, of cells in deeper layers of the epidermis (spongiosis) and the adjacent dermis. In many lesions, mast cells are uniquely prominent in the inflammatory infiltrate. AECD reflects application of a sensitizer to the skin and the rash typically is confined to the area of exposure. Although any portion of the skin surface may become affected, hairless areas, especially the eyelids, are more commonly involved. Reactions of contact sensitivity occur rarely on the oral, vaginal, and anal mucous membranes.

Contact sensitizers are highly reactive substances which often have quite simple chemical structures. Studies in laboratory animals suggest that these materials, on application to skin, penetrate to the deeper epidermal layers where they complex, as haptens, with cutaneous proteins. The resulting conjugates are presented to cells of draining lymph nodes where lymphocytes specifically able to recognize conjugates of the hapten and adjacent portions of the protein carrier are

developed. Hapten-protein conjugation is repeated with subsequent contact exposures and sensitized lymphocytes respond, providing direct cytotoxicity and lymphokine-generated inflammation.

AECD should be suspected in highly pruritic erruptions having patterns of distribution that suggest specific topical exposure. Potential offenders are assessed through a comprehensive environmental review with special attention to topical medications, plant oils, cosmetics and perfumes, cleaning supplies, and work-associated materials. Possible sensitizers may be evaluated by attempting to create the disease in miniature through the use of patch tests. With this approach, extracts or solid fragments of test materials are placed on the unabraided skin, covered with a water-repellent patch, and taped in place. After 48 hours, the sites are uncovered and examined for induration and vesicle formation (Fig. 12-7). Positive reactions may be intense with painful skin erosions as a possible result, and subjects should be prepared to remove patches promptly if itching is severe; offending sites then should be washed thoroughly. In addition, patch testing may worsen ongoing dermatitis and should be deferred until the skin is substantially clear. For many substances, concentrations appropriate for testing may be found by consulting standard references. Tests with other materials must be carried out also on normal (control) subjects, who may be expected to respond comparably to primary irritant agents but not consistently to bland but sensitizing materials. Systemic corticosteroid drugs can partially suppress patch reactivity and are withheld, if possible,

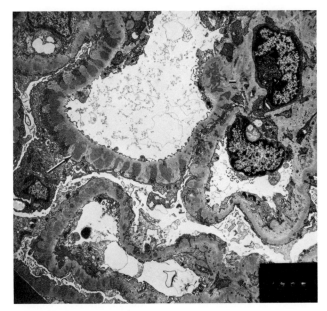

FIGURE 12-5 Antigen-antibody complex (arrow) deposition in the glomerular basement membrane of a nephritic subject. (Electron micrograph courtesy of Dr. Branka Baic.)

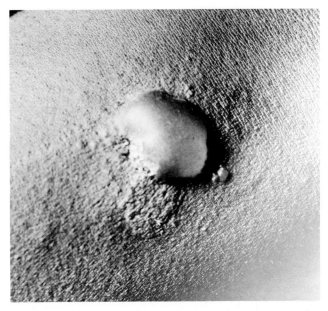

FIGURE 12-6 Large vesicles at the site of application of a crushed leaf of poison ivy 72 hours previously. The subject had had recurrent poison ivy dermatitis for many years.

for at least 24 hours before as well as during testing; antihistaminic drugs and sympathetic agonists appear to have negligible effects. As with wheal-and-flare skin reactions, positive patch tests *cannot* be equated with causation of dermatitis, especially since contact sensitivity to some substances (e.g. specific plant oils) may occur in over one-half of exposed persons. However, test results provide essential correlates for use with clinical data.

Certain substances (i.e., photocontact sensitizers) become allergenic only after skin, to which they are applied, is exposed to visible light or adjacent bands. In the recent past, a family of antimicrobial agents (i.e., halogenated salicylanilides) found in commercial soaps caused widespread skin erruptions in this fashion. The resulting rash—restricted to light-exposed areas—must be distinguished from eruptions caused by wind-borne contact sensitizers (e.g., pollen *oils*) or direct photosensitizers (e.g., tetracyclines, phenothiazines, psoralens, etc.), which produce *phototoxic* reactions (Fig. 12-8).

AECD often develops after several years of unabated exposure, and, through an unexplained "hardening" process, may diminish or resolve completely despite persistent contact with an offending agent. However, since in many persons dermatitis follows exposure indefinitely, avoidance of indicated sensitizers remains essential. A special risk exists in health care personnel who develop contact sensitivity to handled medications (e.g., local anesthetics, penicillin, aminoglycoside antibiotics) that they themselves may receive systemically. Injection of contact sensitive persons with these drugs may provoke a severe erythematous or maculopapular rash, with fever and toxicity, progressing occasionally to extensive exfoliation of skin.

Established dermatitis is managed with soaks when open vesicles predominate and, subsequently, with creams for partially healed lesions. Topical corticosteroids provide substantial though limited benefit, although finite courses of systemic steroids often promote rapid resolution of the dermatitis. At present, no available means of reducing sensitivity is sufficiently safe and effective to justify its recommendation. Patch test reactivity may be reduced during *prolonged* periods of ingestion or injection of specific agents (e.g., poison ivy oils). However the limited results achieved rarely are worth the time, effort, and expense required for such therapy or the substantial risk of inducing local and/or systemic dermatitis.

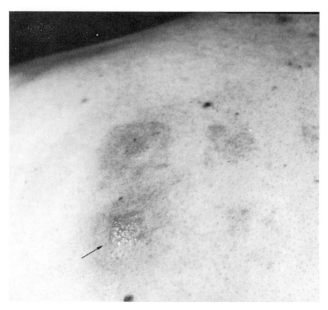

FIGURE 12-7 *Patch test reactions to procaine applied in several concentrations to the back of a sensitive dentist. Vesicles (arrow) denote the strongest grade of reaction.*

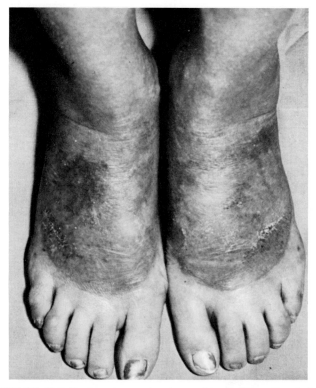

FIGURE 12-8 *Phototoxic reaction in a subject taking dimethylchlortetracycline. (From J. M. Sheldon, R. G. Lovell, and K. P. Mathews, A Manual of Clinical Allergy, 2d ed., Saunders, Philadelphia, 1967.)*

Autoimmune and immune complex-induced diseases—Chap. 12

Directions: Answer the following questions on a separate sheet of paper.

1 What is the significance of the appearance of auto-antibodies?

2 Describe the way in which immune responses to tissue components could arise.

3 Describe Goodpasture's syndrome as an apparent example of antibody-mediated human autoimmunity.

4 What are the usual manifestations (signs and symptoms) of transfusion reactions?

5 List the measures that *must* be employed to prevent or mitigate hemolytic transfusion reactions.

6 What reactions can occur when serums containing potent leukoagglutinins have been infused or when persons deficient in IgA receive whole blood? How can the latter reactions be averted?

Directions: Circle the T for true and the F for false. Correct the false statements.

7 T F Human antibody–dependent, autoimmune disorders affect formed elements of the blood, with neutrophils and eosinophils attacked predominantly.

8 T F Hemolytic transfusion reactions comprise a distinct form of immunohemolytic process occurring usually when a recipient already sensitized to "foreign" human red blood cell antigens receives blood containing these antigens.

Directions: Circle the letter preceding each item below that correctly answers each question. More than one answer may be correct.

9 Increasing evidence has linked the disease idiopathic thrombocytopenic purpura (ITP) with:
a Circulating IgG molecules reactive with platelet surfaces b Prominent decrease in complement levels c Lysis of platelets in the free circulation d Platelets with bound IgG molecules that are more readily removed and destroyed by macrophages in spleen and liver

10 Persistent ITP may be suppressed by:
a Corticosteroid therapy b Splenectomy
c Both *a* and *b* d Neither *a* nor *b*

11 A positive reaction to the indirect Coombs' test is most accurately interpreted as:
a An indicator of unsuspected serum antibody b A sign that the serum contains excessive amounts of immune globulins c An important indicator of pos-

sible danger prior to an intended blood transfusion d Evidence that the concentration of heme pigments is greatly increased

12 Individuals at risk for hemolytic reactions to transfused blood are those sensitized to red blood cell antigens by prior:
a Transfusions b Pregnancy c Both *a* and *b* d Neither *a* nor *b*

13 All of the following spontaneously developing immunohemolytic (IH) phenomena are characteristic of "warm" red blood cell autoantibody reactions EXCEPT:
a Hemolysis may be absent and red cell agglutination minor. b Autoantibodies are usually of the IgG class and are recognized primarily in middle-aged adults. c Hemolysis is evident with rewarming after cold exposure. d The IH disorder may be evident only as a positive Coombs' test (with antihuman IgG).

14 In serum sickness, the pathogenicity of the antigen-antibody complex depends upon the antigen-antibody ratio. Symptoms occur 10 to 14 days after first administration of an antigenic material when this ratio is such that:
a There is a relative antibody excess (three Ab to two Ag). b There is a relative antigen excess (three Ag to two Ab). c The antigen-antibody ratio is equal.

15 The following is true of serum sickness:
a Occurs only after the administration of foreign serums to human beings b Occurs within a few minutes following administration of the offending antigen c May cause joint pain (arthralgia), lymph node enlargement (lymphadenopathy), and neuritis d Requires many previous periods of exposure to an offending antigen before frank disease is seen

16 Mr. J. received an antibiotic injection 12 days previous to his admission to the emergency room. He presents with a fever, angioedema, and is complaining of pain in his hip, antecubital fossa, and knee joints. His diagnosis is serum sickness. Which of the following is true regarding the pathogenesis of this condition?
a It is an immune complex–induced illness. b It is only IgE-mediated. c Circulating antibody-antigen complexes are capable of activating complement components. d It is a delayed hypersensitivity reaction.

17 The treatment of serum sickness may require:
a No medication b Aspirin for fever and rheumatic complaints c Epinephrine to relieve urticaria and angioedema d High doses of corticosteroids for carditis or neurological manifestations e All of the above

18 The following statement(s) is/are true of allergic eczematous contact dermatitis.

a It is exemplified by burns due to caustic detergents.
b It may be appropriately studied by patch tests
applied to unbroken skin. *c* It is exemplified by
poison ivy dermatitis. *d* It is a form of atopic
eczema.

19 Allergic eczematous contact dermatitis is mediated by
which of the following hypersensitivity reactions:

a Immediate-type   *b* Delayed-type   *c* Idiosyncratic
d Anaphylactic

20 An obstetrical nurse has developed an allergic contact dermatitis to penicillin ointment. She last received intramuscular penicillin as a high school
student without ill effect. An injection of penicillin
at this time:

a Can be given with no fear of adverse reaction
b Would almost certainly produce anaphylaxis
c Would almost certainly produce serum sickness
d Would impose a definite risk of a generalized drug
rash

CHAPTER 13   Adverse Reactions to Drugs and Related Substances

---

OBJECTIVES **At the completion of Chap. 13 you should be able to:**

1 Describe at least four mechanisms responsible for adverse reactions to drugs.

2 Identify the significance of a wheal-and-flare reaction at the site of an injection of morphine sulfate.

3 State an example of a (Type I) reaction that is apparently mediated by IgE antibodies and can occur with systemically administered agents.

4 Explain the relationship between IgE-mediated responses to injected antigens and the atopic population.

5 Relate products of penicillin metabolism to types of adverse reaction following administration of the drug.

6 Appreciate for skin testing with penicilloyl polylysine (PPL) the indications for, practical approach to, and information forthcoming from the procedure.

7 List three agents for which an immunologic basis usually can be shown for acute systemic and urticarial reactions.

8 Discuss the signs and symptoms and apparent basis of reactions to local anesthetics.

9 List medications that may induce formation of antinuclear antibodies.

10 Describe the drug-induced reactions that are associated with hemolysis.

11 Identify for drug-associated circulating complexes the type of reactions recognized and examples of responsible drugs.

12 List at least two topically applied agents that are known to elicit contact sensitivity readily.

13 Identify for drug-related fever reactions the postulated basis of the reactions and some associated agents.

14 Identify for nitrofurantoin-induced reactions the organs affected, signs and symptoms, useful diagnostic studies, and prognosis.

15 Describe the characteristic liver changes, clinical syndromes, and courses of adverse reactions to the following therapeutic agents: anabolic steroids, some oral contraceptives, chlorpropamide, isoniazid, Dilantin, and halothane.

16 Describe the skin lesions that are typical of a majority of cutaneous adverse drug reactions.

17 Describe the rashes that may be associated with the administration of penicillin.

18 Discuss the considerations which are helpful in the prevention of adverse drug reactions.

ADVERSE REACTIONS TO DRUGS AND RELATED SUBSTANCES

Well over 10 percent of patients who receive indicated drugs experience unforeseen adverse effects from their medication. Taken together, these events constitute a substantial public health problem and cause a serious waste of human and material resources. Many adverse responses represent unwanted (but recognized) associated effects of drugs or frank toxicity arising from the dose employed or its rate of administration. However some individuals manifest unique and inappropriate reactions, and this propensity is termed *idiosyncrasy.* Both these personal response patterns and instances of readily induced toxicity may arise from inborn deficiencies in drug-metabolizing capability or related *pharmacogenetic* defects. Reactions that mimic immunologic events are seen with drugs that cause direct histamine release from human mast cells (Fig. 13-1). Agents including morphine alkaloids, thiamine, polymyxin, and *d*-tubocurarine share this property and produce wheal-

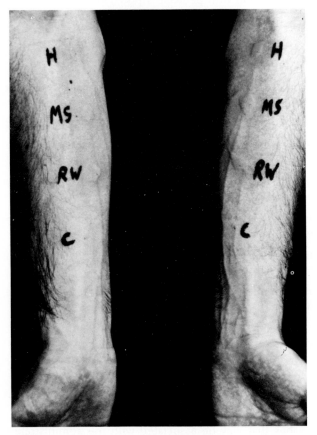

FIGURE 13-1 Skin test sites injected intracutaneously with histamine, morphine sulfate (a histamine releaser), ragweed pollen extract, and a saline control. Several mechanisms have produced similar wheals in this ragweed-sensitive subject.

ing at injection sites or, rarely, generalized hives and flushing following injection. A similar mechanism *may* be responsible for certain occurrences (e.g., flushing, hypotension, urticaria) following intravenous injection of radiopaque contrast media. There remain a large number of reactions involving skin and/or internal organs which are not otherwise explained and are often termed *allergic;* however, a causative immunologic process has been established in only a small fraction of these.

Type I reactions, apparently mediated by IgE antibodies, occur with systemically administered agents (e.g., ACTH, insulin) that serve as complete antigens as well as with those of small molecular size that are capable of stable protein bonding. Adverse reactions to penicillins exemplify the latter mechanism, in which a drug and/or its metabolites serve as haptens. Administration of the sensitizing agent may produce immediately a complete or partial picture of anaphylaxis as well as "late" urticaria with onset after 48 to 72 hours; (with penicillins, immunohemolytic reactions, serum sickness, and allergic eczematous contact dermatitis (AECD) may also occur). Since IgE responses are to be expected to *injected* antigens in most persons, the risk of immediate systemic and urticarial reactions is not confined to, or even concentrated among, the atopic population. In human subjects, penicillin metabolism can proceed along several potential pathways involving many final and intermediate products, some of which are allergenic. Of the resulting substances, the penicilloyl radical appears to be the predominant sensitizer, and antibodies of this specificity are commonly associated with late urticarial and, at times, acute systemic reactions. By contrast, systemic (anaphylactic) responses with serious or, at times, fatal consequences comprise a major proportion of the misadventures referable to native penicillin G, or derivatives including penicilloic and penilloic acids. In view of the *frequency* of associated reactions (rather than their relative *severity*) the penicilloyl radical is often designated as the "major determinant" of penicillin allergy and the others as "minor determinants."

Clarification of the antigens responsible for penicillin sensitivity gave direction to efforts to identify reactive subjects. This goal was attained, however, only after development of a skin-reactive but nonsensitizing "major determinant" reagent, through conjugation of numerous penicilloyl groups to the synthetic peptide, poly-l lysine. Skin testing with the product, penicilloyl polylysine (PPL), is now widely performed and, although minor determinant materials are less readily available, their value is generally acknowledged. Both materials assist the evaluation of reported previous reactions and of the future risk of untoward events. In practice, epidermal skin tests are performed initially with PPL, a mixture of minor determinants, and a saline control. Penicillin G is applied in a strength of 10,000 units/ml unless extreme sensitivity is suggested, when testing is begun at 10 units/ml. Since higher levels may produce skin irritation, 10,000 units/ml is the highest penicillin G concentration employed for testing. If epidermal sites are negative, intracutaneous tests are performed (see

Chap. 9) with 0.02-ml portions of PPL, penicillin G, other minor determinants, and saline control. Persons who react negatively to all of these materials have been shown empirically to tolerate therapeutic doses of penicillin with essentially no danger of *acute systemic* reactions. A small portion of *nonreactors* to PPL may show late urticarial responses or, ultimately, a picture of serum sickness. In addition, there are indications that not *all* positive PPL reactors would have an adverse response to administered penicillin. However, the predictive value of these test procedures is strong, and the high risk associated with positive skin reactivity (especially to minor determinants) is especially noteworthy. Unfortunately, patterns of skin and systemic reactivity to semisynthetic penicillins (e.g., methicillin, ampicillin, carbenicillin) do not always parallel those to penicillin G and its derivatives. These disparities are especially distressing since appropriate test materials for the newer penicillins are available only rarely. Furthermore, even with penicillin G, a single set of negative skin tests cannot ensure lifelong freedom from adverse reactivity when the drug is administered in repeated courses.

An immunologic basis usually can be shown for acute systemic and urticarial reactions to various immunizing biologicals, penicillins, and cephalosporins but rarely for additional agents, including aspirin. Local anesthetics commonly precipitate distressing reactions marked by syncope, hypotension, cardiac rhythm disturbances, and, at times, convulsions. Although reminiscent of anaphylaxis, these reactions are more probably a direct toxic effect of the large doses of drug commonly required for local infiltration. High blood levels may result, especially where these agents are injected with some force into restricted tissue compartments, as is often required for dental procedures.

In rare instances, autoimmune phenomena are clearly related to the administration of specific medications. Several drugs, for example, including hydralazine, procainamide, diphenylhydantoin, and certain ovulatory suppressants may promote formation of antinuclear antibodies. Furthermore, in some affected persons, manifestations mimicking systemic lupus erythematosus have become evident, receding slowly only after the offending drug has been withdrawn. Additional agents, most notably alpha methyldopa, in some way induce red blood cell autoantibodies which underlie positive direct Coombs' tests and, in a minority, bring on spherocytosis and frank hemolysis. Drug-associated hemolysis also has occurred in persons receiving large intravenous doses of penicillin due to acquired sensitivity to a penicillin-conjugated red blood cell substance. Responsible IgG molecules participate in the direct and indirect Coombs' reactions using, respectively, patients' cells and "penicillinized" normal cells. Hemolysis characteristically begins 1 to 2 weeks after initiation of high-dose penicillin treatment but ceases shortly after the drug has been stopped.

Although hemolysis is not a feature of classical serum sickness, drug-associated circulating complexes are known to facilitate red blood cell, leukocyte, and platelet destruction in certain cases. These occurrences have been associated prominently with quinidine, the antituberculous drugs (para-aminosalicylic acid and isoniazid), and sulfonamides, although other medications have been indicated. Initially, complexes of host IgG or IgM and drug (or drug-protein conjugate) become attached to one or more blood cell types. Complement components are localized to the cell surface as a result, and their interaction results in discrete membrane lesions or rapid removal from the circulation, the formed elements being injured as "innocent bystanders" rather than as direct participants. Following fixation of complement factors, the immune complexes often dissociate from affected membranes. Such cells show Coombs' reactivity using antiserums specific for human complement (i.e., positive "nongamma" Coombs' tests) alone.*

Many *additional* forms of adverse drug reactivity are encountered with some frequency; however, of these, only AECD also has a well-defined immunologic basis (see Chap. 12). A remarkably high proportion of topically applied agents are known to elicit contact sensitivity; among the foremost offenders are penicillin, aminoglycoside antibiotics, antihistaminic drugs, and local anesthetics.

Fever is a feature of many drug reactions and occasionally is the sole manifestation of an adverse response. Since both granulocytes and monocytes release substances that indirectly elevate body temperature, it is not surprising that fever accompanies a variety of processes. Drug-related fever has been noted particularly with penicillin, sulfonamides, iodide, streptomycin, Dilantin, and additional agents.

Nitrofurantoin, a drug commonly employed to treat urinary tract infections, has been associated, almost uniquely, with adverse effects centered in the respiratory tract. Affected persons manifest fever, cough, and variable chest discomfort—often with a marked increase in peripheral blood eosinophil leukocytes. Chest x-rays obtained during these reactions often are abnormal, showing diffuse lung infiltrates and, at times, fluid in the pleural spaces. These rapidly developing changes are thought to resolve completely if nitrofurantoin is promptly discontinued; however, a chronic increase in fibrous connective tissue may occur *without* acute manifestations in those receiving the drug over long periods.

Many drugs are directly nephrotoxic (i.e., cause kidney dysfunction and/or damage). In addition, several of the penicillins—especially methicillin—have been implicated in diffuse renal inflammatory reactions, or "interstitial nephritis." Kidney damage has been associated with fever and skin rashes frequently and may result from immune-complex deposition.

The liver is a principal site of drug metabolism and

*Nongamma Coombs' test reactions are obtained using antisera to human serum components other than the gamma globulin fraction or specific immunoglobulin classes that it comprises.

commonly bears the brunt of adverse reactions to therapeutic agents. A spectrum of tissue effects is recognized with certain agents characteristically leading to cholestasis (a failure of bile transport) with little or no inflammation, while others mimic florid viral hepatitis with necrosis of liver cells and collapse of supporting tissues. Bland cholestasis is an infrequent complication of treatment with certain anabolic steroids as well as some oral contraceptives, erythromycin estolate,* chlorpropamide, etc. Bile stasis and jaundice also occur in reactions to chlorpromazine; however, pathologically, dense infiltration of portal areas with neutrophils, eosinophils, and macrophages is an additional feature, and progression to permanent liver damage is seen rarely. Frank hepatitis has resulted during treatment with isoniazid, alpha methyldopa, Dilantin, thiazide diuretics, and additional drugs including the anesthetic agents halothane and methoxyfluorane. These drugs may be associated with acute fatal reactions or may lead to a picture of chronic liver inflammation and scarring (viz., a form of cirrhosis). In some instances, evidence of liver involvement may be preceded by fever, joint pains, peripheral blood eosinophilia, and/or any of a variety of skin rashes. Although such manifestations have led to increased speculation concerning an "allergic" basis for these reactions, the case for immune causation is preliminary, at best.

By far the largest proportion of adverse drug reactions affect the skin. The resulting lesions generally are transient and only rarely provide clues to the responsible agent(s) because of their morphology. A majority of "drug rashes" consist of macules (flat red spots) or

*But not other salts of erythromycin.

papules (raised red spots) which are highly pruritic and tend to coalesce into a measleslike (morbilliform) eruption. In the case of penicillin, maculopapular rashes may be associated with abundant specific IgM antibodies; however, similar correlations have not been suggested for other drugs. Failure to withdraw the responsible medication can, at times, lead to an exfoliative dermatitis in which the skin literally is shed, leading to serious infection as well as heat and fluid losses. Additional common skin manifestations of systemic medication include eruptions that are erythematous (diffuse flush), eczematous, vesicular (small blisters), bullous (large blisters), petechial (tiny hemorrhagic spots), purpuric (large hemorrhagic patches), and urticarial. *Firm* hemorrhagic spots often accompany inflammatory lesions of small blood vessels (vasculitis) with involvement of diverse organs. Reactions to iodides (and bromides) may consist of pustules or merely a worsening of facial and upper-dorsal-area lesions of acne vulgaris. Skin reactions occasionally are confined to discrete patches of rash (viz., "fixed drug eruptions") which become active with each administration of the responsible agent.

The prevention of adverse drug reactions is a serious responsibility which all health care personnel share. An effective approach to this problem requires knowledge of the potential complications of medication and a willingness to consider adverse drug reactivity as a possible cause of *any* unexpected clinical event. Since untoward responses usually are repetitive, no drug should be given without first reviewing the individual's past experience with that agent. Similarly, the clinical data base requires no less than a comprehensive assessment of past drug reactivity. Health care personnel must also be prepared to accept, on face value, reports of previous problems arising from medication until these have been disproven conclusively.

Close surveillance can reveal the earliest stigmata of drug reactions, facilitating prompt withdrawal of the

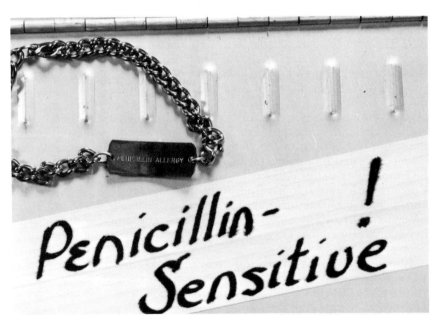

FIGURE 13-2 *Adverse drug reactivity may be minimized by clearly stigmatizing those at risk. Well-marked health records and personal identification, as shown, complement patient education.*

offender and, often, abbreviating morbidity. Once recognized, adverse reactivity must be clearly indicated in the clinical record (Fig. 13-2) and, if possible, the sensitivity identified for the patient or responsible family members. Documentation is aided, for practical purposes, if the patient can carry a card, bracelet, or medallion indicating medication(s) to be avoided. Exhaustive instruction is necessary also where a risk of reaction from related agents exists or when, like aspirin, the offender has many readily available and poorly identified sources.

QUESTIONS

Adverse reactions to drugs and related substances—Chap. 13

Directions: Circle the letter preceding each item below that correctly answers each question. More than one answer may be correct.

1 Which of the following statements are true regarding drug reactions?
  a Toxicity may arise through inborn deficiencies in drug-metabolizing capability. *b* A causative immunologic process has been established in the majority of reactions involving the skin and/or internal organs. *c* *Idiosyncrasy* is an adverse drug reaction that is unrelated to the expected pharmacological effect. *d* Over 10 percent of patients who receive indicated drugs experience adverse reactions from their medication.

2 Wheal-and-flare reactions are readily produced by local:
  a Injection of histamine into most normal persons *b* Injection of ragweed pollen extract into most normal persons *c* Injection of morphine into most normal persons *d* Application of local anesthetics to the skin of a person with a specific allergic eczematous contact dermatitis to these agents

3 Type I reactions apparently mediated by IgE occur with systemically administered agents that serve as:
  a Complete antigens *b* Haptens that are capable of stable protein binding *c* Both *a* and *b* *d* Neither *a* nor *b*

4 Regarding the predictive value of the results of skin testing with penicilloyl polylysine (PPL) which of the following statements are true?
  a There are indications that not all positive PPL reactors would have adverse responses to subsequently administered penicillin. *b* Persons with negative reactions have been shown to tolerate therapeutic doses of penicillin with no danger of acute systemic reactions. *c* This test accurately predicts skin and systemic reactions to semisynthetic penicillins. *d* A single set of negative skin tests can predict lifelong freedom from adverse reactivity when the drug is administered in repeated doses.

5 An immunologic basis usually can be shown for acute systemic and urticarial reactions to all of the following EXCEPT:

  a Certain biologicals *b* Aspirin *c* Penicillin *d* Cephalosporins

6 Autoimmune phenomena are clearly related to the administration of which of the following medications that may induce formation of antinuclear antibodies:
  a Alpha methyldopa *b* Aspirin *c* Hydralazine *d* Procainamide

7 Adverse drug reactions to nitrofurantoin are manifested by:
  a Fever *b* Diffuse lung infiltrates and fluid in the pleural spaces *c* Decrease in eosinophil leukocytes *d* Jaundice

Directions: Circle the T for true and the F for false. Correct the false statements.

8 T F The risk of IgE-mediated responses (immediate systemic and urticarial reactions) to injected antigens is usually confined to atopic individuals.

9 T F Drug-associated circulating complexes are known to facilitate red blood cell, leukocyte, and platelet destruction in certain cases.

10 T F Drug-related fever has been associated with penicillin, sulfonamides, iodide, streptomycin, Dilantin, and additional agents.

Directions: Match the medication in col. A with its characteristic reaction in col. B. More than one item from col. B may be used in col. A.

Column A	Column B
11 ____ Chlorpropamide	a Bile stasis and jaundice
	b Hepatitis
12 ____ Isoniazid	c Maculopapular rashes
13 ____ Iodides	d May lead to chronic liver
14 ____ Halothane	inflammation and scarring
15 ____ Penicillin	e Pustules or a worsening of facial and upper-dorsal lesions of acne vulgaris

Directions: Answer the following questions on a separate sheet of paper.

16 Explain the basis of the adverse reactions observed with drug-associated circulating complexes that affect blood elements.

17 List the reactions commonly associated with the administration of local anesthetics. What is the probable mechanism of these reactions?

18 Discuss the considerations which are helpful in reducing the prevalence of adverse drug reactions.

CHAPTER 14 Approaches to Immune Deficiency States

Current views of immune function emphasize the complex integration of antigen-specific components and effector systems required for normal humoral and cellular hypersensitivity. Both inborn and acquired defects have been recognized at many points in this usually well-coordinated system. The resulting flaws in immune competence may have no clinical consequences or may open the way for catastrophic infection or neoplastic disease. No attempt will be made to describe or catalog the various immunodeficiency disease states. Instead, this section will focus briefly on methods of evaluating immune function, as they relate to deficiency states of several major types.

Deficits in humoral (i.e., antibody-mediated) immu-nity commonly undermine defenses against virulent, pus-forming bacteria, many of which are encapsulated. Impaired hosts are prone to suffer recurrent infections of the skin, middle ear, and meninges as well as of the paranasal sinuses and bronchopulmonary structures. Repeated attacks by bacteria of a *single* antigenic type are often demonstrable, and, in those with the greatest impairment, naturally acquired viral infections and *live* viral vaccines also may cause grave illness.

Assay of serum immunoglobulins by radial immuno-diffusion (Fig. 14-1) provides a widely available, direct measurement of circulating molecules having potential antibody activity. In this procedure, test serums and samples of known immunoglobulin (Ig) content are placed in separate wells cut into agar containing antiserums, derived from other species, to IgA, IgG, IgM, or IgD. As human serum diffuses outward, a line of precipitation forms at the forward edge where a favorable ratio of antiserum and specific human immunoglobulin (Ig) is achieved; within this perimeter, an excess of the Ig (i.e., the antigen) suppresses precipitation. The ring diameter around each well is proportional to the Ig content of the serum added, and absolute levels are derived by referring to the assayed "known" samples. Determination of IgE content requires alternative techniques employing radioactive markers, due to the relatively lower range in which levels of this Ig fall. Normal total values for specific Ig classes are indicated in Table 14-1.

Several methods are available to evaluate *antigen-specific* antibody activity associated with one or more Ig classes; these include:

1 Determination of naturally occurring (IgM) antibodies to ABO blood group substances which are absent from the subjects' red blood cells. Normal persons consistently demonstrate such *isohemagglutinins* by the age of 1 year.
2 Schick testing of persons previously immunized with diphtheria toxoid. If adequate levels of (IgG) specific antibody have been produced, tissue breakdown at the site of toxin injection is prevented.
3 Determination of antibody titers before and after *nonviable* immunizing materials such as tetanus toxoid and typhoid or influenza vaccines.

In addition, estimates of circulating B-lymphocyte numbers may be made by immunofluorescent staining

of the Ig molecules that are prominent on their cell surfaces. In the blood of normal persons, approximately 20 to 25 percent of lymphocytes bear such markers.

The most frequently encountered form of continuing immunodeficiency is a selective deficit of IgA, which is observed in 1 in every 500 to 1000 persons. Serum levels of IgA are below 5 mg/dl in this condition and, at mucosal surfaces, the normal preponderance of IgA commonly is replaced by IgG and IgM. Some affected persons remain free of evident illness, but most manifest recurrent paranasal sinus and pulmonary infections. In addition, increased risks of atopic allergic problems as well as certain rheumatic and gastrointestinal diseases exist in this condition. Replacement of deficient serum IgA is not feasible, and systemic reactions due to anti-IgA antibodies may follow transfusion of human blood products (see Chap. 12).

Males with X-linked hypogammaglobulinemia of infancy exhibit the most severe selective deficiency of humoral immune function, with virtual absence of circulating immunoglobulins and B-cells. In addition, these individuals have marked reduction in the size and structural organization of lymph nodes and lymphoid tissues of pharynx and gut. Recurrent purulent (viz., pus-forming) infections usually begin after 4 to 6 months of age, when transplacentally acquired levels of maternal IgG are no longer protective. Otitis media, bronchitis, pneumonitis, meningitis, and skin infections are prominent and often lead to permanent organ damage (e.g., bronchiectasis). In addition, viruses, including hepatitis B and attenuated strains present in certain vaccines, may produce severe illnesses at times, with central nervous system damage. Rapidly progressive tooth decay and chronic conjunctivitis often add to the patients' discomfort, and an eczematous dermatitis, arthritis resembling rheumatoid disease, and intestinal malabsorption are frequently associated. The administration of commercial gamma globulin by intramuscular injection controls many of these problems and complements appropriate antibiotic treatment; adequate doses usually approx-

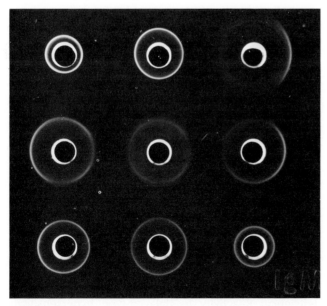

FIGURE 14-1 Determination of immunoglobulin levels by radial immunodiffusion. The agar plate shown contains goat anti-human IgM. The IgM content of samples added to the wells is evidenced by the diameters of the resulting circles of precipitation. The uppermost row of wells contain known serums of increasing IgM content (from left to right).

TABLE 14-1
Normal serum immunoglobulin levels at various ages*

AGE	IgG, mg/dl	IgA, mg/dl	IgM, mg/dl	IgE, IU/ml†
At birth	650–1250	1–6	5–35	1–3
1– 3 yr	250–1320	15–160	15–115	10–500
5–10 yr	550–1450	20–220	30–135	15–600
10–15 yr	620–1450	30–230	35–150	20–750
Adult	720–1800	60–300	45–160	25–900

*Values are approximations of expected ranges derived from several sources.
†IU (international unit) = 2.3 nanograms IgE.

imate 0.2 ml/kg every 2 to 4 weeks. These preparations contain no IgA or IgM, and, possibly as a result, fail to control infection in some persons despite maximum doses. Better results may follow regular plasma infusions from hepatitis antigen–free single donors providing a humoral "buddy system."

Persons of either sex with low Ig levels and infections beginning after infancy are seen with some frequency. This group with acquired, "common, variable hypogammaglobulinemia" have prominent lymph nodes and intestinal lymphoid aggregates as well as normal numbers of circulating B-cells. However, they experience recurrent and sustained sinopulmonary infections as well as intestinal malabsorption, often augmented by infection with the protozoan Giardia lamblia. In both affected persons and their relatives, an increased risk of autoantibodies and related diseases (including ITP, immunohemolytic anemia, pernicious anemia, systemic lupus, and rheumatoid arthritis) are noted. Laboratory evidence of impaired T-cell function also has been obtained in some patients. Appropriate antibiotic therapy and Ig replacement using gamma globulin or suitably screened plasma provides substantial benefit in most cases.

Humoral immunodeficiency is especially prominent in certain malignant states such as multiple myeloma and chronic lymphocytic leukemia and is part of the deficits occurring whenever tumor cells infiltrate lymphoreticular structures. Similar infectious problems may develop in persons deficient in one or more serum complement factors or with inadequate leukocyte numbers or function. Serum levels of C3 may be assayed by radial immunodiffusion.* In addition, overall complement activity is sometimes inferred from the ability of test serums to facilitate hemolysis of optimally sensitized red blood cells; this capacity is expressed as "CH_{50} activity." Defects in leukocyte function may affect the random movement, directed movement (chemotaxis), phagocytosis, formation of enzymatically active vacuoles, and intracellular killing by white blood cells. These modalities can be examined individually with acceptable precision in a minority of laboratories. More generally, available studies include the white blood cell count, leukocyte morphology in peripheral blood smears, and peroxidase stain to confirm the content of myeloperoxidase, a leukocyte enzyme required for intracellular killing of certain ingested organisms. In addition, the quantitative assay of nitroblue tetrazolium (NBT) dye reduction provides a valuable clue to the diagnosis of chronic granulomatous disease (of childhood). Recurrent infection by Staphylococcus aureus (Micrococcus pyogenes), Pseudomonas species, and Escherichia coli as well as organisms normally of low virulence (e.g., Serratia, Staphylococcus epidermidis, Candida, etc.) are

*This technique may be used for additional complement components although the necessary reagents are not available universally.

typical of this X-linked disorder.* Offending organisms are ingested normally but escape death and can multiply intracellularly, ultimately destroying the inept phagocytes; a clinical picture of recurrent abscesses, indolent draining lymph nodes, osteomyelitis, pneumonia, and persistent diarrhea is the result. Defective killing appears to reflect impaired leukocyte metabolism with decreased generation of hydrogen peroxide and related substances, which participate in a microbicidal system. The metabolic defect also precludes the normal reduction of NBT to a readily visible blue-black form, a deficit easily quantitated by colorimetric assay.

Cell-mediated immune function is inadequate in many disease states either as a "primary defect" or secondary to disorders including sarcoidosis, Hodgkin's disease, certain non-Hodgkin's neoplasms, and uremia; therapy with corticosteroids or cytotoxic drugs (e.g., cyclophosphamide) is also a frequent factor. In addition, cellular immunity may be impaired transiently by viral infections such as rubeola (measles). Of the steadily growing list of conditions associated with abnormalities of T-cell function, a large majority also display aberrant humoral (i.e., B-cell) immunity. Overall, victims of these disorders are prone to infection by characteristic spectra of organisms which may include bacteria, viruses, protozoa (especially Pneumocystis carinii), and fungi. Lymphoreticular malignancies are common terminal complications of many of these disorders.

Relatively complete absence of T-cell function occurs when the thymus fails to develop (viz., the DiGeorge syndrome), and affected infants have been restored immunologically to normal with grafts of early fetal thymus tissue. The most compromised individuals are those with severe combined immunodeficiency, who totally lack B- as well as T-cell function, and frequently succumb within the first year of life. Transplantation of bone marrow from optimally matched donors has permitted survival, and partial reconstitution has been achieved with early fetal liver or thymus grafts. Bone marrow recipients often have developed severe "graft versus host" disease due to cytotoxicity of donor lymphocytes reacting against transplantation antigens of the host. A variety of other conditions with combined immunodeficiency are recognized; most often observed are the Wiskott-Aldrich syndrome (eczema, platelet deficiency, low IgM level) and ataxia telangiectasia (ataxia, spontaneous movements, vascular malformations of skin and conjunctiva, mental retardation), both of which are familial.

Although numerous correlates and functional components of cell-mediated immunity are recognized, only a few are widely tested at present. T-cell defects may be reflected in decreased numbers of peripheral blood lymphocytes, and counts consistently below 1200 per μl (2000 per μl in infancy) suggest cellular immunodeficiency. Reactivity to delayed-type hypersensitivity (DTH) skin tests provides a readily available indicator of cellular immune competence. For this purpose, intradermal injections are performed with 0.1-ml portions of

*A variant form in females is known to occur rarely.

substances that elicit DTH and to which a previous sensitizing exposure may be assumed; commonly used materials include PPD (of the tubercle bacillus); streptokinase and streptodornase, enzymes of beta-hemolytic streptococci; and antigens from *Candida albicans,* mumps virus, *Histoplasma capsulatum,* and fungi of superficial skin infections. Test sites are observed and palpated after 48 hours, and an indurated area with a diameter of 10 mm or larger generally is regarded as a positive reaction. Using a "battery" of such materials, at least one positive test should be evident in the vast majority of normal individuals (excluding infants). For nonreactors, a more stringent test of cellular competence is provided by attempting contact sensitization with dinitrochlorobenzene (DNCB). This potent material, which is *absent* elsewhere in the environment, is applied (usually as a 30% solution in acetone) to a small skin area and sensitivity tested with a 1% solution at a distant site 14 days later.* Over 95 percent of normal persons acquire contact allergy by this procedure, confirming (at least partial) T-cell function. DNCB in *30%* solution is also a strong primary irritant, and patients should recognize that a small scar may develop at its point of application. Additional tests reflecting T-cell function may include:

1 Response of lymphocytes in short-term tissue culture to antigens and nonspecific agents (e.g., phytohemagglutinin) that stimulate cell division and associated nucleic acid synthesis. An increase in the incorporation of added thymidine tagged with tritium is observed normally in response to these agents.
2 Peripheral aggregation of sheep red blood cells (i.e., "rosette formation") around human peripheral (T-) lymphocytes when the two are mixed and incubated (Fig. 14-2). Normally, over 60 percent of lymphocytes demonstrate rosetting, although a teleological basis for the sheep cell receptor is unknown.

*Usually a 1 percent solution also is applied initially to detect the rare person previously sensitized to DNCB.

3 Assays of lymphokines produced in response to appropriate antigens added to lymphocyte preparations (see Chap. 5). To date, most studies have focused on the macrophage inhibiting factor (MIF), and defects at several stages prior to its release have been described (Fig. 14-3).

Antigen-specific defects in cell-mediated immunity also are recognized; perhaps the best studied example is chronic mucocutaneous candidiasis (Fig. 14-4). This condition is characterized by indolent *Candida albicans* infections of the skin, nails, and mucous membranes with granuloma formation. Although systemic dissemination is almost unknown, oral candidiasis (thrush), esophageal involvement with dysphagia (difficulty in swallowing), and *Candida vaginitis* may cause severe stress. In addition, affected individuals often show autoantibodies reactive with endocrine tissues and defects in endocrine function—especially adrenal and parathyroid deficiencies—as a possible result. Although cell-mediated immunity to *Candida* is ineffective in this condition, other T-cell functions usually are found to be intact. Defective responses to *Candida* antigens vary among patients, being total in some, while others show intact lymphocyte mitogenic responses and/or MIF production despite negative skin tests at 48 hours; in a few, circulating inhibitors of *Candida*-directed cellular immunity occur. Although treatment with amphotericin B can provide temporary improvement, drug toxicity and the expectation of posttreatment relapse limit its usefulness. Repeated injection of transfer factor (see Chap. 5) prepared from lymphocytes of persons with strong DTH to *Candida* has led to prolonged remissions in some cases.

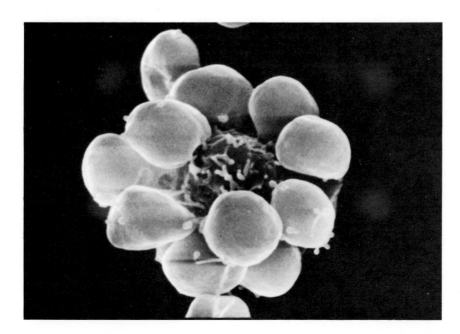

FIGURE 14-2 Human T-cell rosette. A central T-lymphocyte is shown surrounded by adherent sheep red blood cells. (Scanning electron micrograph courtesy of Drs. Michael Deegan and Bertram Schnitzer.)

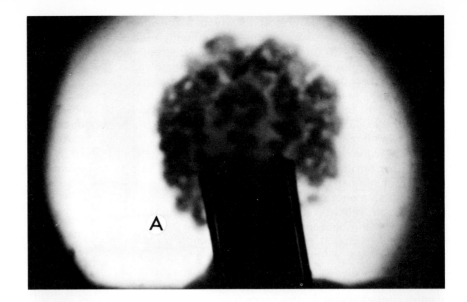

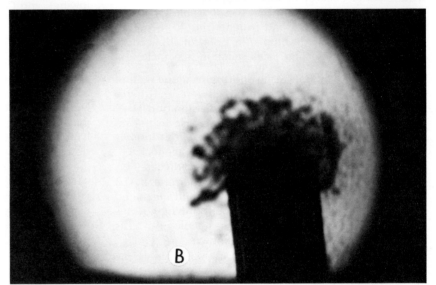

FIGURE 14-3 Macrophage inhibitory factor (MIF) effects as seen in a capillary tube assay. Both tubes contain macrophages plus lymphocytes from a tuberculin-sensitive donor. Tuberculin has been added to the tissue culture medium for B, but not A. The restricted "fan" of migrating cells in B may be measured as an indicator of MIF production by lymphocytes.

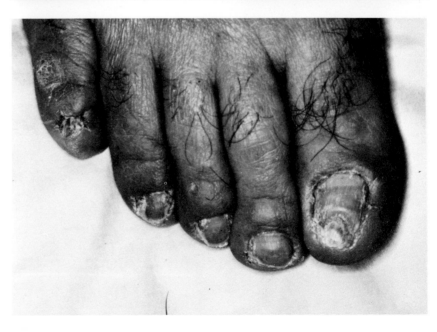

FIGURE 14-4 Skin and nail lesions on the foot of a patient with chronic mucocutaneous candidiasis. (Photo courtesy of Dr. Jeffrey Callen.)

Approaches to immune deficiency states—Chap. 14

Directions: Circle the letter preceding each item below that correctly answers each question. More than one answer may be correct.

1 Deficits in humoral immunity commonly impair defenses against:
   a Tubercle bacilli   b Herpes simplex
   c Giardia lamblia   d Virulent pus-forming bacteria

2 Which of the following characteristics are true of acquired, common variable hypogammaglobulinemia?
   a Virtual absence of circulating B-cells   b Involves only males   c Normal number of circulating B-cells   d Low Ig levels

3 The usual treatment of X-linked hypogammaglobulinemia includes:
   a The administration of commercial gamma globulin
   b Appropriate antibiotic therapy   c Both a and b
   d Neither a nor b

4 Cell-mediated immune function is inadequate in or may be impaired transiently by:
   a Cytotoxic drugs   b Viral infections
   c Adrenal corticosteroids   d Streptococcal pharyngitis

Directions: Circle the T for true and the F for false. Correct the false statements.

5 T F Assay of serum immunoglobulins by radial immunodiffusion provides a widely available, direct measurement of circulating molecules having potential antibody activity.

6 T F The most frequently encountered form of continuing immunodeficiency is a selective deficit of IgG.

7 T F Some persons with a deficit of IgA (level below 5 mg/dl) remain free of evident illness, but most manifest recurrent paranasal sinus and pulmonary infections.

8 T F Humoral immunodeficiency is present as an isolated immunological deficit in non-Hodgkin's lymphoma and uremia.

9 T F Patients with DiGeorge syndrome totally lack B- as well as T-cell function because the thymus fails to develop.

10 T F Chronic mucocutaneous candidiasis is an example of an antigen-specific defect in cell-mediated immunity and is characterized by indolent *Candida albicans* infections of the skin, nails, and mucous membranes with granuloma formation.

Directions: Answer the following questions on a separate sheet of paper.

11 List three methods used to evaluate antigen-specific antibody activity associated with one or more Ig classes.

12 Explain the significance of delayed-type hypersensitivity (DTH) skin tests as an indicator of cellular immune competence.

13 Describe three additional laboratory tests reflecting lymphocyte function.

REFERENCES

AMMANN, A. J. and D. W. WARA: "Evaluation of Infants and Children with Recurrent Infections," *Current Problems in Pediatrics*, **5**(11), 1975.

BEALL, G. N.: "Asthma: New Ideas about An Old Disease," *Annals of Internal Medicine*, **78**: 405, 1973.

BLAYLOCK, W. K.: "Atopic Dermatitis: Diagnosis and Pathobiology," *Journal of Allergy and Clinical Immunology*, **57**: 62, 1976.

DESWARTE, R. D.: "Drug Allergy," in R. Patterson (ed.), *Allergic Diseases*, Lippincott, Philadelphia, 1972.

FISHER, A. A.: *Contact Dermatitis*, Lea & Febiger, Philadelphia, 1974.

FUDENBERG, H. H., D. P. STITES, J. L. CALDWELL, and J. V. WELLS: *Basic and Clinical Immunology*, Lange, Los Altos, Calif., 1976.

KOHLER, P.: "Clinical Immune Complex Disease," *Medicine*, **52**: 419, 1973.

LIEBERMAN, P. and R. PATTERSON: "Immunotherapy for Atopic Disease," *Advances in Internal Medicine,* **19**: 391, 1974.

MATHEWS, K. P.: "A Current View of Urticaria," *Medical Clinics of North America*, **58**: 185, 1974.

MIDDLETON, E., JR., C. E. REED, and E. F. ELLIS: *Allergy: Principles and Practice*, Mosby, St. Louis, (in press).

PARKER, C. W.: "Drug Allergy," *New England Journal of Medicine*, **292**: 511, 732, 957, 1975.

SCHLUETER, D. P.: "Response of the Lung to Inhaled Antigens," *American Journal of Medicine*, **57**: 476, 1974.

SHEFFER, A. L.: "Treatment of Anaphylaxis," *Postgraduate Medicine*, **53**: 62, 1973.

PART III Hematologic Disorders

KENNETH A. STOUTENBOROUGH

Hematology is the study of blood, its nature, function, and diseases. Adult blood disorders are emphasized, although some pediatric hematologic problems are discussed.

This part includes a discussion of the red blood cell, including its function and what happens when you have too many, not enough, or abnormal red blood cells; the white blood cell, its function, morphology, and disease processes; and the basic principles of blood clotting.

OBJECTIVES

At the completion of Part III you should be able to:

1 Identify the component parts of the blood.

2 Describe how pathologic hematologic conditions are manifested as disease processes.

3 Describe the sequence of events in the mechanism of blood clotting.

4 Develop skill in identifying etiology, pathogenesis, and treatment of hematologic disorders.

CHAPTER 15 The Composition of the Blood and Lymphoreticular System

OBJECTIVES   **At the completion of Chap. 15 you should be able to:**

1 Define *hematology*.

2 Describe the characteristics of the two components of the blood.

3 List the major types of cells found in the particulate matter of blood.

4 Identify and describe briefly nine methods used to examine blood.

5 State the "normal" values for the following: red cell count, hemoglobin concentration, mean corpuscular volume (MCV), mean corpuscular hemoglobin concentration (MCHC), total white cell count, platelet count, reticulocyte count.

COMPONENTS OF NORMAL BLOOD

Blood is a suspension of particulate material in an aqueous solution of colloid and electrolytes. It serves as a medium of exchange for the fixed cells of the body between themselves and the exterior and possesses properties protective to the organism as a whole and to itself in particular.

The blood contains basically two components. One is a liquid that is a suspension of colloid, electrolytes, proteins, and many other substances called plasma. The other component consists of particulate matter in the form of both whole cells and parts of cells. The particulate component contains, in particular, red blood cells (also called erythrocytes, red corpuscles, or RBCs) and several different kinds of white blood corpuscles, or leukocytes (WBCs). Platelets, which are parts of the cytoplasm of cells, are also contained in the particulate component of blood. Platelets play a role in the blood clotting mechanism.

The particulate material (cells of the blood) is all thought to be derived from a single, pluripotential "stem" cell (Fig. 15-1) which goes through a series of divisions and maturation changes to result in the mature cells found in the circulating blood. No one has ever seen a stem cell, but there is an increasing body of evidence that such a cell must exist. The mechanisms by which this cell is made to undergo various forms of differentiation leading to cells with vastly different functions, properties, and characteristics are poorly understood at present.

For our purposes *blood* will also include the entire reticuloendothelial system. The reticuloendothelial system of the body includes cells derived from primitive mesenchyme that persist as multipotential cells throughout life.

METHODS FOR STUDYING BLOOD

There are many methods for attempting to quantitate the various constituents of blood. Counting the number of red blood cells in a cubic millimeter (mm^3) of blood is one way of measuring these cells. This method is referred to as the red cell count, and is expressed in terms of millions of cells per cubic millimeter.

The amount of hemoglobin in blood is another measurement made on blood, and is expressed in grams percent (g%), or grams of hemoglobin per hundred millimeters of blood. Another measure, the hematocrit, indicates the volume of the whole blood which is made up of red blood cells. This measurement is determined by spinning a sample of blood in a centrifuge until all the red blood cells are packed on the bottom of the hematocrit tube and the plasma is on the top. A simple percentage of the total height of the column versus the height of the red blood cells is the hematocrit. It is important to remember that the hematocrit is expressed in terms of volumes percent (vol%).

Other measures involve examining the red blood cell itself. Size of the red blood cell is one important factor. The relative size of the red blood cell can be determined by looking at the mean corpuscular volume, which is a simple division of the hematocrit by the red cell count. The mean corpuscular volume is expressed in cubic micrometers (μm³). Table 15-1 indicates the normal value for mean corpuscular volume.

The mean corpuscular hemoglobin concentration, which indicates the amount of the hemoglobin in the cells, is another measure of the blood. Even though a cell may be of abnormal size, it may contain the right amount of hemoglobin. The mean corpuscular hemoglobin concentration is determined by dividing the hemoglobin by the hematocrit and is expressed in grams percent (g%).

A count of the number of white blood cells in a cubic millimeter of blood also indicate abnormalities. Since the red blood cells and white blood cells are mixed, a count of the white blood cells can only be made when the red blood cells have been eliminated from the blood. To obtain this measure, blood is placed in a solution which breaks up all the red blood cells but does not break up the white blood cells. The solution is then transferred to a counting device that determines the number of white blood cells in a cubic millimeter of blood.

Another method for determining the nature of blood involves extracting blood via a finger prick or an ear prick, making a film of blood on a slide, and then strain-ing it. Generally Wright's stain, a Romanovasky tri-chrome stain which stains structures in the cell different colors according to their pH, is used. Colors range from blue to pink or red. The various types of white blood cells—granulocytes, which include the PMNs (poly-morphonuclear leukocytes—also called segmented cells, or segs, neutrophils, or polys), eosinophils, and baso-phils—can be differentiated according to the color they stain (for the differential count). The cytoplasm of eosinophils is eosinophilic (has an affinity for the red stain eosin) when stained with Wright's stain. Basophils have large basophilic granules in the cytoplasm, meaning these granules stain blue. Monocytes cytoplasm stains gray-blue, and lymphocytes stain a light blue. These cells are contained in the normal peripheral blood.

The number of platelets in a cubic millimeter of blood can also be an indication of blood abnormality. A suit-able dilution of whole blood is counted in a counting chamber to obtain the number of platelets in a cubic millimeter of blood.

A blood film can be made just as it is for a differential count, but can be stained with a supravital stain. This supravital stain picks up living RNA within the cell and stains it blue so that there is a group of cells with no color in them at all (mature RBCs) and another group of immature cells (known as reticulocytes) stained with little blue, speckled patterns (reticulin). The developing red blood cells in the bone marrow have nuclei in them. However, the nucleus is extruded before the cell is released into the peripheral blood. Residual RNA is lost

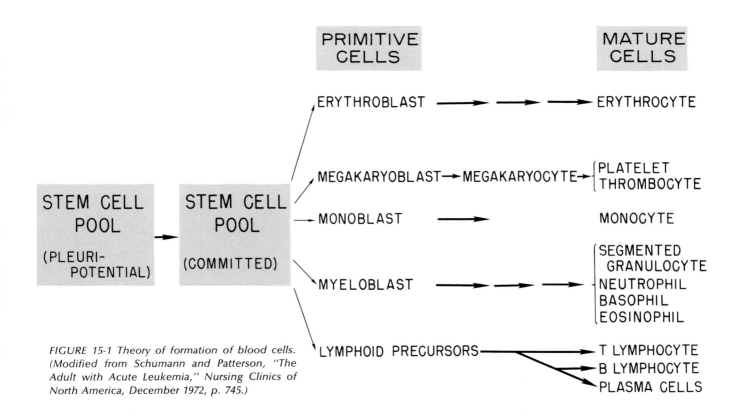

FIGURE 15-1 Theory of formation of blood cells. (Modified from Schumann and Patterson, "The Adult with Acute Leukemia," Nursing Clinics of North America, December 1972, p. 745.)

TABLE 15-1
Methods for examining blood

MEASUREMENT	DESCRIPTION
Red cell count	The number of RBCs in 1 mm³ of blood (millions/mm³)
Hemoglobin concentration	The amount of hemoglobin in a given volume of blood (expressed as g%)
Hematocrit	The percent of blood which is made up of RBCs (vol%)
Mean corpuscular volume (MCV)	The volume of each individual RBC (μm³) $MCV = \dfrac{hematocrit}{red\ cell\ count}$
Mean corpuscular hemoglobin concentration (MCHC)	The amount of hemoglobin in each individual RBC (g Hb/100 ml of erythrocytes) $MCHC = \dfrac{hemoglobin}{hematocrit}$
White cell count	The number of WBCs in 1 mm³ of blood
The differential count	The percent of the various types of WBCs seen on examination of a peripheral film (granulocytes—PMNs, eosinophils, basophils; monocytes; lymphocytes)
Platelet count	The number of platelets in 1 mm³ of blood
Reticulocyte count	The percent of the RBCs which stain positively for reticulin with a supravital stain

TABLE 15-2
Normal blood cell values

	MEN	WOMEN
Red cell count, cells in millions/mm³	4.7–6.1	4.2–5.2
Hemoglobin, g%	13.4–17.6	12.0–15.4
Hematocrit, vol%	42–53	38–46
MCV, μm³	81–96	
MCHC, g%	30–36	
Total white cell count, cells/mm³	4–10,000	
Granulocytes		
PMNs, %	38–70	
Eosinophils, %	1–5	
Basophils, %	0–2	
Monocytes, %	1–8	
Lymphocytes, %	15–45	
Platelets, cells/mm³	200,000–400,000	
Reticulocyte count, %	1–2	

within the first day or two outside of the bone marrow, but until that time, the cells will appear speckled when stained. The reticulocyte count determines the numbers of the cells that were most likely released into the blood within the past day or two. This count gives an approximation of the rate at which the red blood cells are being produced and released into peripheral blood.

In summary, Table 15-1 indicates the methods used to examine blood. In Table 15-2 a chart of "normal" blood cell values is given. There is a wide range for all of these, which makes determining abnormalities somewhat of a challenge. Notice that there are certain differences, particularly in the levels of the red count, hemoglobin concentration, and hematocrit, between men and women.

QUESTIONS

Components of normal blood—Chap. 15

Directions: Answer the following questions on a separate sheet of paper.

1 Define *hematology*.

2 List the three major types of cells found in the particulate component of blood.

Directions: Circle the letter preceding each item below that correctly answers the question. Choose the ONE best answer.

3 The fluid portion of blood, in which cellular elements are suspended, is referred to as the:
   a Cytoplasm of cells   *b* Platelets   *c* Plasma

Directions: Match each descriptive statement in col. A to its appropriate measurement in col. B by placing the letter from col. B in the appropriate blank in col. A.

Column A	Column B
4 ____ Red cell count	*a* Percentage of packed RBCs in a sample of blood (vol%)
5 ____ Hematocrit	*b* Grams of hemoglobin in 100 ml of blood (g%)
6 ____ Mean corpuscular volume (MCV)	*c* Number of WBCs in 1 mm³ of blood
7 ____ Hemoglobin concentration	*d* Number of RBCs in 1 mm³ of blood (millions/mm³)
8 ____ Mean corpuscular hemoglobin concentration (MCHC)	*e* The amount of hemoglobin in each individual RBC
	f Number of platelets in 1 mm³ of blood

The approximate normal values for the following are:

9 _____ Reticulocyte count

10 _____ White cell count

11 _____ Platelet count

12 _____ Differential count

g Volume of each individual RBC (μm³)

h Percentage of the different types of WBCs seen on examination of a peripheral film

i Percentage of RBCs which stain positively for reticulin with a supravital stain

13   T   F   Red cell count (millions/mm³): 3.04–4.0 (*men*); 2.0–3.0 (*women*).

14   T   F   Hematocrit (vol%): 42–53 (*men*); 38–46 (*women*).

15   T   F   Hemoglobin (g%): 13.0–17.0 (*men*); 12.0–15.0 (*women*).

16   T   F   Total white cell count (cells/mm³): 1–3000

17   T   F   Platelets: 50,000–100,000

18   T   F   Reticulocyte count (%): 1–2

Directions: Circle T for true, F for false. Correct the false statements in the space below each question.

CHAPTER 16   The Red Blood Cell

OBJECTIVES   **At the completion of Chap. 16 you should be able to:**

1 Recognize a red blood cell.

2 Describe two functions of the normal red blood cell.

3 Define *anemia*.

4 List the classic signs and symptoms of anemia.

5 Differentiate between morphological and etiologic classification of anemia.

6 Differentiate between the three morphological classifications for anemia.

7 Describe the two major etiologic classifications of anemia.

8 Identify for sickle-cell anemia the etiology, signs, symptoms, and treatment.

9 List the principles involved in the treatment of anemia.

10 Define *polycythemia*.

11 Distinguish between relative and absolute polycythemia and primary and secondary forms of polycythemia.

12 Given a case study, identify the type of anemia evident in the patient.

MORPHOLOGY AND FUNCTION OF THE NORMAL RED BLOOD CELL

A red blood cell is a biconcave disc when viewed from the side. When looked at head on, it appears to have a lighter center, as shown in Fig. 16-1. Though there will not be a hole through the center, it will appear thicker on the outer perimeter and thinner in the middle. The shape of the biconcave disc is the most stable configuration for hemoglobin; if the hemoglobin is unstable, the cell may not assume this shape. The shape of the red blood cell will also change with varying thicknesses of the cell membrane and with different volumes inside the red blood cell. A good example of blood cell changes is found in the case of sickle-cell anemia. Sickle hemoglobin is unstable, and when sickle hemoglobin is deoxygenated, it assumes an abnormal configuration, and the red blood cells assume the shape of a sickle.

The major functions of red cells are to carry oxygen from the lungs to the tissues and carry carbon dioxide from the tissues back to the lungs. They also help to maintain the normal pH of blood through a series of intracellular buffers.

ABNORMALITIES OF RED BLOOD CELL PRODUCTION

Anemia

When there are too few red cells, the condition known as anemia develops. There are many different kinds of anemias, just as there are many different ways of studying anemia. By definition, anemia is a reduction below the normal level in the number of red blood cells, the quantity of hemoglobin, and the volume of packed red cells per hundred milliliters of blood. In other words, the hemoglobin is lower than normal, the hematocrit is lower than normal, and the number of red blood cells in a cubic milliliter of blood is below normal when anemia exists.

The general signs and symptoms of anemia include pallor, or pale appearance of the skin, mucous membranes, conjunctiva, skin folds, and nail beds. The skin itself appears very pale and may, in extreme cases, appear yellow due to the lack of the reddish pigment added to skin by the presence of blood in the subcutaneous tissues and skin.

In anemia the tissues do not receive enough oxygen.

The body attempts to compensate by increasing cardiac output and respiration. Consequently, one of the major symptoms is shortness of breath upon exertion. In addition to shortness of breath, patients with anemia may have headaches. Vertigo or dizziness may also be a result of anemia. Anemic patients can feel weak or faint. Generally, the first symptom that many patients recognize when they become anemic is that they tire easily. They are unable to do the same amount of work without resting.

CLASSIFICATION OF ANEMIAS

Anemia can be classified according to the way cells look (morphological classification) or according to the cause of the anemia (etiologic classification).

Morphological classification

If the red blood cells are of normal size and normal shape, contain the normal amount of hemoglobin (meaning that the mean corpuscular hemoglobin concentration [MCHC] and the mean corpuscular volume [MCV] are normal) but the patient is anemic, this represents a *normocytic normochromic* anemia. *Cytic* refers to size of the red blood cells, and *chromic* to their color. The most frequent cause of this type of anemia would be chronic infection, cancer, or any condition that would cause a patient to be generally debilitated.

The second major category of anemia is known as a *macrocytic normochromic* anemia. *Macrocytic* means the red blood cells are too large; *normochromic* means they contain a normal amount of hemoglobin. Deficiency of either vitamin B_{12} or folic acid is the most common cause of macrocytic normochromic anemia. Both vitamin B_{12} and folic acid are important in the synthesis of the nucleic acid DNA, particularly as it relates to single-carbon metabolism.

The last broad category of anemias are the *microcytic hypochromic* anemias. *Microcytic* means small, *hypochromic* means containing less than the normal amount of pigment, or hemoglobin. In these red blood cells the MCV is decreased and the MCHC is decreased. The most common example of this is iron-deficiency anemia. In fact, iron-deficiency anemia is probably the most common cause of anemia throughout the world.

Etiologic classification

There are many ways in which one can become anemic. One way is through removal of red blood cells from the circulation; this happens most frequently through blood loss. An example of an acute form of blood loss would be a bleeding ulcer. Chronic blood loss occurs in people who have polyps in the colon which are often irritated and bleed small amounts of blood over a long period of time. Menstrual blood loss is another form of chronic blood loss.

A reduction in the number of red blood cells also occur when red blood cells are lost while in the circulatory system. The destruction of red blood cells while in the circulatory system is known as *hemolysis*. Hemolysis can occur as the result of hereditary problems, such as sickle-cell anemia, or it can be due to acquired problems, which are generally related to an immune response. An *isoimmune* response is a response within the same species, but involving different individuals. An isoimmune acquired hemolytic anemia would result from receiving a transfusion with incompatible blood. Hemolysis can also occur when patients make antibodies against their own red blood cells; this is called auto-immune hemolytic anemia. It can occur without any known cause (an idiopathic response) and also as a secondary autoimmune hemolytic anemia. This secondary type of anemia occurs in a wide variety of diseases, such as lymphoma and Hodgkin's disease. Certain drugs will also induce autoimmune hemolytic anemias. A drug used for hypertension called alpha methyldopa can cause autoimmune hemolytic anemia. Hemolysis may also occur as the result of severe burns, especially when the microcirculation is badly disrupted.

A decreased number of red blood cells can also be the result of insufficient production of red blood cells. There are many reasons why either suddenly or chronically over a long period of time one would not produce enough red blood cells. One reason would be the deficiency of a vitamin, particularly B_{12}, or of folic acid. Pernicious anemia is an example of vitamin B_{12} deficiency due to an inability to absorb vitamin B_{12}. As mentioned previously, iron deficiency would produce a microcytic hypochromic anemia.

Anemia may also result from the production of abnormal hemoglobins or red blood cells. These problems are usually the result of inherited abnormalities. The abnormalities may result in inadequate production of red blood cells or hemoglobin (thalassemia) or enhanced destruction of red blood cells (hereditary spherocytosis, sickle-cell anemia).

SICKLE-CELL ANEMIA

Sickle-cell anemia refers to a hereditary hematologic disorder associated with the presence of a defective hemoglobin S in the erythrocyte. It is a recessive disease,

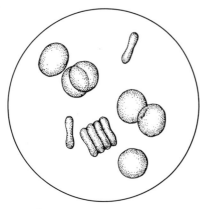

FIGURE 16-1 Erythyrocytes.

requiring a homozygous state to produce the disease. The inheritance of hemoglobin S is classified as autosomal codominant.

Abnormalities in the globin fraction of the hemoglobin molecule have been demonstrated to be responsible for the condition. Hemoglobin S differs from the normal type of hemoglobin A in the substitution of one amino acid for another (β,6-glutamic acid for valine) (Comings, 1972).

As mentioned previously, the formation of sickle-shaped cells follows exposure to lowered oxygen tension in the tissue. Sickle cells are very fragile. Early destruction by hemolysis leads to shortened red blood cell life span.

The most common form of sickle-cell disease is sickle-cell anemia (SS). This disease occurs almost exclusively in blacks. Infants with this disease tend to be asymptomatic because of the temporary presence of normal fetal hemoglobin F. The diagnosis is generally made during the preschool period.

Signs and symptoms of children under 2 years of age include recurrent infection, failure to thrive, fever, swelling of hands and feet, abdominal distension, pallor, nausea, and vomiting. The most common complaints in children over 2 years are joint, back, and abdominal pain. Physical findings may include pallor of the mucous membranes, lymphadenopathy, cardiac enlargement, ascites, joint swelling, enuresis, nocturia, and splenic enlargement. A characteristic appearance of children with sickle-cell anemia is that they are asthenic and have an increased arm span, disproportion between the length of the trunk and the legs, and long, tapering fingers. They also exhibit frontal bossing, prominent upper and central incisor teeth, and a usually frail appearance (Jackson, 1972).

Therefore, the diagnosis should be considered in young black patients who have pale mucous membranes and conjunctival icterus. Some patients are poorly developed with a degree of retardation of secondary sex characteristics. Tortuous, dilated vessels are frequently seen in the ocular field. The heart is enlarged, and there is an impaired ability to concentrate urine. Normochromic anemia is accompanied by laboratory signs of hemolysis with increased erythropoiesis. Oval, cigar-shaped, sickled cells are usually seen on a stained blood smear.

Sickle-cell crisis refers to any new syndrome that develops rapidly in sickle-cell patients that is due to the basic genetic abnormality. The painful crisis is due to the intertwining of sickle cells resulting in the clogging of the small capillaries. The pain may occur spontaneously or may be precipitated by stress. This pain usually has its onset in the morning and occurs in the bones or joints of the extremities. It is usually severe and migratory in nature. The temperature is frequently elevated to 100°F to 104°F with leukocytosis. The duration of these attacks is usually from 4 to 6 days (Comings, 1972).

No consistent therapy is available for this pain crisis. Oxygen therapy may be given but does not cause amelioration of the pain. Narcotics should be avoided since addiction may result. Intravenous fluid therapy with 5% dextrose has been effective in alleviating pain crisis in some patients. Vasodilating drugs, alkaloids, and anticoagulants have also been used. However, the treatment is supportive and symptomatic. For example, in acute crisis it is necessary to maintain adequate hydration and electrolyte balance, and the monitoring of the blood pH. At present, there are no chemotherapeutic agents universally accepted that reverse sickling.

BONE MARROW DEFICIENCIES

Deficiencies can also result from some process going on within the bone marrow itself which would cause a decrease in the production of red blood cells (RBCs). One functional problem would be a destruction of the bone marrow itself which would cause a decrease in the number of stem cells producing red blood cells. An outside agent might also destroy the stem cell and limit the production of RBCs. One of the antibiotics, chloramphenicol, rarely may destroy stem cells and cause a form of drug-induced aplastic anemia. Chloramphenicol can also destroy both the white blood cells and the platelets so that particulate matter is markedly decreased in the peripheral blood. Patients with this condition do not usually survive unless the bone marrow recovers. Certain tumors of the thymus gland can also destroy the stem cell. In this case, whatever it is that destroys the stem cell (perhaps antibodies) destroys only the red blood cell precursors, which causes pure red blood cell aplasia. In this condition, there are normal numbers of white blood cells, normal numbers of platelets, but no red blood cells being produced. Patients with this condition have to be supported with blood transfusions periodically.

Displacement of the marrow cavity can also reduce blood cell production. Probably the most common condition causing replacement of the bone marrow is widely disseminated cancer. Breast cancer patients with bone metastases may have the bone marrow completely replaced with tumor, so that normal development of the cells ceases.

Outside factors not related primarily to the marrow can cause a depression in the rate of red blood cell production. For example, there are hormones produced in the kidney which are essential for normal red blood cell production. In patients with renal failure, the kidney is often destroyed or removed, and the hormone erythropoietin is no longer produced. This condition causes normal red blood cell production to occur at a much slower rate.

Chronic illness is probably the most common cause for depression of red blood cell production, but the reason for this is not clear. It may be that erythropoietin is no longer produced. When the body must curtail production of certain proteins, the glycoprotein molecule erythropoietin is one of the first proteins to stop being produced. The body will tend to conserve muscle protein, for example, much longer than it will preserve the production of the protein portion of the erythropoietin molecule. Thus, a patient who is chronically ill will often become mildly anemic. Such patients usually do not need blood transfusions, but their hemoglobin will go down to 9 or 10 g%.

TREATMENT OF ANEMIA

Successful treatment depends upon finding what caused the anemia and correcting that condition. It would be very simple to give a patient who is iron-deficient an iron supplement which would correct the anemia, but it is very important to find out the reasons for iron deficiency before recommending this treatment. (Only after a specific cause for the anemia has been identified should treatment be instituted.)

Polycythemia

Thus far, discussion has centered on conditions resulting from too few red blood cells. A condition also exists where there are too many red blood cells. This condition is called polycythemia; *poly* meaning too many, *cythemia* meaning red blood cells. Polycythemia is defined as an increase above the normal number of red blood cells in the circulating blood which results in increased whole-blood viscosity and increased blood volume.

There are both relative and absolute forms of polycythemia. *Relative* polycythemia occurs when, for poorly understood reasons, the volume of circulating plasma is decreased. The hematocrit is higher than normal, but the total blood volume of circulating red cells is normal.

In addition to relative polycythemia there is also *absolute* polycythemia. Absolute polycythemia refers to a condition in which there is an actual increase in the circulating red blood cell mass.

In addition to being classified as relative and absolute, polycythemia can also be classified as primary and secondary. For example, absolute polycythemia may be secondary to some underlying medical problem such as lung disease.

On occasion, polycythemia can be due to a primary defect in the red blood cell production. This is referred to as *primary* polycythemia, or polycythemia vera.

Case studies of anemia

The following case studies discuss clinical examples of the various types of anemia that were previously discussed.

Mr. M. is a 56-year-old man who has been drinking steadily since his wife died 1 year ago. In this past year his meals consisted mainly of hamburgers eaten in bars. He came to the hospital because of weakness and syncopal episodes.
Physical exam: Pale, white male
        Tongue smooth, slightly red
        Pale mucous membranes and nail beds
        Liver enlarged as the result of alcoholism
His diagnosis is megaloblastic anemia.

The laboratory data obtained on this patient is shown below:

As shown below, on admission to the hospital, the patient's hematocrit was 17; hemoglobin was 6.2. Vitamin B_{12} and serum folate levels were drawn, but since the test results would not be available for several days, immediate therapy had to be directed without this information. Once these values were obtained, long-range therapy could be determined. As you can see, vitamin B_{12} levels were normal, but serum folate levels were very, very low. This means that the megaloblastic anemia was not due to vitamin B_{12} deficiency but to folate deficiency. Since the patient had an abnormal ECG (suggesting coronary artery disease) and fainting spells, he was given 2 units of blood before the results were obtained. He was treated with folic acid since it was strongly suspected that folate deficiency was his problem. As you can see, in a period of time his hematocrit rose toward normal, his hemoglobin concentration rose toward normal, and the marked macrocytosis as characterized by the mean corpuscular volume (MCV) reading of 115 gradually declined toward normal. The amount of hemoglobin in the cell, the mean corpuscular hemoglobin concentration (MCHC), was normal in the beginning and did not change. Again this points out the fact that this was a macrocytic normochromic anemia. You can see that his reticulocyte count rose, although not

Megaloblastic Anemia

DATE	RBC 10^6/mm³	Hct, vol%	Hgb, g%	MCV, μm³	MCHC, g%	RETICU- LOCYTES, %	OTHERS
7/15		17	6.2				B_{12} 343 (200–900) ⎫ (normal values) Folate 1.0 (3–15) ⎭
7/16							Two units of blood given. Folate therapy begins.
7/18	2.41	27	6.8	115	31	7.3	
7/24		31	8.4			6.5	
8/19	4.0	36	12.4	92	34	6.0	

as dramatically as it might have had he not received a transfusion, but was well above normal for several weeks during which time his hemoglobin concentration and hematocrit improved.

Figure 16-2 depicts the patient's peripheral blood as it was obtained on admission. The polymorphonuclear leukocyte (PMN) in the center of the figure is interesting because it contains at least six segments, though normal PMNs usually contain five or less. This is an example of the hypersegmented neutrophils which are one characteristic of a macrocytic anemia such as Mr. M.'s. In the upper right, note that the red blood cells are not all uniformly round as they were in Fig. 16-1 and are many different sizes. Most of the cells are of normal size or too large, and several are large, oval, red cells called ovalomacrocytes. Ovalomacrocytes are also characteristic of the vitamin B_{12} and folate deficiencies. In the lower left, there are several very large, oval-shaped macrocytes.

The bone marrow of a patient with megaloblastic anemia is shown in Fig. 16-3. In the upper right, there is one red blood cell precursor which is near normal with a condensed nuclear chromatin pattern. The remaining cells are very large and have an open nuclear chromatic pattern. These large cells are also red blood cell precursors, but they are 2 to 3 times normal size. In the lower left, is a large white blood cell precursor (metamyelocyte) which is 2 to 3 times normal size. This finding demonstrates that all cell lines develop abnormally in this condition.

Mrs. C. is a 36-year-old woman, in the second trimester of her third pregnancy. Before becoming pregnant she had been having menorrhagia (excessive menstrual bleeding) aggravated by an intrauterine device. The intrauterine device was removed, and she become pregnant.

On physical exam she was a pale-appearing white woman with pale mucous membranes.

A summary (see chart, p. 172) of Mrs. C.'s hematologic values are as follows: hematocrit, 21; hemoglobin, 5.8. The MCV (normal around 90) was 78, indicating that her red blood cells were too small. Her MCHC was 25, indicating that the cells did not contain enough hemoglobin. The reticulocyte count was essentially normal. The serum iron level (FE) was 36, while the lower normal limit of serum iron concentration is around 50. The total iron-binding capacity (TIBC) was elevated at 450. This is a measure of the ability of the plasma to carry iron from the gut to the bone marrow and is characteristically elevated in iron-deficiency anemia. Thus, iron saturation in the blood was less than 10 percent, indicating that this was iron-deficiency anemia. Other causes of chronic blood loss were looked for, and none was found. The patient was begun on iron replacement, and over a period of time, her hematologic values returned toward normal.

Figure 16-4 demonstrates the marked variation in the size and shape of red blood cells seen in the hypochromic anemias discussed in the previous case study. The pale area of the red blood cell is much larger than

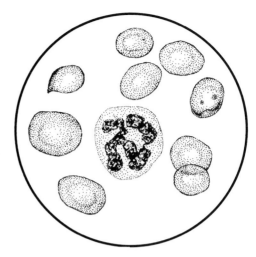

FIGURE 16-2 Peripheral blood characteristic of macrocytic anemia.

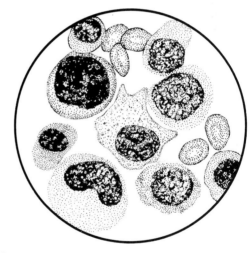

FIGURE 16-3 Bone marrow characteristic of megaloblastic anemia.

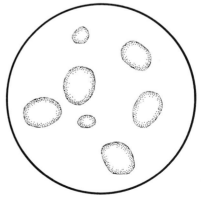

FIGURE 16-4 Erythrocytes characteristic of hypochromic anemia.

it is in a normal red blood cell, and the dark rim of hemoglobin around the edge of the cell is much narrower. There are cells that are too small, and the cells are not uniformly round. This appearance is characteristic of hypochromic anemias in general, and iron-deficiency anemia in particular.

QUESTIONS

The red blood cell—Chap. 16

Directions: Answer the following questions on a separate sheet of paper.

1 What are the two major functions of the normal red blood cell?

2 Why is the term "a lack of blood" a misleading definition for anemia? What is a better definition of anemia?

3 List the classical signs and symptoms of anemia.

4 State two etiologic factors related to anemia and give at least two examples of each type.

5 What are three major principles to consider when treating anemia?

6 What is polycythemia?

7 Describe the two classifications of absolute polycythemia. (Include an example of each type.)

8 Draw a normal red blood cell in the space provided below.

Directions: Complete the following statement by filling in the blank.

9 An anemia in which the MCV and MCHC are normal is referred to as _____ .

Directions: Circle the letter next to each item which correctly answers the following questions. More than one answer may be correct.

10 A macrocytic normochromic anemia is usually caused by a deficiency of:
   a Vitamin B_{12} b Iron   c Folic acid   d Potassium

11 Mrs. B., a 36-year-old female, was diagnosed to have iron-deficiency anemia. Which one of the following red blood cell characteristics is most commonly found in anemia due to iron deficiency?
   a Normocytic normochromic   b Microcytic hypochromic   c Macrocytic normochromic

12 A 4-year-old black female presents with pale mucous membranes and conjunctival icterus. Further examination revealed lymphodenopathy, cardiac enlargement, ascites, joint swelling, and splenic enlargement. Oval, cigar-shaped sickled cells were seen on a stained blood smear. Her diagnosis is sickle-cell anemia. The patient developed severe bone and joint pain in her extremities; and an elevated temperature of 102°F with leukocytosis. This syndrome is referred to as:
   a Chronic sickle-cell anemia   b Sickle-cell thalassemia disease   c Sickle-cell crisis   d Chronic normochromic anemia

13 The principles of treatment for the syndrome described in the above question include:
   a Monitoring of the blood pH   b Administration of narcotics   c Administration of chemotherapeutic agents to reverse the sickling process   d Maintenance of adequate hydration and electrolyte balance

Directions: Circle T if true, F if false. Write a rationale for your selection.

14   T   F   Relative polycythemia is characterized by a normal total red blood cell mass.

15   T   F   Absolute polycythemia refers to an increase in red blood cell mass.

Iron-Deficiency Anemia

DATE	RBC, $10^6/mm^3$	Hct, vol%	Hgb, g%	MCV, μm^3	MCHC, g%	RETICU-LOCYTES, %	OTHER
8/15	3.0	21	5.8	78	25	0.5	FE 36, TIBC 450
8/16		25	7.6			5.0	Ferrous sulfate begun.
8/17		35	12.0	85	34	3.0	

CHAPTER 17   The White Blood Cell

OBJECTIVES   **At the completion of Chap. 17 you should be able to:**

1 List the five types of white blood cells normally found in peripheral blood.

2 Distinguish between the three types of granulocytes, and the monocytes and lymphocytes normally found in the circulation.

3 Describe the functions of each of the cells listed in objective no. 2.

4 Describe leukocytosis by identifying the type of cells and types of disease conditions related to leukocytosis.

5 List the possible etiologic factors of neutropenia.

6 Differentiate between multiple myeloma and Waldenstrom's macroglobulinemia by identifying the location of neoplasm, presenting symptoms, diagnosis, treatment, and prognosis for each.

7 Differentiate between acute or chronic lymphocytic or nonlymphocytic leukemia in relation to clinical course, degree of immaturity of the white blood cells, treatment, and prognosis.

8 Differentiate between Hodgkin's disease and non-Hodgkin's lymphoma according to the type of cells involved, signs and symptoms, complications, staging, treatment, and prognosis.

9 Given case studies, identify the type of plasma cell dyscrasia, leukemia, or lymphoma evident in each patient.

MORPHOLOGY AND FUNCTION OF THE NORMAL WHITE BLOOD CELL

There are three different types of granulocytes (cells with granules in the cytoplasm) contained in the peripheral blood: the polymorphonuclear leukocyte (also known as a neutrophil or a PMN), the eosinophil, and the basophil. The name given to a granulocyte depends on the type of granules contained in the cytoplasm. If there are just faint pink, acidophilic granules, then the cell is a normal segmented neutrophil, or polymorphonuclear leukocyte. If the granules are refractile, eosinophilic granules, the cell is an eosinophil. If the granules are large and blue (or basophilic), they are called basophils. These three types of cells are illustrated in Fig. 17-1. They are all called granulocytes even though they have different functions and occur in different numbers in the peripheral blood.

Lymphocytes are also found in the peripheral blood. They vary in size but are generally smaller than a granulocyte. The lymphocyte has a single, round nucleus, and

the cytoplasm is faintly basophilic. The nuclear chromatin pattern is heavily clumped with a network of inner connections.

The third major cellular element is a monocyte. The nucleus of a monocyte is folded or indented and often looks lobulated. The monocyte also has a clumped nuclear chromatin pattern, but it is a looser clumping than is seen in the lymphocyte. The cytoplasm of the monocyte is a bluish gray or a very light sky blue (Fig. 17-2).

The main function of segmented neutrophils is fighting bacterial infections. They do this through a process of phagocytosis. This process refers to ingestion of material from outside the cell that is then digested by the cell. PMNs also digest foreign particulate matter in the blood, such as breakdown products from cells. Neutrophils are present in the early, acute phase of an inflammatory reaction.

The eosinophils also have a phagocytic function similar to the polymorphonuclear leukocytes, but their role in combating infection is not clear-cut. It has not been demonstrated that the eosinophils are particularly important in digesting bacteria as a defense mechanism. Their levels are not elevated during infections like those of the segmented forms, but they do have the ability to ingest bacteria. Eosinophils appear to play a role in combating allergic reactions.

The function of the basophils is not well understood. The basophils contain many different enzymes which can be released into the blood, but the function of these enzymes is not clear. However, it is thought that the basophils play a role in combating acute systemic allergic reactions.

The monocytes are an extremely interesting group of cells, which are primarily concerned with the phagocytosis of dead red and white blood corpuscles in the blood. They also are important in the processing of antigenic information. (It appears that in the early stage of defense the PMNs are most important in fighting infection, with the monocytes following to clean up the remains.)

The lymphocytes are primarily concerned with the production of antibodies and the maintenance of tissue immunity.

Leukocytosis

Leukocytosis is an elevation in the white cell count. Any of the normal white blood cells can be elevated. An elevation in the number of PMNs is usually due to an acute bacterial infection. Eosinophilia can result as a response to an allergic disorder. Worm infestation can cause very high eosinophil counts. Since the function of basophils is not very well understood, it is not clear why they are increased in certain diseases. However, there are a broad group of diseases known as the *myeloproliferative diseases* (such as chronic granulocytic leukemia, polycythemia vera, and other disease states where the regulation of production of white blood cells seems to be abnormal) that demonstrate an increased number of basophils.

Lymphocytosis and monocytosis

Lymphocytosis refers to an elevation in the number of lymphocytes. The lymphocyte shown in Fig. 17-3 does not look much like a lymphocyte because it is abnormal. This is the type of lymphocyte seen in infectious mononucleosis. It looks much more like a monocyte than a lymphocyte. Similar types of lymphocytic abnormalities are also seen in other viral illness.

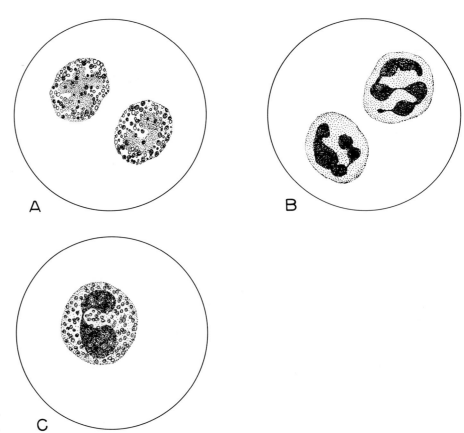

FIGURE 17-1 Granulocytes. A. Basophil. B. Neutrophils. C. Eosinophils.

Monocytosis, a condition where there are too many monocytes, can also occur. Tuberculosis causes monocytosis.

Leukopenia

Just as there are conditions where there are too many white blood cells, there are disease states where there are too few white blood cells (leukopenia). Probably the most frequent cause of neutropenia (decreased numbers of neutrophils) is viral infection. Patients with an acute upper respiratory infection may have a normal or only slightly depressed total white blood cell count, while the total number of neutrophils or segmented forms may be depressed well below normal. Agranulocytosis, a total absence of segmented forms in the peripheral blood, is another condition that can occur. Patients with agranulocytosis are usually quite ill and very vulnerable to sepsis and death. Agranulocytosis can be caused by drugs such as chloramphenicol.

Leukemia

CLASSIFICATION OF LEUKEMIAS

Leukemia is a neoplastic disease associated with an uncontrollable proliferation of any one of the types of white blood corpuscles (granulocytes, lymphocytes, and

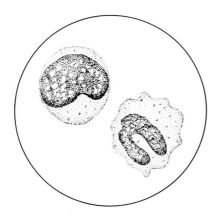

FIGURE 17-2 Monocytes.

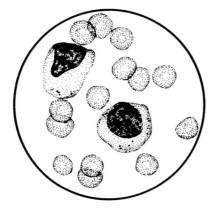

FIGURE 17-3 Abnormal lymphocyte seen in infectious mononucleosis.

monocytes). The type of problem and the type of treatment varies with the type of cell involved. The symptoms of leukemia are related to those of bone marrow failure, anemia, bleeding, and infection.

Leukemias can be classified by the type of cell involved in the malignant process; that is, lymphocytic, granulocytic, or monocytic. The disease can also be classified by the clinical course of the patient and the maturity of the white blood cell; the more primitive the cells look, the more rapidly progressive is the disease.

Listed below in Table 17-1 is an example of one type of classification of the leukemias. It is by no means a complete list.

As indicated above, leukemias can be categorized broadly on the overall course of the disease. Chronic leukemia has a fairly long clinical course. Acute leukemia, untreated, has a rapidly progressive course.

In *chronic lymphocytic leukemia* there is an accumulation of abnormal lymphocytes in the bone marrow and peripheral blood. A patient can have chronic lymphocytic leukemia for many years requiring no treatment. The median survival of patients with newly discovered chronic lymphocytic leukemia is 5 years, and one-third live more than 10 years. However, not all patients with chronic lymphocytic leukemia progress this well. Patients that are very ill at the time of diagnosis have a median survival rate of 1.5 years.

Figure 17-4 shows a normal-looking mature lymphocyte. Though these are relatively normal-looking lymphocytes, there may be several hundred thousand of these in the peripheral blood as opposed to the normal level of two or three thousand. *Chronic granulocytic leukemia* is a disease characterized by the presence of excessive granulocytes in the peripheral blood, including immature forms. The disease usually occurs in patients aged 25 to 60. Median survival is 3.5 years.

The aim of treatment is to control the abnormal proliferation of the granulocytes. It is not clear that the length of survival after diagnosis is improved by this kind of therapy. Most patients with chronic granulocytic

TABLE 17-1
Classification of the leukemias

CHRONIC
Chronic lymphocytic leukemia
Chronic granulocytic leukemia

ACUTE
Acute lymphoblastic leukemia
Acute nonlymphocytic leukemia
Acute granulocytic
Acute myelomonocytic
Acute histiomonocytic
Unclassifiable

leukemia develop an accelerated or an acute blastic phase. Generally, survival is very short after blastic transformation occurs.

The chart below is from a case history of a patient with chronic granulocytic leukemia. She presented with a high white cell count on a routine physical examination. Her physical examination was unremarkable; this patient did not exhibit the enlarged spleen that is often seen in these patients. The white cell count was very high (about 73,000). The patient was placed on busulfan, and over a period of time her white cell count approached normal. The differential count on the peripheral blood showed that there were many of the normal types of cells, but, in addition, there were increased numbers of immature cells as demonstrated by the percentage of metamyelocytes, myelocytes, and progranulocytes. These immature white blood cells which are in various stages of development are normally contained within the bone marrow. Finding these cells in the peripheral blood is distinctly abnormal.

Figure 17-5 demonstrates a number of basophils which are typically increased in chronic granulocytic leukemia. Two or three basophils in one field is distinctly abnormal. The granules are very dense, basophilic, and almost obscure the nucleus.

Figure 17-6 shows the bone marrow of a patient with chronic granulocytic leukemia. All the types of granulocyte precursors are demonstrated in this field. Morphologically there is nothing abnormal about these cells, but the numbers of these cells in the bone marrow are dramatically increased. The marrow appears to be hypercellular.

ACUTE LEUKEMIAS

The acute leukemias can be broadly divided into the lymphoblastic and the nonlymphocytic depending on whether the malignant cell originated from the lymphocytic or granulocytic series.

Acute lymphoblastic leukemia (ALL) occurs primarily in children. Improved survival of children has been dramatic in ALL. Median survival has been increased

from 3 months before modern therapy was available to the point that now 90 to 95 percent of children achieve a complete remission (no evidence of disease), and 40 to 50 percent of these are alive and still in their first remission at 5 years after diagnosis. These dramatic results are achieved with complex multi-drug and interdisciplinary programs including radiation and immunotherapy.

The same disease, from all appearances, occurs in adults, but results of treatment are not as good, with less than 75 percent achieving complete remissions; the median survival is still only around 2 years.

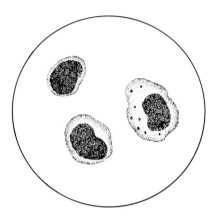

FIGURE 17-4 Mature lymphocyte.

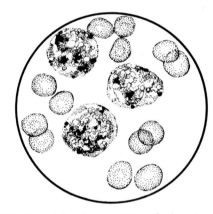

FIGURE 17-5 Basophils characteristic of chronic granulocytic leukemia.

C.S.:	63-year-old female				
Dx:	Chronic granulocytic leukemia (CGL) May, 1975				
Hx:	High WBC count on routine check-up				
PE:	Unremarkable				
Lab:			5/72	6/72	1/73
	Hgb, g%		13.1	12.1	14.3
	Hct, vol%		39.5	37.1	46.1
	WBC, cells/mm³		73,600	6300	19,200
Differential count (%) at Dx:	PMN	50	Progranulocytes	13	
	Band	7	Lymphocytes	7	
	Metamyelocytes	11	Eosinophiles	5	
	Myelocytes	7	Nucl RBC	1	

Figure 17-7 shows a lymphoblast. There is much less cytoplasm than normal, and the nuclear chromatin pattern is very homogeneous in this distinctly abnormal, primitive-looking cell.

The following chart is from a case history of a patient with acute lymphoblastic leukemia. This 18-year-old boy presented with a 3-week history of fatigue, headache, and easy bruising (due to decreased numbers of platelets) evidenced by ecchymoses over his body and enlargement of both the liver and spleen. He was markedly anemic; his white count and platelet count were low, and his differential count showed 11 percent lymphoblasts. The bone marrow was hypercellular with almost

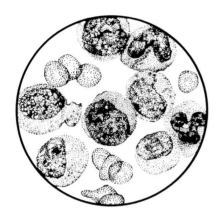

FIGURE 17-6 Bone marrow characteristic of chronic granulocytic leukemia.

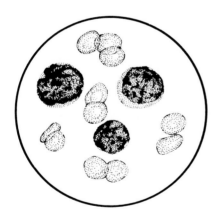

FIGURE 17-7 Lymphoblast.

complete replacement of the bone marrow with lymphoblasts. Treatment with chemotherapy consisting mainly of vincristine and prednisone resulted in a complete remission. The patient was in remission on three different occasions, but succumbed to his disease about 3.5 years after diagnosis. Each succeeding remission was harder to obtain and lasted a shorter period of time.

The nonlymphocytic leukemias include all types of leukemia which are not lymphocytic. The majority of these are granulocytic, and are called acute granulocytic leukemias. Some types of nonlymphocytic leukemias are unclassifiable. Diseases in this category cannot be classified by light microscopy.

The *acute nonlymphocytic leukemias* occur primarily in adults. Treatment requires the use of much more toxic drugs with significant morbidity. Even with the use of these more toxic agents, results of treatment are not as good. Only about 50 percent of patients respond to treatment. Median survival of all patients is still less than 1 year. Remissions, when obtained, generally last less than a year, and second remissions are rare. Even those patients who initially respond to treatment rarely live beyond 2 years after diagnosis.

On those rare occasions when children develop acute nonlymphocytic leukemia, their survival is about the same as adults and is much worse than for children with ALL.

Figure 17-8 demonstrates the bone marrow of a patient with acute histiomonocytic leukemia. The cells shown here are less homogenous in appearance, there are many different sizes and shapes, the nucleus can be folded, and these cells have many characteristics of very early immature monocytes.

PLASMA CELL DYSCRASIAS

Multiple myeloma

The first group of diseases discussed here are the plasma cell dyscrasias. This is the general term for a variety of diseases of which two are described here. The first of the plasma cell dyscrasias to be discussed is multiple

D.H.:	18-year-old male			
Dx:	Acute lymphoblastic leukemia (ALL) June, 1971			
Hx:	3 weeks fatigue, headache, bruises			
PE:	Ecchymoses, hepatosplenomegaly			
Lab:	Hgb, 7.1 g%	Diff (%):	PMN	20; young 6
	Hct, 18.5 vol%		Lymphocytes	33
	WBC, 2850 cells/mm³		Lymphoblasts	11
	Plt, 60,000 cells/mm³		Broken cells	30
Bone marrow:	Hypercellular with 99% lymphoblasts			
Course:	Complete remission with three subsequent relapses in the bone marrow			
	Currently in partial remission			

myeloma, or plasma cell myeloma. This is a malignant neoplasm that arises in the bone marrow and involves primarily bone. This neoplasm usually does not metastasize outside the bone. Examination of the bone marrow is essential for the diagnosis of myeloma. In multiple myeloma, the marrow typically contains at least 15 percent plasma cells with a large proportion of immature and multinucleated forms. These abnormal "myeloma" cells are 15 to 40 μm in diameter and have an eccentrically placed nucleus. When the plasma cells in the bone marrow become malignant and lose the ability to regulate their own division, they begin to form tumors inside bone. This erodes the bone, causing definite holes in the bones which can be seen by x-ray examination. The most frequent presenting complaint in multiple myeloma is bone pain, which may be severe and debilitating. Often these patients become lethargic and lose weight. The bones become so fragile that a hip or an arm can be broken by simply rolling over in bed. A simple cough can cause the patient's ribs to break.

It should also be noted that, because of bony involvement, calcium metabolism may be abnormal, causing some patients to have an elevated level of serum calcium. The plasma cells produce abnormal globulins including cryoglobin, which can produce a variety of symptoms including Raynaud's phenomenon (blanching of the hands on exposure to cold). Renal damage can be caused by the abnormal globulins as well as causing increased viscosity of the blood leading to central nervous system ischemia, congestive heart failure, and bleeding problems.

In recent years, the prognosis in multiple myeloma has improved, but the median survival is still only 3 to 4 years.

Treatment of multiple myeloma consists of using chemotherapeutic agents. Melphalan either alone or with prednisone is most frequently employed, with radiation therapy as an adjunct to the chemotherapy. Radiation therapy can be used to provide relief of bone pain and promote healing of pathologic fractures.

Figure 17-9 is a peripheral blood film from a patient who has multiple myeloma. The background of this figure appears dirty. That is not a technical artifact. The dark, dirty-looking background is caused by the protein that is present in the peripheral blood, which has precipitated out on the field and has darkened with the staining material. The red blood cells demonstrate a phenomenon known as *rouleau* where the cells stack up like coins. They stick together abnormally because of the increased protein content of the blood.

A relatively normal plasma cell is seen in the upper right field of Fig. 17-10, while the other cells shown are abnormal (malignant) plasma cells. These cells are seen in patients with multiple myeloma.

Waldenstrom's macroglobulinemia

The second plasma cell dyscrasia (dysproteinemia) discussed here, Waldenstrom's macroglobulinemia, is rare. Instead of the localized areas of bony abnormality common to multiple myeloma, patients with Waldenstrom's macroglobulinemia have profuse infiltration of the bone marrow with cells which have characteristics of both plasma cells and lymphocytes. The exact origin of these cells remains uncertain, but they are probably lymphocytes.

The course of Waldenstrom's macroglobulinemia is different from that of multiple myeloma in that the major problem is increased protein production by the abnormal cells. The protein content of the blood can get quite high, leading to such things as congestive failure and renal failure. These patients produce tremendous quantities of nonfunctional immunoglobulin, causing the body to stop producing normal immunoglobulin. Patients with this disease become markedly susceptible to infection. In particular, patients with Waldenstrom's macroglobulinemia or multiple myeloma are susceptible to the gram-positive organisms like pneumococci, and they often die from pneumonia rather than from the underlying disease.

The treatment of Waldenstrom's macroglobulinemia

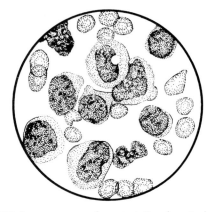

FIGURE 17-8 Bone marrow characteristic of acute histiomonocytic leukemia.

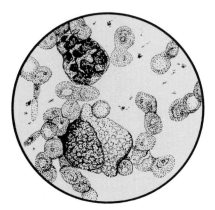

FIGURE 17-9 Peripheral blood characteristic of multiple myeloma.

is generally not very satisfactory. Plasmapheresis, replacement of the plasma which contains the abnormal proteins with saline, is frequently tried. Chemotherapeutic agents have also been used, but they are generally unsuccessful. These patients rarely live beyond a year after diagnosis. Some success recently has been achieved with multiple-drug chemotherapy, offering some hope to people suffering from this disease.

LYMPHOMA

General considerations

Lymphoma is a malignancy found primarily in lymph nodes. This is different than leukemia, because in leukemia the malignant cells are found primarily in the bone marrow. The lymphomas can be divided into two broad groups: one is Hodgkin's disease and the other is non-Hodgkin's lymphoma. The difference between the two types of lymphoma is evident from the pathologic interpretation of the lymph node. If a Reed-Sternberg cell is present in the material, the condition is called Hodgkin's disease. A Reed-Sternberg cell is an abnormal cell which appears to be a malignant histiocyte. Figure 17-11 de-

picts a large cell with two very large pale nuclei which is a Reed-Sternberg cell. If there are not Reed-Sternberg cells in the lymph nodes, then the condition is called a non-Hodgkin's lymphoma. There is an entire classification scheme for non-Hodgkin's lymphomas, but it is not necessary to look at this classification in detail. Patients with non-Hodgkin's lymphomas can have extensive disease and have no symptoms at all. However, if they do have symptoms these often include fever, chills, night sweats, weight loss, and loss of appetite.

Table 17-2 illustrates the Ann Arbor staging classification which is used for Hodgkin's disease and lymphoma. In Stage I the disease is localized to one single group of nodes, either above or below the diaphragm. In Stage II the disease is localized above or below the diaphragm, but it can be in two noncontiguous areas of lymph nodes. Stage III disease is still limited to the lymph nodes, but it occurs in the nodes both above and below the diaphragm. Stage IV disease involves the invasion of other tissues other than the lymph nodes, most notably bone marrow or liver. These four stages are subdivided into A and B groups according to the presence or absence of symptoms. A patients have *no* symptoms at all. Patients with B disease have at least one of the following: fever, chills, night sweats, or weight loss (at least 10 percent of the original body weight). Night sweats are not just a slight sweating at night, but represent drenching sweating at night which requires changing of bed clothes and sheets. There is also a minor subclassification of E patients who have minor extranodal involvement. For example, a patient with Hodgkin's disease located in the chest and with little extension out of the lymph node into the lung would not be classified in Stage IV but as an E patient. It would only be if there was a definite metastasis distally in the lung that the patient would be classified as in Stage IV. It is possible to have limited involvement near involved lymph nodes and outside of lymph nodes and still be an E patient. If the spleen is involved, the patient belongs in the subclassification S. Each of these classifications is used to determine the appropriate therapy.

Itching of the skin is another symptom of Hodgkin's disease and lymphoma. These patients are also prone to

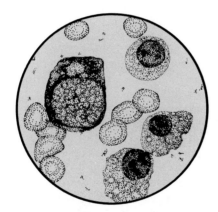

FIGURE 17-10 Plasma cells typical of multiple myeloma.

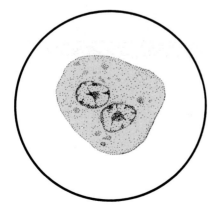

FIGURE 17-11 Reed-Sternberg cell.

TABLE 17-2
Ann Arbor staging classification of Hodgkin's disease and lymphoma

Stage I	Localized disease of a single group of nodes and/or adjacent nodes
Stage II	Disease located above *or* below the diaphragm extending beyond adjacent nodes without extranodal involvement
Stage III	Disease extending above *and* below the diaphragm but limited to lymph nodes (including spleen)
Stage IV	Extranodal disease

develop herpes zoster, a viral infection where very painful vesicles or bubbles on the skin develop. The lesions continue to be painful after they heal.

Hodgkin's disease

Hodgkin's disease occurs primarily in young adults and in late middle age. Its incidence at other times is much less common. Generally, the younger patients do better with treatment. Treatment is determined by the extent of involvement (stage classification) at the time of diagnosis (see Table 17-2). The more limited forms are treated with radiation therapy, and those with more extensive disease receive multiple-drug chemotherapeutic regimens.

Survival is excellent in those with more limited involvement and has been improved with drug therapy in the more advanced stages of the disease.

Non-Hodgkin's lymphoma

Non-Hodgkin's lymphoma occurs with increasing frequency with advancing age. It generally tends to be widespread (advanced in stage) at the time of diagnosis. Treatment of the early stages is with radiation therapy; and more advanced stages are treated primarily with chemotherapy. While response to therapy occurs frequently, it is less obvious that this leads to increased survival, although palliative benefit (relief of symptoms, improved clinical condition) is experienced as a result of response to therapy.

M.M.: 22-year-old male	*Dx:* Hodgkin's disease
Hx: Asymptomatic mass in neck	April, 1971
Evaluation: Stage IA	*Treatment:* Irradiation
April, 1973: 3 months' fever, abdominal pain, weight loss	
Hgb: 9.9 g%	Splenomegaly
Hct: 27.6 vol%	Laparotomy: Nodes positive, spleen negative
WBC: 2900 cells/mm³	IVP: Abnormal
Plt: 153,000 cells/mm³	Extent of disease: Stage IIIB
Rx: MOPP × 6 courses	
May, 1973: Complete remission	

The above chart is from a case of a 22-year-old man who presented with Hodgkin's disease in April, 1971. He was classified Stage IA (meaning disease was present in only one lymph node bearing area), was given irradiation, and did well until 1973 when the disease recurred. At that time he had splenomegaly (enlargement of the spleen) with positive involvement in nodes and the spleen of the abdomen. His x-rays of the kidney were

abnormal due to the involvement of nodes in the abdomen, and he was reclassified as Stage IIIB. At this point a four-drug regimen consisting of nitrogen mustard, vincristine, procarbazine, and prednisone (MOPP) was begun, and a complete remission was obtained. The patient continues to do well to the present day.

DRUGS FREQUENTLY USED IN TREATMENT OF HEMOTOLOGIC MALIGNANCIES

Table 17-3 lists some of the more frequently used chemotherapeutic agents used in the treatment of hematologic malignancies. Their adverse effects are divided into acute and chronic toxicity. Acute toxicity refers to an immediate reaction, that is, within minutes or hours after giving the medication. Chronic toxicity refers to a reaction which is cumulative over a long period of time.

Nitrogen mustard is administered only in the vein, and if the medication is not given "cleanly" in the vein, it can cause an ulcer or marked reaction around the injection site. Almost all patients treated with nitrogen mustard exhibit vomiting. The emesis occurs anywhere from 1 to 3 hours after the injection and lasts anywhere from several hours to 24 hours. The vomiting occurs almost every time the patient is given this medication.

Cylophosphamide is another alkylating agent. High dosages of this drug may cause nausea and vomiting. Alopecia (hair loss) is a sign of chronic toxicity. This can be total or almost total hair loss including the eyebrows and eyelashes. Bone marrow depression causes the white blood and platelet counts to drop when this drug is used. Another sign of toxicity is hemorrhagic cystitis. This is a very serious complication and, on occasion, patients have to have surgical removal of the bladder in order to control the hemorrhage. For this reason, if any patient on cyclophosphamide develops any hematuria, it is an *absolute* necessity to stop the drug until the etiology of the hemorrhage is known.

Although melphalan is usually tolerated well, it can cause anorexia, nausea, vomiting, and bone marrow depression.

Chlorambucil can cause nausea and vomiting, although this is an unusual side effect. There can also be dermatitis (skin eruptions) from this medication.

Mild nausea is not uncommon with busulfan, although vomiting is usually not so severe as with nitrogen mustard. Again, bone marrow depression is a problem, and amenorrhea can occur. Increased skin pigmentation very similar to Addison's disease can occur with this medication after years of treatment with it. Pulmonary fibrosis or scarring of the lungs has been observed.

Antimetabolites are drugs which interfere with the normal metabolism of the cell, particularly as it relates to vitamin B_{12} and folic acid metabolism. Antimetabolites are frequently used in treating leukemia. An example of this type of drug is methotrexate, for which there is little evidence of acute toxic reactions. Chronic toxicities include oral ulcers, diarrhea, alopecia, and cirrhosis after long periods of treatment. The major problem with treatment using methotrexate is ulceration of the gastro-intestinal tract. When this drug is being given, the mouth must be carefully examined for ulcers before a dose of methotrexate is administered. If there are any indications of ulceration of the oral mucosa, the medication must not be given. This is extremely serious, for administration of methotrexate to a patient who already has ulcerations can cause slouching of the entire gastro-intestinal tract from mouth to anus, and fatal hemorrhage can occur.

Cytosine arabinoside is a drug which is used primarily in the treatment of acute leukemia. The major acute toxic effects are nausea, vomiting, headaches, and fever. Mild nausea is very common; fever occurs frequently. Occasional patients have developed marked febrile reactions to this drug, with temperatures up to 105°F and 106°F, which has necessitated stopping the medication. The major long-term effect is bone marrow depression.

Several other antimetabolites such as 6-mercapto-purine and 6-thioguanine are very similar to cytosine arabinoside in their toxicities; both can cause mild nausea and/or vomiting; both can cause bone marrow depression and liver damage.

Two drugs, vincristine and vinblastine, which are called mitotic spindle poisons, are also used in treating leukemia. These drugs damage the apparatus which separates newly divided chromosomes while they are still in the parent cell. Their acute toxicity is mainly a local reaction, causing marked ulceration in the skin if not given cleanly in the vein. Chronic toxicity includes alopecia and peripheral neuropathy, which can be severe. There have been instances of patients who have developed paraplegia after the administration of this drug. Hives, constipation, and muscle wasting or muscle weakness also occur. The toxicities of these two drugs are very similar. Vinblastine happens to cause more severe damage to the bone marrow than vincristine, but otherwise these drugs have very similar side effects.

QUESTIONS

The white blood cell—Chap. 17

Direction: Match the white blood cells listed in col. A with their appropriate function in col. B. More than one letter may be used in col. A.

Column A	Column B
1 ____ PMNs	a Phagocytosis of dead red and white corpuscles; processing of antigenic information
2 ____ Eosinophils	b Chief source of antibody production
3 ____ Basophils	c Present later in the inflammatory process
4 ____ Monocytes	d Present early in the acute phase of an inflammatory reaction
5 ____ Lymphocytes	e Phagocytosis, killing, and/or digestion of bacteria
6 ____ Plasma cells	f Phagocytic function, also appear to be important in allergic reactions
	g Appear to function in combating acute systemic allergic reactions

TABLE 17-3
Chemotherapy agents frequently used in hemotology

DRUG	ACUTE TOXICITY	CHRONIC TOXICITY
Alkylating agents		
Nitrogen mustard	Local reaction, anorexia, nausea, vomiting	Bone marrow depression
Cyclophosphamide	Nausea, vomiting	Alopecia, bone marrow depression, cystitis
Melphalan	Anorexia, nausea, vomiting	Bone marrow depression
Chlorambucil	Nausea, vomiting	Dermatitis
Busulfan	Nausea	Bone marrow depression, amenorrhea, increased pigmentation, wasting syndrome, pulmonary fibrosis
Antimetabolites		
Methotrexate		Oral ulcers, diarrhea, alopecia, liver damage
Cytosine arabinoside	Nausea, vomiting, headache, fever	
6-Mercaptopurine	Nausea, vomiting	Bone marrow depression
6-Thioguanine	Nausea, vomiting	Bone marrow depression
Mitotic spindle poisons		
Vincristine	Local reaction	Alopecia, peripheral neuropathy, hives, constipation, myopathy
Vinblastine	Local reaction, nausea, vomiting	Stomatitis, bone marrow depression, diarrhea, constipation, neuropathy

Directions: Circle T if the statement is true, F if it is false. Correct the false statements on a separate sheet of paper.

7   T   F   Plasma cells are normally found in the peripheral blood.

8   T   F   The most frequent cause of neutropenia is a reaction to a drug such as chloramphenicol.

9   T   F   Agranulocytosis is a total absence of segmented forms in the peripheral blood.

Directions: Complete the following statement by filling in the blanks.

10 _____ refers to an elevation in the white blood count.

11 The cells characteristic of Hodgkin's disease are called _____.

12 _____ is a decrease below normal in the leukocyte count.

13 List what type of white blood cell is elevated in the following conditions:

Condition	Type of cell
Acute bacterial infection	_____
Allergic rhinitis	_____
Myeloproliferative disorders	_____

Directions: Circle the letter next to each item which correctly answers the following questions. More than one answer may be correct.

14 Which of the following are frequent complications encountered in patients with multiple myeloma that must be considered when planning treatment and care?
a Pathologic fractures   *b* Pulmonary infections
c Hypocalcema   *d* Increased bleeding tendencies

15 Mr. B. has been complaining of weight loss, weakness, and repeated episodes of pneumonia. Lab tests show very high levels of an abnormal globulin and nasal bleeding. The most likely diagnosis of Mr. B.'s condition is:
a Chronic lymphocytic leukemia   *b* Lymphoma

c Multiple myeloma   *d* Waldenstrom's macroglobulinemia

16 Which of the following reactions are seen in patients with leukemia?
a Growth of leukemic cells in abnormal areas   *b* Destruction of normal bone marrow   *c* Increased metabolic rate   *d* Production of abnormal protein

17 Your patient is an adult who complains of increasing weakness and fatigue. He has recently noticed abnormal bruising and epitaxis (nosebleeds). On admission he developed fever and pneumonia. The spleen is not palpable. Laboratory studies reveal immature-appearing cells of the neutrophilic series. The most likely diagnosis is:
a Acute lymphocytic leukemia   *b* Acute granulocytic leukemia   *c* Chronic granulocytic leukemia
d Chronic lymphocytic leukemia

18 Hodgkin's disease, a lymphoproliferative disease, will usually be diagnosed by a:
a Blood test   *b* Tissue biopsy   *c* Both *a* and *b*
d Neither *a* nor *b*

19 Sites of spread of Hodgkin's disease may include:
a Lymph nodes   *b* Liver   *c* Spleen
d Bone marrow

Directions: Answer the following questions on a separate sheet of paper.

20 In a sentence or two, write a definition for leukemia.

21 Name the two criteria used to classify leukemia.

Directions: Match the type of drug in col. A with the associated toxic reaction(s) in col. B. More than one letter may be used in col. A. Items may be used more than once.

Column A	Column B
22 ___ Nitrogen mustard	*a* Alopecia, bone marrow depression, hemorrhagic cystitis
23 ___ Cyclophosphamide	*b* Ulceration occurs around injection site if this drug is not properly administered in the vein.
24 ___ Methotrexate	*c* Chromosomal division is damaged by the drug.
25 ___ Vincristine	*d* Emesis almost always occurs after administration of this drug.
	e Interferes with vitamin B_{12} and folic acid metabolism.
	f Major side effect is oral ulcers.

CHAPTER 18 Coagulation

OBJECTIVES

At the completion of Chap. 18 you should be able to:

1 Review the two major functions of platelets.

2 State the purpose of blood clotting.

3 List the 13 plasma clotting factors.

4 Describe the role of the liver as the major site of synthesis of plasma factors.

5 Describe the sequence of events that occurs when a blood vessel is injured by (a) identifying what enzyme is released, (b) identifying the plasma factors shared by both the extrinsic and intrinsic systems, (c) listing the common plasma factors in both systems, (d) explaining what causes a platelet plug, (e) identifying which factors platelets release, (f) explaining the purpose of clot resolution.

6 Explain the difference between prothrombin time and partial thromboplastin time.

7 Differentiate between three broad groups of coagulation abnormalities—primary vascular, primary platelet, and plasma factor deficiencies.

8 Differentiate between thrombocytosis and thrombocytopenia with regard to etiology, diagnosis, and treatment.

9 Describe hemophilia with regard to types, etiology, diagnosis, and treatment.

10 State the rationale for the treatment of diffuse intravascular coagulation.

THE NORMAL COAGULATION PROCESS AND PLASMA CLOTTING FACTORS

Blood coagulation refers to reactions which lead to the formation of a fibrin clot. Plasma factors and platelets are involved in this process.

Platelets, or thrombocytes, are anucleate, disc-shaped fragments of large marrow cells, megakaryocytes. They function to maintain capillary integrity (fill the spaces between the endothelial cells of the capillary bed); to initiate coagulation; and to retract clots.

Table 18-1 lists the plasma clotting factors which have been identified to date and summarizes their functions. They are referred to by both names and Roman numerals since they were found in different labs at different times with each researcher selecting a name for the factor independently. When it was discovered that one

factor had many different names, an international conference convened to identify each factor by Roman numerals. This standardization of naming has resulted in a more coherent body of literature. It should be noted that there is no factor VI since the factor that was originally assigned this number was really just the activated form of factor V. Factor IV is calcium, which is one of the cations that is required for these various reactions, and factor III, thromboplastin, is a tissue factor and does not occur in the circulating blood. All the remaining factors listed in the table do occur in the blood. With the exception of calcium, all the plasma coagulation factors are proteins.

The liver has been shown to be the site of synthesis of some of the plasma coagulation factors. This has been demonstrated by several studies to be the case with fibrinogen (factor I). Vitamin K is necessary for the maintenance of normal blood levels or prothrombin (factor

II) and factors VII, IX, and X. The available evidence suggests the liver, spleen, reticuloendothelial systems (RES), and kidney are possible sites of factor VIII synthesis. There is little evidence to indicate the source of factors XI and XII. Recent studies leave uncertain the role of the liver in factor XIII production (Williams, 1972).

There are various theories regarding how prothrombin is converted to thrombin (discussion of the role of thrombin in clotting follows) in the presence of the various clotting factors. One theory is referred to as a "waterfall," or a "cascade," theory, which postulates that the plasma coagulation factors (with the exception of fibrinogen, which is converted to insoluble fibrin) circulate as a proenzyme which is converted to an enzyme during the clotting process (Williams, 1972). Another theory states that prothrombin evolves into active derivatives termed autoprothrombin I and II and autoprothrombin C, and an immediate precursor of the thrombin molecule, prethrombin (Hiss and Penner, 1969).

Clot formation

The end product of the process of blood clotting is a blood clot. Ordinarily, the clot serves the purpose of stopping bleeding at the site of vascular injury. All of the examples in this chapter will use this situation as a model of clotting action, but it is important to remember that there are other times when blood clotting occurs. In fact, it is believed that blood coagulation is a continuing process, since interruption of this mechanism causes people to bleed uncontrollably at all sites, as evidenced by examining teeth, mucous membranes, urine, stool, skin, the whites of the eyes, and so forth. From these reactions it is evident that the clotting mechanism is part of the general body homeostatic mechanism. In the following discussion, however, emphasis will be placed on understanding clotting at the site of a vascular injury.

The fibrin plug is the essential element of clotting at the site of vascular injury. There are two ways of producing this plug. In both cases, prothrombin is converted to an active proteolytic enzyme, thrombin, which catalyzes the conversion of fibrinogen to fibrin. When this reaction occurs, peptides are released. Fibrinogen is a long monomer (simplest molecular form of a substance), while fibrin is a polymer. In changing fibrinogen to fibrin, strands of protein combine to form multiple strands of protein which, in turn, form a clot. As mentioned previously, this reaction can occur in two ways according to the method by which thrombin is produced.

As indicated in Fig. 18-1, thrombin can be produced through the *extrinsic clotting mechanism* or through the *intrinsic clotting mechanism*. There are different factors involved in each case. The extrinsic system requires a tissue factor which is released at the site of tissue injury and is called tissue thromboplastin (factor III). In the presence of calcium, factors II, V, VII, and factor X, prothrombin is converted to thrombin. The tissue thromboplastin (factor III) is the critical factor; without tissue thromboplastin present, prothrombin cannot form thrombin. The key initiating step in the extrinsic system is the release of tissue thromboplastin by the injured tissues. The system is referred to as being "extrinsic" because the clotting begins outside (or extrinsic to) the vascular tree.

In the intrinsic system (called "intrinsic" since clotting occurs within the blood vessel) platelets and a platelet factor (platelet factor III) are released. In the presence of platelet factor III, calcium, and factors V, VIII, IX, X, XI, and XII, prothrombin is again converted to thrombin.

The enzyme thrombin catalyzes the conversion of fibrinogen to fibrin in the process of clot formation. When the fibrinogen is polymerized, a fibrin gel is formed. This fibrin gel, in the presence of platelets and some factors released by platelets, is stabilized, and a fibrin clot is formed. Thus, fibrinogen is the sol form, and fibrin is the gel form in this reaction. Once the fibrin clot has been formed, hemostasis is usually effected, and the bleeding stops.

Clot resolution

After the vascular injury has occurred, the body must have a mechanism for getting rid of the clot since the clot is no longer needed. There is a system in the body that is activated to dissolve the clot. This is the *fibrinolytic system*. There are preactivators that circulate in the

TABLE 18-1
Plasma clotting factors

I	Fibrinogen—precursor of fibrin (polymerized protein)
II	Prothrombin—precursor of the proteolytic enzyme thrombin and perhaps other accelerators of prothrombin conversion
III	Thromboplastin—a tissue lipoprotein activator of prothrombin
IV	Calcium—necessary for prothrombin activation and fibrin formation
V	Plasma accelerator globulin—a plasma factor which accelerates the conversion of prothrombin to thrombin
VII	Serum prothrombin conversion accelerator—a serum factor that accelerates prothrombin conversion
VIII	Antihemophilic globulin (AHG)—a plasma factor associated with platelet factor III and Christmas factor (IX); activates prothrombin
IX	Christmas factor—serum factor associated with platelet factor III and AHG (VIII); activates prothrombin
X	Stuart-Power factor—a plasma and serum factor; accelerator of prothrombin conversion
XI	Plasma thromboplastin antecedent (PTA)—a plasma factor that is activated by Hageman factor (XII); accelerator of thrombin formation
XII	Hageman factor—a plasma factor; activates PTA (XI)
XIII	Fibrin stabilizing factor—plasma factor; produces stronger fibrin clot that is insoluble in urea

FIGURE 18-1 Plasma clotting mechanism (simplified).

blood and have no activity in dissolving fibrin. However, when the preactivators are in the presence of certain tissue enzymes called kinases, they change to an activated or enzymatic form called fibrinolysin. In the presence of a fibrin clot, the fibrinolysin breaks the fibrin polymer back down to a monomer. This process results in fibrin split products and fibrinolysin. Thus, there are a group of factors circulating in the blood which when activated will enhance blood clotting, and, conversely, there are a group of factors circulating in the blood which when activated will dissolve the clot.

Phases of coagulation

There is an orderly sequence of events that occurs at the site of tissue injury. These events are referred to as the phases of coagulation. The first phase of coagulation occurs at the site of injury and is referred to as the *vascular phase* since it occurs at the blood vessel wall. During this phase, platelets adhere to the collagen (essentially, broken fragments of protein) that is exposed at the site of injury. Tissue thromboplastin is released at the site of injury, and the adhering platelets release adenosine diphosphate (ADP). As mentioned previously, tissue thromboplastin activates the *extrinsic* system causing the conversion of prothrombin to thrombin, which, in turn, acts as a catalyst for fibrinogen to form a fibrin plug. ADP and thrombin cause more platelet aggregation to occur, and a platelet plug is formed at the injured site. During the second phase of coagulation, thrombin causes platelet membrane disruption and release of a substance known as platelet factor III, a clotting factor found in platelets but not in plasma as were the factors previously discussed. The release of this factor into the plasma begins the final phase of coagulation: Platelet factor III activates the *intrinsic* system which causes additional thrombin to be formed. The thrombin that has been released as the result of the action of both the intrinsic and extrinsic systems acts upon the fibrinogen in the surrounding plasma, producing a fibrin clot that becomes attached to, and eventually encloses, the platelet plug. It is essential that all coagulation factors be present at peak concentrations for the sequence to begin. These activated substances may go into the circulating blood; however, inhibitors in the plasma neutralize the coagulation factors to prevent blood clotting away from the injury site.

Figure 18-2 shows how the fibrin polymer is stabilized. Fibrinogen (a monomer) goes to fibrin aggregates (polymers) and in the presence of a fibrin-stabilizing factor, which is factor XIII, and thrombin results in further organization of the fibrin polymer and stabilization.

Figure 18-3 is a diagrammatic picture of the fibrinolytic system, that is, the system that disposes of the clot once it is formed. Again, we have the profibrinolysins (circulating in the blood), which in the presence of activators (kinases) produce fibrinolysin, causing the fibrin polymer to break down into monomers.

Figure 18-4 is a graphic presentation of the sequence of events of the clotting process as previously discussed.

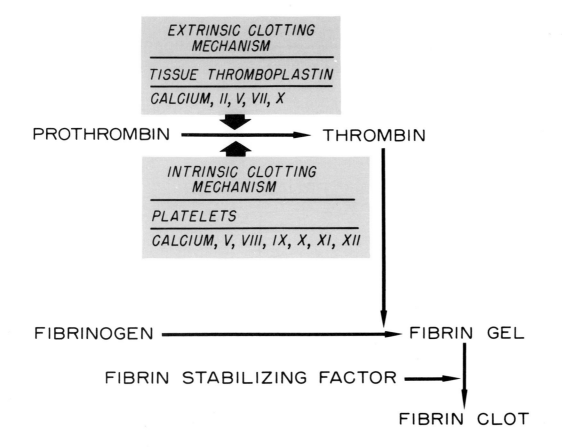

PROTHROMBIN AND PARTIAL THROMBOPLASTIN TIMES

The extrinsic system is measured in the laboratory by the prothrombin time (PT). The intrinsic system is assayed by the partial thromboplastin time (PTT). The normal prothrombin time is 11 to 13 seconds. In the partial thromboplastin time determination a phospholipid mixture is usually added to the plasma. This mixture normally clots in 60 to 90 seconds. However, if this mixture is incubated with a physical or chemical agent such as kaolin cephalin, the PTT is shortened to 30 to 48 seconds. This is called activated PTT. It should be noted that normal values may vary with each individual laboratory. Factor VII and tissue thromboplastin (factor III) are unique to the extrinsic system. Factors VIII, IX, XI, and XII are unique to the intrinsic system. Factors V, X, pro-

thrombin, and fibrinogen are common to both pathways. Assuming normal levels of fibrinogen, if only the PT were prolonged, a deficiency of factor VII could be assumed. If only the PTT were prolonged, a deficiency of a factor inclusive of the intrinsic system could be presumed (VIII, IX, XI, or XII). If both were prolonged, a deficiency of a factor common to both pathways (usually V or X) can be presumed (Fig. 18-5).

ABNORMALITIES OF COAGULATION

There are a variety of abnormalities that can occur within the clotting system. Obviously, there can be problems at any level of the process. The first level at which an abnormality may occur is the vascular level. There are a tremendous number of vascular disorders characterized by bleeding (primarily in the skin and mucous membranes) in which the abnormality occurs in the vascular system rather than in the blood clotting mechanism.

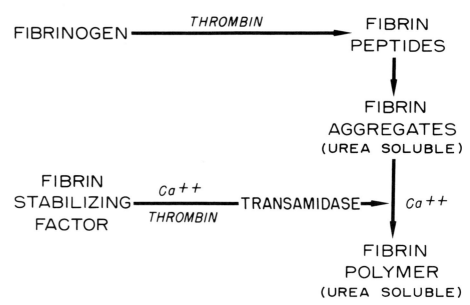

FIGURE 18-2 Stabilization of fibrin polymer.

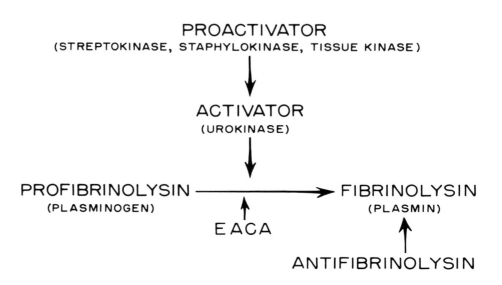

FIGURE 18-3 Fibrinolytic system.

Two examples of this kind of vascular disorder are allergic purpura and nonallergic purpura. Henoch-Schönlein purpura, an allergic purpura, is a disease that occurs primarily in children. The mechanism of this disease is not well understood, but the patients develop vasculitis, an irritation of the vascular tree, at the capillary and venous level. Extensive bleeding into the skin, as evidenced by petechiae, occurs when the blood vessel itself breaks down or small hemorrhages occur in skin and mucous membranes.

There are many forms of nonallergic purpura, diseases where no true allergy has been shown, but where various forms of vasculitis develop. The most common of the nonallergic purpuras is systemic lupus erythematosis. This is a collagen-vascular disease in which the patients develop autoantibodies. Vasculitis, or inflammation of vessels, occurs and destroys the integrity of the vessels, and purpura occurs.

Thrombocytosis and thrombocytopenia

There can be coagulation problems at the platelet level as well. The platelets adhering to the exposed collagen, contracting, and releasing ADP and platelet factor III are all very important in the initiation of the clotting mechanism. There are a number of problems with platelets that will interfere with blood coagulation. Too many

or too few platelets can cause bleeding. The condition characterized by too many platelets is known as thrombocytosis (cytosis = too much). Thrombocytosis is generally defined as an increase in platelet counts above the level of about 400,000 per cubic millimeter. This increased level of platelets does not usually cause any particular problem. However, a count of over 1 million platelets per cubic millimeter tends to cause increased clotting and bleeding in the same patient. The mechanism by which the bleeding occurs is thought to be that when the platelet concentration reaches this high level, spontaneous aggregates of platelets occur. These aggregates block off tiny capillaries. In the process, the wall of the capillary is damaged, resulting in bleeding into the tissues. Causes of thrombocytosis are many, but generally it is a condition that is secondary to other problems. For instance, many patients with myeloproliferative disorders such as polycythemia and chronic granulocytic leukemia, also show a marked increase in the platelet count. Increased numbers of platelets are also evident in patients in whom the spleen has been surgically removed since the spleen is the primary site of destruc-

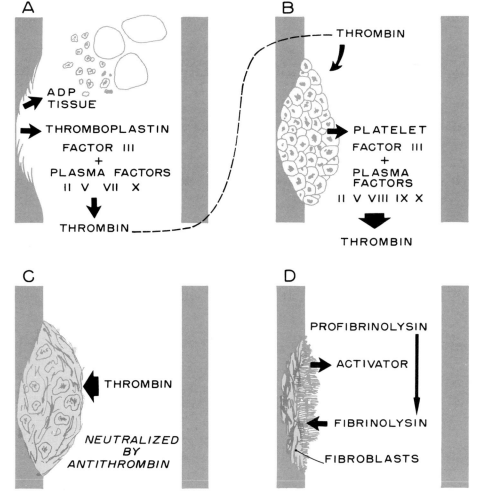

FIGURE 18-4 Sequence of events in the clotting process. (Modified from Hiss and Penner, "The Before and After of Blood Clotting," Medical Clinics of North America, vol. 53, no. 6, November, 1969.)

tion of platelets. Removal of the site of platelet destruction without an accompanying decrease of production causes thrombocytosis. It is not uncommon after removing a patient's spleen to see a platelet count of over 1 million. These patients must sometimes be given anticoagulants in order to keep them from clotting off vessels and having problems with bleeding.

The condition of thrombocytopenia (too few platelets) is defined as a decrease in the platelet level to below 200,000 per cubic millimeter. At this level, there are no particular problems, but reduction in the count to below 100,000 per cubic millimeter can cause problems. It is difficult to predict the level at which a decrease in the number of platelets will cause trouble with bleeding. The "rough" figure that may be used clinically is a count of 100,000 per cubic millimeter. At this level, there is a certain amount of inherent danger in doing any major surgery. Below 50,000 per cubic millimeter there can be problems with bruising or slight injury. So, ordinarily, a count of over 50,000 platelets per cubic millimeter with minor trauma does not cause too much difficulty. When levels fall below 20,000 per cubic millimeter, such as in many patients with leukemia, the chance of spontaneous hemorrhage is much higher. When this spontaneous hemorrhage occurs in a closed space such as the brain that cannot expand, the result is usually death within a few hours. So, patients with platelet counts of less than 20,000 per cubic millimeter run tremendous risks of bleeding and can die of spontaneous hemorrhage very quickly.

Thrombocytopenia can be caused by decreased production or increased destruction of platelets. Examples of the cause of poor production would be marrow replacement problems such as in acute leukemias. The various cancer chemotherapeutic agents that are used may have bone marrow suppression as one of their toxicities. Chemotherapeutic agents can cause marked thrombocytopenia due to destruction of cells in the bone marrow which produce the platelets.

However, there are conditions in which the bone marrow is producing more platelets than usual, but there is still a low platelet count in the peripheral blood. This can be caused by too many platelets being removed from the circulation; the spleen is the primary place where this removal occurs. Immune thrombocytopenic purpura (ITP) is an example of a disease characterized by excessive platelet removal from the blood. In this condition the body produces antibodies against its own platelets. The platelets are coated with antibody and destroyed in the spleen at a very brisk rate. The platelet count can be quite low (5000 or 10,000 platelets per cubic millimeter) causing these patients to be at very high risk of spontaneous hemorrhage. Treatment consists of the use of steroids (prednisone) and, if this fails, splenectomy.

Inherited plasma factor deficiencies

The best-known congenital absence of a clotting factor is hemophilia. Hemophilia is a sex-linked recessive disease which is divided into two classes, hemophilia A and hemophilia B. In patients with true hemophilia A factor VIII is nearly absent. Hemophilia B is characterized by a deficiency of factor IX, or Christmas factor. The ability to produce thrombin, and, therefore, fibrin, by the intrinsic mechanism is severely impaired by the absence of key factors.

The partial thromboplastin time (PTT) is abnormal in hemophilia because factor VIII or factor IX levels are

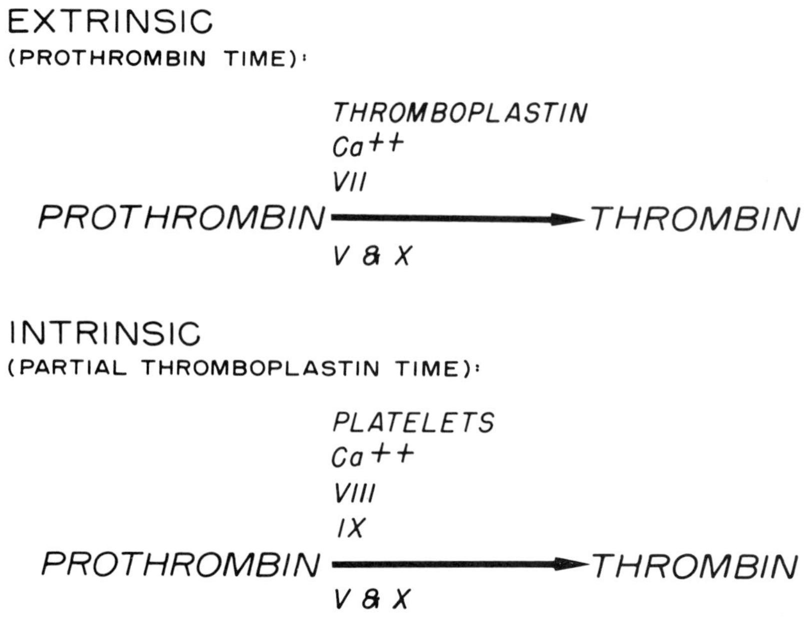

EXTRINSIC
(PROTHROMBIN TIME):

$$PROTHROMBIN \xrightarrow[V\ \&\ X]{\substack{THROMBOPLASTIN \\ Ca++ \\ VII}} THROMBIN$$

INTRINSIC
(PARTIAL THROMBOPLASTIN TIME):

$$PROTHROMBIN \xrightarrow[V\ \&\ X]{\substack{PLATELETS \\ Ca++ \\ VIII \\ IX}} THROMBIN$$

FIGURE 18-5 Conversion of prothrombin to thrombin by the extrinsic (extravascular) and intrinsic (intravascular) mechanisms.

absent or very low. The measurement of the prothrombin time (PT) is normal in hemophilia because the test by-passes the intrinsic system so that only factors VII, X, and V, prothrombin, and fibrinogen affect the test results.

Hemophilia is usually transmitted from an affected male through a daughter carrier to an affected grandson. Females do not have the disease if they are heterozygous. There have been cases of homozygous females as the result of an affected male and a female carrier having a child, but this is very rare.

The severity of the hemophilia varies from person to person. The bleeding tendencies usually appear in infancy or early childhood. Bleeding may occur from minor trauma. More difficult to control are hemorrhages into joint spaces. Many hemophiliac individuals function relatively normally during routine daily living but begin to bleed when some major trauma such as a broken bone or a surgical procedure occurs. Although the blood clotting mechanism in these patients is impaired, it is not so severely impaired that they are unable to function. Bleeding is treated by transfusing factor VIII from normal plasma into the patient with hemophilia.

The vast majority of hemophilia patients do not ever become resistant to the various preparations that are transfused. There are patients (about 1 or 2 percent of the population of hemophiliacs) who develop antibodies (called inhibitors) against the factor which is administered to them. Preparations such as prothrombin complexes go beyond the chain reaction of events which will stimulate prothrombin to thrombin, but do not require factor VIII and are used to treat patients with inhibitors.

Acquired plasma factor deficiency

The most common example of acquired deficiency of the plasma factors is severe liver diseases. Production of all of the factors which are produced in the liver (factors II, VII, IX, and X) can be decreased as the result of cirrhosis of the liver. Decreased levels of the plasma factors can also occur when the body uses the factors faster than they can be produced. This condition is referred to as diffuse intravascular coagulation, or DIC. There are many things that can cause DIC, with some of the most frequent being abruptio placentae (premature separation of the placenta), retained placenta in the uterus after delivery, or retained dead fetus. The placenta is extremely rich in tissue thromboplastin and is probably the richest source of tissue thromboplastin in the body. Therefore, if there is anything that destroys or causes necrosis of the placenta, large amounts of tissue thromboplastin are released into the circulating blood and clotting and resolution of the clots goes on continually throughout the entire vascular tree. Other things that initiate diffuse intravascular coagulation are less well understood and include sepsis, hypotension, and malignancy. Sometimes the specific factor or factors in these clinical situations which is responsible for initiating the DIC is known, and sometimes it is not. DIC can cause the plasma clotting factors to be rapidly depleted. Diffuse hemorrhage and death can occur.

If the initiating cause (i.e., abruptio placentae) can be corrected or removed, the body can compensate very rapidly, and often only supportive treatment with platelets and plasma factors is required. However, sometimes this condition must be interrupted by using anticoagulants, such as heparin, which prevent the tissue thromboplastin from activating the clotting mechanism. The body then is able to produce enough of the various plasma factors and bring their concentration up to high enough levels to stop the hemorrhage.

QUESTIONS

Coagulation—Chap. 18

Directions: Circle T if the statement is true, F if it is false. Correct the false statements on a separate sheet of paper.

1   T   F   Platelets are the primary source of immunoglobulins.

2   T   F   The liver plays a vital role in the synthesis of certain plasma coagulation factors such as prothrombin and factors I, VIII, X, and V.

3   T   F   The purpose of blood clotting is to stop bleeding at the site of injury.

Directions: Circle the letter next to each item which correctly answers the following questions. More than one answer may be correct.

4   Which of the following statements describes what occurs in blood clotting?
    a Tissue thromboplastin is released at the site of vascular injury. b Platelets which have aggregated release factors which stimulate the extrinsic system. c Fibrinolysin causes the release of factor III. d Prothrombin unites with fibrinogen to form fibrin.

5   The key initiating step in the extrinsic system is the release by tissue injury of a substance known as:
    a Prothrombin b Thrombin
    c Tissue thromboplastin d Platelet factor

Directions: Answer the following questions on a separate sheet of paper.

6   List in proper sequence the three ways that platelets contribute to blood coagulation.

7   What two plasma coagulation factors are shared by both the extrinsic and intrinsic systems?

8   State a possible mechanism for the fact that bleeding could occur with thrombocytosis.

Directions: Circle the letter next to each item which correctly answers the following questions. More than one answer may be correct.

9 Thrombocytopenia may result from:
a Vitamin K deficiency b Disseminated intravascular coagulation (DIC) c Chronic liver disease d Antiplatelet antibodies

10 Thrombocytopenia may be considered severe and the risk of hemorrhage great when the platelet count is below:
a 20,000 b 100,000 c 125,000 d 250,000

11 A patient with classic hemophilia A has deficiency of:
a Prothrombin b Factor VII C Christmas factor IX d Factor VIII

12 A hemophiliac person cannot initiate clotting at which of the following levels?
a Extrinsic b Intrinsic c Vascular d Platelet

13 In classic hemophilia A which laboratory findings would you expect?
a Normal prothrombin time (PT), abnormal partial thromboplastin time (PTT) b Abnormal PT, normal PTT c Abnormal PT, abnormal PTT

14 A 30-year-old primipara (woman having her first child) was admitted to the hospital as an obstetrical emergency with an abruptio placentae. She had been hemorrhaging profusely. An anticoagulant (heparin) was ordered. This treatment is expected to:
a Release tissue thromboplastin to prevent the production of thrombin b Block the effect of tissue thromboplastin in the clotting mechanism c Inactivate the intrinsic system d Interrupt the coagulation process so that production of plasma factors is increased

BIBLIOGRAPHY

COMINGS, DAVID E.: "Sickle Cell Disease and Related Disorders," in William J. Williams, E. Beuther, A. Erselv, and R. Rundles (eds.), *Hematology*, McGraw-Hill, New York, 1972, pp. 413–416.

HISS, R. G. and J. PENNER: "The Before and After of Blood Clotting," *Medical Clinics of North America*, **53**(6): 1309–1320, 1969.

HUGHES-JONES, NEVIN C.: *Lecture Notes on Hematology*, Blackwell, Oxford, England, 1970.

JACKSON, DOLORES E.: "Sickle Cell Disease: Meeting a Need," *Nursing Clinics of North America*, **7**(4): 727–741, 1972.

LANGLEY, L. L. and IRA TELFORD: *Dynamic Anatomy and Physiology*, McGraw-Hill, New York, 1974, pp. 373–397.

LEAVELL, BYRD S., and OSCAR A. THORUP: *Fundamentals of Clinical Hematology*, Saunders, Philadelphia, 1971.

OSSERMAN, ELLIOTT: "Multiple Myeloma," *Hospital Medicine*, **5**: 19–30, 1969.

PATTERSON, PHYLLIS: "Hemophilia: The New Look," *Nursing Clinics of North America*, **7**(4): 777–785, 1972.

SCHUMANN, DOLORES and PHYLLIS PATTERSON: "The Adult with Acute Leukemia," *Nursing Clinics of North America*, **7**(4): 743–761, 1972.

SCHUMANN, DOLORES, and PHYLLIS PATTERSON: "Multiple Myeloma," *American Journal of Nursing*, **75**(1): 78–81, 1975.

WILLIAMS, WILLIAM J.: "Production of Plasma Coagulation Factors," in William J. Williams, E. Reuther, A. Erslev, and R. Rundles (eds.), *Hematology*, McGraw-Hill, New York, 1972, pp. 1072–1075.

WIDMANN, FRANCES K.: *Goodale's Clinical Interpretation of Laboratory Tests*, Davis, Philadelphia, 1974.

PART IV Gastrointestinal Disorders

DANIEL J. FALL

Gastrointestinal disorders make up a large proportion of the illnesses which cause patients to seek medical help and are the leading cause of hospitalization in the United States. Although gastrointestinal disorders are not the direct cause of death as frequently as are cardiovascular disorders, they are among the top five causes. Cancer of the gastrointestinal tract accounts for nearly one-third of all the deaths resulting from cancer. Hepatic failure also accounts for a substantial number of deaths. Unlike the treatment for renal failure, science and technology have not advanced sufficiently to allow the liver to be transplanted successfully nor to simulate its complex vital functions with an "artificial liver machine."

The gastrointestinal tract is especially vulnerable to transient disorders which produce violent symptoms but which subside within a short period of time and leave no ill effects. This feature is undoubtedly caused by the ingestion of food and drink contaminated with bacteria or various chemical substances.

This unit follows the conventional approach of gastroenterology by an anatomical classification of disease. Progressing down the alimentary canal, the discussion begins with the esophagus and ends with anorectal disease. The accessory digestive organs are discussed separately.

OBJECTIVES

At the completion of Part IV you should be able to:

1 Describe the relationship between normal gastrointestinal anatomy and physiology and the alterations produced by disease.

2 Develop an understanding of the etiology, pathogenesis, and treatment of the various gastrointestinal diseases or disorders.

CHAPTER 19 The Esophagus

NORMAL ANATOMY AND PHYSIOLOGY

The esophagus is a hollow cylindrical organ about 25 cm long and 2 cm in diameter and extends from the hypopharynx to the cardiac portion of the stomach. It lies posterior to the heart and trachea, anterior to the vertebrae, and passes through a hiatus in the diaphragm just anterior to the aorta. The esophagus functions primarily to transport ingested material from the pharynx to the stomach.

Each end of the esophagus is guarded by a sphincter. The cricopharyngeus forms the upper esophageal sphincter and consists of skeletal muscle fibers. It is normally in a tonic or contracted state except during swallowing. The lower esophageal sphincter, though not anatomically distinct, behaves as a sphincter and serves as a barrier to reflux of stomach contents into the esophagus. It is normally closed except when food passes into the stomach or during belching or vomiting (see Fig. 19-1).

The wall of the esophagus consists of four layers. The inner mucosal layer is made up of stratified squamous epithelium which is continuous with the pharynx at the upper end and undergoes a sharp transition at the esophogastric junction (z-line) to form the simple columnar epithelium of the stomach. The esophageal mucosa is normally alkaline and is not able to tolerate the highly acid contents of the stomach. The submucosal layer con-

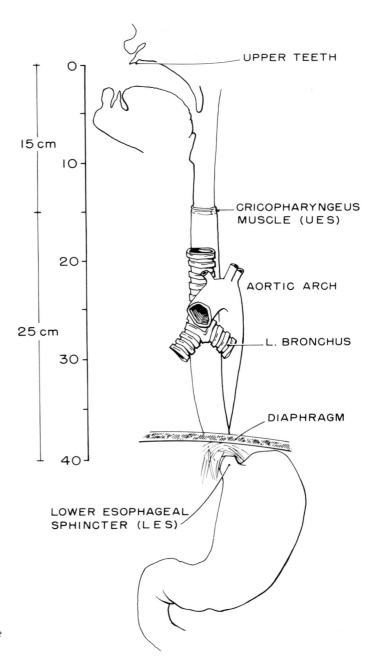

FIGURE 19-1 Gross structure and anatomic relations of the esophagus.

tains secretory cells which produce mucus. The mucus facilitates the passage of food during swallowing and protects the mucosa from chemical injury. The muscle layer is arranged in outer longitudinal and inner circular layers. The muscles of the upper one-third of the esophagus are striated, while those of the lower one-third are smooth. A transitional zone exists in the middle and contains both striated and smooth muscle. The outer layer of the esophagus, unlike the remainder of the gastrointestinal (GI) tract, is not composed of serosa but of thickened fibrous tissue.

The major innervation of the esophagus is supplied by the sympathetic and parasympathetic fibers of the autonomic nervous system. The parasympathetic fibers are carried by the vagus nerve, which is considered to be the motor nerve of the esophagus. The function of the sympathetic fibers is poorly understood. In addition to the above extrinsic innervation, an intrinsic intramural meshwork of nerve fibers exists (Auerbach's plexus) between the circular and longitudinal muscle layers, and it appears to be involved in coordinating normal esophageal peristalsis.

Blood distribution to the esophagus follows a segmental plan. The upper portion is supplied by branches from the inferior thyroid and subclavian arteries. The midportion is supplied by segmental branches from the aorta and from bronchial arteries, while the subdiaphragmatic portion is supplied by the left gastric and inferior phrenic arteries.

Venous drainage also follows a segmental pattern. The cervical esophageal veins drain into the azygos and hemiazygos veins, and below the diaphragm the esophageal veins enter the left gastric vein. Communication between the portal and systemic veins allows for a bypass of the liver in cases of portal hypertension. Collateral flow through the esophageal veins causes the formation of esophageal varices (varicose veins of the esophagus). These enlarged veins may rupture, causing life-threatening hemorrhage which may be fatal. This complication is frequent in cirrhosis of the liver and will be discussed in detail in Chapter 23.

Swallowing

Swallowing is a complex physiologic act whereby food or liquid passes from the mouth to the stomach. It is a highly coordinated muscular sequence which is initiated by a voluntary movement of the tongue and is completed by a series of reflexes in the pharynx and esophagus. The afferent side of this reflex arc involves fibers in the Vth, IXth, and Xth cranial nerves. A swallowing or deglutition center is present in the medulla. Under the coordination of this center, impulses pass outward in a flawlessly timed sequence via the Vth, Xth, and XIIth cranial nerves to the muscles of the tongue, pharynx, larynx, and esophagus.

Although swallowing is a continuous process, it occurs in three phases—oral, pharyngeal, and esophageal. In normal swallowing, a mouthful of chewed food, called a *bolus*, is thrown backwards against the posterior wall of the pharynx by a voluntary movement of the

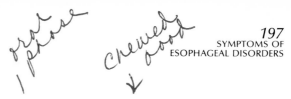

tongue. The impact of the bolus against the pharynx is the stimulus that sets off the reflex movements of swallowing.

During the pharyngeal phase, the soft palate and uvula move reflexly to close off the nasal cavity, at the same time the larynx is elevated and closed off from the pharynx. Respirations are simultaneously inhibited to decrease the possibility of aspiration. In fact, it is almost impossible voluntarily to inhale and swallow at the same time.

The esophageal phase begins as the cricopharyngeus muscle relaxes briefly and allows the bolus to enter the esophagus. Following this brief relaxation, a *primary peristaltic wave*, beginning in the pharynx, is transmitted to the cricopharyngeus, causing it to contract. The peristaltic wave continues throughout the body of the esophagus, propelling the bolus to the lower esophageal sphincter, which relaxes briefly to allow entry into the stomach. The primary peristaltic wave moves at the rate of 2 to 4 cm/second, so that swallowed food reaches the stomach within 5 to 15 seconds. Beginning at the level of the aortic arch, a *secondary peristaltic wave* occurs if the primary wave fails to empty the esophagus. It is triggered by distention of the esophagus from remaining food particles. The primary peristaltic wave is essential for conveying food and liquids through the upper esophagus but is less important in the lower esophagus. The upright posture and the force of gravity are important factors in facilitating lower esophageal transport, but peristalsis makes it possible to drink water while standing on one's head.

During swallowing there are pressure changes within the esophagus which reflect the motor function of the esophagus. In the resting state pressure in the body of the esophagus is slightly below atmospheric pressure, reflecting intrathoracic pressure. In the upper and lower esophageal sphincter regions, areas of high pressure exist. These high-pressure zones function to prevent aspiration and reflux of the gastric contents. The pressure decreases when each sphincter area relaxes during swallowing and then increases when the peristaltic wave passes through.

It is evident that the complex series of movements that together make up the act of swallowing may be upset by a number of pathologic processes. These processes involve interference either with transport or with the prevention of gastric reflux.

SYMPTOMS OF ESOPHAGEAL DISORDERS

Dysphagia, or the subjective awareness of an impairment in the active transport of ingested material from the pharynx, is a major symptom of disease of the pharynx or esophagus. Dysphagia should not be confused with *glo-*

bus hystericus (the feeling of a "lump in the throat"), which may be emotional in origin and present during the absence of swallowing.

Dysphagia occurs most often in nonesophageal disorders which result from muscular or neurologic disease. These diseases include cerebral vascular accidents, myasthenia gravis, muscular dystrophy, and bulbar polio.

Esophageal dysphagia may be of obstructive or motor origin. Obstructive causes include esophageal stricture and tumors extrinsic or intrinsic to the esophagus, resulting in narrowing of the lumen. Motor causes of dysphagia may result from diminished, absent, or disordered peristalsis or dysfunction of the upper or lower esophageal sphincters. Common motor disorders which produce dysphagia are achalasia, scleroderma, and diffuse esophageal spasm.

Pyrosis (heartburn) is another common symptom of esophageal disease. It is characterized by a hot, burning sensation usually felt high in the epigastrium or behind the xyphoid and radiates upward. Heartburn may be caused by reflux of gastric acid or bile secretions into the lower esophagus, both of which are very irritating to the mucosa. Persistent reflux is caused by incompetence of the lower esophageal sphincter and may occur with or without hiatus hernia or esophagitis. Heartburn is a common complaint during pregnancy.

Odynophagia is defined as pain induced by swallowing and may occur with dysphagia. It may be experienced as a sensation of tightness or as a burning pain, indistinguishable from heartburn, in the midchest. It may result from esophageal spasm induced by acute distention, or it may be secondary to inflammation of the esophageal mucosa.

Waterbrash refers to the regurgitation of gastric contents into the oral cavity. It differs from vomiting in that it is effortless and not accompanied by nausea. It is felt in the throat as a sour or bitter-tasting hot liquid. This effortless regurgitation is quite common in infants as a result of incomplete development of the lower esophageal sphincter. In adults, regurgitation reflects both lower esophageal sphincter incompetence and failure of the upper esophageal sphincter to serve as a regurgitation barrier.

INVESTIGATIONAL PROCEDURES

In addition to a careful history and physical examination, special diagnostic measures which are helpful in detecting esophageal disease are the barium x-ray, esophagoscopy with biopsy and possible cytologic studies, manometric or motility studies, and acid reflux tests.

Barium x-ray

Radiologic examination of the esophagus as a routine is usually combined with that of the stomach and duodenum (upper GI tract x-ray series) using barium sulfate in a liquid or creamy suspension which is swallowed. The swallowing mechanism may be directly visualized by fluoroscopy, or the x-ray image may be recorded using motion picture techniques (cineradiography). When esophageal disease is suspected, the radiologist may place the patient in various positions to bring out in greater detail alterations in form and function. Tumors, polyps, diverticulitis, strictures, hiatus hernia, large esophageal varices, uncoordinated swallowing, and weak peristalsis may all be detected using this method.

Esophagoscopy

The direct inspection of the esophageal mucosa is an important procedure in the diagnosis of esophageal disorders. Flexible fiberoptic instruments have made this procedure much simpler and safer for the patient. Inflammation, ulcers, tumors, and esophageal varices may be visualized, photographed, and biopsied. Cell washings may be obtained for cytologic studies which can be highly accurate in the diagnosis of esophageal carcinoma.

Preparation for esophagoscopy includes six hours of fasting and various forms of premedication, including spraying the throat with a local anesthetic. Endoscopic examination of the esophagus, stomach, and duodenum are often combined in one examination.

Motility studies

Motor function of the esophagus may be studied by the use of pressure-sensitive catheters or miniature balloons placed in the stomach and then drawn back in increments. The measurement of pressure changes in the esophagus and stomach at rest and during swallowing have greatly increased understanding of esophageal activity both in health and in disease.

Figures 19-2A and 19-2B show a normal motility recording of the esophagus in the resting state and during swallowing. The function of the lower esophageal sphincter is of particular interest to the gastroenterologist. Normally there is a zone of high pressure (15 to 30

FIGURE 19-2 A, esophageal manometric recordings. The pressure is recorded by three catheters spaced 5 cm apart. The catheters are pulled from the stomach into the esophagus. Note: the zone of high resting pressure at the junction between stomach and esophagus (gastroesophageal sphincter or LES). B, normal swallowing. Swallowing produces a single contraction. At the same time, the sphincter zone relaxes. C, diffuse esophageal spasm. Repetitive nonprogressive contractions occur independent of water swallowing (w.s.). D, Scleroderma. The contractions produced by swallowing (s) are low in amplitude.

cm water above that of the intragastric pressure) in this region which prevents reflux of gastric contents into the esophagus. Reflux may occur if the sphincter fails to maintain a pressure above the intra-abdominal pressure.

Acid reflux tests

The acid perfusion test (Bernstein test) is used to differentiate between chest pain which is cardiac in origin and pain resulting from esophageal spasm, since symptoms may be identical. If the pain is caused by esophageal spasm secondary to reflux esophagitis, the acid perfusion test will be positive.

In the acid perfusion test, 0.1 N HCl is permitted to drip through a catheter at 6 to 15 ml/minute into the distal esophagus (the hydrochloric acid is of the same concentration as normal gastric acid). The patient has esophageal pain or heartburn if the test is positive. Rapid cessation of the pain after instillation of a neutral or alkaline solution confirms the esophageal mucosa as the site of acid-induced pain. The most common finding in a posi-

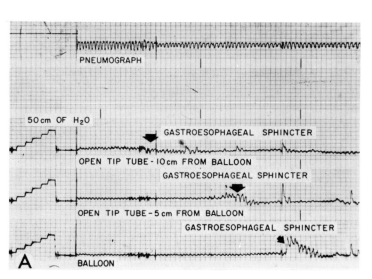

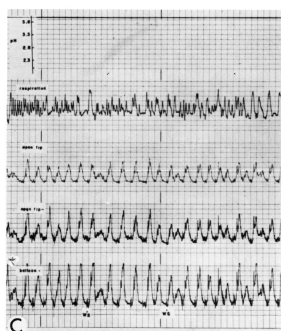

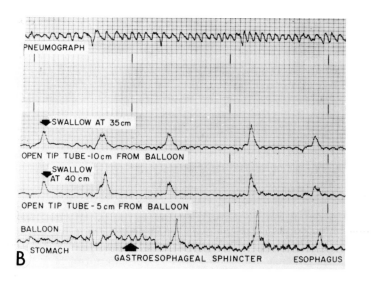

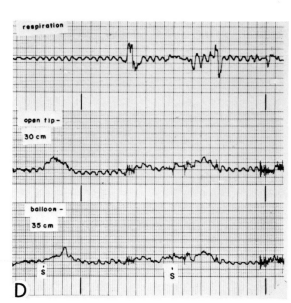

tive test is reflux esophagitis, but any disease which causes a break in mucosal continuity could cause a positive test.

Other reflux tests include monitoring of the pH within the esophagus to detect reflux of acid contents from the stomach, fluoroscopic observation of the esophagus to detect reflux of barium from the stomach into the esophagus, and fluoroscopic observation of the esophagus during the ingestion of a mixture of hydrochloric acid and barium to detect momentary disorders in peristaltic activity. All the currently available tests for acid reflux have both false positives and false negatives; therefore, a combination of two or more of these studies is used for a diagnosis in difficult cases.

DISORDERS OF ESOPHAGEAL MOTILITY

Achalasia

Achalasia, formerly called cardiospasm, is an uncommon hypomotility disorder characterized by weak and uncoordinated peristalsis or aperistalsis within the body of the esophagus and by failure of the lower esophageal sphincter to completely relax during swallowing. Consequently, food and fluids accumulate in the lower esophagus and may then slowly empty as the hydrostatic pressure increases. The body of the esophagus loses its tone and may become greatly dilated (see Fig. 19-3).

The exact etiology of achalasia is unknown, but there is evidence that degeneration of Auerbach's plexus causes the loss of neurologic control. Chagas' disease is

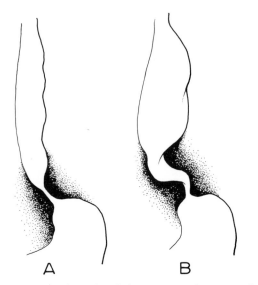

FIGURE 19-3 Esophageal achalasia. A, early stage showing tapering of lower esophagus; B, advanced stage showing dilated, tortuous esophagus.

a clinical syndrome similar to achalasia and occurs as a result of a parasitic infection (*Filaria*). As a result, primary peristaltic waves do not reach the lower esophageal sphincter to stimulate relaxation.

Achalasia is more common in adults than in children. The onset is usually insidious, and the most prominent symptom is dysphagia for both liquid and solid foods. Meals may be interrupted by the necessity to regurgitate. Nocturnal regurgitation may result in aspiration, resulting in chronic pulmonary infections or sudden death. The stasis of food in the esophagus may lead to inflammatory changes, erosions, and in some cases, cancer of the esophagus, although this is usually a late complication.

The diagnosis is made on the basis of the history and the characteristic appearance on x-ray. When barium is swallowed, the peristaltic wave is weak, and the collection of barium in the lower esophagus gives it a funnel-like appearance. The administration of small doses of methacholine (Mecholyl), a cholinergic or parasympathomimetic drug, causes marked contraction and emptying of the esophagus and confirms the diagnosis. Esophageal motility studies may be helpful in the early diagnosis of achalasia. Manometric measurements in these studies reveal that the lower esophageal sphincter fails to relax with swallowing. The resting pressure of the lower esophageal sphincter may be normal or slightly elevated.

Treatment of achalasia is palliative and consists of measures to relieve the obstruction of the lower esophagus. There is no known method of restoring normal peristalsis to the body of the esophagus. Two forms of therapy that effectively relieve symptoms are dilatation of the lower esophageal sphincter and esophagomyotomy. Dilatation may be achieved by passage of a mercury-filled tube called a *bougie* or, more commonly, by dilatation with a pneumatic bag which is placed in the area of the lower esophageal sphincter and forcefully dilated. When dilatation fails to relieve the symptoms, surgical intervention may be indicated.

The surgery most commonly performed for achalasia or esophageal stricture is the Heller myotomy which consists of division of the muscle fibers of the gastroesophageal junction. A pyloroplasty (enlargement of gastric outlet) frequently accompanies this procedure to allow rapid emptying of stomach contents and prevent reflux into the esophagus (see Fig. 19-4).

Other helpful measures to minimize symptoms include slow eating and avoidance of alcohol and hot, cold, or spicy foods. Patients should be instructed to sleep with their head elevated to avoid aspiration.

Diffuse esophageal spasm

Diffuse esophageal spasm is a fairly common condition and is characterized by uncoordinated, nonpropulsive contractions (tertiary peristalsis) of the esophagus in response to swallowing. It is most prominent in the lower two-thirds of the organ but may involve the entire esophagus. The two sphincters operate normally. It is a disease of unknown cause and is seen more frequently in older patients. Similar motility disturbances may be secondary to reflux esophagitis or obstruction of the lower esophagus such as in carcinoma (usually manometric studies in early carcinoma are normal).

Primary diffuse spasm of the esophagus usually occurs in patients over 50 years of age. Nonperistaltic responses to swallowing are common findings on barium x-ray and increase with aging. These x-ray findings are referred to as "corkscrew esophagus," "rosary bead esophagus," "curling," and a variety of other descriptive names which are usually of little clinical significance.

The pathogenetic basis for the diffuse spasm is poorly understood. It may represent a degeneration of local neurons, since some patients have a positive response to the Mecholyl test as in achalasia.

Diffuse esophageal spasm is usually asymptomatic, but in a few cases the contractions may give rise to symptoms. The most common symptoms are those of intermittent dysphagia and odynophagia, which are aggravated by ingestion of cold foods and large boli and by nervous tension. When there is intermittent chest pain, diffuse esophageal spasm may be confused with angina pectoris, especially if symptoms are not associated with eating. To add to this confusion, the pain caused by diffuse spasm is often relieved by nitroglycerin. Consequently, some patients with diffuse esophageal spasm have been misdiagnosed as having cardiac disease.

Motility studies reveal a hypermotile pattern of nonperistaltic contractions and aid in the diagnosis (see Fig. 19-2C).

Treatment consists of dietary manipulations (small meals and avoidance of cold foods), antacids, sedatives, and nitroglycerin to relieve the spasm. If symptoms are persistent and distressing, esophageal dilatation may be recommended. As a last resort, a longitudinal myotomy of the distal esophagus may be performed.

Scleroderma

Esophageal motor dysfunction occurs in over two-thirds of patients with progressive systemic sclerosis (scleroderma). The basic abnormality in the GI tract is atrophy of the smooth muscle of the lower portion of the esophagus.

The diagnosis is suspected on barium swallow x-ray examination but is confirmed by manometric findings. Aperistalsis or weak peristalsis of the distal one-half to two-thirds of the esophagus and diminished pressure of the lower esophageal sphincter characterize the disease (see Fig. 19-2D).

Incompetence of the lower esophageal sphincter often leads to reflux esophagitis with subsequent stricture formation in the lower esophagus. Although gastroesophageal reflux and esophagitis are common, heartburn is not a common symptom. Dysphagia becomes a prominent symptom when esophagitis has led to stricture formation (see below).

ESOPHAGITIS

Inflammation of the esophageal mucosa may be acute or chronic and is seen in a variety of circumstances including the motility disorders just discussed. An innocuous type of esophagitis follows the ingestion of hot liquids. The substernal burning sensation is usually of short duration and may be associated with superficial edema and

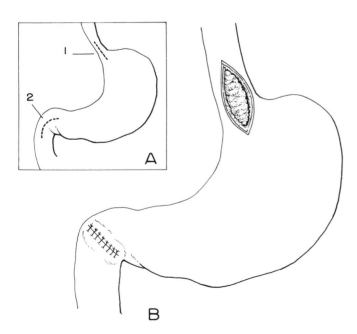

FIGURE 19-4 Surgical treatment of esophageal achalasia. A, longitudinal incision for (Heller) esophagomyotomy (1) and pyloroplasty (2); B, the esophageal incision is made through the muscle layers to allow pouching of the mucosa, thus relieving the esophageal obstruction. A gastric drainage procedure (pyloroplasty) frequently accompanies the esophagomyotomy to prevent esophageal reflux. The pyloric incision is sutured in the opposite direction to enlarge the gastric outlet.

esophagospasm. The most common significant form of esophagitis is caused by acid reflux from the stomach, often in association with hiatus hernia. There are also infectious forms of esophagitis, including monilial esophagitis and, rarely, infections with herpes viruses.

An acute severe form of esophagitis follows the ingestion of strong alkalis or acids. Strong alkalis are commonly found in most households in the form of drain cleaners which, if ingested, will produce a severe liquefying necrosis of the mucosa. Accidental ingestion of these substances occurs most commonly in small children, but occasionally, these substances are used in suicide attempts. Immediate symptoms include severe odynophagia, fever, toxicity, and possible esophageal perforation with consequent infection of the mediastinum and death. Long-term effects include scarring and esophageal stricture which requires periodic dilatations with bougies for the remainder of the patient's life. Treatment must be prompt and vigorous and includes the use of antibiotics, steroids, intravenous fluids, and possibly surgery.

Chronic reflux esophagitis and hiatus hernia

Chronic reflux esophagitis is the most common form of esophagitis encountered clinically. It is caused by incompetence of the lower esophageal sphincter and reflux of acid gastric or alkaline intestinal juice into the esophagus over a long period of time. The sequelae of reflux is inflammation, ulcer formation, bleeding, and scarring with stricture formation. Chronic reflux esophagitis is often associated with hiatus hernia. There is little correlation between the severity of symptoms and the degree of esophagitis. Some patients with heartburn have minimal evidence of esophagitis, while others with chronic reflux may be asymptomatic until there is stricture formation.

MECHANISMS PREVENTING REFLUX

Figure 19-5 illustrates the mechanisms which normally prevent reflux of gastric contents into the esophagus. The high-pressure zone at the gastroesophageal junction (or lower esophageal sphincter) is probably the most important mechanism for preventing reflux. The tone of this sphincter is affected not only by a variety of drugs but also by hormonal influences such as gastrin and secretin, which may play a very important role in maintaining the integrity of the sphincter. The acute angle between the esophagus and stomach may also be an important mechanism for preventing reflux, since this creates a flap-valvelike arrangement which would prevent material from regurgitating. It has also been suggested that the short segment of the esophagus below the diaphragm is kept closed by the intra-abdominal pressure. Displacement of this lower esophageal segment into the chest, such as occurs in hiatus hernia, would eliminate this barrier to reflux and may well explain why there seems to be an association with reflux esophagitis.

HIATUS HERNIA

Hiatus hernia is defined as a herniation of a portion of the stomach into the chest through the esophageal hiatus of the diaphragm. There are two distinct types of hiatus hernia (see Fig. 19-6). The most common form is the *direct* or *sliding hiatus hernia* in which the gastroesophageal junction slides into the thoracic cavity, especially when the patient assumes a supine position. The competency of the lower esophageal sphincter may be destroyed, resulting in reflux esophagitis. Often it is asymptomatic and is discovered only accidentally during a search for the cause of a variety of epigastric symptoms

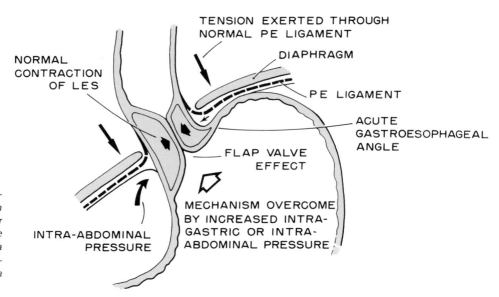

FIGURE 19-5 Mechanisms preventing esophageal reflux: high pressure zone at the lower esophageal sphincter (LES); acute gastroesophageal angle causing a flap-valve effect; phrenoesophageal (PE) ligament causing a pinchcock valve effect.

or on routine GI tract x-rays. In *paraesophageal* or *rolling hiatus hernia,* part of the gastric fundus rolls through the hiatus, and the gastroesophageal junction remains below the diaphragm. There is no insufficiency of the lower esophageal sphincter mechanism, and consequently reflux esophagitis does not occur. The major complication of paraesophageal hernia is strangulation.

Sliding and rolling hiatus hernias are diagnosed with x-ray or endoscopy. The important clinical question is whether or not there is esophageal reflux, since this has serious consequences.

Treatment of sliding hiatus hernia is directed toward the prevention of reflux. The patient is instructed to eat small, frequent meals and take antacids. If overweight, the patient is instructed to reduce. Anticholinergic drugs should not be given because they cause a delay of gastric emptying and relaxation of the lower esophageal sphincter. The patient should avoid activities which involve stooping forward, especially after meals. The head of the bed should generally be elevated during sleep to prevent reflux. Surgical repair may be indicated if medical treatment fails and there is evidence of persistent reflux esophagitis or stricture formation.

TUMORS

The most common benign tumor of the esophagus is a leiomyoma (smooth muscle tumor), although it is rare. Leiomyomas may occasionally bleed but are usually of little clinical significance and are discovered incidentally.

Cancer of the esophagus, however, is not rare. It causes approximately 4 percent of all cancer deaths in the United States. Males between the ages of 50 and 70 years are affected most frequently. Predisposing factors include heavy smoking, alcohol abuse, and esophageal

obstruction. Squamous cell carcinoma is the most common type of tumor, and it is highly malignant. Tumors can occur in any part of the esophagus, but the majority are in the lower two-thirds.

Barium x-ray, cytologic studies, and esophagoscopy with biopsy are all important in the diagnosis. The 5-year survival rate is less than 10 percent. The reason for the poor prognosis is the early lymphatic spread and the late development of symptoms. The first symptom is generally dysphagia, but this does not generally occur until the tumor involves the entire circumference of the esophagus.

Irradiation and surgical resection are the major forms of treatment. Lesions in the upper portion of the esophagus may be impossible to resect and are treated by irradiation. Bougies may be passed to dilate the lumen, or a plastic prosthesis may be inserted to enable the patient to continue eating.

QUESTIONS

The esophagus—Chap. 19

Directions: Answer the following questions on a separate sheet of paper.

1 Describe the function of the esophagus.

2 Why is regurgitation more common in infants than in adults?

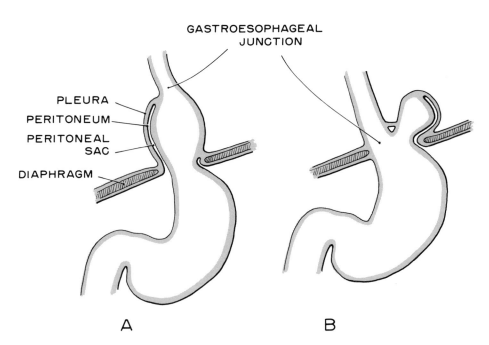

GASTROESOPHAGEAL JUNCTION

PLEURA

PERITONEUM

PERITONEAL SAC

DIAPHRAGM

A   B

FIGURE 19-6 A, sliding or direct hiatus hernia; B, rolling or paraesophageal hiatus hernia.

3 What are esophageal varices and why are they often associated with cirrhosis of the liver? Why is this condition important?

4 What is an esophagomyotomy? What is a pyloroplasty? Why are these two procedures often combined? What condition is commonly treated by esophagomyotomy and pyloroplasty?

5 What kind of instructions would you give to patients with the following conditions to minimize symptoms and prevent complications: diffuse esophageal spasm, scleroderma, sliding hiatus hernia?

6 Sketch the anatomic relations of the gastroesophageal junction and briefly describe the three mechanisms preventing reflux.

7 Describe the consequences of chronic esophageal reflux.

8 Why do patients with achalasia and sliding hiatus hernia often have chronic pulmonary infections?

9 Why is chronic reflux esophagitis sometimes difficult to identify? What test is used to assist in the diagnosis?

Directions: Circle the letter preceding each item that correctly answers the questions. Only one answer is correct unless otherwise noted.

10 Which of the following statements concerning esophagesl anatomy is false?
a Passes through the esophageal hiatus of the diaphragm b Lies posterior to the heart c Length is about 25 cm d An anatomically distinct sphincter is present at the gastroesophageal junction

11 The muscle which functions as the upper esophageal sphincter is the:
a Palatopharyngeus b Phrenoesophageal
c Cricopharyngeus d Palatine

12 The lower esophageal sphincter is:
a A well-differentiated zone of muscle b A zone of high pressure near the gastroesophageal junction c Normally located above the level of the diaphragm d A diaphragmatic muscle band externally compressing the esophagus

13 Which of the following types of epithelium is present throughout most of the length of the esophagus?
a Simple columnar b Pseudostratified ciliated columnar c Stratified squamous

14 The extrinsic motor nerve which coordinates esophageal peristalsis is the:
a Vagus b Auerbach's c Hypoglossal

15 The normal pH of esophageal secretions is:
a Slightly acid b Slightly alkaline c Identical with the pH of gastric secretions

16 The terminal one-third of the muscularis of the esophagus is composed of:
a Smooth muscle fibers b Skeletal muscle fibers
c Both skeletal and smooth muscle fibers

17 The second stage of swallowing is characterized by: (More than one answer is correct)
a Inhibition of respiration b Being under voluntary control c Closure of the vocal cords d Relaxation of the cricopharyngeus muscle

18 All of the following cranial nerves are involved in the control of swallowing *except:*
a III b V c IX d X e XII

19 Transportation of a bolus of food through the esophagus is a function of:
a Primary peristaltic wave b Secondary peristaltic wave c Tertiary peristaltic wave d All of the above

20 After being swallowed, food or liquids normally enter the stomach within:
a 5 to 15 seconds b 30 to 40 seconds c 60 seconds d 2 minutes

21 Which of the following are required for the diagnosis of achalasia? (More than one answer is correct)
a Findings of weak, uncoordinated peristalsis on motility study b Rosary bead esophagus on barium x-ray c Positive Mecholyl test d Narrowed gastroesophageal junction

22 Achalasia is thought to be caused by:
a Stress and nervous tension b Degeneration of Auerbach's plexus c Gastric reflux d Failure of the cricopharyngeus muscle to relax e Infection with a parasite (*Filaria*)

23 Which of the following is the treatment of choice in achalasia?
a Dilatation with bougies (bougienage) b Pneumatic dilatation c Heller esophagomyotomy
d Anticholineric drugs e Psychotherapy

24 Which of the following tests is most helpful in differentiating cardiac and esophageal pain?
a Electrocardiogram b Relief of pain by nitroglycerin confirms cardiac origin of pain c Mecholyl test d 0.1 N HCl acid perfusion test

25 The portion of the esophagus primarily affected in scleroderma is the:
a Body b Upper one-third c Lower esophageal sphincter d Upper esophageal sphincter

26 The most effective early treatment measures for an alkali burn of the esophagus include: (More than one answer is correct)
a Corticosteroid drugs b Immediate induction of vomiting c Broad-spectrum antibiotics d Immediate pneumatic dilatation

27 Which of the following statements about hiatus hernia is true?
a There are two distinct types b The paraesophageal type is the most common c All require surgery d All are associated with gastric reflux

28 Which of the following statements concerning sliding hiatus hernia is true?
  a Most frequent complication is strangulation
  b Presence of gastric reflux is principal indication for surgery   *c* Should always be treated by surgery
  d Gastric fundus rolls through the hiatus, and gastroesophageal junction remains below the diaphragm

29 Which of the following statements concerning cancer of the esophagus are true? (More than one answer may be correct)
  a Very rare form of cancer   *b* More common in males   *c* Associated with alcohol abuse and heavy smoking   *d* More often located in the upper esophagus   *e* Prognosis is generally good

Directions: Match each of the following symptoms in col. A with its proper definition or description in col. B.

Column A	Column B
30 ___ Dysphagia	*a* Hot, burning sensation usually felt high in the epigastrum
31 ___ Regurgitation	
32 ___ Odynophagia	
33 ___ Pyrosis	*b* "Lump in the throat" present during the absence of swallowing
34 ___ Globus hystericus	
	c Subjective awareness of difficulty in swallowing
	d Pain in midchest induced by swallowing
	e Effortless welling up of esophageal or gastric contents into the mouth

Directions: Match each of the following esophageal motor disorders in col. A with its common findings in motility studies in col. B.

Column A	Column B
35 ___ Diffuse esophageal spasm	*a* Loss of contractile power in lower distal portion of esophagus
36 ___ Achalasia	*b* Characterized by a hypermotile pattern of ineffective contractions
37 ___ Scleroderma	
	c Absence of peristalsis in body of esophagus and incomplete relaxation of the lower esophageal sphincter
	d Characterized by lower than normal resting pressures at the lower esophageal sphincter
	e Characterized by higher than normal resting pressure at the lower esophageal sphincter

Directions: Circle T if the statement is true and F if it is false.

38   T   F   Nonperistaltic responses to swallowing increase with age.

39   T   F   Secondary peristalsis is important in removing food particles that remain in the esophagus after the primary peristaltic wave has passed.

40   T   F   The aid of gravity is essential to swallow liquids.

41   T   F   Cell washings for cytologic study is one of the most accurate ways to identify early cancer of the esophagus.

42   T   F   Endoscopic examination of the esophagus with a fiberoptic instrument requires general anesthesia.

43   T   F   Tertiary peristalsis consists of uncoordinated, nonpropulsive contractions of the esophagus.

44   T   F   Long-term effects of lye ingestion may include esophageal stricture and the necessity of periodic bougienage.

REFERENCES

BOGOCH, ABRAHAM (ed.): *Gastroenterology,* McGraw-Hill, New York, 1973, pp. 15–17, 172–245.

BROOKS, F. P. (ed.): *Gastrointestinal Pathophysiology,* Oxford University Press, New York, 1974, pp. 53–80.

GIVEN, B. A. and S. J. SIMMONS: *Gastroenterology in Clinical Nursing,* 2d ed., C. V. Mosby, St. Louis, 1975, pp. 94–112.

GREENBERGER, N. J. and D. H. WINSHIP: *Gastrointestinal Disorders: A Pathophysiologic Approach,* Yearbook, Chicago, 1976, pp. 2–43.

NASH, J. M. and A. E. A. READ: *Basic Gastroenterology,* 2d ed., Yearbook, Chicago, 1974, pp. 17–36.

NETTER, FRANK H.: *Ciba Collection of Medical Illustrations: Vol. 3, Digestive System, Part I, Upper Digestive Tract,* Ciba Pharmaceutical Co., Summit, N. J., 1959, pp. 35–45, 145–156.

SKINNER, D. B.: "The Esophagus," in W. A. Sodeman, Jr. and W. A. Sodeman (eds.), Pathologic Physiology, 5th ed., Saunders, Philadelphia, 1974, pp. 697–708.

CHAPTER 20 Stomach and Duodenum

OBJECTIVES   **At the completion of Chap. 20, you should be able to:**

1 Identify the anatomic divisions of the stomach.

2 Identify the various types of gastric glands and their secretions.

3 Describe the layers of the stomach wall.

4 Describe the innervation of the stomach.

5 Explain the significance of the retroduodenal location of the gastro-duodenal and pancreaticoduodenal arteries.

6 Describe the secretory, digestive, and motor functions of the stomach.

7 Outline and explain the three regulatory phases of gastric secretion.

8 List at least five effects of the hormone gastrin.

9 Explain the purpose of the various tests used in gastric analysis (basal analysis, stimulation analysis, and insulin hypoglycemia tests).

10 Contrast acute superficial and chronic atrophic gastritis (etiology, types of lesions, significance, symptoms, and treatment).

11 Differentiate among gastric erosions, acute ulcers, and chronic ulcers.

12 Identify the components of the gastric mocosal barrier, factors which may disturb this barrier, and the pathophysiologic consequences.

13 Explain the purpose of Brunner's glands.

14 Compare gastric and duodenal ulcers (prevalence, incidence, sex and age groups affected, pathogenesis, common sites, clinical features, and common complications).

15 Describe the complications of gastric and duodenal ulcers.

16 Describe and explain the purpose of vagotomy, antrectomy, and partial gastrectomy in the surgical treatment of peptic ulcers.

17 Differentiate between Curling's and Cushing's ulcers based on probable pathogenetic mechanisms.

18 Describe the treatment of stress ulcers complicated by hemorrhage.

19 Describe gastric carcinoma (sex and age group most commonly affected, predisposing factors, three types of lesions, symptoms, treatment, and prognosis).

ANATOMIC CONSIDERATIONS

The stomach lies obliquely from left to right across the upper abdomen between the liver and the diaphragm above and the transverse colon below. Its shape, size, and position vary a great deal depending on body build, posture, and degree of gastric distention. When empty, the stomach resembles a J-shaped tube and when full, a giant pear. The normal capacity of the stomach is 1 to 2 liters.

The *fundus,* the *body,* and the *pyloris* are the three anatomic divisions of the stomach (see Fig. 20-1). The fundus is the enlarged portion to the left and above the opening of the esophagus into the stomach. The body is the central portion, and the pyloric antrum is the lower portion. The stomach ends with the pyloric sphincter. There are two curvatures of the stomach. The upper right border presents as the concave *lesser curvature* and the lower left border as the convex *greater curvature.*

Both ends of the stomach are guarded by sphincters which regulate inflow and outflow. The *cardiac sphincter* or lower esophageal sphincter guards the opening of the esophagus into the stomach and prevents backflow of material into the esophagus, as discussed in Chap. 19. This area is known as the *cardiac region* of the stomach. The *pyloric sphincter* guards the opening between the pyloric portion of the stomach and the first portion of the small intestine (duodenum) and prevents backflow of intestinal contents into the stomach. The pyloric sphincter is of particular clinical interest, since obstructive narrowing (stenosis) may occur as a complication of peptic ulcer disease. *Pylorospasm* is another abnormality which is very serious in infants. Spasms of these muscle fibers do not allow food to enter the duodenum properly, so that the baby vomits the food instead of digesting and absorbing it. The condition is corrected by smooth muscle relaxants or by surgery.

The stomach is composed of four layers. The outer serous coat is formed by the peritoneum, which covers both surfaces of the stomach and is reflected off the lesser and greater curvature as the *lesser* and *greater omenta.* The lesser omentum is composed of the hepatogastric and hepatoduodenal ligaments attached to the liver, which suspend the stomach along its lesser curvature.

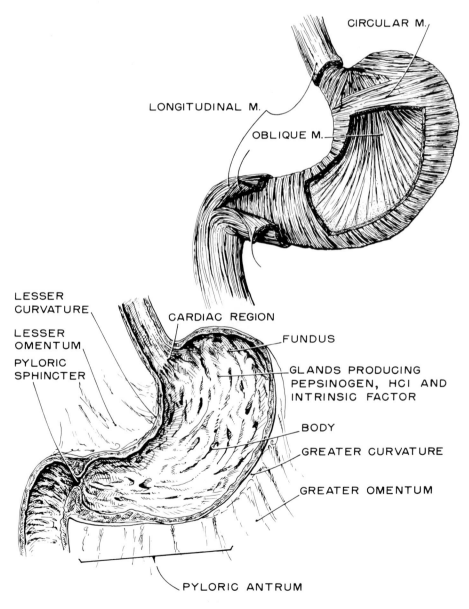

FIGURE 20-1 Anatomy of the stomach.

The three layers of muscle in the wall of the stomach are composed entirely of smooth muscle. The outermost longitudinal muscle layer extends down from the esophagus and passes mainly along the lesser and greater curvatures. The middle circular muscle layer is the most continuous and strongest of the three layers, and as it approaches the pyloris, it becomes thicker to form the muscle of the pyloric sphincter. The innermost oblique muscle is continuous with the circular muscle layer of the esophagus, is thickest in the region of the fundus, and extends to the pyloris.

The submucosa is composed mainly of loose areolar tissue and connects the muscle and mucosal layers of the stomach. It permits the mucosa to move with peristaltic motion. This layer also contains the nerve plexuses, blood, and lymph channels.

The inner mucosal layer of the stomach is arranged in temporary longitudinal folds called rugae, which allow for distention. Several types of glands are located in this layer and are categorized according to the anatomic portion of the stomach in which they lie. Cardiac glands lie near the cardiac orifice and secrete mucus. The fundic or gastric glands are located in the fundus and over the greater part of the body of the stomach. Fundic glands have three main types of cells. Zymogenic or chief cells secrete pepsinogen, which is converted into pepsin in an acid environment. Parietal cells secrete hydrochloric acid and water. The neck cells are found in the gland neck and secrete mucus. The pyloric glands are located in the pyloric region of the stomach and produce gastrin. Other substances secreted in the stomach include enzymes and various electrolytes, especially sodium, potassium, and chloride. Intrinsic factor is secreted by the parietal cells. Intrinsic factor combines with vitamin B_{12}, enabling it to be absorbed in the small intestine. A lack of intrinsic factor results in pernicious anemia.

The stomach receives its nerve supply entirely from the autonomic nervous system. The parasympathetic nerve supply for the stomach and duodenum is conveyed to and from the abdomen through the vagus nerves (see Fig. 20-2). The vagal trunks give off gastric, pyloric, hepatic, and celiac branches. This anatomy is especially important to understand, since selective vagotomy is of primary importance in the surgical treatment of duodenal ulcers and will be discussed in greater detail later in this chapter.

Sympathetic innervation is supplied via the greater splanchnic nerves and the celiac ganglia. The afferent fibers conduct pain impulses which are stimulated by distention, muscle contraction, and inflammation and are felt in the epigastric region of the abdomen. Efferent sympathetic fibers inhibit gastric motility and secretion. Auerbach's and Meissner's nerve plexuses form the intrinsic innervation within the wall of the stomach and function to coordinate the motor and secretory activity of the gastric mucosa.

The entire blood supply of the stomach and pancreas (as well as the liver, gallbladder, and spleen) is derived mainly from the celiac artery or trunk, which gives off branches supplying the lesser and greater curvatures. Two arterial branches of particular clinical significance are the gastroduodenal and the pancreaticoduodenal (retroduodenal) arteries, which course along the posterior duodenal bulb (see Fig. 20-3). Ulcers of the posterior duodenal wall may erode into these arteries and cause hemorrhaging. The venous blood from the stomach and duodenum, as well as that from the pancreas, spleen, and the remainder of the intestinal tract, is conveyed to the liver by the portal vein.

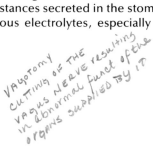

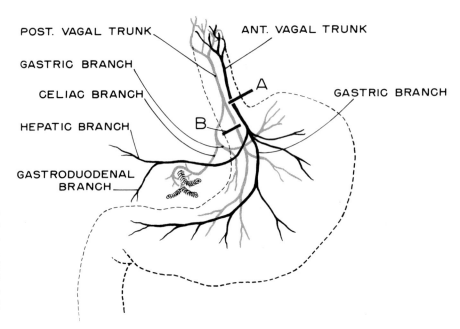

FIGURE 20-2 Parasympatetic (vagal) innervation of the stomach. It is possible to sever the vagal nerve branches supplying the stomach at points A and B, leaving intact those branches supplying other abdominal structures (selective vagotomy). Selective vagotomy is an important aspect of the surgical treatment of duodenal ulcers.

The digestive and motor functions of the stomach are summarized in Table 20-1. The types of secretions have already been discussed. Motor functions include storage, mixing, and emptying *chyme* (food mixed with gastric secretions) into the duodenum. Understanding the regulation and control of gastric secretions is essential for a rational understanding of the pathogenesis and treatment of peptic ulcer disease.

The control of gastric secretion

The regulation of gastric secretion may be subdivided into the cephalic, gastric or hormonal, and intestinal phases. The *cephalic phase* of gastric secretion occurs even before food enters the stomach. It results from the sight, smell, thought, or taste of food. It is mediated entirely by the vagus nerve and is eliminated by vagotomy. Neurogenic signals causing the cephalic phase may originate in the cerebral cortex or in the appetite center. Efferent impulses are then transmitted via the vagus nerve to the stomach. As a result, the gastric glands are stimulated to secrete acid, pepsinogen, and increased mucus. This phase of secretion accounts for about 10 percent of the gastric secretions normally associated with a meal.

The *gastric* or *hormonal phase* begins when food reaches the pyloric antrum. The hormone gastrin is released from the antrum and then carried by the bloodstream to the gastric glands, causing secretions. Gastrin release occurs when the vagus nerve is stimulated mechanically by distention of the antrum [causes local and vasovagal reflexes (impulses travel to the medulla over vagal afferents and then back again to the stomach over vagal efferents which stimulates gastrin release and directly stimulates the gastric glands)]. Gastrin release is

the primary stimulus to acid secretion. Its release is also stimulated by an alkaline pH, bile salts in the antrum, and especially by protein foods and alcohol. Table 20-2 lists the effects of gastrin.

The gastric phase of secretion accounts for more than two-thirds of the total gastric secretion after eating a meal and thus accounts for most of the total daily gastric secretion of about 2000 ml. The gastric phase can be affected by surgical resection of the pyloric antrum, since this is the site of gastrin production.

The *intestinal phase* occurs when food enters the duodenum and causes the stomach to secrete small amounts of gastric juice. This phase is probably almost exclusively hormonal. Gastric secretion is probably mediated by the release of intestinal gastrin, which is probably neurally mediated. However, the role of the small intestine as an inhibitor of gastric secretion is of much greater importance.

Distention of the small intestine initiates the *enterogastric reflex* mediated through the mysenteric plexus, sympathetic nerves, and vagus, which inhibit gastric secretion and emptying. The presence of acid (pH less than 2.5), fat, and protein breakdown products causes the release of several intestinal hormones. Secretin and cholecystokinin–pancreozymin both have a moderate inhibitory effect on gastric secretion.

During the *interdigestive period* when digestion is not occurring in the gut, hydrochloric acid secretion continues at the low rate of 1 to 5 meq/hr. This is called the basal acid output (BAO) and may be measured by a 12-hour fasting gastric analysis of the secretions. The normal gastric secretions during the interdigestive period are mainly composed of mucus and contain very little pepsin

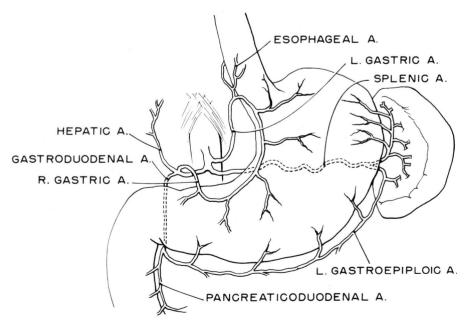

FIGURE 20-3 Blood supply of the stomach and duodenum.

and acid. Strong emotional stimuli, however, can increase the BAO via the parasympathetic (vagus) nerves and is believed to be one of the factors in the development of peptic ulcers.

DIAGNOSTIC MEASURES

Diagnostic procedures that are helpful in identifying the presence of gastric and duodenal disease include the barium x-ray, gastric analysis, and endoscopy using a flexible fiberoptic gastroscope. Photographs, biopsies, and exfoliative cytology may all be performed through the gastroscope. Exfoliative cytology, or collection of cells by lavage with normal saline, is a valuable technique for the identification of malignancies which may not be directly visible through the gastroscope. Malignant cells exfoliate (slough off) more readily than do normal cells. The collected solution should be placed on ice and taken to the lab immediately for analysis. Delay will result in

destruction of the exfoliated cells by the digestive enzymes. Cytologic washings have about 90 percent accuracy rates in the diagnosis of cancer of the stomach.

Gastric analysis of acid secretion is another important technique in the diagnosis of gastric disease. A nasogastric tube is inserted into the stomach and the fasting contents aspirated for analysis. The *basal analysis* measures BAO in the absence of stimulation. This test is valuable in the diagnosis of Zollinger-Ellison syndrome (a tumor of the pancreas that secretes large amounts of gastrin which, in turn, causes marked hyperacidity and multiple recurrent peptic ulcers). Duodenal ulcers are usually associated with a high BAO, while the BAO is normal to low in gastric ulcer and carcinoma.

Stimulation analysis may be performed by measurement of maximum acid output (MAO) after the administration of a drug such as histamine, betazole hydrochloride (Histalog), or pentagastrin (synthetic gastrin), which stimulates acid secretion. *Achlorhydria* is defined as a lack of acid secretions after a maximum dose of one of the stimulating drugs (providing the analysis is accurate and there has been no reflux of duodenal contents into the stomach which would neutralize the acid). If a patient is achlorhydric and has a gastric ulcer, the ulcer probably represents cancer and is not related to acid secretions. Patients with pernicious anemia are also achlorhydric as a result of atrophy of the secretory cells in the stomach and loss of intrinsic factor. Without intrinsic factor, vitamin B_{12} absorption is impaired, and the serum levels of the vitamin B_{12} will be low.

TABLE 20-1
Functions of the stomach

Motor functions	*Reservoir* function. Stores food until it can be partially digested and moved on in GI tract. Adapts to increased volume without an increase in pressure by receptive relaxation of the smooth muscle; mediated by the vagus nerve and induced by gastrin.
	Mixing function. Breaks food into small particles and mixes it with gastric juice through contractions of muscular coat. Peristaltic contractions controlled by a basic intrinsic electrical rhythm.
	Gastric emptying function. Controlled by opening of pyloric sphincter, which is influenced by viscosity, volume, acidity, osmotic activity, physical state, as well as by emotions, drugs, and exercise. Gastric emptying is controlled by nervous and hormonal factors.
Digestive, secretory functions	*Digestion of protein* by pepsin and HCl is begun. Digestion of starches and fats by gastric amylase and lipase is of little importance in the stomach.
	Gastrin synthesis and release affected by ingestion of protein, distention of the antrum, alkalinization of the antrum, and vagal stimuli.
	Intrinsic factor secretion enables the absorption of vitamin B_{12} from the distal small bowel.
	Mucus secretion, which forms a protective shell for the stomach as well as contributing to lubrication of food for easier transport.

TABLE 20-2
Actions of gastrin

ACTIONS	PHYSIOLOGIC SIGNIFICANCE
Stimulates acid and pepsin secretion	Promotes digestion
Stimulates secretion of intrinsic factor	Promotes vitamin B_{12} absorption in small intestine
Stimulates pancreatic enzyme secretion	Promotes digestion
Stimulates increase in the flow of hepatic bile	Promotes digestion
Stimulates the release of insulin	Promotes glucose metabolism
Stimulates gastric and intestinal motility	Promotes mixing and propulsion of ingested food
Promotes receptive relaxation of stomach	Stomach can greatly increase volume without increasing pressure
Increases resting tone of the lower esophageal sphincter	Prevents gastric reflux during active mixing and churning
Inhibits gastric emptying	Allows time for thorough mixing of gastric contents before delivery to intestine

Hypoglycemic analysis (Hollander test) is performed by inducing hypoglycemia through the injection of insulin. The gastric secretory response to insulin hypoglycemia may be used to determine the completeness of vagotomy and the likelihood of recurrent ulcers after surgery for duodenal ulcer. A drop in blood glucose to less than 50 mg% without an increase in free hydrochloric acid indicates that the vagotomy was complete and fibers were not missed. The significance of the surgical treatment will be discussed later in this chapter.

GASTRITIS

Gastritis is an inflammation of the gastric mucosa which may be acute, chronic, diffuse, or localized. The two most common types of gastritis—acute superficial and chronic atrophic gastritis—will be discussed.

Acute superficial gastritis

Acute gastritis is a very common, usually benign, and self-limiting disease which represents the response of the gastric mucosa to a variety of local irritants. The most common cause of acute superficial gastritis is alcohol. When ingested in combination with aspirin, the effect is more deleterious than the effect of either taken alone. Diffuse hemorrhagic erosive gastritis is known to occur with heavy alcohol and aspirin abuse and may lead to the necessity of gastric resection. This serious condition will be considered with stress ulcers, since there are many similarities between the two. Destruction of the gastric mucosal barrier is believed to be the pathogenetic mechanism responsible for the injury and will be considered later.

Other causes of acute superficial gastritis include drugs such as caffeine, digitalis, iodine, aureomycin, ferrous sulfate, cinchophen, and cortisone. Some spicy foods, such as those that include pepper, vinegar, or mustard, may cause symptoms suggestive of gastritis.

In superficial gastritis, the mucosa is reddened, edematous, and covered with adherent mucus; small erosions and hemorrhages are common. The degree of inflammation is highly variable.

In most cases, the diagnosis is based on the patient's history of a self-limited disorder accompanied by epigastric pain, nausea, vomiting, anorexia, and belching. In some cases, when symptoms are prolonged and resistant to treatment, additional diagnostic measures, such as endoscopy, mucosal biopsy, and gastric analysis, may be needed to clarify the diagnosis.

Acute superficial gastritis usually disappears when the offending agent is removed. Food and fluids should be withheld until the inflammation and vomiting subsides. If vomiting is persistent, it may be necessary to correct fluid and electrolyte imbalance with intravenous infusions. Antiemetic drugs may help relieve the nausea and vomiting. Antispasmodics may be given to relieve smooth muscle spasm. A bland diet and antacids may also be helpful.

Chronic atrophic gastritis

Chronic atrophic gastritis is characterized by progressive atrophy of the glandular epithelium with loss of parietal and chief cells. Consequently, there is decreased production of hydrochloric acid, pepsin, and intrinsic factor. The gastric wall becomes thin, and the mucosa presents an unusually smooth surface. This form of gastritis is frequently seen in association with pernicious anemia, gastric ulcer, and cancer.

The etiology and pathogenesis of chronic atrophic gastritis is unknown. It is more common in the elderly. Heavy alcohol intake, hot tea, and smoking may predispose to the development of atrophic gastritis.

In the case of pernicious anemia the pathogenesis may be related to a disturbance of immunologic mechanisms. Many of these patients have circulating antibodies against parietal cells. It is not known whether the antibodies are the cause or the effect of the gastritis.

It is believed that chronic atrophic gastritis predisposes to the development of gastric ulcers and carcinoma. The incidence of gastric cancer is particularly high in patients with pernicious anemia (10 to 15 percent).

Symptoms of chronic gastritis are generally varied and vague; they include a feeling of fullness, anorexia, and vague epigastric distress. The diagnosis is suspected when there is achlorhydria or a low BAO or MAO and is confirmed by the typical histologic changes on biopsy.

The treatment of chronic atrophic gastritis varies, depending on the suspected cause of the disorder. Alcohol and drugs known to irritate the gastric mucosa are avoided. Iron deficiency anemia (due to chronic bleeding), if present, is corrected. Vitamin B_{12} and other appropriate therapy is given in the case of pernicious anemia.

PEPTIC ULCER DISEASE

Peptic ulcers are circumscribed breaks in the continuity of mucosa extending below the epithelium. Strictly speaking, breaks in the mucosa not extending below it are called erosions, although they are often referred to as ulcers (e.g., stress ulcers). Chronic ulcers, as opposed to acute ulcers, have scar tissue at their base (see Fig. 20-4).

By definition, peptic ulcers can be located in any part of the gastrointestinal tract exposed to the acid-peptic gastric juice, including the esophagus, stomach, duodenum, and after gastroenterostomy, the jejunum. Although the peptic digestive activity of gastric juice is an important etiologic factor, there is evidence that this is only one of many factors in the pathogenesis of peptic ulcer disease. Because there are many similarities and differences between gastric and duodenal ulcers, some aspects of these two entities will be considered together for convenience, while special problems relating to each will be considered separately. Gastric erosions or stress ulcers will be considered last. Table 20-3 lists some of the differences between the various types of peptic ulcers.

Pathogenesis of peptic ulcer disease

Since pure acid gastric juice is capable of digesting all living tissues, one of the major questions is why doesn't the stomach digest itself. Two factors seem to protect the stomach from autodigestion: the gastric mucus and the epithelial barrier.

THE GASTRIC MUCOSAL BARRIER

According to Hollander's "two-component mucus barrier theory," the thick, tenacious layer of gastric mucus constitutes the first line of defense against autodigestion. It provides protection against mechanical trauma and chemical agents. Both cortisone and aspirin produce qualitative changes in the gastric mucus which may facilitate its degradation by pepsin. However, no deficiency or abnormality of mucus has been demonstrated in patients with chronic peptic ulcer.

Davenport has emphasized the importance of a gastric mucosal barrier (see Fig. 20-5). Although the exact nature of this barrier is not understood, it probably involves the mucus lining, the lumen of the columnar epithelial cells, and the tight junctions at the apices of these cells. Normally this mucosal barrier allows very little back diffusion of H^+ from the lumen to the blood, even though there is a tremendous concentration gradient (gastric acid pH of 1 versus blood pH of 7.4).

DESTRUCTION OF THE GASTRIC MUCOSAL BARRIER

Aspirin, alcohol, bile salts, and other substances injurious to the gastric mucosa alter the permeability of the epithelial barrier, allowing back diffusion of hydrochloric acid with resultant injury to underlying tissues, especially blood vessels (see Fig. 20-5). Histamine is liberated, stimulating further acid and pepsin secretion and increased capillary permeability to proteins. The mucosa becomes edematous, and large amounts of plasma proteins may be lost. The mucosal capillaries may be damaged, resulting in interstitial hemorrhage and bleeding. The mucosal barrier is unaffected by vagal inhibition or atropine, but back diffusion is inhibited by gastrin.

Destruction of the gastric mucosal barrier is believed to be an important factor in the pathogenesis of gastric ulcers. It is known that the antral mucosa is more susceptible to back diffusion than the fundus, which explains why gastric ulcers are often located in this area. It has also been suggested that the reason for the low level of acid recovered in gastric analysis of patients with gastric ulcer is increased back diffusion, not lower production. This pathogenetic mechanism may also be important in patients with acute hemorrhagic gastritis caused by alcohol, aspirin, and severe stress.

The resistance of the duodenum to peptic ulceration is believed to be a function of *Brunner's glands* (located in the intestinal wall), which produce a highly alkaline (pH of 8), viscid, mucoid secretion which neutralizes the acid chyme. Patients with duodenal ulcer often have excessive acid secretion, which seems to be the most important pathogenetic factor. It is possible that the normal mucosal defense mechanisms are overwhelmed. The factor of decreased tissue resistance is implicated in both gastric and duodenal ulcers, although it seems to be more important in gastric ulcer.

In addition to the mucosal and epithelial barriers, tissue resistance also depends on an abundant vascular supply and continued, rapid regeneration of epithelial cells (normally replaced every 3 days). Failure of this mechanism may also play a role in the pathogenesis of peptic ulcer.

OTHER FACTORS

Duodenal ulcers comprise about 80 percent of all peptic ulcers, and about 10 to 12 percent of the population is affected. Duodenal ulcers generally occur in a much younger age group than do gastric ulcers. The much lower incidence of peptic ulcers in women seems to indicate a sex-linked influence.

It has been suggested that certain drugs such as aspi-

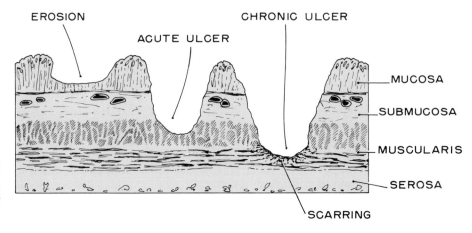

FIGURE 20-4 Peptic ulcers illustrating an erosion, acute ulcer, and chronic ulcer. Both the acute and chronic ulcer may penetrate the entire wall of the stomach.

rin, alcohol, indomethecin, phenylbutazone, and corticosteroids may have a direct irritating effect on the gastric mucosa and produce ulceration. If they do have an effect, it is probably caused by a disruption of one of the protective barriers in the stomach. Other drugs, such as caffeine, will increase acid production. Emotional stress presumably also plays a role in the pathogenesis of peptic ulcers, probably by increasing acid production as a result of vagal stimulation.

Most peptic ulcers occur "downstream" from the source of acid secretion. More than 90 percent of duodenal ulcers are located on the anterior or posterior wall of the first part of the duodenum, within 2 cm of the pyloric ring. Although gastric ulcers may occur anywhere in the stomach, 90 percent are situated along the lesser curvature and in the pyloric gland region.

Individuals with blood group O are 35 percent more susceptible to doudenal ulcer, indicating that genetic

factors are involved. The incidence of gastric ulcers does not seem to be related to blood group.

A number of diseases seem to be associated with peptic ulcer formation, including alcoholic liver cirrhosis, chronic pancreatitis, chronic lung disease, hyperparathyroidism, and the Zollinger-Ellison syndrome.

Finally, abnormal pyloric sphincter function resulting in bile reflux has been proposed as a pathogenetic mechanism in the development of gastric ulcer. The bile disrupts the gastric mucosal barrier, causing gastritis and increased susceptibility to ulcer formation. The damaged mucosa is ultimately eroded and digested by the action of acid and pepsin.

TABLE 20-3
Differentiating features of duodenal, gastric, and stress ulcers

	DUODENAL ULCER	GASTRIC ULCER	STRESS ULCER
Incidence	Duodenal/gastric ulcer—4:1 Prevalence 10–12% population; Age 25–50 yr; Men/women—4:1	Age: Usually over 50 yr Men/women—3.5:1	Related to severe stress, trauma, sepsis, burns, head injuries; No sex difference
Pathogenesis	Hyperacidity important factor; Associated diseases: hyperparathyroidism, chronic pulmonary disease, chronic pancreatitis, alcoholic cirrhosis; Ulcerogenic drugs, alcohol, tobacco;	Disruption of mucosal barrier seems to be an important factor. Normal to low HCl production; Presence of gastritis; Ulcerogenic drugs, alcohol, tobacco; Chronic bile reflux	Head injuries: hypersecretion of HCl; All others: ischemia of the gastric mucosa, disruption of the mucosal barrier, back diffusion of HCl, acute gastritis
	Blood group O—higher frequency; Higher frequency in those subject to stress, responsibility: e.g., executives, leaders	Not related to blood group; More common in laboring groups	Hemorrhagic gastric erosions may be drug-induced; alcohol and aspirin most common offenders
Pathology	90% in duodenal bulb	90% in antrum and lesser curvature	Usually multiple, diffuse erosions; more commonly located in stomach
Complications			
Intractability	About 10%; most respond to medical therapy	More common	
Hemorrhage	Common in posterior wall of duodenal bulb	Less common	Most frequent complication, high mortality
Perforation	More common when located in anterior wall of duodenum	More common in anterior wall of stomach	Common
Obstruction	Common	Rare	
Malignancy	Almost never	Incidence about 7%	
Clinical features	Pain–food–relief pattern of pain; Usually well-nourished; Seasonal exacerbations (more common in spring and fall); Night pain common	Pain–food–relief pattern or food–pain pattern; Anorexia, weight loss common; Night pain uncommon	May be asymptomatic until serious complication such as hemorrhage or perforation

Clinical features

Although duodenal and gastric ulcers possibly arise from different pathologic processes, the signs and symptoms with which they commonly present are sometimes indistinguishable. The principal symptom is upper abdominal pain. This is usually located in the epigastrum and is described as a gnawing, boring, or nagging sensation. The pain usually begins about 2 hours after meals and is relieved by food or antacids. The symptoms may last for a few days, weeks, or months and then disappear for varying periods of time. The periodic nature of the symptoms is so characteristic that constant upper abdominal pain is frequently not caused by peptic ulcer. Although the food–pain–relief pattern also occurs with gastric ulcers, the symptoms seem to be more variable. In fact, with gastric ulcer, food sometimes aggravates the pain. Patients with duodenal ulcer frequently have pain in the middle of the night, although this is not as common in pa-tients with gastric ulcer. Weight loss is frequent in pa-tients with gastric ulcer, but persons with duodenal ulcer usually maintain their normal weight.

Diagnosis

The most important criterion in the diagnosis of duodenal ulcer is a history of the typical pain–food–relief pattern. The history is not as informative in patients with gastric ulcer, since vague symptoms of epigastric distress are more common. It is not usually possible to distinguish between gastric and duodenal ulcer on the basis of history alone.

The diagnosis of peptic ulcer is usually confirmed by barium meal x-ray (see Fig. 20-6). When barium x-ray fails to reveal an ulcer in the stomach or duodenum but characteristic symptoms persist, endoscopic examination is indicated.

BENIGN VERSUS MALIGNANT ULCERS

Although duodenal ulcers are almost never malignant, about 7 percent of gastric ulcers turn out to be carcinoma of the stomach. It is therefore important for the gastro-

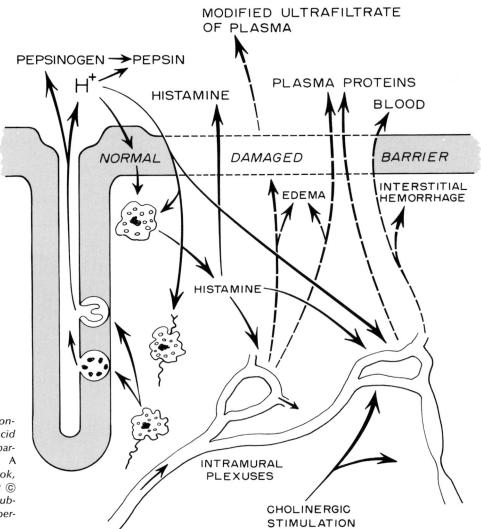

FIGURE 20-5 Pathophysiologic consequences of back diffusion of acid through the damaged mucosal barrier. (From H. W. Davenport, A Digest on Digestion, Yearbook, Chicago, 1975, p. 54.) Copyright © 1975 by Year Book Medical Publishers, Inc., Chicago. Used by permission.

enterologist to differentiate between a benign and malignant gastric ulcer. In general, malignant ulcers have a shaggy, necrotic base, while benign ulcers have a smooth, clean base with a distinct margin (see Fig. 20-7). Biopsy and cytologic studies are also helpful in distinguishing a benign from a malignant ulcer.

Medical treatment

The primary objectives in the medical treatment of peptic ulcer are to inhibit or buffer acid secretions in order to relieve symptoms and promote healing. Measures that achieve these ends are antacids, dietary management, anticholinergics, and physical and emotional rest.

Antacids are given to neutralize the acid gastric contents by keeping the pH high enough so that pepsin is not activated, thus protecting the mucosa and relieving the pain. Small, frequent meals are also important in neutralizing the gastric contents. Stimulants of acid secretion, such as alcohol and caffeine, are avoided. Anticholinergic drugs, such as propantheline (Pro-Banthine)

and atropine (*Atropa belladonna*), inhibit the direct affect of the vagus nerve on the acid-secreting parietal cells. Anticholinergics also inhibit gastric motility and emptying time, and for this reason many physicians do not prescribe this drug for patients with gastric ulcer.

Physical and emotional rest are promoted by a quiet environment, listening to the patient's problems, and offering emotional support. Small doses of sedatives are frequently prescribed.

About 80 to 90 percent of patients with duodenal ulcer have a benign course interrupted by the necessity for medical therapy. An unknown number of patients undoubtedly treat themselves successfully with diet and antacids which are available without a prescription. The response of gastric ulcers to medical therapy is not quite as successful. These remaining patients may develop complications.

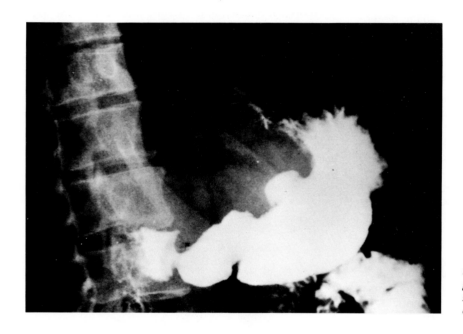

FIGURE 20-6 Barium x-ray appearance of gastric ulcer. Note the large nodular-shaped protrusion on the lesser curvature of the stomach.

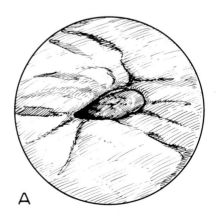
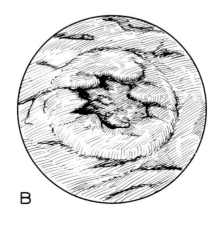

A   B

FIGURE 20-7 Gastroscopic appearance of (A) a benign gastric ulcer and (B) a malignant gastric ulcer (carcinoma). The benign ulcer has a sharp, well-defined margin. The malignant ulcer has an irregular margin which fades into the surrounding tumor mass.

Complications

Complications of peptic ulcer disease include intractability, hemorrhage, perforation, and pyloric obstruction. Any of these complications are indications for surgical treatment, which will be discussed subsequently.

INTRACTABILITY

The most common complication of peptic ulcer disease is intractability, which simply means that the medical therapy has failed to control the symptoms adequately. Patients may have their sleep interrupted by pain, lose time from work, require frequent hospitalization, or just be unable to follow the medical regimen. Intractability is the most common reason for recommending surgery. Malignant transformation is not an important consideration in either gastric or duodenal ulcer. Those ulcers which are malignant started out as malignant, and at least by current knowledge, those that started out as benign remain benign without undergoing malignant degeneration.

HEMORRHAGE

Bleeding is a very common complication of peptic ulcer and occurs in at least 25 percent of the cases at some time during the course of the disease. Although ulcers in any site may bleed, the most common site of hemorrhage is in the posterior wall of the duodenal bulb, since in that location erosion into the pancreaticoduodenal or gastroduodenal arteries may occur.

The symptoms associated with bleeding ulcer depend on the rapidity of blood loss. Mild, chronic blood loss may lead to iron deficiency anemia. The stools may be positive for occult blood (positive guaiac test) or may be black and tarry (melana). Massive bleeding may lead to hematemesis (vomiting blood) and the development of shock and may require blood transfusions and emergency surgery. Relief of pain often follows bleeding as a result of the buffering effect of blood. The mortality in these patients is from 3 to 10 percent, which represents about 25 percent of the total deaths attributable to peptic ulcer disease.

PERFORATION

Approximately 5 percent of all ulcers perforate, and this complication accounts for about 65 percent of deaths from peptic ulcer disease. The ulcers are usually on the anterior wall of the duodenum or stomach, since this area is only covered by peritoneum.

The majority of patients present in a characteristically dramatic fashion. There is a sudden onset of excruciating pain in the upper abdomen. Within minutes a chemical peritonitis develops from the escaping gastric acid, causing intense pain. The patient fears to move or breathe. The abdomen becomes silent to auscultation and assumes a boardlike rigidity to palpation. Acute perforation can usually be diagnosed on the basis of the symptoms alone. The diagnosis is confirmed by the presence of free gas within the peritoneal cavity, presenting as a translucent crescent between the liver and diaphragm shadows. The air, of course, entered the peritoneal cavity through the perforated ulcer. The treatment is immediate surgery with gastric resection or simple suture of the perforation, depending on the patient's condition.

Occasionally a gastric or duodenal ulcer breaks through the wall but remains sealed off by a contiguous structure and is called a *penetrating ulcer*. A classic example of a penetrating ulcer is a duodenal ulcer of the posterior wall which penetrates into the pancreas and is walled off (see Fig. 20-8). Clinically, the pain becomes intractable and may radiate to the back. The patient may present with the finding of pancreatitis.

OBSTRUCTION

Obstruction of the gastric outlet as a result of inflammation and edema, pylorospasm, or scarring occurs in about 5 percent of patients with peptic ulcer. It is more common in patients with duodenal ulcer but occasionally occurs when a gastric ulcer is located close to the pyloric sphincter.

Anorexia, nausea, and bloating after eating are common symptoms. Weight loss is common. When the obstruction becomes severe, pain and vomiting may occur.

Treatment is directed toward restoring fluids and electrolytes, decompressing the stomach by insertion of a nasogastric tube, and surgical correction of the obstruction (pyloroplasty).

Surgical treatment

Patients who do not respond to medical therapy or who develop other complications such as perforation, hemorrhage, or obstruction are treated surgically. In general,

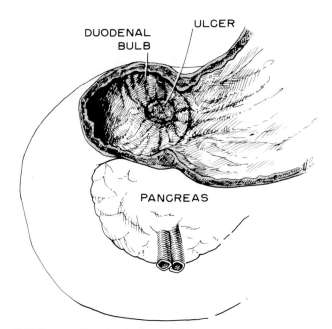

FIGURE 20-8 Duodenal ulcer of the posterior wall penetrating into the head of the pancreas resulting in a walled-off perforation.

surgical treatment is effected by one of two procedures: vagotomy or gastrectomy or sometimes both. There are many variations of these two procedures, and the type of surgery elected depends on many factors, including the nature of the pathology and the patient's age and general condition.

The common aim in the surgical treatment of duodenal ulcers is to permanently reduce the capacity of the stomach to secrete acid and pepsin. This can be achieved in at least four ways:

1 *Vagotomy* is the division of the vagus nerve branches to the stomach, thus eliminating the cephalic phase of gastric secretion. Vagotomy not only diminishes gastric secretions but also decreases gastric motility and emptying. Consequently a "drainage" procedure is required to prevent gastric retention—either a gastrojejunostomy or pyloroplasty.
2 *Antrectomy* is the removal of the entire antrum of the stomach, thus eliminating the hormonal or gastric phase of gastric secretion.
3 *Vagotomy plus antrectomy* eliminates both the cephalic and gastric phases of gastric secretion. Thus, neural stimulation is interrupted, drainage is en-

hanced, and the major site of gastrin production is removed. It is thought to be superior to some of the more extensive surgical procedures.

4 *Partial gastrectomy* is the removal of the distal 50 to 75 percent of the stomach, thus removing a substantial portion of the acid- and pepsin-secreting mucosa. Following gastric resection, gastrointestinal continuity may be restored by anastomosing the gastric remnant to the duodenum (gastroduodenostomy or Billroth I procedure) or to the jejunum (gastrojejunostomy or Billroth II procedure).

Figure 20-9 illustrates some of the common surgical procedures for treating peptic ulcers.

Most surgeons treat gastric ulcer by partial gastrectomy and a gastroduodenal anastomosis. The line of resection is usually proximal to the gastric ulcer. A vagotomy is usually not performed, since these patients have normal to low gastric acid production.

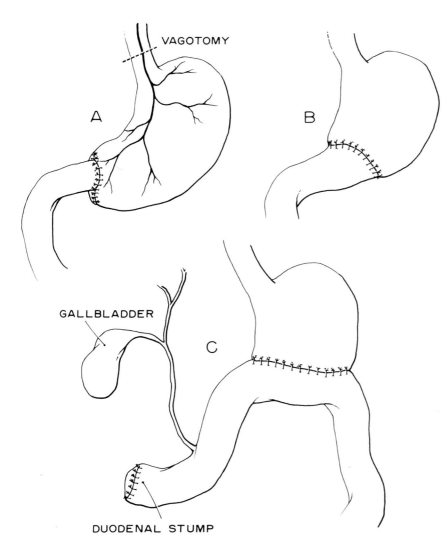

VAGOTOMY

A

B

GALLBLADDER

C

DUODENAL STUMP

FIGURE 20-9 Common surgical procedures for treating peptic ulcers. A, vagotomy + antrectomy (removal of the pyloric antrum); B, Billroth I procedure (gastroduodenostomy anastomosis after resection); C, Billroth II procedure (gastrojejunostomy anastomosis after resection).

Acute stress and drug-induced ulcers

The term "stress ulcer" has been used to describe gastric or duodenal erosions which occur as a sequel to prolonged psychological or physiologic stress. The stress may take many forms, such as hypotensive shock following traumatic injury and major surgery, sepsis, hypoxia, severe burns (Curling's ulcers), or cerebral trauma (Cushing's ulcers). Any seriously ill patient in an intensive care setting is susceptible to the development of a stress ulcer. Acute erosive and hemorrhagic gastritis induced by an alcoholic bout, aspirin or other ulcerogenic drugs, and bile reflux are often grouped with stress ulcers, since the lesions are similar.

Acute stress ulcers are usually shallow, irregular, punched-out lesions which may be large in size, multiple, and often located in the stomach. The lesions may bleed slowly, causing melana, and are often asymptomatic or are overshadowed by the serious illness in the patient. Because these lesions are superficial, they are not usually evident on x-ray examination.

Stress ulcers are clinically apparent when there is mas-sive gastric hemorrhage or perforation. In fact, stress ulcers account for 5 percent of all cases of peptic ulcer bleeding. Massive bleeding resulting from alcohol-induced acute erosive gastritis is also a common problem.

PATHOGENESIS

Stress ulcers are generally divided into two different groups based on probable pathogenetic mechanisms. Cushing's ulcers associated with serious brain injury are characterized by marked hyperacidity, which is possibly mediated by vagal stimulation (cerebral injury → vagal stimulation → hyperacidity → acute peptic ulcer).

On the other hand, stress ulcers associated with shock, sepsis, burns, and drugs are not characterized by gastric acid hypersecretion. The studies of Silen and Skillman (1974) suggest that disruption of the mucosal barrier function of the stomach, especially in the presence of ischemia resulting from poor vascular perfusion, may be important in the pathogenesis (see Fig. 20-10).

TREATMENT

Recent studies reveal that the presence of erosive gastritis (stress ulcers) is a common finding in critically ill patients. About 80 percent of the severely burned pa-

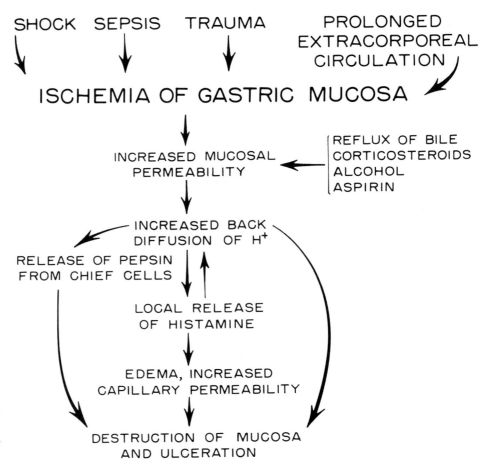

FIGURE 20–10 Pathogenesis of "stress" ulcers. (Adapted from W. Silen and J. J. Skillman, Stress Ulcer, Active Erosive Gastritis and the Gastric Mucosal Barrier, in G. H. Stollerman (ed.): Advances in Internal Medicine, Year Book, Chicago, 1974, vol. 19.) Copyright © 1974 by Year Book Medical Publishers, Inc., Chicago. Used by permission.

tients have evidence of occult blood in their stools. Other studies have revealed an even higher incidence of stress ulcers identified by gastroscopy in critically ill patients. Most of these patients do not have symptoms until there is massive bleeding, which occurs in about 5 percent. The other 95 percent heal with little or no residual effects.

When bleeding occurs, attempts are made to treat the condition conservatively by blood transfusions and by ice-water lavage. When bleeding is serious, some patients have been treated successfully by continuous intra-arterial perfusion with vasopressin, a powerful vasoconstrictor.

Vasopressin infusion is accomplished by inserting a catheter via the femoral artery, through the aorta and celiac trunk, and out the right or left gastric artery. The bleeding site is identified by arteriography, after which a vasopressin infusion is started. Newer and as yet experimental methods include electrocoagulation, photocoagulation (laser coagulation), and application of polymers.

When these conservative methods of treatment fail, surgery may be the only method of treatment, even though these patients are critically ill and poor surgical risks. The most effective surgical procedure is total gastrectomy, since these erosions are multiple or diffuse and tend to rebleed.

CANCER OF THE STOMACH

Carcinoma of the stomach is the most common form of gastric neoplasm and accounts for about 5 percent of all cancer deaths. Males are more frequently affected and most cases occur after the age of 40.

The cause of stomach cancer is unknown, but certain predisposing factors are recognized. Genetic factors seem to be important, since gastric cancer is more common in persons with blood group A. Geographic or environmental factors appear to be important, since gastric cancer is very common in Japan, Chile, and Iceland. For unknown reasons gastric cancer has been declining in the United States during the past 30 years. It is more common in lower socioeconomic groups. One of the most important predisposing factors is the presence of atrophic gastritis or pernicious anemia as previously discussed.

About 50 percent of gastric cancers are located in the pyloric antrum. The remainder of the lesions are distributed throughout the body of the stomach.

There are three general forms of gastric carcinoma. *Ulcerating carcinoma* is the most common type and must be differentiated from a benign gastric ulcer. *Polypoid carcinoma* appears as a cauliflowerlike mass protruding into the lumen and may arise from an adenomatous polyp. *Infiltrating carcinoma* may penetrate the entire thickness of the stomach wall and is responsible for the inflexible "leather bottle stomach" (linitis plastica) (see Fig. 20-11).

Carcinoma of the stomach is seldom diagnosed in an early stage because symptoms develop late or are vague and indefinite. Early symptoms may include a mild feeling of discomfort in the upper abdomen or a feeling of fullness after eating. Eventually there is anorexia and weight loss. When the tumor is located near the cardia, dysphagia may be the first major symptom. Vomiting from pyloric obstruction may occur when the tumor is near the gastric outlet.

Radiologic studies, exfoliative cytology, and endos-

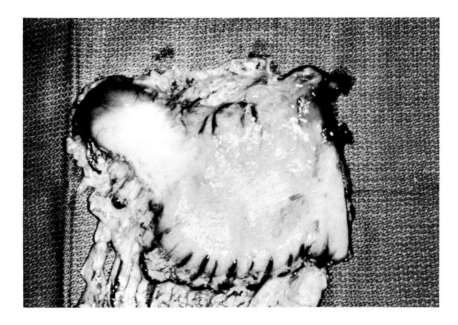

FIGURE 20-11 *Surgical specimen of gastric infiltrative carcinoma. The entire wall is cartilaginous and stiff.*

copy with biopsy are all important methods in the diagnosis of gastric cancer. Surgical excision is the only effective therapy. Because of the usual late diagnosis, the prognosis is poor, with a 10 percent 5-year survival rate.

QUESTIONS

Stomach and duodenum—Chap. 20

Directions: Answer the following questions on a separate sheet of paper.

1 Sketch the stomach and indicate the location of the following: fundus, body, pyloric antrum, pyloric sphincter, cardiac region, lesser curvature, greater curvature, glands secreting HCl and pepsin, intrinsic factor, and gastrin.

2 What are the lesser and greater omenta? Where are they located?

3 What are rugae and what is their purpose in the stomach?

4 How is pepsinogen activated in the stomach? What is the action of pepsin?

5 Describe the extrinsic and intrinsic innervation of the stomach and the function of each.

6 Name the truncal artery and its major branches supplying the stomach.

7 Why is hemorrhage a more frequent complication in duodenal ulcers of the posterior wall?

8 List three motor functions of the stomach.

9 What is the normal capacity of the adult stomach? What prevents an increase in intragastric pressure during a moderate-sized meal?

10 Why do patients become anemic when there is a deficiency or absence of intrinsic factor?

11 What controls the mixing and emptying activities of the stomach?

12 What prevents the stomach from digesting itself? Explain your answer using the theories of gastric mucosal defense formulated by Hollander and Davenport. What drugs or chemicals may alter mucosal defense? What protects the duodenum from the actions of acid and pepsin?

13 List five effects of gastrin and the physiological significance of each.

14 What is acute superficial gastritis? Do you think you have ever had this condition? What are the symptoms?

15 Explain how gastric secretions are controlled during the three phases of gastric secretion.

Directions: Circle the letter preceding each item below that correctly answers the questions. Only one answer may be correct unless otherwise noted.

16 Gastrin is a hormone produced by:
   a Pancreas b Brunner's glands c Duodenum
   d Gastric antrum e Gastric fundus

17 Which of the following agents have been associated with an increased incidence of ulcer disease? (More than one answer may be correct)
   a Aspirin b Ethyl alcohol c High doses of corticosteroids d Phenylbutazone

18 Achlorhydria or hypochlorhydria is commonly seen in: (More than one answer may be correct)
   a Pernicious anemia b Zollinger-Ellison syndrome
   c Atrophic gastritis d Carcinoma of the stomach

19 Which of the following is known to cause an elaboration of gastrin from the gastric antrum? (More than one answer may be correct)
   a Distention of the antrum b Alkalinization of the antrum c Acidification of the antrum d Distention of the fundus e Stimulation of the vagus

20 Which of the following phases accounts for the largest volume of gastric acid secretion?
   a Cephalic b Hormonal c Intestinal
   d Interdigestive

21 The enterogastric reflex: (More than one answer may be correct)
   a Is mediated via the mysenteric nerve plexus
   b Stimulates gastric emptying c Inhibits gastric emptying d Inhibits gastric secretion

22 The gastric secretory pattern in duodenal ulcer is commonly in which range?
   a Achlorhydria b Normal to low c Normal to high
   d Marked hyperacidity

23 Which of the following foods has the greatest acid secretory effect?
   a Proteins b Fats c Carbohydrates

24 Theories regarding the pathogenesis of gastric ulcers include: (More than one answer may be correct)
   a Overactivity of the vagus b Hypersecretion of acid
   c Impaired mucosal resistance d Reflux of bile into the stomach

25 Duodenal ulcer disease is:
   a More common in women than in men b Always responsive to medical treatment c Very common, affecting more than 10 percent of the population
   d Associated with blood group A

26 When bleeding complicates peptic ulcer disease, pain:
   a No longer responds to antacids b Radiates to the back c Becomes more severe d Usually disappears

27 Signs, symptoms, and findings indicating acute perforation of a peptic ulcer include: (More than one answer may be correct)

a Boardlike rigidity of abdomen to palpation
b Relief from pain c Severe pain in upper abdomen
d Subphrenic air bubble evident on x-ray

28 Which of the following contiguous structures would most likely be involved in a confined perforation of a peptic ulcer?
a Liver b Gallbladder c Pancreas d Lesser omentum

29 Recurrent ulcer following peptic ulcer surgery: (More than one answer may be correct)
a Is related to the preoperative level of gastric acid secretion b Occurs most commonly after gastric ulcer c Is less common if vagotomy is performed

30 Which of the following statements applies to the surgical treatment of duodenal ulcer?
a Billroth I procedure is the surgery of choice
b Billroth II procedure is the surgery of choice
c A vagotomy and 75 percent gastric resection should be performed d Some form of vagotomy should be performed

31 Which of the following mechanisms would be the most probable to explain the development of stress ulcers in a patient who developed hypotensive shock following cardiac surgery?
a Excess vagal stimulation → hyperacidity b Gastric ischemia → disruption of the gastric mucosal barrier → increased back diffusion of H^+

32 Carcinoma of the stomach: (More than one answer may be correct)
a Is most frequent after the age of 40 b Is more common in persons with pernicious anemia c Generally has a good prognosis d Most commonly presents as an ulcerative lesion e Commonly infiltrates the stomach wall, causing it to become inflexible

33 Methods of treating acute hemorrhagic gastritis include:
a Electrocoagulation b Intra-arterial vasopressin infusion c Ice-water lavage d Total gastrectomy
e All of the above

Directions: Match the following gastric acid analysis tests in col. A with their diagnostic value in col. B.

Column A
34 _____ Basal acid output (BAO)
35 _____ Maximum acid output (MAO)
36 _____ Insulin hypoglycemia test

Column B
a Especially useful in the diagnosis of the Zollinger-Ellison syndrome
b Used to assess completeness of vagotomy
c May be used to determine if true achlorhydria is present

Directions: Match the following differentiating features of gastric and duodenal ulcers in col. B to the type of peptic ulcer in col. A.

Column A
37 _____ Gastric ulcer
38 _____ Duodenal ulcer

Column B
a Symptomatically improves on antacids

b Pain in the middle of the night more common
c Always should be treated surgically
d Obstruction an infrequent problem
e More common in persons with blood group O
f Higher frequency in persons subjected to stress

Directions: Circle T if the statement is true and F it if is false.

39 T F The chief cells of the stomach secrete HCl.

40 T F The neck cells of the gastric glands secrete mucus.

41 T F Chronic ulcers, as opposed to acute ulcers, have scar tissue at their base.

42 T F A break in the gastric mucosa which does not extend beyond the mucosal layer is called an erosion.

REFERENCES

BOGOCH, ABRAHAM (ed.) *Gastroenterology,* McGraw-Hill, New York, 1973, pp. 296–309, 345–350, 353–380, 394–396, 435–450, 481–492.

BROOKS, FRANK P.: *Gastrointestinal Pathophysiology,* Oxford University Press, New York, 1974, pp. 83–100, 307–310.

DAVENPORT, H. W.: "Salicylate Damage to the Gastric Mucosal Barrier," *New England Journal of Medicine,* **276**:1307, 1967.

———: *Physiology of the Digestive Tract,* 3rd ed., Yearbook, Chicago, 1971.

———: "Mechanisms of Gastric and Pancreatic Secretion," in E. D. Frohlich (ed.), *Pathophysiology,* Lippincott, Philadelphia, 1972, pp. 407–420.

———: *A Digest on Digestion,* Yearbook, Chicago, 1975.

ENGLERT, E. E. JR.: "Cancer, Gastritis, and other Diseases of the Stomach," in *Harrison's Principles of Internal Medicine,* 7th ed., McGraw-Hill, New York, 1974, pp. 1447–1456.

GILLESPIE, I. E. and T. J. THOMSON, (eds.): *Gastroenterology* Churchill Livingstone, London, 1972, pp. 33–71.

GIVEN, B. A. and S. J. SIMMONS: *Gastroenterology in Clinical Nursing,* 2d ed., C. V. Mosby, St. Louis, 1975, pp. 113–150.

GREENBERGER, N. J. and D. H. WINSHIP: *Gastrointestinal Disorders: A Pathophysiologic Approach,* Yearbook, Chicago, 1976, pp. 45–101.

HOLLANDER, F.: "The Two-Component Mucus Barrier, Its

Activity in Protecting the Gastrointestinal Mucosa Against Peptic Ulceration," *Archives of Internal Medicine*, **93**:107, January 1954.

KIRSNER, J. B.: "The Stomach," in W. A. Sodeman, Jr. and W. A. Sodeman (eds.), *Pathologic Physiology*, 5th ed., Saunders, Philadelphia, 1974, pp. 709–732.

NAISH, J. M. and A. E. A. READ: *Basic Gastroenterology*, Yearbook, Chicago, 1974, pp. 47–79.

NETTER, FRANK H.: *Ciba Collection of Medical Illustrations: Vol. 3, Digestive System, Part I, Upper Digestive Tract*, Ciba Pharmaceutical Co., Summit, N. J., 1959, pp. 49–65, 164–187.

ROBBINS, S. L. and M. ANGELL: *Basic Pathology*, Saunders, Philadelphia, 1971, pp. 404–420.

SILEN, WILLIAM: "Peptic Ulcer," in *Harrison's Principles of Internal Medicine*, 7th ed., McGraw-Hill, New York, 1974, pp. 1431–1447.

—— and J. J. SKILLMAN: In G. H. Stollerman (ed.), *Advances in Internal Medicine*, Yearbook, Chicago, 1974, vol. 19.

CHAPTER 21 Small Intestine

OBJECTIVES At the completion of Chap. 21, you should be able to:

1 Describe the following gross and microscopic anatomic features of the small intestine:
   a Length, major divisions, inlet and outlet, position in abdomen, and anatomic relation to the ligament of Treitz
   b Major folds of the peritoneum: mesentery and greater and lesser omenta (describe position and function)
   c The three structural features which greatly increase the absorptive surface
   d Major blood supply and innervation
   e Structure and function of a villus: types of cells and their life cycle, microvilli, crypts of Lieberkühn, and blood and lymphatic supply
   f Location of appendix in relation to small and large bowel

2 List the five principal organs which produce digestive secretions and the approximate volume of their secretions.

3 List the principal digestive enzymes including their source, action, and approximate optimal pH for activity.

4 Describe the function of bile in the digestion and absorption of fats and fat-soluble vitamins.

5 Identify and describe the actions of two hormones important in the regulation of intestinal digestion.

6 List the principal sites of absorption of the following nutrients: fats, sugars, amino acids, folic acid, vitamin B_{12}, and bile salts.

7 Describe and state the significance of the enterohepatic recirculation of bile salts.

8 Differentiate between maldigestion and malabsorption.

9 List at least four basic causes of the malabsorption syndrome.

10 Explain the pathophysiologic basis of the following signs and symptoms of malabsorption:
   a Weight loss
   b Diarrhea
   c Steatorrhea
   d Flatulence, abdominal distention
   e Nocturia
   f Weakness and easy fatigability
   g Edema
   h Amenorrhea
   i Anemia
   j Glossitis, cheilosis, peripheral neuropathy
   k Bruising, bleeding tendency
   l Bone pain, tetany, paresthesias

11 Describe each of the following diagnostic tests of malabsorption and indicate what each one can detect:

a Quantitative stool fat determination
b D-xylose test
c Schilling test
d Culture of small bowel contents
e Barium x-ray of small bowel
f Biopsy of small bowel

12 Describe the gross appearance and characteristics of stool in severe steatorrhea.

13 Identify the substance which causes the toxic reaction in nontropical sprue.

14 Contrast tropical and nontropical sprue with respect to proposed etiology, intestinal biopsy changes, population affected, clinical features, and treatment.

15 Identify a genetic enzyme deficiency disease common in American blacks and explain the pathophysiologic basis of the diarrhea in this condition.

16 Give four reasons why malabsorption may be a problem following extensive gastric resection.

17 Explain why postgastrectomy patients may develop vitamin B_{12} deficiency and ineffective action of bile salts.

18 Explain the basis of the theory that regional enteritis may represent a hypersensitivity reaction similar to the mechanism producing tissue damage in tuberculosis.

19 Describe regional enteritis (lesions and their distribution, clinical features, complications, treatment, and prognosis).

20 Locate the normal position of the appendix at McBurney's point.

21 Describe the anatomic features of the appendix which make it especially vulnerable to obstruction, necrosis, and perforation.

22 Describe the signs and symptoms of a classical case of acute appendicitis and explain why difficulties may be encountered in establishing the diagnosis.

23 Explain why early surgery for acute appendicitis is important.

24 Describe the reaction of the peritoneum to invasion by bacteria.

25 Differentiate between adynamic ileus and mechanical obstruction of the bowel and list the general causes of each.

26 Define the following conditions related to bowel obstruction and indicate the most common site of occurrence, relative frequency, and age groups commonly affected:

a Adhesions
b Volvulus
c Intussusception
d Malignant tumor
e Incarcerated hernia
f Strangulated bowel

27 Describe the pathophysiologic events leading to death from complete obstruction of the small bowel.

28 Describe the signs and symptoms of bowel obstruction.

29 Explain why early diagnosis and surgical intervention are important in mechanical obstruction of the small bowel.

The small intestine is a complex, folded tube extending from the pylorus to the ileocecal valve. It is about 12 ft long in life (22 ft in the cadaver as a result of relaxation) and is contained in the central and lower part of the abdominal cavity. The proximal end is about 3.8 cm in diameter, but it gradually diminishes to about 2.5 cm at the lower end.

The small intestine is divided into the *duodenum, jejunum,* and *ileum.* This division is rather imprecise and is based on slight modifications in structure and relatively more important differences in function. The duodenum is about 25 cm long and extends from the pylorus to the jejunum. The division between the duodenum and jejunum is marked by the *ligament of Treitz,* a musculofibrous band which originates from the right crus of the diaphragm near the esophageal hiatus and attaches to the junction of the duodenum and jejunum, acting as a suspensory ligament. Approximately two-fifths of the remaining intestine is the jejunum, and the terminal three-fifths is ileum. The jejunum lies in the left midabdominal region, while the ileum tends to lie in the right lower abdominal region. Entry of chyme into the small intestine is controlled by the pyloric sphincter, and exit of digested materials into the large intestine is controlled by the ileocecal valve. The ileocecal valve also prevents reflux of large intestinal contents into the small intestine.

The *vermiform appendix* is a blind tube about the size of the little finger located in the ileocecal region at the apex of the cecum. Inflammation or rupture of this structure is an important cause of morbidity in young persons, although it is a less frequent cause of death now than in the preantibiotic era.

The wall of the small intestine is composed of four basic layers. The outer, or serous, coat is formed by the peritoneum. The peritoneum has a visceral and parietal layer, and the potential space between these layers is called the peritoneal cavity. The peritoneum is reflected over and almost completely envelops the abdominal viscera.

Special names have been given to the folds of the peritoneum. The *mesentery* is a broad, fanlike fold of peritoneum which suspends the jejunum and ileum from the posterior abdominal wall and allows considerable motion of the bowel. The mesentery supports the blood and lymph vessels supplying the intestine. The *greater omentum* is a double layer of peritoneum which hangs from the greater curvature of the stomach and descends in front of the abdominal viscera like an apron. The omentum usually contains fat in considerable amounts and lymph nodes, which aid in protecting the peritoneal cavity against infection. The *lesser omentum* is the fold of peritoneum which extends from the lesser curvature of the stomach and upper duodenum to the liver, forming the hepatogastric and hepatoduodenal suspensory ligaments. One of the important functions of the peritoneum is to prevent friction between contiguous organs by secreting a serous fluid which acts as a lubricant. Inflammation of the peritoneum is called *peritonitis* and

may be a serious sequel to inflammation or perforation of the bowel. Adhesions (fibrous bands) may develop following peritonitis or abdominal surgery, sometimes causing obstruction of the bowel.

The muscular coat of the small intestine has two layers: an outer, thinner layer of longitudinal fibers and an inner one of circular fibers. This arrangement aids the peristaltic action of the small intestine. The submucosal layer is composed of connective tissue, and the inner mucosal layer is thick, vascular, and glandular.

The small intestine is characterized by three structural features which greatly increase its surface area and aid in its primary function of absorption. The mucosal and submucosal layers are arranged in circular folds called *valvulae conniventes* (Kerckring's folds) which project into the lumen of the tube about 3 to 10 mm. These folds are prominent in the duodenum and jejunum and disappear near the midileum. They are responsible for the feathery appearance of the small intestine on barium x-ray. The *villi* are fingerlike projections of mucosa numbering about four or five million and are present in the entire length of the small intestine. The villi are 0.5–1.5 mm long (just visible to the naked eye) and account for the velvetlike appearance of the mucosa. The *microvilli* are fingerlike projections about 1.0 μm in length along the outer surface of each individual villus. They are visible by electron microscopy and appear as a *brush border* on light microscopy. If the lining of the small intestine were smooth, the surface area would be about 2000 cm². The valvulae conniventes, villi, and microvilli together increase the total absorbing surface to 2 million square centimeters, which is a thousandfold increase. Diseases of the small intestine, such as sprue, which cause atrophy and flattening of the villi greatly reduce the surface area for absorption, resulting in malabsorption.

Structure of the villus

Figure 21-1 illustrates the structure of a villus, which is the functional unit of the small intestine. Each villus consists of a central lymph channel called a *lacteal* surrounded by a network of blood capillaries held together by lymphoid tissue. This, in turn, is surrounded by columnar epithelial cells. After the food has been digested, it passes into the lacteals and capillaries of the villi. The villous epithelium consists of two cell types: *goblet cells,* which produce mucus, and *absorptive cells* (with microvilli projecting from their surface), which are responsible for absorption of digested foodstuffs. Enzymes are located on the brush border and complete the process of digestion as absorption is taking place.

Surrounding each villus are several small pits called the *crypts of Lieberkühn.* These crypts are intestinal glands which produce secretions containing digestive enzymes. Undifferentiated cells in the crypts of Lieberkühn proliferate rapidly and migrate upward toward the tip of the villus where they become absorptive cells. At the tip of the villus, they are shed into the intestinal lumen. Maturation and migration from the crypts to the tip of the villus requires only 5 to 7 days. It is estimated that 20 to 50 million epithelial cells are extruded into the intestinal lumen each minute. Because of this very high cell turnover rate (fastest in the body), the intestinal epithelium is especially vulnerable to alterations in cell proliferation. Cytotoxic drugs given for cancer or leukemia inhibit cell division, resulting in mucosal atrophy and shortening of both crypts and villi. Patients receiving these drugs often develop ulcerations of the gastrointestinal mucosa. Villi may be flattened or absent in sprue.

Blood supply and innervation

The *superior mesenteric* artery, arising from the aorta just below the celiac artery, supplies all of the small intestine except the duodenum, which is supplied by the gastroduodenal artery and its branch, the superior pancreaticoduodenal artery. Blood is returned by the superior mesenteric vein, which unites with the splenic vein to form the portal vein.

The small intestine is innervated by both branches of the autonomic nervous system. Parasympathetic stimulation stimulates secretory activity and motility and sympathetic stimulation inhibits motility. Sensory fibers of the sympathetic system relay pain, while those of the parasympathetic regulate intestinal reflexes. The intrinsic nerve supply, which initiates motor function, passes through Auerbach's plexus located in the muscular layer and Meissner's plexus in the submucosal layer.

PHYSIOLOGIC CONSIDERATIONS

The small intestine has two primary functions: digestion and absorption of ingested nutrients and water. All other activities either regulate or facilitate this process. The digestive process is initiated in the mouth and stomach by the actions of ptyalin, hydrochloric acid, and pepsin on the ingested food. The process is continued in the duodenum primarily by the action of pancreatic enzymes, which hydrolyze carbohydrates, fats, and proteins into simpler substances. The presence of bicarbonate in the pancreatic secretion helps to neutralize the acid and provide an optimum pH for the action of the enzymes. The secretion of bile from the liver aids the digestive process by emulsifying fats so that a greater surface area is presented for the action of pancreatic lipase.

The action of bile results from the detergent proper-

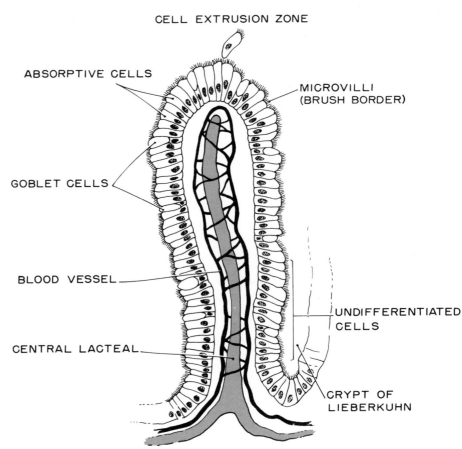

CELL EXTRUSION ZONE

ABSORPTIVE CELLS

MICROVILLI (BRUSH BORDER)

GOBLET CELLS

BLOOD VESSEL

UNDIFFERENTIATED CELLS

CENTRAL LACTEAL

CRYPT OF LIEBERKUHN

FIGURE 21-1 Structure of a villus of the small intestine.

ties of conjugated bile acids which solubilize lipid material by the formation of micelles. *Micelles* are aggregates of bile acids and fat molecules. Fats form the hydrophobic core, and the bile acids, being polar molecules, form the surface of the micelles, with their hydrophobic end pointing inward and their hydrophilic end pointing outward toward the aqueous medium. The center of the micelle also dissolves fat-soluble vitamins and cholesterol. Thus, free fatty acids, glycerides, and fat-soluble vitamins are kept in solution until they can be absorbed by the epithelial cell surface.

The process of digestion is completed by a number of enzymes present in the intestinal juice (succus entericus). Many of these enzymes are located on the brush border of the villi and digest food substances as they are being absorbed. Table 21-1 lists the principal digestive enzymes.

TABLE 21-1
The principal digestive enzymes

ENZYME	SOURCE	SUBSTRATE	PRODUCTS	OPTIMAL pH	VOLUME OF SECRETION*
Salivary amylase (ptyalin)	Salivary glands	Starch	Maltose (a disaccharide and smaller carbohydrate polymer); minor physiologic role	6–7	1–1½ liters daily
Pepsin	Chief cells of stomach	Protein	Proteoses, peptones	1.5–2.5	2–4 liters daily
Gastric lipase	Stomach	Fat	Fatty acids, glycerides (minor physiologic role)		
Enterokinase	Duodenal mucosa	Trypsinogen	Trypsin		
Trypsin		Denatured proteins and polypeptides	Small polypeptides (also activates chymotrypsinogen to chymotrypsin)	8.0	
Chymotrypsin	Exocrine pancreas	Proteins and polypeptides	Small polypeptides	8.0	0.6–0.8 liters daily
Carboxypeptidases		Polypeptides	Smaller polypeptides (removes C-terminal amino acid)		
Nucleases		Nucleic acids	Nucleotides		
Pancreatic lipase		Fat	Glycerides, fatty acids, glycerol	8.0	
Pancreatic amylase		Starch	Disaccharides	6.7–7	
Bile acids (not an enzyme)	Liver	Unemulsified fats	Emulsified fats (formation of micelles; action is physical)	7.5	0.8–1.0 liters daily
Aminopeptidases		Polypeptides	Smaller polypeptides (removes N-terminal amino acid)	8.0	
Dipeptidase		Dipeptides	Amino acids		
Maltase		Maltose	Glucose		
Lactase	Intestinal glands	Lactose	Glucose + galactose } All monosaccharides	5.0–7	2–3 liters daily
Sucrase		Sucrose	Glucose + fructose		
Intestinal lipase		Fat	Glycerides, fatty acids, glycerol	8.0	
Nucleotidase		Nucleotides	Nucleosides, phosphoric acid	8.0	

*All secretions are reabsorbed except about 100 ml water normally excreted in stool per day.

Two hormones are important in the regulation of intestinal digestion. Fat, in contact with the duodenal mucosa, causes the gallbladder to contract, which is mediated by the action of *cholecystokinin*. Products of partially digested proteins in contact with the duodenal mucosa stimulate the secretion of pancreatic juice rich in enzymes and is mediated by the action of *pancreozymin*. Pancreozymin and cholecystokinin are now believed to be the same hormone having two different effects and are called *CCK-PZ*. This hormone is produced by the duodenal mucosa.

Acid in contact with the intestinal mucosa causes the release of another hormone, *secretin*, and the amount released is proportional to the amount of acid flowing through the duodenum. Secretin stimulates the secretion of the bicarbonate-containing juice from the pancreas and bile from the liver. Secretin potentiates the action of CCK-PZ.

Segmental movements of the small intestine mix ingested materials with pancreatic, hepatobiliary, and intestinal secretions, and peristaltic movements propel the contents from one end to the other at a rate suitable for optimal absorption and continuing entry of gastric contents.

Absorption is the transfer of the end products of carbohydrate, fat, and protein digestion (simple sugars, fatty acids, and amino acids) across the intestinal wall to the vascular and lymphatic circulation for use by the body cells. In addition, water, electrolytes, and vitamins are absorbed. Absorption of the various substances takes place by both active and passive transport mechanisms which are for the most part poorly understood.

Although many substances are absorbed throughout the entire length of the small bowel, there are principal sites of absorption for specific nutrients. Knowledge of these absorption sites is necessary in order to understand how disease of the intestine may cause specific nutritional deficiencies (see Fig. 21-2).

Iron and calcium are largely absorbed in the duodenum, and calcium requires vitamin D. The fat-soluble vitamins (A, D, E, and K) are absorbed in the duodenum and require bile salts. Folic acid and the other water-soluble vitamins are absorbed in the duodenum. The absorption of sugars, amino acids, and fats is largely completed by the time the chyme reaches the jejunum. The absorption of vitamin B_{12} takes place in the terminal ileum by a special transport mechanism requiring gastric intrinsic factor. Most of the bile acids released by the gallbladder into the duodenum to aid in the digestion of fats are reabsorbed in the terminal ileum and recirculated to the liver. This circuit is termed the *enterohepatic circula-*

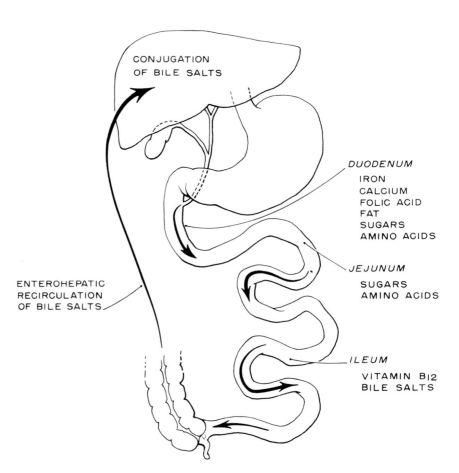

FIGURE 21-2 Absorption sites of the major nutrients and the enterohepatic recirculation of bile salts for reconjugation by the liver.

tion of bile salts and is very important in maintaining the bile pool. The bile acids or salts thus perform their action in relationship to fat digestion many times before being excreted in the feces. Disease or resection of the terminal ileum may thus cause deficiency of bile salts and interference with fat digestion. The entry of large amounts of bile salts into the colon causes colonic irritation and diarrhea.

MALABSORPTION

Diseases of the small intestine are often accompanied by alterations in function manifested by the malabsorption syndrome. Malabsorption is the condition in which there is impaired intestinal mucosal absorption of single or multiple nutrients, resulting in their excretion in the stool.

It is important to distinguish between malabsorption and maldigestion since increased loss of nutrients in the stool may be a reflection of either process. Maldigestion is failure to absorb one or more nutrients due to inadequate digestion.

TABLE 21-2
Some causes of the malabsorption syndrome

Following gastric surgery	Disease of the small intestine
Total gastrectomy	Primary disease of small bowel
Billroth II gastrectomy	Nontropical sprue
Pyloroplasty	Tropical sprue
Vagotomy	Regional enteritis
	Massive bowel resection
Pancreatic disorders	Bacterial overgrowth from
Chronic pancreatitis	stasis in afferent loop fol-
Pancreatic cancer	lowing Billroth II gastrec-
Cystic fibrosis	tomy
Pancreatic resection	Ischemic bowel disease
Zollinger-Ellison syn-	Mesenteric atherosclerosis
drome	Chronic congestive heart
	failure
Hepatobiliary disease	Infections and infestations
Biliary tract obstruction	Acute enteritis
Cirrhosis and hepatitis	Giardiasis
Biliary fistula	Systemic disease involving
	small bowel
	Whipple's disease
	Lymphosarcoma, Hodgkin's
	disease
	Amyloidosis
	Sarcoidosis
	Scleroderma
	Hereditary disorders
	Primary lactase deficiency
	Drug-induced malabsorption
	Neomycin
	Dilantin

Causes of malabsorption syndrome

Table 21-2 lists some of the more common causes of the malabsorption syndrome. The basic causes of maldigestion are included in the first three categories. Gastrectomy, especially the Billroth II procedure, causes poor mixing of chyme with gastric secretions. Hepatobiliary disease may result in insufficiency of intraluminal bile acids. Failure of the pancreas to produce or release sufficient enzymes may result from a number of pancreatic disorders. Failure of CCK-PZ release, which stimulates pancreatic secretion, may occur in the Zollinger-Ellison syndrome as a result of excessive acidification of the duodenum or may result from disease of the intestinal mucosa itself, as in sprue. Disease of the terminal ileum or ileal resection for treatment of regional enteritis may cause insufficient bile salts by interfering with ileal resorption. Bacterial overgrowth in the duodenal stump (blind or afferent loop) causes vitamin B_{12} malabsorption by utilizing this vitamin and causes fat maldigestion by deconjugating bile salts. Unconjugated bile salts are less effective in forming micelles and are absorbed less in the ileum. Pernicious anemia (a gastric disease) causes malabsorption of vitamin B_{12} in the terminal ileum because of the lack of the intrinsic factor for transport. A hereditary lack of lactase causes selective malabsorption of lactose (a milk protein) and is very common in American blacks. Mesenteric atherosclerosis (abdominal angina) may cause malabsorption and is a source of discomfort in elderly persons, but it is infrequently diagnosed. Chapter 23 will deal with pancreatic and hepatobiliary disorders, and this chapter will discuss a few of the more common intestinal disorders associated with malabsorption.

Signs and symptoms of the malabsorption syndrome

The signs and symptoms of malabsorption may be divided into two groups: those resulting from abnormal content in the intestinal lumen and those resulting from deficiency of dietary nutrients. Weight loss, diarrhea, steatorrhea, flatulence, and nocturia are the most common signs and symptoms and are all caused by abnormal intestinal luminal content. The signs and symptoms of malabsorption and their pathophysiologic basis are listed in Table 21-3.

Detection of malabsorption

Most of these tests useful in the diagnosis of malabsorption indicate the presence of malabsorption or maldigestion. Only a few of the tests suggest a specific diagnosis.

STOOL FAT

The oldest and most reliable test for documenting the presence of steatorrhea and thus malabsorption is the quantitative determination of stool fat. Normal persons

TABLE 21-3
Signs and symptoms of the malabsorption syndrome

SIGN OR SYMPTOM	PATHOPHYSIOLOGY
Weight loss and generalized malnutrition	Impaired absorption of carbohydrate, fat, and protein → loss of calories
Diarrhea	Excess load of fluids and electrolytes introduced into colon which may exceed its absorptive capacity; bile acids and fatty acids in colon cause decreased colonic absorption of sodium and water and laxative effect from colonic irritation
Steatorrhea (bulky, frothy voluminous stools)	Excess fat content of feces
Flatulence, abdominal distention	Undigested lactose → fermentation → gas formation; Undigested lactose → osmotic effect → shift of extracellular fluid into gut → diarrhea (may be due to primary lactase deficiency or secondary damage to brush border from intestinal lesions)
Nocturia	Delayed absorption and excretion of water (may be pooled in gut during day)
Weakness and easy fatigability	Anemia; electrolyte depletion due to diarrhea (hypokalemia, hypomagnesemia)
Edema	Impaired absorption of amino acids → protein depletion → hypoproteinemia
Amenorrhea	Protein depletion → secondary hypopituitarism
Anemia	Impaired absorption of iron, folic acid, and vitamin B_{12}
Glossitis, cheilosis	Deficiency of iron, folic acid, vitamin B_{12}, and other vitamins
Peripheral neuropathy	Deficiency of vitamin B_{12}
Bruising, bleeding tendency	Vitamin K malabsorption, hypoprothrombinemia
Bone pain	Calcium malabsorption → hypocalcemia; Protein depletion → osteoporosis; Vitamin D malabsorption → impaired calcium absorption
Tetany, paresthesias	Calcium malabsorption → hypocalcemia; Magnesium malabsorption → hypomagnesemia
Eczema	Cause uncertain

excrete less than 6 g of fat in the stool per day. Fat excretion in excess of 6 g is considered excessive and is termed *steatorrhea*. In severe cases the stools are abnormal to the naked eye and appear pale, greasy, frothy, and floating. They may stick to the side of the toilet and not flush away easily.

A 72-hour stool collection for quantitative fat determination is routinely used to eliminate errors resulting from daily variations. Testing stools for fat is essential in the diagnosis of nontropical sprue, following extensive gastrectomy, and in other malabsorptive disorders. This test does not differentiate between maldigestion as in pancreatic disorders and malabsorption due to an intestinal disease such as nontropical sprue. However, there is a marked increase in undigested meat fibers in the stool in pancreatic insufficiency that is not usually present in nontropical sprue.

D-XYLOSE ABSORPTION TEST

D-xylose is a relatively inert pentose which is absorbed in the proximal bowel without digestion, passes through the liver, and is then totally excreted by the kidneys. Measurement of the amount of D-xylose excreted in the urine therefore gives an indication of the absorptive capacity of the proximal bowel.

The test is carried out after the patient has fasted for 12 hours. At least 20 percent should be excreted in the urine in 5 hours provided renal function is normal. Excretion of less than this amount or blood levels less than 30 mg% indicates malabsorption. An abnormal D-xylose test is found most frequently in disorders affecting the proximal bowel such as sprue. This test is normal in maldigestive disorders such as chronic pancreatitis.

SCHILLING TEST FOR VITAMIN B_{12} ABSORPTION

The Schilling test is a valuable measure of vitamin B_{12} absorption and is frequently carried out in stages to determine the specific cause of the malabsorption. If urine collection is adequate, low excretion of ^{60}Co tagged vitamin B_{12} indicates failure of absorption as a result of a lack of intrinsic factor (pernicious anemia), bacterial overgrowth in the proximal small bowel following Billroth II gastrectomy, diseased ileal mucosa as in regional enteritis, or pancreatic insufficiency. Correction of the malabsorption with intrinsic factor confirms intrinsic factor deficiency (often due to pernicious anemia). If the Schilling test returns to normal after antibiotic therapy, this helps to confirm the diagnosis of malabsorption as a result of bacterial overgrowth in the proximal bowel following Billroth II gastrectomy (the bacteria can actually take up vitamin B_{12}, thus preventing its absorption). Malabsorption of vitamin B_{12} as a result of pancreatic insufficiency may be corrected by the administration of pancreatic enzymes. Vitamin B_{12} malabsorption resulting from regional enteritis involving the terminal ileum is not corrected by any of the above measures.

CULTURE OF DUODENAL AND JEJUNAL CONTENTS

The most reliable test for confirming the presence of bacterial overgrowth in the proximal bowel is aspiration and culture of the contents, but this is technically difficult and seldom used. The proximal small bowel normally contains less than 10^5 organisms per milliliter, and these are generally of the oropharyngeal variety. The most important mechanisms keeping the proximal bowel bacteriologically sterile is the normal peristalsis which sweeps bacteria distally, the gastric acid, and the secretion of immunoglobulin A (IgA) into the gut. Consequently, any condition which causes stasis of proximal intestinal contents, such as the blind loop following Billroth II surgery, may result in macrocytic anemia (utilization of vitamin B_{12} by organisms), diarrhea, and steatorrhea (deconjugation of bile salts by bacteria). Gastric achlorhydria and hypogammaglobulinemia are other conditions which may cause bacterial overgrowth.

GASTROINTESTINAL BARIUM X-RAY STUDIES

The x-ray appearance of the small bowel may be nonspecific or diagnostic. Characteristic features in the malabsorption syndrome are the loss of the feathery pattern of the barium and increased flocculation of the barium with segmentation and clumping. This finding is common in sprue but is also found in other malabsorptive disorders. In regional enteritis, the ileal lumen may be narrowed (string sign).

BIOPSY OF THE SMALL INTESTINE

The most useful test specific for the diagnosis of sprue is a biopsy of the intestinal mucosa, which reveals atrophy of villi. The biopsy may be performed through a capsule which is swallowed, located by x-ray, and fired.

PRIMARY SMALL INTESTINAL DISORDERS ASSOCIATED WITH MALABSORPTION

Nontropical sprue (celiac disease)

Idiopathic steatorrhea in adults and celiac disease in children are the most important causes of severe malabsorption in nontropical areas. Both these conditions are considered phases of the same disease. The disease is characterized by marked atrophy of the villi in the proximal small intestine induced by ingestion of gluten-containing foods.

PATHOPHYSIOLOGY

Gluten is a high molecular weight protein found in rye, oats, barley, and especially wheat. It is, of course, found in bread, bread products, beer, and many other processed foods. Gluten and/or gluten breakdown products (especially gliadin) are toxic to patients with this disease. Symptoms disappear when gluten is withdrawn from the diet and reappear when it is reintroduced. The characteristic lesion of the bowel mucosa induced by gluten is blunting or loss of the villi and elongation of the crypts, which causes the mucosa to appear flat. The loss of villi causes a marked reduction of absorptive surface.

Although the mechanism of gluten toxicity is not understood, it has been suggested that these patients lack a specific peptidase which would normally detoxify a noxious peptide of gluten. This hypothesis is supported by the fact that there is a strong family tendency in occurrence. It has also been proposed that gluten or its metabolites cause a hypersensitivity reaction in the intestinal mucosa. This theory is supported by the fact that circulating antibodies to gliadin have been found in patients with this disease and that partial improvement of symptoms is provided by corticosteroid therapy.

CLINICAL FEATURES

Patients with nontropical sprue are presumably born with the disease tendency but may not develop symptoms for many years even though they include gluten in their diet. Factors which precipitate the clinical onset are unknown. The onset generally occurs in infants between the ages of 6 months and 2 years and in adults between the ages of 20 and 50 years. The symptoms seldom begin during childhood or adolescence.

In infants, anorexia, irritability, and diarrhea with pale, bulky stools are soon followed by weight loss. If not treated, the failure to grow is soon obvious. Lassitude, weakness, and diarrhea are the most common symptoms in adults, but patients may present with any of the signs and symptoms of malabsorption syndrome listed in Table 21-3. Adults frequently give a history suggesting sprue during childhood.

The diagnosis is established by evidence of malabsorption, typical small bowel biopsy changes, and clinical improvement on a gluten-free diet.

TREATMENT

The treatment of nontropical sprue by a gluten-free diet is generally very successful, provided the patient adheres to the diet.

Tropical sprue

Tropical sprue occurs in such tropical regions as Puerto Rico, India, and the Far East. The signs and symptoms are similar to nontropical sprue, and the biopsy changes are similar but less severe. The cause is not known. It is believed to be caused by an infectious agent, although one has not yet been identified. Most patients improve after treatment with broad-spectrum antibiotics (tetracycline).

Lactase deficiency

As indicated in the previous discussion, hydrolysis of disaccharides to monosaccharides occurs within the brush border of the intestinal mucosa. Deficiency of specific enzymes which hydrolyze disaccharides may be present as a result of a genetic defect or may be secondary to disease of the mucosa such as sprue.

Bayless and Christopher estimate that 70 percent of American blacks have a significant decrease in the activity of the enzyme lactase. Since lactose is the principal carbohydrate of milk, many persons showing milk intolerance will prove to be lactase-deficient. Orientals and African Bantus are also significantly affected, while only 5 percent of the white population is lactase-deficient.

Typical symptoms of lactase deficiency are abdominal cramps, bloating, and diarrhea following milk ingestion. The pathogenetic mechanism explaining the diarrhea is as follows. When unhydrolyzed lactose enters the large intestine, it produces an osmotic effect causing the insorption of water into the colonic lumen. Colonic bacteria also ferment the lactose, producing lactic and fatty acids which are irritating to the colon. The result is increased motility due to colonic irritation and an explosive diarrhea.

The condition is diagnosed by the history of milk intolerance and a positive lactose tolerance test. The fecal pH is also very acid (<6.0). Stool normally has a pH of 7.0 to 7.5.

Treatment consists of elimination of milk and milk products from the diet.

Postgastrectomy malabsorption

Malabsorption and weight loss is a well-recognized feature after a gastrectomy. It is the rule following total gastrectomy, common after the Billroth II procedure, and rare after the Billroth I procedure. Increased fat loss in the stools occurs in many patients after the Billroth II procedure, especially if the duodenal stump (afferent or blind loop) is long. The principal causes of the steatorrhea are the following: (1) poor mixing of food and enzymes due to rapid emptying of the gastric remnant (food particles too large for enzymes); (2) reduced pancreatic output because the duodenum is bypassed and has less stimulation by the acid chyme to release secretin and CCK-PZ; (3) stasis of intestinal contents in the afferent loop resulting in abnormal bacterial proliferation which, in turn, uses up vitamin B_{12} and deconjugates bile salts; (4) the loss of stomach reservoir function may result in a more rapid intestinal transit time with resultant diarrhea.

If the malabsorption is severe, the patient may develop anemia and symptoms as a result of any of the nutrient deficiencies listed in Table 21-3. The proper treatment of postgastrectomy malabsorption depends on identification of the responsible mechanism of the malabsorption. Broad-spectrum antibiotics (tetracycline) are given when the cause is bacterial overgrowth. Pancreatic enzyme therapy may be helpful with functional pancreatic deficiency. Smaller meals, low in carbohydrates, and taken without fluids, may help delay rapid gastric emptying (dumping syndrome).

Regional enteritis (Crohn's disease)

Regional enteritis or Crohn's disease is a chronic, relapsing granulomatous inflammatory disease of the intestinal tract. Classically the terminal ileum is affected, although any portion of the gastrointestinal tract may be involved. It usually develops in young adults and affects men and women about equally.

The etiology of regional enteritis is unknown. Although no autoantibodies have been demonstrated, it has been speculated that regional enteritis represents a hypersensitivity reaction or may be caused by an infectious agent which has not yet been identified. These theories are suggested by the granulomatous lesions, which are similar to those found in fungal and tubercular lesions of the lung.

There are some interesting similarities between regional enteritis and ulcerative colitis. Both are inflammatory diseases, although the lesions of each are distinct. Both diseases have extragastrointestinal manifestations, including uveitis, arthritis, and skin lesions which are identical. Some of these similarities and differences will be discussed under ulcerative colitis in Chap. 22.

PATHOLOGY

The terminal ileum is involved in regional enteritis in about 80 percent of the cases. In about 35 percent of the cases, lesions occur in the colon. The esophagus and stomach are less frequently affected. In some instances, "skip" lesions occur; that is, portions of diseased bowel are separated by areas of normal bowel by a few inches or several feet.

Lesions are believed to begin in lymph nodes next to the small bowel, with eventual obstruction of the lymphatic channels of drainage. The submucous coat of the intestine becomes markedly thickened as a result of the hyperplasia of the lymphoid tissue and lymphedema. With progress of the pathologic process the affected segment of the bowel becomes thickened to such a degree that it is as stiff as a garden hose (see Fig. 21-3). The lumen of the bowel may become markedly narrowed, so that it admits only a thin stream of barium, giving rise to the "string sign" on x-ray. The *entire* wall of the bowel is involved. The mucosa is commonly inflamed and ulcerated with a grayish white exudate.

CLINICAL FEATURES

The signs and symptoms of regional enteritis vary a great deal according to whether the disease is early or late and according to what parts of the gastrointestinal tract are involved. Mild intermittent diarrhea (two to five stools per day), colicky pain in the lower abdomen, and malaise increasing over a period of years is usual. Sometimes there is blood in the stool. Some patients develop steatorrhea, weight loss, anemia and other manifestations of malabsorption. Low-grade fever is common.

Certain complications are typical of regional enteritis. The development of stenosis may cause symptoms of vomiting and other signs of intestinal obstruction. An ulcerous lesion may perforate through the intestinal wall, causing peritonitis. More commonly the perforation is closed, and fistulae are formed between loops of bowel and less commonly involve the bladder or vagina. Ulcers, abscesses, and fistulae often occur in the perianal and perirectal regions. External fistulae to the anterior abdominal wall may also occur. High fever is usually associated with extensive inflammation or complications such as fistulae and abscesses.

Extragastrointestinal manifestations of the disease, such as arthritis, uveitis, and skin lesions occur, but are less frequent than in ulcerative colitis.

The diagnosis is established on the basis of the clinical presentation, the characteristic x-ray changes, and in the case of colonic or rectal involvement, biopsy changes showing granulomatous lesions.

TREATMENT AND PROGNOSIS

There is no specific or curative treatment for regional enteritis. The initial management of most patients is medical, supportive and palliative, and aimed at attaining remission of the disease. Corticosteroids, azathioprine, and Azulfidine are used to promote remission and con-

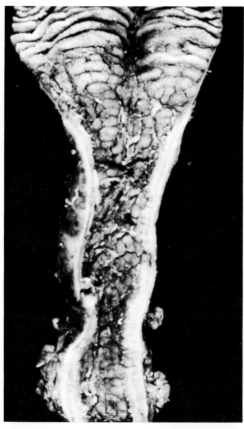

FIGURE 21-3 Regional enteritis (Crohn's disease). The gut wall has been thickened by inflammation and scarring, causing marked narrowing of the lumen. At the top is more normal mucosa. Extending downward are longitudinal ulcers which cross the transverse folds, giving the mucosa a cobblestone appearance. (Courtesy of Dr. Henry D. Appleman, Associate Professor of Pathology, University of Michigan.)

trol suppurative complications. Anticholingeric drugs, such as Pro-Banthine, and antidiarrheal drugs, such as Metamucil and Lomotil, may help reduce cramping, abdominal pain, and diarrhea. Nutrient deficiencies and steatorrhea are treated by the appropriate replacements and a low-fat, low-residue diet.

Surgical treatment is generally avoided because recurrence and spread of the lesion is usual following surgical resection. Nevertheless, surgical intervention is usually necessary sometime during the course of the disease to treat complications.

When regional enteritis is characterized by an acute onset, about half the patients achieve a permanent spontaneous remission. However, regional enteritis has an insidious onset in 90 percent of patients, and the likelihood of permanent remission is only about 10 percent. Although the mortality as a direct result of the disease is low, most patients live out a miserable life with a remitting–relapsing course with intermittent hospitalization for complications.

APPENDICITIS

Appendicitis is the most common major surgical disease. Although it may occur at any age, it is most frequent in young adults. Prior to the era of antibiotics the mortality from this disease was high.

Pathogenesis

The vermiform appendix is the remnant of the apex of the cecum and has no known function in humans. It is a long, narrow tube (about 6 to 9 cm). It contains the appendicular artery which is an end-artery.

In the usual position, it is located on the abdominal wall under McBurney's point. *McBurney's point* is located by drawing a line from the right anterior superior iliac spine to the umbilicus. The midpoint of this line locates the root of the appendix (see Fig. 21-4).

Appendicitis is an inflammation of the appendix involving all layers of the wall of the organ. The usual inciting event is obstruction of the lumen, usually by a *fecalith* (hardened stool). Obstruction of the outflow of mucus secretions results in swelling, infection, and ulceration. The increased intraluminal pressure may cause occlusion of the appendicular end-artery. If the condition is allowed to progress, necrosis, gangrene, and perforation are the usual results.

Clinical features

In the classical case of acute appendicitis, the initial symptoms are mild periumbilical pain or discomfort followed by anorexia, nausea, and vomiting. These symptoms generally develop over a period of 1 or 2 days. Within hours the pain shifts to the lower right quadrant, and there may be tenderness to palpation over McBurney's point. Later, muscle spasm and rebound tenderness may be present. A low-grade fever and moderate leukocytosis are usual findings. When rupture of the appendix occurs, there is commonly a temporary dramatic relief from pain.

Diagnostic problems

The diagnosis of even the classic case of appendicitis is complicated by the fact that many disorders present a similar clinical picture of an acute abdomen which must be differentiated from acute appendicitis. Some of these conditions are (1) acute gastroenteritis (probably the most common); (2) mesenteric lymphadenitis in children; (3) ruptured ectopic pregnancy; (4) mittelschmerz (pain due to rupture of ovarian follicle during ovulation); (5) inflammation of Meckel's diverticulum (persistence of a duct which in the fetus extends from the ileum to the umbilicus; present in about 2 percent of the population); and (6) regional enteritis.

Further diagnostic difficulties result from the fact that some individuals, particularly infants and the very elderly, deviate from the classic presentation. When there is doubt, it is usually safer to perform surgery, since the penalty of delay may be a ruptured appendix and peritonitis. Hospitalization is prolonged, and some patients may die from the peritonitis.

Treatment

Once the diagnosis of appendicitis is made, the patient is prepared for surgery, and the appendix is promptly removed at any time of the day or night. If surgical removal is carried out before rupture and the signs of peritonitis occur, the postsurgical course is generally uncomplicated, and the patient is discharged from the hospital within a few days.

PERITONITIS

Inflammation of the peritoneum is a serious complication which commonly results from spread of infection from abdominal organs (e.g., appendicitis, salpingitis), rupture of the alimentary tract, or from penetrating abdominal wounds. The most frequent infecting organisms are the colon group in the case of a ruptured appendix, whereas staphylococci or streptococci are commonly introduced from without.

The initial reaction of the peritoneum to invasion by bacteria is the outpouring of a fibrinous exudate. Pockets of pus (abscesses) form between the fibrinous adhesions, which glue together the surrounding surfaces and thus localize the infection. The adhesions usually disappear when the infection disappears but may persist as fibrous bands which may later lead to intestinal obstruction.

If the infecting material is distributed widely over the surface of the peritoneum or if the infection spreads, generalized peritonitis may result. As generalized peritonitis develops, peristaltic activity diminishes until a state of paralytic ileus results; the intestine then becomes atonic and distended. Fluids and electrolytes are lost into the lumen of the bowel, leading to dehydration, shock, circulatory embarrassment, and oliguria. Adhesions may form between the distended loops of intestine and may impede the return of intestinal motility and result in intestinal obstruction.

Symptoms vary with the extent of the peritonitis, its severity, and the type of organisms responsible. The principal symptoms are abdominal pain (usually continuous); vomiting; and a tense, rigid, tender, and silent abdomen. Fever and leukocytosis are usual.

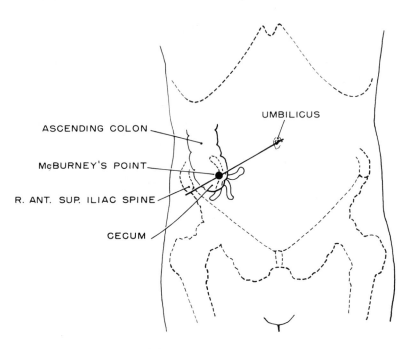

FIGURE 21-4 McBurney's point showing several common positions of the appendix.

The prognosis is good in localized and mild forms of peritonitis and grave in generalized peritonitis due to virulent organisms.

The general principles of treatment include administration of a suitable antibiotic, decompression of the gastrointestinal tract by nasogastric or intestinal suction, intravenous repletion of fluid and electrolyte losses, removal of the septic focus (appendix, etc.) or other cause of inflammation, if possible, with drainage of pus to the outside, and measures to relieve pain.

INTESTINAL OBSTRUCTION

Intestinal obstruction may be defined as an interference (from whatever cause) with the normal flow of intestinal contents through the intestinal tract. Intestinal obstruction may be acute or chronic, partial or complete. Chronic bowel obstruction usually involves the colon as a result of a carcinoma and is slow in development. Most obstructions involve the small bowel. Complete obstruction of the small bowel is a very grave condition which requires early diagnosis and emergency surgical intervention if the patient is to survive.

There are two types of intestinal obstruction: (1) paralytic ileus (adynamic ileus) in which intestinal peristalsis is inhibited as a result of toxic or traumatic affectation of autonomic control of motility; and (2) mechanical obstruction, in which there is intraluminal obstruction or mural obstruction due to extrinsic pressure.

Mechanical obstruction is further classified as *simple mechanical obstruction,* in which there is only one point of obstruction, and *closed loop obstruction,* in which there are at least two points of obstruction. Because a closed loop obstruction cannot be decompressed, there is a rapid increase in intraluminal pressure leading to compression of blood vessels, ischemia, and infarction (strangulation). Figure 21-5 illustrates some of the mechanical causes of bowel obstruction.

Etiology

Nonmechanical obstruction or adynamic ileus commonly follows abdominal surgery in which there is reflex inhibition of peristalsis due to handling of the abdominal viscera. This reflex inhibition of peristalsis is often called paralytic ileus, although there is not complete paralysis of peristalsis. Another condition which is a common

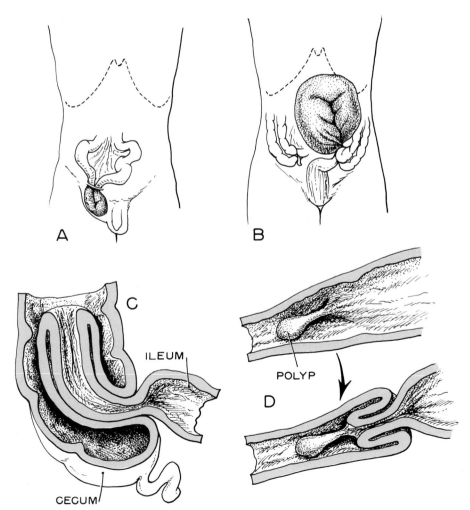

FIGURE 21-5 Mechanical causes of bowel obstruction. A, strangulated inguinal hernia. B, volvulus of the sigmoid colon. C, ileocecal intussusception. D, enteroenteric intussusception due to pedunculated polyp.

cause of adynamic ileus is peritonitis. Intestinal atony and gaseous distention accompany a wide variety of traumatic conditions, especially following rib fracture and fracture of the spine.

The causes of mechanical obstruction are related to the age group affected and the site of the obstruction. About 50 percent of all obstructions occur in middle-aged and older people and result from adhesions from previous surgery. Malignant tumors and volvulus are the most common causes of large intestinal obstruction in middle-aged and older people. Cancer of the colon accounts for 80 percent of the obstructions. *Volvulus* is twisting of the intestine on itself. It occurs most frequently in elderly men and usually involves the sigmoid colon. Incarceration of a loop of bowel in an inguinal or femoral hernia is a very common cause of small bowel obstruction. *Intussusception* is invagination of one section of the intestine into the next section and is a cause of obstruction encountered almost exclusively in infants and young children. A common site for intussusception is the terminal ileum into the cecum. Foreign bodies and congenital anomalies are other common causes of obstruction in infants and children.

Pathophysiology

The pathophysiologic events which occur following intestinal obstruction are similar, whether they result from mechanical or functional causes. The main difference is that in paralytic obstruction, peristalsis is inhibited from the start, while in mechanical obstruction, peristalsis is accentuated at first, is then intermittent, and is finally absent.

The obstructed bowel lumen becomes progressively distended with fluid and gas (70 percent from swallowed air) as a result of the effects of rising intraluminal pressure, which leads to a decreased flux of water and sodium from intestinal lumen to blood. Since about 8 liters of fluid are secreted into the gastrointestinal tract each day, nonabsorption can lead to rapid intraluminal accumulation. Vomiting and intestinal suction after treatment has begun is a major source of fluid and electrolyte loss. The net effect of these losses is contraction of the extracellular fluid compartment leading to shock, that is, hypotension, reduced cardiac output, decreased tissue perfusion, and metabolic acidosis. Continuing bowel distention results in a vicious cycle of decreased fluid absorption and increased fluid secretion into the bowel. The local effects of bowel distention is ischemia from distention and increased permeability due to necrosis, with absorption of bacterial toxins into the circulation.

Signs and symptoms

The cardinal symptoms of small bowel obstruction are pain, vomiting, absolute constipation, and abdominal distention. Pain is usually not as prominent as in ady-

namic ileus, although the abdomen may be tender. The pain is usually cramplike, coming in waves, and is usually located at the umbilicus. The frequency of vomiting varies with the site of obstruction. If the obstruction is high in the small bowel, vomiting is more prevalent than if the obstruction is in the ileum or large intestine. Absolute constipation is likely to occur early in large bowel obstruction, but flatus and feces may be passed early during the course of small bowel obstruction.

The abdominal x-ray is extremely important in the diagnosis of intestinal obstruction. Mechanical small bowel obstruction is characterized by air in the small intestine but not in the colon, while colonic obstruction is characterized by gas throughout the colon but with little or no gas in the small intestine. When the plain films are inconclusive, a barium x-ray may be performed to locate the site of obstruction.

Treatment

Treatment principles of bowel obstruction include correction of fluid and electrolyte imbalances, relief of distention and vomiting by intubation and decompression, control of peritonitis and shock if present, and removal of the obstruction to restore normal bowel continuity and function.

Many cases of adynamic ileus are cured by tubal decompression alone. A small bowel obstruction is much more serious and rapid in development than colonic obstruction. Mortality for simple obstruction is 1 to 2 percent, provided surgical intervention occurs soon enough. Delay in surgical intervention or the development of strangulation or other complications raises the mortality to about 35 or 40 percent.

QUESTIONS

Small intestine—Chap. 21

Directions: Answer the following questions on a separate sheet of paper.

1 Why is the gastrointestinal mucosa especially vulnerable to side effects such as ulceration and bleeding from the administration of such cytotoxic drugs as cyclophosphamide (Cytoxan) and mercaptopurine?

2 Describe the function of bile in the digestion and absorption of fats and fat-soluble vitamins.

3 Differentiate between maldigestion and malabsorption.

4 Describe the appearance and characteristics of stool from a patient which would cause you to suspect steatorrhea.

5 What are the characteristics of regional enteritis which have led theorists to suspect that hypersensitivity might be responsible in its pathogenesis?

6 Name the three structures which greatly increase the absorptive surface area of the small bowel.

7 List four causes of steatorrhea in a patient following total gastrectomy or gastrojejunostomy.

8 Describe the pathophysiologic events leading to death from small bowel obstruction. Explain why early diagnosis and surgical intervention are important in mechanical obstruction of the small bowel.

Directions: Fill in the blanks with the correct word(s) in the following questions.

9 The major artery supplying the small bowel (except the duodenum) is the _____ artery.

10 The _____ sphincter controls the entry of chyme into the small bowel, and the _____ valve controls the exit of digested material into the large intestine.

11 The fanlike fold of peritoneum which suspends the jejunum and ileum from the posterior abdominal wall is called the _____.

12 The fold of peritoneum which drapes over the small bowel like an apron is called the _____ _____. This structure has sometimes been called the policeman of the abdomen, because one of its important functions is to localize _____.

13 The musculofibrous band extending from the diaphragm to the duodenojejunal juncture which acts as a support for this portion of the small bowel is called the _____ of _____.

14 The structures which are responsible for giving the barium x-ray of the small bowel a feathery appearance are the _____.

15 The structures which account for the velvetlike appearance of the small bowel are the _____.

16 The source of the succus entericus is from the _____ of _____.

17 The lymphatic vessel of the villus where fat absorption takes place is called the central _____.

18 McBurney's point is located at the midpoint on a line between the _____ and the anterior superior _____ spine. It is the point where the _____ is normally located.

Directions: Match each of the following enzymes in col. A with its secretory source in col. B and with its substrate in col. C.

Column A	Column B	Column C
19 ___ Lactase	a Duodenal mucosa	e Denatured
20 ___ Ptyalin	b Exocrine pancreas	proteins and
21 ___ Entero-	c Salivary glands	polypeptides
kinase	d Intestinal glands	f Lactose
22 ___ Trypsin		g Starch
		h Trypsinogen

Match each of the following nutrients in col. A with its major site of absorption in col. B. (Items may be used more than once.)

Column A	Column B
23 ___ Iron	a Stomach
24 ___ Vitamin B_{12}	b Duodenum
25 ___ Sugars	c Duodenum and jejunum
26 ___ Fats	d Terminal ileum
27 ___ Amino acids	e Large intestine
28 ___ Bile salts	

Match each of the following symptoms of malabsorption in col. A to its pathophysiologic basis in col. B.

Column A	Column B
29 ___ Edema	a Impaired absorption of amino acids
30 ___ Peripheral neuropathy	b Vitamin K malabsorption
31 ___ Bleeding tendency	c Deficiency of vitamin B_{12}
32 ___ Diarrhea	d Bile salts in colon
33 ___ Tetany, paresthesias	e Lactase,deficiency
34 ___ Nocturia	f Calcium malabsorption
	g Delayed absorption of fluid in gut

Match each of the following terms related to bowel obstruction in col. A with the proper descriptive statements from col. B.

Column A	Column B
35 ___ Adhesions	a Twisting of a loop of bowel on itself
36 ___ Volvulus	b Only one point of obstruction
37 ___ Simple bowel obstruction	c Fibrous bands which form as a result of a fibrinous exudate from peritoneum
38 ___ Strangulated hernia	d Obstruction of the blood supply to a loop of bowel protruding through muscle wall
39 ___ Intussusception	e Almost exclusively a condition of infants and young children
	f Commonly occurs in the sigmoid colon in elderly men
	g Telescoping of the bowel
	h Most common cause of bowel obstruction in adults

Match each of the following descriptions in col. A with the correct entity from col. B.

Column A	Column B
40 ___ Usually responds to broad spectrum antibiotics	a Nontropical sprue (celiac disease)
41 ___ During exacerbation is associated with very low D-xylose excretion	b Tropical sprue
42 ___ Usually responds to gluten withdrawal	c Both
43 ___ Characterized by atrophy and flattening of villi	d Neither

Directions: Circle the letter preceding each item that correctly answers the questions. Only one answer is correct, unless otherwise noted.

44 Which of the following hormones has the primary effect of stimulating the bicarbonate component of the pancreatic juice?
  a CCK-PZ *b* Cholecystokinin *c* Pancreozymin *d* Secretin

45 Hydrolysis of lactose into glucose and galactose takes place:
  a In the stomach *b* Along the brush border *c* Within the lumen of the duodenum *d* Within the lumen of the jejunum

46 Mechanisms which normally keep the proximal bowel relatively sterile include which of the following? (More than one answer may be correct.)
  a Peristalsis *b* Acid chyme entering duodenum *c* Alkalinity of the pancreatic bicarbonate secretion *d* Secretion of IgA into the gut

47 The length of the small bowel in the living person is about:
  a 22 ft *b* 12 ft *c* 10 ft *d* 6 ft

48 The greatest portion of gastrointestinal gas (air) is derived from:
  a Food breakdown *b* Bacterial fermentation *c* Swallowed air

49 The diagnosis of gluten-induced enteropathy must include:
  a History of weight loss *b* Steatorrhea *c* Abnormal small bowel biopsy *d* Abnormal D-xylose excretion

50 Administration of intrinsic factor caused the Schilling test to return to normal after an initial low value in a 56-year-old woman. The probable cause of this patient's problem is:
  a Bacterial overgrowth in the proximal small bowel *b* Regional enteritis *c* Chronic pancreatitis *d* Atrophic gastritis

51 The afferent loop syndrome is characterized by: (More than one answer may be correct.)
  a Malabsorption of vitamin B_{12} *b* Megaloblastic anemia *c* Heavy growth of colonic bacteria *d* Amelioration with administration of broad-spectrum antibiotics

52 The earliest sign on examination in acute appendicitis is:
  a Periumbilical hyperesthesia *b* Abdominal distention *c* Localized tenderness in the lower right quadrant *d* Rebound tenderness

53 Which of the following conditions may present difficulties in differentiation from acute appendicitis? (More than one answer may be correct.)
  a Acute gastroenteritis *b* Ruptured ectopic pregnancy *c* Regional enteritis *d* Inflammation of Meckel's diverticulum *e* Mittelschmerz

54 Bile salts are conjugated in the liver and deconjugated by bacteria in conditions of duodenal stasis.
  a First statement is true but second is false *b* First statement is false but second is true *c* Both statements are true *d* Both statements are false

55 Lactase deficiency is: (More than one answer may be correct.)
  a Always congenital *b* Only found in the Western hemisphere *c* Common in the American blacks *d* A brush border disease *e* Relatively uncommon in Caucasians

56 The secretion of CCK-PZ is stimulated by: (More than one answer may be correct.)
  a Contact of the acid chyme with the duodenal mucosa *b* Fat in contact with the duodenal mucosa *c* Alkaline chyme in contact with duodenal mucosa *d* Denatured proteins in contact with the duodenal mucosa

57 Which of the following may be a cause of intestinal malabsorption? (More than one answer may be correct.)
  a Acute enteritis *b* Chronic hepatitis *c* Whipple's disease *d* Mesenteric atherosclerosis

Directions: Circle T if the statement is true and F if it is false.

58 T F The lumen of the bowel is open and the obstruction is functional in paralytic ileus.

59 T F Parasympathetic fibers supplying the small bowel relay pain.

60 T F The daily total volume of the digestive secretions is about 8 liters.

61 T F Most of the enzymes of the succus entericus would be inactivated by a pH of 5.0.

62 T F Two factors which account for frequent obstruction and ischemic necrosis of the appendix is its narrow lumen ending in a blind pouch and its blood supply from an end-artery.

REFERENCES

BAYLESS, T. M. and N. L. CHRISTOPHER: "Disaccharide Deficiency," *American Journal of Clinical Nutrition,* **22**: 181–190, 1969.

BOGOCH, ABRAHAM (ed.): *Gastroenterology,* McGraw-Hill, New York, 1973, pp. 538–598, 1152–1167.

BROOKS, F. P. (ed.): *Gastrointestinal Pathophysiology,* Oxford University Press, New York, 1974, pp. 286–297.

DAVENPORT, H. W.: *A Digest on Digestion,* Yearbook, Chicago, 1975.

FROLICH, EDWARD D. (ed.): *Pathophysiology,* Lippincott, Philadelphia, 1972, pp. 407–450.

GIVEN, B. A. and S. J. SIMMONS: *Gastroenterology in Clinical Nursing,* 2d ed., C. V. Mosby, St. Louis, 1975, pp. 198–218.

GREENBERGER, N. J. and K. J. ISSELBACHER: "Disorders of Absorption," in *Harrison's Principles of Internal Medicine,* 7th ed., McGraw-Hill, New York, 1974, pp. 1456–1474.

——— and D. H. WINSHIP: *Gastrointestinal Disorders: A Pathophysiologic Approach,* Yearbook, Chicago, 1976, pp. 104–172.

JACOB, S. W. and C. A. FRANCONE: *Structure and Function in Man,* 3d ed., Saunders, Philadelphia, 1974.

MENDELOFF, A. I.: "Diseases of the Small Intestine," in *Harrison's Principles of Internal Medicine,* 7th ed., McGraw-Hill, New York, 1974, pp. 1475–1482.

——— and A. M. SELIGMAN: "Acute Intestinal Obstruction" and "Acute Appendicitis," in *Harrison's Principles of Internal Medicine,* 7th ed., 1974, pp. 1483–1487.

NETTER, FRANK H.: *Ciba Collections of Medical Illustrations, Vol. 3, Digestive System, Part II, Lower Digestive Tract* Ciba Pharmaceutical Co., Summit, N.J., 1962, pp. 47–53.

ROBBINS, S. L. and M. ANGELL: *Basic Pathology,* Saunders, Philadelphia, 1971, pp. 412–414, 422–426.

WATSON, D. W. and W. A. SODEMAN, JR.: "The Small Intestine," in W. A. Sodeman, Jr. and W. A. Sodeman (eds.), *Pathologic Physiology,* 5th ed., Saunders, Philadelphia, 1974, pp. 697–708.

CHAPTER 22 Large Intestine

OBJECTIVES

At the completion of Chap. 22, you should be able to:

1 Identify the gross anatomic features and subdivisions of the large bowel.

2 Compare the small and large intestine with respect to size, length, sphincter control, morphologic layers, motility, and digestive and absorptive functions.

3 Describe the blood supply and innervation of the large bowel.

4 Identify the most important function of the large bowel.

5 Describe the actions of colonic bacteria.

6 Identify the source and components of flatus.

7 Explain the function of haustral churning and mass peristalsis.

8 Describe the act of defecation, including reflex and voluntary control mechanisms and factors which might interfere with control.

9 List five common anorectal disorders.

10 Explain why repeated suppression of the defecation reflex often results in chronic constipation.

11 List the important diagnostic procedures for detection of large bowel disease.

12 Define diverticulosis and diverticulitis.

13 Describe the probable pathogenetic mechanism involved in diverticulosis, including the influence of dietary factors.

14 Explain why a barium enema x-ray is generally contraindicated during an attack of acute diverticulitis.

15 Discuss the signs, symptoms, comparisons, and treatment of diverticulosis and diverticulitis.

16 Compare Crohn's disease and ulcerative colitis with respect to their pathologic and clinical characteristic features.

17 Describe the pathologic and clinical features of acute fulminating, chronic intermittent, and chronic continuous ulcerative colitis.

18 Describe the most common complications of ulcerative colitis (including three serious ones) and their treatment.

19 Describe the following types of colonic polyps: pedunculated, juvenile, familial, and villous adenoma (gross and microscopic characteristics, common, sites, relative frequency, malignant potential, and treatment).

20 Rank cancer of the colon and rectum as a cause of gastrointestinal cancer and as a cause of all cancer deaths in men and women.

21 Explain why rectal digital or proctosigmoidoscopic examination is important in middle-aged and older individuals.

22 List three routes of metastasis for cancer of the large bowel.

23 Identify three predisposing factors in the pathogenesis of cancer of the large bowel.

24 Relate Burkitt's hypothesis concerning the relationship of diet to the development of cancer of the large bowel.

25 Contrast the clinical features of right- and left-sided cancer of the bowel.

26 Describe the pathologic and clinical features of internal and external hemorrhoids (including site, frequency in population, predisposing factors, symptoms, complications, and treatment).

27 Differentiate between first-, second-, and third-degree internal hemorrhoids.

28 Explain the relationship of anal fissures to the skin tags of chronic external hemorrhoids.

29 Identify four common sites of anorectal abscess formation, common causes, infecting organisms, and treatment.

30 Explain the relationship of anal cryptitis and Crohn's disease to anorectal fistulae.

31 Describe the treatment of anorectal abscesses and fistulae.

ANATOMIC AND PHYSIOLOGIC CONSIDERATIONS

The large intestine is a hollow muscular tube about 5 ft in length extending from the cecum to the anal canal. The diameter of the large intestine is noticeably larger than that of the small intestine. Its average diameter is about 2.5 in but decreases toward the lower end of the tube.

The large intestine is divided into the cecum, colon, and rectum as illustrated in Fig. 22-1. The *cecum*, with the appendix attached to its apex and containing the ileocecal valve, comprises the first 2 or 3 in of the large intestine. The colon is subdivided into the *ascending, transverse, descending,* and *sigmoid* colon. The points at which the colon makes a sharp turn at the right and left upper abdomen are called the *hepatic* and *splenic flexures,* respectively. The sigmoid colon begins at the level of the iliac crest and describes an S-shaped curve. The lower part of the curve bends toward the left as it joins the rectum and is the anatomic reason for placing a patient on the left side when giving an enema. In this position, gravity aids the flow of water from the rectum into the sigmoid flexure. The last major portion of the large intestine is called the *rectum* and extends from the sigmoid colon to the *anus* (opening to the outside of the body). The terminal inch of the rectum is called the *anal canal* and is guarded by internal and external sphincter muscles. The length of the rectum and anal canal is approximately 15 cm.

The large intestine exhibits throughout most of its length the four morphologic layers seen in the remainder of the gut. Several features, however, are peculiar to the large intestine. The longitudinal muscle coat is incomplete, being collected into three bands called the *taenia coli.* The taenia coalesce in the distal sigmoid, so that the rectum has a complete longitudinal muscle coat. The taenia are shorter than the intestine, causing it to pucker and form small sacs called *haustra.* The *epiploic appendages* are small fat-filled sacs of peritoneum attached along the taenia. The mucosal layer of the large intestine is much thicker than that of the small intestine and contains no villi or rugae. The crypts of Lieberkühn (intestinal glands) are deeper and have more goblet cells than those of the small intestine.

The large intestine is clinically divided into right and left halves based on the blood supply. The superior mesenteric artery supplies the right half (ascending and transverse colon), and the inferior mesenteric supplies the left half (descending and sigmoid colon and proximal part of rectum). Additional blood supply to the rectum is provided by the middle sacral and middle and inferior hemorrhoidal arteries, which arise from the abdominal aorta and internal iliac arteries.

Venous return from the colon and superior rectum is via the superior and inferior mesenteric veins and superior hemorrhoidal veins, which become a part of the portal system delivering blood to the liver. The middle and inferior hemorrhoidal veins drain into the iliac veins and consequently are part of the systemic circulation. There are anastomoses between the superior and the middle and inferior hemorrhoidal veins, so that increased portal pressure may cause backflow into these veins, resulting in hemorrhoids.

The nerve supply to the large intestine is supplied by the autonomic nervous system with the exception of the external sphincter, which is under voluntary control. Parasympathetic fibers travel via the vagus to the mid-transverse colon, and pelvic nerves of sacral origin supply the distal part. Sympathetic fibers leave the spinal cord via the splanchnic nerve to reach the colon. Sympathetic stimulation causes inhibition of secretion and contraction and stimulates the rectal sphincter, while parasympathetic stimulation has the opposite effect.

The large intestine has a variety of functions all related to the final processing of intestinal contents. The most important function is the absorption of water and electrolytes, which is largely completed in the right side of the colon. The sigmoid colon functions as a reservoir for the dehydrated fecal mass until defecation takes place.

The colon absorbs about 600 ml of water per day compared to about 8000 ml absorbed by the small intestine. The absorption capacity of the large intestine, however, is about 2000 ml/day. When this amount is exceeded by excessive delivery of fluid from the ileum, diarrhea results. The final daily excreted feces weighs about 200 g, of which about 75 percent is water. The remainder is made up of nonabsorbed food residue, bacteria, desquamated epithelial cells, and unabsorbed minerals.

Very little, if any, digestion takes place in the large intestine. The secretion of the large intestine contains much mucus, shows an alkaline reaction, and contains no enzymes. The mucus acts as a lubricant and protects the mucosa. In inflammatory conditions of the bowel, greatly increased mucus secretion of the bowel may be responsible for protein loss in the stool.

The bacteria of the large intestine perform many functions, including the synthesis of vitamin K and several vitamins of the B group. There is constant putrefaction of whatever proteins are left as a result of not having been digested in the small intestine. The list of simple substances resulting from putrefaction is long and includes various peptides, amino acids, indole, skatole, phenol, and fatty acids. Ammonia, CO_2, H_2, H_2S, and CH_3 are the most important gases produced. Some of these substances are given off in the feces, while others are absorbed and carried to the liver where they are changed to less toxic compounds and excreted in the urine.

About 1000 ml of "gas" or flatus is normally expelled from the anus each day. An excess of gas occurs with aerophagia (excessive swallowing of air common in neurotic persons as well as in a variety of upper GI tract diseases) and when there is an increase in intraluminal gas production, which is commonly related to the diet. "Gassy foods" are those with a high content of indigestible carbohydrates. The colon bacteria attack the carbohydrates and release H_2, CO_2, and in some persons, methane (CH_3). Presumably the gas production as a result of eating beans is due to the presence of a carbohydrate component.

In general, the movements of the large intestine are slow. A movement characteristic of the large intestine is

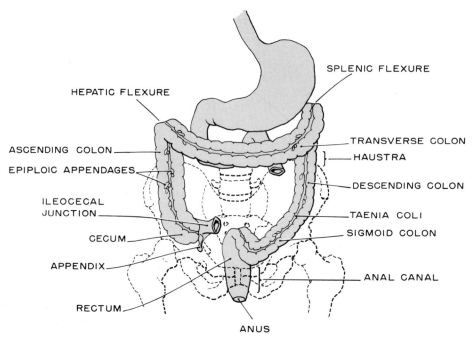

FIGURE 22-1 Anatomic relationships of the large intestine.

haustral churning. The pouches or haustra become distended, and from time to time the circular muscles contract and cause them to empty. The movements are not progressive but cause the contents to move back and forth in a kneading action, thus allowing time for absorption. There are two types of propulsive peristalsis: (1) slow, irregular contractions which arise in a proximal segment and move forward, obliterating a few haustra; and (2) *mass peristalsis,* which is a contraction involving a large segment of the colon. Mass peristalsis moves the fecal mass from the right or transverse colon to the sigmoid colon. It occurs two or three times a day and is stimulated by the gastrocolic reflex after eating, particularly following the first meal of the day.

The act of defecation is a reflex involving the voluntary and involuntary muscles of the anal canal and terminal bowel. Figure 22-2 illustrates the basic anatomy of the rectum and anus. The entry of feces into the rectum distends its walls and stimulates mass peristaltic movements of the bowel. The principal reflex center is in the parasympathetic nerve center in the 2nd to 4th sacral segments of the spinal cord. As the balloon-shaped rectum contracts, the levator ani muscle relaxes, causing the anorectal ring and angle to disappear. The internal and external spincter muscles relax as the anus is pulled up over the fecal mass. The act of defecation is facilitated by an increase in intra-abdominal pressure brought about by voluntary contraction of the chest muscles on a closed glottis and simultaneous contraction of the abdominal muscles (Valsalva's maneuver or straining). Parasympathetic fibers reach the rectum via the pelvic splanchnic nerves and are responsible for contraction of the rectum and relaxation of the internal sphincter.

Voluntary inhibition of defecation can be effected by contraction of the levator ani and external sphincter muscles.

The rectum and anus are the site of the most common diseases known to humans. A common cause of simple constipation is failure to empty the rectum when mass peristalsis occurs. When defecation is not completed the rectum relaxes and the desire to defecate disappears. Water continues to be absorbed from the fecal mass, causing it to become hard, so that subsequent defecation is more difficult. Excessive straining at the stool causes congestion of the internal and external hemorrhoidal veins and is one of the important causes of hemorrhoids (varicose veins of the rectum). Incontinence of stool may result from damage to sphincter muscles or from damage to the spinal cord. The anorectal area is a frequent site of abscesses and fistulae. Cancer of the colon and rectum is the most frequent site of cancer of the gastrointestinal tract.

DIAGNOSTIC PROCEDURES

Diagnosis of pathology associated with the large intestine relates mainly to symptoms associated with elimination. Constipation, diarrhea, alteration in size or color, or the presence of blood in the stools are all important

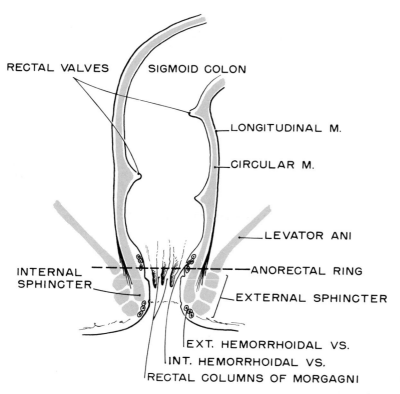

RECTAL VALVES   SIGMOID COLON

LONGITUDINAL M.

CIRCULAR M.

LEVATOR ANI

INTERNAL SPHINCTER

ANORECTAL RING

EXTERNAL SPHINCTER

EXT. HEMORRHOIDAL VS.

INT. HEMORRHOIDAL VS.

RECTAL COLUMNS OF MORGAGNI

FIGURE 22-2 Anatomy of the rectum and anus.

symptoms which focus attention on the colon and rectum. Pain of colonic origin is lateralized to the left or right sides of the abdomen, as opposed to pain of small intestinal origin, which is usually periumbilical.

History and physical exam are important diagnostic procedures. Abdominal masses may be palpated, and digital examination is very important, since about half of all rectal carcinomas are within reach of the examining finger. Examination of the stools, sigmoidoscopy, and radiologic exam are required for a complete assessment in cases of suspected colonic disease.

The barium enema x-ray is the most common test carried out on patients with disorders of the colon. Preparation or prior cleansing of the intestine is important for a proper examination, but in the presence of an obstructing lesion or active ulcerative colitis, the use of strong cathartics may be hazardous or life-threatening to the patient. Neoplasms, strictures, diverticulosis, and polyps may all be visualized. The cecum and ascending colon may be visualized 3 to 5 hours after a barium swallow. The barium enema x-ray should always precede the barium swallow.

Direct visualization of the terminal 25 cm of the large intestine is possible through the rigid proctosigmoidoscope. Sixty percent of all the tumors of the large intestine can be visualized directly with this instrument. In addition to visual inspection of the area, bacteriologic, parasitologic, and cytologic studies can be made on washings through the instrument, and biopsy of suspicious lesions is easy to perform. The flexible fiberoptic colonoscope allows visualization and biopsy of lesions of the entire colon. Experienced examiners may be able to insert the instrument as far as the terminal ileum.

DIVERTICULAR DISEASE OF THE COLON

Diverticulosis is a condition of the colon characterized by herniation of the mucosa through the muscularis, forming flask-shaped saccules. If one or more of the saccules become inflamed, the condition is called diverticulitis.

Pathophysiology

The overall incidence of diverticulosis is high and affects about 10 percent of the population according to most necropsy studies. It is rare below the age of 35 years but increases with age, so that at age 85 two-thirds of the population is afflicted.

The most common site for diverticula to occur is in the sigmoid colon, which is involved in about 90 percent of the cases.

Although the etiology of diverticulosis is unknown, recent motility and pressure studies have done much to support the possibility that diverticular disease may result from a disordered motility pattern of the colon. Figure 22-3 illustrates the normal motility pattern in the colon and the proposed pathogenetic mechanism of diverticulosis. Diverticula-bearing zones of the colon are prone to strong contractions of the circular muscles which build up very high intraluminal pressures. It seems likely that these high pressures are responsible for herniations of the mucosa through the muscle coat, which become diverticula. The usual position for the diverticula is at the mesenteric attachment of the colon, where the entry of blood vessels weakens the wall. The pressure changes in diverticular disease are similar to those found in spastic or irritable colon syndrome, which is believed by many to have a basis in anxiety and emotional tension.

A factor of even greater importance in the etiology of diverticular disease relates to the amount of roughage in the diet. Diverticulosis is rare in those who eat a diet high in roughage but is very common in Europeans and North Americans (all races) who eat a low-roughage diet. The tension or strain on the wall of a hollow organ is related to the pressure within and to the diameter of the organ. Therefore, if a tube such as the colon is habitually of narrow bore (as the result of a low-fiber diet), then the strain on the wall from a buildup of pressure will be greater than if it were filled with feces.

Clinical features and complications

The majority of patients with diverticulosis suffer no symptoms and will remain unidentified unless a barium enema x-ray is performed in the investigation of some unrelated condition. When diverticula are discovered, it is important for the physician to rule out carcinoma. This differentiation is made by the x-ray appearance, colonoscopic exam, and biopsy. A barium enema x-ray is more dangerous during an attack of acute diverticulitis because of the danger of perforation.

In many patients, symptoms are mild and consist of flatulence, intermittent diarrhea or constipation, and discomfort in the lower left quadrant of the abdomen. These symptoms can usually be attributed to the irritable colon syndrome which may precede the development of diverticulosis in some patients.

The complications of diverticular disease are the result of acute or chronic diverticulitis, which may result in bleeding, perforation and peritonitis, abscess and fistula formation, or intestinal obstruction from stricture (see Fig. 22-4).

In the case of acute diverticulitis, there is fever,

FIGURE 22-3 Pathogenesis of diverticular disease. A, normal motility pattern. B, abnormal motility pattern in which there is failure of relaxation and buildup of high intraluminal pressure resulting in the formation of a diverticulum. C, cross-section of colon showing that the weak point is the circular muscle where the blood vessels pierce the muscle. Herniation of the lining mucosa and the formation of diverticuli form at these points.

leukocytosis, and pain and tenderness in the lower left quadrant of the abdomen. During a bout of acute inflammation, bleeding may occur from vascular granulation tissue and is usually minor. In rare instances, bleeding may be massive as a result of erosion of the large penetrating blood vessel next to the diverticula. Bleeding is usually treated conservatively, but on rare occasions a bowel resection has been necessary.

Sometimes, acutely inflamed diverticula rupture. If the perforation is small, the result may be abscess formation next to the perforated diverticulum. If the perforation is large, fecal material may enter the peritoneum and cause a most severe form of peritonitis with a high mortality. Symptoms of perforation are similar to those of perforated ulcer except that pain, rigidity, and tenderness are most marked in the lower left quadrant.

Chronic diverticulitis applies to a bowel which is subjected to repeated attacks of inflammation. The result may be fibrosis and adhesions of the surrounding structures. When chronic inflammation has caused significant narrowing of the lumen, chronic incomplete bowel obstruction may result, giving rise to symptoms of constipation, ribbonlike stools, intermittent diarrhea, and abdominal distention. The final obstructive picture may be precipitated by a superimposed acute attack, leading to a pericolic abscess which narrows the already oc-

cluded lumen. A fistula may also form as a complication of a pericolic abscess. The most common type is the vesicocolic fistula. The flow is always from the colon to the bladder, and the complaint is *pneumaturia* or the passage of air bubbles in the urine.

Treatment

If diverticula are discovered incidentally and the patient is asymptomatic, they are not generally treated. However, 90 percent of the cases of diverticulitis are treated medically. Mild cases without signs of perforation are treated by a liquid diet, stool softeners, bed rest, and a broad-spectrum antibiotic. Antibiotics effective against gram-negative anaerobic bacteria may be given to patients with suspected perforation or abscess. Incision and drainage of abscesses may be necessary.

Surgical intervention is only needed for severe and extensive disease or in the event of complications. The essential surgical treatment is resection of the diseased colon with anastomosis to restore continuity. In the

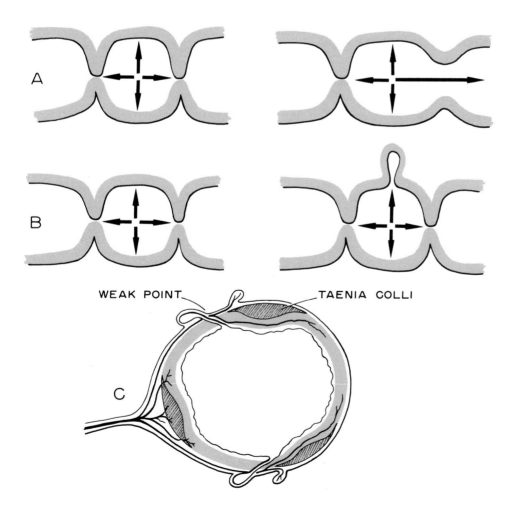

WEAK POINT   TAENIA COLLI

absence of complications the surgery may be carried out in one stage. In other cases a temporary colostomy may be performed with diversion of feces to the abdominal surface (colostomy). Anastomosis and closure is then carried out at a later date.

INFLAMMATORY DISEASE OF THE LARGE INTESTINE

Chronic inflammatory disease of the large bowel is divided into two major entities—nonspecific ulcerative colitis and Crohn's disease of the large bowel (granulomatous colitis). Although these two conditions have many features in common, there are enough differences to separate them into two distinct clinical entities. Table 22-1 lists the differentiating features of these two diseases. There are enough overlapping features to lead some investigators to believe that both these diseases may represent variations in response to the same etiologic agent.

Ulcerative colitis

Ulcerative colitis is a nonspecific inflammatory disease of the colon generally following a prolonged course with alternating periods of remissions and exacerbations. Abdominal pain, diarrhea, and rectal bleeding are the cardinal signs and symptoms. The essential lesion is an inflammatory reaction of the subepithelial zone developing at the base of the crypts of Lieberkühn, which may eventually produce ulceration of the mucosa. The peak onset of the disease is between the ages of 20 and 40 years, and it is equally distributed between the sexes. The incidence of ulcerative colitis is about 1 per 10,000 white adults per year. Crohn's disease is about one-fifth as common.

ETIOLOGY AND PATHOGENESIS

The etiology of ulcerative colitis like Crohn's disease is unknown. Genetic factors seem to be involved in the etiology, since there is a definite familial relationship between ulcerative colitis, Crohn's disease, and ankylosing spondylitis.

There is also evidence to suggest that autoimmunity is involved in the pathogenesis of ulcerative colitis. Anticolon antibodies have been found in the serum of patients with this disease. Lymphocytes from patients with ulcerative colitis damage normal colon epithelial cells in tissue culture.

The psychological aspects of ulcerative colitis have been the subject of much controversy. It now seems that psychological stress only plays a secondary role in provoking overt disease.

The initial pathologic lesion is confined to the mucosal layer and consists of abscess formation in the crypts, as opposed to Crohn's disease, which involves the entire thickness of the bowel wall. Early in the disease, edema and congestion of the mucosa occur. The edema may lead to extreme friability, so that bleeding occurs from any minor trauma, such as lightly rubbing the surface.

In more advanced stages of the disease, the crypt abscess breaks through the wall of the crypt and spreads in the submucosa, undermining the mucosa. The mucosa is then shed into the bowel lumen, leaving areas of denuded mucosa (ulcers). Ulceration is at first scattered and shallow, but at a later stage the mucosal surface is lost over wide areas, leading to considerable loss of tissue, protein, and blood.

CLINICAL FEATURES

There are three common clinical types of ulcerative colitis related to frequency of symptoms. The *acute fulminating* ulcerative colitis is characterized by an abrupt onset, with severe, bloody diarrhea, nausea, vomiting, and fever which causes a rapid depletion of fluids and electrolytes. The entire colon may be involved with undermining and stripping of the mucosa,

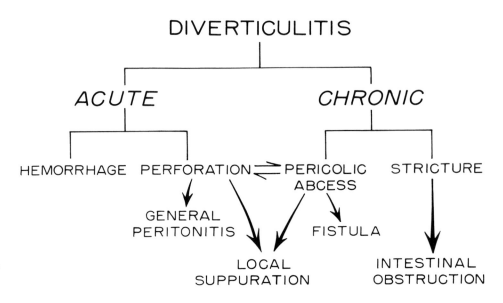

FIGURE 22-4 Complications of diverticulitis.

causing loss of considerable blood and mucus. This type of colitis occurs in about 10 percent of the patients. The prognosis is poor, and toxic megacolon is a frequent complication.

The majority of patients with ulcerative colitis have the *chronic intermittent (recurrent)* type of colitis. The onset tends to be insidious, occurring over a period of months to years. The mild form of the disease is characterized by short attacks occurring at intervals of months to years and lasting 1 to 3 months. There may be little or no fever or constitutional symptoms, and usually only the distal colon is affected. Fever and systemic symptoms may accompany the more severe form, and the attack may last 3 or 4 months, sometimes passing into the *chronic continuous* type of disease. In the chronic continuous disease, the patient continues to have diarrhea after the initial attack. Compared to the intermittent type, more of the colon tends to be involved, and complications are more frequent.

In mild forms of ulcerative colitis, diarrhea may be mild, and bleeding is intermittent and slight. In severe disease there are more than six stools per day with considerable blood and mucus. The chronic loss of blood and mucus may lead to anemia and hypoproteinemia. Severe colicky pain may be present in the lower abdomen and is relieved somewhat by defecation. Very few deaths occur directly from this disease, but it may be mildly or severely disabling.

The diagnosis of ulcerative colitis is usually straightforward. There is diarrhea with passage of blood, and sigmoidoscopy reveals a friable and intensely inflamed mucosa with exudate. In 95 percent of the cases the rectosigmoid area of the colon is involved. It may extend from this area but always in a continuous fashion, as contrasted to Crohn's disease, which tends to skip. X-ray studies of the colon aid in determining the extent of more proximal changes but should not be done during an acute attack, since it may precipitate toxic megacolon and perforation. Colonoscopy and biopsy can often differentiate ulcerative colitis from granulomatous colitis.

COMPLICATIONS

Complications of ulcerative colitis may be local or systemic. Rectal fistulae, fissures, and abscesses are not as common as in granulomatous colitis. Occasionally a rectovaginal fistula forms. A few patients may have narrowing of the bowel lumen as a result of fibrosis, which is generally mild compared to Crohn's disease.

One of the more serious complications is *toxic dilata-*

TABLE 22-1
Differentiating features of ulcerative colitis and Crohn's disease

CHARACTERISTIC FEATURE	ULCERATIVE COLITIS	CROHN'S DISEASE
Depth of involvement	Mucosa and submucosa	Transmural
Granulomatous inflammatory response	Rare	Common
Rectal involvement	95%	50%
Small bowel involved	Usually normal	80%
Right colon involved	Occasionally	Frequent
Distribution of lesion	Continuous with rectum	Discontinuous "skip" lesions
Inflammatory mass	Rare	Commonly palpable
Diarrhea	Common	Common
Rectal bleeding	Common, continuous	Rare
Internal fistulae	Rare	Common
Anal abscess	Occasional	Common
Anorectal fissures and fistulae	Rare	Common
Cobblestone appearance of mucosa	Unusual (pseudopolyps, granular, shaggy)	Common
Toxic megacolon	Occasionally	Rare
Malignant potential	High after 10 years	Very low
Extragastrointestinal manifestations (arthritis, eye and skin involvement, etc.)	Occasionally	Less frequent than in ulcerative colitis
Strictures	Occasionally, mild	Common
Finger clubbing	Rare	Common
Relative frequency	Five times more common than Crohn's disease	
Familial and Jewish association	Yes	Yes
Autoantibodies	Frequent	Not found

tion or *megacolon* in which there is paralysis of the motor function of the transverse colon, with rapid dilatation of that segment of the bowel. Toxic megacolon is most frequently associated with pancolitis. The mortality is about 30 percent, and perforation of the bowel frequently results. The treatment for this complication is emergency colectomy. Massive hemorrhage is another complication sometimes requiring emergency colectomy.

Carcinoma of the colon is another significant complication which occurs with increasing frequency after the patient has had the disease for more than 10 years. After patients have had total colon involvement with ulcerative colitis for 25 years, the probability of cancer is increased to 40 percent.

The systemic complications are diverse, and it is difficult to relate some of them causally to the colonic disease. These include pyoderma gangrenosum, episcleritis, uveitis, arthritis, and ankylosing spondylitis. Disordered hepatic function is common in ulcerative colitis, and established hepatic cirrhosis is an accepted complication. The presence of severe systemic complications may be an indication for surgical treatment of the colitis, even when the colonic symptoms are mild (see Fig. 22-5).

TREATMENT

There is no cure or specific medical treatment for ulcerative colitis. The aims of therapy are to control the inflammation, maintain the patient's nutritional status, give symptomatic relief, and prevent infection and other complications.

Corticosteroid drugs are given to reduce inflamma-tion and induce clinical remission. Sulfonamide drugs are given, but their mechanism of action is poorly understood. A low-residue diet causes diminution in the number of stools and thereby makes the patient more comfortable. The diet must also be high in protein to compensate for that lost in the exudative lesions and high in vitamins as well. During exacerbations, tincture of opium and paregoric are sometimes given to control diarrhea. Anticholingeric drugs also help relieve the abdominal cramps and diarrhea. Emotional support and reassurance is an important aspect of treatment.

When medical management fails and when the condition becomes intractable, surgical intervention is indicated. The most common procedure performed is total colectomy and the creation of a permanent ileostomy. Some physicians also recommend a colectomy for all patients who have had total colon involvement for more than 10 years, since the incidence of carcinoma of the colon is so high. Cancer of the colon is difficult to diagnose in these patients, since such symptoms as weight loss or bloody stools may be regarded as another exacerbation of the ulcerative colitis rather than as signs of cancer.

NEOPLASMS OF THE LARGE INTESTINE

Neoplasms of the colon and rectum may be benign or malignant. True benign neoplasms (lipomas, carcinoid tumors, and leiomyomas) are rare in the colon. Colonic polyps, however, are very common and occupy an intermediate position between benign and malignant neoplasms.

Colonic polyps

A polyp is a growth which arises from a mucosal surface and extends outward. There are three recognized pat-

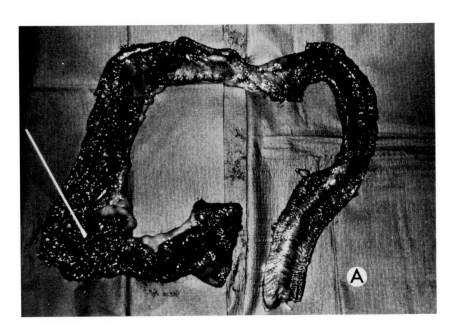

FIGURE 22-5 Some complications of ulcerative colitis. A, hemorrhage—surgical specimen of large intestine removed from a patient with ulcerative colitis to control bleeding. The probe is at the site of a small perforation. B, toxic megacolon. The large dilated colon is protruding through a surgical inicision. C, pyoderma gangrenosum. This is a necrotic skin ulcer found in association with inflammatory bowel disease.

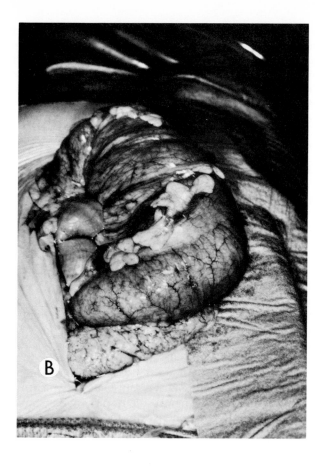

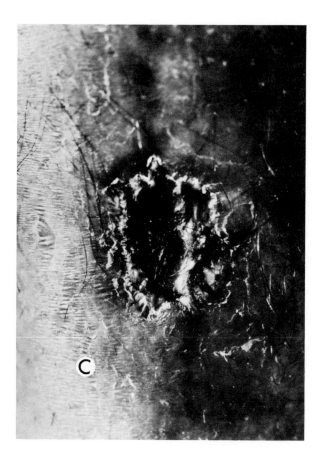

terns of colonic polyps: pedunculated adenomas, villous adenomas, and familial polyposis.

Pedunculated adenomas (also called adenomatous polyps or polypoid adenomas) are globelike structures attached to the mucous membrane by a thin stalk. This type of polyp occurs in both sexes and in all age groups, although they become increasingly common with advancing age. Autopsy and sigmoidoscopy studies show that 7 to 10 percent of the population over the age of 45 years is afflicted. Although pedunculated polyps may occur in any part of the colon, they are more frequently located in the distal 25 to 30 cm. Pedunculated polyps may be singular or multiple; they are usually 0.5 to 1.0 cm in diameter but may be as large as 4 or 5 cm. Histologically, these polyps consist of proliferating glands. The relationship of adenomatous polyps to cancer of the colon is a subject of great controversy, since they have much the same distribution in the colon as cancer and are often associated with cancer. The prevailing opinion is that they are harmless. However, if the polyps are multiple or if the head is greater than 1.0 cm in diameter, the chances of malignancy are higher.

Another form of pedunculated polyp occurring most frequently in children under the age of 10 years is the *juvenile polyp*. Juvenile polyps are often large, vascular, and have long pedicles. They are believed to be inflammatory in origin and may present by bleeding or prolapse through the anus. Juvenile polyps occasionally occur in adults.

The *villous adenoma* (villous papilloma, sessile adenoma), in contrast to the pedunculated adenoma, is a sessile (broad-based) tumor. The surface is distinctly papillary to the naked eye and appears as a nodular mass. Histologically, the lesion is composed of fingerlike (villous) projections. It is usually solitary and located in the sigmoid colon or rectum. Villous adenomas are generally large (greater than 5 cm) and are about one-eighth as frequent as pedunculated adenomas. Malignancy is much more likely to occur in these tumors (25 percent chance) than in the pedunculated adenomas.

Familial polyposis is a rare disorder transmitted genetically as a dominant trait and characterized by the presence of hundreds of adenomatous polyps, both pedunculated and sessile, throughout the entire large intestine. Both sexes are affected equally. The polyps are not present at birth but usually make their appearance about the time of puberty. The probability of the development of cancer increases with age and is almost 100 percent by the age of 40.

CLINCIAL FEATURES

Most adenomatous polyps are asymptomatic and are found incidentally on examination by sigmoidoscopy, barium enema, or on autopsy. When polyps do give rise to symptoms, these generally consist of overt or occult bleeding. Occasionally a large polyp may initiate an intussusception and cause bowel obstruction (see Fig. 21-5D). Diarrhea and mucus discharge may be associated with large villous adenomas and familial polyposis.

TREATMENT

The treatment of colonic polyps is influenced by the debate concerning their malignant potential. Since there is no question about the malignant potential in familial polyposis, this condition is treated by total proctocolectomy and permanent ileostomy or subtotal resection with ileorectal anastomosis. When the rectum is preserved, it is examined periodically for cancer.

The guidelines for the treatment of pedunculated or villous adenomas are not as clear. In general, polyps which are greater than 2 cm in diameter, multiple or villous, are regarded with a high degree of suspicion and should be removed. Polyps which are pedunculated, singular, and less than 1.0 in diameter are rarely malignant and can be observed periodically.

Polyps may be excised from below through the sigmoidoscope or colonoscope. Larger lesions and villous adenomas are treated by laporotomy and segmental resection.

Carcinoma of the colon and rectum

The colon (including rectum) is the most common site for malignancy of the gastrointestinal tract. Cancer of the colon is the second leading cause of all cancer deaths in both men and women in the United States and is led only by cancer of the lung and breast. Cancer of the large intestine is usually a disease of older people, and the peak incidence is in the sixth and seventh decades. It is rare below the age of 40, except in persons with a history of ulcerative colitis or familial polyposis. The sexes are affected about equally, although cancer of the colon is more common in women, while the lesion is more common in the rectum in males. Nearly three-fourths of all the cancers of the bowel occur in the rectosigmoid portion, so that they may either be palpated during a rectal exam or viewed with a sigmoidoscope. The cecum and ascending colon is the next most common site. The transverse colon and flexures are least likely to be affected.

The tumor may present as a *polypoid,* bulky fungating mass projecting into the lumen which becomes ulcerated very quickly or may extend around the bowel as an *annular,* ringlike stricture. Annular lesions are more common in the rectosigmoid portion of the bowel, while the polypoid or flat lesion is more common in the cecum and ascending colon. Histologically, almost all of the large bowel cancers are adenocarcinomas (composed of glandular epithelium) and may secrete mucus to a varying degree. The tumor may spread (1) by direct infiltration of adjacent structures, such as into the bladder;

(2) by lymphatics to the pericolic and mesocolic lymph nodes; and (3) by the bloodstream, usually to the liver, since the colon is drained by the portal system. The prognosis is relatively favorable when the lesion is confined to the mucosa and submucosa at the time of surgical resection and much less favorable when lymph node metastasis has occurred.

ETIOLOGY

Although the causes of cancer of the large bowel, as with other cancers, have not been established, certain predisposing factors have been identified. The relationship between ulcerative colitis, certain types of colonic polyps, and cancer of the bowel has already been discussed.

Another important predisposing factor may relate to dietary habits, since cancer of the bowel (like diverticulosis) is about 10 times more common in Western populations, which eat foods high in refined carbohydrates and low in roughage, than in primitive populations (Africa), which eat foods high in roughage. Burkitt has proposed that a low-fiber, highly refined carbohydrate diet leads to alterations in fecal flora and changes in the degradation of bile salts or of the breakdown products of protein and fat, some of which may be carcinogenic. The net result is prolonged contact time of potential carcinogens with the bowel mucosa.

CLINICAL FEATURES

The most common symptoms of cancer of the bowel are changes in bowel habits, bleeding, pain, anemia, anorexia, and weight loss. The signs and symptoms vary according to the location and are commonly divided into those affecting the right and left halves of the large bowel.

Carcinoma of the left colon and rectum tends to cause a change in bowel habits as a result of irritation and reflex responses. Diarrhea, crampy pain, and distention are common. Since lesions of the left colon tend to encircle, obstruction is a common problem. Stool may be narrow and ribbonlike in shape. Both mucus and gross blood are often visible on the feces. Anemia may result from chronic blood loss. A sigmoid or rectal growth may involve nerve roots, lymphatics, or veins, producing symptoms in the legs or perineum. Hemorrhoids, low back pain, rectal urgency, or urinary frequency may develop as a result of pressure on these structures.

Carcinoma of the right colon, where the bowel contents are liquid, tends to remain occult until far advanced. There is little tendency to obstruct, since the bowel lumen is larger and the feces is liquid. Anemia due to bleeding is common, but the blood is occult and can only be detected by a guaiac test (a simple test which may be performed on the clinical unit). Mucus is likewise not visible, as it is well mixed in the stool. In the thin person a tumor of the right colon may sometimes be palpated, but this is not usual at an early stage. The patient may suffer from vague abdominal discomfort which is sometimes epigastric.

The treatment of carcinoma of the colon and rectum is surgical removal of the tumor and its lymphatic drainage. The most common procedures performed are the right hemicolectomy, transverse colectomy, left hemicolectomy or anterior resection, and abdominoperineal resection. The results of surgical excision are fairly good compared to cancer in other areas of the body. The overall 5-year survival rate is approximately 50 percent.

ANORECTAL DISORDERS

Hemorrhoids

Hemorrhoids, or "piles," are varicose veins of the anal canal. They are usually arbitrarily divided into two classes, internal and external. Internal hemorrhoids are varices of the superior and middle hemorrhoidal veins, and external hemorrhoids are varices of the inferior hemorrhoidal veins. As the terms imply, the external hemorrhoids appear external to the sphincter ani muscles, and the internal hemorrhoids appear behind the sphincters.

Both types of hemorrhoids are very common and are present in about 35 percent of the population over the age of 25 years. Although the condition is not life-threatening, it may cause considerable discomfort.

Hemorrhoids result from venous congestion caused by interference with venous return from the hemorrhoidal veins. Several etiologic factors have been implicated, including constipation or diarrhea, straining, pelvic congestion associated with pregnancy, enlargement of the prostate, uterine fibroids, and tumors of the rectum. Chronic liver disease associated with portal hypertension frequently results in hemorrhoids, since the superior hemorrhoidal veins drain into the portal system (see Fig. 23-2). In addition, the portal system is valveless, so that backflow readily occurs.

External hemorrhoids are classified as acute or chronic. The acute form presents as a bluish, rounded swelling at the anal verge and is actually a hematoma, although it is referred to as an acute external thrombosed hemorrhoid. They are often quite painful and pruritic because the nerve endings in the skin are pain receptors. Sometimes it is necessary to evacuate the clot under local anesthesia, or it may be treated by hot sitz baths and analgesics. A chronic external hemorrhoid or skin tag is usually the sequel to an acute hematoma. Anal skin tags consist of one or more folds of anal skin composed of connective tissue and a few blood vessels.

Internal hemorrhoids are classified as first, second, and third degree. First-degree (early) internal hemorrhoids do not protrude through the anal canal and can only be detected by proctoscopy. They are usually located in the right and left posterior and right anterior positions, following the distribution of the tributaries of the superior hemorrhoidal vein, and appear as globular reddish swellings. Second-degree hemorrhoids may prolapse through the anal canal after defecation; they may recede spontaneously or can be reduced manually. Third-degree hemorrhoids are permanently prolapsed. The most common symptom of internal hemorrhoids is painless bleeding, since there are no pain fibers in this area. Most cases of hemorrhoids are of the mixed variety rather than being strictly internal or external.

The most common complications of hemorrhoids are bleeding, thrombosis, and strangulation. A strangulated hemorrhoid is a prolapsed one in which the blood supply is cut off by the anal sphincter.

Diagnosis of hemorrhoids is made by inspection and proctoscopy. When hemorrhoids and rectal bleeding occur in a middle-aged or older patient, it is important for the physician to rule out cancer.

The majority of patients with hemorrhoids need not undergo surgery. Medical treatment includes sitz baths or other forms of moist heat, bed rest, stool softeners to prevent constipation, and the use of suppositories. Surgical excision may be indicated when there is persistent bleeding, prolapse, or intractable pruritis and anal pain.

Anal fissure (fissure in ano)

An anal fissure (fissure in ano) is a crack in the lining of the anus caused by stretching from the passage of hard fecal matter; therefore, constipation is a common cause. The most prominent symptom is severe burning pain following defecation, and the bowel movement is usually accompanied by a small amount of bright red blood. These patients are nearly always constipated, and since the bowel movement is so very painful, the constipation becomes progressively worse, since they fear to have a bowel movement. Anal fissures are often seen in association with the skin tags of external hemorrhoids. Treatment is surgical excision of the tract if local dilatations, ointments, and cleansing do not help.

Anorectal abscess and fistula in ano

An anorectal abscess is a localized infection, with the collection of pus in the anorectal area. The infecting organisms are usually *Escherichia coli*, staphylococci, or streptococci. A fistula in ano is a chronic granulomatous tract that goes from the anal canal to the skin outside the anus or from an abscess to the anal canal or the perirectal area. An anorectal fistula is often preceded by abscess formation. The sites of abscess and fistula formation are illustrated in Fig. 22-6. The parianal abscess is the most common type of anorectal abscess, followed by the ischiorectal, submucous, and pelvirectal locations. The perianal abscess is usually obvious as a red, painful swelling close to the anal verge. The pain is aggravated by sitting or coughing. A submucous or ischiorectal abscess may be palpated as a swelling on rectal examination. A pelvirectal abscess may be more difficult to identify. Discharge of pus from an anorectal fistula may be the first sign. Sometimes a fistula may be palpated or its course determined by the gentle passage of a probe from the external opening, with a finger of the other hand in the anal canal.

Anorectal abscesses commonly begin as an inflammation of the anal crypts, which are located at the lower end of the columns of Morgagni. The anal glands open into these crypts. Obstruction or trauma to their ducts gives rise to stasis and predisposes to infection. Mucosal tears from hard, constipated stools may be a predisposing factor. In a few cases a predisposing local lesion such as ulcerated hemorrhoids or anal fissure may be present.

When symptoms of diarrhea are associated with recurrent anorectal fistulae, it is important to suspect Crohn's disease, since 75 percent of patients with Crohn's disease confined to the large bowel develop a fistula in ano. Twenty-five percent of patients develop a fistula in ano when Crohn's disease is confined to the small intestine.

The treatment of anorectal abscesses and fistulae is incision and drainage of the abscess and excision of any associated fistulae.

QUESTIONS

Large intestine—Chap. 22

Directions: Answer the following questions on a separate sheet of paper.

1 Draw a picture of the large intestine in the abdominal and pelvic cavities and label the parts with the following terms: appendix; cecum; ascending, transverse, descending, and sigmoid colon; rectum; anal canal; anus; hepatic and splenic flectures; haustra; and taenia coli.

2 What are the most important functions of the large bowel?

3 Discuss the differences in structure between the small and large bowel. How do these lead to differences in function?

4 Briefly summarize the mechanical operation of the large bowel (haustral churning, mass peristalsis).

5 List five common anorectal disorders.

6 List the most common diagnostic procedures used for the detection of disease of the large bowel. What can be detected with each?

7 Do all cases of acute diverticulitis require surgical intervention? If not, what is the medical treatment for acute diverticulitis?

8 Identify three predisposing factors in the pathogenesis of cancer of the colon or rectum.

9 What is Burkitt's hypothesis concerning the relationship of diet to the development of cancer of the bowel?

10 Why are hemorrhoids a frequent manifestation of hepatic cirrhosis and portal hypertension?

11 Define fissure in ano and fistula in ano. Is there any relationship between these two disorders and hemorrhoids? What disease of the gastrointestinal tract is often associated with anorectal fistulae?

Directions: Circle the letter preceding each item that correctly answers each question. Only one answer is correct, unless otherwise noted.

12 The right half of the colon receives its blood supply from the:

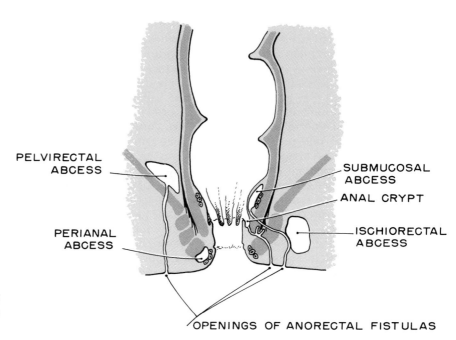

FIGURE 22-6 Common sites of anorectal abscesses and fistulae. Inflammation often begins in the anal crypts.

a Superior mesenteric artery   *b* Splenic artery
c Inferior mesenteric artery   *d* Left colic artery

13 The superior hemorrhoidal veins are part of the:
a Portal circulation   *b* Systemic circulation

14 The major reservoir for feces is in which segment of the large bowel?
a Cecum   *b* Transverse colon   *c* Ascending colon
d Descending colon   *e* Sigmoid colon

15 In which segment of the colon is the greatest amount of water absorbed?
a Cecum and ascending colon   *b* Descending and sigmoid colon   *c* Rectum

16 Which of the following statements are true about colonic mucus? (More than one answer may be correct.)
a It is under autonomic control   *b* Parasympathetic stimulation causes an increase in mucus production
c The colonic mucosa maintains a layer of mucus on its surface   *d* The presence of visible mucus in the stools indicates overproduction

17 Variations in intestinal gas normally depend on: (More than one answer may be correct.)
a How much air is swallowed   *b* Variations in diet
c Type of intestinal bacteria   *d* Weight of the individual

18 The desire to defecate is initiated by:
a Contraction of the external anal sphincter   *b* Contraction of the internal anal sphincter   *c* Contraction of the rectum   *d* Distention of the sigmoid colon
e Distention of the rectum

19 Substances produced by bacterial putrefaction in the large intestine:
a Indole   *b* Skatole   *c* Phenol   *d* Amino acids and fatty acids   *e* All of these

20 The cecum and ascending colon may be visualized on x-ray within how many hours after a barium meal?
a One-half   *b* 1 to 2   *c* 3 to 5   *d* 10 to 12

21 Approximately what percentage of rectal and large bowel tumors may be visualized or palpated on rectal digital or proctosigmoidoscopic examination?
a 100 percent   *b* 60 to 70 percent
c 25 to 35 percent   *d* 10 to 20 percent

22 Which of the following statements concerning diverticulosis is true? (More than one answer may be correct.)
a It is a common condition in persons over the age of 50 years in the United States.   *b* It occurs more frequently in Africans who eat a high-fiber diet.   *c* It is frequently associated with or preceded by the irritable colon syndrome.   *d* Disordered colonic motility with generation of high intraluminal pressures in the colon is important in the pathogenesis.
e Diverticula of the colon form most frequently at the point where arterioles penetrate the muscularis.

23 Diverticula are most common in which segment of the colon?
a Cecum   *b* Ascending colon   *c* Transverse colon
d Descending colon   *e* Sigmoid colon

24 The most common symptom of an attack of acute diverticulitis is:
a Pain in the lower left quadrant of the abdomen
b Pain in the lower right quadrant of the abdomen
c Vomiting   *d* Massive bleeding from the rectum

25 The most common complications of acute or chronic diverticulitis are: (More than one answer may be correct.)
a Massive bleeding requiring emergency colectomy
b Perforation   *c* Stricture causing partial bowel obstruction   *d* Vesicocolic fistula

26 The most common site of fistula formation as a result of a perforated diverticulum is the:
a Peritoneum   *b* Small intestine   *c* Urinary bladder
d Vagina

27 Which of the following is the most common clinical course of ulcerative colitis?
a Acute fulminating   *b* Acute onset with full recovery   *c* Chronic continuous   *d* Chronic continuous with full recovery after 5 to 10 years   *e* Chronic intermittent (relapsing–remitting course)

28 Patients with ulcerative colitis may reveal abnormalities in which of the following organ systems? (More than one answer may be correct.)
a Joints   *b* Heart   *c* Eyes   *d* Lungs   *e* Skin

29 The rectosigmoid segment of the large bowel is involved in what percentage of cases of ulcerative colitis?
a 15 percent   *b* 45 percent   *c* 75 percent
d 95 percent

30 Which of the following statements are true concerning toxic megacolon? (More than one answer may be correct.)
a It is often associated with pancolitis.   *b* The motor function of a bowel segment is paralyzed.   *c* The transverse colon is frequently affected.   *d* It is usually treated medically.   *e* It is associated with a high mortality.

31 A cardinal symptom or sign of ulcerative colitis is:
a Constipation   *b* Diarrhea with blood and mucus in the stool   *c* Ribbon-shaped stools   *d* Periumbilical pain

32 Some of the known extracolonic manifestations of ulcerative colitis are: (More than one answer may be correct.)
a Uveitis   *b* Pyoderma gangrenosum   *c* Episcleritis
d Arthritis   *e* Ankylosing spondylitis

33 Skin manifestations are associated with which of the following disorders? (More than one answer may be correct.)
a Diverticulosis   *b* Ulcerative colitis   *c* Cancer of the colon   *d* Granulomatous colitis   *e* Regional enteritis

34 The role of adrenal steroid drugs in the treatment of ulcerative colitis is to:
a Cure the active disease b Induce clinical remission c Prevent recurrence completely

35 The most common surgical treatment for intractible ulcerative colitis is:
a Right hemicolectomy b Left hemicolectomy
c Total colectomy with permanent ileostomy
d Cecostomy

36 Cancer of the bowel involving which of the following sites is frequently diagnosed late in its course?
a Cecum b Descending colon c Sigmoid colon
d Rectum

37 The most common cause of death secondary to gastrointestinal cancer in the United States is from cancer of the:
a Esophagus b Stomach c Small intestine
d Colon and rectum

38 The most common symptom of cancer of the right colon is:
a Change in bowel habits b Pain c Constipation
d Gross blood in the stools e Diarrhea

39 Symptoms which commonly accompany cancer of the left colon include: (More than one answer may be correct.)
a Change in bowel habits b Melana
c Back pain d Abdominal cramps

40 Which statements are true with respect to adenomatous polyps? (More than one answer may be correct.)
a It is the most common type of benign tumor in the colon. b They are most frequently located in the distal 25 to 30 cm of the bowel. c They are familial.
d They occur more frequently in patients with cancer of the large bowel. e Generally benign when singular or less than 1 cm in diameter.

41 Familial polyposis of the colon is characterized by: (More than one answer may be correct.)
a Densely packed polyps throughout the colon b An inheritable recessive trait c Marked predisposition to cancer of the large bowel d Alopecia

42 The most common site of malignant lesions of the large bowel:
a Rectosigmoid area b Descending colon
c Cecum d Transverse colon

Directions: Fill in the blanks with the correct word(s) or circle the correct option.

43 _____ is a condition in which there is herniation of the mucosa through the muscularis of the large bowel to form flask-shaped saccules. The condition is called _____ when the saccules become inflamed.

44 A _____ adenoma or adenomatous polyp is a globelike structure on a pedicle arising from a mucosal surface. _____ polyps have very long pedicles and often occur in children.
A _____ adenoma is a broad-based tumor composed of villous projections. _____
_____ is a hereditary disease characterized by the presence of hundreds of polyps throughout the colon.

45 An encircling or _____ form of cancer growth is more common in the left colon, while the _____ shape is more likely to be _____ in the cecum.

46 Three routes of metastasis from cancer of the bowel are_____, _____
_____, and _____.

47 Internal hemorrhoids are varicosities of the _____
_____ and _____ hemorrhoidal veins and are located (inside or outside) the anal sphincters. The _____ hemorrhoidal veins are involved in external hemorrhoids.

48 Three common complications of hemorrhoids are
_____, _____,
and _____.

Directions: Match each of the following characteristic features of inflammatory bowel disease in col. A with the correct disorder in col. B.

Column A	Column B
49 ____ Caused by a specific infectious agent	a Crohn's disease
50 ____ Granulomatous inflammation	b Ulcerative colitis
51 ____ Familial and Jewish association	c Both
52 ____ Transmural lesion common	d Neither
53 ____ Internal fistulae common	
54 ____ Lesions continuous with rectum	
55 ____ High malignant potential after 10 years	
56 ____ Most commonly associated with toxic megacolon	
57 ____ Most common disease of the two	
58 ____ "Skip" lesions common	
59 ____ May represent an immunologic disorder	
60 ____ Anorectal abscesses, fissures, and fistulae common complications	

61 Rank the following types of colonic polyps according to malignant potential, with 1 being the highest:
a Villous adenoma b Familial polyposis c Pedunculated polyp less than 1.0 cm in diameter

Directions: Circle T if the statement is true and F if it is false. Correct the false statements.

62 T F Fecal incontinence results from destruction of the 2nd to 4th sacral segments of the spinal cord.

63 T F The external anal sphincter is under autonomic nervous control.

64 T F Diverticulitis almost always requires surgical resection.

65 T F Vitamin D is synthesized in the large bowel by the action of colonic bacteria.

66 T F Normally, about 1000 ml of flatus is expelled from the anus daily.

67 T F Barium enema x-ray is generally contraindicated during acute diverticulitis because of the danger of perforation.

68 T F First-degree internal hemorrhoids are permanently prolapsed.

69 T F Second-degree hemorrhoids prolapse following straining at the stool but recede spontaneously or can be reduced manually.

70 T F Approximately 5 percent of the population over the age of 25 years suffer from hemorrhoids.

71 T F The parianal and ischiorectal areas are the most common sites of anorectal abscess formation.

72 T F The formation of an anorectal abscess or fistulae is often preceded by an anal cryptitis initiated by a mucosal tear from hard feces.

73 T F Successful treatment of anorectal abscess or fistulae usually requires surgery.

74 T F Medical treatment of hemorrhoids includes stool softeners, moist heat, and the use of suppositories.

REFERENCES

BOGOCH, ABRAHAM (ed.): *Gastroenterology,* McGraw-Hill, New York, 1973, pp. 602–618, 636–683, 695–699.

BROOKS, F. P. (ed.): *Gastrointestinal Pathophysiology,* Oxford University Press, New York, 1974, pp. 21–26, 249–268.

BURKITT, D. P.: "Epidemiology of the Colon and Rectum," *Cancer,* **28**: 3–13, 1971.

GIVEN, B. A. and S. J. SIMMONS: *Gastroenterology in Clinical Nursing,* 2d ed., C. V. Mosby, St. Louis, 1975, pp. 219–234.

GREENBERGER, N. J. and D. H. WINSHIP: *Gastrointestinal Disorders: A Pathophysiologic Approach,* Yearbook, Chicago, 1976, pp. 174–205.

MENDELOFF, A. I., J. T. LaMONT, and K. J. ISSELBACHER: "Diseases of the Colon and Rectum," in *Harrison's Principles of Internal Medicine,* 7th ed., McGraw-Hill, New York, 1974, pp. 1488–1509.

NAISH, J. M. and A. E. A. READ: *Basic Gastroenterology,* 2d ed., Yearbook, Chicago, 1974, pp. 329–338.

NETTER, FRANK H.: *Ciba Collection of Medical Illustrations, Vol. 3, Digestive System, Part II, Lower Digestive Tract,* Ciba Pharmaceutical Co., Summit, N.J., 1962, pp. 54–60, 77, 86–87, 170, 173.

ROBBINS, S. L. and M. ANGELL: *Basic Pathology,* Saunders, Philadelphia, 1971, pp. 425–433.

CHAPTER 23 Liver, Biliary Tract, and Pancreas

OBJECTIVES   **At the completion of Chap. 23, you should be able to:**

1 Describe the anatomic relation of the liver to the biliary tract, stomach, duodenum, and pancreas.

2 Describe the gross structure, size, and shape of the liver.

3 Describe the structure and function of the liver lobule.

4 Explain why blood circulation through the liver is unusual.

5 Identify the capillary beds which drain into the portal circulation and clinically significant points of anastomosis between the portal and systemic circulations.

6 List and describe the eight major functions of the liver.

7 Identify the major components of bile.

8 Identify the major plasma proteins and coagulation factors synthesized by the liver.

9 Describe the circulatory, defense, and detoxification functions of the liver.

10 Describe the gross structure and function of the gallbladder.

11 Identify the following structures of the biliary tract: right hepatic duct, common hepatic duct, cystic duct, common bile duct, ampulla of Vater, and sphincter of Oddi.

12 Describe the gross structure of the pancreas: size, shape, divisions, and ducts.

13 Describe the histology of the pancreas in relation to its functions.

14 Identify the three types of pathologic changes in diseases of the liver, gallbladder, and pancreas.

15 Explain the clinical significance of the following tests in the evaluation of liver, biliary, and pancreatic function: serum and urine bilirubin, urobilinogen, bromosulphalien (BSP) test, serum proteins, prothrombin time, blood ammonia, serum and urine amylase, serum lipase, cholesterol, enzymes, and hepatitis B antigen.

16 Identify the radiographic techniques used in the diagnosis of liver, biliary, and pancreatic disorders and describe what each may reveal.

17 Describe a liver biopsy (preparation, contraindications, procedure, aftercare, and possible complications).

18 Describe the methods of portal pressure measurement and the significance of an elevation.

19 Define jaundice and indicate the sites of earliest detection.

20 Outline the steps of normal bilirubin metabolism.

21 Differentiate between unconjugated and conjugated bilirubin.

22 Identify the four general pathogenetic mechanisms of hyperbilirubinemia and jaundice; describe disorders associated with each.

23 Define kernicterus.

24 Explain the pathogenesis of transient jaundice common in the newborn.

25 Differentiate between intrahepatic and extrahepatic cholestasis and list the common causes of each.

26 Compare the following features of hemolytic, hepatocellular, and obstructive jaundice: skin, urine and stool color, pruritis, serum and urine bilirubin, and urine urobilinogen.

27 Contrast hepatitis A and hepatitis B with respect to the following features: common synonyms, transmission, incubation, presence of hepatitis antigens in serum, population affected, seasonal incidence, clinical features and general prognosis, and complications.

28 Describe the morphologic changes in the liver in a mild case of hepatitis.

29 Describe the clinical features of hepatitis during the prodromal, icteric, and recovery phases.

30 Differentiate between chronic persistent and chronic active hepatitis.

31 Describe the treatment of hepatitis.

32 Describe the value of gamma globulin in the prevention and treatment of hepatitis A and B.

33 List public health and clinical measures to reduce the incidence of hepatitis.

34 Define cirrhosis of the liver and describe its consequences.

35 Identify the single most important cause of cirrhosis.

36 Distinguish among Laennec's, postnecrotic, and biliary patterns of cirrhosis on the basis of prevalence, gross and microscopic pathology, pathogenesis, and prognosis.

37 Describe the relationship between malnutrition, alcoholism, and fatty infiltration of the liver.

38 Describe alcoholic hepatitis and its possible relationship to cirrhosis.

39 Explain the relationship of primary cancer of the liver to cirrhosis.

40 Distinguish between primary and secondary biliary cirrhosis.

41 Explain the pathophysiologic basis of the following clinical manifestations of cirrhosis: jaundice, peripheral edema, hepatic coma, gynomastia, spider angiomas, testicular atrophy, altered hair distribution, hypoalbuminemia, increased bleeding tendency, anemia, leukopenia, thrombocytopenia, and splenomegaly.

42 Define portal hypertension and identify the basic mechanism responsible for its development in cirrhosis of the liver.

43 Define ascites and identify key factors responsible for its development.

44 Explain the development of esophageal varices, prominent superficial abdominal veins, and internal hemorrhoids in cirrhotics.

45 Discuss possible complications from esophageal varices, including the treatment and prognosis.

46 Describe possible complications in the treatment of ascites with diuretics or a large paracentesis.

47 Identify the basic characteristics of hepatic encephalopathy.

48 Identify the primary source of ammonia in the body, its normal metabolism, and excretion.

49 Describe the relationship of liver cell failure and/or portal-systemic shunting to the development of hepatic encephalopathy.

50 Identify several endogenous or exogenous factors which may precipitate hepatic encephalopathy.

51 Describe the major signs, symptoms, and electroencephalogram findings of the four stages in the progression of hepatic encaphalopathy to coma.

52 Describe asterixis, how it is tested, and its significance.

53 Describe constructional apraxia and its significance in monitoring the progression of hepatic encephalopathy.

54 Explain why it is important to detect hepatic encephalopathy in its early stages.

55 Describe the treatment of hepatic encephalopathy, including measures to prevent its recurrence.

56 Explain why dietary protein restriction, removal of blood from the intestinal tract, and intestinal sterilization are important measures in the treatment of hepatic encephalopathy.

57 Compare the characteristics of bilirubin, cholesterol, and mixed cholesterol gallstones.

58 Describe cholelithiasis and cholecystitis (incidence, population affected, etiology, pathogenesis, clinical features, diagnosis, complications, and treatment).

59 Define the identifying characteristics of acute and chronic pancreatitis.

60 Describe the mechanisms which protect the normal pancreas from autodigestion.

61 List the two primary etiologic factors in acute and chronic pancreatitis.

62 Describe the range of injury in acute pancreatitis and possible mechanisms causing the injury.

63 Describe the signs, symptoms, diagnosis, and treatment objectives for acute pancreatitis.

64 Differentiate between a pancreatic abscess and a pseudocyst.

65 Describe the primary features of chronic pancreatitis (pathology, etiology, clinical course, diagnosis, and treatment).

66 Discuss the prevalence, types, and general prognosis of primary cancer of the liver, gallbladder, and pancreas.

67 Explain the relationship of gallstones and cirrhosis of the liver to cancer of the gallbladder and liver.

68 Identify possible reasons why the liver is such a common site of malignant tumor metastasis.

69 Explain why cancer of the gallbladder or pancreas is usually diagnosed in an advanced stage.

The liver, biliary tract, and pancreas all develop as off-shoots of the fetal foregut in a region which later becomes the duodenum and are intimately associated with the physiology of digestion. It is reasonable to consider these structures together because of their anatomic proximity, their closely related functions and the similarity of the symptom complexes induced by many of their disorders.

Liver

The liver is the largest gland in the body, averaging about 1500 g, or 2.5 percent of the body weight in a normal human adult (see Fig. 23-1). It is a soft plastic organ which is molded by the surrounding structures. The superior surface is convex and lies beneath the right dome of the diaphragm and part of the left. The lower portion of the liver is concave and provides a roof over the right kidney, stomach, pancreas, and intestines. There are two principal lobes, the right and the left. The right lobe is divided into anterior and posterior segments, and the left is divided into medial and lateral segments by the falciform ligament. The *falciform ligament* passes from the liver to the diaphragm and the anterior abdominal wall. The surface is covered by visceral peritoneum, except for a small area on its posterior surface which is attached directly to the diaphragm. Several ligaments which are reflections of the peritoneum help to support the liver. Beneath the peritoneum is a dense connective tissue layer called the *capsule of Glisson,* which covers the surface of the entire organ, and at the hilum or *porta hepaticus* on the inferior surface, it is continued into the liver substance, forming a framework for the branches of the portal vein, hepatic artery, and bile ducts.

MICROSCOPIC STRUCTURE

Each lobe of the liver is divided into structures called *lobules,* which are the microscopic and functional units of the organ (see inset of Fig. 23-1). Each lobule is a hexagonal body composed of plates of cuboidal hepatic cells arranged radially around a central vein that drains it. Between the plates of hepatic cells are capillaries called *sinusoids*, which are branches of the portal vein and hepatic artery. The sinusoids, unlike other capillaries, are lined with phagocytic or *Kupffer cells*. Kupffer cells belong to the reticuloendothelial system, and their main function is to engulf bacteria and other foreign particles in the blood. Only the bone marrow exceeds the liver in the mass of reticuloendothelial cells; thus it is one of the principal organs of defense against bacterial invasions and toxic agents. In addition to branches of the portal vein and hepatic artery encircling the periphery of the liver lobule, bile ducts are also present. The interlobular bile ducts form very small bile capillaries called *canaliculi* (not shown), which course within the center of the liver cell plates. Bile formed in the hepatocytes is excreted into the canaliculi, which join to form larger and larger bile ducts until the common bile duct is reached.

CIRCULATION

The liver has a dual blood supply: from the digestive tract and the spleen via the *portal vein* and from the aorta via the *hepatic artery*. About one-third of the incoming blood is arterial and about two-thirds is venous from the portal vein. A total volume of 1500 ml passes through the liver each minute and is drained via the right and left *hepatic veins,* which empty into the inferior vena cava (see Fig. 23-2).

The portal vein is unique in that it is interposed between two capillary beds: one in the liver and the other in the digestive area which it drains. Upon entering the liver, the portal vein divides into branches which come into contact with the circumference of the liver lobule. These branches then give off interlobular veins, which run between the lobules. These give rise to the sinusoids, which run between the plates of hepatocytes to enter the central veins. Central veins from several lobules join to form the sublobular veins, which in turn join to form the hepatic veins (refer back to inset of Fig. 23-1). The finest branches of the hepatic artery also empty into the sinusoids, making the blood composition unique in that it is a mixture of arterial blood from the hepatic artery and venous blood from the portal vein. Figure 23-2 illustrates the origin of blood flowing into the portal system; increased pressure in this system is a common manifestation in liver disorders, with serious consequences involving the vessels in which the portal blood originates. Several points of portacaval anastomosis are of clinical significance. In cases of obstruction to flow in the liver, portal blood may be shunted around the liver to the systemic venous system. The consequences of portal hypertension and shunting are discussed in greater detail later in this chapter.

LIVER FUNCTION

In addition to ranking first in size as a parenchymal organ, the liver also ranks first in the number, complexity, and variety of its functions. The liver is essential for the maintenance of life and is involved in almost every metabolic function of the body and is specifically responsible for more than 500 separate activities. Fortunately, it has a large reserve capacity and needs only 10 to 20 percent functioning tissue to sustain life. Complete destruction or removal of the liver results in death within 10 hours. The liver has an impressive regenerative ability. Partial surgical removal will, in most cases, initiate a rapid replacement of dead or diseased cells with new liver tissue.

Table 23-1 lists the major functions of the liver.

Understanding these functions is a prerequisite to understanding its pathophysiology.

The formation and excretion of bile is a major function of the liver; the bile ducts transport and the gallbladder stores and releases bile into the small intestine as needed. The liver secretes about 1 liter of yellow bile each day. The basic components of bile are water (97 percent), electrolytes, bile salts, phospholipids (mainly lecithin), cholesterol, and bile pigments (mainly conjugated bilirubin). Bile salts are essential for fat digestion and absorption in the small intestine. After being acted upon by bacteria in the small intestine, most of the bile salts are reabsorbed in the ileum, recirculated to the liver, and reconjugated and resecreted (see Chap. 21). Although bilirubin (bile pigment) is a metabolic end product and has no physiologically active role, it is nonetheless important as an indicator of

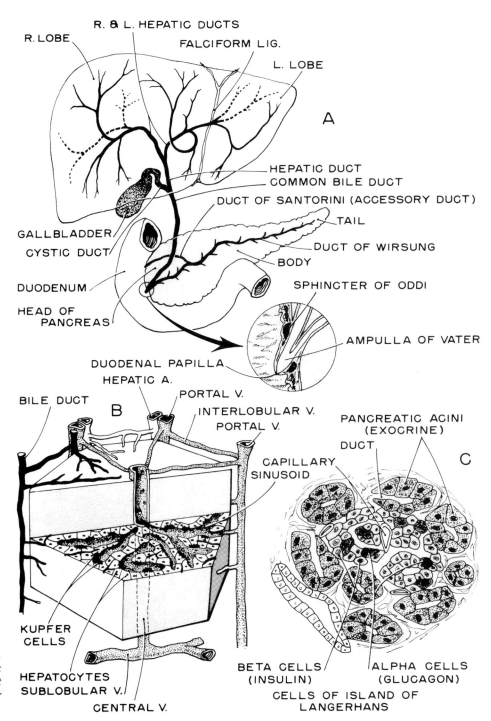

FIGURE 23-1 A, liver, gallbladder, and pancreas. B, microscopic structure of hepatic functional unit (liver lobule). C, pancreatic acinar units.

liver and biliary tract disease, since it tends to color tissues and fluid with which it comes in contact. Normal bilirubin metabolism and jaundice as a sign of disease are discussed later in this chapter.

The liver plays an essential role in the metabolism of three types of foodstuffs delivered by the portal vein after absorption from the intestines. These are carbohydrates, proteins, and fats. Monosaccharides from the small intestine are converted into glycogen and stored as such in the liver (glycogenesis). From this storage depot of glycogen, a constant supply of glucose is released into the blood (glycogenolysis) to meet the changing body requirements. Some of the glucose is metabolized in the tissues to produce heat and energy, and the remainder is converted either into glycogen and stored in the muscles or into fat and stored in the subcutaneous tissues. The liver is also capable of synthesizing glucose from proteins and fat (gluconeogenesis). The role of the liver in protein metabolism is essential to survival. The plasma proteins, except gamma globulin, are synthesized by the liver. These include albumin, which is necessary for the maintenance of the colloid osmotic pressure, and prothrombin, fibrinogen, and other clotting factors. In addition, most degradation of amino acids begins in the liver with deamination, or the removal of an amino group (NH_3). The ammonia released is then synthesized into urea and excreted by the kidneys and intestines. Ammonia formed in the gut by the action of bacteria on protein is also converted to urea in the liver. Other metabolic functions of the liver include fat metabolism; vitamin, iron, and copper storage; the conjugation and excretion of adrenal and gonadal steroids;

and the detoxification of numerous endogenous and exogenous substances. The detoxification function is very important and is accomplished by liver enzymes which oxidize, reduce, hydrolyze, or conjugate the potentially harmful substance, rendering it physiologically inactive. Endogenous substances, such as indol, skatol, and phenol, which are produced by the action of bacteria on amino acids in the large intestine, and exogenous substances, such as morphine, phenobarbital, and other drugs, are detoxified in this manner.

Finally, the liver functions as a "flood chamber" and "filter" because of its strategic position between the intestinal and general circulation. In cases of right heart failure, the liver may become passively congested with a large amount of blood. The Kupffer cells in the sinusoids filter the portal blood of bacteria and other injurious materials by phagocytosis.

Gallbladder

The gallbladder is a pear-shaped hollow sac resting directly beneath the right lobe of the liver (see Fig. 23-1). Bile, which is being secreted continuously by the liver, enters the small bile ducts within the liver. The small bile ducts join to form two larger ducts which emerge from the undersurface of the liver as the *right* and *left hepatic ducts* but which immediately join to

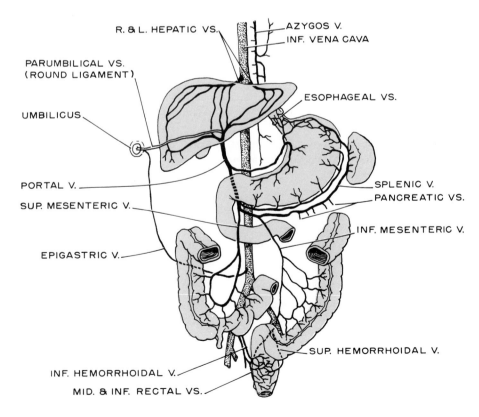

R. & L. HEPATIC VS.
AZYGOS V.
INF. VENA CAVA
PARUMBILICAL VS.
(ROUND LIGAMENT)
UMBILICUS
ESOPHAGEAL VS.
PORTAL V.
SUP. MESENTERIC V.
SPLENIC V.
PANCREATIC VS.
INF. MESENTERIC V.
EPIGASTRIC V.
SUP. HEMORRHOIDAL V.
INF. HEMORRHOIDAL V.
MID. & INF. RECTAL VS.

FIGURE 23-2 Hepatic-portal system. Blood is carried from the stomach, intestines, spleen, and pancreas into the liver sinusoids. Hepatic veins convey it to the inferior vena cava. Clinically significant sites of anastomosis between the hepatic and systemic circulations are (1) through the esophageal veins (portal tributary) which anastomose with the azygos veins (systemic tributary); (2) the paraumbilical veins in the round ligament originate in the left branch of the portal vein and connect with the superficial veins of the anterior abdominal wall (systemic tributaries) in the area of the umbilicus; (3) the superior rectal or hemorrhoidal veins (portal tributary) anastomose with the middle and inferior rectal veins (systemic tributaries); (4) the portal tributaries to the intestines, pancreas, and liver anastomose with the phrenic, renal, and lumbar veins (systemic tributaries not shown). In portal hypertension and chronic liver disease, blood may back up in these veins and shunted around the liver through the points of anastomoses.

form the *common hepatic duct*. The hepatic duct merges with the *cystic duct* from the gallbladder, forming the *common bile duct*. In many persons, the common bile duct merges with the pancreatic duct to form the *ampulla of Vater* (dilated portion in common channel) before opening into the small intestine. The terminal parts of both ducts and the ampulla are surrounded by circular muscle fibers, known as the *sphincter of Oddi*.

The principle function of the gallbladder is the storage and concentration of bile. It is capable of holding about 45 ml of bile. Hepatic bile may not immediately enter the duodenum; instead, after passing down the hepatic duct, it may be diverted into the cystic duct and gallbladder. In the gallbladder, the lymphatics and blood vessels absorb water and inorganic salts, so that gallbladder bile is about 10 times as concentrated as hepatic bile. At intervals the gallbladder contents are emptied into the duodenum by simultaneous contraction of the muscular coat and relaxation of the sphincter of Oddi. The normal stimulus of gallbladder contraction and emptying is the entry of acid chyme into the duodenum. The presence of fatty foods is the strongest stimulus to contraction. The hormone CCK-PZ mediates the contraction.

Pancreas

The pancreas is a long slender organ about 6 in in length and 1.5 in in width. It lies retroperitoneal and is divided into three major segments—the head, body, and tail (see Fig. 23-1). The head lies in the concavity formed by the duodenum, and the tail touches the spleen.

The pancreas is made up of two basic types of cells having entirely different functions (see inset of Fig. 23-1). The exocrine cells, called *acini*, produce the components of the pancreatic juice (see Table 21-1). The endocrine cells, or islets of Langerhans, produce the endocrine secretions insulin and glucagon, which are important for carbohydrate metabolism.

TABLE 23-1
Major functions of the liver

FUNCTION	COMMENTS
Formation and excretion of bile Bile salts metabolism	Bile salts are essential for the digestion and absorption of fats and fat-soluble vitamins in the intestine.
Bile pigment metabolism	Bilirubin, the main bile pigment, is a metabolic end product from the processing of old red blood cells. It is conjugated in the liver and excreted in bile.
Carbohydrate metabolism Glycogenesis Glycogenolysis Glyconeogenesis	Liver plays an important part in maintaining the normal blood glucose level and providing energy for the body. Carbohydrate is stored in the liver as glycogen.
Protein metabolism Protein synthesis	Serum proteins synthesized by the liver include albumin, and the alpha and beta globulins (except gamma globulin).
	Blood-clotting factors synthesized by liver include fibrinogen (I), prothrombin (II), and factors V, VII, VIII, IX, and X. Vitamin K is a necessary cofactor in the synthesis of II, V, IX, and X.
Urea formation	Urea is formed exclusively in the liver from NH_3, which is then excreted in the urine and feces. NH_3 is formed from deamination of amino acids and action of intestinal bacteria on amino acids.
Protein (amino acid) storage	
Fat metabolism Ketogenesis	Hydrolysis of triglycerides, cholesterol, phospholipids, and lipoproteins (absorbed from intestine) to fatty acids and glycerol.
Cholesterol synthesis Fat storage	Liver plays major role in cholesterol synthesis, most of which is excreted in the bile as cholesterol or cholic acid.
Vitamin and mineral storage	Fat-soluble vitamins (A, D, E, K) stored in liver; also vitamin B_{12}, copper, and iron.
Steroid metabolism	Liver inactivates and excretes aldosterone, glucocorticoids, estrogen, progesterone, and testosterone.
Detoxification	Liver responsible for biotransformation of substances that are potentially harmful into harmless substances which are then excreted by kidneys (e.g., drugs).
Flood chamber and filter action	Liver sinusoids provide depot for blood backed up from venae cavae (right heart failure); phagocytic action of Kupffer cells remove bacteria and debris from blood.

The pancreas is a compound tubuloalveolar gland. As a whole, it resembles a bunch of grapes, the branches of which are the ducts terminating in the main pancreatic duct (duct of Wirsung). Small ducts from each acinus empty into the main ducts. The main duct, extending throughout the length of the gland, often joins the common bile duct at the ampulla of Vater before entering the duodenum. An accessory duct, the *duct of Santorini*, is frequently found extending from the head of the pancreas into the duodenum, about an inch above the duodenal papilla.

OVERVIEW

Pathologic changes in diseases of the liver, gallbladder, and pancreas may be broadly categorized into three types: inflammatory, fibrotic, and neoplastic. Hepatitis, cholecystitis, and pancreatitis show evidence of acute or chronic inflammation of the involved tissues. Gallstones and biliary tract obstruction are frequently associated with cholecystitis and pancreatitis. Fibrotic changes occur with cirrhosis of the liver and in chronic inflam-

matory conditions. Primary tumors of the liver, pancreas, or gallbladder, whether benign or malignant, are rare. Widespread destruction of parenchymal cells resulting from inflammation, fibrosis, neoplasms, or obstruction interferes with secretory and excretory functions. Jaundice (yellow coloration of the body tissues) is a common symptom and results from interference with the excretion of bilirubin. Portal hypertension, ascites, esophageal varices, and hepatic encephalopathy are common complications in advanced cirrhosis and hepatic failure.

DIAGNOSTIC TESTS

Table 23-2 lists some of the most common diagnostic tests used to detect disordered function of the liver, gallbladder, and pancreas. It should be emphasized that

TABLE 23-2
Tests of liver, biliary, and pancreatic function

TEST	NORMAL	CLINICAL SIGNIFICANCE
Biliary excretion		Measures the ability of the liver to conjugate and excrete bile pigment.
Direct serum bilirubin (conjugated)	0.1–0.4 mg%	Direct bilirubin elevated with impaired excretion of conjugated bilirubin.
Indirect serum bilirubin (unconjugated)	0.1–0.5 mg%	Indirect bilirubin elevated in hemolytic conditions and Gilbert's syndrome.
Total serum bilirubin	0.2–0.9 mg%	Both direct and total serum bilirubin elevated in hepatocellular disease.
Urine bilirubin	0	Conjugated bilirubin excreted in urine when elevated in serum, suggesting liver cell or biliary tract obstruction. Urine appears brown, and foam appears yellow when shaken—simple bedside test.
Urine urobilinogen	0–4 mg/24 h	Decreased with impaired bile excretion; increased when amount produced exceeds ability of liver to reexcrete it as in hemolytic jaundice.
Dye excretion Bromsulphalien test (BSP) Indocyanine green (less commonly used)	<5% retention in 1 h	Nontoxic dye removed from blood, stored, conjugated, and then excreted in the bile. Excretion dependent on functional liver cells, patent biliary ducts, and hepatic blood flow. BSP test is a very sensitive index of liver function, useful in detecting early liver cell damage and recovery from infectious hepatitis.
Protein metabolism Total serum protein Serum albumin Serum globulin	6–8 g% 3.5–5.5 g% 1.5–3 g%	Most of the serum proteins and coagulation proteins are synthesized by the liver and are therefore decreased in a variety of liver impairments.
Prothrombin time	11–16 sec	Increased with decreased synthesis due to liver cell damage or decreased vitamin K absorption in biliary obstruction. Vitamin K essential for prothrombin synthesis.

TABLE 23-2 (continued)

Blood ammonia	30–70 μg%	Liver converts NH_3 to urea. Rises in hepatic failure or in large portal-systemic shunts.
Carbohydrate metabolism Serum amylase	60–180 units /100 ml	Obstruction and inflammatory disease of the pancreas interfere with normal flow of amylase into intestinal tract and result in increased serum levels. Marked increase in acute pancreatitis (also increased in parotid gland disease and many other conditions).
Urine amylase	<260 units/h	Urinary amylase increased longer than serum amylase (1 wk); >300 units/h indicates pancreatitis.
Fat metabolism Serum lipase Serum cholesterol	<1.5 units 150–280 mg%	Pancreatic digestive enzyme released into blood with breakdown of acinar cells in obstructive or inflammatory conditions of pancreas. Cholesterol increased in bile duct obstruction; decrease in liver cell damage.
Serum enzymes SGOT SGPT LDH	5–40 units/ml 5–35 units/ml 90–200 milliunits/ml (varies with units used)	Enzymes serum glutamic oxaloacetic transaminase (SGOT), serum glutamic pyruvic transaminase (SGPT), and lactic dehydrogenase (LDH) are concentrated, especially in heart, liver, and skeletal muscle. Released from damaged tissue (necrosis or altered cell permeability). Increased in liver cell damage and in other conditions especially myocardial infarction.
Alkaline phosphatase	2–5 Bodansky units	Manufactured in bone, liver, kidneys, intestine, and excreted in bile. Increased in biliary obstruction. Also increased in bone disease, liver metastasis.
Immunologic tests		Key diagnostic test in detecting hepatitis B antigen (HBAg or Australia antigen) in long-incubation or serum hepatitis.

TABLE 23-3
Radiologic methods in the diagnosis of liver, biliary, and pancreatic disorders

TEST	COMMENTS
Plain film of abdomen	May reveal calcific densities in the gallbladder, biliary tree (gallstones), pancreas, and liver. May also reveal splenomegaly.
Barium meal (see Fig. 23-3A)	Esophageal varices are revealed in 70–90% of the cases. Tumors of the head of the pancreas often produce a displacement or irregularity of the second portion of the duodenum (reverse 3 sign common).
Oral cholecystogram	Conjugation and excretion of the dye by the liver allows visualization of the gallbladder and bile ducts, thus revealing gallstones. Poor or nonvisualization of the contrast media may be caused by liver cell disease or biliary obstruction.
Intravenous cholecystogram	Used to visualize the bile ducts and for localization of obstructive lesions of the major ducts.
Transhepatic cholangiogram (see Fig. 23-3B)	Dye given by percutaneous puncture and blind probing for a bile duct into which dye is injected. May help to distinguish hepatic from posthepatic jaundice. Hazards involve bile leakage and hemorrhage.
Endoscopic retrograde cholangiopancreatography (ERCP) (see Fig. 23-3B)	Endoscopic insertion of a catheter into the duodenal papilla—injection of contrast medium through catheter into pancreatic or biliary ductiles allows visualization of these structures.
Radioisotope liver scan with radio-tagged iodinated rose bengal, gold, or technetium (see Fig. 23-3C)	Reveals anatomic changes in liver tissue; lesions appear as filling defects (tumors, cysts, abscesses).
Selective celiac axis angiography (see Fig. 23-3D)	Visualization of pancreatic, hepatic, and portal circulation possible, revealing tumor masses, disruption as in cirrhosis, and portal collateral circulation.
Portal pressure measurement (see Fig. 23-3E)	Principal procedures are percutaneous splenic pulp manometry, transhepatic puncture, and catheterization of the hepatic vein or the umbilical-portal vein. Portal pressure elevated in cirrhosis. Procedures often combined with injection of contrast medium.
Splenoportogram (see Fig. 23-3E)	Demonstrates size and patency of portal and splenic collaterals.

no single test or procedure is capable of measuring the total function of the liver, since it is involved in nearly every metabolic process in the body and has a large functional reserve. Usually a battery of diagnostic tests is utilized.

Radiologic methods useful in the diagnosis of disorders of the liver, biliary system, and pancreas are summarized in Table 23-3. Other diagnostic methods include esophagoscopy, allowing direct visualization of esophageal varices; duodenoscopy, allowing visualization of the papilla of Vater and insertion of a catheter in order to inject contrast medium directly into the biliary or pancreatic system; peritoneoscopy (insertion of peritoneoscope through an abdominal stab wound), allowing direct visualization of the anterior surface of the liver and gallbladder; and an electroencephalogram, which may be abnormal in hepatic encephalopathy. Finally, percutaneous liver biopsy is a common proce-

dure performed at the bedside and is described in greater detail below.

Percutaneous liver biopsy is a valuable method of diagnosing diffuse parenchymal disease such as cirrhosis, hepatitis, and drug reactions. Prior to performing the procedure, the patient's capacity to clot blood is evaluated, and cross-matched blood is provided in case of need. The procedure itself is brief. The skin is cleansed and anesthetized. As the patient holds his or her breath in expiration to bring the liver and diaphragm to the highest position, the needle is inserted into the liver in the eighth or ninth intercostal or subcostally and withdrawn (see Fig. 23-3F). The specimen is

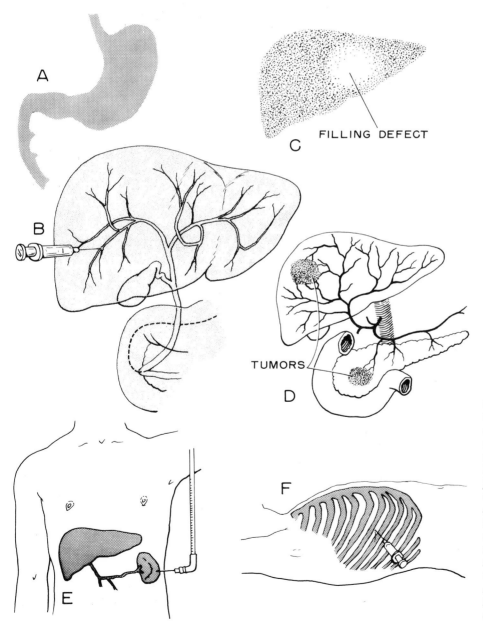

FILLING DEFECT

TUMORS

FIGURE 23-3 Illustrations of diagnostic tests useful in the diagnosis of liver, biliary, and pancreatic disorders. A, barium x-ray of the GI tract. B, transhepatic cholangiogram in which contrast material is injected percutaneously. The hepatic or pancreatic ductal systems may also be approached from below by inserting a catheter into the papilla of Vater and injecting contrast material (ERCP). C, liver scan. D, selective celiac axis angiography. E, splenoportogram and measurement of portal pressure. F, liver biopsy. (See Table 23-3 and text for explanation of tests.)

then expelled into formalin for later histologic examination. It is vitally important that patients understand that they are to hold their breath and not move during the procedure to prevent laceration of the liver. The procedure is contraindicated in patients who cannot meet this requirement.

After the procedure the patient lies on the right side for about 2 hours to splint the chest and remains in bed for 24 hours. Although rare, complications of liver biopsy may be dangerous. The chief danger is intraperitoneal hemorrhage (0.2 percent), which results from penetration of a large blood vessel. Bile peritonitis is a rare but serious complication requiring immediate surgical intervention. Vital signs are checked every 15 minutes until stable and then every 1 or 2 hours for the first 24 hours after the procedure. The dressing is checked frequently for local bleeding, and a pressure dressing is applied if necessary. Severe abdominal pain may indicate bile peritonitis and should be carefully evaluated. Figure 23-3 illustrates some of the diagnostic procedures useful in the diagnosis of liver, biliary, and pancreatic disorders.

BILIRUBIN METABOLISM AND JAUNDICE

The accumulation of bile pigments in the body causes yellow discoloration of the tissues called *jaundice*. Jaundice can usually be detected in the sclerae (whites of eyes), skin, or by a darkening of the urine when the serum bilirubin reaches 2 to 3 mg%. The normal serum bilirubin is 0.2 to 0.9 mg%. Surface tissues richest in elastin, such as the sclerae and the under surface of the tongue, usually become stained first.

A consideration of the mechanisms of jaundice involves an understanding of the formation, transportation, metabolism, and excretion of bilirubin.

Normal bilirubin metabolism

In the normal individual, bilirubin formation and excretion proceeds smoothly through the steps outlined in Fig. 23-4. About 85 percent of the bilirubin is produced by the breakdown of senescent red blood cells in the reticuloendothelial system. The average life span of a red blood cell is 120 days. Each day about 50 ml of blood is destroyed, producing 200 to 250 mg of bilirubin. It is now known that about 15 percent of total bile pigment does not depend on this mechanism but is derived from destruction of maturing erythroid cells in the bone marrow (ineffective hematopoiesis) and from other hemoproteins, notably in the liver.

In the catabolism of hemoglobin (largely occurring in the spleen), globin is first dissociated from heme, after which the heme is converted to biliverdin. Unconjugated

bilirubin is then formed from biliverdin. Unconjugated bilirubin, loosely bound to albumin, is transported in the blood to the liver cells. Bilirubin metabolism by the liver cell involves three steps—uptake, conjugation, and excretion. Uptake by the liver cell involves two cytoplasmic or acceptor proteins, which have been designated as Y and Z proteins. Conjugation of bilirubin with glucuronic acid takes place in the endoplasmic reticulum of the liver cell. This step is dependent on the presence of glucuronyl transferase, an enzyme which catalyzes the reaction. Conjugation of the bilirubin molecule greatly changes its characteristics. Conjugated bilirubin is lipid-insoluble, water-soluble, and capable of being excreted in the urine. In contrast, unconjugated bilirubin is lipid-soluble, water-insoluble, and incapable of being excreted in the urine. Transport of conjugated bilirubin across the cell membrane and secretion into the bile canaliculi by an active process is the final step of bilirubin metabolism in the liver. In order to be excreted in the bile, bilirubin must be conjugated. Conjugated bilirubin is then excreted via the biliary tree into the small intestine.

Intestinal bacteria reduce conjugated bilirubin to a series of compounds called stercobilin or urobilinogen. These substances account for the brown color of stool. About 10 to 20 percent of the urobilinogen undergoes enterohepatic circulation, while a small fraction is excreted in the urine.

Pathophysiologic mechanisms in jaundice states

There are four general mechanisms by which hyperbilirubinemia and jaundice can occur: (1) excess production of bilirubin; (2) impaired hepatic uptake of unconjugated bilirubin; (3) impaired conjugation of bilirubin, and (4) decreased excretion of conjugated bilirubin into bile due to both intrahepatic and extrahepatic factors which may be functional or due to mechanical obstruction. The first three mechanisms result in predominantly unconjugated hyperbilirubinemia, while the fourth results in predominantly conjugated hyperbilirubinemia.

EXCESS BILIRUBIN PRODUCTION

Hemolytic disease, or an increased rate of red blood cell destruction, is the most common cause of excess bilirubin production. The resultant jaundice is customarily called *hemolytic jaundice*. Conjugation and transfer of bile pigment proceeds normally, but the supply of unconjugated bilirubin is greater than the liver can handle. Consequently, the level of unconjugated bilirubin in the blood rises. The serum bilirubin level, however, rarely exceeds 5 mg% in patients with severe hemolysis, and the jaundice is a mild pale yellow. Since unconjugated bilirubin is water-insoluble, it cannot be excreted in the urine, and bilirubinuria does not occur. There is, however, increased production of urobilinogen (due to the increased bilirubin load presented to the

FIGURE 23-4 Normal bilirubin metabolism.

liver and increased conjugation and excretion), which in turn results in increased fecal and urinary excretion. The urine and stool may thus be darker.

Some common causes of hemolytic jaundice are abnormal hemoglobins (hemoglobin S in sickle cell anemia), abnormal red blood cells (hereditary spherocytosis), antibodies in the serum (Rh or transfusion incompatibility or as a result of autoimmune hemolytic disease), administration of some drugs, and some lymphomas (enlarged spleen and increased hemolysis). In some cases hemolytic jaundice may result from increased destruction of red blood cells or their precursors in the bone marrow (thalassemia, pernicious anemia, porphyria). This process is referred to as ineffective erythropoiesis.

In the adult, chronic overproduction of bilirubin may lead to the formation of gallstones predominantly composed of bilirubin; otherwise the mild hyperbili-

rubinemia is not generally harmful. Treatment is directed toward correction of the hemolytic disease. However, in infancy unconjugated bilirubin levels over 20 mg% may lead to *kernicterus,* a condition in which bilirubin is deposited in the lipid-rich basal ganglia of the brain, causing damage.

IMPAIRED UPTAKE OF BILIRUBIN

Gilbert's syndrome is a benign familial condition characterized by mild unconjugated hyperbilirubinemia (<5 mg%) and jaundice. The degree of jaundice fluctuates, and it is often aggravated by prolonged fasting, infec-

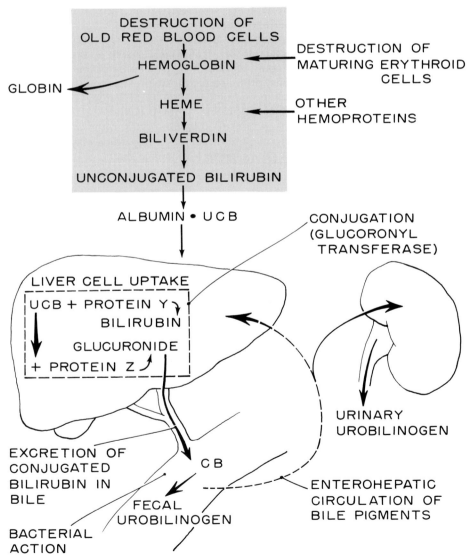

tion, stress, or trauma. The onset is most common during adolescence, and the condition is reported to affect about 5 percent of the male population. Liver function tests and fecal and urinary urobilinogen levels are normal. Bilirubinuria is absent. The underlying defect is considered to be a deficiency of the hepatic uptake of bilirubin, although impaired conjugation may also play a role. One of the most important aspects of Gilbert's syndrome is its recognition so that the affected individual can be reassured that the condition is benign.

Impaired uptake of bilirubin resulting from immaturity of the Y and Z acceptor proteins may play a role in neonatal jaundice. In other conditions, damage to these proteins by certain drugs such as novobiocin, infection, or malnutrition may also account for elevation of unconjugated serum bilirubin.

IMPAIRED CONJUGATION OF BILIRUBIN

The Crigler-Najjar syndrome is a rare hereditary disease in humans in which there is a complete deficiency of glucuronyl transferase from birth. Since conjugation of bilirubin cannot take place, the bile is colorless, unconjugated serum bilirubin generally exceeds 20 mg%, and kernicterus is common. The prognosis is poor, and death usually occurs during infancy or early childhood. In a milder form of the disease in which there is only a partial deficiency of glucoronyl transferase, jaundice may not be manifested until adolescence, and the prognosis is good. Phenobarbital, which is able to induce increased gluceronyl transferase activity, often causes jaundice to disappear in these patients.

The transient unconjugated hyperbilirubinemia which develops during the second and fifth day of life in the newborn is believed to result from immaturity of the hepatic enzyme system.

DECREASED EXCRETION OF CONJUGATED BILIRUBIN

Impaired excretion of bilirubin, whether due to functional or obstructive factors, results in predominantly conjugated hyperbilirubinemia. Because conjugated bilirubin is water-soluble, it is excreted in the urine, giving rise to bilirubinuria and dark urine. Fecal and urinary urobilinogen are commonly decreased, so that the stools are pale. Elevated conjugated bilirubin levels may be accompanied by other evidence of hepatic excretory failure, such as elevated serum levels of alkaline phosphatase, SGOT, cholesterol, and bile salts. The presence of elevated bile salts in the blood adds the new dimension of itching to the jaundice. Jaundice resulting from conjugated hyperbilirubinemia is usually deeper than that resulting from unconjugated hyperbilirubinemia. The color change ranges from a mild or deep orange-yellow to a yellow-green in cases of complete

obstruction of biliary outflow. These changes are evidence of *cholestatic jaundice,* which is another name for *obstructive jaundice.* Cholestasis may be either *intrahepatic* (involving the liver cell, canaliculi, or cholangioles) or *extrahepatic* (involving bile ducts outside the liver). Similar biochemical disturbances are present in both.

The most common causes of intrahepatic cholestasis are *hepatocellular diseases* in which the hepatic parenchymal cells are damaged by viral hepatitis and the various types of cirrhosis. In these diseases, swelling and disorganization of the liver cells can compress and block the canaliculi or cholangioles. Hepatocellular disease usually interferes with all phases of bilirubin metabolism—uptake, conjugation, and excretion—but since excretion is usually impaired to the greatest extent, conjugated hyperbilirubinemia predominates. Other less common causes of intrahepatic cholestasis include certain drugs and the rare hereditary disorders of the Dubin-Johnson and Rotor syndromes. In these conditions, there appears to be interference with transfer of bilirubin across the hepatocyte membrane. Common offending drugs include halothane (anesthetic), oral contraceptives, estrogens, anabolic steroids, isoniazid, and chlVDpromazine.

The most common causes of extrahepatic cholestasis are impaction of a gallstone, usually at the lower end of the common bile duct; carcinoma of the head of the pancreas, producing extrinsic pressure on the bile duct; and carcinoma of the ampulla of Vater. Less common causes are strictures from previous inflammation or surgery and enlarged lymph nodes in the porta hepatis. Intrahepatic lesions such as a hepatoma may sometimes obstruct the right or left hepatic ducts.

Intrahepatic versus extrahepatic cholestasis

The most important diagnostic decision for the physician and surgeon in conjugated hyperbilirubinemia is to decide whether the obstruction to bile flow is intrahepatic or extrahepatic. Extrahepatic cholestasis may benefit from surgery, while surgery on a patient with hepatocellular disease (intrahepatic cholestasis) may enhance the illness and even lead to death. The differentiation is not easy, since all forms of cholestasis produce the same clinical syndrome of jaundice, itching, increased transaminases, increased alkaline phosphatase, defective excretion of cholecystographic dyes, and nonvisualization of the gallbladder. Although the ultimate judgment is a clincial one, help in making the differentiation comes from evaluating the degree of obstruction. Intrahepatic obstruction is seldom as complete as extrahepatic obstruction. Consequently, intrahepatic cholestasis generally results in only moderate elevations of alkaline phosphatase, and small amounts of pigment appear in the stools or urobilinogen in the urine when compared to extrahepatic cholestasis. Liver biopsy or duodenal or transphepatic cholangiography may be utilized to clarify difficult cases. Table 23-4 lists some of the differentiating features of the common types of jaundice.

Acute viral hepatitis is an infectious disease which is generalized in its distribution within the body, although the predominant effect is on the liver. The best known forms of hepatitis are hepatitis A and hepatitis B. These terms are preferred to the former terminology of infectious and serum hepatitis, since both diseases may be transmitted through parenteral and nonparenteral routes. Other synonyms and the differential features of hepatitis A and B are listed in Table 23-5 and are discussed in the following pages. Newer immunologic techniques are being developed to identify other forms of viral hepatitis (non-A and non-B hepatitis).

Hepatitis has become an important public health problem not only in the United States but also throughout the world. More than 60,000 cases are reported to the Center for Disease Control each year in the United States, and each year the number steadily increases. Although mortality from viral hepatitis is relatively low, extensive morbidity and economic loss are associated with the disease.

Etiology and epidemiology

Numerous studies in human volunteers have clearly shown that hepatitis can be transmitted between persons by a bacteria-free filtrate. Although the virus causing hepatitis has not yet been propagated in tissue

TABLE 23-4
Differentiating features of hemolytic, hepatocellular, and obstructive jaundice

FEATURE	HEMO-LYTIC	HEPATO-CELLULAR	OBSTRUC-TIVE
Skin color	Pale yellow	Mild or deep orange-yellow	Mild to deep yellow-green
Urine color	Normal (may darken urobilin)	Dark (conjugated bilirubin)	Dark (conjugated bilirubin)
Stool color	Normal or dark ($\uparrow$ stercobilin)	Pale (less stercobilin)	Clay-colored
Pruritis	None	Not persistent	Usually persistent
Serum bilirubin: (Indirect or unconjugated)	Increased	Increased	Increased
(Direct or conjugated)	Normal	Increased	Increased
Urine bilirubin	Absent	Increased	Increased
Urine urobilinogen	Increased	Slight increase	Decreased

culture or in experimental animals, recent significant discoveries have provided new insights which may eventually lead to better control of the disease. Two types of circulating antigen are present in the majority of patients with type B hepatitis. Hepatitis B surface antigen (HB_sAg), previously referred to as the Australia antigen or hepatitis-associated antigen, is believed to be the outer coat of the hepatitis B virus. Hepatitis B core antigen (HB_cAg) is believed to be the core of the virus that is produced and replicates in the hepatocyte nucleus, causing tissue damage. In addition, antibodies to both the surface and core antigens exist (anti-HB_s, and anti-HB_c). Neither the antigens nor the antibodies exist in the serum of patients with documented infections with hepatitis A. HBAg appears in the serum of patients during the incubation period before the signs and symptoms of hepatitis appear and usually disappears within 3 to 12 weeks. Studies of HBAg-positive blood donors have clearly shown a high frequency of hepatitis in recipients of HBAg-positive transfusions. In addition, HBAg has been found in urine, feces, saliva, nasopharyngeal washings, and semen, indicating that infection may be transmitted by nonparenteral routes. Since the presence of HBAg is the mark of infectivity, an HBAg-positive patient should be regarded as potentially infectious. HBAg occurs in about 0.1 percent of the normal population and in 5 to 10 percent of patients following recovery from hepatitis B infection. It is not clear whether these persons are carriers or have chronic anicteric hepatitis.

Classically, the incubation period for hepatitis A was believed to range from 30 to 60 days (short incubation) and that of hepatitis B from 50 to 180 days (long incubation). Recent data, however, show that the incubation period for hepatitis A ranges from 28 to 94 days and that patients with hepatitis B become HBAg-positive 17 to 98 days after exposure to the infecting agent. Viremia occurs during the incubation period and during the early phase of the illness in both hepatitis A and B. Recent studies reveal that fecal excretion of the virus occurs in hepatitis B as well as in A.

Hepatitis A occurs mainly in the fall and early winter, affecting children more often than adults. Fecal–oral transmission, primarily by person-to-person contact, is the most common mode of transmission. It is transmitted by human carriers and persons who are incubating the disease. Sporadic cases occur, and epidemics may arise from spread by contaminated water or food, especially in institutional settings. Other modes of transmission include the ingestion of uncooked clams, oysters, and other shellfish which may harbor the virus. Hepatitis A may also be transmitted parenterally.

Hepatitis B occurs all year round and affects all age groups. Parenteral transmission seems to be the major mode of spread, although recent evidence implicates fecal–oral transmission as well. Contamination of needles, syringes, lancets, and tattooing instruments has been associated with outbreaks. Drug addicts who share common needles and syringes are at high risk. Patients on chronic hemodialysis, as well as the staff who care for them, are also at high risk. The virus has been transmitted in as little as 0.00004 ml of blood. It was hoped that the elimination of HBAg-positive blood donors would eliminate the problem of posttransfusion hepatitis, but it now appears that hepatitis A (or other viruses) may also be responsible. A test for the detection of hepatitis A virus is badly needed. Whole blood and blood products, with the exception of immuno-globulins, treated albumin, and the plasma protein fraction, may be contaminated with the hepatitis virus.

Pathology

The morphologic changes in the liver are identical in hepatitis A and B. In the classic case, the liver appears normal in size and color but is sometimes slightly edematous, enlarged, and bile-stained. Histologically,

there is hepatocellular disarray, varying degrees of liver cell injury and necrosis, and periportal inflammation. These changes are completely reversible when the acute phase of the disease subsides. In a few cases, sub-massive or massive necrosis may lead to fulminant hepatic failure and death.

Clinical features

Infection with a hepatitis virus can result in a range of effects from fulminant hepatic failure to anicteric sub-clinical hepatitis. The latter is more common in type A infections, and the patient often mistakes it for the "flu." Type B infections tend to be more severe than type A infections, and the incidence of massive necrosis and fulminant hepatic failure is more common.

The vast majority of both hepatitis A and B infections are mild with complete recovery, and the clinical features are similar. Prodromal symptoms occur in all patients and may be present for a week or so before the onset of jaundice (although not all patients develop jaundice). The main features at this time are malaise, lassitude, anorexia, headache, low-grade fever, and the loss of desire to smoke. Many patients experience arthralgias, arthritis, urticaria, and transient skin rashes.

TABLE 23-5
Differential features of viral hepatitis

	HEPATITIS A	HEPATITIS B
Synonyms	Infectious hepatitis Short-incubation hepatitis	Serum hepatitis Long-incubation hepatitis
Tests for hepatitis antigens and antibodies (i.e., HB_sAg, HB_cAg, anti-HB_s, anti-HB_c)	Negative	Positive
Incubation period	28 to 94 days	17 to 98 days
Age groups	More common in young children and in institutional settings	All age groups affected. Drug addicts, patients on chronic hemodialysis, and medical personnel are at high risk
Season	Fall and early winter	All year round
Transmission	Usually fecal to oral route among persons living in close contact; contaminated water supply; shellfish; also transmitted by parenteral route	Usually by transfusion of blood and blood products or some other form of inoculation, especially parenteral drug abuse; also transmitted by the fecal–oral route
Clinical features	Majority of type A infections mild and anicteric; patient simply thinks it is the "flu"	Type B hepatitis tends to be more severe and sometimes requires hospitalization for extended periods
	Fatigue, anorexia, low-grade fever, abdominal discomfort, arthralgias, skin rashes, enlarged tender liver, light stools, dark urine, jaundice	Similar changes in hepatitis B
	Elevated SGOT, SGPT (early), hyperbilirubinemia, abnormal liver function tests	
Mortality	Less frequent	More frequent
Incidence of chronic aggressive hepatitis as a complication	Very low	Somewhat higher

Rarely, glomerulonephritis occurs. These extrahepatic manifestations of viral hepatitis may represent a syndrome similar to serum sickness and may be caused by circulating immune complexes. In addition, there may be discomfort in the right upper quadrant, usually attributed to stretching of the liver capsule.

The prodromal phase is followed by the icteric phase and the onset of jaundice. This phase usually lasts 4 to 6 weeks. During this phase, there is generally an improved feeling of well-being. Appetite returns and the fever subsides as the urine becomes darker and the stool somewhat paler. The liver is moderately enlarged and tender, and the spleen is palpably enlarged in about one-fourth of the patients. A tender lymphadenopathy is often present.

The earliest biochemical abnormality is an elevation of SGOT and SGPT levels, which precedes the onset of jaundice by 1 or 2 weeks. Urine examination at the onset will reveal the presence of bilirubin and an excess of urobilinogen. The bilirubinuria persists throughout the illness, but the urobilogen may disappear temporarily if there is an obstructive phase due to cholestasis; this clears during the recovery phase.

The icteric phase is associated with hyperbilirubinemia (both conjugated and unconjugated fractions), which is usually less than 10 mg%. The serum alkaline phosphatase level is usually normal or only moderately elevated. A mild leukocytosis is usually found in viral hepatitis, and the prothrombin time may be prolonged. HBAg is found in the serum during the prodromal phase and definitely establishes type B hepatitis.

In the uncomplicated case, recovery begins 1 or 2 weeks from the onset of jaundice and lasts from 2 to 6 weeks. Easy fatigability is a common complaint. The stools rapidly regain their normal color, the jaundice lessens, and urine color lightens. Splenomegaly, if present, rapidly subsides, but hepatomegaly may return to normal only some weeks later. Liver function tests may be abnormal for 3 to 6 months.

Complications

Not every patient with viral hepatitis pursues an uneventful course. A few patients (less than 1 percent) show rapid clinical deterioration following the onset of jaundice due to fulminant hepatitis and massive liver necrosis. Death may occur within days in some patients, while others may survive for weeks if the damage is less extensive. Many of these patients are obese, middle-aged females, and there is frequently an associated acute renal failure. Fulminant viral hepatitis is more common in type B infections contracted through the parenteral route than in type A infections contracted through the fecal–oral route.

The most common complication of viral hepatitis is a more prolonged course lasting 4 to 8 months. This is called *chronic persistent hepatitis,* and it occurs in 5 to 10 percent of patients. Despite the delayed convalescence in chronic persistent hepatitis, patients almost always recover.

Approximately 5 percent of patients with viral hepatitis have a relapse following recovery from the initial episode. This is usually associated with the ingestion of alcohol or undue physical exertion. Commonly, the jaundice is not as marked, and the liver function tests do not show the same degree of abnormality. Further bed rest is usually followed by an uneventful recovery.

Following acute viral hepatitis, a few patients may develop *chronic active* or *aggressive hepatitis* in which there is piecemeal destruction of the liver and the development of cirrhosis. The condition is distinguished from chronic persistent hepatitis by liver biopsy. Corticosteroid therapy may retard the progression of hepatic injury, but the prognosis is poor. Death usually occurs within 5 years as a result of hepatic failure or the complications of cirrhosis. Chronic active hepatitis is more common following type B infections than type A. There is persistence of HBAg in the serum in about one-third of the patients, which may be related to the development of chronic active hepatitis. It is possible that the chronicity or activity of the hepatitis may be related to immunologic mechanisms initiated by the acute hepatitis. Not all cases of chronic active hepatitis follow acute viral hepatitis. Drugs may be involved in the pathogenesis of this disorder. Specific drugs implicated include alphamethyldopa or Aldomet, isoniazid, sulfonamides, and aspirin.

Treatment

There is no specific treatment for viral hepatitis. Bed rest during the acute phase and a diet that is both acceptable and nutritious are the usual general measures. Intravenous feeding may be necessary during the acute phase if the patient has persistent vomiting. Some limitation of physical activity is usually necessary until symptoms have subsided and the liver function tests return to normal.

Prevention

If individuals have been in contact with or are liable to be exposed to cases of viral hepatitis, the use of human gamma globulin is recommended. The recommended dose is 0.01 ml/lb body weight by intramuscular injection. If given early enough, gamma globulin is highly effective in reducing the incidence of hepatitis A. In cases of exposure to type B virus, there is at least some possibility that the globulin may contain sufficient quantities of hepatitis B antibody to be helpful. Gamma globulin is of no value in the treatment of overt hepatitis.

Community measures important in the prevention of hepatitis include the provision of a safe food and water supply as well as effective sewage disposal. Careful attention to general hygiene, handwashing, and safe disposal of the urine and feces of infected patients are important. Personnel engaged in high-risk contact, such as in hemodialysis, exchange transfusions, and parenteral therapy, need to exercise great care in the handling of equipment and the avoidance of needle puncture. The use of disposable catheters, needles, and syringes eliminates an important source of infection. All blood donors should be screened for the presence of HBAg before being accepted on the donor panel.

CIRRHOSIS OF THE LIVER

Cirrhosis is a chronic disease of the liver characterized by distortion of the normal hepatic architecture by bands of connective tissue and by nodules of regenerating liver cells unrelated to the normal vasculature. The regenerating nodules may be small (micronodular) or large (macronodular). Cirrhosis may interfere with intrahepatic blood circulation, and in far advanced cases it causes gradual failure of liver function.

The incidence of this disease has increased significantly since World War II, establishing cirrhosis as one of the most prominent causes of death in the adult male. This increase is due in part to a corresponding increase in the incidence of viral hepatitis but more significantly to an enormous increase in the intake of alcohol. Alcoholism is the single most important cause of cirrhosis.

Etiology, pathology, and pathogenesis

Although the etiology of many forms of cirrhosis is poorly understood, three characteristic patterns account for the majority of cases—Laennec's, postnecrotic, and biliary cirrhosis.

LAENNEC's CIRRHOSIS

Laennec's cirrhosis (also called alcoholic, portal, and nutritional cirrhosis) is a peculiar pattern of cirrhosis associated with chronic abuse of alcoholic beverages. It accounts for 50 percent or more of the cases of cirrhosis.

The exact relationship between alcohol abuse and Laennec's cirrhosis is not known, although there is a clear and unmistakable association. The first change in the liver caused by alcohol is the gradual accumulation of fat within the liver cells (fatty infiltration). A similar pattern of fatty infiltration is also seen in kwashiorkor (a disorder common in backward nations as a result of severe protein deficiency), hyperthyroidism, and diabetes. Most authorities agree that alcoholic beverages exert a direct toxic affect on the liver. The accumulation of fat reflects a number of metabolic disturbances, including excess formation of triglycerides, their de-

creased utilization in the formation of lipoproteins, and decreased oxidation of fatty acids. It is also possible that the person ingesting excess alcohol does not eat properly and fails to consume enough protein to provide a sufficient quantity of lipoprotein agents (choline and methionine) needed for the transport of fat. It is known that low-protein diets depress the activity of alcohol dehydrogenase, the principal enzyme which metabolizes alcohol. However, the primary cause of liver damage is believed to be the direct effect of alcohol on the liver cell, which is increased by malnutrition.

Uncomplicated fatty degeneration of the liver, such as might be seen in early alcoholism, is reversible provided the person ceases ingestion of alcohol; very few cases of this relatively benign condition progress to cirrhosis. Grossly the liver is enlarged, fragile, and greasy in appearance and may be functionally deficient because of the large accumulation of fat.

If the habit of alcohol abuse persists, particularly when it becomes more severe, something may occur (it is not known for sure what does it) to tip the whole process in favor of widespread scar formation. Some authorities (Helman et al., 1971), believe that the critical lesion in the development of cirrhosis of the liver may be alcoholic hepatitis. Alcoholic hepatitis is characterized histologically by hepatocellular necrosis and polymorphonuclear neutrophil leukocyte (PMN) infiltration of the liver. However, not all patients who develop the lesion of alcoholic hepatitis progress to full-blown cirrhosis of the liver.

In far-advanced cases of Laennec's cirrhosis, thick fibrous bands form at the periphery of many lobules, partitioning the parenchyma into fine nodules. These nodules may enlarge somewhat as a result of regenerative activity as the liver attempts to replace damaged cells. The liver appears to consist of tightly packed nests of degenerating and regenerating liver cells encased in thick fibrous capsules. On this basis the condition is often referred to as fine nodular cirrhosis. In the final stages the liver is shrunken, hard, and almost devoid of normal parenchyma, resulting in portal hypertension and hepatic failure.

POSTNECROTIC CIRRHOSIS

Postnecrotic cirrhosis presumably follows patchy necrosis of liver tissue, resulting in large and small degenerative nodules surrounded and partitioned by scar and interspersed with normal liver parenchyma. About 75 percent of the cases tend to progress and result in death within 1 to 5 years. Postnecrotic necrosis accounts for about 20 percent of the cases of cirrhosis. About 25 percent of the cases have a prior history of viral hepatitis. Many patients have positive test results for HBAg, indicating that chronic active hepatitis may be an essential event. A small percentage of cases stem from documented intoxication with industrial chemicals, poisons, or drugs, such as phosphorus, chloroform, carbon tetrachloride, or poison mushrooms.

A peculiar feature of postnecrotic cirrhosis is that it appears to predispose the patient to the occurrence of a primary hepatic neoplasm of the liver (hepatoma). This is seen to a somewhat lower degree in Laennec's cirrhosis also.

BILIARY CIRRHOSIS

Liver cell destruction that begins around the bile ducts gives rise to a pattern of cirrhosis known as biliary cirrhosis. It accounts for about 15 percent of the cases of cirrhosis.

The most common cause of biliary cirrhosis is post-hepatic biliary obstruction. Stasis of bile causes its accumulation within the liver substance with destruction of liver cells. Fibrous bands begin forming around the periphery of the lobule, but rarely do they transect a lobule as in the pattern of Laennec's cirrhosis. The liver is enlarged, firm, finely, granular, and has a green hue. Jaundice is always an early and primary part of the syndrome, as is pruritis, malabsorption, and steatorrhea.

Primary biliary cirrhosis presents a pattern somewhat similar to the secondary biliary cirrhosis just described, but it is much more rare. The cause of this condition associated with lesions of the intrahepatic bile ductules is unknown. The bile capillaries and ductules contain bile plugs, and the liver cells frequently contain a green pigment. The extrahepatic biliary tract is not involved. Portal hypertension as a complication is rare.

Clinical manifestations

The clinical features and complications of cirrhosis are common to all forms of the disease regardless of the cause, although individual types of cirrhosis may have additional distinctive clinical and biochemical features. The period during which cirrhosis presents as a clinical problem is generally only a small fraction of the total life history of the disease. For many years, cirrhosis is latent, the pathologic changes progressing slowly until major symptoms induce awareness of the disease. During the long latent period, there is a gradual deterioration of liver function.

Early symptoms are vague and nonspecific and include lassitude, anorexia, dyspepsia, flatulence, a change in bowel habits (either constipation or diarrhea), and slight weight loss. Nausea and vomiting, especially in the morning, are common. A dull ache or heavy feeling in 'the epigastrum or right upper quadrant is present in about half of the patients. In most cases the liver is hard and palpable regardless of whether it is enlarged or atrophied.

The major and late manifestations of cirrhosis develop as a result of two types of disordered physiology: liver cell failure and portal hypertension. Manifestations of hepatocellular failure include jaundice, peripheral edema, bleeding tendencies, palmar erythema, spider angiomas, fetor hepaticus, and hepatic encephalopathy. Clinical features that depend primarily on portal hypertension are splenomegaly, esophageal and gastric varices, and other evidence of abnormal collateral circulation. Ascites (fluid in the peritoneal cavity) can be considered as a manifestation of both hepatocellular failure and portal hypertension. Figure 23-5 illustrates the primary clinical manifestations of cirrhosis discussed in the following pages.

HEPATOCELLULAR FAILURE MANIFESTATIONS

Jaundice occurs in at least 60 percent of patients at some time during the course of the disease and is usually minimal. Hyperbilirubinemia without jaundice is more common. The patient may become jaundiced during a phase of decompensation with reversible deterioration of liver function. For example, the patient with cirrhosis may become jaundiced after a heavy drinking bout. Intermittent jaundice is a characteristic feature of biliary cirrhosis and occurs when there is active inflammation of the liver bile ductules (cholangitis). Patients dying from hepatic failure are usually jaundiced.

Endocrine disturbances are common in cirrhosis. Hormones of the adrenal cortex, testes, and ovaries are normally metabolized and inactivated by the liver. Spider angiomas are seen on the skin, particularly around the neck, shoulders, and chest. They consist of a central arteriole from which many small vessels radiate. Spider angiomas, testicular atrophy, gynecomastia, pectoral and axillary alopecia, and palmar erythema (red palms) are all considered to be caused by an excess of circulating estrogen. Increased pigmentation of the skin is believed to result from excessive activity of melanin-stimulating hormone (MSH).

Hematological disorders common in cirrhosis include bleeding tendencies, anemia, leukopenia, and thrombo-cytopenia. Nosebleeds, gingival bleeding, menstrual bleeding, and easy bruising are not uncommon, and the prothrombin time may be prolonged. These manifestations are the result of decreased hepatic production of the clotting factors. The anemia, leukopenia, and thrombocytopenia are believed to be the resultants of hypersplenism. Not only is the spleen enlarged (splenomegaly) but it is also more active in the removal of blood cells from the circulation. Other mechanisms contributing to the anemia include folate deficiency, vitamin B_{12} deficiency, and iron deficiency secondary to blood loss, and increased hemolysis of red blood cells. The patient is also more susceptible to infection.

The peripheral edema which generally occurs after the development of ascites may be explained by the hypoalbuminemia and abnormal salt and water retention. The failure of the liver cells to inactivate aldosterone and antidiuretic hormone contributes to sodium and water retention.

Hepatic fetor is a musty sweetish odor which may be detected on the patient's breath, especially in hepatic coma, and is believed to result from the liver's inability to metabolize methionine.

The most serious neurological disorder in advanced cirrhosis is hepatic encephalopathy (hepatic coma). It is believed to result from abnormalities in the metabolism of ammonia and increased cerebral sensitivity to toxins. The development of hepatic encephalopathy is often a terminal event in cirrhosis and will be discussed in greater detail later.

PORTAL HYPERTENSION MANIFESTATIONS

Portal hypertension is defined as a sustained elevation of pressure in the portal vein above the normal level of 6 to 12 cm of water. The primary mechanism for inducing portal hypertension, regardless of the disease, is increased resistance to blood flow through the liver. In addition, there is usually an increase in splanchnic arterial flow. The two factors of decreased outflow through the hepatic vein and increased inflow combine to overload the portal circuit. This overload of the portal circuit stimulates the development of collateral channels which circumvent the hepatic obstruction (varices). The back pressure in the portal system causes splenomegaly and is partly responsible for the accumulation of ascites.

Ascites is an intraperitoneal accumulation of watery fluid containing small amounts of protein. Key factors in the pathogenesis of ascites are the increased hydrostatic pressure in the intestinal capillary bed (portal hypertension) and the decreased colloid osmotic pressure from hypoalbuminemia. Other contributing factors include the abnormal sodium and water retention and the increased synthesis and flow of hepatic lymph.

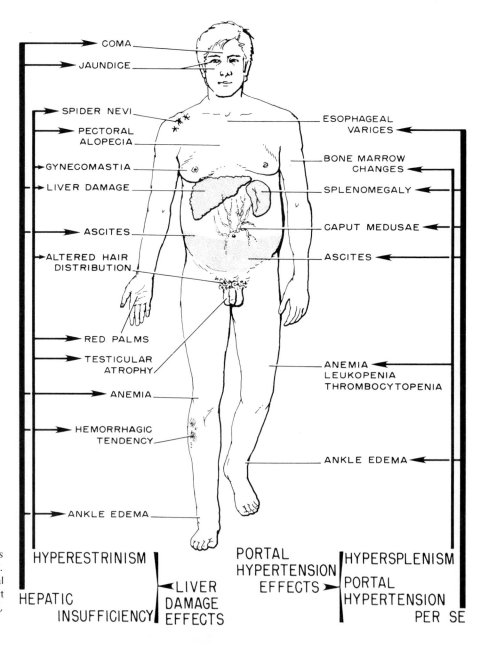

FIGURE 23-5 Clinical manifestations of cirrhosis. (Modified from F. H. Netter, Ciba Collections of Medical Illustrations, Digestive System, Part III, Biliary Tract and Pancreas, 1964, vol. 3.)

The important collateral channels which develop as a result of cirrhosis and portal hypertension are found in the lower esophagus. The shunting of blood through this circuit to the venae cavae causes dilatation of these veins (esophageal varices). These varices occur in about 70 percent of patients with advanced cirrhosis. Bleeding from these varices is a common cause of death (see Fig. 23-6).

The collateral circulation also involves the superficial veins of the abdominal wall, and its development leads to dilated veins around the umbilicus (caput medusae). Dilatation of anastomoses between the branches of the inferior mesenteric vein and the rectal veins often leads to the development of internal hemorrhoids (see Fig. 23-2 to review points of anastomoses). Serious hemorrhage from the rupture of hemorrhoids does not usually occur, since the pressure is not as high as in the esophagus because of the greater distance from the portal vein.

Splenomegaly in cirrhosis can be explained on the basis of chronic passive congestion due to backup and higher pressure of blood in the splenic vein.

Complications and treatment

The treatment of cirrhosis is unsatisfactory. There are no pharmacologic agents which either arrest or reverse the fibrotic process. Therapy is aimed first at dealing with any underlying cause such as alcohol abuse or bile duct obstruction and then at treating the various complications, including gastrointestinal hemorrhage, ascites, and hepatic encephalopathy.

GASTROINTESTINAL BLEEDING

The most common and the most serious cause of gastrointestinal bleeding in cirrhosis is bleeding from esophageal varices and accounts for about one-third of all deaths. Other causes of bleeding include gastric and duodenal ulcers (there is an increased incidence in cirrhotics), acute gastric erosions, and a generalized bleeding tendency (as a result of prolonged prothrombin time and thrombocytopenia).

The patient presents with either melana or hematemesis. Occasionally the first sign of bleeding is hepatic encephalopathy. Depending on the amount and speed of the blood loss, there may be hypovolemia and hypotension.

A variety of measures have been used for the immediate control of bleeding. Tamponade with an apparatus such as the Sengstaken-Blakemore tube, when properly used, will stop the hemorrhage, at least temporarily (see Fig. 23-7).

Vasopressin (Pitressin) has been used to control bleeding. The drug decreases portal pressure by decreasing splanchnic blood flow, although the effect is only temporary. In spite of these emergency measures, about 70 percent of patients die during their first episode of bleeding.

If the patient recovers from the bleeding, either spontaneously or after emergency treatment, a portacaval shunt operation may be considered. This surgery reduces the portal pressure by anastomosing the portal vein (high pressure) to the inferior vena cava (low pressure). The shunt procedure represents drastic therapy of a major complication of cirrhosis. It lessens the chance of further esophageal bleeding but at the price of an increased risk of hepatic encephalopathy. The patient's life expectancy is not increased but depends on the progress of the liver disease.

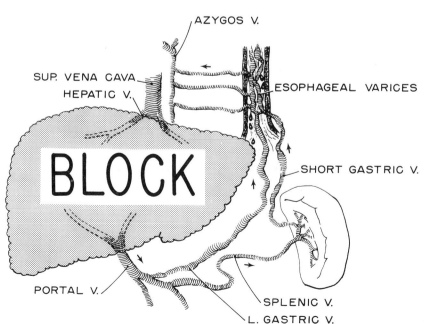

FIGURE 23-6 Hemodynamic changes in liver cirrhosis leading to the development of esophageal varices.

Gastrointestinal bleeding is one of the important precipitating causes of hepatic encephalopathy. The encephalopathy results when ammonia and other toxins enter the systemic circulation. The source of the ammonia is the bacterial breakdown of protein in the gastrointestinal tract. Hepatic encephalopathy will follow if the blood is not removed by gastric aspiration, saline cathartics, and cleansing enemas and if the bacterial breakdown of the blood protein is not prevented by the administration of neomycin or a similar antibiotic. These measures are discussed further in a later section.

ASCITES

A large abdominal paracentesis is no longer considered desirable treatment for ascites because of its deleterious effects. There is danger of inducing hypovolemia, hypokalemia, hyponatremia, hepatic encephalopathy, and renal failure. Since the ascites fluid also contains 10 to 30 g of protein in each liter of fluid, there is further depletion of serum albumin, promoting the reaccumula-

tion of the fluid. Paracentesis is only performed when ascites causes prominent respiratory difficulty or for diagnostic purposes. Some patients with ascites also develop pleural effusions, especially in the right hemithorax. The fluid is thought to enter the chest through tears which develop in the tendinous portion of the diaphragm because of the increased abdominal pressure.

Salt restriction is a major method of treating ascites. Diuretics may also be used in conjunction with a low-sodium diet. There are a variety of diuretics and diuretic programs, but the essential feature is to introduce the diuretics gradually to avoid too brisk a diuresis. Electrolyte imbalance must be avoided, and even then diuretics may precipitate hepatic encephalopathy.

HEPATIC ENCEPHALOPATHY

Hepatic encephalopathy (hepatic coma) is a neuropsychiatric syndrome in a patient with severe liver disease. It is characterized by mental confusion, muscle tremors, and a peculiar flapping tremor called asterixis. The mental changes may begin with mild mental clouding and progress to death in a deep coma. Hepatic encephalopathy ending in coma is the mechanism of death in about one-third of the fatal cases of cirrhosis.

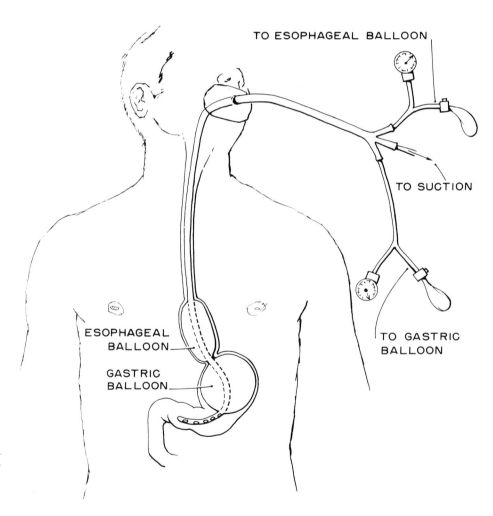

FIGURE 23-7 Sengstaken-Blakemore tube in place for the emergency treatment of hemorrhage from esophageal varices. The tube has three openings: one for gastric aspiration, one for inflating the esophageal balloon, and one for inflating the gastric balloon. The esophageal balloon is inflated to a pressure of 20 to 40 mmHg (the pressure is monitored by attachment to a gauge or a sphygmomanometer) which compresses the esophageal veins. The gastric balloon inflated with 250 ml of air applies pressure to the fundal veins when slight traction is applied.

In simplest terms, hepatic encephalopathy can be described as a form of cerebral intoxication caused by intestinal contents that have not been metabolized by the liver. This condition may occur when there is liver cell damage due to necrosis or shunting (pathological or surgically created), which permit large amounts of portal blood to reach the systemic circulation without traversing the liver.

The metabolites responsible for the encephalopathy have not been identified with certainty. The basic mechanism appears to be intoxication of the brain by breakdown products of protein metabolism produced by bacterial action in the gut. These products are able to bypass the liver because of liver cell disease or shunting. Ammonia, normally converted into urea by the liver, is one of the known toxic substances and is believed to interfere with brain metabolism (see Fig. 23-8).

Hepatic encephalopathy in chronic liver disease is usually precipitated by such events as GI bleeding, excessive protein intake, diuretics, paracentesis, hypokalemia, acute infections, surgery, azotemia, and the administration of morphine, sedatives, or ammonia-containing drugs. The harmful effects of many of these

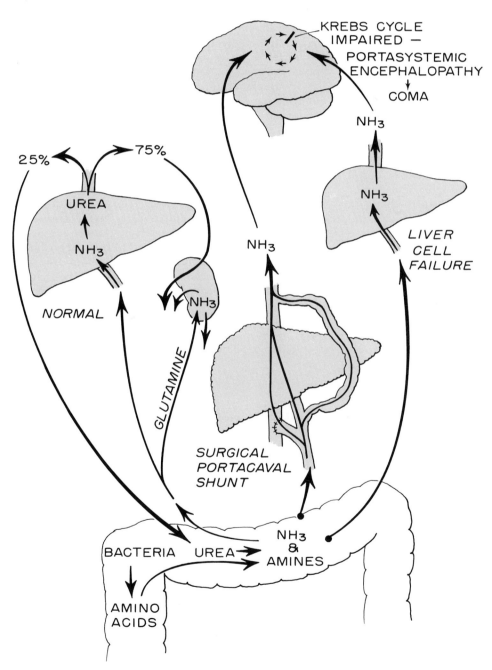

FIGURE 23-8 Normal and abnormal circulation of ammonia.

can be traced to mechanisms that result in the formation of large amounts of ammonia in the bowel. Encephalopathy that follows potassium depletion or paracentesis is probably related to the formation of excessive ammonia by the kidneys and alterations of acid/base balance.

Clinical features

Clinical signs and symptoms of hepatic encephalopathy may arise very quickly and progress to coma when hepatic failure occurs in a fulminating hepatitis. In cirrhotic patients the progress is usually much slower and reversible in the early stages if detected in time. Progression of hepatic encephalopathy to coma is commonly divided into four stages.

The signs in stage I are very subtle and may be easily missed. Danger signals include slight personality and behavioral changes. These may include an unkempt appearance, vacant stare, slurred speech, inappropriate laughter, forgetfulness, and inability to concentrate. However, patients may appear to be perfectly rational but uncooperative or disrespectful at times. Careful observation may reveal that they are more lethargic or sleep more than usual or that their sleep rhythms are reversed. Because of close association with such a patient, the nurse is in a strategic position to notice these changes and should enlist the help of the family to detect subtle personality changes.

The signs in stage II are more prominent and are easily detected. Generalized muscle twitching and asterixis are characteristic findings. Asterixis, or flapping tremor, is elicited by having the patient raise both arms with forearms fixed and fingers extended. This maneuver causes involuntary rapid flexion and extension movements of the wrists (flapping) and metacarpophylangeal joints. Asterixis is a peripheral manifestation of impaired cerebral metabolism. It may also occur in the uremic syndrome. During this stage the lethargy and personality and behavioral changes become more marked.

Constructional apraxia is another prominent feature of hepatic encephalopathy. The patient cannot write clearly or draw figures such as stars or houses. A serial record of handwriting or figure construction is a useful method of determining the progress of the encephalopathy.

In stage III the patient may become noisy, abusive, and violent, so that restraints may become necessary. If the patient is given a sedative at this time rather than treatment to reverse the toxic process, coma will probably ensue, and the outcome may be fatal. During this stage the patient may sleep much of the time. The electroencephalogram begins to change in stage II and is definitely abnormal in stages III and IV.

In stage IV the patient fades into a coma from which he or she cannot be aroused. Hyperactive reflexes and a positive Babinski's sign appear. At times a musty sweetish odor (hepatic fetor) may be detected on the patient's breath or by just entering the room. Hepatic fetor is a grave prognostic sign, and the intensity of the odor correlates very well with the degree of somnolence and confusion. Elevation of the blood ammonia level is an additional laboratory finding which may be helpful in the detection of encephalopathy.

Treatment

The steps in treatment of hepatic encephalopathy have been suggested in discussing the mechanisms that cause it. It is most important to look for any precipitating factors, such as GI bleeding or overenthusiastic diuretic therapy, and give corrective treatment.

The initial treatment is to exclude all protein from the diet and inhibit the action of bacteria on protein substances in the bowel, since the breakdown of protein in the bowel is the source of ammonia and other nitrogenous substances. Neomycin, a nonabsorbable antibiotic, is usually the drug of choice for the inhibition of gut bacteria. The usual dose is about 4 g/day. If the patient has had recent GI bleeding (source of protein), magnesium sulfate or enemas may be given to purge the bowel. It is important to correct fluid and electrolyte imbalance, especially hypokalemia, which enhances the encephalopathy. Barbiturates and narcotics are avoided. Nourishment is given in the form of sweetened fruit juices or intravenous glucose. These measures are usually successful if instituted early in the course of precoma and if the liver damage is not too far advanced.

A number of measures are used to prevent encephalopathy in the patient with a portocaval shunt or in one who has recovered from encaphalopathy. These measures include a modest protein diet, maintenance doses of neomycin, avoidance of potassium-depleting diuretics and ammonia-containing medication, avoidance of sedatives and narcotics, avoidance of constipation, and prohibition of all dietary protein if the symptoms should recur.

CHOLELITHIASIS AND CHOLECYSTITIS

The two most prominent diseases of the biliary tree, from the standpoint of frequency, are stone formation (cholelithiasis) and an associated chronic inflammation (cholecystitis). Although either of these conditions may occur alone, they are commonly associated and will be discussed together.

Pathology

Gallstones are essentially precipitates of one or more components of bile: cholesterol, bilirubin, bile salts, calcium, and protein. Of these substances, cholesterol is nearly insoluble in water and bilirubin is poorly soluble. Gallstones may be composed of pure bilirubin, pure cholesterol, or may be mixed cholesterol stones.

The latter may also contain calcium. Pure bilirubin stones are usually small, multiple, black, and associated with hemolytic disorders. These gallstones are uncommon. Pure cholesterol stones usually present as a large, solitary, round or oval structure which is pale yellow in color. Mixed cholesterol stones are the most common and are multiple and dark brown in color. Gallstones of mixed composition are frequently visible on x-ray, while those of pure composition may be translucent.

Etiology and pathogenesis

Gallstones are unusually common in the United States, with 10 to 20 percent of the adult population affected. Each year, several hundred thousand of these patients undergo biliary tract surgery. Gallstones are uncommon during the first two decades of life. Racial and familial factors seem to be associated with a higher incidence of gallstones. American Indians have an unusually high incidence, followed by Caucasians and finally Negroes. Clinical conditions associated with a higher incidence of gallstones include diabetes, cirrhosis of the liver, pancreatitis, cancer of the gallbladder, and ileal disease or resection.

Gallstones are almost invariably formed in the gallbladder and rarely in other parts of the biliary tree. The etiology of gallstones is still incompletely understood; however, the most important predisposing factors appear to be metabolic disturbances causing changes in the composition of bile, bile stasis, and gallbladder infection.

Changes in the composition of bile is probably the most important factor in gallstone formation. A number of studies have indicated that the livers of patients with cholesterol gallstone disease secrete a bile that is supersaturated with cholesterol. This excess cholesterol is precipitated in the gallbladder in a manner that is not yet fully understood.

Stasis of bile in the gallbladder can lead to progressive supersaturation, changes in the chemical composition, and precipitation of the constituents. Disordered contractility of the gallbladder or spasm of the sphincter of Oddi or both could cause stasis. Hormonal factors, especially during pregnancy, may be related to delayed gallbladder emptying and account for the higher incidence in this group.

Bacterial infection within the biliary tract can play a part in stone formation by increasing cellular desquamation and mucus production. Mucus increases the viscosity, and the cellular elements or bacteria may serve as a nidus for precipitation. It is probable, however, that infection is more commonly a result of the formation of gallstones than a cause of them.

Clinical features

Patients with gallstones often present with symptoms of acute or chronic cholecystitis. The acute form is characterized by the sudden onset of agonizing pain in the upper abdomen, mostly in the midepigastrium; it may radiate to the back and right shoulder. The patient may break out in a profuse sweat or walk the floor or roll from side to side in the bed. Nausea and vomiting are common. The pain may last for several hours or may recur after a partial remission. As the pain subsides, tenderness may be noted over the gallbladder. Acute cholecystitis is often associated with impaction of a stone in the cystic duct and is frequently referred to as *biliary colic*.

The symptoms of chronic cholecystitis are similar to those of acute cholecystitis, but the severity of the pain and the presence of physical signs is less marked. Often there is a history of vague dyspepsia, fat intolerance, heartburn, or flatulence over a prolonged period of time.

Once formed, gallstones may lie quietly in the gallbladder and cause no trouble, or they may cause complications. The most common complications are infection of the gallbladder (cholecystitis) and obstruction of the cystic or common bile ducts by a stone. Such obstruction may be temporary, intermittent, or permanent. Rarely, stones may slough through the wall of the gallbladder and cause severe inflammation, often leading to peritonitis, or cause the walls to become thin and rupture.

Diagnosis and treatment

The diagnosis of both the acute and chronic forms of cholecystitis and cholelithiasis often rests on cholecystography to reveal the presence of stones or malfunctioning of the gallbladder (see Fig. 23-9).

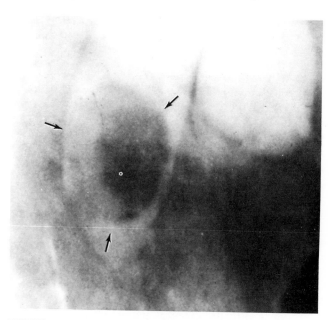

FIGURE 23-9 Gallstone.

The common treatment of these two conditions is surgical removal of the gallbladder (cholecystectomy) and/or removal of stones from the common bile duct (choledocholithotomy), which can be expected to effect a cure in about 95 percent of the cases. In cases of acute cholecystitis with severe symptoms and suspicion of pus formation, some surgeons operate at once, while others operate only if improvement does not occur within a few days. In cases of empyema or if the patient is in poor condition, the gallbladder may not be removed but merely drained (cholecystostomy).

PANCREATITIS

The range of diseases of the pancreas is unusual in that this organ functions both as an endocrine and exocrine gland. The chief endocrine disorder is diabetes and will be discussed in the endocrinology section of this book. The exocrine products of the pancreas contain powerful enzymes which normally digest proteins, fats, and carbohydrates in ingested food. However, these potent enzymes which are so effective in digestion in the lumen of the small intestine also serve as a source of great danger to the organism if they are activated within the substance of the pancreas itself. This is essentially what happens in pancreatitis. Pancreatitis is commonly divided into the acute and chronic forms.

Acute pancreatitis

Acute pancreatitis is an acute inflammatory process involving the pancreas and characterized by varying degrees of edema, hemorrhage, and necrosis of the acinar cells and blood vessels. The mortality and clinical symptoms vary with the degree of the pathologic process. When there is only pancreatic edema, mortality may be from 5 to 10 percent, while massive hemorrhagic necrosis has a mortality of 50 to 80 percent.

ETIOLOGY AND PATHOGENESIS

The main etiologic factors in acute pancreatitis are biliary tract disease and alcoholism. Less common causes include trauma, especially bullet or knife wounds, penetrating duodenal ulcer, hyperparathyroidism, hyperlipidemia, viral infection, and certain drugs such as corticosteroids and thiazide diuretics. Many times a precipitating cause cannot be found.

Pancreatitis is fairly common in adults but is rare in children. In men it is more frequently associated with alcoholism, while in women it is associated more often with gallstones.

There is virtually universal agreement that the common pathogenetic mechanism in pancreatitis is autodigestion, but the process by which the pancreatic enzymes become activated is not clear. In the normal pancreas, there are a number of protective mechanisms which act as safeguards against inadvertent activation of enzymes and autodigestion. First, the enzymes which digest protein are secreted as inactive precursors (zymogens) which must be activated by trypsin. Trypsinogen, the inactive form of trypsin, is normally converted into trypsin by the action of enterokinase in the small intestine. Once trypsin is formed, it is the key that activates all the other proteolytic enzymes. Trypsin inhibitors are present in the plasma and in the pancreas, which can bind and inactivate any trypsin inadvertently produced, so that proteolytic digestion is unlikely to occur in the normal pancreas.

Reflux of bile and duodenal contents into the pancreatic ducts have been proposed as possible mechanisms for the activation of pancreatic enzymes. This could occur when there is a common channel present and a gallstone becomes impacted at the ampulla of Vater. Atony and edema of the sphincter of Oddi might permit duodenal reflux. Obstruction of the pancreatic ducts and pancreatic ischemia may also play a role.

The two activated enzymes which are believed to play a critical role in pancreatic autodigestion are elastase and phospholipase A. Phospholipase A may be activated by trypsin or bile acids. It digests the phospholipids of cell membranes. Elastase is activated by trypsin and digests the elastic tissue of blood vessel walls, producing hemorrhage. The activation of kallikrein by trypsin is believed to play a role in the development of local damage and systemic hypotension. Kallikrein causes vasodilatation, increased vascular permeability, invasion of white blood cells, and pain.

CLINICAL FEATURES

The most prominent symptom of acute pancreatitis is severe abdominal pain which is sudden in onset and continuous. It is usually felt in the epigastrum but may be accentuated to the right or left of the midline. Radiation of the pain to the back is common, and the patient may obtain some relief by sitting forward. Nausea and vomiting often accompany the pain. The pain is usually severe for about 24 hours and then passes off over a period of days.

Physical examination may reveal varying degrees of shock, tachycardia, leukocytosis, and fever. There is tenderness and guarding of the abdominal muscles, but rigidity and other evidence of peritonitis occur only when the inflammation involves the peritoneum. Bowel sounds may be reduced or absent. Severe retroperitoneal bleeding may manifest as bruising in the flanks or around the umbilicus.

The diagnosis of acute pancreatitis is usually established by the finding of an increased serum amylase level. The serum amylase level is elevated during the first 24 to 72 hours and values may be five times greater than normal. Urinary amylase levels are elevated up to 2 weeks after an episode of acute pancreatitis. Other biochemical changes include elevation of the serum lipase level, hyperglycemia, hypocalcemia, and hypokalemia. Hypocalcemia is a common finding caused by marked fat necrosis with the formation of calcium soaps. It may be severe enough to cause tetany.

Complications of acute pancreatitis include the development of diabetes mellitus; severe tetany; pleural effusion, especially in the left hemithorax; and a pancreatic abscess or pseudocyst.

Abscesses are defined as collections of liquid secretory and necrotic products within the pancreas, while collections which occur outside the gland are called pseudocysts. Pancreatic abscesses and pseudocysts commonly occur during the second or third week after the onset of pancreatitis. A common site of a pancreatic pseudocyst is within the lesser omental sac. Secondary infection of these collections of fluid are common.

The most common sequelae of acute pancreatitis are recurrent acute attacks and the development of chronic pancreatitis.

TREATMENT

The primary early treatment of acute pancreatitis is medical, with surgical treatment limited to biliary obstruction or the treatment of specific complications such as a pancreatic pseudocyst. Treatment objectives include relief of pain, reduction of pancreatic secretions, prevention or treatment of shock, restoration of fluid and electrolyte balance, and treatment of secondary infection. Shock and hypovolemia are treated with plasma and electrolyte infusions using the hemotocrit, central venous pressure, and urine output as indices of adequate volume replacement. Demerol, rather than opiates, is used to relieve the pain, since it causes less spasm of the sphincter of Oddi. Elimination of all oral intake and constant gastric suction reduce intestinal distention and prevent acid contents from entering the duodenum and stimulating pancreatic secretion. Antibiotic treatment of established infection is essential, and it may be given during the first 2 weeks in the hope of preventing pancreatic abscess.

Pancreatic abscesses are treated by surgical drainage through the anterior abdominal wall or flank. Pseudocysts are managed by internal drainage between the anterior wall of the cyst and the posterior wall of the gastric antrum.

Once the acute phase of the illness subsides, oral feedings may be given beginning with carbohydrates, which stimulate pancreatic secretions least. Attempts are made to determine the cause of the inflammation. The patient is advised against alcohol for at least 3 months, and if the pancreatitis is believed to be alcohol induced, there should be permanent and total abstinence.

Chronic pancreatitis

Chronic pancreatitis is characterized by progressive destruction of the gland, with fibrotic replacement that may result in stricture and eventual calcification. The etiologic factors are the same as in acute pancreatitis—about one-third to one-half of patients are alcoholics.

The clinical course may be one of recurrent episodes of acute pain, each leaving the patient with less functioning pancreatic mass, or a slow advance. Steatorrhea, malabsorption, weight loss, and diabetes are manifestations of advanced destruction. Chronic pancreatitis may follow acute pancreatitis, but in many patients it begins insidiously.

The most sensitive test for detecting chronic pancreatitis is the determination of bicarbonate concentration and output in the duodenum after stimulation with secretin. Other useful diagnostic measures include fecal fat determination, fasting blood glucose levels to determine islet cell damage, and arteriography and x-ray examination to detect fibrosis and calcification. Unfortunately, invasive pancreatic carcinoma can produce the same pathophysiologic findings as chronic pancreatitis and consequently presents a major problem for the physician in the differential diagnosis.

The treatment of chronic pancreatitis is taxing and unsatisfactory. Relief of pain is difficult and may require large and frequent doses of analgesics. Narcotic addiction becomes a serious problem. Steatorrhea is managed with a low-fat diet and oral administration of pancreatic enzymes. Diabetes requires control either with oral hypoglycemic agents or with insulin. Alcohol ingestion is contraindicated.

CANCER OF THE LIVER, GALLBLADDER, AND PANCREAS

Primary cancer of the liver and gallbladder are relatively uncommon tumors in the United States. However, primary cancer of the liver is quite common in Africa and Japan. Both of these malignancies have a very poor prognosis.

Malignant tumors primary to the liver arise from either parenchymal cells or bile duct epithelium. The former is known as *hepatoma* and comprises 90 percent of primary liver malignancies; the latter is called *cholangiocarcinoma*. About 75 percent of patients who develop hepatoma have underlying cirrhosis of the liver, especially the alcoholic and postnecrotic types. The most important diagnostic cues are unexplained deterioration in a cirrhotic and rapid enlargement of the liver.

The most common tumor of the liver is a malignant tumor which has metastasized from some other site. Metastasis to the liver can be detected in more than 50 percent of all cancer deaths. This is particularly true of gastrointestinal malignancies, but many others also show this tendency (e.g., breast, lung, uterus, and pancreas).

Most cancers of the gallbladder are adenocarcinomas, and 80 percent of these patients have gallstones. Diagnosis is generally late, since the early symptoms are insidious and resemble those of chronic cholecystitis and cholelithiasis.

Cancer of the pancreas is a relatively common tumor now approaching the incidence of cancer of the stomach. This tumor is more common in males than in females by a ratio of 2:1 or 3:1. The peak incidence is in the advanced years. About 60 percent arise in the head of the pancreas, usually obstructing the biliary tract and causing jaundice and a palpably enlarged gallbladder, whereas those arising in the body and tail often remain silent until far advanced. Other signs and symptoms include abdominal pain, weight loss, anorexia, and nausea. Differential diagnosis from chronic pancreatitis may be difficult. Because of the difficulties in diagnosis, the tumor is usually not discovered until it has already spread beyond hope of local resection.

The average life expectancy after establishing the diagnosis of cancer of the liver, gallbladder, or pancreas is less than 1 year.

QUESTIONS

Liver, biliary tract and pancreas—Chap. 23

Directions: Answer the following questions on a separate sheet of paper.

1 Explain why blood circulation through the liver is unusual.

2 Briefly describe the structure and function of the gallbladder and pancreas. What hormones control the release of bile and the exocrine pancreatic secretions?

3 List the eight major functions of the liver. Why is the liver a major organ of defense? Why is the liver called a flood chamber? How does the liver perform its detoxification functions (mechanisms involved)? What is the role of the liver in carbohydrate, fat, and protein metabolism?

4 List the four general pathogenetic mechanisms of jaundice.

5 What is kernicterus? What is its significance?

6 Why do newborn babies often have a slight transient jaundice during the first few days after birth?

7 Does gamma globulin have any value in the treatment of existing hepatitis?

8 Enumerate measures which might help prevent the spread of viral hepatitis in the community, in the home, and in the clinical unit.

9 What percentage of liver destruction is still compatible with life? How long could you live after a total hepatectomy?

Directions: Fill in the blanks with the correct words or circle the correct word option when indicated below.

10 The liver is roughly _____ in shape, weighs about (150) or (1500) g, and is located in the _____ _____ quadrant of the abdomen. The right lobe forms a roof over the right _____ and the _____, and the left lobe forms a roof over two important digestive organs, the _____ and _____. The _____ ligament divides the medial and lateral segments of the left lobe and is attached to the anterior abdominal wall. The liver is enveloped by dense connective tissue called the capsule of _____, and the stretching of this capsule in cases of hepatic enlargement is believed to cause tenderness or dull pain.

11 The chief secretory product of the liver is _____ _____, which exits from the liver through the right and left _____ duct, which immediately merge to form the common _____ duct; this secretory product enters the gallbladder through the _____ duct and enters the duodenum through the common _____ duct. This terminal bile duct joins with the main _____ duct before entering the duodenum. The sphincter of _____ encircles the common channel and controls the entry of secretions into the duodenum.

12 Blood is supplied to the liver by the _____ artery and the _____ vein and is drained by the right and left _____ veins, which enter the inferior _____ _____. The paraumbilical veins form a potential pathway from the umbilicus to the _____ vein, allowing passage of a catheter and direct measurement of pressure in this vein. In cases of right heart failure, blood may back up through the _____ veins, causing passive congestion of the liver but rarely cirrhosis. When blood flow through the liver is blocked in cirrhosis, blood may back up in the splenic vein, causing enlargement of the _____, or may be shunted around the liver through the _____ veins, causing varices, or through the _____ veins, causing internal hemorrhoids.

13 The structural and functional unit of the liver is called the _____, which is hexagonal in shape and composed of plates of liver cells. Mixed arterial and portal venous blood flows through liver capillaries called _____, which are lined with phagocytic cells called _____ cells and drains into a central vein at the center of the structural unit. Bile capillaries course between the hepatocytes and are called _____.

Directions: Circle the letter preceding each item which correctly answers each question. Only one answer is correct, unless otherwise noted.

14 Which of the following clotting factors is not synthesized by the liver?
a Prothrombin b Factor IV c Factor V
d Factor VII e Factor X

15 All of the following serum proteins are synthesized by the liver except:
a Albumin *b* Alpha globulins *c* Beta globulins *d* Gamma globulins *e* Fibrinogen

16 Which of the following hormones are catabolized by the liver? (More than one answer may be correct.)
a Estrogen *b* Testosterone *c* Cortisone *d* Aldosterone

17 Which of the following is *not* a basic liver function?
a Synthesis of albumin *b* Detoxification of chemicals by oxidation, reduction, and conjunction *c* Synthesis of urea from ammonia *d* Catabolism of bile *e* Phagocytosis of bacteria in portal blood

18 Which of the following functions is evidence that the liver plays a central role in lipid metabolism?
a Chief site of bile formation *b* Synthesis of fatty acids from carbohydrate *c* Cholesterol synthesis *d* Phospholipid formation *e* Lipoprotein formation

19 The greatest value of liver scanning is in the detection of:
a Hepatitis *b* Cirrhosis *c* Circumscribed hepatic lesions *d* Portal hypertension

20 Which of the following statements is *not* true concerning percutaneous liver biopsy?
a The procedure is contraindicated in persons with a prolonged prothrombin time. *b* The patient must hold his or her breath and not move during needle insertion. *c* The patient must lie on the left side for 2 hours following the procedure. *d* Postbiopsy care includes frequently monitoring vital signs. *e* Significant hemorrhage is a rare complication.

21 *Direct* measurement of portal vein pressure may be achieved by:
a Percutaneous measurement of intrasplenic pressure *b* Catheterizing the hepatic vein and measuring wedged pressure *c* Passing a catheter through the umbilical vein to the left branch of the portal vein *d* Percutaneous measurement of pressure in the liver ductules

22 The *chief* source of bilirubin is:
a Senescent red blood cells *b* Red blood cell precursors in the bone marrow *c* Hemoproteins from the liver *d* Spleen

23 Bilirubin is formed in the reticuloendothelial system by the reduction of:
a Hemoglobin *b* Globin *c* Biliverdin *d* Urobilinogen

24 The primary site of free (unconjugated) bilirubin formation:
a Liver *b* Kidneys *c* Spleen *d* Gastrointestinal tract

25 Unconjugated bilirubin is transported in the blood to the liver bound to:
a Globulins *b* Red blood cell membranes *c* Fibrinogen *d* Albumin

26 The enzyme responsible for the final step in bilirubin conjugation:

a Glucuronyl transferase *b* SGOT *c* Alkaline phosphatase *d* Lactic dehydroginase

27 Conjugated bilirubin is:
a Excreted in the bile *b* Water-soluble *c* Characterized by its great affinity for lipids *d* Capable of being excreted in the urine

28 A 21-year-old male college student is seen with the chief complaint of jaundice. His friend, a nursing student, noticed that his eyes were yellow, although he had been completely asymptomatic. He also remembered that a younger brother had been icteric on several occasions. The physical exam was negative. SGOT, alkaline phosphatase, CBC, and liver scan were all normal. The test for urine bilirubin was negative. Total serum bilirubin was 4.8 mg% (conjugated portion 0.5 mg%). His most likely problem is:
a Viral hepatitis *b* Infectious mononucleosis *c* Hemolytic anemia *d* Gilbert's syndrome

29 The prognosis for the condition in question 28 is:
a Poor *b* Good

30 The most likely pathogenetic mechanism causing the condition in question 28 is:
a Transport failure of bilirubin due to defective binding to albumin *b* Excessive load of bilirubin presented to liver due to hemolysis *c* Impaired excretion of conjugated bilirubin *d* Impaired uptake of bilirubin by hepatocyte

31 Ms. B has been admitted to the hospital for evaluation of her jaundice. Additional findings include clay-colored stools, dark urine which forms a yellow-tinted foam when shaken, pruritis, and a predominantly conjugated hyperbilirubinemia. These findings are compatible with:
a Hemolytic jaundice *b* Intrahepatic cholestasis *c* Extrahepatic cholestasis *d* Only *b* and *c* *e* All of the above

32 In hemolytic jaundice increased bilirubin will not be present *because* it is all unconjugated.
a Both statement and reason are true *b* Statement is true, reason is false *c* Both statement and reason are false *d* Statement is false, reason is true

33 Pathologic changes common to diseases of the liver, gallbladder and pancreas include:
a Fibrosis *b* Inflammation *c* Neoplasms *d* All of the above

34 Common findings during the prodromal phase of hepatitis include:
a Malaise *b* Icterus *c* Anorexia and loss of desire to smoke *d* Periportal inflammation revealed by biopsy *e* Low-grade fever

35 Match each of the features in col. A to the two types of hepatitis in col. B.

Column A	Column B
____ Transmitted by fecal–oral route	*a* Hepatitis A
____ Positive test for hepatitis antigen	*b* Hepatitis B
____ Seasonal incidence	*c* Both A and B
____ Higher mortality and complications	*d* Neither A nor B
____ Higher incidence among institutionalized	
____ Especially common in drug addicts	
____ Longer incubation period	
____ A constant threat to patients and staff in hemodialysis units	
____ Epidemics common when water supply contaminated	
____ Synonym—serum hepatitis	
____ Synonym—infectious hepatitis	

36 Match each of the following altered lab tests of liver, biliary, and pancreatic function in col. A to their possible clinical significance in col. B.

Column A	Column B
____ Marked increase of serum amylase	*a* Hepatic failure or large portosystemic shunt may be present
____ Marked increase of serum alkaline phosphatase	*b* May indicate biliary obstruction; also increased in bone disease
____ Prolonged prothrombin time	*c* Results in increased bleeding tendency; may indicate liver cell damage
____ Hypoalbuminemia	
____ Increased blood ammonia	*d* Common in acute pancreatitis
____ BSP test	*e* Normally absent from urine; presence indicates hepatocellular disease or biliary obstruction
____ Urine bilirubin	
____ Hyperbilirubinemia (unconjugated)	*f* Possible hemolytic process
____ Urine urobilinogen	*g* Most sensitive index of liver function
	h Decreased in biliary obstruction
	i Related to edema formation in hepatic insufficiency.

Directions: Answer the following questions on a separate sheet of paper.

37 What is alcoholic hepatitis and what is its significance in relation to cirrhosis of the liver?

38 Why is cirrhosis of the liver usually not diagnosed until it is advanced?

39 What is portal hypertension? What is the basic mechanism involved in its development?

40 Describe two emergency methods of treatment for bleeding esophageal varices. Why is it so important to remove the blood from the GI tract? Describe the surgical treatment of esophageal vertices to prevent recurrent bleeding. Why does the patient often develop hepatic encephalopathy after this type of surgery?

41 What is hepatic encephalopathy? How is it related to portal-systemic shunting and liver cell failure? Why is it important to detect hepatic encephalopathy in its early stages?

42 What is asterixis? How is it tested?

43 What is constructional apraxia? Significance?

44 Make a table which includes the four progressive stages of hepatic encephalopathy and the major clinical features of each stage.

45 Compare the clinical features of acute and chronic cholecystitis.

46 Why is the liver such a common site of metastasis for malignant tumors?

Directions: Circle the letter preceding each item that correctly answers each question. More than one answer may be correct.

47 Pathological changes present in cirrhosis of the liver include:
a Distortion of the liver architecture *b* Fibrosis *c* Necrosis *d* Regenerative nodules *e* Fatty infiltration

48 The single most important cause of cirrhosis in the United States is:
a Cholecystitis *b* Cholestasis *c* Chronic alcoholism *d* Viral hepatitis

49 The major body site for the metabolism of alcohol:
a Gastrointestinal tract *b* Kidneys *c* Brain *d* Liver

50 The first morphologic change in the liver associated with alcohol abuse is:
a Fatty infiltration *b* Cholestasis *c* Necrosis *d* Fibrosis

51 The hepatic lesion in severe kwashiorkor is:
a Cirrhosis of the postnecrotic type *b* Laennec's cirrhosis *c* Hepatitislike picture *d* Fatty infiltration

52 Possible pathogenetic mechanisms accounting for fatty infiltration of the liver include:
a Excess formation of triglycerides *b* Excess formation of urea by the liver cell *c* Decreased oxidation of fatty acids by the liver cell *d* Decreased synthesis of lipoproteins

53 The two most serious consequences of liver cirrhosis are: (Choose *two*)

a Hepatocellular failure *b* Fatty infiltration of the liver *c* Portal hypertension *d* Increased production of alcohol dehydrogenase

54 The most common cause of biliary cirrhosis is:
a Chronic active hepatitis *b* Posthepatic biliary obstruction *c* Alcoholism *d* Primary inflammatory disease of the bile ductiles

55 Postnecrotic cirrhosis is characterized by:
a Prior intoxication with chemicals in a few cases *b* A pattern of patchy necrosis *c* An enlarged firm liver with a green hue *d* An increased incidence of hepatoma

56 The incidence of esophageal varices in advanced Laennec's cirrhosis:
a 20 percent *b* 50 percent *c* 70 percent *d* 100 percent

57 Possible causes of anemia associated with some cases of cirrhosis include:
a Blood loss *b* Folate and vitamin B_{12} deficiency *c* Increased hemolysis in the spleen *d* All of the above

58 Common physical signs in cirrhosis include:
a Ascites *b* Vascular spiders *c* Palmar erythema *d* Prominent superficial abdominal veins *e* All of the above

59 What percentage of cirrhotic patients die during their first episode of bleeding from esophageal varices?
a 5 percent *b* 25 percent *c* 50 percent *d* 70 percent

60 The most important source of ammonia in the human body is the:
a Kidney *b* Liver *c* Digestive tract *d* Central nervous system

61 In hypokalemia, there is increased production of ammonia by the:
a Liver *b* Kidney *c* Digestive tract *d* Central nervous system

62 Asterixis may be seen in:
a Hypoglycemic states *b* Hyperglycemic states *c* Hepatic encephalopathy *d* Uremia

63 Characteristics of hepatic encephalopathy include all of the following *except:*
a Mental confusion *b* Deterioration of ability to write and construct figures *c* Abnormal EEG *d* Increased blood urea nitrogen

64 The treatment of hepatic encephalopathy usually includes:
a High-protein diet *b* Oral neomycin *c* Intravenous penicillin *d* Corticosteroids

65 Hepatic fetor has been related to the metabolism of:
a Bilirubin *b* Cholic acid *c* Methionine *d* Alpha-ketoglutaric acid

66 Hepatic encephalopathy may be precipitated by:
a Vigorous diuretic therapy *b* Infection *c* Constipation *d* Paracentesis *e* Gastrointestinal bleeding

67 Prominent veins across the lateral walls of the abdomen suggest:
a Portal hypertension *b* Inferior vena caval obstruction *c* Hepatic vein thrombosis *d* Thrombosis at the bifurcation of the iliac veins

68 Marked elevation of serum amylase (fivefold) almost invariably signifies:
a Parotitis *b* Cancer of the pancreas *c* Intestinal obstruction *d* Pancreatitis

69 Pancreatitis may be caused by:
a Chronic alcohol abuse *b* Common duct gallstones *c* Excess coffee ingestion *d* Trauma to the pancreas

70 Mechanisms which protect the normal pancreas from autodigestion include:
a Proteolytic enzymes secreted in inactive form *b* Key enzyme trypsin must be activated by enterokinase *c* Trypsin inhibitors present in plasma *d* Secretion of bicarbonate

Directions: Circle T if the statement is true and F if it is false. Correct the false statements.

71 T F Ascites is the accumulation of fluid within the pleural cavity.

72 T F Reflux of bile and/or duodenal contents into the pancreatic ducts causing activation of enzymes within the pancreas are possible mechanisms in the development of pancreatitis.

73 T F Hemorrhagic pancreatitis may be characterized by shock, hypovolemia, paralytic ileus, and tetany.

74 T F Chronic pancreatitis is most frequently associated with cholelithiasis and cholecystitis in males.

75 T F Abdominal pain is the most prominent symptom of pancreatitis.

76 T F Kallikrein, when activated within the pancreas, causes vasodilitation, increased vascular permeability, and pain.

77 T F Mixed cholesterol gallstones are frequently associated with hemolytic disorders.

78 T F A pancreatic pseudocyst is a collection of liquid secretory and necrotic products which forms within the pancreas itself during the course of acute pancreatitis.

79 T F Cancer of the liver and gallbladder are common tumors in the United States, are generally detected in the early stages, and have a good prognosis.

80 T F The majority of patients with cancer of the gallbladder have gallstones.

81 T F Cancer of the head of the pancreas may be difficult to differentiate from chronic pancreatitis.

82 T F Steatorrhea, malabsorption, weight loss, and diabetes are manifestations of advanced destruction of the pancreas.

83 T F Surgical removal of the gallbladder is called choledocholithotomy.

84 Match each of the following clinical features of cirrhosis in col. A to the most likely mechanism causing them in col. B.

Column A

_____ Peripheral edema
_____ Jaundice
_____ Spider angiomas
_____ Leukopenia
_____ Clotting abnormalities
_____ Hemorrhoids

Column B

a Increased circulating levels of estrogens due to failure of liver cell to inactivate

b Hypersplenism

c Impaired uptake, conjugation, and excretion of bilirubin

d Portal hypertension → increased flow and pressure through points of portal-systemic anastomoses.

e Decreased hepatic production of fibrinogen, factor V, and other vitamin K-dependent clotting factors

f Liver cell failure → hypoalbuminemia → decreased colloid osmotic pressure; increased sodium and water retention

REFERENCES

Bockus, H. L.: *Gastroenterology*, 3d ed., Saunders, Philadelphia, 1974, vol. 3.

Bogoch, Abraham (ed.): *Gastroenterology*, McGraw-Hill, New York, 1973, pp. 722–839, 844–916, 923–960.

Brooks, F. P. (ed.): *Gastrointestinal Pathophysiology*, Oxford University Press, New York, 1974, pp. 105–205.

Davidson, Charles S.: *Liver Pathophysiology*, Little, Brown, Boston, 1970.

Frolich, Edward D. (ed.): *Pathophysiology*, Lippincott, Philadelphia, 1972, pp. 455–484.

Given, B. A., and S. J. Simmons: *Gastroenterology in Clinical Nursing*, 2d ed., C. V. Mosby, St. Louis, 1975, pp. 152–196, 266–308.

Gocke, D. J.: "Current Status of Viral Hepatitis," *Hospital Medicine*, March 1975, pp. 8–17.

Greenberger, N. J., and D. H. Winship: *Gastrointestinal Disorders: A Pathophysiologic Approach*, Yearbook, Chicago, 1976, pp. 214–352.

Helman, R. A. et al.: "Alcoholic Hepatitis," *Annals of Internal Medicine*, **74**: 311–321, 1971.

Iber, F. L.: "Normal and Pathologic Physiology of the Liver," in W. A. Sodeman, Jr. and W. A. Sodeman (eds.), *Pathologic Physiology*, 5th ed., Saunders, Philadelphia, 1974, pp. 790–815.

Isselbacker, K. J.: "Diagnostic Procedures in Liver Disease," in *Harrison's Principles of Internal Medicine* 7th ed., McGraw-Hill, New York, 1974, pp. 1517–1521.

Isselbacher, K. J.: "Disturbances in Bilirubin Metabolism," in *Harrison's Principles of Internal Medicine*, 7th ed., McGraw-Hill, New York, 1974, pp. 1521–1527.

Koff, R. S., and K. J. Isselbacher: "Acute Hepatitis," in *Harrison's Principles of Internal Medicine*, 7th ed., McGraw-Hill, New York, 1974, pp. 1528–1536.

Mikkelson, W. P.: "Portal Hypertension," *Hospital Medicine*, November 1973, pp. 56–70.

Monroe, L. S.: "Cholangitis," *Hospital Medicine*, October 1969, pp. 111–121.

Naish, J. M., and A. E. A. Read: *Basic Gastroenterology*, Yearbook, Chicago, 1974, pp. 168–244.

Netter, Frank H.: *Ciba Collection of Medicine Illustrations, Vol. 3, Digestive System, Part III, Liver, Biliary Tract and Pancreas*, Ciba Pharmaceutical Co., Summit, N.J., 1964.

Sleisenger, M., and G. Fordtran: *Gastrointestinal Disease*, Saunders, Philadelphia, 1973.

Snodgrass, P. J.: "Disease of the Pancreas," in *Harrison's Principles of Internal Medicine*, 7th ed., McGraw-Hill, New York, 1974, pp. 1568–1579.

Swartz, S. I.: "Liver," in S. I. Swartz (ed.) *Principles of Surgery*, 2d ed., McGraw-Hill, New York, 1974, pp. 1178–1217.

Tumen, H. J.: "Pitfalls in the Management of Advanced Cirrhosis," *Hospital Medicine*, April 1971.

Tumen, H. J.: "Alcoholic Liver Disease," *Hospital Medicine*, September 1974.

PART V Normal Cardiovascular Function and Cardiovascular Pathophysiology

PENNY J. FORD

The devastating impact of cardiovascular disease upon American society cannot be overstated. Cardiovascular disease is epidemic in proportion. Approximately 27 million Americans are afflicted with some disease of the heart or blood vessels; over 1 million deaths per year are attributable to a cardiovascular disorder. Disease of the heart and blood vessels is the leading cause of death in the country, claiming more lives than do all other causes combined.

Heart attack is the major cause of cardiovascular mortality and morbidity. Approximately, 700,000 deaths per year are attributable to heart attacks; many of these deaths affect middle-aged males. Of great concern is the fact that heart attack often occurs with little or no warning; the incidence of sudden death is high. Over half of the deaths from myocardial infarction occur during the first few hours after the onset of symptoms prior to hospitalization. With the advent of coronary care units in the early 1960s, the hospital mortality from lethal disturbances of the cardiac rhythm has decreased significantly. However, the mortality from mechanical pump failure and shock is relatively unchanged. Efforts to mechanically assist the ventricle and reduce the size of the infarct are currently under investigation in an attempt to decrease shock mortality.

Additional cardiovascular diseases with significant morbidity and mortality include rheumatic heart disease, stroke, arteriosclerosis, hypertension, and congenital heart disease. The major therapeutic thrust for the control of these diseases must be primary prevention. Each disease entity is associated with demonstrable precursors or risk factors that increase an individual's susceptibility to the development of disease. Despite the fact that the precise pathogenesis of many of these diseases remains unknown, control of risk factors by effective screening and public education can effect a substantial reduction in cardiac morbidity and mortality. The emphasis must be upon prophylaxis rather than upon treatment of established disease; the lethal and disabling sequelae of cardiovascular disease are too pronounced to await evidence of disease.

The subsequent chapters present a detailed discussion of coronary atherosclerotic disease, valvular heart disease, and peripheral vascular disease. Rheumatic fever and hypertension as they relate to the aforementioned disease entities are also considered.

OBJECTIVES

At the completion of Part V you should be able to:

1 Correlate the pathophysiology of cardiovascular disease entities with the signs and symptoms of disease and the rationale for therapy.

2 Describe the influences predisposing cardiovascular structures to the development of specific disorders.

CHAPTER 24 Anatomy of the Cardiovascular System

The apparent simplicity in the design of the cardiovascular system belies the intricate, yet logical, interdependence of circulatory structure and function in health and disease. Each portion of the cardiovascular system is uniquely adapted to contribute to highly integrated cardiovascular responses to disease processes. Hence, an understanding of cardiovascular anatomy is prerequisite to the examination of cardiovascular disease mechanisms and the capabilities and limitations of circulatory compensatory responses.

ANATOMIC RELATIONSHIPS

The heart lies within the mediastinal space of the thoracic cavity between the lungs. The pericardium encloses the heart and is composed of two layers: the inner layer, or *visceral pericardium*, and the outer layer, or *parietal pericardium*. The two pericardial layers are separated by a small amount of lubricating fluid, which reduces the friction created by the pumping action of the heart. The parietal pericardium is attached anteriorly to the sternum, posteriorly to the vertebral column, and inferiorly to the diaphragm; the visceral pericardium is in direct contact with the surface of the heart. The heart itself is composed of three layers: the outer layer, or *epicardium;* the middle, muscular layer, or *myocardium;* and the inner, endothelial layer, or *endocardium* (see Fig. 24-1).

Functionally, the heart is divided into right- and left-sided pumps, which respectively propel venous blood into the pulmonic circulation and oxygenated blood into the systemic circulation. This functional division facilitates conceptualization of the anatomic sequence of blood flow: venae cavae, right atrium, right ventricle, pulmonary artery, lungs, pulmonary veins, left atrium, left ventricle, aorta, arteries, arterioles, capillaries, venules, veins, venae cavae (see Fig. 24-2).

The schematic conception of the right and left sides of the heart shown in Fig. 24-2 is anatomically misleading however. In actuality, the heart is rotated to the left with its apex tilted anteriorly. This rotation places the right side of the heart anteriorly beneath the sternum, with the left side of the heart relatively posterior. The apex of the heart can be palpated at the midclavicular line at the fourth or fifth intercostal space (see Fig. 24-3).

CARDIAC CHAMBERS

Right atrium

The thin-walled right atrium functions as a reservoir and a conduit for systemic venous blood flowing to the right ventricle and lungs. Venous blood enters the right atrium via the superior vena cava, the inferior vena cava, and the coronary sinus. There are no true valves within the orifices of the venae cavae; only rudimentary valvular folds or muscular bands separate the venae cavae from the atrial chamber. Therefore, elevation in right atrial pressure as a result of right-sided congestion will be reflected backward into the systemic venous circulation.

Approximately 80 percent of the venous return to the right atrium flows passively into the right ventricle through the tricuspid valve. An additional 20 percent of ventricular filling occurs during atrial contraction; this active contribution to ventricular filling is called the atrial

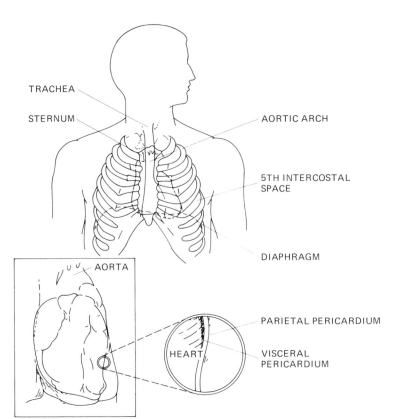

FIGURE 24-1 Anatomic relation of the heart to the surrounding structures. Inset shows the two layers of pericardium separated by pericardial fluid. (From G. H. Whipple, et al., Acute Coronary Care, *Little, Brown, Boston, 1972, p. 22.)*

kick. Loss of the atrial kick in certain cardiac arrhythmias can reduce ventricular filling and consequently decrease ventricular output.

Right ventricle

During ventricular contraction, each ventricle must generate adequate force to propel the blood received from the atrium into either the pulmonic or the systemic circulation. The right ventricle is designed in a unique crescent shape to generate a low-pressure, bellowslike contraction sufficient to propel blood into the pulmonary artery. The pulmonic circulation is a low-pressure system, offering considerably less resistance to blood flow from the right ventricle than the high pressure systemic circuit offers to blood flow from the left ventricle. Therefore, the work load of the right ventricle is much lighter than that of the left ventricle. Consequently, the wall thickness of the right ventricle is only one-third that of the left ventricle (see Fig. 24-4).

In the face of gradually increasing pulmonary pressures, as with progressive pulmonary hypertension, the right ventricle undergoes muscular hypertrophy to increase its pumping force to overcome the elevated pulmonary resistance to ventricular emptying. However, in the event of an acute elevation in pulmonary resistance (such as in massive pulmonary embolization), the pumping capability of the right ventricle could be overwhelmed and death might result.

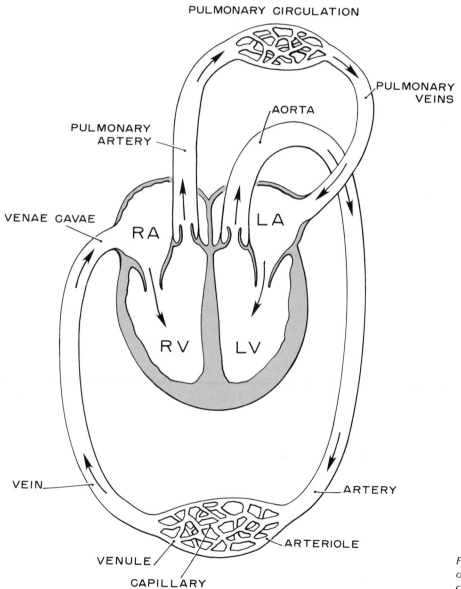

FIGURE 24-2 Schematic representation of blood flow through the cardiovascular system.

Left atrium

The left atrium receives oxygenated blood from the lungs via the four pulmonary veins. No true valves separate the pulmonary veins from the left atrium. Therefore, alterations in left atrial pressure are readily reflected retrograde into the pulmonary vasculature, and acute elevations in left atrial pressure will cause pulmonary congestion. The left atrium is a thin-walled, low-pressure chamber. Blood flows from the left atrium into the left ventricle through the mitral valve.

Left ventricle

The left ventricle must generate high pressures to overcome the resistance of the systemic circulation and sustain blood flood to peripheral tissues. The thick musculature and circular configuration of the left ventricle facilitate the development of high pressure during ventricular contraction. Even the interventricular septum separating the ventricles contributes to the powerful compression exerted by the entire ventricular chamber during contraction.

Left ventricular pressure exceeds right ventricular pressure by approximately fivefold during contraction; if an abnormal communication exists between the ventricles (as with rupture of the interventricular septum after myocardial infarction), blood will be shunted from left to right through the defect. As a result, normal forward blood flow from the left ventricle through the aortic valve to the aorta will be decreased.

CARDIAC VALVES

The four cardiac valves function to maintain unidirectional blood flow through the chambers of the heart. These valves are of two types: the *atrioventricular valves* (or AV valves), which separate the atria from the ventricles, and the *semilunar valves*, which separate the pulmonary artery and aorta from the corresponding ventricle. The valves open and close passively in response to pressure and volume changes within the cardiac chambers and vessels.

Atrioventricular valves

The leaflets of the atrioventricular valves are delicate, yet durable. The *tricuspid valve*, located between the right atrium and right ventricle, contains three leaflets. The *mitral valve* separating the left atrium and left ventricle is a bicuspid valve with two valve cusps or leaflets.

The cusps of both valves are attached to thin strands of fibrous tissue called *chordae tendinae*. The chordae tendinae extend to *papillary muscles*, which are muscular projections arising from the ventricular wall (see Fig. 24-5). The chordae tendinae support the valves during ventricular contraction to prevent eversion of the valve cusps into the atria. Rupture or malfunction of the chordae tendinae or papillary muscles would permit backflow or regurgitation of blood into the atrium during ventricular contraction.

Semilunar valves

Both semilunar valves are of similar configuration, consisting of three symmetrical cuplike cusps secured to a fibrous ring. The *aortic valve* is situated between the left

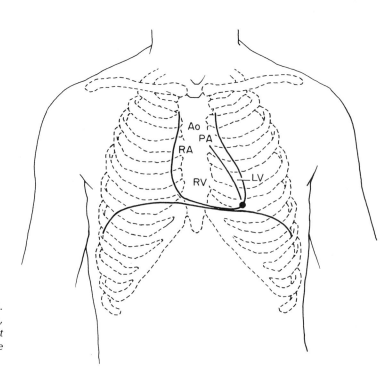

FIGURE 24-3 Orientation of the heart within the thorax. Ao = aorta, RA = right atrium, PA = pulmonary artery, RV = right ventricle, LV = left ventricle. The black dot marks the normal location of the apical impulse in the fifth left intercostal space near the midclavicular line.

ventricle and the aorta, whereas the *pulmonic valve* is positioned between the right ventricle and pulmonary artery. The semilunar valves prevent backflow from the aorta or pulmonary artery into the ventricles during ventricular relaxation.

Immediately above the cusps of the aortic valve there are three outpouchings of the aortic wall called the *sinuses of Valsalva* (see Fig. 24-6). The orifices to the coronary arteries are located within these outpouchings. These sinuses protect the coronary orifices from occlusion by the valve leaflets when the aortic valve opens.

CONDUCTION SYSTEM

To ensure rhythmic and synchronized excitation and contraction of the heart muscle, specialized conduction pathways exist within the myocardium (see Fig. 24-7). This conduction tissue exhibits the following properties:

1 Automaticity—the ability to spontaneously generate impulses.
2 Rhythmicity—the regularity of impulse generation.
3 Conductivity—the ability to transmit impulses.
4 Excitability—the ability to respond to stimulation.

As a consequence of these properties, the heart spontaneously and rhythmically initiates impulses that are transmitted throughout the conduction system to excite the myocardium and stimulate muscular contraction.

The cardiac impulse normally originates in the *sino-*

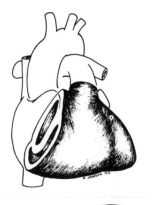
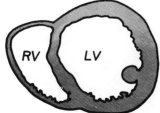

FIGURE 24-4 *Schematic drawings of the heart to illustrate the differences in shape of the right and left ventricles. A, ventricles in approximate anatomic position. B, cross section illustrating the greater wall thickness and nearly circular dimensions of the left ventricle. (From J. W. Hurst,* The Heart, *3d ed., McGraw-Hill, New York, 1974, p. 25.)*

atrial (SA) node. The SA node is therefore referred to as the natural pacemaker of the heart. The SA node is located in the posterior wall of the right atrium near the entrance to the superior vena cava.

The cardiac impulse then spreads from the SA node to specialized atrial conduction pathways and to the atrial muscle. An interatrial pathway, Bachman's bundle, facilitates impulse spread from the right to the left atrium. Internodal pathways—the anterior, middle, and posterior pathways—connect the SA node with the atrioventricular node.

The electrical impulse then reaches the *atrioventricular (AV) node* positioned at the top of the interventricular septum in the right atrium near the opening of the coronary sinus. The AV node is the normal route for impulse transmission between the atria and ventricles and performs two critical functions. First, the cardiac impulse is delayed here for 0.08 to 0.12 seconds to allow for ventricular filling during atrial contraction. Second, the AV node controls the number of atrial impulses reaching the ventricles; normally, no more than 180 impulses per minute are permitted to reach the ventricles. This protective effect is critical during certain abnormal cardiac rhythms in which atrial rates can exceed 400 beats per minute (bpm). If the ventricles were not protected from this excessive impulse bombardment, ventricular filling time would suffer and cardiac output would fall dramatically. Excessive delay or failure of impulse transmission at the AV node is known as heart block.

The wave of electrical excitation spreads from the AV node to the *bundle of His,* a thick bundle of fibers extending down the right side of the interventricular septum. The bundle divides into the *right bundle branch* and the *left bundle branch,* which descend on opposite sides of the interventricular septum. The left bundle branch bifurcates into a thin anterior and thick posterior division. The bundle branches terminate in a complex branching network of fibers, the *Purkinje system,* which spreads throughout the inner surface of both ventricles. Spread of the wave of excitation through the Purkinje fibers is extremely rapid.

While these specialized conduction pathways speed the transmission of the cardiac impulse throughout the heart, the arrangement of myocardial cells outside the conduction system further ensures rapid impulse spread. Adjacent cells lie in close approximation, joined at sites called intercalated discs. Within these discs are points of intercellular membrane fusion or nexuses. These nexuses facilitate rapid cell-to-cell transmission of electrical excitation, resulting in virtually simultaneous activation and contraction of the myocardial cells.

Therefore, the normal sequence of excitation through the conduction system is SA node, atrial pathways, AV node, bundle of His, bundle branches, Purkinje fibers. Excitation normally originates in the SA node because the SA node exhibits the fastest intrinsic rate of impulse generation, approximately 60 to 100 bpm. However, in the event of SA node failure or inability to generate impulses at an adequate rate, other sites can assume the role of pacemaker. The AV node is capable of generating impulses at a rate of approximately 40 to 60 bpm, and ventricular sites can generate impulses at rates of approximately 20 to 30 bpm. These lower, or "escape," pacemakers serve a critical function in the prevention of cardiac standstill (asystole) if the natural pacemaker fails.

SYSTEMIC CIRCULATION

The structural characteristics of each portion of the systemic vasculature determines its physiologic role in the integration of cardiovascular function. The vessel wall consists of three layers: the outer layer, or *adventitia;* the muscular middle, or *medial layer;* and the inner endothelial layer, or *intima.* The systemic circulation can be subdivided into five anatomic and functional categories: (1) arteries, (2) arterioles, (3) capillaries, (4) venules, and (5) veins (see Fig. 24-8).

Arteries

The walls of the aorta and major arteries are composed of much elastic tissue and some smooth muscle. The left ventricle ejects blood into the aorta under high pressure. This sudden expulsion of blood distends the elastic arterial walls; during ventricular relaxation the elastic recoil of the walls propels blood forward throughout the circulatory system.

Peripherally, the branches of the arterial system proliferate and subdivide into smaller vessels, resulting in two important alterations in flow. First, the relative increase in the cross-sectional area of the arterial system reduces the velocity of blood flow. Second, the compression effect of the arterial walls progressively converts the pulsatile, phasic arterial flow into steady, continuous flow. This reduction in velocity of flow and conversion into steady flow facilitates the eventual exchange of nutrients and metabolites at the capillary level. The arterial bed contains approximately 15 percent of the total blood volume at one time. Therefore the arterial system is considered a low-volume–high-pressure circuit. Because of these volume–pressure characteristics, the arterial tree is called a *resistance circuit.*

Arterioles

At the arteriole level, the vascular wall is primarily smooth muscle with some elastic fiber. The muscular wall of the arteriole is highly responsive and can dilate

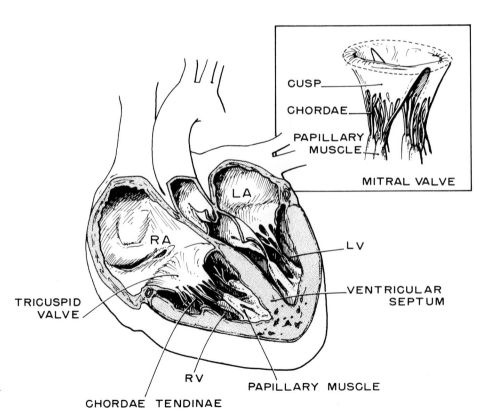

FIGURE 24-5 Anatomy of the atrioventricular valves.

or constrict to control the flow of blood to the capillary bed. The arterioles are the major sites of resistance to flow in the arterial tree as a result of this ability to significantly alter the radius of the vessel. At the junction between the arteriole and capillary, there is a *precapillary sphincter* subject to intricate physiologic control.

Capillaries

The capillary wall is thin, consisting of a single layer of endothelial cells. Nutrients and metabolites diffuse across this thin, semipermeable membrane from areas of high concentration to areas of lower concentration. Oxygen and nutrients therefore leave the vessel to enter the interstitial space and the cell; carbon dioxide and metabolites diffuse in the opposite direction. Net fluid movement between the blood vessel and the interstitial space is dependent upon the relative balance between hydrostatic and osmotic pressures at the capillary bed.

Venules

The venules function as collecting tubules and are composed of a relatively weak, yet responsive muscle wall. At the juncture between the capillary and venule, there is a *postcapillary sphincter.*

Veins

The veins are relatively thin-walled conduits for transport of blood from the capillary bed through the venous system to the right atrium. Venous flow to the heart is unidirectional as a result of valves strategically located within the venous channels. The veins can accommodate large volumes of blood under relatively low pressure. Because of these low-pressure–high-volume characteristics, the venous system is referred to as a *capacitance system.* Approximately 50 percent of the blood volume lies within the venous system at a given time. However, the capacity of the venous bed can be altered. Venoconstriction reduces the capacity of the venous bed, forcing blood forward to the heart and thereby increasing venous return. The movement of blood from the capillary bed toward the heart is influenced by two

factors: (1) venous compression by skeletal muscles and (2) alterations in thoracic and abdominal pressures. The venous system terminates in the inferior and superior venae cavae.

CORONARY CIRCULATION

The efficiency of the heart as a pump depends on adequate oxygenation and nourishment of the heart muscle. The coronary circulation courses over the surface of the heart, carrying oxygen and nutrients to the myocardium via small intramyocardial branches. The distribution of the coronary arteries to the heart muscle and to the conduction system must be understood to recognize the consequences of coronary heart disease. The morbidity and mortality associated with myocardial infarction depends upon the degree of both mechanical and electrical dysfunction.

The coronary arteries are the first branches of the systemic circulation. The coronary orifices are located within the sinuses of Valsalva in the aorta immediately above the aortic valve. The coronary circulation consists of the *right coronary artery* and the *left coronary artery.* The left coronary artery has two major branches: the *left anterior descending artery* and the *left circumflex artery* (see Fig. 24-9).

The arteries course around the heart in two external anatomic grooves: the *atrioventricular groove,* encircling the heart between the atria and ventricles, and the *interventricular groove,* separating the two ventricles. The juncture of these two grooves on the posterior surface of the heart is a critical anatomic landmark known as the *crux of the heart.* The AV node is located at this juncture; therefore, whichever vessel crosses the crux nourishes the AV node. The terms "right dominance" and "left dominance" simply designate whether the right or the left coronary artery, respectively, crosses the crux.

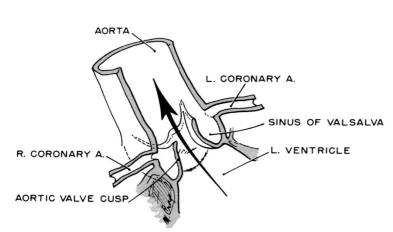

FIGURE 24-6 Sinuses of Valsalva.

The right coronary artery courses laterally around the right side of the heart in the right atrioventricular groove. In 90 percent of all hearts, upon reaching the posterior surface of the heart, the right coronary artery extends to the crux, then descends toward the apex of the heart in the posterior interventricular groove. The main left coronary artery branches shortly after its origin in the aorta. The left circumflex artery extends laterally around the left side of the heart in the left atrioventricular groove. This circumferential distribution corresponds to its designation as the "circumflex" artery. Similarly the term "left anterior descending artery" describes the anatomic pathway of this arterial branch. The left anterior descending artery courses down the surface of the heart in the anterior interventricular groove. It crosses the apex of the heart, reversing direction and extending upward along the posterior surface of the interventricular groove to meet the distal branches of the right coronary artery. Each major vessel gives off characteristic epicardial and intramyocardial branches.

The anatomic pathways result in the following correlations between coronary arteries and nutrient supply of cardiac muscle. Basically, the right coronary artery supplies the right atrium, right ventricle, and a portion of the posterior wall of the left ventricle. The left circumflex artery supplies the left atrium and the lateral and posterior walls of the left ventricle. The left anterior descending artery nourishes the massive anterior wall of the left ventricle.

The nutrient supply of the conduction system is another critical correlation determined by anatomic pathways. The SA node, despite its position in the right atrium, is supplied 55 percent of the time by the right coronary artery and 45 percent of the time by a branch of the left circumflex artery. The AV node, supplied by the artery crossing the crux, is nourished 90 percent of the time by the right coronary artery and 10 percent of the time by the left circumflex artery.

These correlations have significant clinical implications. For instance, a lesion of the right coronary artery would be expected to be associated with the highest incidence of AV nodal conduction disturbances, whereas a lesion of the left anterior descending artery would be more likely to interfere with the pumping function of the left ventricle.

Anastomoses between arterial branches exist within the coronary circulation. These anastomoses are of critical import as potential routes for collateral or alternative circulation to nourish myocardial regions deprived of flow by lesions obstructing normal pathways in the coronary vasculature (see Fig. 24-10).

Cardiac veins

The distribution of the coronary veins essentially parallels that of the coronary arteries. There are three subdivisions of the venous system of the heart: (1) the *thebesian veins* comprise the smallest system, draining a portion of the right atrial and right ventricular myocardium; (2) the *anterior cardiac veins* are intermediate in importance, emptying a large portion of the right ventricular venous drainage directly into the right atrium; (3) the *coronary sinus and its branches* compose the largest, most significant venous system, draining the bulk of myocardial venous return into the right atrium through the coronary sinus ostium beside the orifice to the inferior vena cava.

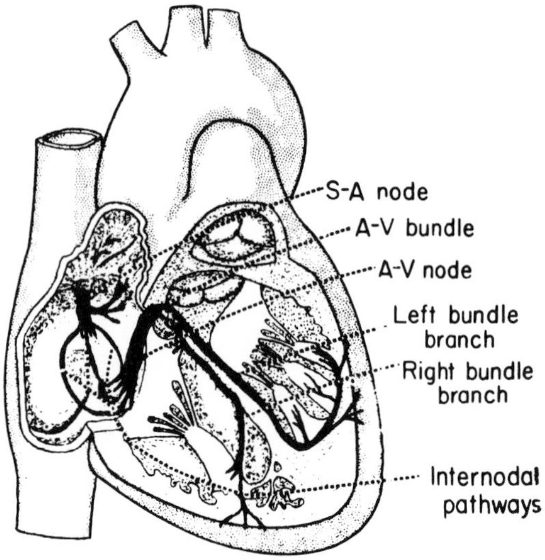

LYMPHATIC CIRCULATION

The lymphatic capillary network in the interstitial spaces collects excess fluid and protein filtered through the systemic capillaries. This capillary filtrate is then returned to the systemic circulation via collecting vessels located in close approximation to the veins. Lymph is propelled upward through unidirectional valves by a combination of two dynamic influences: (1) external compression by muscles and arterial pulsations and (2) intrinsic peristaltic action. The terminal thoracic duct and right lymphatic duct empty into the subclavian veins.

PULMONIC CIRCULATION

The pulmonic circulation is described in depth in Part VI. However, significant differences between the systemic and the pulmonic circulation warrant mention. The pulmonic vasculature has thinner walls and less smooth

FIGURE 24-7 The conduction system of the heart (From A. C. Guyton, Textbook of Medical Physiology, *5th ed., Saunders, Philadelphia, 1976, p. 177.)*

S-A node
A-V bundle
A-V node
Left bundle branch
Right bundle branch
Internodal pathways

muscle. The pulmonary circuit is therefore more distensible and offers less resistance to flow. Pressure in the pulmonic circuit is approximately one-sixth that of the systemic circuit. The walls of the pulmonary vasculature are much less reactive to autonomic and humoral influences, whereas alterations in oxygen and carbon dioxide content of the blood and alveoli profoundly alter flow through the pulmonary vasculature. These differences make the pulmonary circuit particularly well suited to fulfill its physiologic function of oxygen uptake and carbon dioxide liberation.

INNERVATION OF THE CARDIOVASCULAR SYSTEM

The cardiovascular system is richly innervated by fibers of the autonomic nervous system. The two divisions of the autonomic nervous system are the parasympathetic and sympathetic systems which exhibit opposite effects

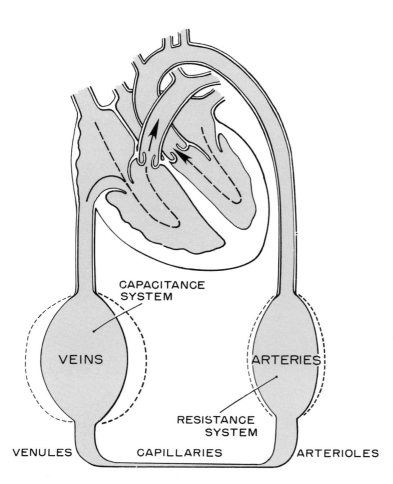

FIGURE 24-8 Schematic illustration of the systemic circulation. The arterial system may be considered as a resistance circuit (low volume, high pressure) whereas the venous system may be considered as a capacitance circuit (high volume, low pressure).

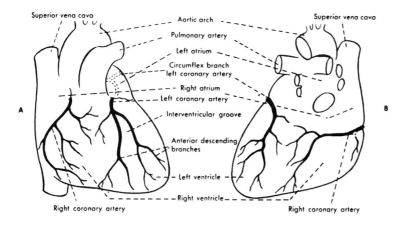

FIGURE 24-9 A, coronary arteries supplying the anterior aspect of the heart. B, coronary arteries supplying the posterior aspect of the heart. (From K. G. Andreoli, V. H. Fowkes, D. P. Zipes, and A. G. Wallace, Comprehensive Cardiac Care, 3d ed., Mosby, St. Louis, 1975, p. 3.)

and operate reciprocally. For instance, stimulation of the sympathetic system is coupled with inhibition of the parasympathetic system; conversely, parasympathetic stimulation and sympathetic inhibition are concurrent events. This reciprocal action increases the precision of neural regulation by the autonomic nervous system.

Autonomic nervous system regulation of the cardio-vascular system requires the following components: (1) sensors, (2) afferent pathways, (3) an integration center, (4) efferent pathways, and (5) receptors.

There are two primary groups of sensors: the *baro-receptors* and the *chemoreceptors*. The baroreceptors, located in the aortic arch and carotid sinus, are sensitive to the stretch or distortion of the vessel wall caused by alterations in arterial pressure. Stimulation of these receptors by elevation of arterial pressure signals the cardioregulatory center to inhibit cardiac activity; conversely, reduction of arterial pressure initiates reflex augmentation of cardiac activity. The chemoreceptors, located in the carotid body and aortic arch, are stimulated by reduction in arterial oxygen concentration, elevation of carbon dioxide tension and elevation in

hydrogen ion concentration (reduced blood pH). Activation of the chemoreceptors stimulates the cardioregulatory center to augment cardiac activity. Other receptors, which are sensitive to stretch resulting from alterations in blood volume, are located in the great veins and right atrium. Two reflex responses occur upon stimulation of these receptors: an increase in heart rate (Bainbridge reflex) and diuresis.

Afferent pathways in the vagus and glossopharyngeal nerves carry the neural impulses from the receptors to the brain. The integration center or cardioregulatory center is located in the upper medulla and lower pons. The cardioregulatory center receives impulses from the baroreceptors and chemoreceptors and transmits impulses to the heart and vessels via the parasympathetic and sympathetic nerve fibers. Higher centers of the brain, such as the cerebral cortex and hypothalamus, can also influence autonomic nervous activity via the medulla. The efferent pathway from the cardioregulatory center to the heart is chiefly via the vagus nerves for the parasympathetic fibers, whereas the sympathetic fibers travel via the cardiac nerves. Receptors are located in the conduction system of the heart, the myocardium, and the smooth muscle of the blood vessels. Stimulation of the receptors alters the heart rate, the strength of myocardial contraction, and the diameter of blood vessels.

The parasympathetic fibers innervate the SA node, the

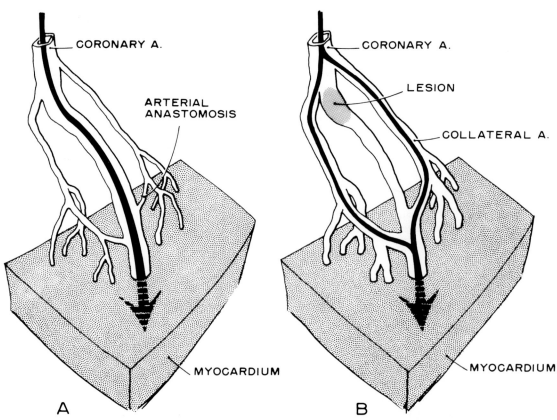

FIGURE 24-10 Collateral circulation to the myocardium. A, the bulk of blood flow to an area of myocardium is through the coronary blood vessel with minimal flow through arterial anastomoses. B, a lesion (e.g., an atherosclerotic plaque) in the coronary artery causes the development of increased collateral circulation which may allow an adequate blood supply to the compromised area of myocardium.

atrial musculature, and the AV node via the vagus nerves. Parasympathetic fibers also extend to the ventricular muscle, but the functional significance of these pathways seems limited. Stimulation of parasympathetic fibers causes the release of acetylcholine. Acetylcholine mediates the transmission of the neural impulse to the cardiac receptors. Parasympathetic stimulation restrains cardiac action by reducing the heart rate, the speed of impulse conduction through the AV node, and the force of atrial and perhaps ventricular contraction. This response to parasympathetic stimulation is also referred to as a *cholinergic response* or a *vagal response*.

The sympathetic fibers extend to the entire conduction system and myocardium, as well as to the smooth muscle of the vasculature. Norepinephrine is the sympathetic neurotransmitter. Sympathetic stimulation causes the release of epinephrine and norepinephrine from the adrenal medulla. Sympathetic stimulation accelerates the heart by increasing heart rate, speed of impulse conduction through the AV node, and the force of myocardial contraction. This sympathetic response is also called the *adrenergic response*. The response of the heart to sympathetic stimulation is mediated by cardiac receptors called beta receptors. The vasculature contains two types of receptors, alpha and beta receptors. Sympathetic stimulation of vascular alpha receptors results in vasoconstriction; vascular beta receptor stimulation results in vasodilation. Selective stimulation of these receptors, combined with variations in the intensity of sympathetic activity, regulates the degree of vasoconstriction, thereby controlling the capacity of the vascular bed and influencing the vascular resistance to blood flow and consequently arterial pressure. For example, arterial constriction would increase arterial pressure and the peripheral resistance to blood flow. Venoconstriction would reduce the capacity of the venous bed and increase venous return to the heart.

This cardiovascular reflex arc operates to stabilize arterial pressure and cardiac output and to mediate alterations relative to body needs (see Fig. 24-11). Cardiac output and arterial pressure can be increased by sympathetic stimulation and parasympathetic inhibition, resulting in an elevation of heart rate, increased force of contraction, and vasoconstriction. Conversely, abnormal elevations in blood pressure will result in reflex slowing of heart rate, reduced contractility, and vasodilation.

QUESTIONS

Anatomy of the cardiovascular system—Chap. 24

Directions: Answer the following questions on a separate sheet of paper.

1 Trace the anatomic sequence of blood flow through the cardiovascular system naming the structures traversed.

2 Describe the two critical functions of the AV node.

3 Discuss the differences in the wall thickness of the right and left ventricles in terms of function. Relate the relative wall thicknesses to differences in the systemic and pulmonary circulations.

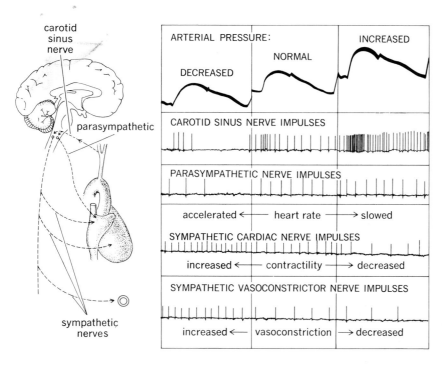

FIGURE 24-11 *The carotid sinus reflexes are the major blood-pressure-regulating reflexes. A decrease in arterial pressure causes a decrease in the rate of discharge of the carotid sinus baroreceptors, which causes a reflex inhibition of the parasympathetic nerves to the heart and stimulation of the sympathetic nerves to the heart, arterioles, and veins; the net result is an increased cardiac output and peripheral resistance, both of which cause the arterial blood pressure to increase. Precisely the opposite events occur in response to an increase in the blood pressure. (From A. J. Vander, J. H. Sherman, and D. S. Luciano,* Human Physiology, *2d ed., McGraw-Hill, New York, 1975.)*

4 What is the function of the chordae tendinae and papillary muscles.

5 How many valve cusps are there on the valve between the left ventricle and aorta? Name this valve. Name the outpouchings above the valve cusps. What is the function of these outpouchings?

6 Identify the layers of the pericardium. What does the space between the layers contain and what is its function?

7 How is lymph propelled in lymphatic vessels?

8 Contrast the vascular effects of sympathetic stimulation of the alpha and beta receptors.

Directions: Circle the letter preceding each item that correctly answers each question. Only one answer is correct unless otherwise noted.

9 The portion of the heart lying directly beneath the sternum is the:
a Cardiac apex *b* Left atrium *c* Crux of the heart
d Right ventricle

10 The apex of the heart is normally palpated in the:
a Fifth intercostal space to the right of the sternum at the midclavicular line *b* Fifth intercostal space to the right of the sternum at the anterior axillary line
c Fifth intercostal space to the left of the sternum at the midclavicular line *d* Fifth intercostal space to the left of the sternum at the anterior axillary line

11 All the valves of the heart have three cusps *except:*
a Pulmonic *b* Aortic *c* Mitral *d* Tricuspid

12 Oxygenated blood is contained within the:
a Pulmonary artery *b* Pulmonary veins
c Superior vena cava *d* Inferior vena cava

13 In order to generate high pressure to propel blood through the systemic circulation, the configuration of the left ventricle is:
a Cresent-shaped *b* Circular *c* Elliptical

14 The outermost layer of the wall of a blood vessel is called the:
a Intima *b* Media *c* Adventitia *d* Serosa

15 The primary reason that blood flow through the capillaries is slow is because:
a Capillaries are very small *b* Capillary pressure is low *c* Precapillary resistance is high *d* Total capillary cross-sectional area is great

16 The SA node is the pacemaker of the heart because:
a It is the only structure capable of spontaneously generating impulses *b* It is richly innervated by sympathetic nerves *c* It has the fastest intrinsic rate of impulse generation *d* It is anatomically the point of impulse origin

17 Cardiac impulse conduction is slowest through the:
a Purkinje fibers *b* Interatrial pathways
c Bundle branches *d* AV node

18 At any given time, most of the blood in the circulatory system is in the:
a Arteries *b* Veins *c* Capillaries *d* Heart

19 An increase in the mean arterial pressure causes: (More than one answer may be correct)
a Activation of baroreceptors *b* Decreased sympathetic outflow to the heart *c* Increased parasympathetic outflow to the heart *d* Increased sympathetic outflow to vascular receptors

20 The response resulting from the above would be: (More than one answer may be correct)
a A decrease in the blood pressure *b* An increase in the total peripheral resistance *c* A decrease in the heart rate *d* Reduced contractility of the heart

21 Which of the following statements concerning the cardiovascular chemoreceptors is *not* true?
a They are located in the carotid sinus and aortic arch. *b* Afferent impulses from the chemoreceptors are carried to the cardioregulatory center via the glossopharyngeal and vagus nerves. *c* Chemoreceptors are stimulated by a reduction in the arterial oxygen concentration. *d* Chemoreceptors are stimulated by an elevation of CO_2 tension. *e* Activation of the chemoreceptors stimulates the cardioregulatory center to increase parasympathetic outflow to the heart.

Directions: Match each of the coronary arteries in col. A with appropriate items in col. B.

Column A	Column B
22 ___ Right coronary artery	*a* Divides into two main branches
23 ___ Left coronary artery	*b* One of its branches supplies the anterior wall of the left ventricle
	c Supplies the AV node 90 percent of the time
	d Supplies the SA node more than 50 percent of the time

24 Arrange the following structures to represent the normal sequence of cardiac conduction:
a Bundle of His *b* Purkinje fibers *c* SA node
d Bundle branches *e* Interatrial pathways
f AV node

Directions: Match each of the cardiovascular structures in col. A with its location in col. B.

Column A	Column B
25 ___ Chordae tendinae	*a* Separates right and left ventricles into two chambers
26 ___ Interventricular septum	*b* Muscular layer of heart
27 ___ Endocardium	*c* Attached to AV valve leaflets on one end and to papillary muscles at the other end
28 ___ Epicardium	

29 _____ Myocardium
30 _____ Sinuses of Valsalva

d Outer layer of the heart
e Inner layer of the myocardial wall
f Contains orifices of coronary arteries

Directions: Fill in the blanks with the correct word or phrase.

31 The conduction tissue of the heart exhibits the following properties: _____, the ability to spontaneously generate impulses; _____, the ability to respond to stimulation; _____, the ability to transmit impulses; _____, the regularity of impulse generation.

32 Elevations of right atrial pressure or left atrial pressure readily result in neck vein distention and pulmonary congestion, respectively, because the venae cavae and pulmonary veins, unlike most systemic veins, have no true _____.

33 In cases of coronary artery occlusion, _____ circulation may protect the involved muscle tissue from ischemia or necrosis.

34 Lesions of the _____ _____ artery are associated with the highest incidence of AV nodal conduction disturbances. Lesions of the _____ _____ _____

artery are more apt to interfere with the pumping function of the left ventricle.

35 The intrinsic rate of the SA node is _____; the rate of the AV node is _____; and the ventricular rate is _____.

BIBLIOGRAPHY

BERNE, ROBERT and MATTHEW LEVY: *Cardiovascular Physiology*, Mosby, St. Louis, 1972.

GUYTON, ARTHUR C.: *Textbook of Medical Physiology*, Saunders, Philadelphia, 1976.

HURST, J. WILLIS (ed.): *The Heart*, McGraw-Hill, New York, 1974.

RUSHMER, ROBERT: *Cardiovascular Dynamics*, Saunders, Philadelphia, 1970.

SODEMAN, WILLIAM A., and WILLIAM A. SODEMAN JR.: *Pathologic Physiology: Mechanisms of Disease*, Saunders, Philadelphia, 1974.

VANDER, ARTHUR, JAMES SHERMAN, and DOROTHY LUCIANO: *Human Physiology*, McGraw-Hill, New York, 1970.

CHAPTER 25 Physiology of the Cardiovascular System

CARDIAC CYCLE

Each cardiac cycle consists of a sequence of interdependent electrical and mechanical events. The wave of electrical excitation spreading from the SA node through the conduction system and to the myocardium stimulates muscular contraction. This electrical excitation is referred to as *depolarization*, followed by electrical recovery or *repolarization*. The mechanical responses are *systole*, or muscular contraction, and *diastole*, or muscular relaxation.

The electrical activity of the cell, recorded graphically via intracellular electrodes, exhibits a characteristic configuration, the *action potential* (see Fig. 25-1A). The summated electrical activity of all myocardial cells can be visualized in an *electrocardiogram* (see Fig. 25-1B). The waves on the electrocardiogram correlate with the spread of electrical excitation through the conduction system and myocardium. The significance of the waveforms are discussed in subsequent chapters.

Cardiac pacemaking cells possess the ability to depolarize spontaneously, thereby initiating the wave of excitation that is propagated throughout the conduction system and myocardium. This wave of excitation stimulates muscular contraction. The correlation between ventricular depolarization and ventricular contraction is illustrated in Fig. 25-2.

Immediately following myocardial depolarization, there is a brief interval, known as the "absolute refractory period," during which the myocardium is incapable of responding to any stimulus. A "relative refractory period" follows when the myocardium will respond only to strong stimulation. Tetanic contracture of the myocardium as a result of repetitive stimulation is therefore impossible.

Electrophysiology

In the resting state, the cardiac cell exhibits a difference in electrical potential or voltage across the cell membrane. The inside of the cell is negative, and the outside of the cell is positive; thus the cell is polarized (see Fig. 25-3A). This difference in polarity results from the relative permeability of the cell membrane to positively charged sodium and potassium ions. Potassium is the dominant intracellular cation, whereas sodium concentration is highest extracellularly. In the resting state,

the cell membrane is more permeable to potassium than to sodium; therefore small amounts of potassium ions seep out of the cell, where the potassium concentration is high, to the extracellular fluid, where the potassium concentration is low. This intracellular loss of positive potassium ions leaves the inside of the cell relatively negative in electrical charge.

Depolarization of the cell is the result of greatly increased membrane permeability to sodium. Extracellular sodium ions rush into the cell propelled by the sodium concentration gradient. This influx of positive sodium ions reverses the relative charges along the cell membrane; the outside of the cell becomes negative, and the inside becomes positive (see Fig. 25-3B).

Repolarization occurs when the cell membrane again becomes more permeable to potassium and loses its permeability to sodium. Potassium moves out of the cell, reducing the positive charge within the cell; eventually the inside of the cell regains its relative negativity, and the outside of the cell its relative positivity (see Fig. 25-3C). Finally, the initial ionic distribution is restored by the active transport mechanism of the sodium–potassium pump moving potassium intracellularly and sodium extracellularly.

Thus the electrical activity of the heart is the result of alterations in cell membrane permeability which create ionic fluxes across the cell membrane that shift the relative electrical charge across the cell membrane. Derangements of cardiac rhythm and conduction can be traced to alterations in cellular electrophysiology. The potassium and sodium ions are of critical significance in the regulation and stabilization of the electrical events of the cardiac cycle. For example, potassium depletion increases tissue excitability and can lead to abnormal cardiac impulse formation.

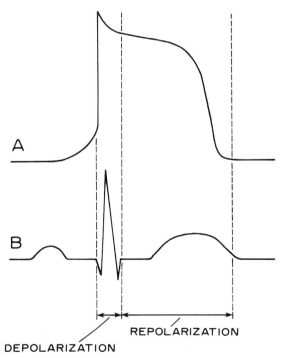

FIGURE 25-1 Electrical activity of the heart. A, recording of the intracellular potential of a single cardiac cell during a complete cardiac cycle. B, illustration of a standard electrocardiographic recording from the body surface representing the summated electrical activity of all the myocardial cells. The time periods within the dashed lines represent depolarization and repolarization of the ventricles.

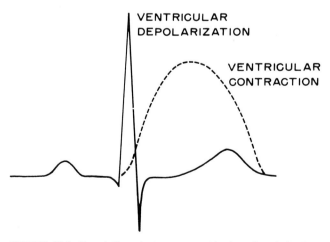

FIGURE 25-2 Correlation between ventricular depolarization and ventricular contraction. (Modified from A. J. Vander, J. H. Sherman, and D. S. Luciano, Human Physiology, 2d ed., McGraw-Hill, New York, 1975, p. 238.)

contractile force by reducing the amount of overlap and subsequent linkage formation between the actin and myosin filaments.

Muscle ultrastructure

The electrical excitation of the myocardial cell initiates muscular contraction by stimulating the release of calcium from the sarcoplasmic reticulum. The calcium diffuses through the sarcoplasm to the sarcomere, the basic contractile unit of the myocardial cell. Calcium then binds to the troponin protein, inactivating the inhibitory effect of the troponin–tropomyosin system upon the contractile proteins, actin and myosin. The actin and myosin myofilaments then interact to form linkages or cross-bridges that generate force to slide these overlapping myofilaments past each other, thereby shortening the sarcomere (see Fig. 25-4). The shortening of multiple sarcomere units produces muscular contraction. Relaxation of the muscle is the result of calcium uptake by the sarcoplasmic reticulum dissociating the actin–myosin cross-bridges.

The force of myocardial contraction is dependent upon the interaction between sarcomere myofilaments. Administration of calcium can increase contractile force by increasing calcium availability to the sarcomere. Conversely, extreme dilation of the myocardium reduces

Phases of the cardiac cycle

The phases of the cardiac cycle can most easily be conceptualized in the following sequence: (1) mid-diastole (2) late diastole (3) early systole (4) late systole (5) early diastole (see Fig. 25-5).

1 Mid-diastole: This is the phase of slow ventricular filling, or "diastasis." The atrial and ventricular chambers are relaxed. Blood entering the atria through venous channels flows passively into the ventricles through the open AV valves. The semilunar valves are closed.
2 Late diastole: The wave of depolarization spreads through the atria and pauses at the AV node. The atrial muscle contracts, contributing an additional 20 percent to the ventricular volume.
3 Early systole: Depolarization spreads from the AV node through the bundle branches to the ventricular myocardium. As ventricular contraction begins, the pressure within the ventricles rises above that of the atria, causing the AV valves to close, which generates the first heart sound. The ventricular chambers continue to develop higher pressures; however, during

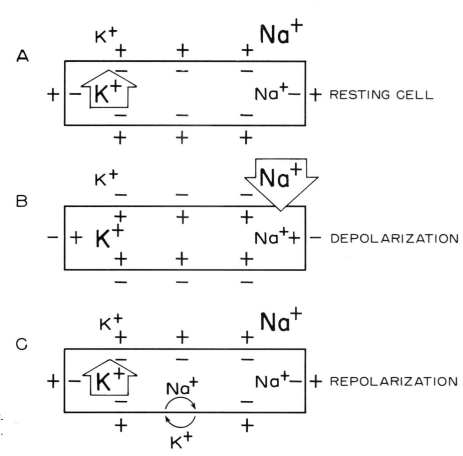

FIGURE 25-3 Cellular electrophysiology. A, resting state. B, depolarization. C, repolarization.

this phase the pressures within the aorta and pulmonary artery exceed the ventricular pressures keeping the semilunar valves closed. This is termed *isovolumetric contraction,* since the ventricular volumes remain constant.

4 Late systole: As soon as the ventricular pressures exceed the pressures within the vessels, the semilunar valves open and ventricular ejection into the pulmonic and systemic circulation occurs.

5 Early diastole: The wave of repolarization then spreads through the ventricular myocardium and the ventricular chambers relax. As the muscle relaxes, the ventricular pressures drop below the arterial pressures, causing the semilunar valves to close, which produces the second heart sound. Relaxation continues until the ventricular pressures drop below that of the atrial pressures, causing the AV valves to open. As the valves open the ventricles fill rapidly with the venous blood that has accumulated in the atria. Almost 80 percent of ventricular filling occurs during this phase.

CARDIAC OUTPUT

Definitions

The result of the synchronized, rhythmic myocardial contraction is the ejection of blood into the pulmonic and systemic circulations. The volume of blood ejected by each ventricle per minute is the *cardiac output.* An average cardiac output is 5 liters/minute. However, cardiac output varies to meet the needs of the peripheral tissues for oxygen and nutrients. Since cardiac output requirements also vary according to body size, a more accurate indicator of cardiac function is the *cardiac index.* The cardiac index is the cardiac output divided by body surface area and ranges from 2.8 to 3.3 liters/minute.

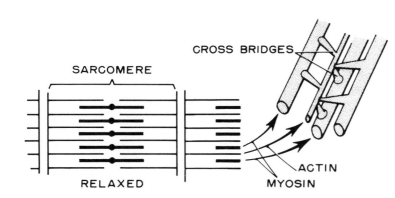

FIGURE 25-4 Muscle ultrastructure. The myofibrils are composed of thick myosin filaments and thin actin filaments. Cross-bridges are observed at regular intervals between the actin and myosin filaments, forming linkages during muscle contraction. The amount of overlap between the actin and myosin filaments is decreased during muscle relaxation and increased during contraction. This causes a corresponding increase or decrease in the sarcomere length.

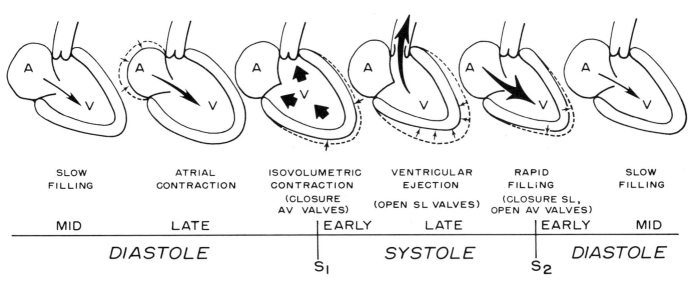

FIGURE 25-5 Phases of the cardiac cycle. (Modified from M. O. Vinsant, M. I. Spense, and M. E. Chapell, A Commonsense Approach to Coronary Care: A Program, Mosby, St. Louis, 1975, p. 6.)

Stroke volume is the volume of blood ejected by each ventricle per beat. Approximately two-thirds of the volume of blood in the ventricle at the end of diastole (end-diastolic volume) is ejected during systole. This portion of blood ejected is known as the *ejection fraction;* the residual ventricular volume at the end of systole is referred to as the *end-systolic volume* (see Fig. 25-6A). Depression of ventricular function impairs the ability of the ventricle to empty, thereby reducing stroke volume and the ejection fraction with a consequent elevation of residual ventricular volumes (see Fig. 25-6B).

Determinants of cardiac output

Cardiac output is dependent upon the relationship between two variables: heart rate and stroke volume.

cardiac output = heart rate × stroke volume

Cardiac output can be held remarkably constant despite alterations in one variable by compensatory adjustments in the other variable. For instance, if the heart rate slows, the period of ventricular relaxation between heart beats is longer, thereby increasing ventricular filling time. Consequently, ventricular volumes are greater and more blood can be ejected per beat. Conversely, if stroke volume drops, cardiac output can be stabilized by increasing the heart rate. Obviously, these compensatory adjustments can only maintain cardiac output within limits. The alteration and stabilization of cardiac output depends upon control mechanisms regulating heart rate and stroke volume.

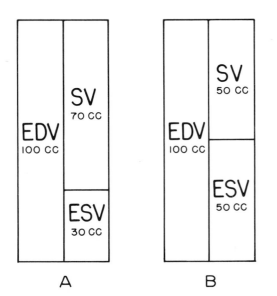

FIGURE 25-6 Relationship between end-diastolic volume (EDV), systolic volume (SV), and end-systolic volume (ESV). A, normal ventricular function. B, depressed ventricular function.

CONTROL OF HEART RATE

Heart rate is largely under the extrinsic control of the autonomic nervous system; parasympathetic and sympathetic fibers innervate the SA node and the AV node, influencing the rate and speed of impulse conduction. Stimulation of the parasympathetic fibers decreases the heart rate, whereas sympathetic stimulation increases it. In the normal resting heart, the influence of the parasympathetic system seems to dominate in maintaining the heart rate at approximately 80 bpm. If all neural and hormonal influences upon the heart were blocked, the intrinsic rate would be about 100 bpm. However, in the presence of heart disease, the sympathetic system predominates in the control of heart rate and the maintenance of cardiac compensation. Endogenous myocardial stores of norepinephrine augment the catecholamine supply available from neural sympathetic fibers and the adrenal medulla. These endogenous stores eventually become depleted in chronic heart failure.

CONTROL OF STROKE VOLUME

Stroke volume is dependent upon three variables: (1) preload, or Starling's law of the heart, (2) contractility, and (3) afterload.

Starling's law of the heart states that stretching the myocardial fibers during diastole will increase the force of contraction during systole (see Fig. 25-7). An analogous example is that of increasing the stretch on a rubber band to increase the force of elastic recoil upon release. Myocardial fibers can be stretched by increasing ventricular diastolic volumes. The degree of stretch is expressed in terms of *preload* (i.e., diastolic fiber length prior to contraction).

The degree of fiber stretch or preload is determined by the ventricular volume. The volume of blood contained within the ventricles during diastole depends upon the amount of venous return. Venous return is influenced primarily by circulating blood volume and the venous tone. Increasing venous return and consequently ventricular volumes stretches the myocardial fibers. Stretching the sarcomere maximizes the number of interaction sites available for actin–myosin linkage by increasing the overlap between the myofilaments. Consequently, the force of contraction rises.

Normally, the sarcomere is stretched to 2.0 μm during diastole (see Fig. 25-8A). The optimal sarcomere length is 2.2 μm (see Fig. 25-8B). Therefore a reserve in sarcomere length and resultant force of contraction exists. Starling's law is functional within limits determined by the myocardial ultrastructure described earlier. Stretching the sarcomere above 2.2 μm will reduce the strength of contraction by reducing the number of available interaction sites (see Fig. 25-8C).

The relationship between myocardial fiber length and force of contraction is referred to as the *ventricular function curve* (see Fig. 25-9). Increasing ventricular end-diastolic volumes will initially increase force of contraction and stroke volume. Subsequently, further increments in ventricular volumes and myocardial fiber stretch will depress stroke volume. Thus the curve

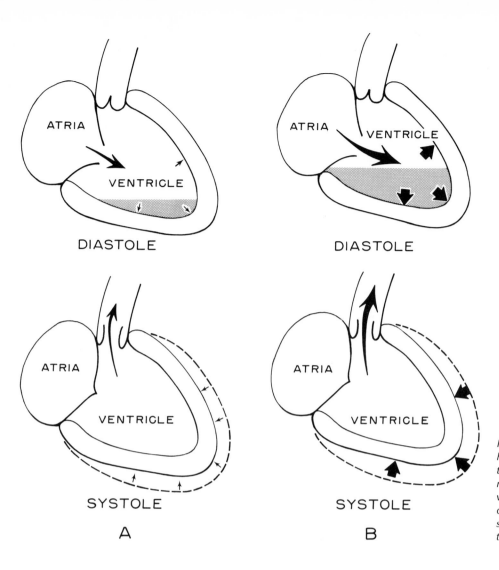

ATRIA

VENTRICLE

DIASTOLE

ATRIA

VENTRICLE

DIASTOLE

ATRIA

VENTRICLE

SYSTOLE

A

ATRIA

VENTRICLE

SYSTOLE

B

FIGURE 25-7 Starling's law of the heart. A, normal filling during diastole causes normal fiber stretch, normal contractile force and stroke volume. B, increased filling during diastole causes increased fiber stretch, increased force of contraction and increased stroke volume.

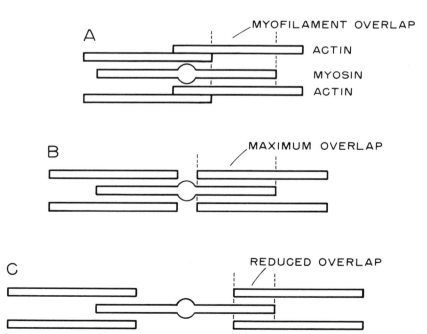

A

MYOFILAMENT OVERLAP

ACTIN

MYOSIN

ACTIN

B

MAXIMUM OVERLAP

C

REDUCED OVERLAP

FIGURE 25-8 Effect of sarcomere length upon myofilament overlap. A, usual sarcomere length 2.0 μm. B, optimal sarcomere length 2.2 μm. C, excessive sarcomere length 2.5 μm.

demonstrates an ascending limb of improved function and a descending limb of reduced function. As illustrated in Fig. 25-9, there is a considerable cardiac reserve ability to improve myocardial function by increasing end-diastolic volumes. However, excessive ventricular volumes and myocardial fiber stretch precipitates cardiac failure. In summary, increased preload will, within limits, increase the force of contraction and, consequently, the volume of blood ejected from the ventricle.

Contractility is the second determinant of stroke volume. Contractility by definition refers to alterations in the force of contraction occurring independent of myocardial fiber length. Increased contractility is the result of intensification of the interactions at the actin–myosin cross-bridges in the sarcomere. Clinically, the terms "contractility" and "contractile force" are used interchangeably. Administration of certain substances, such as calcium or epinephrine, will increase contractility, as would sympathetic nervous system stimulation. Increased contractility elevates stroke volume by increasing ventricular emptying during systole.

Afterload is the third determinant of stroke volume. Afterload is the amount of tension the ventricle must develop during systole to open the semilunar valve and eject blood. It is a function of arterial pressure and ventricular size. The relationship between ventricular tension, arterial pressure, and ventricular radius is expressed in this simplified version of the Laplace relationship:

ventricular tension = arterial pressure
× ventricular radius

The Laplace equation indicates that an increment in either arterial pressure or ventricular radius elevates the amount of tension the ventricle must develop to eject blood. In order to generate a given pressure, the ventricle must develop more tension as the ventricular radius or size increases. Therefore, a dilated ventricle must develop more tension than a normal ventricle to generate the same systolic pressure of 120 mmHg (see Fig. 25-10).

Similarly, elevation of arterial pressure will increase the resistance to ejection, thereby necessitating the development of increased ventricular tension. Thus an increment in afterload will result from either increased arterial pressure or ventricular dilation. Excessive increases in afterload may adversely affect ventricular emptying, reducing stroke volume and, consequently, cardiac output.

In summary, the integration of the mechanisms controlling heart rate and stroke volume determine ventricular function and cardiac output. Heart rate is primarily under extrinsic neural control. Control of stroke volume is a function of the interaction of three variables: preload, contractility, and afterload (see Fig. 25-11).

BLOOD FLOW TO THE PERIPHERY

The dynamics of peripheral blood flow is perhaps the most critical element of circulatory physiology for two reasons. First, the distribution of the cardiac output within the periphery depends upon properties of the vascular bed. Second, the volume of cardiac output depends upon the amount of blood returning to the heart. Essentially, the heart will eject a volume of blood equivalent to its venous return.

Principles of blood flow

Blood flow is dependent upon two opposing variables: (1) the pressure propelling blood and (2) the resistance to flow. Blood flow increases as the pressure propelling blood increases; inversely, flow decreases as resistance increases.

A pressure difference or pressure gradient must exist between two points for blood to flow between the points. The greater the pressure gradient, the greater the flow. Blood flows throughout the systemic circulation from the arterial to the venous end in response to pressure gradients. The mean arterial pressure, or average driving pressure at the arterial end of the circulation, is approximately 100 mmHg. Capillary pressure averages 25 mmHg. Pressure at the venous end of the circulation or right atrium is close to 0 mmHg. Therefore, pressure progressively declines throughout the systemic circulation. The pressure gradient between the arterial

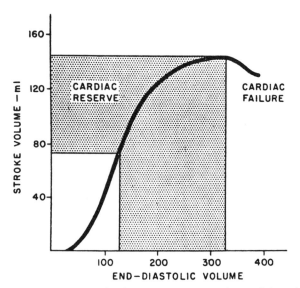

FIGURE 25-9 Ventricular function curve. As the end-diastolic volume increases, so does the force of ventricular contraction. Thus the stroke volume becomes greater up to a critical point after which stroke volume decreases (cardiac failure). (From L. L. Langley, *Review of Physiology,* 3d ed., *McGraw-Hill, New York, 1971, p. 264.)*

and venous ends of the systemic circulation is approximately 100 mmHg (mean arterial pressure – central venous pressure).

Alterations in either the *mean arterial pressure* or the *right atrial pressure* will influence blood flow by changing the pressure gradient between the two points. Mean arterial pressure will change if either the vascular contents (cardiac output) or the vascular capacity (total peripheral resistance) is altered.

mean arterial pressure = cardiac output
× total peripheral resistance

Either massive hemorrhage or extensive vasodilation (as in gram-negative sepsis) can profoundly reduce arterial pressure. However, the pressure alteration is sensed by the baroreceptors, and reflex compensatory responses mediated by the autonomic nervous system ensue to stabilize arterial pressure. Right atrial pressure depends upon the balance between venous return to the atria and the ability of the right atria to empty. Disease of the tricuspid valve and impaired right ventricular function can both reduce right atrial output and abnormally elevate right atrial pressure.

Resistance, the second determinant of blood flow, is primarily determined by the radius of the blood vessel. Other factors, such as blood viscosity and vascular length, also alter resistance to flow. However, since these properties are relatively constant, their influence is normally insignificant. Resistance is extremely sensitive to alterations in the lumen of the blood vessel. Poiseuille's law demonstrates that resistance is inversely proportional to the fourth power of the radius of the blood vessel.

$R \propto 1/r^4$

Hence, reduction of the radius by one-half will increase the resistance to flow 16-fold. The arteriole is the major site of vascular resistance. Alterations in the smooth muscle tone of the arteriolar wall regulates resistance to flow and, consequently, the amount of flow to the capillary bed.

In summary, flow is directly proportional to the pressure gradient and inversely proportional to the vascular resistance:

$$F = \frac{\Delta P}{R}$$

The pressure gradient is determined by pressures at the arterial and venous ends of the circulation. Resistance is primarily a function of the radius of the blood vessels, altered most significantly at the arteriolar level.

Distribution of blood flow

Blood flow is distributed among the multiple organ systems according to the metabolic needs and functional demands of the tissues. Since tissue needs are continually changing, blood flow must continually be readjusted. As tissue metabolism increases, blood flow must increase to supply oxygen and nutrients and to remove the end products of metabolism. For instance, during strenuous exercise, flow to the exercising skeletal muscle must increase. Dual control of the distribution of cardiac output is possible through extrinsic and intrinsic regulatory mechanisms.

EXTRINSIC CONTROL

Blood flow to a given organ system can be increased either by increasing cardiac output or by shunting blood from a relatively inactive organ system to the more active organ. The activity of the sympathetic nervous system can produce both responses. First, sympathetic stimulation augments cardiac output by increasing heart rate and force of contractility. Second, sympathetic adrenergic fibers also extend to the peripheral vasculature, particularly the arteriole. Selective alterations in sympa-

PRESSURE DEVELOPED

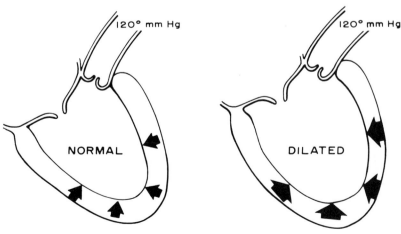

NORMAL

DILATED

TENSION GENERATED

FIGURE 25-10 Effect of ventricular size on afterload. The dilated ventricle on the right must generate more tension than the normal ventricle on the left to generate the same systolic pressure of 120 mmHg.

thetic discharge will stimulate alpha and beta receptors, preferentially constricting some arterioles and dilating others to redistribute blood to capillary beds according to need. Within any capillary bed, there is considerable reserve for increased flow, since only a portion of the capillaries are perfused at a given time. Therefore, flow can be increased by opening nonperfused capillaries as well as by further arteriolar dilation of perfused capillaries.

Skeletal muscle vasculature is uniquely capable of vasodilation because sympathetic cholinergic fibers originating in the cerebral cortex innervate these vessels. These fibers release acetylcholine, resulting in relaxation of vascular smooth muscle. Parasympathetic cholinergic fibers innervate only selected, small portions of the peripheral vasculature; therefore, parasympathetic activity does not significantly influence the distribution of cardiac output or total peripheral resistance.

In addition to neural control, humoral agents exert an extrinsic influence upon peripheral resistance and flow. The adrenal medulla secretes catecholamines, epinephrine and norepinephrine, in response to sympathetic activity. These hormones elicit sympathetic responses in the peripheral vasculature. Other bloodborne agents—vasopressin, angiotensin, serotonin, bradykinin, and histamine—are currently under investigation to establish their role in peripheral vascular control.

INTRINSIC CONTROL

An extremely potent stimulus for vasodilation is tissue ischemia. The logic of this compensatory response is obvious, although the exact mechanism is unclear. Perhaps the vasodilation is a direct response to the oxygen lack, or the lack may trigger the release of chemical vasodilators, such as adenosine. The direct vasodilatory effect of metabolites, elevated PCO_2, and low pH offers another explanation.

The relative strength of extrinsic and intrinsic control mechanisms varies among organ systems. In vital, flow-dependent organs, such as the heart and brain, the intrinsic mechanisms predominate, whereas in less dependent areas, such as the skin, autonomic control predominates.

In addition to these control mechanisms designed to increase oxygen delivery to the tissues, the tissues can increase oxygen supply by extracting more oxygen from the arterial blood. In most organs, with the notable exception of the heart, only a small proportion of the oxygen available in the arterial blood is extracted by the tissue. When an oxygen deficit develops in the tissues, the concentration gradient of oxygen between the arterial blood and the tissue increases. This causes more oxygen to diffuse from the intravascular to the extravascular space, thereby increasing oxygen delivery to the cells.

When compensatory mechanisms are unable to sustain adequate peripheral perfusion, as in shock, flow must be distributed according to priority. Blood will be shunted away from "nonvital" areas, such as the skin and kidney, to maintain perfusion of the brain and heart. Consequently, early signs of shock or inadequate tissue perfusion are decreased urine output and cold, pale skin. Significant alterations in mentation and cardiac function occur much later in the shock state when flow is compromised even to the vital organs.

CARDIAC RESERVE

Normally, the heart possesses the ability to increase its pumping capacity significantly above resting levels. This cardiac reserve enables the normal heart to increase output approximately fivefold. The increase in cardiac

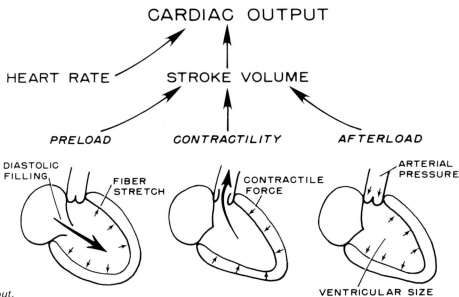

FIGURE 25-11 Control of cardiac output.

output can occur through increments in heart rate or stroke volume (cardiac output = heart rate × stroke volume).

Heart rate can normally increase from resting levels of between 60 to 100 bpm to approximately 180 bpm, primarily through sympathetic stimulation. Rates above this can be deleterious for two reasons. First, as heart rate increases, the duration of diastole shortens and ventricular filling time is reduced; eventually stroke volume will fall, negating the advantage of further rate increments. Second, rapid heart rates can adversely affect myocardial oxygenation because cardiac work is increased while the diastolic period, during which most coronary flow occurs, is reduced.

Stroke volume can increase either by increased ventricular emptying due to increased contractility or by increased diastolic filling and a subsequent rise in ejection volume. However, both increased force of contraction and increased ventricular volumes will elevate cardiac work and oxygen demand. In addition, the effect of increased diastolic filling upon contractility and stroke volume is limited by the degree of myocardial fiber stretch. Excessive fiber stretch will reduce the force of contraction as the descending limb of the ventricular function curve is approached.

If the heart is subjected to chronic volume or pressure overload, the ventricular muscle may *dilate* to increase contractile force, according to Starling's law, or *hypertrophy* to increase muscle mass and pumping force. Both responses, although compensatory in nature, eventually contribute to further cardiac decompensation. Dilation increases cardiac work by increasing the amount of tension the ventricle must develop to generate a given pressure according to the law of Laplace. Furthermore, excessive dilation will eventually reduce contractile force. Hypertrophy increases the muscle mass requiring nutrient supply, thereby increasing oxygen demand.

QUESTIONS

Physiology of the cardiovascular system—Chap. 25

Directions: Answer the following questions on a separate sheet of paper.

1 What are the two major mechanical phases of the cardiac cycle and what does each represent? What does an electrocardiogram represent and how is it different from an action potential? What is the relationship between the electrical and mechanical events of the cardiac cycle?

2 State Starling's law of the heart. What is the relationship of Starling's law to the ventricular function curve?

3 State Poiseuille's law as it applies to blood circulation. How would you calculate the systemic blood pressure gradient?

4 Hemodynamic measurements on a 46-year-old woman with a body surface area of 1.5 m² reveal the following data: cardiac output (CO) 4.5 liters/minute; left ventricular end-diastolic volume (EDV) 100 ml; left

ventricular end-systolic volume (ESV), 30 ml. What is her left ventricular stroke volume (SV)? What is her cardiac index (CI) and left ventricular ejection fraction (EF)? Are these values normal?

Directions: Circle the letter preceding each item that correctly answers each question. Only one answer is correct, unless otherwise noted.

5 The depolarizing phase of an action potential in heart muscle is caused by a:
a Sudden increase in the permeability of the membrane to sodium   b Decrease in the permeability of the membrane to potassium   c Decrease in the sodium–potassium pumping rate   d Sudden increase in the permeability of the membrane to potassium

6 Which of the following substances is released from the sarcoplasmic reticulum and diffuses to the sarcomere to produce myocardial contraction?
a Na^+ b K^+ c Ca^{2+} d ATPase

7 Expected changes resulting from severing both vagi include: (More than one answer may be correct)
a Interruption of the afferent pathways from the aortic arch baroreceptors   b Increase in the heart rate to approximately 100 bpm   c Increase in the cardiac output   d Increase in the mean arterial pressure

8 When a patient was given a certain drug, the mean arterial pressure increased and the total peripheral resistance decreased. This drug probably caused:
a Vasoconstriction and an increase in cardiac output   b Vasoconstriction and a decrease in the cardiac output   c Vasodilation and an increase in the cardiac output   d Vasodilation and a decrease in the cardiac output

9 Within limits, an increase in the end-diastolic volume of the ventricle will: (More than one answer may be correct)
a Increase the stroke volume of the ventricle   b Decrease the stroke volume of the ventricle   c Increase the force of contraction   d Decrease the cardiac work

10 The ventricular function curve reveals that cardiac reserve, or the ability to increase cardiac output, is normally increased about:
a Twofold   b Threefold   c Fivefold   d Tenfold

11 Cardiac muscle cannot be tetanized because:
a The refractory period lasts throughout the period of contraction   b The impulse spread through the conduction system is too rapid   c The muscle fibers are relatively ischemic after each contraction   d Intracardiac calcium levels are too low

12 The volume of blood ejected by the ventricle depends on: (More than one answer may be correct)
a Preload   b Afterload   c Contractile state

13 Which of the following statements concerning the Laplace relationship between wall tension, arterial pressure, and ventricular radius is *not* true? (More than one answer may be correct)
a The ventricle must generate increased tension to empty if ventricular size increases. *b* The ventricle must generate increased tension if the ventricular size decreases. *c* The ventricle must generate increased tension if arterial pressure increases. *d* The ventricle must generate increased tension if arterial pressure decreases.

14 The most important extrinsic control mechanism affecting the distribution of cardiac output is:
a The parasympathetic system *b* The sympathetic system *c* Circulating neurohormones *d* Tissue ischemia

15 Distribution of blood flow to vital organs such as the heart and brain is predominantly controlled by:
a Extrinsic mechanisms such as neural control and humoral agents *b* Intrinsic mechanisms or autoregulation

16 Coronary perfusion takes place:
a Primarily during systole *b* Primarily during diastole *c* Equally during systole and diastole

17 Stretching myocardial fibers to the optimum sarcomere length increases the force of contraction by:
a Increasing the overlap of the myofilaments *b* Intensifying the cross-bridge interactions *c* Increasing the volume of blood to be ejected

18 Factors that affect cardiac output include: (More than one answer may be correct)
a Circulating levels of hormones *b* Stimulation of the cardiac sympathetic nervous system *c* Exercise *d* Stroke volume

Directions: Match each of the hemodynamic parameters in col. A with its equivalent in col. B.

Column A
19 ____ Cardiac output
20 ____ Mean arterial pressure
21 ____ Stroke volume
22 ____ Ejection fraction
23 ____ Cardiac index
24 ____ Blood flow

Column B
a End-diastolic volume–end-systolic volume
b $\dfrac{\text{Cardiac output}}{\text{Body surface area}}$
c Cardiac output × total peripheral resistance
d Heart rate × stroke volume
e $\dfrac{\text{Stroke volume}}{\text{End-diastolic volume}}$
f $\dfrac{\text{(Mean arterial pressure} - \text{central venous pressure)}}{\text{Resistance}}$

25 Arrange the mechanical events of the cardiac cycle in the proper time sequence beginning with (*a*), the closure of the AV valves.
a AV valves close *b* AV valves open *c* Semilunar valves close *d* Semilunar valves open *e* Ventricular filling *f* Ventricular ejection *g* Ventricular relaxation *h* First heart sound *i* Second heart sound

Directions: Fill in the blanks with the correct words or circle the correct option.

26 The _____ _____ period is that time during the cardiac cycle when the myocardium will not respond to any stimulus. The myocardium is capable of responding to a strong stimulus during the _____ _____ period.

27 In the resting state the inside of the cell is _____ charged with respect to the outside. During the repolarization of a cell the sodium-potassium pump moves _____ into the cell and _____ out of the cell.

28 During the ventricular filling phase of the cardiac cycle the AV valves are (open) (closed) and the semilunar valves are (open) (closed).

29 During the ventricular ejection phase of the cardiac cycle the AV valves are (open) (closed) and the semilunar valves are (open) (closed).

30 During the phase of ventricular filling the cardiac impulse is delayed at the _____.

BIBLIOGRAPHY

BERNE, ROBERT, and MATTHEW LEVY: *Cardiovascular Physiology*, Mosby, St. Louis, 1972.

BRAUNWALD, EUGENE: "Regulation of the Circulation: Parts I and II," *New England Journal of Medicine*, **290**: 1124–1129, 1420–1425, May 16, 1974 and June 20, 1974.

GUYTON, ARTHUR C.: *Textbook of Medical Physiology*, Saunders, Philadelphia, 1976.

HURST, J. WILLIS (ed.): *The Heart*, McGraw-Hill, New York, 1974.

RUSHMER, ROBERT: *Cardiovascular Dynamics*, Saunders, Philadelphia, 1970.

SODEMAN, WILLIAM A., and WILLIAM A. SODEMAN JR.: *Pathologic Physiology: Mechanisms of Disease*, Saunders, Philadelphia, 1974.

SONNENBLICK, EDMUND H.: "Myocardial Ultrastructure in the Normal and Failing Heart," *Hospital Practice*, **5**: 35–43, April 1970.

VANDER, ARTHUR, JAMES SHERMAN, and DOROTHY LUCIANO: *Human Physiology*, McGraw-Hill, New York, 1970.

WARNER, HOWARD F., MARGARET W. RUSSELL, and JAMES F. SPANN JR.: "Heart Muscle: Clinical Applications of Basic Physiology and Cellular Anatomy," *Heart and Lung*, **1**: 494–507, July-August, 1972.

CHAPTER 26 Diagnostic Procedures

OBJECTIVES At the completion of Chap. 26 you should be able to:

1 Define each of the following signs and symptoms of heart disease and state its physiologic basis: angina, dyspnea, orthopnea, paroxysmal nocturnal dyspnea, palpitations, peripheral edema, syncope, and weakness and fatigue.

2 Define the four functional categories of the New York Heart Association classification of heart disease.

3 Describe and explain the possible significance of the following findings during examination of the arterial system: pulse deficit, bounding pulse, thready pulse, irregular pulse, slow upstroke, waterhammer pulse, and alterations in pulse pressure.

4 Name and locate the peripheral pulses commonly palpated in the physical exam; explain the significance of absent, diminished, or unequal peripheral pulses.

5 Correlate the auscultated sounds of Korotkoff with arterial systolic and diastolic blood pressures.

6 State the formula for estimation of the mean arterial pressure.

7 Describe the procedure for estimation of central venous pressure by examination of the jugular veins; explain the significance of deviations from normal.

8 Explain the significance of Kussmaul's sign and a positive hepatojugular reflux test.

9 Explain the significance of the jugular venous a, c, and v waveforms and the possible significance of deviations from normal.

10 Outline the types of information that may be obtained in examination of the precordium.

11 Explain the possible significance of lateral displacement of the point of maximum impulse, a substernal heave, and precordial thrills.

12 Define and explain the possible significance of the following observations related to precordial auscultation: physiological and paradoxical splitting of the second heart sound, ventricular and atrial gallops, opening snap, and systolic and diastolic murmurs.

13 State the standard method of grading murmur loudness.

14 Name and locate on the chest the four standard areas for heart sound auscultation.

15 Identify the waveforms of a normal electrocardiogram and give examples of abnormalities which may be detected using this diagnostic technique.

16 State the recording sites utilized for each lead of the 12-lead electrocardiogram, including the polarity of each.

17 Define vector and electrical axis.

18 Explain how the hexaxial reference system is derived.

19 Describe the following diagnostic procedures and give examples of cardiovascular abnormalities which may be detected using each technique:
a Vectorcardiogram
b Echocardiogram
c Phonocardiogram
d Chest x-ray
e Nuclear imaging
f Cardiac catheterization
g Coronary arteriography

20 Identify five categories of data obtainable during cardiac catheterization.

21 Describe the anatomic approach for catheterization of the right and left sides of the heart.

22 Contrast the diagnostic approach for obtaining evidence of valvular stenosis and valvular regurgitation.

23 State the indications for performing coronary angiography and the characteristics of a bypassable lesion.

24 List four hemodynamic parameters measured at the bedside with intravenous catheters.

Increasingly sophisticated diagnostic techniques are available to detect heart disease and its clinical sequelae. However, the utilization of these techniques and the interpretation of test results are adjuncts to the systematic clinical assessment of the patient, not substitutes for a thorough history and physical examination. Thus a brief overview of the systematic bedside assessment of the patient with heart disease must precede a description of common diagnostic procedures.

CLINICAL ASSESSMENT

A systematic clinical assessment includes a complete history and physical examination utilizing the techniques of inspection, palpation, percussion, and auscultation. Examination of the cardiovascular system must include the heart and the peripheral vascular system. A detailed discussion of the peripheral vascular examination and related diagnostic tests is presented in Chap. 29.

History

The history must include an assessment of the individual's life-style and the impact of heart disease upon the activities of daily living if the patient rather than the disease is to be treated. The following signs and symptoms of heart disease are commonly elicited during the history of the patient with heart disease: (1) *angina*, or chest pain, a consequence of myocardial oxygen lack or ischemia; (2) *dyspnea*, or difficulty breathing, due to increased respiratory effort associated with pulmonary vascular congestion and alterations in lung distensibility; *orthopnea*, or difficulty breathing in the recumbent position; *paroxysmal nocturnal dyspnea*, or an attack occurring at rest during the night as a result of left ventricular failure; (3) *palpitations*, or an awareness of the heartbeat, due to changes in the rate, regularity, or force of cardiac contraction; (4) *peripheral edema*, or swelling caused by fluid accumulation in the interstitial spaces, usually noted in dependent areas as a result of the effect of gravity and preceded by weight gain; (5) *syncope*, or transient loss of consciousness, a result of inadequate cerebral blood flow; and (6) *fatigue and weakness*, commonly a consequence of low cardiac output and reduced peripheral perfusion.

It must be determined what factors precipitate symptoms and what relieves the symptoms. Angina is commonly precipitated by exertion and relieved by rest. Dyspnea is commonly associated with exertion; however, changes in body position and the consequent redistribution of body fluid according to the principle of gravity may precipitate dyspnea. Orthopnea, or dyspnea in the recumbent position, can be relieved by elevation of the trunk with pillows. In addition, the degree of disability associated with the elicited symptoms must be determined. The New York Heart Association has developed guidelines for the classification of patients according to the level of physical activity required to produce symptoms (see Table 26.1). The categories range from Class I patients, asymptomatic with ordinary physical exertion, to Class IV patients, symptomatic at rest.

Simple inspection yields a wealth of information regarding the patient's physical and psychological status. Observations, such as color, body build, respiratory pattern, work of breathing, and affect must all be incorporated into the clinical picture. Palpation, coupled with inspection, furthers and substantiates the cumulative data base. Skin temperature, turgor and moistness can be evaluated. Severity of edema can be quantified by the persistence of the indentation left by the palpating finger in an edematous area. The following structures are systematically examined: arteries, veins, and anterior chest wall.

ARTERIAL PULSE AND PRESSURE

The arterial pulse is palpated to elicit the following information: (1) rate, (2) regularity, (3) amplitude, and (4) quality. Certain cardiac arrhythmias can be detected by alterations in the rate or regularity of the arterial pulse. Irregularities of cardiac rhythm are associated with variability in pulse amplitude. If the interval between cardiac impulses is irregular, the ventricular filling time and, consequently, the stroke volume vary for each beat. For instance, shortening the interval between beats reduces filling time and stroke volume; consequently, the amplitude of the peripheral arterial pulsation is reduced for that beat. For this reason, irregular rhythms are occasionally associated with a "radial pulse deficit," or a palpated radial rate slower than the auscultated apical rate. This simply indicates that the ventricular filling time was so short that the volume of blood ejected into the periphery for that beat was too small to be palpated in the peripheral bed.

The quality of the arterial pulses is an important index of peripheral perfusion. A consistently weak, thready pulse may indicate a low stroke volume or increased peripheral vascular resistance. Conversely, a forceful, bounding pulse correlates with high stroke volumes and reduced peripheral resistance. The contour of the arterial pulse can best be appreciated by light palpation of the carotid artery. Palpation of a small pulse with a slow upstroke would characterize aortic stenosis, a lesion which impedes blood flow through the aortic valve. The valvular lesion of aortic regurgitation produces a bounding, rapidly rising and collapsing pulse, referred to as a *waterhammer pulse*.

An impression of the consistency of the arterial wall can best be obtained by rolling a peripheral artery under

TABLE 26.1
New York Heart Association patient classification guidelines

Class I	Asymptomatic with ordinary physical exertion
Class II	Symptomatic with ordinary physical exertion
Class III	Symptomatic with less than ordinary physical exertion
Class IV	Symptomatic at rest

the examining fingers; hardening or thickening of the walls can be detected. A full cardiovascular examination includes palpation of arterial pulsations for quality and equality at multiple sites: (1) dorsalis pedis, (2) posterior tibialis, (3) popliteal, (4) femoral, (5) radial, (6) brachial, (7) carotid, and (8) temporal.

Auscultation of blood pressure concludes the arterial examination. Arterial blood pressure is measured by listening for the onset and disappearance of sounds, referred to as Korotkoff sounds, in an artery occluded by a blood pressure cuff (see Fig. 26-1). The timing of these sounds is correlated with pressure readings on a mercury manometer. Initially, the pressure in the cuff is increased to exceed systolic pressure in the artery so that no flow through the artery occurs and no sound is heard. As pressure in the cuff is gradually reduced below systolic pressure, flow begins. However, the flow is turbulent because it occurs through a constricted lumen; turbulent flow produces sound. The onset of turbulent flow is heard as the first Korotkoff sound and correlates with systolic pressure. Further reductions in cuff pressure produce characteristic alterations in the sound as flow increases through the arterial lumen, until the sound disappears. Either abrupt muffling or disappearance of sound correlates with diastolic pressure.

The normal arterial blood pressure is approximately 120/80. Hypertension is designated as a diastolic pressure over 90 mmHg or a systolic pressure over 140 mmHg. In elderly patients, values up to 160/100 would be considered normal. Hypotension, for a given individual, is best evaluated in terms of adequacy of peripheral perfusion. Early signs of inadequate peripheral perfusion would be a decreased urine output or cold, pale skin with reduced peripheral pulses. The kidneys and skin are relatively nonvital organs; therefore, as arterial pressure falls, blood is shunted from these organs to the more vital organs, the heart and brain.

The *pulse pressure* is the difference between the systolic and diastolic blood pressure. For example, a blood pressure of 120/80 corresponds to a pulse pressure of 40 mmHg. If arterial pressure falls and sympathetic compensatory vasoconstriction occurs, the pulse pressure is reduced or narrowed. A fall in pressure to 105/90 would narrow the pulse pressure to 15 mmHg. The pulse pressure is influenced most significantly by stroke volume and peripheral resistance. A narrow pulse pressure indicates a low stroke volume or a high peripheral resistance or both. A falling blood pressure and narrowing pulse pressure is an ominous sign of left ventricular dysfunction. The *mean arterial pressure* is the average peripheral perfusion pressure. This value is not simply the average of the diastolic and systolic pressures, because the duration of diastole exceeds the duration of systole at normal heart rates. Consequently, mean arterial pressure is estimated by adding the diastolic pressure to one-third of the pulse pressure.

VENOUS PRESSURE AND PULSATIONS

Jugular venous pressure and pulsations reflect the function of the right side of the heart. The cervical veins are examined to estimate central venous pressure and to analyze waveforms. To estimate central venous pressure, the cervical veins are examined with the trunk elevated to approximately 45°. Normally, the cervical veins will ascend no more than 1 to 2 cm of water above the clavicle. Abnormal elevation of the venous pressure, as in right heart failure, can be estimated by measuring the vertical distance between the level of jugular venous distention and the angle of Louis (i.e., the juncture between the manubrium and body of the sternum). With extreme elevations of pressure, usually over 25 cm of water, the cervical veins remain distended to the angle of the jaw with trunk elevations of 90°.

Venous pressure normally fluctuates with respiration; inspiration produces a fall in venous pressure as intrathoracic pressure decreases favoring venous return to the heart. A paradoxical increase in venous pressure with inspiration known as *Kussmaul's sign* indicates an impediment to venous return to the right side of the heart. Severe right heart failure, constrictive pericarditis, or cardiac tamponade would impair the ability of the right side of the heart to fill.

The hepatojugular reflux test is an important diagnostic clue to the presence of right heart failure. Manually sustained pressure is applied for approximately 30 to 60 seconds over the right upper quadrant of the abdomen; the neck veins are observed simultaneously. The abdominal pressure increases venous return to the heart. The normal heart is able to adapt and immediately accept the increased venous return. However, the failing right side of the heart is unable to readily accept this increased load; therefore the distention of the cervical veins will increase and the level of venous pulsations will rise in the neck. This response of the cervical veins is referred to as a positive hepatojugular reflux test.

The pulsations of the cervical veins are also analyzed to evaluate right heart function. At normal venous pressures, maximal venous pulsation can best be observed with trunk elevation of approximately 15 to 30°. The venous waves are gentle and undulating, with three positive components: the a, c, and v waves (see Fig. 26-2A). The a wave is produced by atrial contraction; the c wave correlates with ventricular contraction and seems to result from the bulging of the tricuspid valve into the right atrium; the v wave corresponds to the period of atrial filling prior to opening of the tricuspid valve.

Predictable alterations in waveform configuration result from tricuspid valve disease. Tricuspid stenosis impedes the blood flow from the right atrium into the right ventricle, forcing the right atrium to generate more pressure during contraction and creating "giant a waves" (see Fig. 26-2B). Tricuspid valvular regurgitation during ventricular systole produces a huge retrograde flow wave distorting the a and c waves, referred to as an "exaggerated v wave" (see Fig. 26-2C). Certain cardiac arrhythmias also alter the configuration of the venous waves by disrupting the sequential, synchronized contraction of the atria and the ventricles.

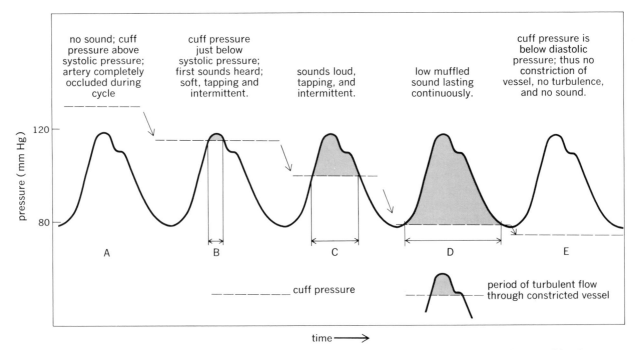

FIGURE 26-1 Korotkoff sounds. Systolic blood pressure is recorded at B when the first sounds are heard during a blood pressure measurement. Diastolic pressure is recorded at the point of sound muffling or disappearance, D or E. (From A. J. Vander, J. H. Sherman, and D. S. Luciano, Human Physiology, *2d ed., McGraw-Hill, New York, 1975, p. 250.)*

Physical examination of the anterior chest involves inspection, palpation, and percussion of the precordium. The thoracic movements are inspected for symmetry and visible pulsations. The chest is then palpated for normal and abnormal pulsations. The apical impulse, produced by the thrust of the heart against the chest wall during systole, is located. Normally, the point of maximal impulse (PMI) can be palpated as a rhythmic, brief tap approximately 2 to 3 cm in diameter, located in the fifth intercostal space at the midclavicular line.

With left ventricular hypertrophy, the apical impulse becomes more sustained, more forceful, and larger. The PMI is displaced laterally to the left and downward. Right ventricular hypertrophy characteristically produces a "substernal heave," or a systolic lift of the sternum, as the contractile force of the anterior right ventricle increases. Abnormal pulsations are also noted with coronary atherosclerotic disease; damaged myocardial fibers with limited or absent contractile force bulge passively outward during systole, creating paradoxical precordial movements. In addition, the turbulent flow associated with heart murmurs can create palpable precordial vibrations, known as "thrills."

Percussion was at one time utilized to estimate the size and contour of the heart and great vessels. This technique distinguished the absolute dullness to percussion of these structures compared to the relative resonance of surrounding structures—in essence, outlining the heart. The heart was considered enlarged if the left boundary extended beyond the midclavicular line. This gross estimation of cardiac size has essentially been replaced by the far superior techniques of chest radiology.

HEART SOUNDS

Auscultation of the chest permits identification of normal heart sounds, abnormal heart sounds, murmurs, and extracardiac sounds. The first and second heart sounds correlate with closure of the AV valves and the semilunar valves, respectively. Thus the first heart sound is heard at the onset of ventricular systole, as ventricular pressures rise above atrial pressures, closing the mitral and tricuspid valves. An abnormal accentuation of the first heart sound is noted in mitral stenosis as a result of the stiffening of the valve leaflets.

The second heart sound is audible at the beginning of ventricular relaxation as ventricular pressure falls below the pressure within the pulmonary artery and aorta, closing the pulmonic and aortic valves. Normally, right ventricular ejection lasts slightly longer than left ventricular ejection, resulting in asynchronous valve closure. Therefore the aortic valve closes before the pulmonic valve, producing a normal physiologic splitting or separation of the valve closure sounds. Inspiration accentuates physiologic splitting because venous return to the right side of the heart increases, thus producing

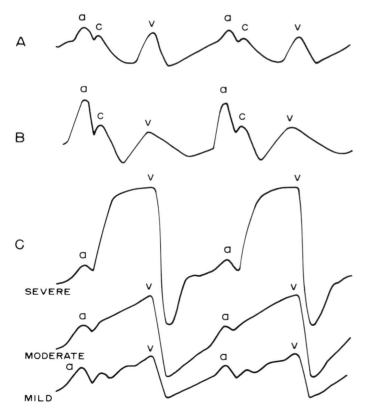

FIGURE 26-2 Jugular venous waveforms. A, normal waves are of low amplitude and undulating. The a wave is produced by atrial contraction, the c wave by ventricular contraction and the consequent bulging of the tricuspid valve into the right atrium, and the v wave is produced during atrial filling prior to the opening of the tricuspid valve. B, giant a waves seen in tricuspid stenosis. C, mild, moderate, and severe tricuspid regurgitation. In severe tricuspid regurgitation, the c and v waves summate into huge v waves. (Modified from J. W. Hurst, The Heart, 3d ed., McGraw-Hill, New York, 1974, pp. 184, 187.)

an increment in the volume of right ventricular ejection. During expiration, splitting becomes less pronounced or disappears.

Abnormal paradoxical splitting signifies closure of the pulmonic valve prior to the aortic valve. A paradoxical response to respiration is noted; that is splitting is most pronounced with expiration and subsides with inspiration. Paradoxical splitting is observed during delayed activation of the left ventricle, as in left bundle branch block, or with prolonged left ventricular ejection, as in aortic stenosis.

Two additional heart sounds, known as *gallop rhythms*, can be heard during ventricular diastole, usually in conjunction with heart disease. The first occurs during the period of rapid ventricular filling. It is referred to as a *ventricular gallop*, or the third heart sound. This sound can occur normally in children and young adults. However, it is usually a pathologic finding produced by cardiac dysfunction, particularly ventricular failure. The term "gallop rhythm" is applicable because the third heart sound occurs close to the second heart sound, simulating the rhythm of a horse's gallop.

The second gallop rhythm occurs during atrial systole. It is referred to as an *atrial gallop*, or the fourth heart sound. Normally it is faint or inaudible, occurring immediately prior to the first heart sound. The atrial gallop is audible when ventricular resistance to atrial filling increases, as a result of either reduced ventricular wall distensibility or increased ventricular volumes.

Heart murmurs are the result of turbulent flow within the cardiac chambers and vessels. Turbulent flow is produced either by flow through structural abnormalities (narrowed valvular orifices, incompetent valves, or dilated arterial segments) or by high velocity flow through normal structures. Murmurs are described according to (1) timing relative to cardiac cycle, (2) loudness, (3) location or region of maximum audibility, and (4) characteristics.

Diastolic murmurs occur after the second heart sound during ventricular relaxation. The murmurs of mitral stenosis and aortic regurgitation occur during diastole. Systolic murmurs are designated as either ejection murmurs, occurring during midsystole after the early phase of isovolumetric contraction, or regurgitant murmurs, occurring throughout systole. Murmurs occurring throughout systole are referred to as pansystolic or holosystolic. The murmur of aortic stenosis would typify an ejection murmur; whereas mitral regurgitation produces a regurgitant murmur.

The loudness of a murmur is graded on a scale of I to VI, with grade I representing a faint murmur and grade VI representing a murmur audible with the stethoscope off the chest wall. Four standard areas of the chest wall, illustrated in Fig. 26-3 as aortic, tricuspid, pulmonic, and apical regions, are commonly utilized to localize the region of maximum murmur audibility. Specification of

unique sound characteristics such as pitch, pattern of intensification and decline, or radiation is also included in the description of a heart murmur.

Finally, identification and description of extracardiac sounds are essential. For instance, the stiff, thickened valve cusps in mitral stenosis produce an audible "opening snap" in early diastole. A pericardial "friction rub," caused by pericardial inflammation, is audible as a rough sandpaper sound.

NONINVASIVE DIAGNOSTIC PROCEDURES

Electrocardiogram

The electrocardiogram (ECG) is the graphic recording of the heart's electrical activity. Characteristic waveforms on the ECG, arbitrarily designated as P, QRS, and T waves, correlate with the spread of electrical excitation and recovery through the conduction system and myocardium (see Fig. 26-4A). These waves are recorded on graph paper with a horizontal time scale and a vertical voltage scale (see Fig. 26-4B). The significance of the waveforms and intervals on the ECG is as follows:

1   *P wave:* The P wave corresponds to atrial depolarization. The normal stimulus for atrial depolarization originates in the sinus node; however, the magnitude of electrical current associated with excitation of the sinus node is too small to be visualized on the ECG. The P wave is normally gently rounded and upright in most leads. Atrial enlargement may increase the amplitude or width of the P wave and alter its configuration. Cardiac arrhythmias can also change the P wave configuration. For instance, rhythms originating near the AV junction may cause inversion of the P wave because the direction of atrial depolarization is reversed.

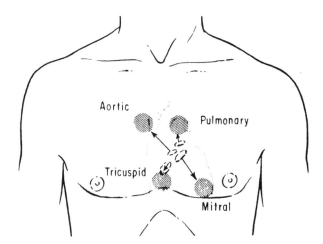

FIGURE 26-3 Positions for auscultation of heart sounds. Illustration shows anatomic location of the heart valves and the points to which their sounds are usually referred. (From K. G. Andreoli, V. H. Fowkes, D. P. Zipes, and A. G. Wallace, Comprehensive Cardiac Care, *3d ed., Mosby, St. Louis, 1975, p. 31.)*

2 *P-R interval:* The P-R interval is measured from the beginning of the P wave to the onset of the QRS complex. This interval includes impulse transmission time through the atria and the delay of the impulse at the AV node. The normal interval is 0.12 to 0.20 seconds. Abnormal prolongation of the P-R interval is indicative of an impulse conduction disturbance, referred to as *first-degree heart block.*

3 *QRS complex:* The QRS complex represents ventricular depolarization. The amplitude of this wave is great as a result of the large muscle mass traversed by the electrical impulse. However, impulse spread is rapid; normally, the duration of the QRS complex is between 0.06 and 0.10 seconds. Prolongation of impulse spread through the bundle branches, known as *bundle branch block,* widens the ventricular complex. Abnormal cardiac rhythms originating in the ventricles, such as ventricular tachycardia, also widen and distort the QRS complex because the specialized

pathways speeding impulse spread through the ventricles are bypassed. Ventricular hypertrophy would increase the amplitude of the QRS complex as the muscle mass enlarges.

Atrial repolarization occurs during the period of ventricular depolarization. However, the magnitude of the QRS complex obscures any electrocardiographic evidence of atrial recovery.

4 *S-T segment:* This interval is interposed between the wave of ventricular depolarization and repolarization. The initial phases of ventricular repolarization occur during this period; however, the changes are too subtle to be apparent on the ECG. Abnormal depression or elevation of the S-T segment is associated

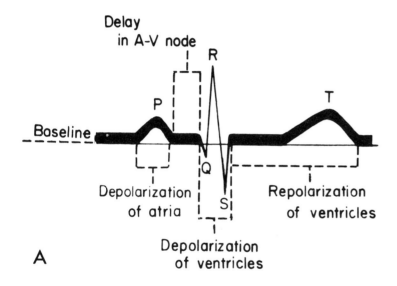

A

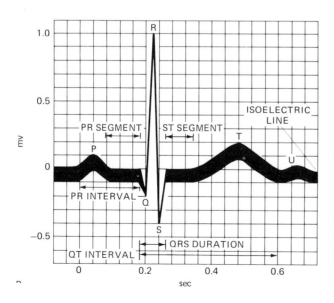

B

FIGURE 26-4 A, correlation between the waves of the electrocardiogram and impulses that spread through the heart. B, the normal recording of the electrocardiogram on graphic paper. Amplitude in millivolts is represented on the vertical axis while the horizontal axis represents time in seconds. Each small square represents 0.04 second with 5 small squares equaling 0.2 seconds. Normal intervals are: P-R, 0.12–0.20 seconds; QRS, 0.06–0.10 second; Q-T, 0.36–0.44 seconds. The ventricular rate may be calculated by counting the number of R waves in 6 seconds and multiplying by 10 or counting the number of small squares between two complexes (R to R) and dividing this number into 1500. (A, from Jules Constant, Learning Electrocardiography, *Little, Brown, Boston, 1973, p. 3; B, reproduced with permission, from W. F. Ganong,* Review of Medical Physiology, *8th ed., Lange Medical Publications, Los Altos, Calif., 1977, p. 405.)*

with myocardial ischemia and infarction, respectively. Digitalis administration characteristically produces sagging of the segment.

5 *T wave:* Ventricular repolarization generates the T wave. Normally, the T wave is slightly asymmetrical, rounded, and upright in most leads. Inversion of the T wave is associated with myocardial ischemia. Hyperkalemia, or serum potassium elevation, will cause peaking and elevation of the T wave.

6 *Q-T interval:* This interval is measured from the beginning of the QRS complex to the end of the T wave, encompassing ventricular depolarization and repolarization. The normal Q-T interval is 0.36 to 0.44 seconds. The Q-T interval is prolonged with the administration of certain antiarrhythmic drugs, such as quinidine.

The electrical currents generated within the heart during depolarization and repolarization are conducted to the body surface where they can be recorded by electrodes in contact with the skin. By convention, nine recording electrodes are placed on the extremities and chest wall with a ground electrode, utilized to reduce electrical interference, attached to the right leg. Varying combinations of these electrodes produce 12 standard leads. Each of the 12 leads records the electrical events

of the entire cardiac cycle; however, each lead views the heart from a slightly different perspective; therefore, waveforms will look slightly different in each lead. Three categories of leads are commonly designated (see Fig. 26-5):

1 *Standard limb leads (leads I, II, III):* These leads measure the difference in electrical potential between two points; thus the leads are bipolar, with one negative and one positive pole. Electrodes are placed on the right arm, left arm, and left leg. Lead I views the heart from the axis connecting the right arm and left arm, with the left arm as the positive pole; lead II, from the right arm and left leg, with the left leg positive; and lead III, from the left arm and left leg, with the left leg positive (Fig. 26-5A).

2 *Augmented limb leads (leads aVR, aVL, aVF):* These leads are electrically adjusted to measure the absolute electrical potential at one recording site, that of a positive electrode placed on the extremities, creating, in essence, a unipolar lead. This is accomplished by electrically canceling out the effect of the negative pole and establishing an "indifferent" electrode at zero potential. Adjustments are made automatically within the ECG machine to join the other limb electrodes creating a common indifferent electrode with essentially no effect on the positive recording electrode. The voltage recorded from the positive electrode is then amplified or "augmented" to produce a selected, unipolar limb lead tracing. There are three augmented limb leads: aVR, recording from the

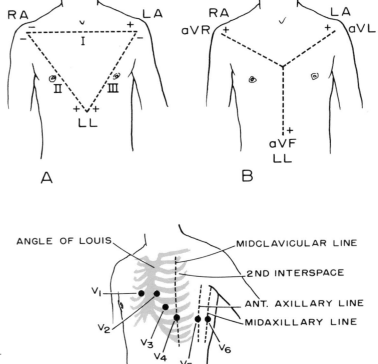

FIGURE 26-5 Electrode positions for the standard 12-lead electrocardiogram. A, standard limb leads (I, II, III). B, augmented limb leads (aVR, aVL, aVF). C, precordial leads (V₁–V₆).

right arm; aVL, from the left arm; and aVF, from the left leg. (The aVF location can be easily remembered by associating the "F" with "foot") (Fig. 26-5B).

3 *Precordial or chest leads* (V₁ *to* V₆): These leads are unipolar leads recording the absolute electrical potential of sites on the anterior chest wall, or precordium.

Identification of the following landmarks facilitates accurate placement of the precordial electrodes: (1) angle of Louis, the sternal protuberance at the juncture between the manubrium and body of the sternum; (2) the second intercostal space, adjacent to the angle of Louis; (3) the left midclavicular line; and (4) the anterior and midaxillary lines (Fig. 26-5C). Electrodes are placed sequentially on the chest wall at six different sites:

a V₁—located in the fourth intercostal space to the right of the sternum.

b V₂—located in the fourth intercostal space to the left of the sternum

c V₃—located midway between V₂ and V₄

d V₄—located in the fifth intercostal space in the midclavicular line

e V₅—horizontal to V₄ in the anterior axillary line

f V₆—horizontal to V₅ in the midaxillary line

The standard limb leads and augmented limb leads view the heart in the frontal plane. The relative perspective of each lead is conceptualized most easily utilizing a schematic diagram, known as *the hexaxial reference system*. This reference system is derived in the following manner (see Fig. 26-6): (1) Connecting the lead axes of leads I, II, and III forms an equilateral triangle, referred to as *Einthoven's triangle*. The heart is considered the electrical center of the triangle. (2) Positioning the lead axes so that each radiates from the center of the triangle creates a second diagram, known as the *triaxial reference system*. (3) Combining the triaxial reference system diagram with the schematic representation of the augmented limb leads radiating from the electrical center of the thorax produces the *hexaxial reference system*. The hexaxial reference system is an invaluable aid to electrocardiographic interpretation, permitting calculation of the average direction of electrical activity within the heart. The average direction of electrical activation, calculated from the ECG is referred to as the *electrical axis* of the heart.

The waveform configurations apparent in each lead will depend upon the orientation of the particular lead relative to the path of cardiac electrical activity. The leads of the hexaxial reference system view the heart in the frontal plane; the six precordial leads offer another perspective from the horizontal plane. Waves will be positive (i.e., deflected upward) if the electrical activity of the heart approaches the positive electrode of a given lead. For example, in Fig. 26-7, the P wave and QRS complex of lead II are positive because the wave of depolarization approaches the positive left leg electrode of lead II. Conversely, the same waves in lead aVR are negative because the path of electrical activity is moving away from the positive right arm electrode. In addition,

the amplitude of waves varies among leads. As a rule, wave amplitude will be greatest in a lead lying parallel to the path of depolarization. Notice that lead II in Fig. 26-7 demonstrates the greatest wave amplitude, indicating that lead II most closely parallels the path of depolarization in this ECG.

The ECG permits detection of abnormalities in cardiac rate and rhythm, chamber enlargement, myocardial ischemia or infarction, drug and electrolyte effects, and shifts in the direction of electrical activation.

Vectorcardiogram

The vectorcardiogram depicts the sequential changes in the direction and magnitude of electrical forces generated within the heart during the cardiac cycle. This technique is based upon the concept of a vector; a *vector* is a force with both magnitude and direction represented by an arrow. The length of the arrow represents the magnitude of the force, and the direction of the force is depicted by the arrowhead.

As the wave of electrical excitation moves through the heart, multiple fibers depolarize virtually simultane-

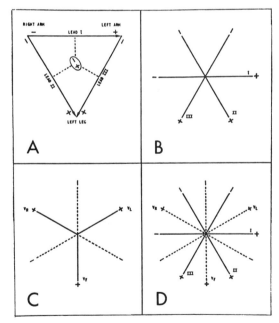

FIGURE 26-6 Derivation of the hexaxial reference system. A, the Einthoven triangle showing the axes of the standard limb leads with the heart at the center of the triangle. B, the axes of the limb leads are moved to the center of the triangle forming a triaxial reference system. C, the axes of the augmented (unipolar) limb leads. D, the axes of the standard and unipolar limb leads are superimposed forming a hexaxial reference system. (From H. H. Friedman, Outline of Electrocardiography, *McGraw-Hill, New York, 1963, p. 28.)*

ously. At any given instant, the average direction and magnitude of the electrical forces generated by these fibers can be represented by a vector, referred to as an *instantaneous vector*. As the depolarization process continues through the heart, a series of instantaneous vectors can be plotted.

For example, the series of instantaneous vectors resulting from the sequential depolarization of the ventricles is illustrated in Fig. 26-8A. The cardiac impulse spreads from the AV node down the bundle branches, initially activating the left side of the ventricular septum with resultant impulse spread from left to right (vector 1). Next, excitation moves toward the cardiac apex, activating the free walls of the ventricles; however, the forces to the left are dominant as a result of the relatively greater muscle mass of the left ventricle (vectors 2, 3, 4, 5, and 6). The final areas to be activated are the high posterior and basal regions of the ventricles (vectors 7 and 8). A "vector loop" is constructed from the instantaneous vectors by sequentially connecting the heads of each vector and the point of origin (see Figs. 26-8B and 26-8C).

The complete vectorcardiogram consists of three loops: the P loop representing atrial activation, the QRS loop of ventricular depolarization, and the T loop of ventricular recovery. The vectorcardiogram is recorded from body surface electrodes arranged to produce three projections: frontal, sagittal, and horizontal.

The vectorcardiogram is an invaluable adjunct to the ECG in the detection and analysis of alterations in conduction patterns resulting from (1) myocardial infarction, (2) abnormal impulse conduction through specialized conduction pathways, and (3) chamber hypertrophy. In Fig. 26-9, notice the difference between the normal vectorcardiogram and that of left ventricular hyper-

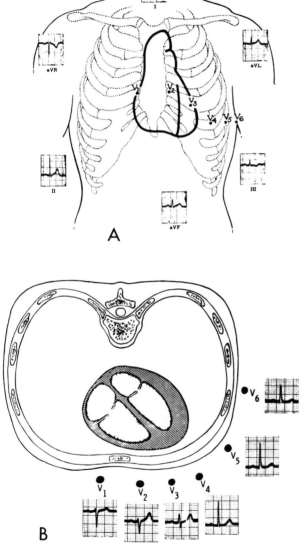

A

B

FIGURE 26-7 A, *normal ECG patterns in the frontal plane (standard leads I, II, and III and augmented unipolar leads aVR, aVL, and aVF). B, normal ECG patterns in the horizontal plane (precordial leads V_1–V_6). (Reproduced with permission, from M. J. Goldman,* Principles of Clinical Electrocardiography, *Lange Medical Publications, Los Altos, Calif., 9th ed., 1976.)*

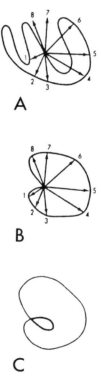

A

B

C

FIGURE 26-8 *Derivation of vector loop. A, instantaneous vectors of ventricular depolarization (longitudinal section of heart with middle section representing the septum). B, derivation of vector loop by connecting vector heads. C, resultant QRS vector loop. (From A. Castellanos, L. Lemberg, B. Berkovits, and B. W. Claxton, "Didactic Vectorcardiography: General Concepts,"* Heart and Lung, **4**: 697, 1975.)

trophy. The increased preponderance of left ventricular muscle mass shifts the direction to the left and amplifies the magnitude of forces.

Echocardiogram

Echocardiography is a cardiac diagnostic technique utilizing ultrasound as the examination medium. A transducer transmitting ultrasonic waves, or high-frequency sound waves beyond the limit of human hearing, is applied to the patient's chest wall and directed at the heart (see Fig. 26-10). As the ultrasonic beam traverses the heart, ultrasonic waves are reflected back to the transducer whenever the beam crosses a boundary between cardiac structures or substances (e.g., blood) with different acoustic impedance. These reflected ultrasonic waves, or "cardiac echoes," are then converted to electrical impulses, amplified, and recorded, documenting the dimensions and motion of cardiac structures.

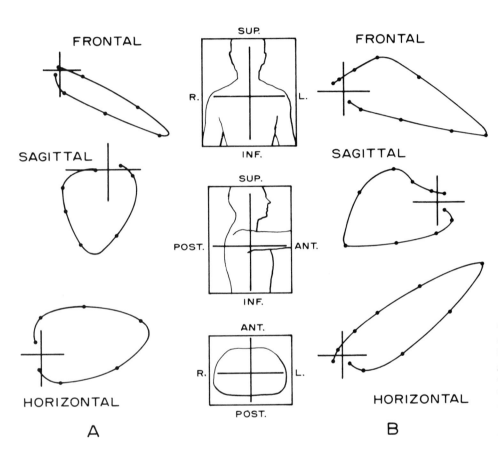

FIGURE 26-9 Vectorcardiogram. A, normal QRS vector loop in the frontal, sagittal and horizontal planes. B, QRS vector loop pattern representing left ventricular hypertrophy. (Modified from Hoechsts Pharmaceuticals. Directions in Cardiovascular Medicine. Vol. I: Book 2, 1973, pp. 17–18.)

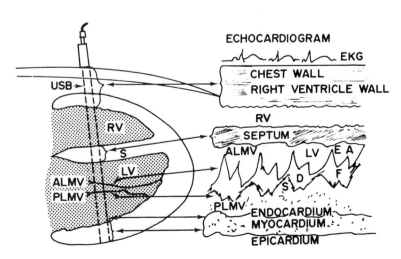

FIGURE 26-10 Normal echocardiogram. Path of ultrasound beam (USB) shown schematically on the left. On the right is a diagram of the corresponding echocardiogram for this direction of the transducer. Abbreviations: RV, right ventricle; S, septum; LV, left ventricle; ALMV, anterior leaflet of the mitral valve; PLMV, posterior leaflet of the mitral valve; S, systole; D, diastole; E, peak of rapid anterior opening of mitral valve during beginning of diastole; A, peak of anterior movement of leaflet into the ventricle produced by atrial systole; F, position of leaflet during rapid ventricular filling. (From Peter C. Gazes, Clinical Cardiology, copyright © 1975 by Year Book Medical Publishers, Inc., Chicago, used by permission.)

The precordium can be scanned by moving the transducer in several directions, aiming at certain structures. Figure 26-11 illustrates the normal motion of the anterior and posterior mitral valve leaflets relative to the restricted motion of stenotic, immobile mitral leaflets.

Phonocardiogram

A phonocardiogram is the graphic recording of the sounds, both normal and abnormal, generated during the cardiac cycle. It is usually recorded in conjunction with the ECG and an external pulse tracing, such as the carotid or apical pulsation (see Fig. 26-12). A microphone positioned on the chest wall receives the sound waves, which are then amplified and recorded. Simultaneously, a pressure transducer senses the external pulsations of the carotid artery or cardiac apex. The ECG is obtained from body surface electrodes.

The phonocardiogram provides documentation and confirmation of auscultated heart sounds and murmurs. Simultaneous recording of the phonocardiogram, ECG, and pulse tracing permits correlation of the timing of recorded sounds with the mechanical and electrical events of the cardiac cycle. This facilitates accurate interpretation of abnormal cardiac sounds.

Chest x-ray

A series of chest x-rays in four standard positions are useful in the cardiac diagnostic workup (see Fig. 26-13): (1) posteroanterior or frontal position; (2) left lateral position with left side forward; (3) right anterior oblique position with the body rotated approximately 60° to the left, placing the right shoulder anterior; and (4) left anterior oblique position with the left shoulder anterior. In each position, a different anatomic perspective of the heart is visible. The contour of the heart contrasts with the radiolucent air-filled lungs.

The following findings can be obtained from the chest x-ray: (1) generalized cardiac enlargement, or cardiomegaly; (2) localized chamber enlargement; (3) calcification in valves or coronary arteries; (4) pulmonary venous congestion; (5) interstitial or alveolar edema; and (6) enlargement of the pulmonary artery or dilation of the ascending aorta.

An impression of generalized cardiac enlargement can be noted in chest x-rays; however, precise estimation of the degree of enlargement is of questionable

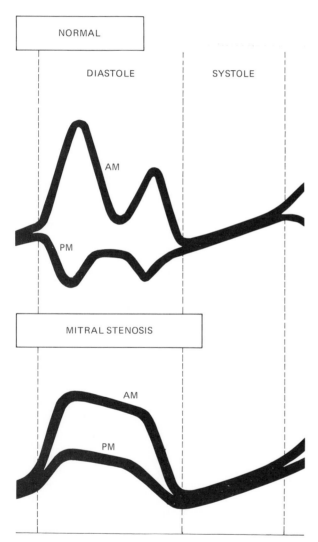

FIGURE 26-11 Mitral valve echocardiogram. A, normal leaflet motion (AM = anterior mitral valve leaflet; PM = posterior mitral valve leaflet). B, abnormal leaflet motion with mitral stenosis. (Adapted from J. M. Duchak, S. Chang, and H. Feigenbaum, "The Posterior Mitral Valve ECHO and the Electrocardiographic Diagnosis of Mitral Stenosis," American Journal of Cardiology, **29**: 631, 1972.)

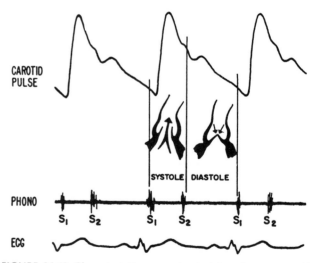

FIGURE 26-12 Characteristic normal arterial pulse wave with simultaneous recording of a phonocardiogram and electrocardiogram. (Adapted from J. Sana and R. D. Judge, Physical Appraisal Methods in Nursing Practice, Little, Brown, Boston, 1975, p. 192.)

accuracy. In contrast, chamber enlargement distinctly alters the contour of the heart, permitting specification of the involved chamber. In the posteroanterior position, the right border of the heart consists of the superior vena cava with the right atrium below. An angle appears at the juncture between the two. The structures comprising the left border, from top to bottom, are the aorta, pulmonary artery, and left ventricle. This projection permits identification of right atrial, left ventricular, and pulmonary arterial enlargement. Right atrial enlargement, for example, displaces the right boundary outward to the right, rounding the curvature of the cardiac contour.

In the left lateral position, the anterior border is primarily the right ventricle, with the posterior border consisting of the left atrium superiorly and the posterior wall of the left ventricle inferiorly. The esophagus lies behind the posterior boundary. Right ventricular and left atrial enlargement are best appreciated in this view. Outlining the esophagus with swallowed barium facilitates the diagnosis of left atrial enlargement, which produces an esophageal indentation with posterior displacement.

Radiologic examination of the lungs demonstrates the effects of cardiac dysfunction upon the pulmonary vasculature. Left-sided heart failure or mitral valve disease increases pulmonary venous congestion, dilating the pulmonary veins in characteristic patterns. Excessive elevation of venous pressure results in transudation of fluid into the interstitial space and eventually into the alveoli. Fluid seepage from the intravascular space, or pulmonary edema, produces a clouding, or haziness, of the vascular shadows, progressively whitening the normally dark shadows of the radiolucent lungs.

Characteristic findings typify particular cardiac lesions. For example, in mitral stenosis, a lesion impeding blood flow from the left atrium to the left ventricle, left atrial enlargement, and pulmonary venous congestion would be noted. Valvular calcification might also be observed.

Nuclear imaging

Nuclear imaging is a relatively new diagnostic adjunct to cardiovascular medicine. Small quantities of radioactive substances, referred to as *tracers*, are injected into a peripheral vein. Within minutes the tracer is distributed throughout the cardiovascular system and selectively taken up by the myocardium or bound to the albumin of the blood. The tracer's affinity for either the myocardium or the blood depends upon properties of the radioactive substance selected. The distribution of the tracer substance can be detected by sensitive nuclear cameras which record a "nuclear image" of the heart in various positions.

Nuclear imaging is most valuable in the assessment of ventricular function. Distribution of a radioisotope within the myocardium depends upon the relative blood flow to myocardial regions. Reduction in tracer concentration within a given area is the result of decreased blood flow. Areas of infarction, beyond obstructive coronary arterial lesions, can thus be delineated by abnormalities in tracer concentration. Myocardial uptake of the tracer also permits estimation of ventricular wall thickness.

Ventricular wall motion can best be appreciated utilizing tracers bound to the blood, thereby outlining the internal dimensions of the cardiac chambers. Blood-bound tracers are also useful to record the sequence and rate of blood flow through the cardiovascular system. This information is obtained by recording on a magnetic tape the timing and pattern of tracer distribution immediately following injection into a peripheral vein.

INVASIVE DIAGNOSTIC PROCEDURES

Cardiac catheterization

Cardiac catheterization is the insertion of catheters into the cardiovascular system to study the anatomy and function of the heart in the presence of suspected or documented heart disease. Depending on the location of a suspected lesion and the degree of myocardial dysfunction, selected studies will be performed, including (1) measurement of pressures in the cardiac chambers and vessels, (2) analysis of the waveform configuration of

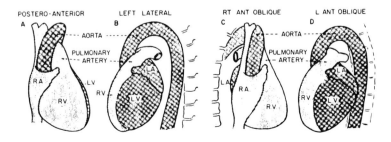

FIGURE 26-13 Orientation of the heart in four standard positions for cardiac roentgenography. A, in the posteroanterior position the borders of the right atrium and left ventricle are displayed. The right ventricle and the left atrium are not visible on the borders of the silhouette. B, in the left lateral position, the silhouette of the right ventricle is seen anteriorly and the left atrium posteriorly. C, in the right anterior position the right ventricle and left atrium are again seen in silhouette. D, in the left anterior oblique the right and left ventricle are seen in silhouette. The left atrium can be discerned in this projection. (From R. F. Rushmer, Cardiovascular Dynamics, 3d ed., Saunders, Philadelphia, 1970, p. 336.)

recorded pressures, (3) sampling of the oxygen content in selected regions, (4) opacification of the cardiac chambers and/or coronary arteries with contrast material, and (5) determination of cardiac output. Normal pressures, waveform configurations, and oxygen contents are illustrated in Fig. 26-14.

Two general approaches to the heart are currently utilized: right heart catheterization and left heart catheterization. Right heart catheterization requires insertion of a catheter into the venous system, usually via an antecubital vein in the right arm or the femoral vein. The catheter is progressively advanced through the peripheral venous system to the vena cava into the right atrium, right ventricle, and pulmonary artery. Advancing the catheter further into a distal segment of the pulmonary arterial bed eventually produces a "wedging," or lodging, of the catheter tip in the vessel lumen. This wedge position is referred to as the pulmonary capillary position. Left heart catheterization involves the retrograde passage of the catheter through the arterial system to the aorta, across the aortic valve, and into the left ventricle. The catheter is commonly inserted in either the brachial or femoral artery. Passage of the catheter into the aorta also permits selective cannulation and study of the coronary arteries.

Catheterization is useful to confirm the presence of valvular stenosis or regurgitation, to estimate the severity of the lesion, and to establish or exclude the presence of associated but clinically unsuspected lesions. The approach to the two lesions—stenosis, or valvular obstruction to blood flow, and regurgitation, or backward flow through the valve—differs.

Valvular regurgitation is documented by injection of contrast material into the chamber beyond the diseased valve; if regurgitation is present, opacification of the chamber proximal to the valve will occur when the valve fails to close securely. For example, with mitral regurgitation, the contrast medium injected into the left ventricle would appear in the left atrium during the next ventricular contraction as blood and contrast material flow backward through the diseased valve. The severity of the regurgitation is estimated according to the degree of left atrial opacification and the time required for the contrast material to disappear from the left atrium. Aortic regurgitation is detected by injection of contrast material into the ascending aorta, with subsequent opacification of the left ventricle during ventricular relaxation.

Regurgitation is also associated with abnormalities in the pressures within the cardiac chambers and alterations in waveform configuration. Mitral regurgitation creates a volume overload for the left atrium, elevating left atrial and pulmonary pressures. In addition, the

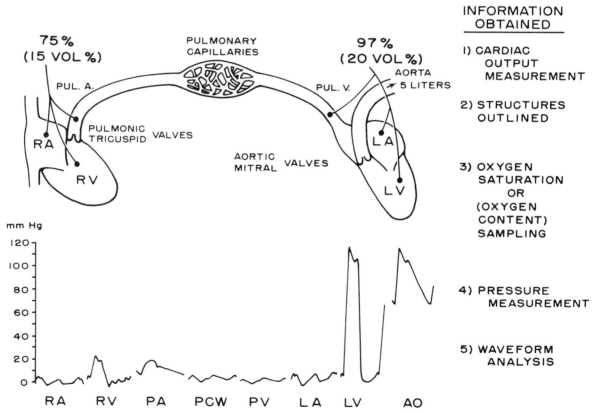

FIGURE 26-14 Data obtained during cardiac catheterization.

typical low-amplitude undulating left atrial waveform exhibits an abrupt increase in amplitude during ventricular contraction as blood flows backward through the valve.

Valvular stenosis can be visualized by injecting contrast material into the chamber proximal to the diseased valve; as the opacified blood flows through the restricted orifice, the valve boundaries are outlined. Typical alterations in pressures and waveforms are seen with valvular stenosis. For instance, the aortic pressure tracing associated with aortic stenosis demonstrates a slow upstroke and delayed peak as a result of the resistance to ventricular ejection into the aorta (see Fig. 26-15). Elevations in pressure in the chambers proximal to a stenotic lesion also occur. For example, mitral stenosis elevates left atrial and pulmonary venous pressures. These pressure elevations are reflected retrograde through the lungs and detected most easily via a catheter in the wedge position in the pulmonary artery. This pressure measurement is known as the "pulmonary capillary wedge pressure" and accurately reflects left atrial pressure.

Valvular stenosis produces a pressure gradient, or difference in pressure, between the chambers on either side of the valve. The pressure gradient results because the chamber proximal to the lesion must generate increased pressure to force blood through the obstructed valve. An example of a pressure gradient resulting from severe aortic stenosis is illustrated in Fig. 26-16. Notice the large pressure discrepancy, with the left ventricle generating pressures up to 200 mmHg to force blood through the aortic valve to sustain an aortic systolic pressure of 80 mmHg. The pressure gradient in this example is 120 mmHg; normally the pressure gradient is less than 5 mmHg.

In addition to the measurement of the pressure gradient, it is necessary to utilize a formula calculating the valve orifice. The determination of the pressure gradient across the valve and estimation of the valve area are the two most critical indices of the severity of stenosis.

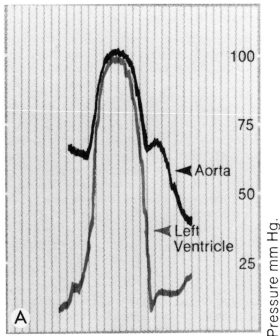

Time Lines: 0.04 secs.

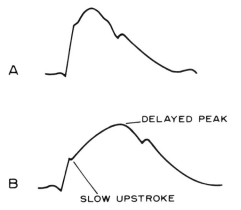

FIGURE 26-15 Carotid artery pressure tracing. A, *normal.* B, *aortic stenosis.*

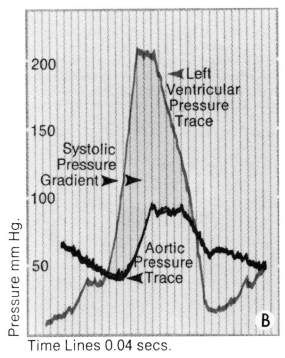

Time Lines 0.04 secs.

FIGURE 26-16 *Pressure gradient across the aortic valve.* A, *normal.* B, *pressure gradient of about 100 mmHg between the aorta and left ventricle in severe aortic stenosis. (From Hoechst Pharmaceuticals, Directions in Cardiovascuiar Medicine, "Cardiac Catheterization," 1973, vol. 3, Book VIII, pp. 4, 5.)*

CATHETERIZATION IN CORONARY ATHEROSCLEROTIC DISEASE

Coronary angiography, or injection of contrast material into the coronary arteries, is most commonly utilized to determine the feasibility and timing of coronary artery bypass grafting for a given patient. Additional indications for coronary angiography include evaluation of atypical angina and coronary revascularization results. The catheterization procedure involves the opacification of both coronary arteries, followed by a left ventriculogram, or injection of the contrast medium into the left ventricle, to evaluate left ventricular function.

Coronary angiography provides the following information: (1) the location of the lesion or lesions, (2) the degree of obstruction, (3) the presence of collateral circulation, and (4) the extent of disease in the distal arterial bed. For surgical intervention to be feasible, the following conditions are desirable: (1) a lesion located proximally so that it can be bypassed, (2) significant obstruction of over 75 percent of the vessel lumen, and (3) a patent artery beyond the lesion for graft anastomosis. Certain lesions, identified at the time of catheterization, are considered high-risk lesions. One example of a high-risk lesion is significant stenosis of the main left coronary artery, which threatens the entire left ventricle; therefore relatively urgent surgery may be advised.

The evaluation of left ventricular function is an important adjunct to coronary angiography. Injection of contrast material into the left ventricle permits visualization of ventricular wall movement and chamber size; areas of absent motion (akinesis), reduced motion (hypokinesis), or asynchronous contraction (dyskinesis) or bulging are noted. Rupture of a necrotic interventricular septum after myocardial infarction would also be detected during left ventriculography. Since the pressures are higher on the left side of the heart than on the right, blood would be shunted through the interventricular defect, opacifying the right ventricle. In addition, oxygen sampling would demonstrate abnormal elevation of oxygen content in the right ventricle as a result of the recirculation of oxygenated blood through the defect. Measurement of left ventricular pressure, arterial pressure, cardiac output, and ejection fraction completes the overall assessment of left ventricular function.

Hemodynamic monitoring

Four hemodynamic parameters, measured at the bedside via intravenous catheters, permit ongoing evaluation of cardiovascular status. These four parameters are (1) central venous pressure, (2) arterial pressure, (3) pulmonary arterial and pulmonary capillary wedge pressures, and (4) cardiac output.

Alterations in central venous pressure correlate most directly with changes in right-sided heart function. For example, right ventricular dysfunction, tricuspid valve disease, or alterations in venous return will influence central venous pressure. Mean arterial pressure is a function of cardiac output and total peripheral resistance.

Bedside techniques to measure pulmonary capillary wedge pressure and cardiac output are invaluable in the evaluation of left ventricular function. To measure pulmonary pressures, a balloon-tipped, flow-directed catheter is advanced into the pulmonary artery via a peripheral vein (see Fig. 26-17). With the balloon deflated, pressures in the pulmonary artery can be measured. Periodically, the balloon is inflated. With inflation of the balloon, blood flow propels the catheter distally into the pulmonary vasculature until the tip "wedges" in a small arterial branch. In this position the pressure transmitted backward from the left side of the heart through the pulmonary vasculature is sensed. Therefore, the pulmonary capillary wedge pressure reflects left atrial and, consequently, left ventricular diastolic pressure.

Cardiac output can be measured at the bedside by

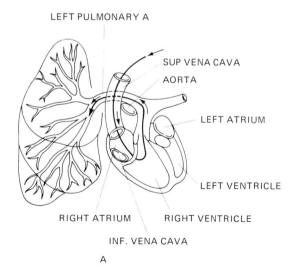

LEFT PULMONARY A

SUP VENA CAVA
AORTA

LEFT ATRIUM

LEFT VENTRICLE

RIGHT ATRIUM   RIGHT VENTRICLE

INF. VENA CAVA

A

LEFT PULMONARY A

SUP. VENA CAVA
AORTA

LEFT ATRIUM

LEFT VENTRICLE

RIGHT ATRIUM   RIGHT VENTRICLE

INF. VENA CAVA

B

two techniques: indicator dilution and thermal dilution. The indicator dilution technique involves the injection of a known quantity and concentration of dye into the venous end of the circulation, usually via a central venous line. The dye mixes with the blood and is progressively diluted. Downstream, a sample of arterial blood is gradually withdrawn and analyzed for dye concentration. A dilution curve is recorded (i.e., dye concentration against time), permitting calculation of cardiac output.

The thermal dilution technique substitutes a known quantity of fluid at a given temperature as the injectate. The temperature change of the blood mixed with the fluid is sensed by a thermistor located downstream. A special thermodilution pulmonary arterial catheter has been designed for cardiac output measurement. This catheter has an additional lumen opening into the right atrium for injection of the cold fluid and a thermistor at the distal tip in the pulmonary artery.

QUESTIONS

Diagnostic procedures—Chap. 26

Directions: Answer the following questions on a separate sheet of paper.

1 Mr. H is a 59-year-old accountant who has been diagnosed as having atherosclerotic heart disease. Recently he found it necessary to resign from the manufacturing firm where he worked because of weakness, fatigue, and inability to climb the stairs to his second-floor office without precipitating an episode of chest pain. At home, Mr. H is able to perform light housework but experiences shortness of breath and/or chest pain if he attempts to mow the lawn with a power mower. How would this patient's heart disease be categorized according to the New York Heart Association guidelines?

2 Palpation of the carotid arteries on a 68-year-old female with a blood pressure of 178/100 reveals that the left carotid has a much lower amplitude than the right. Explain the possible significance of this finding. What is this patient's mean arterial pressure?

3 How is the hepatojugular reflux test performed? How would you determine if the test were positive? What is the possible significance of a positive test?

FIGURE 26-17 Swan-Ganz pulmonary arterial pressure monitoring. A, pulmonary arterial position as it rests in the main pulmonary artery with the balloon deflated. The normal pressure in the pulmonary artery is 25/10 mmHg. B, inflation of the balloon causes the Swan-Ganz catheter to advance to the pulmonary capillary wedge position. The normal mean pulmonary wedge pressure is 5 to 12 mmHg. (From Vicki Bolognini, "The Swan-Ganz Pulmonary Artery Catheter: Implications for Nursing," Heart & Lung, 3: 976, 1974.)

4 What is a hexaxial reference system and how is it derived?

5 Discuss the type of data and evaluation of the cardiovascular status that may be obtained from cardiac catheterization.

6 List the indications for performing coronary angiography and the characteristics of a bypassable lesion.

Directions: Circle the letter preceding each item that correctly answers each question. Only one answer is correct unless otherwise noted.

7 The symptoms of weakness and easy fatigability in patients with myocardial failure are probably a consequence of:
a Low cardiac output b Increased contractility of the heart muscle c Decreased peripheral perfusion d Only a and c e All of the above

8 Hypertension in the young or middle-aged adult is defined as blood pressure greater than:
a 120/80 mmHg b 130/80 mmHg c 140/90 mmHg d 160/90 mmHg

9 A decreased pulse pressure may indicate: (More than one answer may be correct)
a Decreased stroke volume b Decreased peripheral resistance c Increased peripheral resistance d Decreased blood viscosity

10 A slow-rising and sustained carotid pulse is characteristic of:
a Mitral stenosis b Aortic stenosis c Mitral regurgitation d Aortic regurgitation

11 A quick-rising and collapsing (waterhammer) pulse is characteristic of:
a Mitral stenosis b Aortic stenosis c Mitral regurgitation d Aortic regurgitation

12 Jugular venous distention to the level of the jaw angle in a person sitting with the trunk elevated 90° correlates with a central venous pressure of at least:
a 10 cm water b 15 cm water c 20 cm water d 25 cm water

13 In the normal adult lying with the trunk elevated 45°, the pulsation within the jugular vein should rise above the clavicle no more than:
a 1 to 2 cm b 3 to 4 cm c 5 to 6 cm d 7 to 8 cm

14 A large, early v wave in the jugular venous pulse is most likely to be present in:
a Mitral regurgitation b Tricuspid regurgitation c Mitral stenosis d Tricuspid stenosis

15 A giant a wave in the jugular venous pulse is most likely to be present in:
a Mitral regurgitation b Tricuspid regurgitation c Mitral stenosis d Tricuspid stenosis

16 In the cardiovascular examination, the chest is inspected and palpated for: (More than one answer may be correct)
a Apical impulse *b* Thrills *c* Symmetry of thoracic movements *d* Lifts or heaves

17 A thrill is a palpable:
a Pericardial friction rub *b* Heart sound
c Apical impulse *d* Murmur

18 The apical impulse is normally located at:
a The fifth intercostal space near the left midclavicular line *b* Adjacent to the angle of Louis *c* The lower left sternal border in the fourth intercostal space
d The fourth intercostal space at the anterior axillary line

19 In cases of left ventricular hypertrophy, the PMI will: (More than one answer may be correct)
a Comprise an area less than 2 to 3 cm in diameter
b Comprise an area greater than 2 to 3 cm in diameter
c Shift laterally to the left and downward *d* Shift to the mediastinal area producing a substernal heave

20 The precordium refers to the area of the chest overlying the:
a Lungs *b* Sternum *c* Heart *d* Mediastinum

21 A lift or heave is the rise with each heartbeat of the:
a Precordium *b* Cardiac apex *c* Sternum
d Rib cage

22 A heart sound that occurs in early diastole and is considered normal in children and young adults but pathologic in older adults is the:
a First heart sound *b* Second heart sound
c Third heart sound *d* Fourth heart sound

23 Sounds occurring early in systole are most likely:
a Atrial gallops *b* Ventricular gallops
c Systolic ejection murmurs *d* Opening snaps of the mitral valve

24 The heart sound normally heard best over the aortic area is the:
a First heart sound *b* Second heart sound
c Third heart sound *d* Fourth heart sound

25 Murmurs occurring in diastole follow the:
a First heart sound *b* Second heart sound

26 During auscultation of the blood pressure, systolic pressure correlates with the:
a Onset of sound in the occluded artery *b* Abrupt muffling of sound *c* Disappearance of sound
d Persistent tapping

27 The ECG monitor strip represents:
a Mechanical activity of the heart *b* Electrical activity of the heart *c* Both *a* and *b* *d* Neither *a* nor *b*

28 Normally, ventricular depolarization:

a Occurs at the T wave *b* Occurs after ventricular contraction *c* Indicates ventricular diastole
d Stimulates ventricular contraction

29 By convention, a positive wave on the ECG indicates:
a The path of electrical activity is approaching a negative electrode *b* The path of electrical activity is approaching a positive electrode *c* The path of electrical activity is moving away from a negative electrode
d The path of electrical activity is moving away from a positive electrode

30 The ECG leads measuring the horizontal plane of the heart are the:
a Standard limb leads *b* Augmented limb leads
c Precordial leads *d* Bipolar leads

31 In standard lead II of the ECG, the electrical potential difference is recorded between the:
a Right arm and left leg *b* Right arm and left arm
c Right arm and right leg *d* Left arm and right leg

32 Which of the following leads is *not* unipolar?
a aVR *b* aVF *c* V_6 *d* II

33 A normal QRS electrical axis is characterized by:
a Large positive QRS deflections in leads II, III, and aVF *b* Large positive QRS deflections in lead aVR
c Large negative QRS deflections in leads II, III, and aVF *d* Large positive QRS deflections in leads I and aVL

34 A catheter wedged in a branch of the pulmonary artery measures a pressure correlating most directly with:
a Right atrial pressure *b* Right ventricular pressure
c Left atrial pressure *d* Pulmonary arterial pressure

35 Which of the following vessels is commonly used for right heart catheterization?
a Femoral artery *b* Brachial artery
c Jugular vein *d* Antecubital vein

36 The correct identification of the aortic and pulmonic components of the second heart sound on the phonocardiogram is aided by the simultaneous recording of the:
a Electrocardiogram *b* Jugular venous pulse
c Carotid arterial pulse *d* Radial pulse

37 Echocardiography utilizes the principle of:
a Hydrodynamics *b* Ultrasound *c* Radioemission
d Electromagnetic force

38 A noninvasive procedure to analyze cardiac structures and wall motion is:
a Phonocardiography *b* Electrocardiography
c Echocardiography *d* Vectorcardiography

Directions: Match each of the terms in col. A with its definition in col. B.

Column A	Column B
39 ___ Angina	*a* Awareness of increased
40 ___ Palpitations	breathing effort

41 ___ Orthopnea
42 ___ Syncope
43 ___ Dyspnea
44 ___ Edema

b Difficulty breathing in the recumbent position
c Chest pain due to myocardial ischemia
d Heartbeats sensed by the patient
e Accumulation of fluid in the interstitial spaces
f Transient loss of consciousness
g Abnormal chest pulsations noticed by the patient

333
QUESTIONS

Directions: Match each of the jugular venous waveforms in col. A with its cause in col. B.

Column A
45 ___ a wave
46 ___ v wave
47 ___ c wave

Column B
a Produced by bulging of the tricuspid valve into the right atrium during ventricular contraction
b Produced by increased right atrial pressure during atrial filling prior to the opening of the tricuspid valve
c Produced by atrial contraction

Directions: Match each of the abnormal heart sounds in col. A with its probable cause in col. B.

Column A
48 ___ Midsystolic murmur
49 ___ Pansystolic murmur
50 ___ Mid-diastolic murmur
51 ___ Opening snap in early diastole

Column B
a May be produced by aortic stenosis
b May be produced by pulmonic regurgitation
c May be produced by mitral stenosis
d May be produced by mitral regurgitation

Directions: Match each area of transmission of the cardiac valvular sounds in col. A with its anatomic location on the chest in col. B.

Column A
52 ___ Mitral
53 ___ Tricuspid
54 ___ Aortic
55 ___ Pulmonic

Column B
a Second intercostal space, left sternal border
b Second intercostal space, right sternal border
c Fifth intercostal space, midclavicular line
d Lower left sternal border

Directions: Match the ECG waveform in col. A to the electrical events in col. B.

Column A
56 ___ P wave
57 ___ QRS complex
58 ___ T wave

Column B
a Ventricular repolarization
b Atrial depolarization
c Ventricular depolarization
d Atrial repolarization

Directions: Match each of the ECG intervals in col. A with its normal duration in col. B.

Column A
59 ___ P-R interval
60 ___ QRS complex
61 ___ Q-T interval

Column B
a 0.36 to 0.44 seconds
b 0.12 to 0.20 seconds
c 0.06 to 0.10 seconds

Directions: Match each ECG abnormality in col. A with its possible cause in col. B.

Column A
62 ___ Depression of the S-T segment
63 ___ Elevation of the S-T segment
64 ___ Inversion of the P wave
65 ___ Inversion of the T wave
66 ___ Peaking of the T wave
67 ___ Prolonged P-R interval
68 ___ Prolonged Q-T interval

Column B
a Slow conduction time through the AV node
b Myocardial ischemia
c Hyperkalemia
d Myocardial necrosis
e AV nodal arrhythmia
f Quinidine effect

Directions: Match each of the cardiac diagnostic techniques in cols. A with its purpose in col. B.

Column A
69 ___ Flow-directed balloon-tipped catheter
70 ___ Vectorcardiography
71 ___ Phonocardiography
72 ___ Echocardiography
73 ___ Thermodilution pulmonary artery catheter
74 ___ Catheter tip lies in the right atrium or superior vena cava inserted via an antecubital vein
75 ___ Chest roentgenogram
76 ___ Nuclear imaging

Column B
a Provides information about the magnitude and direction of electrical activity during the cardiac cycle
b Murmurs heard during heart auscultation may be documented
c Cardiac output may be calculated at the bedside with data obtained
d Size and location of an area of necrosis may be estimated
e Abnormal valve motion may be detected
f Pulmonary wedge pressure may be measured
g Central venous pressure may be measured
h Enlargement of the heart and great vessels may be detected

Directions: Circle T if the statement is true and F if it is false.

77 T   F   The dorsalis pedis pulse may be palpated in back of the knee.

78 T F Left atrial enlargement is detected best in the lateral view of the chest x-ray.

79 T F An arrow symbol representing both magnitude and direction of force is called a vector.

80 T F Kussmaul's sign is a decrease in the central venous pressure during inspiration.

81 T F A patient with an apical heart rate of 78 and a radial rate of 70 has a pulse deficit.

82 T F Physiologic splitting of the second heart sound is caused by asynchronous closure of the aortic and pulmonic valves and is always considered pathologic.

83 T F Paradoxical splitting of the second heart sound is heard on expiration and disappears on inspiration and may be caused by left bundle branch block.

84 T F The sounds of Korotkoff are produced by turbulent blood flow through the aortic valve during blood pressure measurement.

85 T F Paroxysmal nocturnal dyspnea is a symptom of left ventricular failure.

Directions: Fill in the blanks with the correct words.

86 During cardiac catheterization, contrast material is injected into the heart chamber distal to the diseased valve to confirm the diagnosis of valvular _____ _____.

87 The pressure gradient between the left ventricle and the aorta is normally less than _____ mmHg. A large pressure gradient indicates _____ _____ _____.

88 Heart murmurs are the result of _____ blood flow within the cardiac structures.

BIBLIOGRAPHY

AMERICAN HEART ASSOCIATION: *Examination of the Heart,* American Heart Association, New York, 1967.

ANDREOLI, KATHLEEN, VIRGINIA FOWKES, DOUGLAS ZIPES, and ANDREW WALLACE: *Comprehensive Cardiac Care,* Mosby, St. Louis, 1975.

BOLOGNINI, VICKI: "The Swan-Ganz Pulmonary Artery Catheter: Implications for Nursing," *Heart and Lung,* **3**: 976–981, November-December, 1974.

CASTELLANOS, AGUSTIN JR., LOUIS LEMBERG, BAROUH BERKOVITS, and BRADFORD W. CLAXTON: "Didactic Vectorcardiography: General Concepts," *Heart and Lung,* **4**: 697–723, September-October, 1975.

COATS, KATHYRN: "Non-invasive Cardiac Diagnostic Procedures," *American Journal of Nursing,* **75**: 1980–1986, November, 1975.

CONSTANT, JULES: *Learning Electrocardiography,* Little, Brown, Boston, 1973.

HURST, J. WILLIS: *The Heart,* McGraw-Hill, New York, 1974.

JUDGE, RICHARD, and GEORGE ZUIDEMA: *Physical Diagnosis,* Little, Brown, Boston, 1968.

RISEMAN, JOSEPH: *P-QRS-T: A Guide to Electrocardiogram Interpretation,* Macmillan, New York, 1968.

RUSHMER, ROBERT: *Cardiovascular Dynamics,* Saunders, Philadelphia, 1970.

WAGNER, HENRY N.: "Cardiovascular Nuclear Medicine: A Progress Report." *Hospital Practice,* **11**: 77–83, July, 1976.

CHAPTER 27 Coronary Atherosclerotic Disease

Objectives   **At the completion of Chap. 27, you should be able to:**

1 Describe the interaction between myocardial oxygen supply and demand and identify the determinants of each.

2 Differentiate between myocardial infarction and ischemia and describe the relationship between them; explain why the left ventricle is most vulnerable to ischemia and infarction.

3 Describe the progressive pathological changes in a coronary blood vessel in the development of clinically significant atherosclerotic lesions.

4 Identify the most common sites of coronary atherosclerotic lesions.

5 Identify modifiable and nonmodifiable factors that increase the likelihood of developing coronary atherosclerotic disease.

6 List the metabolic, physiologic, hemodynamic, electrocardiographic, and clinical changes associated with myocardial ischemia.

7 Define and explain the common terms used to describe myocardial infarction: subendocardial, transmural, anterior, and inferior.

8 Describe the sequential changes associated with myocardial healing after myocardial infarction.

9 Describe the functional changes resulting from myocardial infarction and the factors affecting the degree of functional impairment.

10 Define vasovagal response.

11 Identify the characteristic diagnostic triad associated with myocardial infarction.

12 Define and describe the physiologic consequences of the following complications of myocardial infarction:
a Congestive heart failure
b Cardiogenic shock
c Papillary muscle dysfunction
d Rupture of the ventricular septum
e Rupture of the ventricular free wall
f Ventricular aneurysm
g Thromboembolism
h Pericarditis
i Dressler's syndrome
j Arrhythmias

13 Identify seven factors which predispose to arrhythmias in coronary atherosclerotic disease.

14 Explain how abnormal rates of impulse generation resulting in tachycardia or bradycardia compromise cardiac function.

15 Differentiate between premature and escape beats.

16 Identify the most common arrhythmia.

17 Identify and place on a rate continuum atrial and ventricular arrhythmias resulting from myocardial irritability.

18 Differentiate between first-, second-, and third-degree heart block; describe bundle branch block.

19 List eight risk factors which may increase the incidence of atherosclerotic heart disease.

20 Identify three hemodynamic factors which may be modified to reduce oxygen demand in the treatment of myocardial ischemia.

21 Describe the mechanisms of action of the following drugs in the treatment of ischemic heart disease: Inderal, digitalis, antihypertensive agents, vasodilators, and sedatives.

22 Explain why the treatment of myocardial ischemia by increasing the coronary blood flow and oxygen supply is limited.

23 Describe the effects of hypoxemia, hypotension, and arrhythmias on coronary oxygen supply and how these problems are treated.

24 State the rationale for rest in the treatment of acute myocardial infarction.

25 Describe the general principles of treatment for the following arrhythmias: tachycardia, bradycardia, escape rhythms, ventricular irritability, atrial irritability, atrial tachycardia, ventricular fibrillation, and heart block.

26 Describe the treatment for congestive heart failure, acute pulmonary edema, and cardiogenic shock.

27 State the indications, hemodynamic and physiologic effects, and possible complications of intra-aortic balloon pumping.

28 Identify and describe two additional circulatory assist devices.

29 Compare saphenous vein bypass graft as a method of coronary revascularization to a mammary artery bypass graft.

30 List the indications for coronary revascularization, the cardiac catheterization findings indicating operable disease, and the two most important factors affecting the success of surgery.

31 Describe the following cardiac surgical procedures: aneurysmectomy, septal defect repair, infarctectomy, mitral valve replacement, and heart transplant.

32 Explain the importance of rehabilitation in the treatment of patients with atherosclerotic heart disease.

A critical balance exists between myocardial oxygen supply and demand; oxygen supply must equal demand (see Fig. 27-1). A reduction in oxygen supply or an increase in oxygen demand can disturb this balance and threaten myocardial function.

There are four major determinants of myocardial oxygen demand: heart rate, contractile force, muscle mass, and ventricular wall tension (see Table 27-1). Wall tension or afterload is a function of variables identified in the Laplace equation: arterial pressure, or resistance to ejection, and ventricular radius. Therefore, cardiac work and oxygen demand are elevated by tachycardia (rapid heart rates), increased force of contraction, hypertrophy, hypertension, and ventricular dilation.

If myocardial oxygen demand increases, oxygen supply must increase concurrently. To significantly increase oxygen supply, coronary flow must increase, since myocardial oxygen extraction from the arterial blood is almost maximal under resting conditions. The most potent stimulus to dilating the coronary arteries and increasing coronary flow is local tissue hypoxia. The normal coronary vasculature can dilate and increase flow approximately four to five times above resting levels. However, stenotic, diseased vessels are unable to dilate, and therefore a state of oxygen deficit can result when oxygen demand exceeds the capacity of the vasculature to increase flow. *Ischemia* is a transient, reversible state of oxygen lack. Prolonged ischemia will lead to muscle death, or *necrosis*. Clinically, necrosis of the myocardium is referred to as *myocardial infarction*.

The left ventricle is the chamber most susceptible to myocardial ischemia and infarction by virtue of unique myocardial oxygenation characteristics. First, left ventricular oxygen demand is great as a result of the high systemic resistance to ejection and the large muscle mass. In addition, coronary flow is phasic in nature. The branches of the coronary arteries are deeply embedded in the myocardium. During systole, these intramyocardial branches are compressed, increasing the resistance to flow. Coronary flow therefore occurs primarily during diastole. Contraction of the thick left ventricular wall essentially terminates systolic flow through its intramyocardial branches, especially in the innermost or subendocardial region; some systolic flow continues in the vessels of the thinner-walled right ventricle.

PATHOGENESIS

Pathology

Coronary atherosclerosis is the most common cause of coronary artery disease. Atherosclerosis causes a localized accumulation of lipid and fibrous tissue within the

coronary artery, progressively narrowing the lumen of the vessel. As the lumen narrows, resistance to flow increases, and myocardial blood flow is compromised. As the disease progresses, the luminal narrowing is accompanied by vascular changes that impair the ability of the diseased vessel to dilate. Thus the balance between myocardial oxygen supply and demand becomes precarious, threatening the myocardium beyond the lesion.

Considerable controversy has arisen regarding the pathogenesis of coronary atherosclerosis. However, the pathologic changes within the affected vessel can be summarized as follows (Fig. 27-2):

1 Deposition of small amounts of lipid material, apparent as "fatty streaks," in the intima.
2 Accumulation of lipid, especially cholesterol-rich β-lipoprotein, in the intima and inner media.
3 Fibrous encapsulation of the lesion, creating "fibrous plaques."
4 Development of "atheroma" or complex atherosclerotic plaques consisting of lipid, fibrous tissue, collagen, calcium, cellular debris, and capillaries.
5 Degenerative changes in the arterial wall.

Despite this progressive luminal narrowing and the concurrent loss of vascular responsiveness, clinical manifestations of disease do not appear until the atherogenic process is well advanced. This preclinical phase can last 20 to 40 years. Clinically significant lesions, producing myocardial ischemia and dysfunction, usually obstruct over 75 percent of the vessel lumen. The final step in the pathologic process producing the clinical insult can occur in the following ways: (1) progressive luminal narrowing by plaque enlargement; (2) hemorrhage into the atheromatous plaque; (3) thrombus formation initiated by platelet aggregation; (4) embolization of a thrombus or plaque fragment; (5) coronary arterial spasm.

Notably, atherosclerotic lesions usually develop in the proximal, epicardial segments of the coronary artery at sites of abrupt curvature, branching, or attachment. The lesions tend to be localized and focal in distribution; however, in advanced disease, areas of diffuse involvement become pronounced.

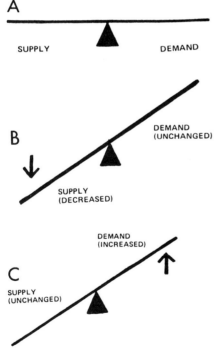

*FIGURE 27-1 Balance between myocardial oxygen supply and demand. A, normally, myocardial oxygen supply and demand are in balance. B, imbalance due to decreased coronary blood supply (e.g., low blood pressure) while the demand for oxygen remains unchanged. C, imbalance due to increased demand (e.g., exercise) while the blood supply to the myocardium remains unchanged (e.g., coronary atherosclerosis limits ability of blood vessels to increase supply). (Adapted from Marie C. Clark, "Chest Pain," Heart & Lung, **4**: 956, 1975.)*

TABLE 27-1
Determinants of myocardial oxygen demand

Heart rate
Contractile force
Muscle mass
Wall tension
Arterial pressure
Ventricular radius

Risk factors

It is no longer contended that atherosclerosis is simply a result of the aging process. The appearance of "fatty streaks" in the coronary arterial wall as early as childhood is a natural phenomenon and does not necessarily progress to atherosclerotic lesions. It is now believed that many factors interact to accelerate the atherogenic process. A number of so-called risk factors have been identified that increase susceptibility to the development of coronary atherosclerosis in a given individual (Table 27-2).

There are four nonmodifiable, biologic risk factors: age, sex, race, and family history. Susceptibility to coronary atherosclerosis increases with age; the development of significant disease before age 40 is unusual. However, the correlation between age and disease onset may simply reflect the longer duration of exposure to other atherogenic factors. Females seem relatively immune until after menopause and then become as susceptible as males. The protective effect of estrogen has been postulated as an explanation for early female immunity. Blacks are more vulnerable to atherosclerosis than whites. Finally, a positive family history for coronary heart disease (i.e., siblings or parents developing disease before age 50) increases the likelihood of the premature development of atherosclerosis. The relative contribution of genetic and environmental influences is unknown. A genetic component can be linked with some pronounced, accelerated forms of atherosclerosis, as in familial lipid disorders. However, family history may also reflect a strong environmental component, perhaps a life-style producing tension or obesity.

Additional risk factors are amenable to modification, potentially retarding the atherogenic process. Major risk factors are elevated serum lipid levels, hypertension, cigarette smoking, impaired glucose tolerance, and diets high in saturated fat, cholesterol, and calories. Elevation of serum lipid levels is a potent determinant of susceptibility; hyperlipidemia is associated with increased severity and prematurity of the disease. Risk seems to correlate most directly with serum cholesterol levels. No specific serum cholesterol level can be cited as the critical "abnormal" threshold; however, the optimal serum cholesterol level is under 200 mg%. According to the American Heart Association, levels over 250 mg% increase risk threefold. The risk increases progressively with further serum cholesterol elevation. The plasma lipids—cholesterol, triglycerides, phospholipids, and free fatty acids—are insoluble in plasma; therefore the lipids are bound to proteins as a mechanism for serum transport. The lipoproteins are soluble in plasma. Epidemiologic studies are examining the predictive validity of lipoprotein levels as indices of disease susceptibility.

Hypertension definitely accelerates atherogenesis; abnormalities in pressure and hemodynamic stress may initiate vascular changes. Both diastolic and systolic elevations (i.e., systolic over 140 mmHg, diastolic over 90 mmHg) are predictive of increased vulnerability; risk is directly related to the degree of elevation. An individual with a systolic pressure over 150 mmHg is twice as susceptible to atherosclerosis as an individual with a systolic pressure under 120 mmHg. The risk of cigarette smoking is related to the number of cigarettes smoked per day, not to the duration of smoking. An individual smoking more than a pack a day is twice as susceptible as a nonsmoker. The effect of nicotine on catecholamine release by the autonomic nervous system seems to be the mechanism responsible. The effect, however, is noncumulative; ex-smokers seem to revert to the low risk of nonsmokers.

Diabetics evidence a greater prevalence, prematurity, and severity of coronary atherosclerosis. The mechanism is as yet unresolved, but perhaps an abnormality in lipid

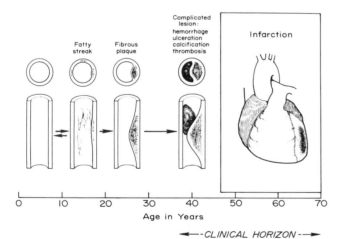

FIGURE 27-2 *Progressive pathologic changes in coronary atherosclerotic disease. Fatty streaks are found as one of the earliest lesions of atherosclerosis. Many fatty streaks regress, whereas others progress to fibrous plaques and eventually to atheromata. These may then become complicated by hemorrhage, ulceration, calcification, or thrombosis and may produce myocardial infarction. (From J. W. Hurst,* The Heart, *3d ed., McGraw-Hill, New York, 1974, p. 989.)*

TABLE 27-2
Risk factors

NONMODIFIABLE	MODIFIABLE
Age	Major
Sex	Elevated serum lipids
Family history	Hypertension
Race	Cigarette smoking
	Impaired glucose tolerance
	Diet high in saturated fat, cholesterol, and calories
	Minor
	Sedentary life-style
	Psychological stress
	Personality type

metabolism or a predisposition to vascular degeneration associated with the impaired glucose tolerance is responsible. The American diet—high in calories, total fat, saturated fat, sugar and salt—contributes to the development of obesity and hyperlipoproteinemia. In addition, cardiac work increases with obesity.

The list of minor risk factors expands as additional biologic–environmental correlates with coronary heart disease are identified. At present, a sedentary life-style and psychosocial stress seem contributory. An intriguing relationship between the so-called type A behavior pattern and accelerated atherogenesis has been popularized by Rosenman and Friedman. The type A personality manifests intense competitiveness, ambition, aggressiveness, and a sense of time urgency. It is commonly acknowledged that catecholamine release accompanies stress; however, the question arises as to whether stress is atherogenic or simply precipitates the attack. A theory of stress-induced atherogenesis might postulate neuroendocrine influences upon circulatory dynamics, serum lipids, and blood clotting.

Hence, the speculation continues. However, the fact remains that coronary atherosclerosis is a multifactorial disease with substantiated evidence that certain risk factors accelerate atherogenesis. The complexity of the process is highlighted by the fact that in the presence of more than one risk factor, the susceptibility to atherogenesis is not simply additive but synergistic. The interaction of factors significantly accelerates the disease process.

PATHOPHYSIOLOGY

Ischemia

Oxygen demand in excess of the capacity of the diseased vessels to supply oxygen results in localized myocardial ischemia. Transient ischemia causes reversible changes at the cellular and tissue level, depressing myocardial function.

The oxygen lack forces the myocardium to shift from aerobic metabolism to anaerobic metabolism. Anaerobic metabolism via glycolytic pathways is a much less efficient means of energy production than aerobic metabolism via oxidative phosphorylation and the Krebs cycle; the production of high-energy phosphate is reduced considerably. The end product of anaerobic metabolism, lactic acid, accumulates, reducing cellular pH.

The combination of hypoxia, reduced energy availability, and acidosis rapidly impairs left ventricular function. The strength of contraction of the affected myocardial region is reduced; the fibers shorten inadequately with less force and velocity. In addition, the wall motion of the ischemic segment is abnormal; the segment passively bulges outward with each ventricular contraction (see Fig. 27-3).

The reduced contractility and impaired wall motion alters hemodynamics. The hemodynamic response is variable, depending upon the size of the ischemic

segment and the degree of reflex compensatory response by the autonomic nervous system. Depression of left ventricular function may lower cardiac output by reducing stroke volume (the amount of blood ejected per beat). Reduction in systolic emptying increases ventricular volumes. As a result, left-sided pressures rise; the left ventricular end-diastolic pressure and pulmonary capillary wedge pressure will be elevated. This pressure elevation is magnified by changes in wall compliance or distensibility induced by ischemia. A reduction in compliance occurs, accentuating the elevation in pressure for a given ventricular volume (see Fig. 27-4).

During ischemia, the manifest hemodynamic pattern is commonly that of mild increments in blood pressure and heart rate prior to the onset of pain. Apparently, this represents a sympathetic compensatory response to the depression of myocardial function rather than a response to subsequent pain and anxiety. Although certainly with the onset of pain, a further catecholamine stimulation could occur. A depression of blood pressure would suggest ischemic involvement of a large area of myocardium.

Myocardial ischemia is typically associated with two characteristic electrocardiographic changes resulting from alterations in cellular electrophysiology: T wave inversion and S-T segment depression (see Fig. 27-5). A variant form of angina, Prinzmetal's angina, is always associated with S-T segment elevation.

Ischemic attacks usually subside within minutes if the imbalance between oxygen supply and demand is corrected. The metabolic, functional, hemodynamic, and electrocardiographic changes are reversible.

Angina pectoris is the chest pain associated with myocardial ischemia. The exact mechanism by which

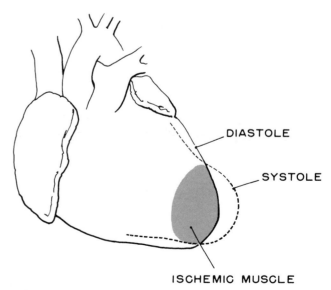

FIGURE 27-3 Ischemic wall bulging during systole.

ischemia produces pain is unclear. It seems that neural pain receptors are stimulated by the accumulated metabolites, by an unidentified chemical intermediary, or by local mechanical stress resulting from abnormal myocardial contraction. Typically, the pain is described as a substernal pressure, occasionally radiating down the medial aspect of the left arm. A clenched fist placed upon the sternum graphically illustrates the classical pattern. However, many patients never experience typical angina; anginal pain may mimic indigestion or a toothache. Angina is precipitated by activities increasing myocardial oxygen demand, such as exercise, and is relieved within minutes by rest or nitroglycerin (see Fig. 27-6).

Infarction

Prolonged ischemia of over 30 to 45 minutes causes irreversible cellular damage and muscle death, or necrosis. Permanent cessation of contractile function occurs in the necrotic or infarcted area of the myocardium. The infarct is surrounded by a zone of ischemic, potentially viable tissue (see Fig. 27-7). The ultimate size of the infarct depends upon the fate of this ischemic zone; necrosis of this marginal area will extend the infarct size, whereas reversal of the ischemia minimizes the residual necrosis.

Myocardial infarction usually affects the left ventricle. A *transmural infarction* involves the full thickness of the wall; a *subendocardial* infarction is limited to the inner half of the myocardium (see Fig. 27-8). Infarctions are described further according to location on the ventricular wall (see Fig. 27-9). For instance, an anterior myocardial infarction involves the anterior wall of the left ventricle. Other commonly designated infarct sites are inferior, lateral, posterior, and septal. Extensive infarctions involving large portions of the ventricle would be described accordingly, that is, anteroseptal, anterolateral, or inferolateral.

Obviously, the infarct location correlates with disease in a particular region of the coronary circulation. For example, anterior wall infarctions result from lesions in the left anterior descending artery. Knowledge of the infarct location and the coronary anatomy is of critical importance in the anticipation of complications associated with myocardial infarction. For example, inferior wall infarction, usually the result of right coronary artery lesions, can be associated with variable degrees of heart block. This is to be expected, because the AV node receives its nutrient supply from the same vessel nourishing the inferior wall of the left ventricle.

The infarcted muscle undergoes a sequence of changes during the healing process. Initially the infarcted muscle appears bruised and cyanotic as a result of regional stagnation of blood. Cellular edema and an inflammatory response with leukocytic infiltration ensue within 24 hours. Cardiac enzymes are released from the cells. Tissue degradation and removal of all necrotic fibers begins by the second or third day. During this phase, the necrotic wall is relatively thin. By about the third week, scar formation begins. Gradually, fibrous connective tissue replaces the necrotic muscle and undergoes progressive thickening. By the sixth week, the scar is well established.

Myocardial infarction significantly depresses ventricular function as a result of the loss of contractility in the necrotic muscle and the impaired contractility in the surrounding ischemic muscle. Functionally, myocardial infarction results in changes similar to those noted with ischemia: (1) reduced contractility, (2) abnormal wall motion, (3) reduced stroke volume, (4) diminished ejection fraction, (5) elevated ventricular end-systolic and end-diastolic volumes, (6) increased left ventricular end-diastolic pressure, and (7) altered ventricular wall compliance.

A wide spectrum of left ventricular dysfunction is apparent after myocardial infarction. The degree of functional impairment depends upon a number of factors:

1 Infarct size—infarcts of over 40 percent of the myocardium are associated with a high incidence of cardiogenic shock.
2 Infarct location—anterior wall infarction is more likely

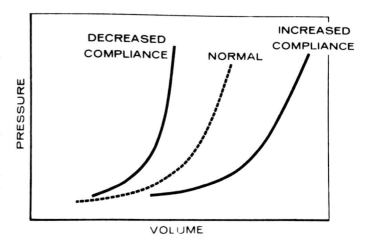

FIGURE 27-4 Ventricular compliance, or the pressure–volume relationship of the ventricles. The dotted line in the center indicates the typical relationship between pressure and volume. As volume is increased initially, there is only a small rise in pressure. As volume increase continues, the rise in pressure is greater. Each solid line indicates an alteration in pressure–volume relationships: decreased compliance on the left and increased compliance on the right. This represents a greater or lesser degree of stiffness of the ventricle in relation to the filling volume. Ventricular compliance is a dynamic phenomenon, and this property can change rapidly. (From W. A. Sodeman, Jr. and W. A. Sodeman (eds.), Pathologic Physiology, 5th ed., Saunders, Philadelphia, 1974, p. 276.)

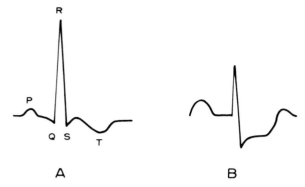

FIGURE 27-5 Classic ECG changes with ischemia. A, T-wave inversion. B, S-T segment depression.

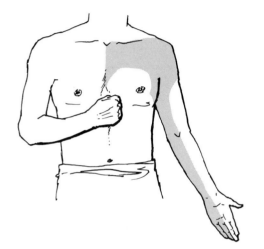

FIGURE 27-6 Typical pattern of referred pain in angina pectoris.

to significantly depress myocardial function than inferior wall damage.

3 Function of uninvolved myocardium—old infarcts would compromise residual myocardial function.

4 Collateral circulation—collateral circulation, either via preexisting arterial anastomoses or new channels, can develop in response to chronic ischemia and regional hypoperfusion, improving blood flow to the threatened myocardium.

5 Cardiovascular compensatory mechanisms—reflex compensatory mechanisms operate to maintain cardiac output and peripheral perfusion.

Reflex sympathetic augmentation of the heart rate and contractility can improve ventricular function. Generalized arteriolar constriction increases total peripheral resistance, thereby increasing mean arterial pressure. Venoconstriction reduces venous capacity, increasing venous return to the heart and ventricular filling. Increased ventricular filling elevates the force of contraction and subsequent ejection volumes. This is best illustrated by comparing the normal ventricular function curve with that of the compromised myocardium (see Fig. 27-10). With depression of ventricular function, higher diastolic filling pressures are necessary to maintain stroke volume. Elevation of diastolic filling pressure and ventricular volume stretches myocardial fibers, increasing the force of contraction according to Starling's law. Circulatory filling pressures can be increased further by renal retention of sodium and water. As a result, myocardial infarction is commonly associated with transient left ventricular enlargement caused by compensatory cardiac dilation. If necessary, compensatory cardiac hypertrophy can also occur to increase the force of contraction and ventricular emptying.

In summary, a battery of reflex responses are available to forestall deterioration of cardiac output and perfusion pressure: (1) augmentation of heart rate and contrac-

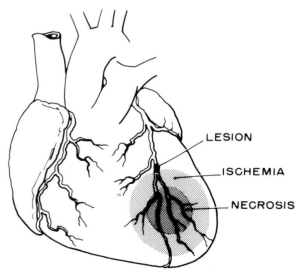

FIGURE 27-7 Zones of necrosis and ischemia.

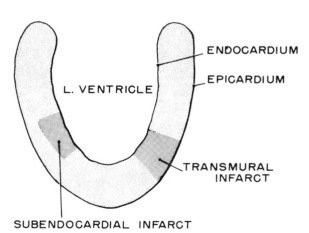

FIGURE 27-8 Transmural and subendocardial infarction.

tility, (2) generalized vasoconstriction, (3) sodium and water retention, (4) ventricular dilation, and (5) ventricular hypertrophy. However, all compensatory responses can eventually contribute to further myocardial deterioration by increasing myocardial oxygen demand.

The hemodynamic presentation after myocardial infarction is variable. Typically, cardiac output may be slightly reduced or maintained at normal levels. Heart rate is usually not persistently elevated unless extensive myocardial depression occurs. Blood pressure is a function of the interaction between myocardial depression and autonomic reflexes. The autonomic response to myocardial infarction is not always the predictable sympathetic support of the compromised circulation. Pain or stimulation of parasympathetic ganglia in the myocardium, especially in the inferior wall, complicates the hemodynamic response. Parasympathetic stimulation reduces the heart rate and blood pressure, adversely affecting cardiac output and peripheral perfusion. This type of response is known as *vasovagal*.

Myocardial infarction is classically associated with a characteristic diagnostic triad. First, there is a clinical picture consisting of severe, prolonged chest pain frequently associated with sweating, nausea, vomiting, and a sense of impending doom. Second, serum levels of the cardiac enzymes released by the necrotic myocardial cells are elevated. Finally, electrocardiographic changes, consisting of pronounced Q waves, S-T segment elevation and inverted T waves, are evident (see Fig. 27-11). These changes are apparent in the leads overlying the area of myocardial necrosis.

Complications of infarction

CONGESTIVE HEART FAILURE

Congestive heart failure is the most common mechanical complication following myocardial infarction, occurring approximately 50 percent of the time. The loss of left ventricular contractile force diminishes the ability of the left ventricle to empty during systole. This reduction in systolic emptying, coupled with increased diastolic filling as a circulatory compensatory mechanism elevates left ventricular volume and pressure. The pressure elevation is reflected backward into the left atrium and pulmonary veins and may cause pulmonary congestion. Fluid transudation into the interstitial space and eventually the alveoli will result if pulmonary capillary hydrostatic pressure exceeds colloid osmotic pressure. Pulmonary edema is discussed in Part VI.

The functional integrity of the right ventricle may remain unaffected by left ventricular failure. However, if reflex pulmonary arteriolar constriction occurs to protect the pulmonary vasculature from further pressure increments, the resistance to right ventricular ejection will rise. Chronic right-sided congestion with elevation of systemic venous and capillary pressures can result. Fluid transudation at the systemic capillary level causes peripheral edema.

CARDIOGENIC SHOCK

Cardiogenic shock results from profound left ventricular dysfunction following massive infarction, usually involving over 40 percent of the left ventricle. A vicious, self-perpetuating cycle of progressively irreversible hemodynamic changes ensues: (1) reduced peripheral perfusion, (2) reduced coronary perfusion, (3) increased pulmonary congestion. Hypotension, metabolic aci-

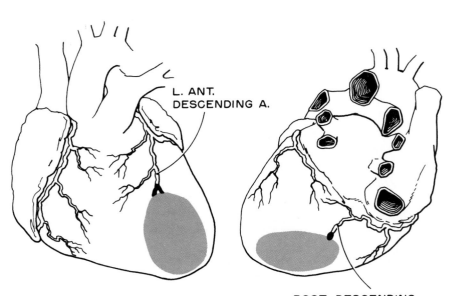

FIGURE 27-9 Localization of infarcts on the ventricular wall. Infarct of the anterior wall due to occlusion of the left anterior descending artery (left). Inferior wall infarction due to occlusion of the posterior descending branch of the right coronary artery (right).

L. ANT.
DESCENDING A.

POST. DESCENDING
BRANCH R. CORONARY A.

dosis, and hypoxemia further depress myocardial function. The incidence of cardiogenic shock is 10 to 15 percent. The associated mortality is approximately 80 to 90 percent.

PAPILLARY MUSCLE DYSFUNCTION

Closure of the mitral valve during ventricular systole is dependent upon the functional integrity of the left ventricular papillary muscles and chordae tendinae. Ischemia or necrotic rupture of the papillary muscle impairs mitral valve function, permitting varying degrees of leaflet eversion into the atria during systole (see Fig. 27-12). Valvular incompetence results in retrograde flow from the left ventricle into the left atrium with two consequences: a reduction in forward aortic flow and an elevation in left atrial and pulmonary venous congestion. The volume of regurgitant flow depends upon the extent of papillary muscle disease; ischemia commonly causes mild to moderate congestive heart failure. However, papillary muscle necrosis and rupture is a catastrophic event that rapidly deteriorates into pulmonary edema and cardiogenic shock.

VENTRICULAR SEPTAL DEFECT

Necrosis of the interventricular septum can result in rupture of the septal wall, creating a ventricular septal defect. Since the septum receives a dual blood supply from arteries descending the anterior and posterior surface of the interventricular groove, septal rupture indicates extensive coronary artery disease involving more than one artery.

Essentially, the rupture establishes a second outflow tract from the left ventricle. During each ventricular contraction, there is competitive outflow through the aorta and septal defect (see Fig. 27-13). Since pressures on the left side of the heart are far greater than pressures on the right side of the heart, blood will be shunted through the defect from left to right, from the area of greater pressure to the area of lesser pressure. Great

volumes of blood can be shunted over to the right side of the heart, reducing the amount of blood available to be ejected via the aorta. Significant reductions in cardiac output with concurrent elevations in right ventricular work and pulmonary congestion result.

CARDIAC RUPTURE

Although rare, cardiac rupture of the ventricular free wall may occur early in the course of transmural infarction during the phase of necrotic tissue removal prior to scar formation. The thin, necrotic wall ruptures, resulting in massive bleeding into the pericardial sac. The relatively inelastic pericardial sac is unable to distend. Thus the blood-filled pericardial sac compresses the heart, producing cardiac tamponade (see Fig. 27-14). Cardiac tamponade reduces venous return and cardiac output. Death usually occurs within a few minutes.

VENTRICULAR ANEURYSM

Although transient paradoxical myocardial bulging of the ischemic myocardium is common, a sustained ventricular aneurysm occurs less than 25 percent of the time. The aneurysm is usually on the anterior or apical surface of the heart. Ventricular aneurysms balloon outward with each systole, passively distended by a portion of the stroke volume (see Fig. 27-15). Ventricular aneurysms can produce three problematic consequences: (1) chronic congestive heart failure, (2) systemic embolization of mural thrombi, and (3) refractory ventricular arrhythmias.

THROMBOEMBOLISM

Necrosis of the ventricular endothelium roughens the endothelial surface, predisposing to thrombus formation. A fragment of an intracardiac mural thrombus can dislodge and embolize systemically. A second potential site of thrombus formation is the systemic venous system; venous embolization would cause pulmonary embolism, a complication discussed in Part VI.

PERICARDITIS

Transmural infarction can roughen the epicardial layer in contact with the pericardium, irritating the pericardial surface and resulting in an inflammatory reaction; rarely, a pericardial effusion, or fluid accumulation between the layers, occurs. Fluid accumulation is rarely significant enough to cause cardiac tamponade.

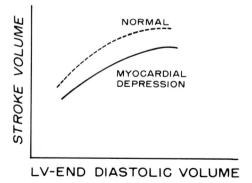

FIGURE 27-10 *Depression of the ventricular function curve. The dotted line represents the relationship of stroke volume to left ventricular end-diastolic volume for the normal heart shown previously in Fig. 25-9. The failing heart (solid line) must increase the end-diastolic volume to maintain stroke volume. Therefore, cardiac dilatation occurs.*

DRESSLER'S SYNDROME

This postmyocardial infarction syndrome is a benign inflammatory response with pleuropericardial pain. It is postulated that the syndrome might represent a hypersensitivity reaction to the necrotic myocardium.

ARRHYTHMIA

A disturbance of cardiac rhythm, or arrhythmia, is the most common complication during myocardial infarction, having an incidence of approximately 90 percent. Arrhythmias result from alterations in myocardial cellular electrophysiology. The electrophysiologic alteration is manifested by a change in the configuration of the action potential, which is the graphic recording of cellular electrical activity. For instance, sympathetic stimulation increases the rate of rise of the action potential, thereby increasing the heart rate (see Fig. 27-16). Clinically, arrhythmia diagnosis is based upon interpretation of the electrocardiogram.

Multiple predisposing factors account for the high incidence of arrhythmias in the setting of coronary atherosclerotic disease: (1) tissue ischemia, (2) hypoxemia, (3) autonomic nervous system influences (e.g., parasympathetic stimulation decreases heart rate), (4) metabolic derangements (e.g., lactic acidosis due to compromised tissue perfusion), (5) hemodynamic abnormalities (e.g., reduction in coronary perfusion associated with hypotension), (6) drugs (e.g., digitalis toxicity), and (7) electrolyte imbalance (e.g., hypokalemia with excessive diuresis).

There are three types of cardiac rhythm abnormalities: abnormal rate of impulse formation, abnormal site of impulse formation, and abnormal impulse conduction.

The normal heart rate is between 60 and 100 bpm. A heart rate under 60 bpm is referred to as a *bradycardia*, whereas a *tachycardia* indicates a heart rate over 100 bpm (see Fig. 27-17). Both rate abnormalities can adversely affect cardiac function. Since heart rate is a primary determinant of cardiac output (CO = HR × SV), extreme increments or reductions in heart rate can lower cardiac output; tachycardias lower it by reducing ventricular filling time and stroke volume, and bradycardias lower it by reducing the frequency of ventricular ejection. As cardiac output falls, arterial pressure and peripheral perfusion decrease. Furthermore, tachycardias can aggravate myocardial ischemia by increasing myocardial oxygen demand while simultaneously reducing the duration of diastole, the period of greatest coronary flow, thereby compromising coronary oxygen supply.

Any cardiac impulse originating outside of the sinus node is considered abnormal and is referred to as an *ectopic beat*. Ectopic beats can originate in the atria, atrioventricular junction, or ventricles under two conditions: (1) failure or excessive slowing of the sinus node and (2) increased automaticity or "irritability" of another cardiac site. Ectopic beats resulting from sinus node failure serve a protective function by initiating a cardiac impulse before prolonged cardiac standstill can occur (see Fig. 27-18). These beats are called *escape beats*. If the sinus node fails to resume normal function, the ectopic site will assume the role of pacemaker and sustain the cardiac rhythm. This is referred to as an *escape rhythm*. Once the sinus node resumes normal function, the escape focus is suppressed.

Irritability of cardiac sites other than the sinus node disrupts the normal cardiac cycle; impulses occur prematurely before the sinus node recovers sufficiently from one beat to initiate another (see Fig. 27-19). These beats are referred to as *premature beats*. Irritable sites can produce isolated premature beats or sustained tachycardias; irritability can develop in the atria, atrioventricular junction, or ventricles and are designated accordingly. For instance, an "atrial premature beat" originates in the atria, whereas "ventricular tachycardia" is ventricular in origin.

Ventricular premature beats are the most common form of arrhythmia (see Fig. 27-20A). However, ventricular irritability can degenerate into life-threatening ventricular tachycardia or ventricular fibrillation (see Figs. 27-20B and 27-20C). *Ventricular tachycardia* severely reduces cardiac output as a result of the rapid rate, usually over 120 bpm, and the loss of mechanical synchrony between atrial and ventricular contraction. *Ventricular fibrillation* results in the abrupt cessation of effective ventricular contraction; the ventricles quiver without coordination.

Atrial irritability can be conceptualized along a continuum of rate acceleration associated with progressive reduction in atrial function: (1) *premature atrial beat*, (2) *atrial tachycardia*—atrial rate approximately 150, (3) *atrial flutter*—atrial rate approximately 300, and (4) *atrial*

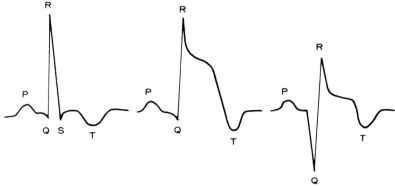

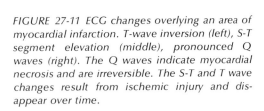

FIGURE 27-11 ECG changes overlying an area of myocardial infarction. T-wave inversion (left), S-T segment elevation (middle), pronounced Q waves (right). The Q waves indicate myocardial necrosis and are irreversible. The S-T and T wave changes result from ischemic injury and disappear over time.

fibrillation—quivering, uncoordinated atrial activity (see Fig. 27-21). To protect the ventricles from responding to extremely rapid atrial stimulation, the AV node does not normally conduct atrial impulses at rates greater than 180 bpm. For instance, in atrial flutter with an atrial rate of 300, only every second or third atrial impulse is conducted; consequently the ventricular rate is 100 to 150. The hemodynamic response to atrial arrhythmias depends upon the ventricular rate and the efficacy of atrial contraction. For instance, in atrial fibrillation, the atrial musculature is unable to contract effectively and actively contribute to ventricular filling; thus, cardiac output may fall.

Delay or interruption of impulse conduction constitutes the final category of rhythm abnormality. The cardiac impulse normally spreads from the sinus node along internodal pathways to the AV node and ventricles

within 0.20 seconds (normal P-R interval); ventricular depolarization occurs within 0.10 seconds (normal QRS duration). *Heart block* is a delay or interruption in impulse conduction through the atria to the ventricles. Heart block occurs in three progressively more serious forms. In *first-degree heart block*, all impulses are conducted through the AV junction; however conduction time is abnormally prolonged. In *second-degree heart block*, some impulses are conducted to the ventricles, but some impulses are blocked. There are two types of second-degree heart block. Wenckebach (Mobitz I) is

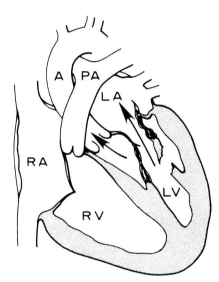

FIGURE 27-12 Papillary muscle rupture.

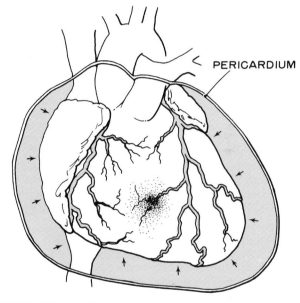

FIGURE 27-14 Cardiac tamponade.

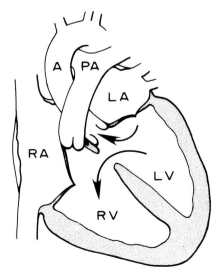

FIGURE 27-13 Ventricular septal defect.

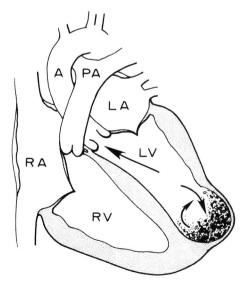

FIGURE 27-15 Ventricular aneurysm.

characterized by repetitive cycles of progressively lengthening AV conduction time, culminating in the nonconduction of one beat. The second type, Mobitz II, involves conduction of some impulses with a constant AV conduction time and nonconduction of other impulses. In *third-degree heart block,* no impulses are conducted to the ventricles. Unless "escape pacemakers," either junctional or ventricular in origin, begin to function, cardiac standstill results (see Fig. 27-22). *Bundle branch block* is an interruption of conduction in the bundle branches which prolongs ventricular depolarization time beyond 0.10 seconds.

THERAPEUTIC INTERVENTION

Primary prevention

The most critical therapeutic intervention in the setting of coronary atherosclerosis is the primary prevention of the disease. Disease prevention is essential for many reasons:

1 Clinically apparent disease is preceded by a long latent period with silent progression of disease, apparently in early adulthood. Lesions considered to be precursors of atherosclerotic disease have been identified in the coronary arterial walls of children and young adults.
2 There is no curative therapy for coronary atherosclerotic disease; once the disease is recognizable clinically, therapy is essentially palliative, undertaken to minimize the severity of clinical sequelae and to potentially slow disease progression.
3 The consequences of coronary atherosclerosis can be catastrophic. Myocardial infarction often occurs with little or no warning; the incidence of sudden death is high. Over half of the deaths associated with myocardial infarction occur during the first few hours of infarction prior to hospitalization.
4 Coronary atherosclerosis is the leading cause of death in the country; approximately 700,000 deaths were attributable to myocardial infarction in 1973.

Since the precise pathogenesis of atherosclerosis is still undefined, the control of risk factors known to increase susceptibility to atherogenesis is the crux of disease prophylaxis. The risk factors amenable to modification are (1) hyperlipidemia, (2) hypertension, (3) smoking, (4) obesity, (5) dietary intake high in calories, total fat, saturated fat, cholesterol, and salt, (6) diabetes, (7) sedentary life-style, and (8) psychosocial stress. Measures should be initiated to eliminate or control these risk factors in every individual, with major emphasis upon the first three.

The question arises of when to initiate risk factor surveillance and control. Currently, the concept of disease prophylaxis has been applied primarily to "coronary-prone" adults, those with identified risk factors, and individuals with evidence of disease. However, control of risk factors earlier in life seems more likely to prevent atherogenesis or retard disease progression so that a substantive reduction in cardiac morbidity and mortality can be achieved. The emphasis must be upon health education with early detection and control of risk factors rather than upon treatment of the clinical sequelae of established disease.

Medical intervention

ISCHEMIA

The therapeutic aim with myocardial ischemia is to correct the imbalance between myocardial oxygen demand and oxygen supply. Restoration of oxygen balance can be accomplished by two mechanisms: reduction of oxygen demand and elevation of oxygen supply (see Table 27-3).

To reduce oxygen demand, the physiologic variables determining myocardial oxygen requirements must be controlled. Three major determinants of oxygen demand are amenable to therapy: (1) heart rate, (2) contractile

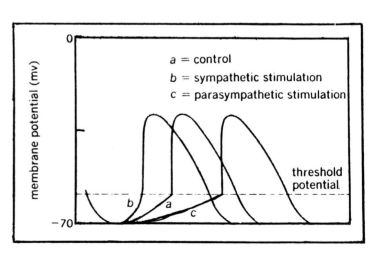

FIGURE 27-16 Effects of sympathetic and parasympathetic stimulation on the slope of the action potential of an SA node cell. (From A. J. Vander, J. H. Sherman, and D. S. Luciano, Human Physiology, *1st ed., McGraw-Hill, New York, 1970, p. 258.)*

force, and (3) afterload (arterial pressure and ventricular size). Reducing heart rate, force of contraction, arterial pressure, and ventricular size reduces cardiac work and oxygen demand.

Nitroglycerin, the therapeutic mainstay for reversal of ischemia, relieves angina primarily by peripheral vasodilation of the arterial and venous beds and secondarily by improving the distribution of coronary blood flow to ischemic areas. Arterial vasodilation reduces arterial pressure, thereby decreasing the systemic resistance to ventricular ejection. Dilation of the veins increases the capacity of the venous bed with pooling of blood in the periphery. As a result, venous return to the heart falls, decreasing ventricular volume and ventricular size. Thus, peripheral vasodilation reduces afterload and, consequently, oxygen demand by a reduction in arterial pressure and ventricular size. Long-acting nitrites, still the subject of controversy, exhibit similar effects.

Propranolol (Inderal), a beta-adrenergic blocking agent, interrupts ischemia by selectively inhibiting the effects of the sympathetic nervous system upon the heart; these effects are mediated by beta receptors. Beta stimulation increases heart rate and force of contraction. Inderal blocks these effects, reducing heart rate and force of contraction and thereby diminishing myocardial oxygen requirements. The reduced contractile force does produce a mild increment in ventricular

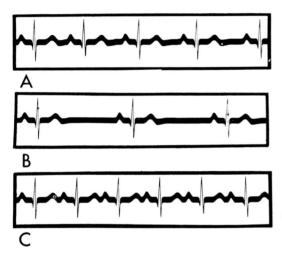

FIGURE 27-17 A, normal sinus rhythm. B, sinus bradycardia. C, sinus tachycardia. (Reprinted with permission of Macmillan Publishing Co. Inc., from P-QRS-T: A Guide to Electrocardiographic Interpretation, 5th ed., copyright © by Joseph E. F. Riseman, 1968, p. 63.)

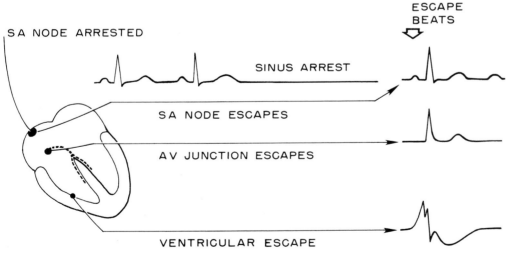

FIGURE 27-18 Escape beats. A period of cardiac asystole may result when the SA node fails to send impulses to the atria unless lower pacemakers or "escape" pacemakers take over to maintain the cardiac rhythm. If the first beat after the sinus arrest originates in the AV node, it is called a junctional escape beat. If the impulse after sinus arrest originates in the ventricles, it is called a ventricular escape beat. (Modified from Frank H. Netter, The Ciba Collection of Medical Illustrations, Vol. 5, The Heart, Ciba Pharmaceutical Company, Summit, N.J., 1969, p. 67.)

size by lowering stroke volume. However, in the absence of heart failure, this slight increment in oxygen demand is greatly outweighed by the reduced demand prompted by blockade of the sympathetic effects upon heart rate and contractility.

Digitalis can relieve angina associated with heart failure by increasing the force of contraction and, as a result, stroke volume. As ventricular emptying increases, ventricular size is reduced. Despite the increased oxygen demand associated with increased contractile force, the net effect of digitalization in heart failure is a reduction of myocardial oxygen demand.

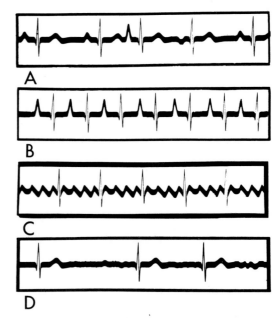

FIGURE 27-21 Atrial arrhythmias. A, atrial premature beats from different foci. B, atrial tachycardia with p superimposed on T. C, atrial flutter (4:1). D, atrial fibrillation. (Reprinted with permission of Macmillan Publishing Co., Inc., from P-QRS-T: A Guide to Electrocardiographic Interpretation, 5th ed., copyright © by Joseph E. F. Riseman, 1968, pp. 67, 71.)

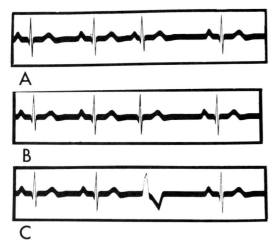

FIGURE 27-19 A, atrial premature beat. B, AV junctional premature beat with p hidden in the QRS. C, ventricular premature beat. (Reprinted with permission of Macmillan Publishing Co., Inc., from P-QRS-T: A Guide to Electrocardiographic Interpretation, 5th ed., copyright © by Joseph E. F. Riseman, 1968, pp. 69, 83.)

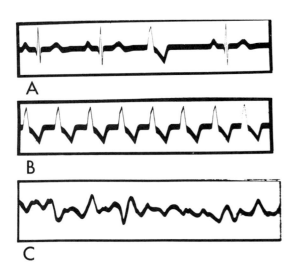

FIGURE 27-20 Ventricular arrhythmias. A, ventricular premature beat. B, ventricular tachycardia. C, ventricular fibrillation. (Reprinted with permission of Macmillan Publishing Co., Inc., from P-QRS-T: A Guide to Electrocardiographic Interpretation, 5th ed., copyright © by Joseph E. F. Riseman, 1968, pp. 69, 71, 99.)

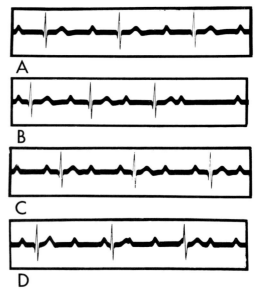

FIGURE 27-22 Heart block. A, first-degree heart block. B, second-degree heart block—Wenckebach or Mobitz I. C, second-degree heart block—Mobitz II. D, third-degree heart block or complete heart block. (Reprinted with permission of Macmillan Publishing Co., Inc., from P-QRS-T: A Guide to Electrocardiographic Interpretation, 5th ed., copyright © by Joseph E. F. Riseman, 1968, p. 81.)

Other pharmacologic interventions similarly act upon the determinants of myocardial oxygen demand to correct the oxygenation imbalance. Diuretics reduce blood volume and venous return to the heart, thereby reducing ventricular volume and size. Antihypertensive agents or vasodilators decrease arterial pressure and resistance to ventricular ejection. Consequently, afterload is diminished. Sedatives and antidepressants can also reduce angina induced by stress or depression.

The impaired ability of the diseased coronary vasculature to dilate and increase blood flow limits the available therapeutic measures to increase coronary oxygen supply. Although nitroglycerin is known to dilate the major epicardial branches of the coronary circulation, total coronary blood flow does not increase. However, nitroglycerin does improve flow to the ischemic area apparently by vasodilation of collateral vessels.

Two potential consequences of myocardial dysfunction that can further the reduction in myocardial oxygen supply are hypoxemia and hypotension. In the setting of hypoxemia, oxygen administration can increase the oxygen content of arterial blood and, consequently, myocardial oxygen delivery. Hypotension reduces coronary perfusion pressure. This is particularly worrisome because diseased coronary vessels, unable to dilate to increase flow, are "pressure-dependent" to maintain flow. A reduction in coronary perfusion pressure can perpetuate the ischemic imbalance. Therefore, vasopressors to maintain arterial pressure or volume administration to maintain adequate ventricular filling pressures and stroke volume may be indicated. Arrhythmias can also adversely affect coronary perfusion by reducing cardiac output and arterial pressure; therefore, antiarrhythmics may be beneficial.

The value of anticoagulants and fibrinolytic agents, such as urokinase, in the dissolution or prevention of coronary thrombi remains the subject of much controversy.

TABLE 27-3
Medical therapy of myocardial ischemia

1 Reduction of oxygen demand
   a Pharmacologic reduction in cardiac work
      (1) Nitroglycerin
      (2) Nitrites
      (3) Inderal
      (4) Digitalis
      (5) Diuretics
      (6) Antihypertensives
      (7) Sedatives
   b Physical reduction in cardiac work
      (1) Bed rest
      (2) Restful environment
2 Increment in oxygen supply
   a Nitroglycerin
   b Oxygen administration
   c Vasopressors
   d Antiarrhythmics
   e Anticoagulants and fibrinolytic agents

INFARCTION AND ITS COMPLICATIONS

After myocardial infarction, rest is the primary therapeutic principle. The objectives are to allow for healing of the infarcted tissue, thus reducing the incidence of complications, and to salvage the ischemic zone surrounding the infarct, thereby reducing the ultimate size of the infarct.

Early detection and prevention of complications is of utmost importance. Two categories of complications must be anticipated: electrical instability or arrhythmias and mechanical dysfunction or pump failure. Electrocardiographic monitoring is initiated immediately. Arrhythmia management follows logical principles:

1 Tachycardias are decelerated by parasympathetic stimulation (e.g., carotid sinus massage), antiarrhythmic drugs, or electrical cardioversion, if necessary. Bradycardias can be accelerated by drugs that either stimulate sympathetic beta receptors, such as Isuprel, or inhibit parasympathetic effects, such as atropine. Electrical pacing may be indicated if hemodynamic deterioration is pronounced and drugs are ineffective.
2 "Escape beats," which result from sinus node failure, must be differentiated from "premature beats," which are caused by tissue irritability, to effectively treat rhythm disturbances originating in sites other than the sinus node. To treat escape rhythms, drugs are administered to speed the normal pacemaker, the sinus node; obviously, drugs must not be given to suppress the escape pacemaker, since cardiac standstill could result.
   Ventricular irritability usually responds to antiarrhythmic agents, such as Xylocaine and Pronestyl. Ventricular fibrillation requires immediate defibrillation with cardiopulmonary resuscitation maneuvers. Atrial irritability is best controlled by administering an antiarrhythmic, such as quinidine, to suppress the irritability. Digoxin administration is required with atrial tachycardias to slow conduction through the AV node and control the ventricular rate response. This combination of drugs may convert the abnormal rhythm to normal. Electrical cardioversion may be indicated to restore the normal rhythm if the arrhythmia persists and is poorly tolerated.
3 Therapy of heart block is directed at restoring or simulating normal conduction, either through the administration of drugs speeding conduction and heart rate, such as atropine or Isuprel, or by electrical pacing.

Mechanical dysfunction produces a clinical spectrum ranging from mild congestive heart failure to cardiogenic shock. Congestive heart failure prompts efforts to (1) reduce intravascular volume and congestion, (2) reduce fluid transudation from the intravascular space into tissues and alveoli, and (3) improve myocardial function. Mild to moderate congestive heart failure is managed with restrictions of fluid and salt intake, diuretics, and digitalis. The development of pulmonary edema necessitates the addition of more aggressive measures. Morphine, in addition to its sedative and respiratory depressant effects, dilates the periphery with pooling of blood in the veins and reduction in venous return. Severe pulmonary edema may require phlebotomy, the withdrawal of 100 to 500 ml of blood, or the application of rotating tourniquets to reduce the volume overload. Aminophylline can be administered to relieve associated bronchospasm and, secondarily, to increase cardiac output by increasing contractile force. Administration of oxygen is required to correct hypoxemia. Positive pressure breathing devices are useful to increase intra-alveolar pressure, thus reducing fluid transudation across the pulmonary capillary membrane.

Progression of left ventricular dysfunction to cardiogenic shock, characterized by inadequate tissue perfusion, is an ominous development. This syndrome, with a mortality approaching 100 percent, remains a therapeutic dilemma. Efforts are directed at the maintenance of tissue perfusion and the simultaneous reduction of cardiac work. Vasopressors are frequently needed to maintain arterial pressure. However, some advocate the administration of vasodilators, such as nitroglycerin or sodium nitroprusside (Nipride) to reduce the resistance to ejection, thereby facilitating ventricular emptying. Peripheral vasodilators would also increase tissue perfusion. Steroids may be suggested to improve metabolic derangements at the cellular level. Metabolic acidosis, caused by lactic acid accumulation, must be reversed by the administration of sodium bicarbonate.

Circulatory assistance

Circulatory assistance was initially utilized to support patients in cardiogenic shock. It was hoped that circulatory assistance would interrupt the vicious cycle of cardiogenic shock by elevating arterial pressure, improving peripheral perfusion, and reducing cardiac work, thereby preserving ischemic, still salvageable zones of myocardium.

The intra-aortic balloon is positioned in the descending thoracic aorta just distal to the left subclavian artery. It is inserted via a femoral arteriotomy and threaded retrograde through the descending abdominal aorta (see Fig. 27-23). The balloon is inflated and deflated in synchrony with the mechanical events of the heart. Obviously, during left ventricular ejection or systole, the balloon must be deflated. During ventricular diastole, the balloon is inflated.

Inflation of the balloon with gas occurs just as the aortic valve closes at the end of systole; balloon inflation raises aortic volume, elevating aortic pressure. This

effect is referred to as *augmentation of diastolic pressure*. The physiologic effect of diastolic augmentation is twofold (see Fig. 27-24): (1) the perfusion pressure at the coronary orifices is increased during diastole, the period of greatest coronary flow, potentially increasing coronary flow; (2) systemic perfusion may also improve through elevation of mean arterial pressure.

Balloon deflation occurs rapidly, immediately prior to systole, just before the aortic valve opens. As gas is removed from the balloon, intra-aortic volume is lowered, and therefore aortic pressure is reduced. This reduction in aortic pressure lowers the resistance against which the left ventricle must eject blood. In other words, balloon deflation *reduces afterload*. The physiologic effects are (see Fig. 27-25): (1) reduction in cardiac work, (2) reduction in oxygen demand and myocardial oxygen consumption (MVO_2), and (3) increased cardiac output.

Balloon pumping is particularly effective in the reversal of cardiogenic shock resulting from mechanical defects, such as ventricular septal defect and mitral regurgitation. Initiation of balloon pumping in these patients reduces aortic pressure and resistance to ejection, thereby increasing forward flow through the aorta and reducing abnormal flow through the defect. Refractory cardiac ischemia is also responsive to balloon pumping: physiologically, the intra-aortic balloon pump can influence both the supply and demand determinants of the myocardial oxygenation balance. Potentially, coronary blood flow increases as myocardial oxygen demand falls as a result of the reduction in afterload.

Obviously, any invasive device carries a degree of risk; associated complications consist of infection, arterial trauma, and thromboembolism. Therefore, non-invasive circulatory assist devices are of interest. External

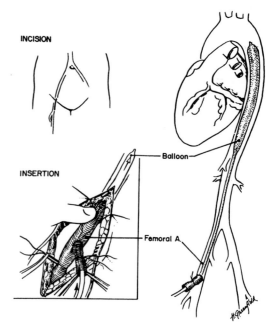

FIGURE 27-23 Insertion and location of the aortic balloon. (From P. J. Ford and R. W. Weintraub, Intra-Aortic Balloon Pumping, *Aristrocrat Press, Cambridge, 1974, p. IV-2.)*

circulatory assistance devices are also available. In one external counterpulsation device, the legs are enclosed in water-filled sleeves. Pressure exerted upon the extremities is varied in synchrony with the cardiac cycle. Pressure alterations result in blood displacement within the peripheral vasculature. During diastole, the sleeves exert a positive pressure, reducing the capacity of the peripheral vasculature; compressing the venous bed increases venous return and ventricular filling, while compression of the arterial bed elevates or augments arterial pressure. During systole, negative pressure is applied to the legs, increasing peripheral vascular capacity, displacing blood into the extremities, and thereby reducing aortic pressure and resistance to ejection (i.e., afterload). However, the reduction in afterload and cardiac work seems less significant than with invasive, intra-aortic balloon pumping.

Left heart assist devices are currently generating much interest as temporary circulatory assist devices. These units are attached to the left side of the heart, either the left atrium or the left ventricle, and to a major systemic artery to shunt blood away from the left ventricle and thereby reduce the volume of blood that the heart must eject. These devices function as auxiliary pumps relieving cardiac work.

Surgical therapy

REVASCULARIZATION

The aim of revascularization is to increase the blood flow and oxygen supply to ischemic regions beyond an obstructive coronary arterial lesion. Two techniques are currently utilized: saphenous vein bypass graft and internal mammary artery bypass graft.

The technique of saphenous vein bypass grafting involves anastomosing a reversed segment of the saphenous vein to the ascending aorta and to the coronary artery beyond the area of obstruction (see Fig. 27-26). Thus, a vascular conduit is created to shunt blood around the lesion to the ischemic myocardium. Internal mammary artery grafting requires anastomosis of the distal segment of the internal mammary artery to the coronary artery.

Vein bypass grafting is the more common procedure. However, a small proportion of these grafts gradually occlude as a result of a fibrous overgrowth of the intimal wall of the vein. It is postulated that this process of "subintimal fibrous hyperplasia" might be the result of subjecting a vein to arterial pressures. Although the internal mammary artery does not seem vulnerable to the same incidence of occlusion, certain disadvantages are associated with this procedure relative to vein bypass grafts: (1) the anterior anatomic location of the internal mammary artery limits its application to lesions of the left anterior descending artery and proximal lesions of other vessels; (2) the diameter of the vessel is smaller, limiting blood flow; (3) arterial responsiveness to sympathetic stimulation may produce graft vasoconstriction and reduced flow during periods of increased sympathetic tone.

The indications for revascularization are not standardized nor is the precise impact of surgical intervention upon the natural history of coronary artery disease known. However, the following indications seem to

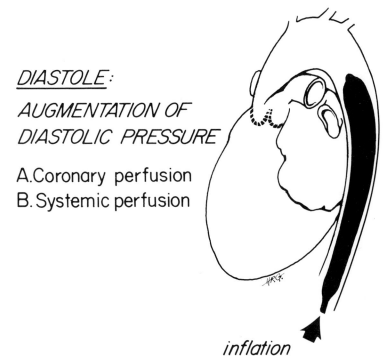

DIASTOLE:

AUGMENTATION OF

DIASTOLIC PRESSURE

A. Coronary perfusion

B. Systemic perfusion

inflation

FIGURE 27-24 *Effect of intra-aortic balloon inflation.*

warrant surgical intervention: (1) disabling angina refractory to medical therapy, (2) unstable or preinfarction angina (i.e., recurrent angina at rest despite maximal medical therapy), (3) ongoing ischemia after myocardial infarction, and (4) lesions threatening major portions of the myocardial wall (i.e., main left coronary artery lesions). Early revascularization after myocardial infarction to salvage the ischemic zone surrounding the infarct is the subject of speculation, as is the value of surgery in cardiogenic shock. It must be emphasized that revascularization cannot reverse necrosis; only ischemic areas of myocardium benefit from the increased blood flow and oxygen supply.

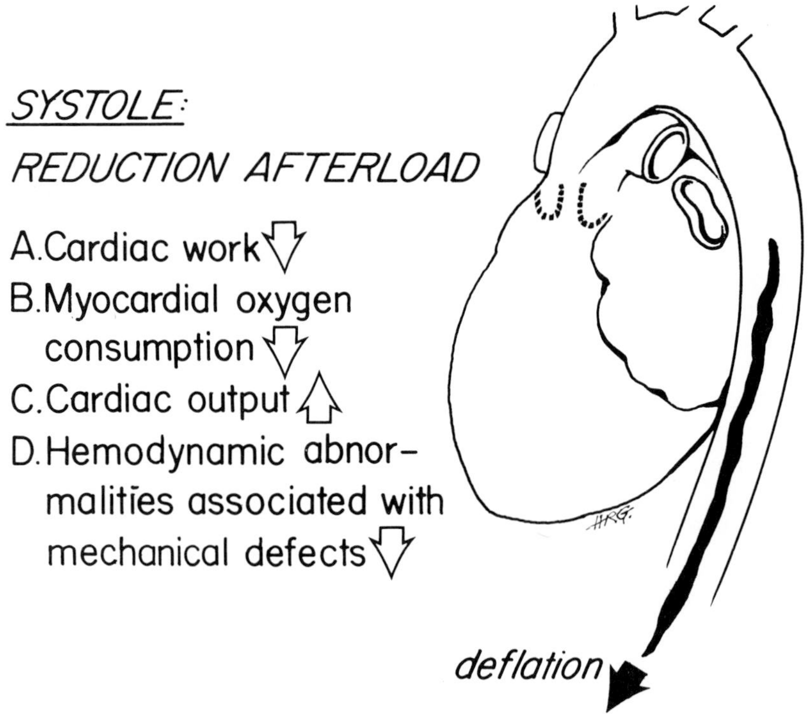

SYSTOLE:
REDUCTION AFTERLOAD

A. Cardiac work ⬇
B. Myocardial oxygen consumption ⬇
C. Cardiac output ⬆
D. Hemodynamic abnormalities associated with mechanical defects ⬇

deflation

FIGURE 27-25 Effect of intra-aortic balloon deflation.

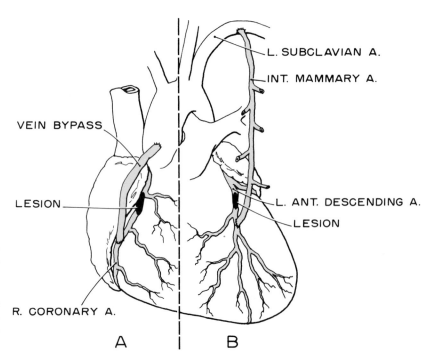

FIGURE 27-26 Coronary artery revascularization procedures. A, saphenous vein bypass graft. The vein is sutured to the ascending aorta and to the right coronary artery at a point distal to the blockage so that flow distal to the blockage is again established. B, in the mammary artery procedure, the mammary artery is shown anastomosed to the anterior descending branch of the left coronary artery bypassing the lesion.

Prior to revascularization, cardiac catheterization is necessary to determine the location and extent of disease. The following findings characterize operable disease: (1) a bypassable lesion (i.e., located proximally in the artery), (2) a significant or "high-grade" lesion (i.e., obstructing over 75 percent of the vessel lumen), and (3) a patent distal vessel, which ensures a site beyond the lesion to anastomose the graft. Revascularization is performed in some patients with endartarectomy of the distal bed if diffuse distal disease is noted. Endartarectomy is the removal of the inner atherosclerotic core of the vascular lumen.

At the time of catheterization, the function of the left ventricle is also assessed. The success of surgery seems to correlate most directly with two factors: the degree of left ventricular dysfunction and the magnitude of flow achieved through the bypass graft.

ANEURYSMECTOMY

Aneurysmectomy is the removal of the noncontractile, paradoxically bulging scar. There are three indications for aneurysm resection: (1) chronic congestive heart failure, (2) systemic embolization of mural thrombi, and (3) recurrent ventricular arrhythmias. Aneurysms are associated with a high incidence of malignant, refractory ventricular arrhythmias, perhaps resulting from the persistent mechanical strain at the boundary between the normal myocardium and the scarred, outpouching segment. The aneurysm is excised through the left ventricular scar with removal of mural thrombi. Removal of the aneurysm and subsequent reduction of ventricular size improves the mechanical efficiency of the heart.

VENTRICULAR SEPTAL DEFECT REPAIR

A ventricular septal defect can be repaired either by simple closure of the hole in the septum or by insertion of a patch graft; access to the septum is gained via the infarct in the ventricle. Upon closure of the left ventricular incision, a portion of the noncontractile left ventricular scar is frequently excised, a procedure referred to as *infarctectomy.*

MITRAL VALVE REPLACEMENT

Dysfunction of the mitral valve resulting from papillary muscle rupture or malfunction necessitates replacement of the mitral valve with excision of the papillary muscles.

TRANSPLANTATION

Cardiac transplantation can be lifesaving for patients considered inoperable or unsalvageable with less aggressive surgical intervention. Patients with end-stage heart disease are considered for cardiac transplantation. The operation involves removal of the diseased heart and replacement with a normal donor heart. Technically, the operation is uncomplicated, requiring reanastomoses of the separated vessels with the donor heart. Currently, the major obstacle to cardiac transplantation is immunologic—the rejection of the donor tissue by the recipient's defense mechanisms. Therapeutic suppression of the immunologic system to facilitate acceptance of the donor heart increases vulnerability to overwhelming sepsis.

REHABILITATION

The ultimate goal of therapeutic intervention in coronary atherosclerotic disease is to restore the cardiac patient to a productive, satisfying existence. The potential long-term consequences of myocardial infarction—physical or psychological invalidism—have long been ignored with devastating impact. The complications of myocardial disease are not restricted to the in-hospital patient setting, nor does the responsibility of health professionals for the ultimate well-being and coping ability of patients terminate upon discharge from the hospital.

Patients must be assisted to progressively resume a level of activity consistent with physical limitations and unhampered by psychological distress. Many patients can resume all normal activities. Explicit, individualized instruction in diet, medication, activity progression, and control of risk factors is mandatory. Every patient and family needs guidance and education during the transition from the dependence of illness to the independence of health.

QUESTIONS

Coronary atherosclerotic disease—Chap. 27

Directions: Answer the following questions on a separate sheet of paper.

1 Explain why the left ventricle is most vulnerable to ischemia and infarction.

2 What are the most common sites of coronary arterial occlusion?

3 Name five factors affecting the degree of functional impairment following an acute myocardial infarction.

4 What is a vasovagal response and what might cause this response following an acute myocardial infarction? How does it affect the compensatory response?

5 Name three important diagnostic findings associated with myocardial infarction.

6 Explain hemodynamically why either tachycardias or bradycardias impair cardiac function.

7 Identify three hemodynamic factors which may be modified to reduce oxygen demand in the treatment of myocardial ischemia.

8 Explain why medical efforts to treat myocardial ischemia by increasing coronary blood flow and oxygen supply are of little value.

9 State the primary objective of rest in the treatment of acute myocardial infarction.

10 Describe the treatment of congestive heart failure, pulmonary edema, and cardiogenic shock.

11 Briefly describe three circulatory assist devices for mechanical dysfunction of the heart.

12 Why is rehabilitation an important aspect of the treatment of patients with atherosclerotic heart disease?

Directions: Circle the letter preceding each item that correctly answers each question. Only one answer is correct unless otherwise noted.

13 The most potent stimulus to increasing coronary blood flow is:
a Systemic lactic acidosis *b* Local myocardial hypoxia *c* Sympathetic stimulation *d* Increased arterial pressure

14 In the normal heart, coronary blood flow can increase _____ times above resting levels.
a 1 to 2 *b* 4 to 5 *c* 8 to 10 *d* 15 to 20

15 The earliest pathologic change apparent in the coronary blood vessel in the development of coronary atherosclerosis is:
a Fibrous encapsulation of the lesion *b* Fatty streaks in the adventitia *c* Fatty streaks in the intima *d* Accumulation of β-lipoprotein in the media

16 Myocardial infarction may result from: (More than one answer may be correct)
a Hemorrhage into the coronary atheromatous plaque *b* Platelet aggregates in the coronary blood vessel *c* Coronary artery spasm *d* Embolization of a thrombus or plaque fragment

17 Major modifiable risk factors for coronary atherosclerotic disease include all of the following *except:*
a Hyperlipidemia *b* Hypertension
c Family history *d* Cigarette smoking

18 Optimal serum cholesterol levels should be no greater than _____ to reduce the risk of coronary atherosclerotic disease:
a 150 mg% *b* 200 mg% *c* 250 mg% *d* 300 mg%

19 A form of angina in which there is S-T segment elevation is:
a Preinfarction angina *b* Prinzmetal's angina
c Dressler's angina *d* Unstable angina

20 Which of the following changes does *not* commonly occur before or during an attack of angina pectoris?
a An increase in blood pressure *b* A decrease in heart rate *c* An increase in myocardial oxygen demand *d* An increase in left ventricular end-diastolic pressure *e* A decrease in myocardial wall compliance

21 Depressed left ventricular function resulting from an area of ischemia or necrosis always necessitates:
a An increase in end-diastolic volume to maintain stroke volume *b* A decrease in end-diastolic volume to maintain stroke volume *c* An increase in heart rate to maintain cardiac output *d* An increase in blood pressure to maintain tissue perfusion

22 Complete occlusion of the left anterior descending coronary artery would result in:
a Anterior wall infarct *b* Inferior wall infarct
c Complete heart block *d* Posterior wall infarct

23 Which of the following functional changes would be least expected in patients with acute myocardial infarction?
a A decrease in cardiac output *b* A decrease in left end-diastolic pressure *c* An increase in pulmonary wedge pressure *d* An increase in the central venous pressure

24 Impending left heart failure following myocardial infarction can be detected earliest by monitoring the:
a Systemic blood pressure *b* Central venous pressure *c* Pulmonary wedge pressure *d* Pulse pressure

25 The earliest stage of lung involvement in left heart failure is:
a Interstitial edema *b* Alveolar edema
c Pleural effusion *d* Pulmonary congestion

26 In patients who develop cardiogenic shock, the percentage of left ventricular mass which is infarcted is generally at least:
a 10 percent *b* 20 percent *c* 40 percent
d 60 percent

27 Characteristic hemodynamic abnormalities in cardiogenic shock include: (More than one answer may be correct)
a Decreased peripheral perfusion *b* Decreased coronary perfusion *c* Hypotension *d* Decreased cardiac output

28 Left ventricular papillary muscle rupture following myocardial infarction results in: (More than one answer may be correct)
a Mitral regurgitation *b* A systolic murmur *c* A diastolic murmur *d* Death in a high percentage of cases *e* Pulmonary congestion

29 Which of the following statements regarding ventricular rupture is *not* correct?
a The peak incidence is during the healing phase of necrotic tissue removal. *b* Rupture is a complication of transmural myocardial infarction. *c* The peak incidence is about 6 weeks following infarction. *d* Rupture is associated with cardiac tamponade.

30 The major effect of cardiac tamponade is to:

a Produce atelectasis   *b* Distend the pericardium
c Compress the heart   *d* Increase the pulse pressure

31 The myocardial scar following myocardial infarction is well established after approximately:
a 3 weeks   *b* 6 weeks   *c* 3 months   *d* 6 months

32 A ventricular aneurysm may give rise to:
a Chronic congestive heart failure   *b* Systemic emboli   *c* Refractory ventricular arrhythmias   *d* All of the above

33 The most frequent complication following myocardial infarction is:
a Congestive heart failure   *b* Cardiogenic shock
c Left ventricular papillary muscle dysfunction
d Dressler's syndrome   *e* Arrhythmias

34 Factors predisposing to the development of arrhythmias in coronary atherosclerotic disease are: (More than one answer may be correct)
a Myocardial ischemia   *b* Lactic acidosis
c Hypokalemia   *d* Digitalis toxicity

35 An ectopic beat may originate in all of the following sites *except:*
a Atria   *b* Ventricles   *c* AV junctional tissue
d SA node

36 Which of the following is the most common arrhythmia associated with myocardial infarction?
a Atrial tachycardia   *b* Atrial fibrillation.
c Ventricular premature beats   *d* Ventricular fibrillation   *e* Left bundle branch block

37 Left bundle branch block results in:
a Absence of all P waves   *b* Absence of every other P wave   *c* Prolongation of the P-R interval   *d* Widening of the QRS complex

38 Which of the following drugs used for the treatment of myocardial ischemia improve cardiac function by decreasing arterial resistance to ventricular ejection? (More than one answer may be correct)
a Inderal   *b* Digitalis   *c* Diuretics
d Vasodilators   *e* Nitroglycerin

39 Which sign or symptom would occur latest in the course of left heart failure?
a Orthopnea   *b* Lung congestion
c Decreased urine output   *d* Distended neck veins

40 Factors which result from and compound the problem of myocardial ischemia include: (More than one answer may be correct)
a Hypoxemia   *b* Hypotension   *c* Arrhythmias
d Acidosis

41 Which of the following statements concerning atherosclerotic heart disease is *not* true?
a Lesion precursors may be found in children and young adults.   *b* The disease begins abruptly in susceptible middle-aged adults.   *c* It is the leading cause of death in the United States.   *d* Hypertension, hyperlipidemia, and smoking are major predisposing factors

42 The arrhythmia with the least effective ventricular action is:
a Atrial flutter   *b* Ventricular tachycardia
c Ventricular fibrillation   *d* Complete heart block

43 Which of the following ECG monitor strip tracings is typical of second-degree heart block?
a P waves without a QRS complex   *b* P-R interval longer than 0.2 seconds   *c* Widening of the QRS complex   *d* Inversion of the T wave

44 Pacemakers are *not* used to:
a Suppress ventricular ectopic beats   *b* Suppress sinus tachycardia   *c* Treat third-degree heart block
d Treat sinus bradycardia

45 During intra-aortic balloon pumping, the balloon is: (More than one answer may be correct)
a Deflated during left ventricular systole   *b* Inflated during left ventricular systole   *c* Inflated during left ventricular diastole   *d* Deflated during left ventricular diastole

46 Physiologic effects of intra-aortic balloon pumping include all of the following *except:*
a Decreased myocardial oxygen demand
b Increased cardiac output   *c* Decreased cardiac work   *d* Increased afterload

47 Coronary bypass surgery is generally indicated for patients with:
a Preinfarction angina   *b* Cardiogenic shock
c Stable angina pectoris   *d* Acute myocardial infarction   *e* Ventricular aneurysm

48 The removal of an atherosclerotic plaque in coronary atherosclerotic disease is called:
a Infarctectomy   *b* Endarterectomy
c Septal defect repair   *d* Aneurysmectomy

Directions: Circle T if the statement is true and F if it is false. Correct the false statements.

49   T   F   Atherosclerotic heart disease is more common in diabetics than in nondiabetics.

50   T   F   In postmyocardial infarction syndrome (Dressler's syndrome), the pain is characteristic of pericarditis rather than of infarction.

51   T   F   An internal mammary artery bypass graft is associated with a significant incidence of subintimal fibrous hyperplasia.

52   T   F   Ventricular hypertrophy decreases myocardial oxygen demand.

53   T   F   Escape beats are caused by myocardial tissue irritability.

Directions: Fill in the blanks with the correct word or circle the correct word.

54 In myocardial infarction, an area of _____ surrounds the area of infarction.

55 A reduction in ventricular wall compliance (increases) (decreases) pressure for a constant ventricular volume.

56 Arrange in correct order the following changes that occur after an acute myocardial infarction.
a Removal of nectoric tissue   *b* Bruised and cyanotic tissue   *c* Scar formation   *d* Polymorphonuclear neutrophil infiltration

Directions: Match the characteristics in col. A with the disorders in col. B.

Column A	Column B
57 _____ S-T segment depression is typical	*a* Myocardial ischemia
58 _____ S-T segment elevation is typical	*b* Myocardial infarction
59 _____ Deep Q waves	
60 _____ Pain relieved by nitroglycerin	
61 _____ Muscle death	
62 _____ Muscle hypoxia	
63 _____ If prolonged, results in necrosis	
64 _____ Reversible	
65 _____ Irreversible	

Directions: Match the type of heart block in col. A with the ECG pattern in col. B.

Column A	Column B
66 _____ First-degree heart block	*a* No impulses conducted
67 _____ Wenckebach or Mobitz I	*b* All impulses conducted with prolonged P-R interval
68 _____ Mobitz II	*c* Some impulses nonconducted in repetitive pattern with progressive prolongation of the P-R interval
69 _____ Complete heart block	*d* Some impulses nonconducted but conducted impulses have a constant P-R interval

Directions: Match each of the arrhythmias in col. A to its possible therapeutic intervention in col. B.

Column A	Column B
70 _____ Sinus bradycardia	*a* Carotid sinus massage
71 _____ Atrial tachycardia	*b* Defibrillation
72 _____ Multiple premature ventricular beats	*c* Xylocaine
73 _____ Ventricular fibrillation	*d* Atropine

Directions: Match each of the drugs used to treat coronary atherosclerotic disease in col. A with its effect in col. B.

Column A	Column B
74 _____ Inderal	*a* Suppression of ventricular irritibility
75 _____ Xylocaine	*b* Increased heart rate
76 _____ Atropine	*c* Decreased heart rate and force of contraction
77 _____ Nitroglycerin	*d* Increased force of myocardial contraction
78 _____ Digitalis	*e* Vasodilation of coronary collaterals and peripheral vessels

BIBLIOGRAPHY

ANDREOLI, KATHLEEN, VIRGINIA FOWKES, DOUGLAS ZIPES, and ANDREW WALLACE: *Comprehensive Cardiac Care*, Mosby, St. Louis, 1975.

BRAUNWALD, EUGENE (ed.): *The Myocardium: Failure and Infarction*, HP Publishing, New York, 1974.

GRIFFITH, GEORGE C.: "The Life Cycle of Coronary Artery Disease," *Heart and Lung*, **1**: 63–67, January-February, 1972.

HURST, J. WILLIS (ed.): *The Heart*, McGraw-Hill, New York, 1974.

NORMAN, JOHN C. (ed.): *Cardiac Surgery*, Appleton-Century-Crofts, New York, 1972.

ROSENMAN, RAY H.: "Observations on the Pathogenesis of Coronary Heart Disease," *Heart and Lung*, **1**: 68–73, January-February, 1972.

RUSSEK, HENRY and BURTON ZOHMAN: *Coronary Heart Disease*, Lippincott, Philadelphia, 1971.

SODEMAN, WILLIAM A., and WILLIAM A. SODEMAN JR.: *Pathologic Physiology: Mechanisms of Disease*, Saunders, Philadelphia, 1974.

SONNENBLICK, EDMUND H., and C. LYNN SKELTON: "Oxygen Consumption of the Heart: Physiological Principles and Clinical Implications," *Modern Concepts of Cardiovascular Disease*, **XL**: 9–15, March, 1971.

WEISS, IRA: *Essentials of Heart Rhythm Analysis*. Davis, Philadelphia, 1973.

WHIPPLE, GERALD, MARY ANN PETERSON, VIRGINIA HAINES, EDWARD LEARNER, and ELIZABETH MACKINNON: *Acute Coronary Care*, Little, Brown, Boston, 1972.

CHAPTER 28 Valvular Heart Disease

OBJECTIVES **At the completion of Chap. 28 you should be able to:**

1 Identify the characteristics of normal valvular function, including the mechanism of opening and closure.

2 Describe the functional effects of valvular stenosis and regurgitation.

3 Identify and briefly describe five causes of valvular heart disease.

4 Compare the frequency of lesions for the four heart valves.

5 Describe the pathogenesis of valvular damage in rheumatic fever.

6 Describe the morphologic changes in valvular stenosis and regurgitation.

7 Define functional regurgitation.

8 Describe the pathophysiology of the following valvular disorders: mitral stenosis and regurgitation, aortic stenosis and regurgitation, tricuspid stenosis and regurgitation.

9 Indicate and contrast the auscultatory, electrocardiographic, roentgenographic, and cardiac catheterization findings for the valvular disorders listed in objective 8.

10 Describe the etiology and functional disturbances in pulmonic valvular disease.

11 Predict and give examples of functional alterations resulting from compound valvular lesions.

12 Describe the preventive therapy for rheumatic fever and bacterial endocarditis.

13 Describe the medical therapy for mitral valve disease.

14 Define mitral commissurotomy.

15 Describe the indications, contraindications, and surgical procedure for a mitral commissurotomy and a mitral valve replacement.

16 Explain how a ball and cage prosthetic heart valve operates.

17 Explain why prompt surgical intervention is important after the onset of symptoms in the treatment of aortic stenosis.

18 Indicate the surgical treatment of aortic stenosis and regurgitation.

19 Describe the operation of a heart-lung machine (cardiopulmonary bypass).

Valvular disease causes abnormalities in blood flow across the cardiac valves. Normal valves demonstrate two critical flow characteristics: unidirectional flow and unimpeded flow. The valves open when the pressure in the chamber proximal to the valve exceeds the pressure in the chamber or vessel beyond the valve. Closure occurs when the pressure beyond the valve exceeds pressure in the proximal chamber. For instance, the atrioventricular valves open when atrial pressures exceed ventricular pressures and close when ventricular pressures exceed atrial pressures. The valve leaflets are so responsive that even a slight pressure difference (less than 1 mmHg) between chambers will open and close the leaflets.

A diseased valve can produce two types of functional derangements: (1) *valvular regurgitation*—the valve leaflets fail to close securely, permitting backward flow ("valvular insufficiency" and "valvular incompetence" are synonymous terms); and (2) *valvular stenosis*—the valve orifice becomes restricted, impeding forward flow. Regurgitation and stenosis can occur together in the same valve as a "mixed lesion," or either one can occur alone as a "pure lesion."

Valvular dysfunction increases cardiac work. Valvular regurgitation forces the heart to pump the additional regurgitant volume of blood, thus producing an increment in "volume work." Valvular stenosis necessitates the generation of increased pressure to overcome the increased resistance to flow, thereby elevating "pressure work." The characteristic myocardial responses to volume work and pressure work are, respectively, chamber dilation and muscular hypertrophy. Myocardial dilation and hypertrophy are compensatory mechanisms intended to increase the pumping capability of the heart.

PATHOGENESIS

Etiology

Valvular heart disease was once considered to be almost entirely rheumatic in origin. Despite the declining incidence of rheumatic fever, rheumatic damage is still the most common cause of valvular deformity. However, other causes of valvular deformity and malfunction are being recognized with increasing frequency. Other significant causes of valvular heart disease are (1) valve destruction by bacterial endocarditis, (2) dysfunction or rupture of the papillary muscles as a result of coronary atherosclerosis, (3) congenital malformations, and (4) inborn defects of connective tissue.

The incidence of valvular disease is highest in the mitral valve, followed by the aortic valve. The predominance of left-sided valvular disease is attributed to the relatively greater hemodynamic trauma experienced by these valves. It is postulated that hemodynamic stress increases the degree of acquired valvular deformity. The incidence of tricuspid disease is relatively low. Pulmonic disease is rare. Disease of the tricuspid or pulmonic valves is usually associated with other valvular lesions, whereas aortic or mitral disease is frequently seen as an isolated lesion.

Certain valvular lesions strongly suggest the underlying cause of dysfunction. Isolated mitral stenosis is usually rheumatic in origin, whereas isolated aortic stenosis usually results from progressive calcification of a congenital bicuspid valve. Isolated tricuspid or pulmonic disease is almost invariably a congenital defect. Combined valvular lesions suggest rheumatic causation.

Pathology

The pathologic changes associated with rheumatic valvular damage are the product of the acute inflammatory insult, the subsequent healing with scar formation, and progressive deformity with aging. Acute rheumatic fever is a systemic inflammatory disease potentially involving all layers of the heart. Endocardial inflammation can afflict the valvular tissue, causing leaflet swelling and erosion of the cusp edges. Beadlike fibrous elevations or vegetations are deposited along the leaflet borders (see Fig. 28-1). Characteristic nodular lesions, called Aschoff's bodies, appear in the cardiac walls. Aschoff's bodies provide histologic evidence of active rheumatic carditis.

Initial attacks of rheumatic fever usually subside with little residual damage. Recurrent attacks produce the characteristic valvular lesions. Valvular stenosis is characterized by cusp thickening and leaflet fusion along the commissures (the juncture between leaflets); the chordae tendinae of the AV valves thicken and fuse (see Fig. 28-2). These changes narrow the valvular orifice and reduce leaflet motion, thus producing an obstruction to forward blood flow.

The lesion associated with valvular regurgitation consists of shrunken, retracted cusps that inhibit cusp contact and shortened, fused chordae tendinae that restrain the AV leaflets (see Fig. 28-3). These changes impair valve closure, thereby permitting backward flow through the valve.

Calcification and sclerosis of valvular tissue with aging contribute to the ultimate deformity in valves with rheumatic or congenital malformation. Chronic disease with ventricular failure and enlargement can disrupt the function of the AV valves. As the ventricular shape alters, the ability of the papillary muscles to approximate the

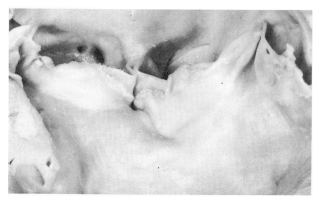

FIGURE 28-1 Acute rheumatic endocarditis of the aortic valve. The vegetations form a beadlike row of deposits which tends to conform to the line of closure. (From J. W. Hurst, The Heart, *3d ed., McGraw-Hill, New York, 1974, p. 795.)*

valvular leaflets during valve closure is reduced. In addition, the valve orifice can enlarge. Valvular regurgitation can result. Regurgitation occurring secondary to chamber enlargement is known as *functional regurgitation*.

PATHOPHYSIOLOGY

Mitral stenosis

Mitral stenosis impedes blood flow from the left atrium to the left ventricle during ventricular diastole (see Fig. 28-4). To adequately fill the ventricle and maintain cardiac output, the left atrium must generate more pressure to propel blood beyond the valvular obstruction. Therefore the pressure difference, or pressure gradient, between the chambers rises; normally the pressure gradient is minimal.

The left atrial musculature hypertrophies to increase its pumping force. The active contribution of atrial contraction to ventricular filling becomes increasingly important. The primary function of the left atrium ceases to be that of a passive reservoir and conduit for blood flowing to the ventricle. Atrial dilation occurs as the left atrial volume rises owing to the inability of the chamber to empty normally.

The rise in left atrial pressure and volume is reflected backward into the pulmonary vasculature; pressure in the pulmonary veins and capillaries rises. A spectrum of pulmonary congestion, ranging from mild venous congestion to interstitial edema with occasional fluid transudation into the alveoli, results.

Pulmonary arterial pressure must rise in response to

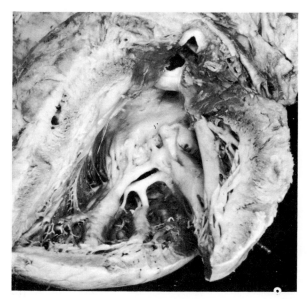

FIGURE 28-2 *Mitral valve from below in a case of mitral stenosis. The valve is converted into a funnel-shaped structure, the apex of which is in the left ventricle. (From J. W. Hurst,* The Heart, *3d ed., McGraw-Hill, New York, 1974, p. 798.)*

the elevated pulmonary venous resistance. This response ensures an adequate pressure gradient for blood flow through the pulmonary vasculature. However, pulmonary hypertension increases the resistance to right ventricular ejection into the pulmonary artery. The right ventricle responds to this increased pressure work with muscular hypertrophy.

Gradually, the pulmonary vasculature undergoes anatomic changes apparently designed to protect the pulmonary capillaries from excessively high right ventricular pressures and pulmonary flow. The mechanism mediating this anatomic response is unclear. Structural changes—medial hypertrophy and intimal thickening—occur in the walls of the small arteries and arterioles. These changes narrow the vessel lumen, elevating pulmonary vascular resistance. Pulmonary pressures can progressively climb to systemic levels.

The right ventricle is ill-suited to perform as a high-pressure pump over long periods of time. Therefore the right ventricle eventually fails as a pump. Right ventricular failure is reflected backward into the systemic circulation, producing systemic venous congestion and peripheral edema. The right-sided failure can be compounded by functional regurgitation of the tricuspid valve as a result of right ventricular enlargement.

Over a period of years the lesion of mitral stenosis narrows the valve orifice. Symptoms characteristically do not appear until the valve orifice has been reduced by approximately 50 percent, from normal dimensions of 4 to 6 cm² to 2 to 3 cm². A diastolic heart murmur, indicative of abnormal flow through the restricted orifice, is usually noted much earlier in the course of the disease.

The earliest symptom is usually dyspnea on exertion. Two hemodynamic changes associated with exertion are poorly tolerated in mitral stenosis: (1) tachycardia (rapid heart rate) and (2) elevated left atrial pressure. Tachycardia reduces the duration of diastole, the period of ventricular filling from the atria. The duration of diastole is critically important in mitral stenosis because the lesion itself impairs ventricular filling and, consequently, atrial emptying. Therefore, cardiac output is essentially "fixed," or unable to be increased because of the valvular obstruction to blood flow into the ventricle. As ventricular filling time falls with tachycardia, cardiac output is reduced further, and pulmonary congestion increases. The elevation of left atrial pressure with exertion further compounds the pulmonary congestion; since forward flow is restricted, the pressure elevation is transmitted backward to the lungs. Thus, dyspnea upon exertion is the result of pulmonary congestion. Weakness and fatigue are also prominent early symptoms as a result of the fixed, and eventually reduced, cardiac output.

As the disease progresses, respiratory symptoms become more pronounced. Susceptibility to pulmonary infection is high. Orthopnea and paroxysmal nocturnal dyspnea at rest may be noted. Transmission of the elevated pulmonary vascular pressures to the bronchial capillaries may result in capillary rupture and mild hemoptysis. Eventually, the lungs become fibrotic and noncompliant. The distribution of blood flow within the lungs shifts. Normally, there is relatively greater perfusion of the lower lobes than of the upper lobes because of the effect of gravity upon blood flow. In mitral stenosis, flow predominates in the upper lobes, presumably as a result of greater pulmonary vascular disease and interstitial edema in the lower lobes.

Atrial fibrillation frequently develops as a result of chronic atrial hypertrophy and dilation. With the onset of atrial fibrillation, severe exacerbation of symptoms can occur. The quivering atrial musculature is incapable of coordinated muscular contraction. This loss of the active "atrial kick" reduces ventricular filling. Ventricular filling is further reduced by the rapid ventricular response to atrial fibrillation (heart rates approximate 150 bpm unless treated). The abrupt onset of rapid atrial fibrillation can result in low cardiac output and pulmonary edema. Hemodynamic adaptation occurs, usually with pharmacologic assistance (i.e., digoxin). However, the stasis of blood in the left atrium predisposes to thrombus formation with the threat of systemic embolization.

End-stage mitral stenosis is associated with right heart failure with consequent systemic venous engorgement, peripheral edema, and ascites. However, mitral stenosis need not progress to this extreme. With the onset of symptoms, the disease can be managed medically, with eventual surgical correction.

The following findings are commonly noted in mitral stenosis: (1) *auscultation:* diastolic murmur and accentuated first heart sound (AV valve closure) and opening snap resulting from the loss of leaflet pliability. (2) *electrocardiogram:* left atrial enlargement (prolonged and notched P-wave, known as "P mitrale"), right

ventricular hypertrophy, and atrial fibrillation; (3) *chest x-ray:* left atrial enlargement, pulmonary venous congestion, interstitial pulmonary edema, and vascular redistribution to upper lobes; (4) *cardiac catheterization:* elevated pressure gradient across the mitral valve; elevated left atrial pressure, pulmonary capillary wedge pressure, and pulmonary arterial pressure; and low cardiac output.

Mitral regurgitation

Mitral regurgitation permits retrograde blood flow from the left ventricle to the left atrium as a result of incomplete valve closure (see Fig. 28-5). During systole, the ventricle simultaneously ejects blood forward into the aorta and backward into the left atrium. The work of both the left ventricle and the left atrium must increase to preserve cardiac output.

The left ventricle must pump a sufficient volume of blood to maintain a normal forward flow into the aorta and the regurgitant flow through the mitral valve. For instance, the normal ventricular output per beat ("stroke volume") is 70 ml. If the regurgitant flow is 30 ml per beat, the ventricle must pump 100 ml per beat to maintain a normal stroke volume. The additional volume load created by the regurgitant valve prompts ventricular dilation. According to Starling's law of the heart, ventricular dilation increases myocardial contractility. Eventually, the ventricular wall hypertrophies to further increase contractile force.

In the early stages of mitral regurgitation, the wall compliance or distensibility of the dilated left ventricle is increased. Increased wall compliance affects the relationship between ventricular volume and pressure (wall compliance = volume/pressure), enabling the ventricle to accommodate increased diastolic volumes without abnormal elevations in pressure. However, when the left ventricle begins to fail, left ventricular diastolic pressure rises, reflecting inadequate ventricular emptying.

Regurgitation creates a volume load not only for the left ventricle but also for the left atrium. The left atrium dilates to accommodate the increased volume and to increase the force of atrial contraction. Subsequently, the atrium hypertrophies to further increase atrial con-

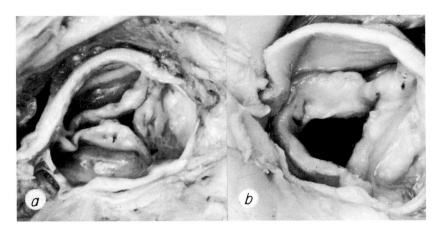

FIGURE 28-3 Two examples of rheumatic endocarditis with aortic insufficiency. A, the valve leaflets are thickened and shortened to a relatively minor degree. The shortening creates a small triangular-shaped orifice in the center of the aortic valve, persisting during diastole. B, the aortic valve leaflets are significantly reduced in size, producing a wide triangular-shaped orifice. (From J. W. Hurst, The Heart, 3d ed., McGraw-Hill, New York, 1974, p. 803.)

tractile force and output. Initially, increased left atrial compliance permits accommodation of increased volume without significant pressure elevation. Thus, for a while, the left atrium buffers the effect of the regurgitant volume, protecting the pulmonary vasculature.

However, mitral regurgitation is a self-perpetuating lesion. As ventricular volumes and dimensions increase, valve function worsens. Chamber enlargement increases the degree of regurgitation by displacement of the papillary muscles and dilation of the mitral orifice reducing leaflet contact during valve closure.

As the lesion worsens, the ability of the left atrium to distend and protect the lungs is exceeded. Left ventricular failure is usually the prelude to accelerated cardiac decompensation. The left ventricle becomes overburdened, and forward flow through the aorta falls, with a simultaneous rise in backward congestion. Gradually, the predictable sequence of pulmonary and right heart involvement ensues: (1) pulmonary venous congestion, (2) interstitial edema, (3) pulmonary arterial hyperten-

sion, and (4) right ventricular hypertrophy. Mitral regurgitation can culminate in right heart failure, although less frequently than does mitral stenosis.

The course of the disease is profoundly altered if the onset of mitral regurgitation is acute, as in papillary muscle rupture, rather than chronic. Acute mitral regurgitation is poorly tolerated. Normally, the left atrium is relatively noncompliant and therefore unable to abruptly distend and accommodate the regurgitant volume (see Fig. 28-6). Thus the sudden increase in volume and pressure is transmitted directly to the pulmonary vasculature. Within hours, fulminating pulmonary edema and shock can develop.

The earliest symptoms of mitral regurgitation are (1) weakness and fatigue caused by the reduction in for-

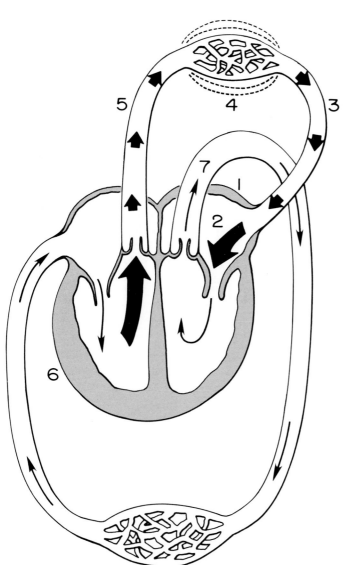

FIGURE 28-4 Pathophysiology of mitral stenosis: 1, left atrial hypertrophy; 2, left atrial dilation; 3, pulmonary venous congestion; 4, pulmonary congestion; 5, pulmonary hypertension; 6, right ventricular hypertrophy; 7, fixed cardiac output.

ward flow, (2) exertional dyspnea, and (3) palpitations. Severe symptoms are precipitated by left ventricular failure with consequent low cardiac output and pulmonary congestion. The following findings are associated with mitral regurgitation: (1) *auscultation:* murmur throughout systole; (2) *electrocardiogram:* left atrial enlargement ("P mitrale"), left ventricular hypertrophy, and atrial fibrillation; (3) *chest x-ray:* left atrial enlargement, left ventricular enlargement, and variable pulmonary vascular congestion; (4) *cardiac catheterization:* opacification of the left atrium during left ventricular injection of contrast material, increased left atrial and left ventricular pressure, and variable elevations of pulmonary pressures.

Aortic stenosis

Aortic stenosis obstructs blood flow from the left ventricle into the aorta during ventricular systole. As the resistance to ventricular ejection increases, the pressure work of the left ventricle rises. In response, the left ventricle hypertrophies to generate more pressure and maintain peripheral perfusion; a marked pressure gradient develops between the left ventricle and the aorta (see Fig. 28-7). Hypertrophy reduces ventricular wall compliance, and the wall becomes relatively stiff. Thus, despite the maintenance of normal cardiac output and ventricular volumes, ventricular diastolic pressure is slightly elevated.

The reserve pumping capability of the left ventricle is considerable. For instance, the left ventricle, which normally generates a systolic pressure of 120 mmHg, can develop pressures up to 300 mmHg during ventricular contraction. Therefore, despite the progressive restric-

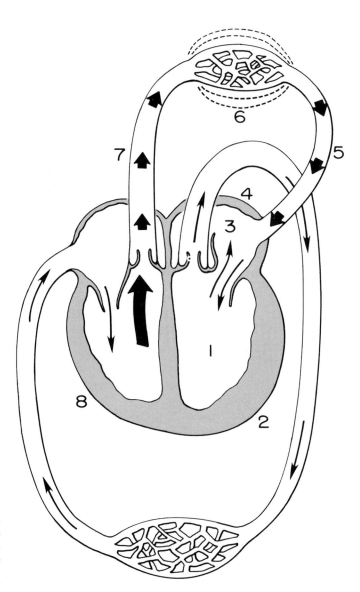

FIGURE 28-5 Pathophysiology of mitral regurgitation: 1, left ventricular dilation; 2, left ventricular hypertrophy; 3, left atrial dilation; 4, left atrial hypertrophy; 5, pulmonary venous congestion; 6, pulmonary congestion; 7, pulmonary artery hypertension; 8, right ventricular hypertrophy.

tion of the aortic orifice and a consequent elevation of ventricular work, the mechanical efficiency of the heart is maintained for long periods. Eventually, however, the adaptive ability of the left ventricle is overwhelmed. The onset of progressive symptoms heralds a critical point in the course of aortic stenosis.

A characteristic triad of symptoms is associated with aortic stenosis: (1) syncope, (2) angina, and (3) left ventricular failure. If unheeded, these symptoms indicate a grave prognosis, with an average survival of less than 5 years. The onset of left ventricular failure, indicating cardiac decompensation, is particularly ominous. Angina is produced by an imbalance in myocardial oxygen supply and demand; demand increases with hypertrophy and increased myocardial work, while supply is potentially reduced by the powerful systolic compression of the coronary arteries by the hypertrophied muscle. In addition, with myocardial hypertrophy, the ratio of capillaries to muscle fibers is reduced. The oxygen diffusion distance is therefore increased, potentially limiting myocardial oxygen supply. Syncope occurs primarily with exertion, either as a result of arrhythmias or an inability to increase cardiac output sufficiently to maintain cerebral perfusion.

Progressive ventricular failure impairs ventricular emptying. Cardiac output falls and ventricular volumes rise. Ventricular dilation, occasionally associated with functional mitral regurgitation, ensues. Advanced aortic stenosis is associated with severe pulmonary congestion. Right ventricular failure and systemic venous congestion are indicative of end-stage disease. Rarely does aortic stenosis progress to this extreme. The rare occurrence of right heart failure is probably caused by the high mortality associated with left heart failure earlier in the course of the disease. In addition, there is a significant incidence of sudden death in symptomatic patients with aortic stenosis. The pathogenesis of sudden death is controversial.

The signs of aortic stenosis are as follows: (1) *auscultation:* systolic murmur; (2) *electrocardiogram:* left ventricular hypertrophy; (3) *chest x-ray:* poststenotic aortic dilation (resulting from local trauma from blood ejected under high pressure striking the aortic wall) and valvular calcification (occasional observation); (4) *cardiac catheterization:* significant aortic gradient (over 80 to 100 mmHg), elevated diastolic ventricular pressure, and normal left atrial and pulmonary pressures.

Aortic regurgitation

Aortic regurgitation produces a reflux of blood from the aorta into the left ventricle during ventricular relaxation (see Fig. 28-8). In essence, the peripheral bed competes with the left ventricle for the blood ejected by the ventricle during systole. The magnitude of forward flow, or "runoff," into the periphery relative to retrograde flow into the ventricle depends upon the degree of valve closure and the relative resistance to flow between the periphery and the ventricle. Characteristically, peripheral vascular resistance is low in aortic regurgitation, apparently to maximize forward flow. However, late in the course of the disease, peripheral resistance rises, increasing retrograde flow through the aortic valve and accelerating the disease progression.

The clinical course of aortic regurgitation is the least understood of the valvular lesions. However, the disease obviously imposes a severe volume load upon the left ventricle. With each contraction, the ventricle must eject a quantity of blood equal to the normal stroke volume plus the regurgitant volume. The left ventricle dilates greatly and eventually hypertrophies, assuming a distinctive "boot shape" with an elongated cardiac apex. An associated increase in wall compliance enables the ventricle to tolerate increased diastolic volumes without abnormal pressure elevations.

The marked left ventricular compensatory ability in combination with a competent mitral valve maintains ventricular function for a long time. Symptoms rarely develop until left ventricular decompensation, occasion-

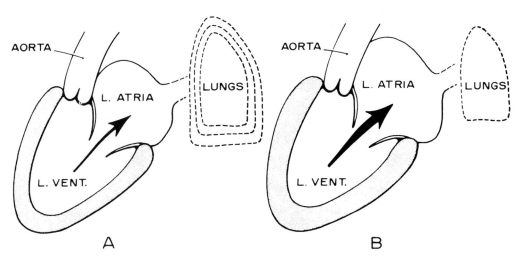

FIGURE 28-6 A, acute, and B, chronic mitral regurgitation. Note that in chronic mitral regurgitation there is greater dilatation and hypertrophy of the left atria and ventricle. Acute mitral regurgitation causes greater pulmonary congestion because the left atrium is less compliant or distensible.

ally compounded by functional mitral regurgitation, occurs. Irreversible left ventricular damage resulting from the prolonged ejection of the volume overload against systemic resistance can be sustained. The point of significant deterioration is ill-defined. Early symptoms are fatigue, dyspnea on exertion, and palpitations. Heart failure precipitates a downhill course of falling cardiac output and rising ventricular volume with retrograde left atrial and pulmonary congestion.

The following signs are associated with aortic regurgitation: (1) *auscultation:* diastolic murmur, characteristic Austin-Flint murmur or diastolic rumble, and systolic murmur caused by increased ejection volume; (2) *electrocardiogram:* left ventricular hypertrophy; (3) *chest x-ray:* boot-shaped elongation of the cardiac apex; (4) *cardiac catheterization:* opacification of the left ventricle during injection of contrast material into the aortic root.

Characteristic findings are noted in the peripheral circulation as a result of the hyperdynamic myocardial action and the low peripheral resistance. The forceful, high-volume, left ventricular ejection followed by the rapid forward runoff of blood into the periphery and backward into the left ventricle through the diseased valve creates a rapid distention of the vasculature followed by a sudden collapse. These cardiovascular dynamics can be manifested by (1) waterhammer, or Corrigan, pulses characterized by a rapid rise and fall of the arterial pulse; (2) pistol-shot pulses, audible upon auscultation of femoral artery; (3) Quincke's capillary pulsation, visible as alternating flushing and paling of the nail-bed capillaries; (4) systolic head bobbing as the collapsed neck vessels fill rapidly; and (5) widened pulse pressure with a low diastolic pressure.

Tricuspid valve disease

Stenosis of the tricuspid valve restricts blood flow from the right atrium into the right ventricle during diastole. This lesion is usually associated with disease of the mitral

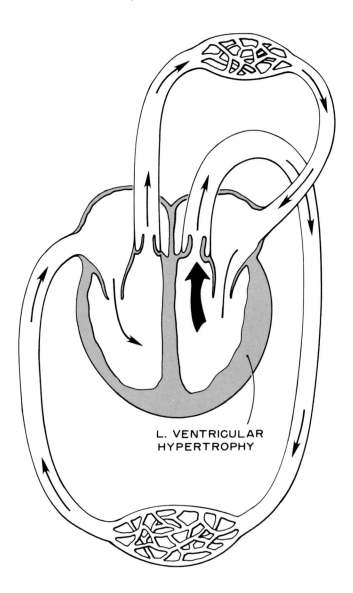

L. VENTRICULAR HYPERTROPHY

FIGURE 28-7 *Pathophysiology of aortic stenosis.*

and aortic valves secondary to severe rheumatic heart disease. Tricuspid stenosis increases the work of the right atrium, forcing the chamber to generate more pressure to maintain flow across the obstructed valve. The right atrium has a limited ability to compensate and therefore dilates rapidly. As right atrial volumes and pressures rise, systemic venous engorgement and pressure elevation result (see Fig. 28-9).

The classic findings of right-sided heart failure ensue: (1) venous distention, (2) peripheral edema, (3) ascites, (4) hepatic enlargement, and (5) nausea and anorexia resulting from gastrointestinal engorgement. The following signs are associated with tricuspid stenosis: (1) *auscultation:* diastolic murmur; (2) *electrocardiogram:* right atrial enlargement (tall, peaked P waves known as "P pulmonale"); (3) *chest x-ray:* right atrial enlargement; (4) *cardiac catheterization:* pressure gradient across the tricuspid valve and elevated right atrial and central venous pressures.

Pure tricuspid regurgitation is usually the consequence of advanced left-sided heart failure or severe pulmonary hypertension resulting in right ventricular

deterioration. As the right ventricle fails and enlarges, functional regurgitation of the tricuspid valve is produced. Tricuspid regurgitation is associated with right-sided heart failure and the following findings: (1) *auscultation:* murmur throughout systole; (2) *electrocardiogram:* right atrial enlargement ("P pulmonale") and right ventricular hypertrophy; (3) *chest x-ray:* right atrial and ventricular enlargement; (4) *cardiac catheterization:* contrast reflux into the right atrium during injection of the right ventricle with contrast material.

Pulmonic valve disease

The incidence of pulmonic valvular lesions is extremely low. Pulmonic stenosis is usually congenital, rather than rheumatic, in origin. Stenosis of the pulmonic valve

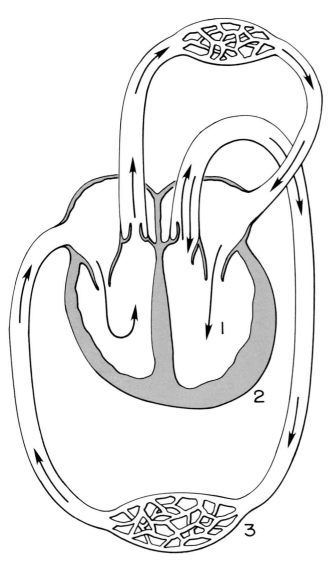

FIGURE 28-8 Pathophysiology of aortic regurgitation: 1, left ventricular dilation; 2, left ventricular hypertrophy; 3, hyperdynamic peripheral circulation.

increases right ventricular pressure work, producing right ventricular hypertrophy. Symptoms result when right ventricular failure occurs, producing systemic venous engorgement and its clinical sequelae.

Functional pulmonic regurgitation can occur as a sequelae to left-sided valvular dysfunction with chronic pulmonary hypertension and dilation of the pulmonic valve orifice. However, this lesion is seen rarely.

Compound valvular disease

"Mixed lesions," consisting of stenosis and regurgitation in the same valve, commonly occur. This is to be expected because a stenotic, immobile valve is often unable to close completely. "Combined lesions," or multivalvular disease, are often seen because rheumatic heart disease commonly afflicts multiple valves.

Mixed lesions and combined lesions compound the valvular dysfunction described for isolated or "pure" lesions, altering to a variable degree the physiologic consequences. Compound lesions can either magnify or buffer a physiologic consequence of a pure lesion. For instance, mixed aortic regurgitation and aortic stenosis increase the volume load and pressure work of the left ventricle and greatly intensify the left ventricular strain. As a result, this combination is associated with a rapidly progressive downhill course.

However, the combination of aortic stenosis and mitral stenosis, in essence, protects the left ventricle from the magnitude of left ventricular strain associated with isolated aortic stenosis. This protective effect results from the reduction in left ventricular filling caused by the restriction to blood flow through the mitral valve. Diminished ventricular filling reduces the volume of the blood that the left ventricle must force through the restricted aortic orifice.

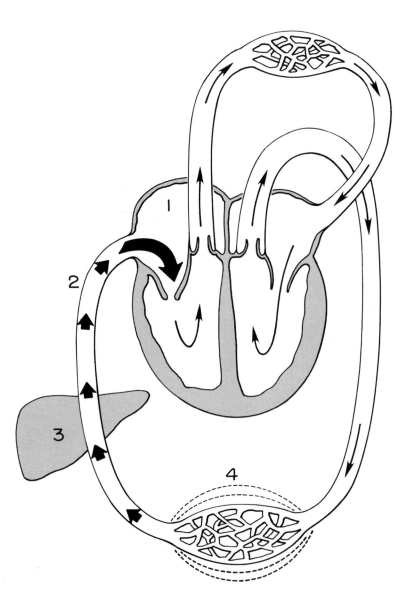

FIGURE 28-9 Pathophysiology of tricuspid stenosis: 1, right atrial dilation; 2, venous congestion; 3, hepatomegaly; 4, systemic congestion.

Rheumatic fever and subacute bacterial endocarditis are two disease processes afflicting the heart valves that can be prevented or controlled, thus reducing the incidence or severity of acquired valvular lesions. Rheumatic fever can be prevented by early detection and appropriate antibiotic prophylaxis of β-hemolytic streptococcal infections. Since rheumatic fever tends to recur, antibiotic prophylaxis may be indicated after the acute attack has subsided. Damaged heart valves are particularly vulnerable to infection, or endocarditis, from systemic bacterial infections or even from the transient septicemia associated with minor surgical procedures (e.g., dental extractions). Appropriate prophylactic antibiotic coverage during substantiated or potential systemic infection is critical to prevent further valvular deterioration. Once valvular damage has been sustained, the course of the disease and medical therapy varies according to the site and severity of the lesion.

Mitral valve disease produces symptoms earlier in the course of the disease than does aortic valve disease. This earlier onset of symptoms results from the fact that the diseased mitral valve imposes a burden primarily upon the left atrium, whereas the diseased aortic valve burdens the left ventricle. The thin-walled left atrium is poorly suited to maintain its pumping capability in the face of an ever-increasing pressure or volume load. In addition, since no true valves separate the pulmonary veins from the left atrium, left atrial congestion is readily transmitted retrograde to the lungs, producing pulmonary symptoms. With aortic valve disease, the left ventricle compensates well for a long period of time, resulting in a long asymptomatic phase. The left atrium is protected from the left ventricular strain as long as the mitral valve remains competent and the left ventricular pumping capability is sustained.

Mitral valve disease

The clinical progression of mitral valve disease is gradual and prolonged. Dyspnea is usually the most prominent and disabling symptom. However, symptoms are initially responsive to medical therapy consisting of (1) diuretics to reduce congestion, (2) digoxin to increase contractile force in the presence of mitral regurgitation, which increases left ventricular work, (3) antiarrhythmics, if atrial fibrillation occurs, and (4) anticoagulants, if systemic embolization becomes a threat. Eventually, surgical intervention becomes necessary to control the progressively disabling symptoms. Occasionally, surgical intervention is precipitated by an abrupt deterioration associated with arrhythmias, embolization, or pulmonary infection.

Selected patients with pure mitral stenosis are considered for mitral commissurotomy, or surgical splitting of the valve leaflets fused along the commissures, when their symptoms have progressed to functional Class II heart disease (i.e., symptomatic with ordinary physical exertion). Mitral commissurotomy is contraindicated in patients with mitral regurgitation or with significant valvular calcification; splitting the commissures under these two conditions would either worsen the regurgitation or prompt calcific embolization.

Mitral commissurotomy (see Fig. 28-10) is performed by introducing a dilator through the apex of the left ventricle that is guided by a finger inserted through the left atrium into the mitral orifice. The commissures are then split by blunt pressure as the dilator tip is opened. This procedure separates the fused leaflets, dilating the mitral orifice. This procedure usually results in relief or reduction of symptoms for a period of years. However, the procedure is palliative; eventually mitral valve replacement is considered as disease progression produces further disability. In carefully selected cases, mitral commissurotomy can be a valuable therapeutic adjunct, postponing the need for valve replacement.

Mitral valve replacement is considered when symptoms have progressed to functional Class III heart

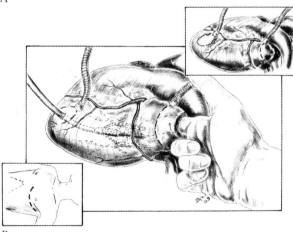

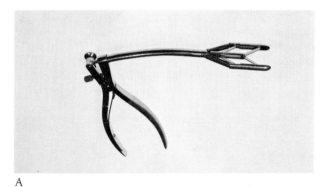

FIGURE 28-10 Mitral commissurotomy. A, Tubb's mitral valve dilator, used for closed mitral commissurotomy. B, transventricular mitral valvulotomy. It is important to advance the dilator into the mitral valve under control by the right index finger. (From J. W. Hurst, The Heart, 3d ed., McGraw-Hill, New York, 1974, p. 973.)

disease (i.e., symptoms with less than ordinary physical exertion). At this point, symptoms are less responsive to medical therapy, and the resultant disability is considered significant. Pulmonary hypertension, indicative of significant disease progression, substantiates the decision to replace the mitral valve. Further disease progression to functional Class IV is associated with a higher operative mortality and morbidity as a result of residual myocardial and pulmonary dysfunction.

Mitral valve replacement involves excision of the valve, chordae tendinae, and papillary muscles. A prosthetic valve, designed to simulate normal valve function, is inserted. One type of prosthetic valve, a ball and cage, is illustrated in Fig. 28-11. During ventricular relaxation, the ball rests in the bottom of the cage, permitting blood to flow from the atrium to the ventricles. During ventricular contraction, as ventricular pressure exceeds atrial pressure, the ball is propelled upward in the cage to seal the mitral orifice preventing backward flow.

Aortic valve disease

The management of aortic valve disease is in distinct contrast to that of mitral valve disease. The onset of significant symptoms—angina, syncope, failure—usually correlates with left ventricular decompensation, signaling a need to consider surgical intervention. The risk of operation for most symptomatic patients is less than the risk of prolonged medical therapy. Once symptomatic, the course of aortic disease is progressively downhill. Severe aortic stenosis is a potentially unpredictable, lethal entity; sudden death can occur without warning. Aortic regurgitation poses somewhat of a therapeutic dilemma; the timing of surgery is less well-defined. Close surveillance of patients with aortic valve disease is essential to detect early signs of clinical deterioration.

Surgical intervention in both aortic regurgitation and aortic stenosis requires replacement of the valve. During heart valve replacement, the oxygenation and systemic circulation of blood is sustained by a heart-lung machine, referred to as cardiopulmonary bypass (see Fig. 28-12). Catheters, or cannulae, are inserted into the superior vena cava and inferior vena cava to shunt venous blood away from the right side of the heart into the bypass machine. The bypass machine oxygenates the blood and propels it into the arterial circulation via cannulae in either the aortic arch or the femoral artery.

QUESTIONS

Valvular heart disease—Chap. 28

Directions: Answer the following questions on a separate sheet of paper.

1 List and briefly describe five causes of valvular heart disease.

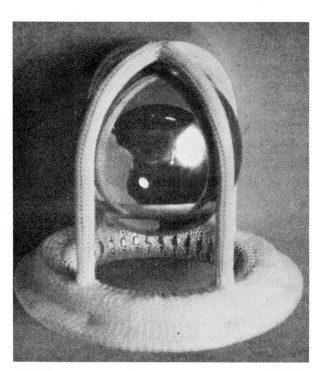

FIGURE 28-11 *Starr-Edwards ball prosthesis model 6320. (From J. W. Hurst, The Heart, 3d ed., McGraw-Hill, New York, 1974, p. 976.)*

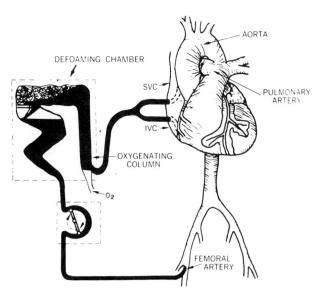

FIGURE 28-12 *Total cardiopulmonary bypass. Desaturated venous blood is drained from the superior and inferior venae cavae to the oxygenating column, defoaming chamber and returned under systemic pressure to the femoral artery. (Reprinted by permission of G. P. Putnam's Sons from Cardiovascular Nursing by J. Kernicki, B. Bullock, and J. Matthews, copyright © 1971 by G. P. Putnam's Sons, 1970, p. 63.)*

2 What is functional AV regurgitation?

3 Comment on the following statement: "Before rendering any treatment that may result in even the slightest release of bacteria into the bloodstream, one is obligated to make absolutely sure that the patient is not affected by any kind of heart deformity. If it is known or suspected that the patient has a deformity of the heart, it is absolutely necessary to administer prophylactic antibiotics."

4 What is the medical treatment for each of the following problems associated with mitral valve disease: pulmonary congestion, atrial fibrillation, and systemic emboli?

5 What is a mitral commissurotomy?

6 What is a heart-lung machine? Under what circumstances would it be utilized?

Directions: Circle the letter preceding each item that correctly answers each question. Only one answer is correct unless otherwise noted.

7 Mitral valve closure occurs when:
a Left ventricular pressure exceeds left atrial pressure
b Left atrial pressure exceeds left ventricular pressure
c Left ventricular pressure exceeds aortic pressure
d Left atrial pressure equals left ventricular pressure

8 Arrange the heart valves in correct order according to their relative frequency of involvement in valvular heart disease.
a Pulmonic *b* Aortic *c* Mitral *d* Tricuspid

9 The organism which precedes the development of rheumatic heart disease is:
a Group A, β-hemolytic streptococcus *b* Streptococcus viridans *c* Staphylococcus aureus *d* Staphylococcus albus

10 Progressive valvular lesions in rheumatic fever are primarily a result of:
a A single episode of rheumatic carditis *b* Chronic infective carditis *c* Recurrent episodes of rheumatic carditis *d* Subacute bacterial endocarditis

11 The primary site of vegetations in rheumatic carditis is:
a On the papillary muscles *b* Diffuse distribution over the endocardium *c* Along the chordae tendinae *d* Along the valve leaflets at their lines of contact

12 Morphologic changes which characterize pure rheumatic valvular stenosis include all of the following *except:*
a Leaflet fusion along the commissures *b* Shrunken, retracted cusps *c* Thickening of the chordae tendinae *d* Thickening of valvular cusps

13 Morphologic changes which characterize pure rheumatic valvular regurgitation include all of the following *except:*
a Shrunken, retracted cusps *b* Shortened, fused

chordae tendinae *c* Rupture of the papillary muscles *d* Enlargement of the valvular orifice

14 Dilation and hypertrophy of the left atrium is the initial compensatory response in:
a Aortic stenosis *b* Tricuspid stenosis *c* Mitral stenosis *d* Acute rheumatic fever

15 Dilation and hypertrophy of the left ventricle occurs in:
a Mitral stenosis *b* Mitral regurgitation *c* Tricuspid regurgitation *d* Pulmonary stenosis

16 Which of the following is the earliest symptom in patients with mitral stenosis?
a Palpitations *b* Dyspnea on exertion *c* Orthopnea *d* Angina

17 Symptoms with mild exertion appear when the orifice of the mitral valve (normally 4 to 6 cm²) is reduced to:
a 3 to 4 cm² *b* 2 to 3 cm² *c* 1 to 2 cm² *d* Less than 1 cm²

18 Which of the following disorders is least likely to result in left ventricular strain?
a Systemic hypertension *b* Aortic regurgitation *c* Mitral stenosis *d* Ventricular aneurysm

19 Atrial fibrillation complicating mitral stenosis creates the following problem or problems: (More than one answer may be correct)
a Loss of atrial contraction *b* Potential systemic embolization *c* Potential right ventricular failure *d* Decreased ventricular filling time

20 Chronic mitral stenosis may result in all of the following *except:*
a Enlargement of the left atrium *b* Increased pressure in the left ventricle *c* Redistribution of pulmonary blood flow to the upper lobes *d* A fixed cardiac output *e* Pulmonary hypertension

21 Mitral valve insufficiency will result in blood regurgitating from the:
a Right ventricle back to the right atrium *b* Pulmonary artery back to the right ventricle *c* Left ventricle back to the left atrium *d* Right atrium back to the superior and inferior vena cavae

22 The most likely cause of *acute* mitral regurgitation would be:
a Recurrent episodes of rheumatic endocarditis *b* Chest trauma *c* Bacterial endocarditis *d* Ruptured papillary muscle complicating myocardial infarction

23 In differentiating acute mitral regurgitation from chronic mitral regurgitation, all of the following statements are correct *except:*
a Fulminating pulmonary edema is more common in acute mitral regurgitation. *b* Left ventricular hyper-

trophy is common in chronic mitral regurgitation. *c* A dilated left atrium is common in acute and chronic mitral regurgitation. *d* Atrial fibrillation is common in chronic mitral regurgitation, but normal sinus rhythm is more likely in the acute form.

24 Isolated aortic stenosis usually results from:
a A congenital bicuspid valve *b* Rheumatic valvular disease *c* Atherosclerotic heart disease *d* Progressive calcification with aging

25 The primary response to aortic stenosis is:
a Right ventricular hypertrophy *b* Left ventricular hypertrophy *c* Pulmonary hypertension *d* Enlargement of the left atrium

26 Atrial fibrillation is least likely to be associated with:
a Mitral regurgitation *b* Mitral stenosis
c Aortic stenosis *d* Coronary atherosclerotic disease

27 Which of the following findings would not be expected in a patient with severe aortic stenosis?
a Paradoxical splitting of the second heart sound *b* Poststenotic dilation of the aorta on chest x-ray *c* Enlarged and sustained apical impulse on palpation *d* A pressure gradient of 100 mmHg between the aorta and left ventricle on cardiac catheterization *e* A widened pulse pressure

28 Potential symptoms and signs in moderate aortic stenosis include all of the following *except:*
a Angina pectoris *b* Effort syncope *c* Peripheral edema *d* Paroxysmal noctural dyspnea

29 In aortic stenosis, life expectancy after the onset of significant symptoms averages:
a Less than 5 years *b* 5 to 8 years *c* 9 to 11 years *d* 12 to 15 years

30 Characteristic signs of severe aortic regurgitation include: (More than one answer may be correct)
a Pistol-shot pulses heard over the femoral artery *b* Corrigan (waterhammer) pulses *c* Austin-Flint murmur *d* Systolic head bobbing *e* Alternating flushing and paling of nail-bed capillaries (Quincke's capillary pulsation)

31 Which of the following statements concerning tricuspid stenosis is *not* true?
a There is an increased pressure gradient between the right ventricle and right atrium on cardiac catheterization. *b* Electrocardiographic findings include tall, peaked P waves and right atrial enlargement. *c* Central venous pressure is usually normal. *d* There is accentuation of the a wave of the jugular venous pulse. *e* Hepatomegaly and ascites are common findings on physical examination.

32 Pure tricuspid regurgitation is usually:
a Associated with rheumatic heart disease *b* A functional disorder associated with right heart failure *c* Associated with acute myocardial infarction *d* A functional disorder associated with left ventricular hypertrophy

33 Which of the following findings is *not* associated with tricuspid regurgitation?
a Positive hepatojugular reflux test *b* Waterhammer pulse *c* Prominent v wave of the jugular venous pulse *d* Distended neck veins *e* Opacification of the right atrium when the right ventricle is injected with contrast media

34 Which of the following combinations of valvular disease would probably be the most lethal?
a Aortic stenosis + mitral stenosis *b* Tricuspid regurgitation + mitral stenosis *c* Aortic regurgitation + mitral regurgitation *d* Aortic regurgitation + aortic stenosis

35 The x-ray findings of right ventricular hypertrophy in the absence of pulmonary arterial hypertension are suggestive of:
a Tricuspid stenosis *b* Mitral stenosis
c Pulmonic stenosis *d* Aortic regurgitation

36 Pulmonic stenosis is usually the result of:
a Rheumatic fever *b* Coronary atherosclerotic disease *c* Congenital deformity of the valve *d* None of the above

37 Subacute bacterial endocarditis in a susceptible host may be prevented by: (More than one answer may be correct)
a Replacement of diseased valves *b* Use of antibiotics prior to and after dental surgery *c* Antibiotic prophylaxis throughout adolescence *d* Antibiotic prophylaxis for genitourinary tract instrumentation

38 Replacement of the mitral valve is indicated when the patient's disability is classified, according to the New York Heart Association, as:
a Class I *b* Class II *c* Class III *d* Class IV

39 A suitable candidate for mitral commissurotomy is a patient with a mitral valve that is:
a Heavily calcified *b* Stenotic and regurgitant *c* Stenotic and flexible *d* Stenotic and immobile

40 Which statements regarding the function of a prosthetic ball and cage heart valve in the mitral position are correct? (More than one answer may be correct)
a During systole the ball is propelled upward to seal the orifice and prevent backflow *b* The prosthetic valve is sutured to the papillary muscles which regulate valve opening and closure *c* During diastole the ball rests on the bottom of the cage *d* The fact that atrial pressure exceeds ventricular pressure accounts for the upward propulsion of the ball

41 Which of the following criteria is an indication for consideration of imminent aortic valve replacement in aortic stenosis?
a Arterial pulse pressure of 50 mmHg *b* Aortic valve calcification on chest x-ray *c* Onset of symptoms of angina pectoris, effort syncope, and left heart failure

d An increased left ventricular end-diastolic pressure at cardiac catheterization

42 Cardiopulmonary bypass would be required for which of the following types of surgery? (More than one answer may be correct)
a Mitral valve replacement *b* Repair of a ventricular septal defect *c* Closed mitral commissurotomy *d* Coronary revascularization

Directions: Match the functional valvular disorder in col. A to its effects in col. B.

Column A
43 _____ Valvular regurgitation
44 _____ Valvular stenosis

Column B
a Increased cardiac volume work
b Increased cardiac pressure work
c Backward flow
d Resistance to forward flow
e Chamber dilation
f Muscle hypertrophy

Directions: Fill in the blanks with the correct words.

45 During cardiopulmonary bypass, venous blood flows through catheters placed in the _____ to an _____ where diffusion of gases takes place and blood is returned to the body by a catheter placed in the _____ or _____.

BIBLIOGRAPHY

FRIEDBERG, CHARLES K.: *Diseases of the Heart,* Saunders, Philadelphia, 1966.

HURST, J. WILLIS (ed.): *The Heart,* McGraw-Hill, New York, 1974.

NORMAN, JOHN C. (ed.): *Cardiac Surgery,* Appleton-Century-Crofts, New York, 1972.

POWERS, MARYANN, and FRANCES STORLIE: *The Cardiac Surgical Patient,* Macmillan, New York, 1968.

ROSS, JOHN, JR., and EUGENE BRAUNWALD: "Aortic Stenosis," *Circulation,* **37** and **38** (Supplement) V-61–V-67, July, 1968.

RUSHMER, ROBERT: *Cardiovascular Dynamics,* Saunders, Philadelphia, 1970.

SELZER, ARTHUR, and KEITH E. COHN: "Natural History of Mitral Stenosis: A Review," *Circulation,* **XLV**: 878–889, April, 1972.

SODEMAN, WILLIAM A., and WILLIAM A. SODEMAN JR.: *Pathologic Physiology: Mechanisms of Disease,* Saunders, Philadelphia, 1974.

CHAPTER 29 Peripheral Vascular Disease

OBJECTIVES **At the completion of Chap. 29, you should be able to:**

1 Define arteriosclerosis, atherosclerosis, Mönckeberg's sclerosis, arteriolosclerosis, and thromboangitis obliterans.

2 Identify four factors affecting the outcome of atherosclerosis.

3 Identify the common sites of atherosclerotic plaque formation in the peripheral vascular system.

4 Enumerate the signs and symptoms of arterial insufficiency to a limb.

5 Describe aneurysms (etiology, types, shapes, common sites, and associated signs, symptoms, and complications).

6 Differentiate between true and false aneurysms.

7 Define thrombosis, thrombus, embolization, and embolus.

8 Identify several conditions predisposing to arterial thrombus and embolization.

9 Identify the signs and symptoms of arterial embolization.

10 Describe the following diagnostic procedures useful in the detection of peripheral vascular disease: arteriography, venography, ultrasonic Doppler flow measurements, impedance plethysmography, thermography, and oscillometry.

11 Describe Raynaud's phenomenon.

12 Describe the Leriche syndrome.

13 Differentiate between thrombophlebitis and phlebothrombosis.

14 List the three major predisposing factors in venous thrombosis.

15 Compare superficial and deep thrombophlebitis with respect to signs, symptoms, and complications.

16 Describe varicose veins (pathogenesis, signs, symptoms, and complications).

17 Describe the principles and procedures for the medical and surgical treatment of peripheral arterial and venous disease.

18 Enumerate methods of preventing recurrent thrombophlebitis.

Disease processes can afflict both systemic arteries and veins, impairing tissue perfusion and interfering with venous return to the heart. Peripheral vascular disease can alter the structural and pressure–volume characteristics of these vascular beds.

ARTERIAL DISEASE

Arteriosclerosis

Arteriosclerosis includes any disease process producing degeneration, hardening, or thickening of the arterial walls. *Atherosclerosis*, the most common form of arteriosclerosis, is characterized by lipid deposition on the intimal layer of the artery, which progressively occludes the vascular lumen. The medial layer of the arterial wall is also susceptible to pathologic alterations. *Medial sclerosis*, or senile arteriosclerosis, occurs with aging. The medial layer gradually loses its elasticity as the elastic and smooth muscle fibers of this layer degenerate; the relative collagen content of the arterial wall increases. *Mönckeberg's sclerosis* is a focal calcification of the media of the smaller arteries. The arterioles can also thicken, usually in association with chronic hypertension, producing *arteriolosclerosis*. Buerger's disease, or *thromboangiitis obliterans*, is an inflammatory process involving the peripheral, small blood vessels of the hands and feet; all vascular layers are affected.

ATHEROSCLEROSIS

Atherosclerotic lesions can occur throughout the arterial system. The localized accumulation of lipid and fibrous tissue within the artery progressively narrows the arterial lumen, increasing the resistance to blood flow. As resistance to flow increases, blood flow to the tissue beyond the lesion is reduced. If the oxygen needs of the tissue exceed the ability of the vessel to supply oxygen, tissue ischemia results. The effects of compromised arterial flow upon peripheral tissues depends upon (1) the site of the lesion, (2) the severity of the lesion, (3) the metabolic demand of the tissue beyond the lesion, and (4) the extent of collateral circulation bypassing the lesion.

Atherosclerotic lesions preferentially develop at points of branching, bifurcation, abrupt curvature, or vessel narrowing. Lesions occur more frequently in the lower extremities than in the upper extremities, frequently occurring at the bifurcation of the aorta, common iliac, or common femoral. Segmental or localized lesions are commonly noted in the main branches of larger caliber vessels, such as proximal iliac, femoral, and popliteal arteries (see Fig. 29-1).

The tendency of atherosclerotic lesions to be localized and to enlarge gradually favors the development of collateral circulation. Localization of the lesion implies that the distal artery is patent; thus alternative routes of arterial flow can bypass the lesion to perfuse the tissue beyond. In addition, as the resistance to flow increases at the site of the obstruction, pressure increases proximal to the lesion with a proportionate drop in pressure distal to the lesion. This pressure gradient across the obstruction promotes flow through collateral vessels, bypassing the lesions because the pressure is similarly elevated at the entrance to the collateral vessel and decreased at the exit of the bypass pathway. The collateral vessels gradually enlarge. Mild, chronic ischemia is also considered to be a stimulus to the development of collateral pathways.

SIGNS AND SYMPTOMS

Irrespective of the underlying pathophysiologic mechanism responsible for progressive arterial occlusion, the signs and symptoms are the result of tissue ischemia in regions beyond the lesion. The earliest symptoms are noted during exercise when metabolic demands increase, exceeding the ability of the diseased vessels to supply oxygen. Characteristically, *intermittent claudication*, ischemic pain occurring with exercise and subsiding with rest, is noted. The location of the pain cor-

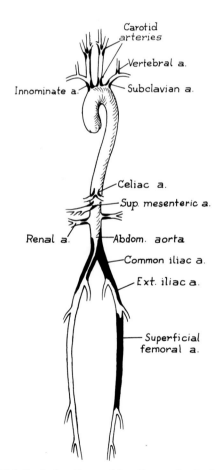

FIGURE 29-1 Typical patterns of location and extent of atherosclerotic disease of the aorta and its major branches. (From J. W. Hurst, The Heart, 3d ed., McGraw-Hill, New York, 1974, p. 1674.)

relates with the location of arterial disease. Pain typically occurs in the calf, thigh, or buttock, correlating respectively with lesions of the superficial femoral, the iliac, and the distal aorta. The correlation between pain and lesion location is approximate in that it indicates the lowest or proximal level of disease.

Pain occurring at rest is indicative of severe ischemia, usually associated with diffuse disease. Intense pain is associated with tissue ulceration and gangrene once arterial insufficiency has progressed to the point of tissue death or necrosis.

The following characteristic tissue changes occur as a result of chronic underperfusion: (1) atrophic changes of skin and nails, with thinning of the skin and thickening of the nails; (2) loss of hair, particularly on the dorsum of the feet and toes; (3) wasting of the leg muscles and soft tissues. Severe underperfusion culminates in ulceration and gangrene, usually of the digits, interdigital surface, heels, or metatarsal heads.

The signs of arterial occlusion are (1) reduced or absent peripheral pulses, (2) coolness of the extremities, (3) auscultated "bruits" over regions of vascular narrowing in major arteries, (4) postural color changes, and (5) pallor, cyanosis, or mottling of skin.

The postural color changes are pallor on elevation and redness, followed by cyanosis, with dependency of the extremity. The elevation pallor is the result of gravitational effects which reduce the arterial pressure and, consequently, the blood volume in the capillary bed. As the extremity is lowered below heart level, the color gradually returns. Redness, or rubor, initially develops as the capillaries fill, with the elevation of arterial pressure. Evidently, the blood flow across the obstruction lesion is extremely pressure-dependent and exquisitely sensitive to the effects of gravity. Color should return within 15 to 30 seconds unless the arterial occlusion is extremely severe. Cyanosis may follow the stage of rubor because the blood flow through the capillary bed is reduced, necessitating increased oxygen extraction from the arterial blood to meet tissue requirements for oxygen. Cyanosis is produced by the increased amount of reduced hemoglobin in the capillary bed.

Aneurysm

An *aneurysm* is an outpouching or dilation of the arterial wall. Aneurysms are usually caused by medial arteriosclerosis, atherosclerosis, syphilis, or trauma. Aneurysms are classified according to type and described according to shape. A *true aneurysm* consists of a dilation enclosed by an intact arterial wall; a *false aneurysm* is an extravascular accumulation of blood, or hematoma, caused by a disruption of all layers of the arterial wall; surrounding tissues comprise the boundary of the aneurysm. A *dissecting aneurysm* indicates a separation of the arterial layers with blood accumulation in the medial layer sec-

ondary to a tear in the intima. The dissecting column of blood can extend varying distances beyond the intimal tear. Aneurysms are fusiform or saccular in shape (see Fig. 29-2); a *fusiform* aneurysm is a uniform circumferential arterial dilation, whereas a *saccular* aneurysm is an outpouching with a small neck adherent to the arterial wall.

Aneurysms can occur in the aorta or peripheral arterial branches. Aortic aneurysms are usually abdominal, located below the renals, or occasionally thoracic. Abdominal aneurysms may be asymptomatic, although a pulsatile mass may be palpable. Symptoms are usually the result of pressure upon adjacent structures, rupture, or dissection. For instance, thoracic aneurysms may produce dysphagia, or difficulty in swallowing, as a result of esophageal compression or hoarseness caused by pressure upon the recurrent laryngeal nerve. Rupture produces rapid exsanguination and fulminating shock. Dissecting aneurysms are associated with excruciating pain and characteristic changes in tissue perfusion as critical aortic branches are obstructed by the advancing column of blood; signs of impaired cerebral, renal, or coronary flow are easily detected.

Aneurysms of the popliteal or femoral arteries are apparent as palpable, pulsating masses. Occasionally the mass will become nonpulsatile as a result of thrombosis of the blood pooling in the aneurysmal sac. Aneurysm thrombosis can give rise to peripheral embolization if a fragment of the thrombus dislodges and lodges peripherally. Peripheral aneurysms may produce pain resulting from compression of adjacent nerve fibers or venous distention resulting from compression of adjacent veins.

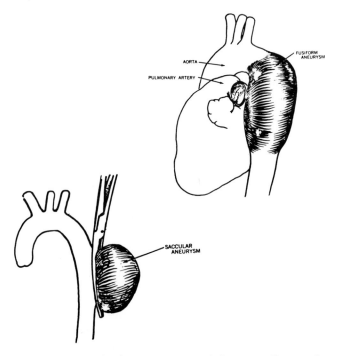

FIGURE 29-2 A, fusiform aneurysm of the aorta. B, saccular aneurysm of the descending aorta. (Reprinted by permission from J. Kernicki, B. Bullock, and J. Mathews, Cardiovascular Nursing, G. P. Putnam's Sons, New York, 1971, pp. 86–87.)

Arterial thrombosis and embolism

Thrombosis is the formation of a blood clot, or *thrombus*, within the vascular system. Arterial thrombosis usually occurs at the site of an atherosclerotic plaque or within an arterial aneurysm. Detachment of the thrombus into the bloodstream is referred to as *embolization*. The *embolus* is propelled downstream to lodge in the smaller branches of the arterial system, occluding the vascular lumen. Most arterial emboli originate in the left side of the heart. Mitral stenosis and atrial fibrillation predispose to the development of atrial thrombi. Transmural myocardial infarction roughens the endothelial lining of the left ventricle, potentiating the formation of mural ventricular thrombi. Depending on the size and destination of the clot, dislodgment of thrombi from the cardiac chambers is a potentially devastating event.

Embolization to the periphery produces the following characteristic signs of arterial occlusion: (1) diminished or absent pulses, (2) skin pallor and cyanosis, (3) pain, (4) muscle weakness and loss of sensation, and (5) collapse of superficial veins as a result of reduced arterial inflow.

The aortic bifurcation is vulnerable to embolic or thrombotic occlusion. Sudden embolic occlusion of the distal aorta is known as *saddle embolism*. Gradual occlusion due to thrombosis is referred to as the *Leriche syndrome*.

Arteriospastic disease

Raynaud's phenomenon is believed to be an exaggerated vasoconstrictive response of the small arteries and arterioles of the skin and subcutaneous tissue, especially the hands. The spasm is usually precipitated by cold or anxiety; the etiology is unknown. The vasospasm produces a paroxysmal pallor of the hands as a result of the reduction in arterial flow; ischemic pain follows. The episode lasts a few minutes and is followed by a hyperemic phase of intense reddening with associated painful throbbing of the digits.

DIAGNOSTIC METHODS USED IN ARTERIAL DISEASE

The diagnosis of peripheral arterial disease is usually based upon the signs and symptoms of arterial occlusion and reduced tissue perfusion. However, the following specialized diagnostic tools are available to determine the exact location and the extent of arterial involvement:

1 *Arteriography*—the injection of contrast material into the arterial tree to visualize the vasculature.
2 *Ultrasonic Doppler flow measurements*—records the velocity of blood flow via an ultrasonic probe placed over the vessel.
3 *Impedance plethysmography*—measures the magnitude of pulsatile arterial flow as manifested by changes in blood volume in the vessel.

4 *Thermography*—records skin temperature via a thermistor, or temperature sensor, applied to the skin.
5 *Oscillometry*—records the arterial pulsations transmitted to a pressure cuff.
6 *Auscultation of the blood pressure* proximal and distal to the suspected lesion to determine the pressure gradient.

THERAPEUTIC INTERVENTION IN ARTERIAL DISEASE

The basic principles of care are to improve tissue perfusion, reduce tissue oxygen demand, prevent complications, retard disease progression, and relieve pain. Tissue perfusion can be maximized by slight dependency of the involved extremity. Dependency increases perfusion pressure, relieving ischemia; elevation of the extremity is contraindicated because arterial flow would be further compromised. Excessive dependency would also impair flow by promoting venous congestion and edema formation. Vasoconstrictive influence, such as cold temperatures and smoking, are also to be avoided.

The application of direct heat is also contraindicated because heat will increase the metabolic rate of the tissue, thus increasing the disparity between oxygen demand and supply. Furthermore, direct heat could burn and injure the ischemic tissue. Arterial insufficiency can interfere with sensory function, retarding detection of noxious, injurious stimulants. Complications are more easily prevented than treated. Care must be taken to protect vulnerable tissue from injury; bed cradles and sheepskin padding may be indicated in severe ischemic states. Careful positioning to prevent pressure ulceration is essential. Application of lanolin or oil for dry skin may be essential to prevent breakdown and infection.

Disease progression of atherosclerosis can best be achieved by controlling risk factors, such as hyperlipidemia, hypertension, and smoking. Anticoagulation or administration of low molecular weight Rheomacrodex may be indicated in thromboembolic states. Relief of pain with analgesics may be necessary.

Surgical intervention in peripheral arterial occlusive disease can take several forms:

1 *Endarterectomy*—removal of an atheromatous vascular core.
2 *Embolectomy*—removal of an embolus through an arteriotomy utilizing a balloon-tipped catheter.
3 *Arterial revascularization*—bypassing the arterial lesion with a graft, usually an autogenous vein graft.
4 *Arterial reconstruction*—arterial repair utilizing synthetic patch grafts or resection of small segments of the artery.
5 *Sympathectomy*—disruption of the sympathetic in-

nervation of the vasculature to reduce vasomotor tone and improve regional blood flow.

6 *Aneurysm resection*—removal of the aneurysm with insertion of a synthetic graft.

7 *Amputation* when all else fails and intractable pain, disability, or gangrene dominate the clinical picture.

VENOUS DISEASE

Thrombophlebitis

Phlebitis signifies vein inflammation; inflammation of the lining of the vein roughens the endothelial surface, increasing the likelihood of clot formation, or thrombosis. *Thrombophlebitis*, by definition, is venous inflammation with thrombosis of the involved vein. *Phlebothrombosis* refers to venous thrombosis without inflammation of the vascular wall. However, clinically undetectable inflammation is a concomitant of phlebothrombosis; therefore, thrombophlebitis is considered the primary clinical entity.

Three primary factors predispose individuals to the development of thrombophlebitis: (1) venous stasis or pooling of blood, (2) damage to the endothelial layer of the vein, and (3) hypercoagulability of blood. Prolonged bed rest or limited mobility promotes venous stasis. The compression of the veins by contracting muscles profoundly influences venous return to the heart against gravity. Loss of the pumping action of the muscles increases venous congestion and pressure in dependent regions of the body. Stagnant blood pooling in these regions has an increased tendency to clot. The intravenous injection of irritating chemicals, sepsis, and direct trauma can damage the lining of the endothelium. Blood dyscrasias and dehydration, which increase the viscosity of the blood, can increase the tendency to clot.

The basic pathophysiologic process underlying thrombophlebitis is an acute inflammatory process with thrombus formation. The greater the inflammatory reaction, the more adherent the thrombus is to the vessel wall. This is significant because the most feared complication of thrombophlebitis is embolization of a thrombus fragment to the lungs. Consequently, phlebothrombosis with minimal vein inflammation has a higher incidence of pulmonary embolism. Once the acute inflammatory process in thrombophlebitis subsides, healing occurs; the vessel lumen eventually opens as the thrombosis undergoes recanalization.

Either the superficial or the deep veins can be affected with differing clinical manifestations and consequences. The superficial veins are connected to the deep veins by perforating or communicating veins. Valves in the communicating vessels shunt some venous blood from the superficial veins to the deep veins, reducing the volume of blood returned to the heart via the superficial venous system (see Fig. 29-3). This redistribution of venous blood increases the efficiency of venous return because the deep veins are surrounded by muscle; therefore venous return can be facilitated by the pumping action of muscular contraction. The superficial veins receive minimal support from surrounding subcutaneous tissues.

Superficial thrombophlebitis presents with no generalized edema, because the deep venous system continues to function, reducing venous engorgement and fluid transudation from the capillary bed into extravascular tissues. The dominant signs and symptoms are those of inflammation along the length of the involved vein: redness, heat, and tenderness are noted. The involved vein may be palpable as a hardened cord. The extremity may ache. Deep thrombophlebitis is characterized by generalized edema of the involved extremity as a result of the obstruction of venous flow. The extremity is tender and painful; systemic signs of inflammation, such as an elevated temperature, may be noted. The superficial veins may be distended as a result of the impaired deep venous drainage. Deep femoral or pelvic thrombophlebitis may be relatively asymptomatic and clinically undetected; pulmonary embolism may be the first indication of venous disease.

The complications of thrombophlebitis are pulmonary embolism, chronic venous insufficiency, and postphlebitic neurosis. Pulmonary embolism is discussed in

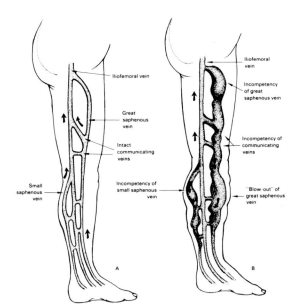

FIGURE 29-3 A, diagram of the venous circulation of the healthy lower limb. Note that the blood ascends in both the superficial and deep systems and in health the blood passes into the deep veins via the communicating veins. B, varicosities produced in the superficial venous system as a result of incompetency of the valves in the communicating veins. In both drawings the arrows indicate the flow of blood in the superficial and deep systems and in the communicating veins. (Adapted from David I. Abramson, Vascular Disorders of the Extremities, 2d ed., Harper & Row, New York, 1974, p. 514.)

Part VI. Chronic venous insufficiency results from destruction of the venous valves. Chronic dependent edema of the ankles with induration of the subcutaneous tissues occurs. The skin around the malleoli assumes a brownish discoloration as a result of deposition of hemosiderin and melanin, products of red blood cell destruction caused by venostasis and subsequent capillary rupture. Postphlebitic neurosis is usually iatrogenic in origin, induced by overemphasis of the hazards of thrombophlebitis and pulmonary embolism in susceptible, suggestible individuals. These individuals react with an exaggerated concern regarding resumption of activity.

Varicose veins

Varicose veins are dilated, tortuous vessels with varying degrees of valvular incompetence. Venous dilation can result from a primary, intrinsic weakness of the vessel wall or can be secondary to venous obstruction or disease somewhere in the venous system, for example in the venae cavae or ileofemoral veins. Venous dilation and valvular incompetence produce venous stasis or pooling which predisposes to the development of thrombophlebitis; conversely, an attack of deep thrombophlebitis can produce valve destruction and, consequently, varicose veins. The superficial veins of the legs are most commonly affected.

Initially, superficial venous engorgement is apparent with varicosities of the extremities. Calf heaviness and aching are experienced and can be relieved by elevation of the involved limb. With disease progression, dependent edema is noted, and skin pigmentation caused by venous stasis may appear. The clinical significance of varicose veins ranges from innocuous cosmetic embarrassment to venous dysfunction predisposing to stasis ulceration and thrombus formation.

DIAGNOSTIC METHODS USED IN VENOUS DISEASE

The relative paucity of definitive signs and symptoms in venous disease, particularly of the deep veins and pelvic vessels, in combination with the lethal nature of potential complications constitutes a diagnostic dilemma. As a result, an emphasis upon prophylaxis and treatment of suspected, although perhaps unconfirmed, thrombophlebitis is necessary.

Invasive and noninvasive diagnostic methods are utilized: (1) venography (visualization of the venous bed utilizing injected contrast material), (2) ultrasonic Doppler flow measurements, (3) impedance plethysmography, and (4) scanning with radioisotope-tagged fibrinogen (detection of venous thrombosis by measuring and locating the isotope incorporated into a thrombus).

The following signs, elicited during the physical exam, are useful: (1) *positive Homan's sign,* or calf pain with sharp dorsiflexion of the foot; this maneuver compresses the calf muscle against the tibia, exerting pressure upon the vein; (2) *changes or asymmetry in limb circumference* may appear if edema or unilateral in-

volvement is present; (3) *increased sensitivity to the application of pressure* to the involved extremity utilizing compression with a blood pressure cuff at pressures between 80 and 120 mmHg. Application of tourniquets at successive points along the extremity to observe variations in the timing and direction of filling of the superficial veins during dependency following elevation permits detection and localization of valve incompetency.

THERAPEUTIC METHODS IN VENOUS DISEASE

Prophylaxis involves the prevention of venous stasis, endothelial injury, and hypercoagulability. Avoidance of prolonged bed rest, early ambulation, leg exercises, elastic stockings, and occasionally anticoagulation are indicated. Once venous disease is suspected or confirmed, the above measures should be continued. Bed rest, with elevation of the affected extremity, may be necessary initially until the signs of inflammation subside. Once the acute phase has subsided, the risk of pulmonary embolism is reduced considerably because the thrombus is organized and adherent to the vascular wall. Warm, moist packs, coupled with elevation of the extremity, promote venous drainage and resolution of the edema.

On occasion, venous thrombectomy is performed. Ligation of the venous system above significant lesions may be indicated to prevent pulmonary embolism; smaller collateral vessels will maintain venous return to the heart.

QUESTIONS

Peripheral vascular disease—Chap. 29

Directions: Answer the following questions on a separate sheet of paper.

1 List two obstructive diseases specific to the arteries.

2 List four factors affecting the outcome of atherosclerosis.

3 Identify several common sites for the formation of atherosclerotic plaques.

4 What are varicose veins and what causes them? Where are they generally located? What are some possible complications? How does a varix differ structurally from an aneurysm?

5 Is deep vein thrombosis or superficial vein throm-

bosis potentially more serious? Why? Why do the superficial veins often become dilated when there is deep vein thrombosis?

6 List several recommendations to prevent recurrent thrombophlebitis.

7 What is an aneurysm and what causes them? What are the dangers of an aneurysm? What is a dissecting aneurysm and what are its consequences?

8 What causes the brownish pigmentation around the ankles and feet in patients with chronic venous insufficiency?

9 Name several conditions predisposing to arterial thrombosis and embolism.

Directions: Circle the letter preceding each item that correctly answers each question. Only one answer is correct unless otherwise noted.

10 Which of the following would *not* be a sign of chronic arterial occlusive disease in the extremities?
a Dependent rubor b Increased pallor of the elevated foot c Thick nails d Absent or diminished pedal pulses e Thin nails

11 Which of the following is usually the earliest sign or symptom of chronic occlusive arterial disease in the extremities?
a Intermittent claudication b Muscle atrophy
c Loss of hair over dorsum of foot d Digital ulceration of the involved extremity e Gangrene of the toes

12 Intermittent claudication resulting from chronic occlusive disease of the superficial femoral arteries commonly causes pain in the:
a Arch of the foot b Calf c Thigh d Buttocks

13 A delayed venous filling time when a leg is moved from an elevated to a dependent position occurs with which of the following conditions?
a Varicose veins b Chronic venous insufficiency
c Peripheral arterial insufficiency d Lymphedema

14 Which of the following physical findings is *not* present in patients with sudden arterial occlusion?
a Absence of one or more arterial pulses b Loss of muscular strength c Decreased skin temperature in the extremity d Dilated superficial veins e Pallor and mottling of skin

15 Which of the following is the most common source of arterial emboli?
a Pulmonary artery b Aorta c Right atrium
d Left atrium e Peripheral artery

16 Gradual occlusion of the bifurcation of the abdominal aorta is called:

a Saddle embolism b Thromboangiitis obliterans
c Leriche syndrome d Raynaud's phenomenon

17 Which of the following statements are true concerning true and false aneurysms? (More than one answer may be correct)
a False aneurysms are caused by entry of blood between the intima and medial layers of the blood vessel causing separation. b A true aneurysm is a dilation enclosed by an intact arterial wall. c A false aneurysm consists of a localized area of clot and blood caused by a gap in the arterial wall. d True aneuryms only form in the aorta.

18 The formation of a blood clot within the vascular system is called:
a Embolization b Embolus c Thrombus
d Thrombosis

19 Which of the following signs and symptoms might indicate that a postoperative patient has thrombophlebitis of the leg? (More than one answer may be correct)
a Decreased hair growth over involved area
b Aching of extremity c Positive Homan's sign
d Pain and tenderness along course of superficial vein e Oral temperature 103°F

20 The initial treatment of an acute thrombophlebitis generally consists of: (More than one answer may be correct)
a Bed rest with the feet elevated b Leg exercises
c Venous thrombectomy d Warm moist compresses to the extremity e Anticoagulant therapy

21 The risk of pulmonary embolism is high: (More than one answer may be correct)
a During the recovery phase of thrombophlebitis
b During the acute phase of thrombophlebitis
c In phlebothrombosis d In deep thrombophlebitis
e In superficial thrombophlebitis

22 Which of the following statements regarding Raynaud's phenomenon is *incorrect*?
a It results from episodic vasoconstriction of the small arteries in an extremity. b Symptoms are more frequent in a warm environment. c Changes in skin color caused by pallor, cyanosis, and hyperemia occur sequentially during an episode. d Ulceration and gangrene of the digits may occur.

23 The presence of deep vein thrombosis can be detected noninvasively by:
a Thermography b Impedance plethysmography
c Venography d Monitoring blood pressure along the affected limb e Monitoring skin color changes

Directions: Match each of the terms in col. A to its best description in col. B.

Column A	Column B
24 ____ Arteriosclerosis	a Focal calcification of the media of smaller arteries
25 ____ Atherosclerosis	
26 ____ Mönckeberg's arteriosclerosis	b General term denoting "hardening of the arteries"

27 _____ Arteriolo-
sclerosis

    c Endothelial lining of artery replaced by patches of fatty material which gradually invade media

    d Thickening of walls of arterioles and small arteries commonly associated with hypertension

Directions: Match each of the diagnostic methods in col. A to the most appropriate statement in col. B.

Column A	Column B
28 _____ Thermography	*a* Measures velocity of flow in vessel noninvasively; useful in detecting arterial occlusion or venous thrombosis
29 _____ Venography	
30 _____ Oscillometry	
31 _____ Ultrasonic Doppler flow detector	*b* Involves injection of contrast media into vascular tree
	c Provides an objective record of the arterial pulsation in a limb; in cases of embolism, level on the limb at which pulsations abruptly stop may be determined
	d Skin temperature recorded which reflects local blood flow

Directions: Fill in the blank with the correct word

32 _____ means inflammation of the vein accompanied by the formation of a clot; _____ means the formation of a clot in a vein in which there is little or no inflammation.

33 An arterial disease which starts in the smaller arteries of the hands and feet and has an intense inflammatory component is _____ _____.

Directions: Circle T if the statement is true and F if it is false. Correct the false statements.

34   T F   Application of external heat to an extremity is an effective method of improving circulation to an extremity in arterial occlusive disease.

35   T F   Patients with occlusive arterial disease of the extremities should not smoke.

36   T F   The insertion of a balloon-tipped catheter into a blood vessel in order to remove a blood clot is called an endarterectomy.

37   T F   Patients with arterial occlusive disease of the lower extremities should keep the extremities slightly elevated to improve circulation.

38   T F   Occlusive arterial disease is a segmental disease of the large- and medium-sized arteries.

BIBLIOGRAPHY

HOLLING, H. EDWARD: *Peripheral Vascular Diseases*, Lippincott, Philadelphia, 1972.

HUME, MICHAEL, and PAUL FREMONT SMITH: "Non-invasive Techniques in the Diagnosis of Leg Thrombosis," *Hospital Practice*, **10**: 57–69, December, 1975.

HURST, J. WILLIS (ed.): *The Heart*, McGraw-Hill, New York, 1974.

KERNICKI, JEANETTE, BARBARA BULLOCK, and JOAN MATTHEWS: *Cardiovascular Nursing*, Putnam, New York, 1970.

ROBERTS, BROOKE: "The Acutely Ischemic Limb," *Heart and Lung*, **5**: 273–276, March-April, 1976.

RUSHMER, ROBERT: *Cardiovascular Dynamics*, Saunders, Philadelphia, 1970.

SODEMAN, WILLIAM A., and WILLIAM A. SODEMAN JR.: *Pathologic Physiology: Mechanisms of Disease*, Saunders, Philadelphia, 1974.

PART VI Normal Respiratory Function and Respiratory Pathophysiology

LORRAINE M. WILSON
SYLVIA A. PRICE

Disorders of the respiratory system are a major cause of morbidity and mortality. Respiratory tract infections are more frequent than infections of any other organ system and range from the common cold with its relatively mild symptoms and inconvenience to a fulminant pneumonia. In 1974, approximately 80,000 persons died of lung cancer. In fact, cancer of the lung is the leading cause of male cancer deaths in the United States; it has increased at an alarming rate and is now about 15 times more prevalent than it was 40 years ago. The incidence of chronic respiratory disease, notably chronic pulmonary emphysema and bronchitis, has also been increasing and is now a leading cause of chronic disability among the male population.

Because of the physical, social, and economic impact of respiratory diseases on the population as a whole, the prevention, diagnosis, and treatment of respiratory disorders is of paramount importance.

This section includes a brief review of respiratory tract anatomy and physiology, a discussion of the common diagnostic tests used to detect respiratory dysfunction, cardinal signs and symptoms of respiratory disease, manifestations of respiratory insufficiency and failure, and a discussion of the common respiratory diseases.

At the completion of Part VI, you should be able to:

1 Describe the relationship between normal respiratory tract anatomy and physiology and the effects of respiratory dysfunction as a disease process.

2 Identify the etiology, pathogenesis, and treatment principles in the various respiratory diseases or disorders.

CHAPTER 30 Normal Respiratory Function

OBJECTIVES

At the completion of Chap. 30, you should be able to:

1 List three disorders of the respiratory system which are a major cause of morbidity and mortality.

2 Define respiration.

3 Name the air-conducting passages.

4 Describe the structure and identify the functions of the epithelial surfaces of the airways.

5 Describe the functions of the larynx.

6 Differentiate anatomically between the right and left mainstem bronchi.

7 Explain the clinical implications of the anatomic differences in the mainstem bronchi.

8 Identify the relationships between the following anatomic structures: lobar and segmental bronchi, terminal bronchioles, acinus, respiratory bronchioles, alveolar ducts, terminal alveolar sacs, alveolar septa, and pores of Kohn.

9 Describe the microscopic structure and function of an alveolar duct and surrounding alveoli.

10 Differentiate between a respiratory bronchiole and a terminal bronchiole on the basis of structure and function.

11 Identify the function of surfactant and the conditions necessary for its production.

12 Identify the relationships between the following anatomic structures of the thoracic cavity: mediastinum, hilus, lobar and segmental divisions of both lungs, apex and base of lungs, diaphragm muscle, pleura and pleural space.

13 Differentiate between the parietal and visceral pleura.

14 Construct and label a diagram showing the relationship between the heart and lungs and the circulation between them.

15 List the unique features of the lung's circulatory system and identify the significance of each feature.

16 Explain the pathogenesis of pulmonary edema.

17 Describe briefly the mechanical process of ventilation.

18 Explain the mechanism of regulation of respiration and identify the important variables.

19 List the defense mechanisms of the respiratory tract.

20 Describe the unique characteristics of the alveolar macrophage.

21 Identify the three main stages whereby oxygen is transferred from the air to the tissues and carbon dioxide is excreted in the expired air.

22 Describe the mechanical process of ventilation including thoracic pressure–volume and air-flow dynamics.

23 Describe the process whereby the diffusion of gases occurs across the alveolar–capillary membrane.

24 State the ventilation–perfusion requirements necessary for the transfer of gas between the alveolus and the pulmonary capillary bed.

25 Differentiate between a dead space and shunt-producing respiratory unit.

26 Compute the volume of anatomic dead space for a given body weight.

27 Identify the two mechanisms whereby oxygen is transported from the lungs to the tissues.

28 Describe oxygen transportation in relationship to the oxyhemoglobin dissociation curve.

29 List the factors which may either increase or decrease the affinity of hemoglobin for oxygen.

30 Describe the process of carbon dioxide transport in the blood.

31 Identify the relationships between ventilation, carbon dioxide homeostasis, and the acid–base balance of the body.

32 State the relationships between hemoglobin concentration, hemoglobin saturation, the partial pressure of oxygen in the arterial blood, and actual oxygen delivered to the tissues.

33 Describe at least three examples of situations which may result in respiratory insufficiency and identify in each case the altered physiologic mechanism that interferes with adequate respiration.

ANATOMIC CONSIDERATIONS

Respiration may be defined as the combined activity of the various mechanisms that are involved in supplying oxygen to all the cells of the body and removing carbon dioxide (the product of cell combustion). The respiratory system accomplishes the task of respiration. Essentially, the respiratory system consists of a series of air passages which bring outside air into contact with a large expanse of specialized respiratory membrane. This membrane lies in close proximity to the capillaries, and the interface between the membrane and the capillaries is the location for exchange of oxygen and carbon dioxide.

Anatomy of the respiratory tract

The air-conducting passages that bring air into the lungs are the nose, pharynx, larynx, trachea, bronchi, and bronchioles (see Fig. 30-1). The respiratory tract from the nose to the bronchioles is lined with ciliated mucous membranes. As air enters the nasal cavity, it is filtered, warmed, and humidified. These three processes are primarily functions of the respiratory mucosa, which consists of pseudostratified ciliated columnar epithelium and goblet cells (see inset, Fig. 30-1B). The epithelial surface is covered by a mucous blanket which is secreted by both the goblet cells and the serous glands. Coarse dust particles are filtered by hair in the nares, while fine

particles are trapped in the mucous blanket. Ciliary action propels the mucous blanket posteriorly in the nasal cavity and superiorly in the lower respiratory tract toward the pharynx from which it is swallowed or expectorated. Water for humidification is given up by the mucous blanket, and heat is supplied to the inspired air by a rich underlying vascular network. Inspired air is thus conditioned so that it reaches the pharynx nearly "dust-free," at body temperature, and 100 percent humidified.

Air passes from the pharynx into the larynx, or voice box. The larynx consists of a series of cartilaginous rings united by muscles and contains the vocal cords. A triangular space between the vocal cords opens into the trachea and is called the *glottis*. The glottis forms the division between the upper and lower respiratory tracts. Although the larynx has been thought of chiefly in relationship to phonation, its protective functions are of much more importance. During swallowing, the rising action of the larynx, the closure of the glottis, and the leaf-shaped *epiglottis*, which has a doorlike action at the entrance of the larynx, all serve to guide food and fluids into the esophagus. If foreign substances do get beyond the glottis, the cough function of the larynx assists in

FIGURE 30-1 The respiratory system. Inset A, acinus or pulmonary functional unit. Insert B, ciliated mucous membrane.

expelling these substances as well as secretions from the lower respiratory tract.

The trachea is supported by horseshoe-shaped cartilaginous rings and is about 5 in long. The structure of the trachea and bronchi is analogous to a tree and is therefore called the tracheobronchial tree. The point where the trachea branches into the right and left mainstem bronchi is known as the carina. The carina is heavily innervated and can produce severe bronchospasms and coughing when stimulated.

Note in Fig. 30-1 that the right and left mainstem bronchi are not symmetric. The right bronchus is shorter, wider, and continues from the trachea in a nearly vertical course. In contrast, the left bronchus is longer, narrower, and continues from the trachea at a more acute angle. This anatomic peculiarity has important clinical implications. An endotracheal tube which

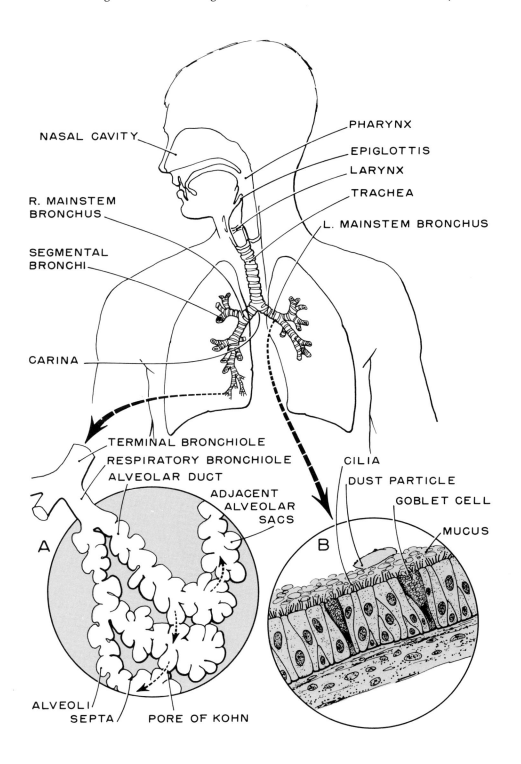

NASAL CAVITY

PHARYNX

EPIGLOTTIS

LARYNX

TRACHEA

R. MAINSTEM BRONCHUS

L. MAINSTEM BRONCHUS

SEGMENTAL BRONCHI

CARINA

TERMINAL BRONCHIOLE
RESPIRATORY BRONCHIOLE
ALVEOLAR DUCT

ADJACENT
ALVEOLAR
SACS

CILIA

DUST PARTICLE

GOBLET CELL

MUCUS

A

B

ALVEOLI
SEPTA
PORE OF KOHN

has been placed to secure a patient airway may easily slip down into the right mainstem bronchus unless well secured at the mouth or nose. If it did slip, air would not be able to enter the left lung, and it would collapse (atelectasis). However, the more vertical course of the right bronchus makes it easier to introduce a catheter for deep suctioning. Also foreign bodies which are aspirated are more apt to lodge in the right bronchial tree because of its vertical course.

The right and left mainstem bronchi divide to become the *lobar* and then the *segmental bronchi*. This branching in ever-decreasing sizes continues down to the *terminal bronchioles*, which are the smallest airways that do not contain alveoli (air sacs). Terminal bronchioles are about 1 mm in diameter. Bronchioles are not supported by cartilaginous rings but are surrounded by smooth muscle, which allows alterations in size. All the airways down to the level of the terminal bronchioles are called conducting airways, since their main function is to serve as air conduits to the gas-exchanging areas of the lung.

Beyond the terminal bronchiole is the *acinus* which is the pulmonary functional unit where gas exchange takes place (see inset Fig. 30-1A). The acinus consists of *respiratory bronchioles*, which have occasional small air sacs or alveoli arising from their walls. The *alveolar ducts*, which are completely lined with alveoli, and the *terminal alveolar sacs* are the final structures of the lung. There are about 23 generations of branching from the trachea to the terminal alveolar sac. The individual alveolus (in the grapelike cluster of alveolar sacs that make up the terminal sac) is separated from its neighbor by a thin wall or *septa*. Small openings in the septa, called the *pores of Kohn*, allow communication between terminal alveolar sacs. The alveolus has only one layer of cells, which is less than the diameter of a red blood cell in thickness. There are about 300 million alveoli in each lung, with a surface area about the size of a tennis court.

Figure 30-2 shows the microscopic structure of an alveolar duct and the surrounding alveoli, which are polygonal in shape. Since the alveolus is essentially a gas bubble surrounded by a capillary network, the liquid–gas interface creates a surface tension which tends to resist expansion on inspiration, and favors collapse on expiration. The alveoli, however, are lined with a lipoprotein substance called *surfactant* which lessens the surface tension and lowers the resistance to expansion on inspiration and prevents collapse of the alveoli on expiration. The production of surfactant by the alveolar lining cells depends on adequate ventilation and blood supply. A deficiency or surfactant is believed to be an important factor in the pathogenesis of a number of lung diseases.

The thoracic cavity

The lungs are elastic, cone-shaped organs which lie within the thoracic cavity or chest. They are separated by the central mediastinum, which contains the heart and great vessels (Fig. 30-3). Each lung has an apex and a base. Pulmonary and bronchial blood vessels, bronchi, nerves, and lymphatics enter each lung at the hilus to form the root of the lung. The right lung is larger than the left and is divided into three lobes by the interlobar fissures. The left lung is divided into two lobes.

Lobes are further divided into segments correspond-

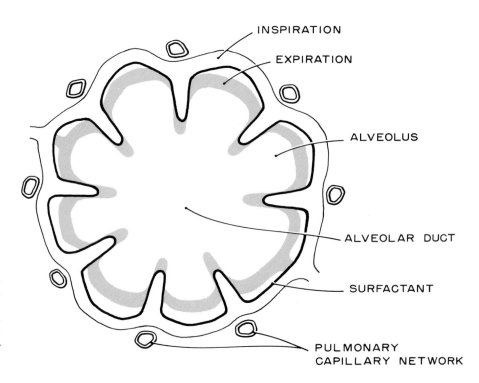

FIGURE 30-2 Structural changes in the terminal alveolar sac (cross section) during the respiratory cycle. (Modified from Louis Gluck, "Pulmonary Surfactant and Neonatal Distress," Hospital Practice, November 1972.)

INSPIRATION

EXPIRATION

ALVEOLUS

ALVEOLAR DUCT

SURFACTANT

PULMONARY
CAPILLARY NETWORK

ing to the segmental bronchi. The right lung is divided into 10 segments and the left lung is divided into 9 (see Fig. 30-3, bronchopulmonary segments). Pathologic processes such as atelectasis and pneumonia are often localized to individual lobes and segments. Knowledge of the segmental anatomy of the lung is important not only for the radiologist, bronchoscopist, and thoracic surgeon but also for the nurse and physical therapist, who must know with accuracy the location of the lesion in order to apply their skills. A continuous thin sheet of

collagen and elastic tissue, known as the pleura, lines the thoracic cavity (parietal pleura) and encases each lung (visceral pleura). Between the parietal and visceral pleura is a thin film of pleural fluid which allows the two surfaces to glide over each other during respiration and

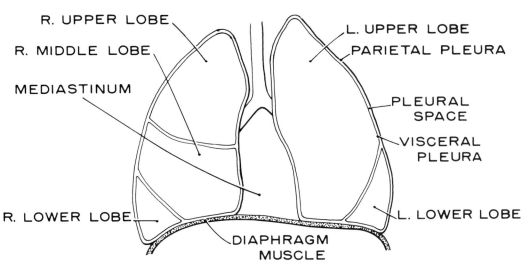

BRONCHOPULMONARY SEGMENTS

RIGHT LUNG SEGMENTS

UPPER LOBE

1 APICAL
2 POSTERIOR
3 ANTERIOR

MIDDLE LOBE

4 LATERAL
5 MEDIAL

LOWER LOBE

6 APICAL
7 MEDIAL BASAL
8 ANTERIOR BASAL
9 LATERAL BASAL
10 POSTERIOR BASAL

LEFT LUNG SEGMENTS

UPPER LOBE

1
2 > APICOPOSTERIOR

3 ANTERIOR
4 SUPERIOR
5 INFERIOR

LOWER LOBE

6 APICAL (SUPERIOR)
7 MEDIAL BASAL (CARDIAC)
8 ANTERIOR BASAL
9 LATERAL BASAL
10 POSTERIOR BASAL

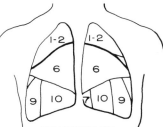

ANTERIOR

POSTERIOR

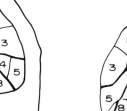

R. LATERAL

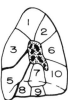

R. MEDIAL

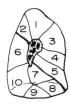

L. MEDIAL

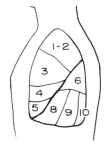

L. LATERAL

FIGURE 30-3 The thoracic cavity and the bronchopulmonary segments.

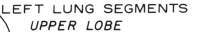
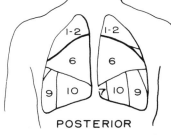

prevents the separation of the thorax and lungs. The pressure within the pleural space is below that of the atmosphere and thus prevents the collapse of the lung. In disease, the pleura may become inflamed or air or fluid may enter the pleural space, causing compression or collapse of the lung. The diaphragm is a dome-shaped muscle that forms the floor of the thoracic cavity and separates it from the abdominal cavity.

Pulmonary circulation

The blood supply to the lungs is unique in several respects. First, the lung has a dual blood supply from the bronchial and pulmonary arteries. The bronchial circulation provides oxygenated blood from the systemic circulation and serves to meet the metabolic needs of the lung tissue. The bronchial arteries arise from the thoracic aorta and travel along the posterior walls of the bronchi. The larger bronchial veins empty into the azygos system, which empties into the superior vena cava and returns blood to the right atrium. The smaller bronchial veins drain into the pulmonary veins. Since the bronchial circulation does not take part in gas exchange, the unoxygenated blood accounts for a shunt which is normally about 2 to 3 percent of cardiac output.

The pulmonary artery arising from the right ventricle provides mixed venous blood to the lungs where the blood is involved in gas exchange. A vast network of pulmonary capillaries surrounds and envelops the alveoli, providing the intimate contact necessary for the exchange of gases between the alveoli and the blood. Oxygenated blood is then returned through the pulmonary veins to the left ventricle, which distributes it to the cells via the systemic circulation. Figure 30-4

shows the functional position of the lungs in the pulmonary circulation.

Another feature of the pulmonary circulation is that it is a low-pressure, low-resistance system in comparison to the systemic circulation. Systemic blood pressure is about 120/80 mmHg, while pulmonary blood pressure is about 25/10 mmHg, with a mean pressure of about 15 mmHg. These features of the pulmonary circulation have several important consequences. The great distensibility and low resistance of the pulmonary vascular beds allows the work load of the right ventricle to be much lighter than that of the left and also allows a great increase in pulmonary blood flow during exercise without significantly increasing the pulmonary blood pressure.

Figure 30-5 illustrates that if the normal mean pulmonary hydrostatic pressure of about 15 mmHg should exceed the colloid osmotic pressure of the blood of about 25 mmHg, fluid would leave the pulmonary capillaries and enter the interstitium or alveoli, causing pulmonary edema. Pulmonary edema interferes with gas exchange by interfering with the diffusion pathway between the alveolus and the capillary. Pulmonary edema is a common complication of congestive heart failure, pneumonia, and many other lung disorders.

Control of respiration

There are a number of mechanisms which contribute to bringing air into the lungs so that exchange of gases can occur. The mechanical function of moving air in and out of the lungs is termed *ventilation* and is accomplished by a number of interacting components. Of particular importance is a reciprocating pump called the *respiratory bellows*. This bellows has two volume-elastic components: the lung itself and the chest wall surrounding the lung. The chest wall consists of the skeleton and tissues of the thoracic cage, as well as the diaphragm, abdominal contents, and abdominal wall. The respiratory

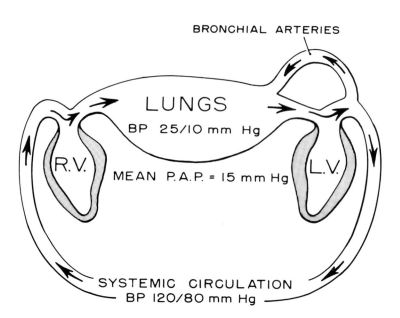

FIGURE 30-4 Functional position of the lungs in the pulmonary circulation.

muscles, which are a part of the thoracic wall, provide the driving force for the operation of the bellows. The diaphragm and the external intercostal muscles are the principal muscles involved in increasing the volume of the lung and thoracic cage during inspiration; expiration is a passive process during quiet breathing. The mechanics of ventilation will be discussed in greater detail in Chap. 31.

The respiratory muscles are controlled by the respiratory center, which is composed of neurons and receptors located in the pons and medulla (see Fig. 30-6). The respiratory center is the part of the nervous system that controls all aspects of breathing. The prime factor in the control of breathing is the response of the central chemoreceptors in the respiratory center to the partial pressure of carbon dioxide (P_aCO_2) and the pH of the arterial blood. An increase in the P_aCO_2 or a decrease in the pH stimulates breathing.

A decrease of the partial pressure of oxygen in the arterial blood (P_aO_2) can also stimulate ventilation. Peripheral chemoreceptors located at the carotid bifurcation (carotid body) and at the arch of the aorta (aortic body) are sensitive to a decrease in the P_aO_2. The P_aO_2, however, must fall from the normal level of about 90 to 100 mmHg to a level of about 60 mmHg before ventilation is significantly stimulated.

There are also mechanisms which control the amount of air taken into the lungs. As the lung is inflated, these receptors signal the respiratory center to stop further inflation. Signals from the stretch receptors cease at the end of expiration when the lung is deflated and the respiratory center is free to initiate another inspiration. This mechanism is known as the *Hering-Breuer reflex*. Movements of joints and muscles (e.g., during exercise) also stimulate an increase in ventilation. Voluntary control input from the cerebrum can modify output from the respiratory centers, thus allowing interruption of the normal breathing cycle for laughing, crying, and speak-ing. The pattern and rhythmic control of breathing is exercised through the interaction of the respiratory centers located in the pons and medulla. Final motor output is transmitted via the spinal cord and phrenic nerve, which supplies the diaphragm, the principal muscle of ventilation. Other major nerves involved are the spinal accessory and thoracic intercostal nerves, which supply the accessory muscles of respiration and the intercostal muscles.

Defenses of the respiratory tract

The large surface area of the lung, which is separated only by a thin membrane from the circulatory system, makes an individual theoretically vulnerable to invasion by foreign bodies (dust) and bacteria in the inhaled air. However, the lower respiratory tract is normally sterile. There are several defense mechanisms which maintain this sterility. We have already mentioned the swallowing or gag reflex, which prevents entry of food or fluid into the trachea, and the action of the "mucociliary escalator," which traps dust and bacteria and transports them to the throat. The cough reflex provides another more forceful mechanism to expel secretions upward so that they may be swallowed or expectorated. The *alveolar macrophage* provides the final and most important defense against bacterial invasion of the lung. The alveolar macrophage is a phagocytic cell with unique migratory and enzymatic characteristics. It moves freely over the alveolar surface and engulfs inert particulate matter and bacteria. After engulfing a microbial particle, lytic enzymes within the macrophage kill and digest the microorganism without producing any obvious inflam-

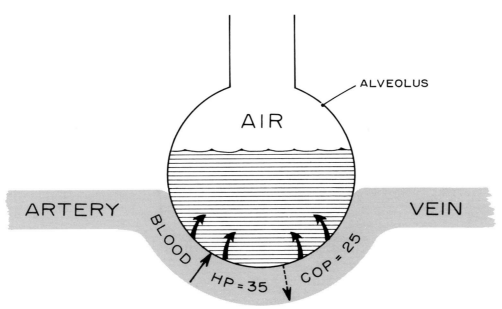

FIGURE 30-5 Pathogenesis of pulmonary edema.

matory reaction. The dust particle or microorganism is then transported by the macrophage to the lymphatics or to the bronchioles where they are removed by the mucociliary escalator. Alveolar macrophages can clear the lung of inhaled bacteria with amazing speed. Ethyl alcohol ingestion, cigarette smoking, and corticosteroid drugs interfere with this defense mechanism.

PHYSIOLOGIC CONSIDERATIONS

The physiologic process of respiration whereby oxygen is transferred from the air to the tissues and carbon dioxide is excreted in the expired air may be divided into three main stages as illustrated in Fig. 30-7. The first stage is ventilation, which is the flow of a mixture of gases into and out of the lungs. The second stage,

transportation, must be considered from several aspects: (1) the diffusion of gases between the alveolus and pulmonary capillary (external respiration) and between the systemic blood and tissue cells; (2) the distribution of blood in the pulmonary circulation and its match with the distribution of air in the alveoli; and (3) the chemical and physical reactions of oxygen and carbon dioxide with the blood. Cell respiration, or internal respiration, is the final stage of respiration, during which metabolites are oxidized to obtain energy, and carbon dioxide is produced as a waste product of cell metabolism and excreted by the lungs.

Ventilation

Air moves in and out of the lungs because pressure gradients are created between the atmosphere and the alveoli by muscular mechanical means. As mentioned previously, the thoracic cage functions as a bellows. The changes in the intrapleural and intrapulmonary (airway) pressures and lung volumes during ventilation may be followed on the graph in Fig. 30-8. During inspiration, the volume of the thorax increases because

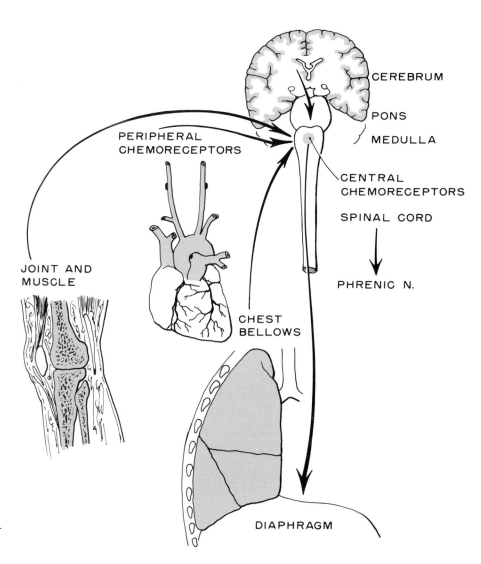

FIGURE 30-6 The control of respiration.

of the descent of the diaphragm and the elevation of the ribs caused by the contraction of the external intercostal muscles. The accessory muscles of ventilation include the scalene muscles, which elevate the first two ribs, and the sternocleidomastoids, which raise the sternum, but there is little activity in these muscles during quiet breathing. This increase in volume causes the intrapleural pressure to decrease from about −4 mmHg (relative to atmospheric pressure) to about −8 mmHg as the lungs are pulled to a more expanded position during inspiration. At the same time intrapulmonary or airway pressure decreases to about −2 mmHg (relative to atmospheric pressure) from 0 mmHg at the beginning of inspiration. The pressure gradient between the airways and the atmosphere causes air to flow into the lungs until airway pressure at the end of inspiration is again equal to atmospheric pressure.

During quiet breathing, expiration is a passive movement produced by the elastic recoil of the chest wall and lungs. As the external intercostal muscles relax, the rib cage is lowered and the dome of the diaphragm ascends into the thoracic cavity, causing the volume of the thorax to decrease. The internal intercostal muscles may forcefully pull the ribs downward and inward during active, forceful expiration, coughing, defecating, or vomiting. In addition, the abdominal muscles may contract, increasing the intra-abdominal pressure and pushing the diaphragm upward. This decrease in volume of the thorax causes both the intrapleural and intrapulmonary pressures to increase. The intrapulmonary pressure now rises to about 1 or 2 mmHg above that of the

atmosphere. The pressure gradient between the airways and the atmosphere is now reversed, causing air to flow out of the lungs until airway and atmospheric pressure are again equal at the end of expiration. Note that intrapleural pressure is always below atmospheric pressure during the respiratory cycle. Alterations in ventilation are assessed by pulmonary function tests. The alterations, their significance, and additional complexities of mechanical ventilation will be discussed in Chap. 31.

Transportation

DIFFUSION

The second stage in the respiratory process involves the diffusion of gases across the thin (less than 0.5 μm in thickness) alveolar–capillary membrane interface. The driving force for this transfer is the partial pressure gradients between the blood and gas phases. The partial pressure of oxygen in the atmosphere at sea level is about 149 mmHg (21 percent of 760 mmHg). By the time oxygen is inspired and reaches the alveoli, its partial pressure is reduced to about 103 mmHg. This decrease in partial pressure is accounted for by the fact that inspired air is mixed with old anatomic dead-space air from

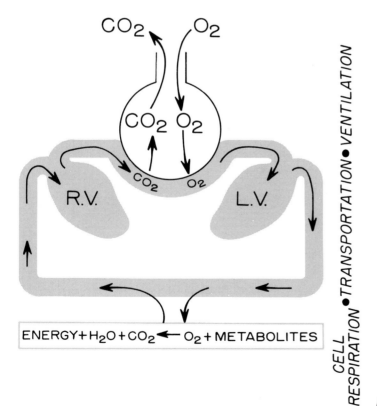

FIGURE 30-7 Principal stages of the respiratory process.

the conducting airways and with water vapor. The anatomic dead space normally holds a volume of about 1 ml of air per pound of body weight (150 ml/150 lb male). Only the fresh air which reaches the alveolus is effective ventilation. As seen in Fig. 30-9, the partial pressure of oxygen in the mixed venous blood (P_vO_2) in the pulmonary capillary is about 40 mmHg. Since the partial pressure of oxygen in the capillary is less than that in the alveolus ($P_AO_2 = 103$ mmHg), oxygen diffuses readily into the bloodstream. A much smaller pressure gradient (6 mmHg) between the blood and alveolar CO_2 causes carbon dioxide to diffuse into the alveolus. The carbon dioxide is then expired into the atmosphere, where its concentration is essentially zero. The carbon dioxide gradient between blood and alveolus, even though very small, is adequate, since it diffuses about 20 times more readily than oxygen across the alveolar–capillary membrane because of its greater solubility.

VENTILATION–PERFUSION RELATIONSHIPS

The effective transfer of gas between the alveolus and pulmonary capillary bed requires an even distribution of air in the lungs and perfusion (blood flow) in the capillaries. In other words, the ventilation and perfusion of a pulmonary unit must be evenly matched. In the normal upright person at rest, ventilation and perfusion are nearly evenly matched except at the apex of the lung. The low-pressure, low-resistance pulmonary circulation results in a greater flow of blood at the base of the lung than at the apex as a result of the influence of gravity. Ventilation, however, is fairly evenly distributed. The mean value for the ratio of ventilation to perfusion ($\dot{V}/\dot{Q}$) is 0.8. This figure is obtained by taking the ratio of the normal rate of alveolar ventilation (4 liters/minute) and dividing it by the normal cardiac output (5 liters/ minute). Figure 30-10 illustrates the normal state of evenly matched ventilation and perfusion in the lung, which is near unity at 0.8.

Ventilation–perfusion inequalities occur in most respiratory diseases. Three theoretical abnormal respiratory units are illustrated in Fig. 30-11. Figure 30-11A depicts a *dead-space unit* in which there is normal ventilation but no perfusion, causing ventilation to be wasted ($\dot{V}/\dot{Q} =$ infinity). The second abnormal respiratory unit (Fig. 30-11B) is a *shunt unit* in which there is normal perfusion but no ventilation, so that perfusion is wasted ($\dot{V}/\dot{Q} = 0$). The last unit (Fig. 30-11C) is a *silent unit* in which there is neither ventilation nor perfusion. There are, of course, variations between the three extremes depending on the overall balance between ventilation and perfusion in the lungs. Lung diseases and functional respiratory disorders may be classified physiologically according to whether they are largely shunt-producing ($\dot{V}/\dot{Q} < 0.8$) or dead space-producing ($\dot{V}/\dot{Q} > 0.8$) diseases.

OXYGEN TRANSPORT IN THE BLOOD

Oxygen can be transported from the lungs to the tissues via two routes: it can be physically dissolved in the plasma or chemically combined with hemoglobin as oxyhemoglobin (HbO_2). The chemical combination of oxygen with hemoglobin is reversible, and the actual amount carried in this form is related in a nonlinear fashion to the P_aO_2 (partial pressure of oxygen in the arterial blood), which is determined by the amount of oxygen physically dissolved in the blood plasma. In turn, the amount of oxygen physically dissolved in the plasma is directly related to the partial pressure of oxygen in the alveolus (P_AO_2). It also depends on the solubility of oxygen in plasma. The amount of physically dissolved oxygen is normally very small because of its low solubility in plasma. Only about 1 percent of the total oxygen transported to the tissues is transported in this manner. This method of transport is not sufficient to support life even at rest. The great bulk of oxygen is carried by hemoglobin, which is located inside the red blood cells. Under certain circumstances (e.g., carbon monoxide poisoning or massive hemolysis in which there is insuf-

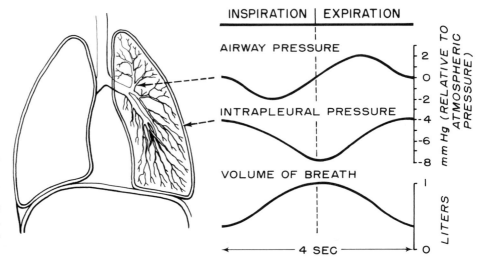

FIGURE 30-8 Changes in intrapleural and intrapulmonary (airway) pressures during inspiration and expiration (Modified from Arthur J. Vander, James H. Sherman, and Dorothy S. Luciano, Human Physiology, 2d ed., McGraw-Hill, New York, 1975, p. 290.)

INSPIRATION | EXPIRATION

AIRWAY PRESSURE

INTRAPLEURAL PRESSURE

2
0
-2
-4
-6
-8

mm Hg (RELATIVE TO ATMOSPHERIC PRESSURE)

VOLUME OF BREATH

LITERS

4 SEC

ficient hemoglobin), sufficient oxygen to support life may be transported in physical solution by subjecting the patient to oxygen under greater than atmospheric pressure (hyperbaric oxygen chamber).

The relationships involved in oxyhemoglobin transportation are illustrated in Fig. 30-12. A gram of hemoglobin can combine with 1.34 ml of oxygen. Since the average hemoglobin concentration in the blood for the adult male is about 15 g/100 ml, 100 ml of blood can carry ($15 \times 1.34 = 20.1$) 20.1 ml of oxygen per 100 ml of blood when it is completely saturated ($S_aO_2 = 100$ percent). However, a small amount of mixed venous blood from the bronchial circulation is added to the oxygenated blood leaving the pulmonary capillaries. This dilution accounts for the fact that only about 97 percent of the blood leaving the lungs is saturated and 19.5 volume percent (vol%) is carried to the tissues.

At the tissue level, oxygen dissociates from hemoglobin into the plasma and diffuses from the plasma into the tissue cells in order to supply tissue needs. Although tissue needs are highly variable, normally about 75 percent of hemoglobin is still combined with oxygen when it returns to the lungs as mixed venous blood. Thus, only about 25 percent of the oxygen in the arterial blood is used to supply the tissues. Hemoglobin which has dissociated from oxygen at the tissue level is called *reduced hemoglobin* (Hb). Reduced hemoglobin is purple in color and accounts for the bluish color of venous blood which is observed in the superficial veins, such as in the hands, whereas oxyhemoglobin (hemoglobin combined with oxygen) is bright red in color and accounts for the color of arterial blood.

Oxyhemoglobin dissociation curve

A clear understanding of the respiratory process requires that one understand the affinity of oxygen for hemoglobin, since tissue oxygen supply, as well as pulmonary oxygen uptake, depends critically on this relationship. This knowledge is necessary in order to interpret blood gas measurements correctly and to apply therapeutic measures for respiratory insufficiency. If whole blood is exposed to different partial pressures of oxygen and the percent saturation of hemoglobin is measured, an S-shaped curve is obtained when these two measurements are plotted. This curve is known as the oxyhemoglobin dissociation curve and demonstrates the affinity of hemoglobin for oxygen at various partial pressures. In Fig. 30-13, the middle curve represents the affinity relationship between oxygen and hemoglobin under normal conditions of body temperature (98.6°F) and a blood pH of 7.4.

One fact of great physiologic importance to be noted about the curve is that there is a flat upper portion, known as the arterial portion (A), and a lower, steeper venous portion (V) which is shifted slightly to the right. At the flat upper portion of the curve, large changes in oxygen tension are associated with very small changes in oxyhemoglobin saturation. This implies that relatively constant quantities of oxygen can be supplied to the tissues even at high altitudes where the PO_2 may be

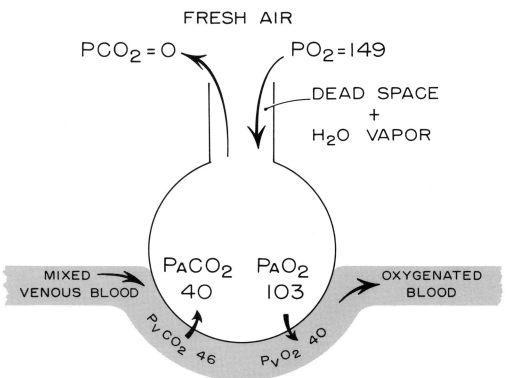

FIGURE 30-9 Diffusion of gases across the alveolar-capillary membrane.

60 mmHg or less. It also implies that the administration of oxygen in high concentrations (normal air = 21 percent) to patients with mild hypoxemia (P_aO_2 60 to 75 mmHg) is wasted, since oxyhemoglobin can only be increased a small amount. In fact, the administration of high concentrations of oxygen may be toxic to the lung tissues and may produce other harmful effects. The release of oxygen to the tissues is augmented by the relationship of the PO_2 to oxygen saturation on the steep venous portion of the curve where large changes in oxyhemoglobin saturation are associated with small changes in the PO_2. The normal differences in oxyhemoglobin saturation and PO_2 between arterial and mixed venous blood are indicated by the arrows on Fig. 30-13.

The affinity of oxygen for hemoglobin is influenced by many other factors which accompany tissue metabolism and which may be modified by disease. A list of some of these factors and their effect on the affinity of hemoglobin for oxygen are given in Table 30-1.

The oxyhemoglobin curve is shifted to the right (see Fig. 30-13) in cases of a decrease in blood pH or a rise in the PCO_2. In this state, hemoglobin has less affinity for oxygen at a given PO_2, so that less oxygen can be transported in the blood. Pathologic conditions which cause metabolic acidosis, such as shock (production of excess lactic acid from anaerobic metabolism) or the retention of carbon dioxide (as is found in many pulmonary diseases), will cause a shift of the curve to the right. A slight shift of the curve to the right, represented by the venous portion of the normal curve (pH 7.38), assists the release of oxygen to the tissues. This shift is called the *Bohr effect*. The slight increase in acidity results from the effect of carbon dioxide being released from the tissues. Other factors causing a shift of the curve to the right are an increase in temperature and increased 2,3-diphosphoglycerate (2,3-DPG), which is an organic phosphate in the red blood cell that binds hemoglobin and decreases its affinity for oxygen. Red cell 2,3-DPG is increased in conditions of anemia and chronic hypoxemia. It is important to appreciate that while the oxygen transport capability of the hemoglobin is decreased with a rightward shift of the curve, hemoglobin release of oxygen to the tissues is facilitated. Therefore, in conditions of anemia and chronic hypoxemia, the rightward shift of the curve is compensatory.

A rightward shift of the curve with a rise in temperature, reflecting increased cell metabolism and a greater need for oxygen, is also adaptive and causes more oxygen to be released to the tissues for a given blood flow.

Conversely, an increase in blood pH (alkalosis) or a decrease in PCO_2, temperature, and 2,3-DPG causes a leftward shift in the oxyhemoglobin dissociation curve (see Fig. 30-13). The shift to the left causes hemoglobin to have a greater affinity for oxygen. Thus, there is increased oxygen uptake in the lung when there is a leftward shift, but release of oxygen to the tissues is impaired. Therefore, it is theoretically possible to have hypoxia (insufficient tissue oxygen to meet metabolic needs) in severe conditions of alkalosis, especially if accompanied by hypoxemia. This condition could occur during mechanical overventilation with a respirator or at high altitudes as a result of hyperventilation. Since hyperventilation is also known to decrease cerebral blood flow as a result of the decrease in the P_aCO_2, cerebral ischemia might also account for symptoms of "light-headedness" common to such persons. Stored blood loses 2,3-DPG activity and causes a greater affinity of hemoglobin for oxygen. Therefore, patients who are transfused with massive amounts of stored blood may also have impaired oxygen release to the tissues because of the leftward shift in the oxyhemoglobin dissociation curve.

Carbon monoxide has an affinity for hemoglobin that is about 250 times greater than that of oxygen. When this gas is inhaled, it combines with hemoglobin to form carboxyhemoglobin. When oxygen combines with carboxyhemoglobin, the reaction is not reversible, so that the amount of hemoglobin available for oxygen transport is reduced. In addition, there is a leftward shift of the remaining normal hemoglobin, resulting in deficient unloading of oxygen to the tissues.

CARBON DIOXIDE TRANSPORT IN THE BLOOD

Carbon dioxide homeostasis is also a necessary aspect of respiratory sufficiency. The transportation of carbon dioxide from the tissues to the lungs for elimination is accomplished in three ways. About 10 percent of the CO_2 is physically dissolved in plasma, because CO_2,

TABLE 30-1
Factors affecting oxyhemoglobin affinity

HbO$_2$ DISSOCIATION CURVE

Shift to left	Shift to right
1 ↑ pH	1 ↓ pH
2 ↓ PCO_2	2 ↑ PCO_2
3 ↓ temperature	3 ↑ temperature
4 ↓ 2,3-DPG	4 ↑ 2,3-DPG

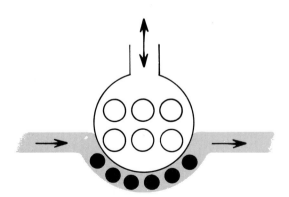

FIGURE 30-10 Even match of ventilation and perfusion in an ideal respiratory unit (normal $\dot{V}/\dot{Q} = 0.8$).

unlike O_2, is highly soluble in plasma. About 20 percent of the CO_2 is combined with the amino groups on hemoglobin (carbaminohemoglobin) in the red blood cell, and about 70 percent is transported as plasma bicarbonate. Carbon dioxide combines with water as shown in the following reaction:

$$CO_2 + H_2O \rightleftharpoons H_2CO_3 \rightleftharpoons H^+ + HCO_3^-$$

This reaction is reversible and is known as the bicarbonate–carbonic acid buffer equation. The acid–base balance of the body is greatly affected by pulmonary function and carbon dioxide homeostasis. (This subject will not be discussed in detail in this book. The reader is referred to the many fine books which explore fluid and electrolyte homeostasis in depth.) In general, *hyperventilation* (alveolar ventilation in excess of metabolic needs) causes alkalosis (increases in blood pH above the normal 7.4) as a result of the excess excretion of CO_2 from the lungs; *hypoventilation* (alveolar ventilation in-

sufficient to meet metabolic needs) causes acidosis (decrease of the blood pH below the normal 7.4) as a result of the retention of carbon dioxide by the lungs. It is evident from examining the buffer equation that lowering the PCO_2, as in hyperventilation, would cause the reaction to proceed to the left with consequent lowering of the H^+ concentration (elevated pH) or that raising the PCO_2 causes the reaction to proceed to the right, producing an increase in H^+ (decreased pH). Hypoventilation occurs in many conditions that affect the respiratory bellows. Carbon dioxide retention is also associated with emphysema and chronic bronchitis caused by trapped air in the lungs.

Just as the amount of O_2 transported in the blood is

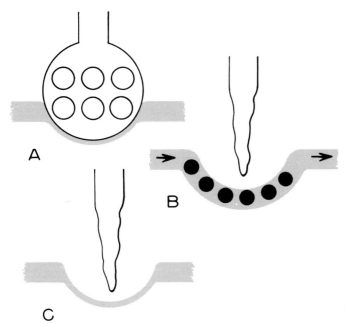

FIGURE 30-11 Three theoretical respiratory units: A, dead-space unit—normal ventilation but no perfusion; B, shunt unit— normal perfusion but no ventilation; C, silent unit—no ventilation, no perfusion.

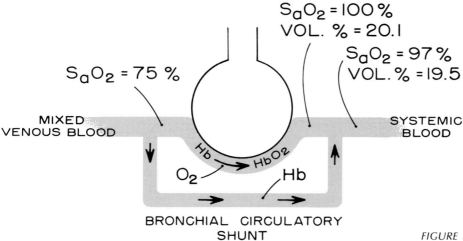

FIGURE 30-12 Oxyhemoglobin transportation.

related to the PO_2 to which the blood is exposed, so the amount of CO_2 in blood is related to the PCO_2. Unlike the S-shaped oxyhemoglobin dissociation curve, the carbon dioxide dissociation curve is nearly linear in the physiologic range of PCO_2. This means that the carbon dioxide content of the blood is directly related to the PCO_2. In addition, there is never any significant barrier to CO_2 diffusion. Therefore, the P_aCO_2 provides a good index of the adequacy of ventilation.

Assessment of the respiratory status

It is important to point out that knowledge of the blood gases (the PO_2, PCO_2, and pH of the arterial blood) alone does not give enough information about the transport of O_2 and CO_2 to be sure that a patient's tissues are being oxygenated properly. Many other factors are involved in the transport process, such as the adequacy of cardiac output and tissue perfusion as well as diffusion of gases at the tissue level. For example, in shock there may be inadequate tissue perfusion as a result of shunting of blood past the tissue cells, stagnation of blood caused by pooling, and inadequate cardiac output. Tissue edema may also interfere with the diffusion pathway at the tissue level. Consequently the detection

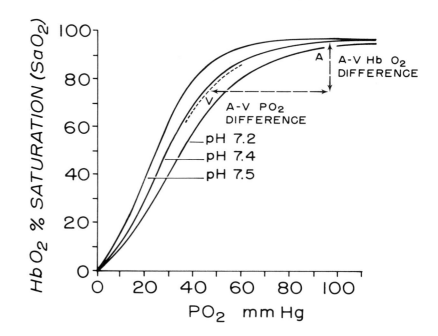

FIGURE 30-13 Oxyhemoglobin dissociation curve.

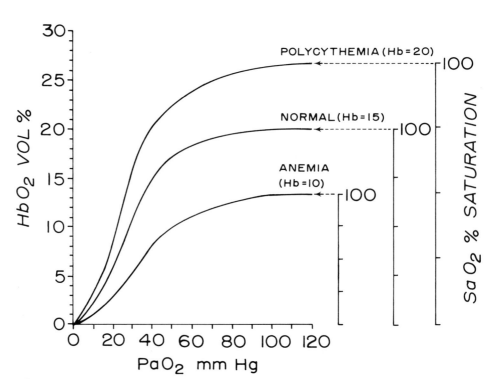

of tissue hypoxia must always involve clinical observations as well as the interpretation of blood gases.

Another important piece of information that is needed for the assessment of a patient's respiratory status is the hemoglobin concentration, as well as the percent saturation of that hemoglobin. The correlation of the P_aO_2, S_aO_2 and the oxyhemoglobin in volume percent for a patient with anemia (Hb = 10 g%), one with a normal Hb of 15 g% and the other with polycythemia (Hb = 20 g%) is shown in Fig. 30-14. All the information illustrated is necessary for a proper assessment of oxygen transport. Note that the percent saturation of hemoglobin is independent of the hemoglobin concentration, while the oxygen content in volume percent is directly related to hemoglobin concentration. The volume percent reveals how much oxygen can be delivered to the tissues at a given P_aO_2. For example, at a P_aO_2 of 100 mmHg and 100 percent saturation of hemoglobin with oxygen, the polycythemic patient can transport 26.8 ml of oxygen in every 100 ml of blood (oxygen content = 26.8 vol%), while the anemic patient can only deliver 13.4 ml at the same oxygen tension and saturation. This is a twofold variation and illustrates the point that knowledge of the blood gases alone is insufficient information for respiratory assessment. Hemoglobin concentration, oxygen saturation, and cardiac status are also vital data.

It is obvious from the previous discussion of the structure and function of the respiratory system that adequate respiration can be prohibited on a number of levels. For example, brain injury or barbiturate overdose in an attempted suicide may interfere with control by the respiratory centers in the central nervous system. A decrease in the PO_2 of inspired air as a result of high altitudes or airway obstruction interferes with respiration. Neuromuscular diseases and skeletal deformities of the chest result in inadequate bellows performance. Respiratory difficulty occurs at the alveolar–capillary interface when there is thickening of the diffusion pathway as in pulmonary fibrosis or edema. Transport of gases in the blood may be interfered with in many respects, including the limiting factor of the amount of hemoglobin. The pulmonary, cardiovascular, and hematologic systems are thus intimately associated with tissue oxygenation.

QUESTIONS

Normal respiratory function—Chap. 30

Directions: Answer the following questions on a separate sheet of paper.

1 List three disorders of the respiratory system which are a major source of morbidity and mortality.

2 Define respiration.

FIGURE 30-14 Relationship of hemoglobin content to oxygen content of blood at various oxygen tensions. (From N. Balfour Slonim and Lyle H. Hamilton, Respiratory Physiology, *3d ed., Mosby, St. Louis, 1976, p. 84.)*

3 Draw and label the epithelial surface of the airways and discuss the function of the mucosal lining in respiration.

4 Why are foreign bodies, when aspirated, usually found in the right mainstem bronchus?

5 What would happen if the pressure within the pleural space were to become equal to that of the atmosphere?

6 Sketch the position of the lungs in the circulatory system and describe some of the unique features of blood supply to the lungs.

7 If the mean pulmonary artery pressure is 30 mmHg and the colloid osmotic pressure of the blood is 20 mmHg, is pulmonary edema likely to occur? Why or why not?

Directions: Complete the following statements by filling in the blanks.

8 The structure which forms the division between the upper and lower respiratory tracts is the _____.

9 The alveoli are lined by a lipoprotein substance called _____. During inspiration, expansion is facilitated, and during expiration, collapse is prevented as this substance functions to lower the _____ _____.

10 The movement of air in and out of the lungs is called _____. To accomplish this function, the thoracic cage and lungs have been compared to a reciprocating pump or _____ _____.
The muscles which provide the main driving force during inspiration are the _____ and _____ muscles.

11 A reflex which controls the amount of air taken into the lungs is known as the _____ reflex.

12 Centers which control the pattern and rhythmicity of breathing are located in the _____ and _____ of the brain.

Directions: Circle the letter preceding each item below that correctly answers the questions. Choose the one best answer.

13 Which of the following factors affects respiration the most?
a Body heat b pH c P_aCO_2 d P_aO_2
e Reflexes from moving limbs

14 The tracheobronchial tree divides repeatedly in a dichotomous fashion and in ever-decreasing sizes until the final pulmonary functional unit is reached. Approximately how many generations of subdivisions are involved?
a 64 b 32 c 23 d 10

15 The right lung has:
a 10 lobes b 8 lobes c 3 lobes d 2 lobes

16 Each bronchus divides into functional subunits which include:
   a Lobar bronchi *b* Segmental bronchi *c* Terminal bronchioles *d* Respiratory bronchioles *e* All of the above

17 The function unit of the lung (acinus) consists of all of the following *except:*
   a Terminal bronchioles *b* Respiratory bronchioles *c* Alveolar duct *d* Alveolar sac *e* Alveoli

18 The pores of Kohn:
   a Are located between pulmonary capillaries *b* May provide collateral ventilation *c* Are artifacts and do not really exist *d* Provide a communication between right and left lungs

19 Alveolar macrophages:
   a Move freely over the alveolar surface *b* Are phagocytic cells *c* Contain lytic enzymes *d* Are inhibited by cigarette smoking, alcohol ingestion, and corticosteroid drugs *e* All of the above

20 The left mainstem bronchus is:
   a Symmetric with the right *b* Shorter and broader than the right *c* Nearer to the vertical in its course than the right *d* More angulated than the right

21 All of the following structures are closely associated with the larynx *except* the:
   a Epiglottis *b* Glottis *c* Carina *d* Vocal cords

22 Protective functions of the larynx include all of the following *except:*
   a Swallowing reflex *b* Cough *c* Major role in humidification of inspired air

23 Label the diagram below (Fig. 30-15) by matching the number of the structure on the diagram with the appropriate term from the list.
   a _____ Diaphragm   *g* _____ Trachea
   b _____ Carina   *h* _____ Mainstem bronchus
   c _____ Epiglottis   *i* _____ Segmental bronchus
   d _____ Mediastinum   *j* _____ Apex of lung
   e _____ Pharynx   *k* _____ Visceral Pleura
   f _____ Larynx   *l* _____ Parietal pleura

24 Label the diagram below (Fig. 30-16) by matching the number of the structure with the appropriate term from the list.
   a _____ Pores of Kohn   *e* _____ Acinus
   b _____ Alveolar duct   *f* _____ Alveolus
   c _____ Respiratory bronchiole *g* _____ Septa
   d _____ Terminal bronchiole

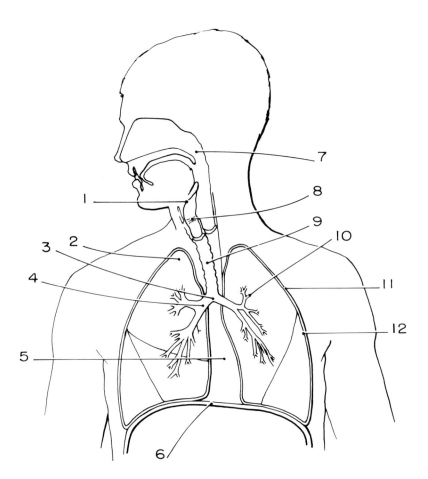

FIGURE 30-15 The respiratory tract.

Directions: Answer the following questions on a separate sheet of paper.

25 Why is the alveolar PO_2 as low as 103 mmHg when it is 149 mmHg in the inspired air?

26 What is the volume of your own anatomic dead space?

27 What is the chief mechanism of gas movement in the respiratory zone of the lung? What provides the driving force?

28 Is ventilation and perfusion perfectly matched in the healthy person at rest in the upright position? Why or why not?

29 If alveolar ventilation is 3 liters/minute and cardiac output (perfusion) is 6 liters/minute, what is the $\dot{V}/\dot{Q}$ ratio? Is this value normal or does an individual with this value have dead-space or shunt-producing disease?

30 What advantage would be gained, if any, by placing an individual with severe hemolytic anemia in a hyperbaric chamber?

31 If a patient is breathing fresh air at sea level, the P_AO_2 is about 103 mmHg, the arterial blood is 97 to 98 percent saturated with oxygen, and the oxygen content is 20 vol%, will it be advantageous to increase the oxygen concentration of the inspired air? Why or why not?

32 Explain why the PO_2 can vary over a wide range and have little effect on the hemoglobin saturation?

33 What is the Bohr effect? What is its significance in terms of tissue oxygenation?

34 When an individual hyperventilates, why is there no significant increase in the O_2 content of the arterial blood, yet there is a significant decrease in the P_aCO_2? Explain this phenomenon in terms of the O_2 and CO_2 dissociation curves.

35 Why does an elevated P_aCO_2 never result from impaired diffusion?

36 Does knowledge of the blood gases alone provide all the information necessary to accurately assess the respiratory status? If not, what other data are necessary?

37 Beginning with inspired air, list at least three altered mechanisms or conditions which may interfere with normal respiration.

38 The respiratory process may be divided into three stages. List and describe each briefly.

39 Which muscles are used during normal quiet inspiration? During inspiration of maximum effort?

40 How many milliliters of oxygen are utilized by tissue cells each minute if the hemoglobin concentration is 12.0 g/100 ml of blood, there is 100 percent saturation of the hemoglobin, cardiac output is 5000 ml/minute, and 25 percent of the oxygen delivered is utilized? (1.34 ml of oxygen combines with each gram of hemoglobin. Ignore the oxygen which is transported physically dissolved in blood plasma.)

41 Account for the fact that hemoglobin is 100 percent saturated with oxygen upon leaving the pulmonary capillary bed yet is 97 to 98 percent saturated in the systemic arteries.

42 If alveolar ventilation doubles and CO_2 production remains constant, what are the effects on arterial PCO_2 and the blood pH? What happens to the oxyhemoglobin dissociation curve and what are the consequences?

43 What is the partial pressure of oxygen in the inspired air of a climber on the summit of Mount Everest if the atmospheric pressure is 247 mmHg and water vapor pressure at body temperature is 47 mmHg? Do you think the mountain climber could walk very far?

Directions: Circle the letter preceding each item below that correctly answers the questions. More than one answer may be correct.

44 In what form is most of the CO_2 carried in the venous blood?
a Bicarbonate   b Physically dissolved in the plasma
c Carbaminohemoglobin

45 Which of the following shift the oxyhemoglobin dissociation curve to the left?
a Decrease in temperature   b Increase in pH
c Decrease in 2,3-DPG   d Increase in PCO_2

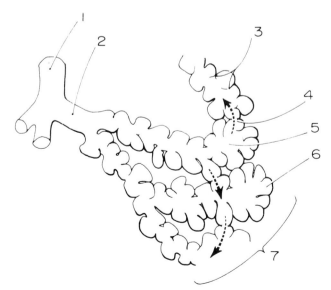

FIGURE 30-16 Pulmonary functional unit.

46 During normal quiet breathing, intrapleural pressure will be:

a Equal to atmospheric pressure b Below atmospheric pressure c Above atmospheric pressure

Directions: Circle the word which correctly completes each sentence.

47 During inspiration, muscular contraction causes the size of the thorax to (increase) (decrease). This size change causes a(n) (increase) (decrease) in the intrapleural pressure. Since pressure in the alveoli is (less) (more) than atmospheric pressure, air moves (into) (out of) the lungs.

48 During expiration, when the diaphragm muscle relaxes, the diaphragm (ascends) (descends), thus (increasing) (decreasing) the volume of the thoracic cavity.

49 During normal quiet expiration, the size change in the thoracic cavity causes a(n) (increase) (decrease) in the intrapleural pressure. Since pressure in the alveoli is now (more) (less) than atmospheric pressure, air moves (into) (out of) the lungs.

50 A person is accidentally exposed to carbon monoxide which combines with half the hemoglobin in the arterial blood. Will the P_aO_2 be (normal) (high) (low)? Will the S_aO_2 be (normal) (high) (low)? Will the arterial oxygen content be (normal) (high) (low)?

51 In general, hyperventilation causes a(n) (increase) (decrease) in the PCO_2, and a(n) (increase) (decrease) in the blood pH, resulting in a condition of (alkalosis) (acidosis).

BIBLIOGRAPHY

AMERICAN CANCER SOCIETY: *Cancer Facts and Figures 1974.*

AMERICAN CANCER SOCIETY: *A Cancer Source Book for Nurses,* 1975.

BATES, D. V., et al.: *Respiratory Function in Disease,* Saunders, Philadelphia, 1971.

BURROWS, B., R. J. KNUDSON, and L. J. KETTEL: *Respiratory Insufficiency,* Yearbook, Chicago, 1975, pp. 50–57.

CHERNIACK, R. M., L. CHERNIACK, and A. NAIMARK: *Respiration in Health and Disease,* 2d ed., Saunders, Philadelphia, 1972, chaps. 1, 3.

HOLMAN, C. W.: "Anatomy" in C. W. Holman and C. Muschenheim (eds.), *Bronchopulmonary Diseases and Related Disorders,* Harper & Row, New York, 1972, vol. 1, pp. 3–40.

LANGLEY, L. L., I. R. TELFORD, and J. B. CHRISTENSEN: *Dynamic Anatomy and Physiology,* 4th ed., McGraw-Hill, New York, 1974, pp. 523–539.

ROBIN, EUGENE D. and L. M. SIMON: "Oxygen Transport and Cellular Respiration," in Edward D. Frohlich (ed.), *Pathophysiology: Altered Regulatory Mechanisms in Disease,* Lippincott, Philadelphia, 1972.

SHAPIRO, B. A.: *Clinical Application of Blood Gases,* Yearbook, Chicago, 1973.

CHAPTER 31 Diagnostic Procedures in Respiratory Disease

OBJECTIVES **At the completion of Chap. 31, you should be able to:**

1 List the six most common methods used to detect pulmonary disease and adequacy of pulmonary function.

2 List the five types of radiologic techniques used to detect pulmonary disease.

3 Describe four aspects of what is depicted on a routine chest x-ray.

4 State the purpose of chest fluoroscopy.

5 Describe a bronchography, including radiopaque materials used, purpose, and potential hazards.

6 Differentiate between angiography of the pulmonary vessels and a lung scan according to material and techniques used, purpose, and major risks involved.

7 Describe bronchoscopy by identifying procedures, purposes, precautions, and potential hazards.

8 Describe the techniques used to obtain lung tissue specimens for biopsy studies.

9 State the purpose and procedure for sputum studies.

10 State the purpose and limitations of ventilatory function tests and blood gas measurements.

11 List and differentiate between the four primary static lung volumes and the four lung capacities.

12 Describe the structure and function of a spirometer.

13 Describe the following indices of ventilatory measurements in terms of the procedures used for measurement, the amount of air being measured, and the calculations required to determine the measurement:
 a Minute volume ($\dot{V}_E$)
 b Respiratory frequency (f)
 c Tidal volume (V_T)
 d Physiologic dead space (V_D)
 e Alveolar ventilation ($\dot{V}_A$)

14 Identify an example that illustrates the relationships between minute ventilation, breathing pattern, and effective alveolar ventilation.

15 State the relationship of the V_D/V_T ratio to effective alveolar ventilation.

16 Define work of breathing.

17 Differentiate between the elastic and nonelastic resistances to ventilation.

18 Define pulmonary compliance and list common causes of decrease.

19 Write the compliance formula and explain each of its components.

20 Differentiate between the forced vital capacity and forced expiratory volume measurements.

21 Describe the significance of the FEV_1/FVC ratio.

22 State the purpose of the maximum breathing capacity (MBC) or maximum voluntary ventilation (MVV) test.

23 Identify the relationship between the mechanical work of breathing and the respiratory pattern in patients with restrictive or obstructive pulmonary disorders.

24 Describe the technique used for the collecting of blood to measure the arterial blood gases by identifying the following: artery of choice, positioning of the patient's arm, procedure for puncture, syringe used, conditions under which specimen should be delivered to the lab.

25 List the normal values for the arterial blood gases.

26 List the causes of hypoventilation and hyperventilation and their relationship to the P_aCO_2.

27 Summarize the acid–base changes that occur in both acidosis and alkalosis.

28 List four mechanisms in respiratory disease which may lead to hypoxemia.

29 Contrast the following in regard to changes in ventilatory function and blood gases in restrictive and obstructive patterns of pulmonary disease: vital capacity, residual volume, functional residual capacity, total lung capacity, forced expiratory volume, forced vital capacity, FEV_1/FVC, maximum breathing capacity, compliance, blood gases.

MORPHOLOGIC METHODS

Diagnostic procedures used for the detection of pulmonary disease may be classified into methods which are primarily morphologic or physiologic. Morphologic methods include radiologic techniques, endoscopy, biopsy studies, and sputum studies. Blood gas measurements and ventilatory function tests are tests which reveal physiologic function.

Radiologic techniques

The thorax is an ideal region for a radiologic examination. The aerated lung parenchyma offers little resistance to the passage of x-rays and therefore produces very radiant shadows. The soft tissues of the chest wall, the heart and great vessels, and the diaphragm do not permit the rays to pass through as readily as the lung parenchyma and therefore appear denser on the x-ray film. The bony structures of the thorax, including the ribs, sternum, and vertebrae, are even less readily penetrated, and their shadows are even denser. Radiologic methods commonly used to detect pulmonary disease include the routine chest x-ray, fluoroscopy, bronchography, angiography, and lung scanning.

ROUTINE CHEST X-RAY

The routine chest x-ray is taken at a standard distance following maximum inspiration and breath-holding to stabilize the diaphragm. Films are taken from the posteroanterior perspective, and sometimes lateral and oblique views are taken as well. These films provide the following information:

1 The status of the thoracic cage including the ribs, pleura, and the contour of the diaphragm and of the upper airway as it enters the chest
2 The size, contour, and position of the mediastinum and hilus of the lung including the heart, aorta, lymph nodes, and the root of the bronchial tree
3 The texture and degree of aeration of the lung parenchyma
4 The size, shape, number, and location of pulmonary lesions including cavitation, fibrous markings, and zones of consolidation.

The appearance of the normal chest x-ray varies somewhat in relationship to sex and age in different subjects to varying conditions of respiration in the same subject. The correct interpretation of a chest film is a skill that takes considerable time to acquire. It is an invaluable aid to the physician when correlated with other observations.

Fluoroscopy is an x-ray technique which enables the roentgenologist to view the thorax and all its contents in motion. Information can be obtained about how various zones of the lung behave during the respiratory cycle. The diaphragm can be studied particularly well using this method. In spite of its usefulness, this type of study is discouraged because of the radiation hazards to the patient and to the examiner.

BRONCHOGRAPHY

An x-ray film of the chest taken after radiopaque material is introduced into the tracheobronchial tree is called a bronchogram. Substances commonly used as radiopaque material are iodized oils and, more recently, tantalum, which is inhaled as a fine powder with the help of positive pressure equipment. The bronchogram reveals in great detail the size and appearance of the tracheobronchial tree and therefore is a particularly useful technique for confirming the diagnosis of bronchiectasis and for detecting other forms of bronchial distortion. Postoperative care is the same as after bronchoscopy (discussed on the following pages). In addition, percussion and postural drainage should be used to assist in the evacuation of the contrast medium.

ANGIOGRAPHY OF THE PULMONARY VESSELS

The pulmonary arterial pattern and flow can be demonstrated by injecting radiopaque fluid through a catheter inserted via an arm vein into the right atrium, right ventricle, and then into the main pulmonary artery. This technique is used to locate the site of a massive embolization or to determine the extent of a pulmonary infarction. Anomalies such as aneurysms and alterations in vascularity common in emphysema are also detectable. However, simpler diagnostic techniques are preferred for the detection of pulmonary disease whenever possible. The major risk during angiography is the development of cardiac arrhythmia as the catheter is passed through the heart chambers.

LUNG SCAN

The isotope lung scan, though a less reliable method for the detection of pulmonary embolism, is a safer procedure. Pulmonary perfusion and sometimes ventilation scanning are carried out. A perfusion scan is obtained by the injection of albumen microspheres, usually labeled with technetium 99m, into a peripheral vein; these particles appear as transient emboli in the pulmonary capillaries in proportion to the active blood flow. The radioactivity distribution is counted with a scintiscanner, and the image is recorded with a camera. The pattern is almost always abnormal in embolism (area with absent radioactivity) but is not highly specific, since abnormalities are also present in other conditions, such as emphysema and pneumonia. The ventilation scan utilizes the inhalation of a bolus of radioactive gas, usually xenon 133. The ventilation lung scan is usually normal in embolism but abnormal in infarction, pneumonia, and emphysema.

Bronchoscopy

Bronchoscopy is a technique which allows direct visualization of the trachea and its major subdivisions. It is used most frequently to confirm the diagnosis of bronchogenic carcinoma but can be used to remove a foreign body. The conventional bronchoscope is a hollow metal tube containing a lighted mirror–lens system which is passed readily into the tracheobronchial tree after administration of local anesthesia. The newer fiberoptic bronchoscope is a flexible instrument which can transmit light and a clear image around corners. Because of its flexibility and smaller diameter, its use causes far less trauma than the conventional metal bronchoscope. The fiberoptic bronchoscope may also be passed through the nose, and inspection of the smaller bronchial subdivisions is possible. Tissue biopsy can be obtained by using a tiny forceps or flexible brush at the tip of the bronchoscope. Suction tubes may also be passed through the bronchoscope to obtain secretions for culture and cytologic studies. The fiberoptic bronchoscopy can be performed at the bedside, although the location of choice is the operating room.

Following bronchoscopy, food and fluids are withheld for at least 2 or 3 hours until the gag reflex returns; otherwise the patient may aspirate material into the tracheobronchial tree. The return of the gag reflex can be tested by touching a cotton applicator to the back of the patient's throat. When this causes the patient to gag, swallowing may be permitted. Other complications which may follow bronchoscopy are bleeding and pneumothorax caused by a ruptured bronchus. Common procedures following bronchoscopy to detect these complications are the monitoring of vital signs for a period of several hours, a chest film, and the collection of all sputum for 24 hours. The nurse should also be aware that laryngeal spasm or edema may be a delayed complication and may require endothracheal intubation and the administration of oxygen.

Biopsy studies

Tissue specimens for biopsy study may be obtained from the upper or lower airways by endoscopic techniques using either the laryngoscope or the bronchoscope. Biopsy specimens of the pleura or lung tissue may also be obtained by either open or closed techniques. The open technique consists of a limited thoracotomy; a small intercostal incision is made after administration of anesthesia, and a tissue specimen is excised under direct visualization. A cylinder of tissue can also be obtained by the newer techniques of percutaneous needle biopsy using an air-turbine drill. The main value of lung biopsy is in diffuse lung disease not diagnosable by other means. Pneumothorax and bleeding are encountered in a substantial number of patients following this procedure.

Sputum studies

Gross, microscopic, and bacteriologic examination of the sputum are important in the etiologic diagnosis of many respiratory diseases. The color, odor, and presence of blood provide valuable clues. Microscopic examination may reveal the causative organism in many bacterial pneumonias, in tuberculosis, and in some fungus infections. Exfoliative cell studies of the sputum may also be helpful in the diagnosis of lung carcinoma. The best time for collection of sputum is shortly after awakening, since abnormal bronchial secretions tend to accumulate during sleep. Sometimes it is necessary to induce sputum production by the use of a nebulizer. Considerable quantities of sputum are also unknowingly swallowed. In such patients, the gastric contents are aspirated in order to obtain sputum. This procedure is carried out shortly after the patient awakens in the morning after a period of fasting.

PHYSIOLOGIC METHODS: PULMONARY FUNCTION TESTS

During the past generation, numerous tests and techniques related to the study of respiratory physiology have evolved. These pulmonary function tests fall into two broad categories: those related to ventilatory func-

tion of the lungs and chest wall and those related to gas exchange. Ventilatory function tests include measurements of lung volumes under static and dynamic conditions as well as pressure measurements. Tests related to gas exchange include analysis of gases in the expired air and in the blood. Blood gas measurements of the arterial blood commonly include the PO_2, PCO_2, and the pH and reflect cardiopulmonary physiology.

Pulmonary function tests are becoming an increasingly important part of routine clinical evaluation and are taking their place among other diagnostic aids such as the chest x-ray and electrocardiogram. It is important to realize, however, that these tests only show the effects of disease on function and cannot be used to give a diagnosis on the basis of a pathologic change. Some diseases, however, do have a characteristic pattern of disordered function, and it is possible to distinguish an obstructive pattern of ventilatory abnormality from a restrictive pattern. Obstructive ventilatory disorders affect the ability to exhale, while restrictive disorders affect the ability to inhale. Two major patterns of functional disorders which also emerge based on blood measurements are disorders in which there is increased dead space or shunting.

It is essential to realize that no single test of pulmonary function can measure all possible attributes. Nevertheless, pulmonary function tests do give valuable information. Ventilatory function tests give quantitative data so that the progress of a lung disease, as well as response to treatment, may be followed. In cases of pulmonary disability in which surgery is planned, such tests help to assess the patient's ability to tolerate

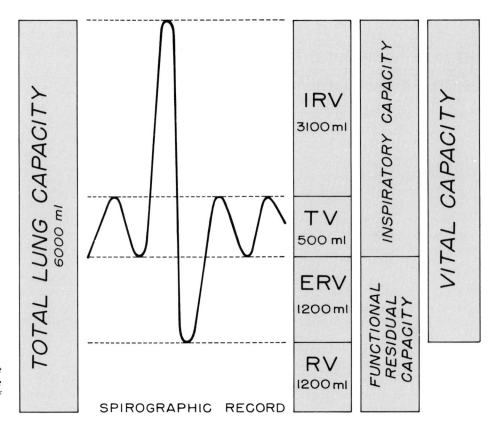

FIGURE 31-1 Relationship on the lung volumes and capacities (see Table 31-1 for explanation of symbols).

anesthetics, narcotics, or the removal of lung tissue and help to prescribe the postoperative care needed. Since only one aspect of pulmonary function may be altered by some diseases, these studies occasionally assist in establishing the diagnosis. Blood gas measurements are an invaluable aid in assessing the severity of respiratory insufficiency and guiding the appropriate therapy. In this chapter, discussion will be confined to those tests of pulmonary function which are most widely used and most helpful in patient management.

Ventilatory function tests

STATIC LUNG VOLUMES

Lung volumes and capacities are anatomic measurements that are affected by exercise and disease. There are four lung volumes and four lung capacities. Lung capacities always consist of two or more lung volumes. The relationships of these measurements and the average values for a young, healthy, adult male are shown in Fig. 31-1. Symbols and a description of the lung capacities and volumes are listed in Table 31-1.

The following five lung capacities and volumes can be measured directly on an instrument called the spirometer: V_T, IRV, ERV, VC, and IC. The FRC is measured by indirect means using helium or nitrogen gases. The TLC and RV are then derived arithmetically (i.e., TLC = FRC + IC and RV = TLC − VC).

A spirometer is a simple instrument containing a bellows or bell which is displaced as the patient breaths into it through a valve and connecting tube as shown in Fig. 31-2. As the spirometer is used, a graphic record of the measurement is made on a rotating drum with a recording pen.

Measurements of the static lung volumes in practice

are used to reflect the elastic properties of the lungs and thorax. The most useful measurements are VC, TLC, FRC, and RV. These volumes are reduced by diseases which limit lung expansion (restrictive disorders). In contrast, diseases which cause airways obstruction may cause an increase in TLC, FRC, and RV as a result of hyperinflation of the lungs.

DYNAMIC LUNG VOLUMES AND THE WORK OF BREATHING

Much more information can be obtained concerning the ventilatory status if the rate of air movement in and out of the lungs is considered as well as the work of breathing. The following definitions will be useful in the discussion of effective ventilation:

Minute volume or *minute ventilation* ($\dot{V}_E$) is the volume of air which is breathed in during inspiration or out during expiration during a 1-minute time period. It may be calculated by multiplying the V_T times respiratory rate. At rest $\dot{V}_E$ is about 6 liters/ minute. The minute volume is measured by collecting expired air in a large rubber balloon and dividing the volume collected by the number of minutes taken to collect the sample. The subscript E in the symbol for minute volume means that the measurement is made of the expiratory phase of the tidal volume, and the dot over the V indicates that it is a timed measurement.

Respiratory frequency (f) is the number of breaths taken per minute. At rest the respiratory rate is about 15 breaths per minute.

TABLE 31-1
Lung capacities and volumes

MEASUREMENT	SYMBOL	ADULT MALE AVERAGE VALUE	DESCRIPTION
Tidal volume	V_T	500 ml	Amount of air inhaled or exhaled with each breath (value listed is for resting conditions)
Inspiratory reserve volume	IRV	3100 ml	Amount of air that can be forcefully inhaled after taking a normal tidal volume inhalation
Expiratory reserve volume	ERV	1200 ml	Amount of air that can be forcefully exhaled after taking a normal tidal volume exhalation
Residual volume	RV	1200 ml	Amount of air left in the lungs after a forced exhalation
Total lung capacity	TLC	6000 ml	Maximum amount of air that can be contained in the lungs after a maximum inspiratory effort: TLC = V_T + IRV + ERV + RV
Vital capacity	VC	4800 ml	Maximum amount of air that can be expired after a maximum inspiration: VC = V_T + IRV + ERV (should be 80% TLC)
Inspiratory capacity	IC	3600 ml	Maximum amount of air that can be inspired after a normal expiration: IC = V_T + IRV
Functional residual capacity	FRC	2400 ml	Volume of air remaining in the lungs after a normal tidal volume expiration: FRC = ERV + RV

Source: J. H. Comroe, Jr., et al., *The Lung*, 2d ed., Yearbook, Chicago, 1962.

Tidal volume (V_T) is the amount of air inhaled or exhaled with each breath. V_T is about 500 ml at rest but may increase to 3000 ml during exercise when deep breaths are taken. It is obtained by dividing the minute volume by the respiratory rate.

Physiologic dead space (V_D) is the volume of inspired air that does not exchange with pulmonary blood; it may be regarded as wasted ventilation. Physiologic dead space is composed of anatomic dead space (the volume of air in the conducting airways, about 1 ml/lb of body weight), alveolar dead space (alveoli being ventilated but not perfused; the alveolar dead space is highly variable), and ventilation in excess of perfusion. In healthy individuals, the physiologic dead space is only slightly greater than the anatomic dead space, but it may be increased if ventilated alveoli are underperfused or not perfused at all, as is the case in pulmonary embolism. The ratio of dead space to tidal volume (V_D/V_T) reflects the portion of the tidal volume that does not exchange with pulmonary blood. In other words, it is a measurement of the percentage of the tidal volume that is physiologic dead space. This ratio is calculated by data collected by measuring the PCO_2 in the expired air and the PCO_2 in the arterial blood. The larger the difference between these two measurements, the greater the physiologic dead space. The V_D/V_T ratio does not exceed 30 to 40 percent in the healthy person. This ratio is frequently used to follow the course of patients receiving mechanical ventilation.

Alveolar ventilation ($\dot{V}_A$) is the volume of fresh air entering the alveoli each minute that exchanges with pulmonary blood; it is the effective ventilation. It is

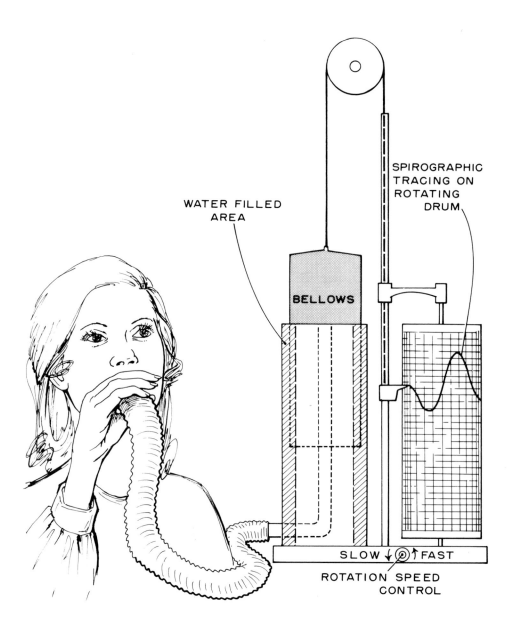

WATER FILLED
AREA

BELLOWS

SPIROGRAPHIC
TRACING ON
ROTATING
DRUM

SLOW ↓ ⊙ ↑ FAST
ROTATION SPEED
CONTROL

FIGURE 31-2 Spirometer.

normally about 4.2 liters/minute at rest. Alveolar ventilation is calculated using this formula: $\dot{V}_A = (V_T - V_D) \times f$.

Alveolar ventilation is a better index of ventilation than minute volume or tidal volume since it takes into account the volume of air wasted in ventilating the physiologic dead space. The calculations in Table 31-2 illustrate the relationships between minute ventilation, breathing pattern, and effective alveolar ventilation. The physiologic dead space for each of the three patients will be assumed to be constant at 150 ml, while the rate and depth of breathing is varied.

Several deductions can be made from the data in Table 31-2. In each case the total amount of air entering and leaving the lungs is the same (the minute volume), although there is great variation in the percentage of the tidal volume which is physiologic dead space and in the effective ventilation. It is evident that rapid, shallow breathing results in less effective ventilation as more is wasted in dead space volume. This fact becomes obvious if one considers the formula for the calculation of alveolar ventilation. As tidal volume approaches the physiologic dead-space volume (150 ml), effective ventilation approaches zero regardless of how rapid the respiratory rate ($0 \times f = 0$). The percentage of the tidal volume which is physiologic dead space also approaches 100 percent as the tidal volume approaches the dead-space volume. When the fact that total physiologic dead space can vary greatly with disease is also considered, it is obvious that clinical observation of ventilatory adequacy has great limitations even though some gross qualitative judgments can be made.

In order for air to move in and out of the lungs, the body must work to overcome the combined resistances of the thorax, lungs, and abdomen. The work (in the form of energy expenditure to move the chest bellows) is referred to as the *work of breathing*. The work of breathing can be expressed as the amount of oxygen consumed by the respiratory muscles. In the normal person at rest, this is a small fraction (less than 5 percent) of the total body oxygen consumption, although in disease the proportion may be much greater.

Expenditure of energy is required to overcome two types of resistances: elastic and nonelastic. The *elastic resistance* is the resistance to stretch caused by the elastic properties of the lungs and thorax. The elastic properties of the thorax result from the stretching properties of the tendons, muscles, and connective tissue. The elastic properties of the lungs are produced by the surface tension of fluid lining the alveoli and by the elastic fibers throughout the lung itself. *Nonelastic*

resistance is the frictional resistance to air flow in the airways and, to a small degree, resistance resulting from the viscosity of the lung tissues. The work of breathing increases if there is an increase in either the elastic resistance (e.g., "stiff lungs" as in pulmonary fibrosis) or in the nonelastic resistance (e.g., turbulent air flow in emphysema as a result of narrowing of the airways).

Compliance (C) is a measure of the elastic properties (distensibility) of the lungs and thorax and is defined as the change in volume per unit change in pressure under static conditions. Total compliance (compliance of the lungs and thorax) or lung compliance alone can be determined. Two manometers are used to measure pressure changes: one is connected to the mouth or nostril (to measure alveolar pressure or the total pressure exerted by the lung-thorax system) and the other is connected to an esophageal balloon (to measure intrapleural pressure). Volume and pressure changes are then measured under various degrees of lung inflation and breath-holding. Compliance is estimated by calculating the slope of the pressure–volume curve which is plotted from the data. Normal lung compliance and thoracic cage compliance are each about 0.2 liter/cmH_2O, and total compliance (lungs and thoracic cage) is about 0.1 liter/cmH_2O.

$$\text{Compliance (C)} = \frac{\Delta V \text{ (change in lung volume in liters)}}{\Delta P \text{ (change in pressure in centimeters of water)}}$$

Compliance is reduced in restrictive patterns of pulmonary disease which increase the stiffness of the lung or thorax and limit expansion. In these cases, a greater force (ΔP) than normal is required to give the same increase in volume (ΔV), causing the compliance to be smaller. Common causes of decreased lung compliance are atelectasis (collapse of alveoli), pulmonary edema, pneumonia, and pulmonary fibrosis. When pulmonary surfactant is decreased, compliance is also decreased because the lung becomes stiffer as a result of the increase in surface tension (surfactant normally reduces surface tension). Chest wall compliance is reduced in obesity, abdominal distention, and bony deformities of the chest cage such as kyphoscoliosis.

The nonelastic airway resistance can be measured by placing an individual in an airtight box (body plethysmograph) and measuring the pressure around the body

TABLE 31-2
Effective ventilation and respiratory pattern

PATIENT	V_D	V_T	f	$\dot{V}_E = V_T \times f$	$\dot{V}_A = (V_T - V_D) \times f$	V_D/V_T
Patient A (rapid, shallow breathing)	150 ml	250 ml	40	10 liters/min	4 liters/min	60%
Patient B (normal rate and depth)	150 ml	500 ml	20	10 liters/min	7 liters/min	30%
Patient C (slow, deep breathing)	150 ml	1000 ml	10	10 liters/min	8½ liters/min	15%

(which reflects the change in alveolar pressure); at the same time the rate of the flow of air at the mouth is measured. More commonly, however, nonelastic resistance is estimated by measuring forced expiratory volumes and flow rates. This measurement is made on a spirometer or by a portable hand unit which can be used at the bedside. The following volumes of air are measured by the spirometer:

Forced vital capacity (FVC) is the vital capacity measurement performed with expiration as forceful and rapid as possible. This volume of air is normally about the same as the vital capacity but may be significantly reduced in patients with airway obstruction because of premature closure of the small airways and the consequent trapping of air.

Forced expiratory volume (FEV) is the volume of air that can be exhaled in a standard time period during the FVC maneuver. Usually the FEV is measured during the first second of the forced exhalation; this is termed FEV_1. The FEV is a very useful index of the impairment of ventilatory capacity and values of less than 1 liter during the first second indicate severe impairment of ventilatory function.

The FEV should always be related to the FVC or VC. Normal individuals can expire about 80 percent of their vital capacity in 1 second, expressed as the FEV_1/FVC ratio. It makes little difference whether FVC or VC is used for the ratio; the result is about the same. This ratio is of great value in differentiating between diseases which cause airway obstruction and those that cause restriction of lung expansion. In obstructive diseases such as chronic bronchitis and emphysema, there is a greater reduction in FEV_1 than in the vital capacity (vital capacity may be normal), so that the FEV_1/FVC ratio is less than 80 percent. In a restrictive disease of the lung parenchyma such as sarcoidosis, both the FEV_1 and the FVC or VC are reduced in about the same proportion, and the FEV_1/FVC ratio remains at about 80 percent or greater.

The overall effects on alterations in the elastic and

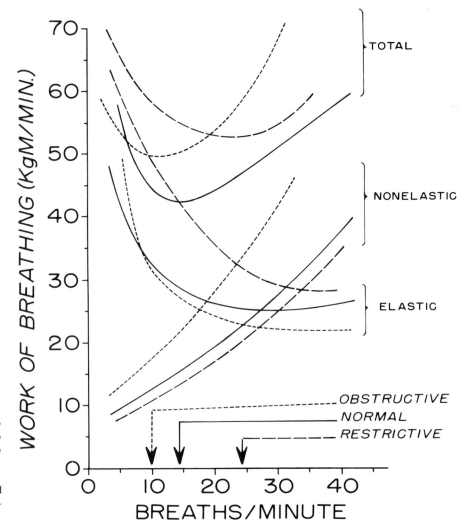

FIGURE 31-3 Relationship between the mechanical work of breathing and the respiratory pattern in health and in pulmonary disease. (Modified from R. M. Cherniack, L. Cherniack, and A. Naimark, Respiration in Health and Disease, 2d ed., Saunders, Philadelphia, 1972, p. 48.)

nonelastic properties of the lungs can be assessed by a simple test which measures the *maximum breathing capacity* (MBC) or the *maximum voluntary ventilation* (MVV). The MVV or MBC can be estimated directly by having the patient breathe as rapidly and deeply as possible for 15 seconds and collecting the expired air in a Douglas bag. This volume is multiplied by 4 to determine the minute volume in liters per minute. MBC can be affected by changes in compliance because of the increased muscular effort required. It is also affected by changes in airway resistance because of the increased turbulence resulting from airway collapse when breathing at high speeds. The healthy, young male adult can move as much as 170 liters of air per minute compared to a minute volume of about 6 liters/minute at rest. The difference represents the pulmonary reserve, which is very large in the young, healthy adult. The pulmonary reserve is reduced in both restrictive and obstructive disease but much more in the latter.

As already stated, less than 5 percent of the total oxygen consumption is expended for the work of breathing in the normal person at rest. The oxygen cost of breathing is greatly increased in both obstructive and restrictive patterns of pulmonary disease. The patient with emphysema (increased airways resistance) or the person who is very obese (restriction of chest movement) may consume 25 percent or more of the total inspired oxygen for the work of breathing. In severe disease, fatigue may be an important factor in the development of respiratory failure because of the increased muscular effort required for the work of breathing.

There is also a relationship between the mechanical work of breathing and the respiratory pattern (rate and depth of breathing). Respiratory physiologists have demonstrated that for any given alveolar ventilation, there is an optimum respiratory rate and tidal volume at which the total work of breathing is minimal. The graphs in Fig. 31-3 show the relationship between the mechanical work of breathing (including the total work and the elastic and nonelastic work), expressed in kilogram-meters, and the respiratory frequency. The principle illustrated is applied to normal persons as well as to those with pulmonary disease. The total work is the sum of the elastic and nonelastic work. (As you should recall, elastic work is expended to overcome the elastic resistances of the lungs and thorax, and nonelastic work is expended to overcome flow resistance and tissue viscous resistance.) In the normal person at rest, at a particular alveolar ventilation, the total work of breathing is least at about 15 breaths per minute (illustrated by the solid lines in Fig. 31-3). At the same alveolar ventilation, rapid, shallow breathing results in the least amount of work for the patient with a restrictive pulmonary disorder (increased elastic work) such as pneumonia or obesity (long dashed lines in Fig. 31-3). This pattern probably occurs because small increments in tidal volume greatly increase the elastic resistance. However, if the pattern of breathing becomes too rapid and shallow, the dead-space volume becomes disproportionately high. On the other hand, the person with an obstructive

pulmonary disorder (increased nonelastic work) such as might occur in emphysema, adopts a slow, deep pattern of respiration (short dashed lines in Fig. 31-3). This pattern is adopted because a higher flow rate is likely to increase the amount of work to overcome resistance to airflow. In fact, if the patient with obstructive disease should voluntarily hyperventilate to blow off more carbon dioxide, the PCO_2 might actually rise as a result of its increased production from the increased mechanical work of breathing.

Blood gas analysis

In order to assess respiratory function adequately, it is necessary to look beyond the lung to the volume and distribution of gas transport by the circulatory system. The factors which affect gas transport and removal between the lungs and tissue cells have already been discussed in Chap. 30. In this chapter, the technique used for the collection of blood to measure the blood gases and some general guidelines for the interpretation of measurements are presented.

Usually a sample of arterial blood is used for the blood gas analysis. Figure 31-4 demonstrates the correct technique for drawing a blood sample. The radial artery is often chosen because of its accessibility. The wrist is extended by positioning it over a rolled towel. After the skin has been sterilized, the artery is stabilized with two fingers of one hand while the arterial puncture is made using a heparinized syringe with the other hand. After drawing up 5 ml of blood into the syringe, air is removed, and the blood is placed on ice and taken immediately to the blood gas laboratory for analysis. This procedure is commonly performed by the intensive care nurse. Table 31-3 lists the normal values for the arterial blood gases.

The P_aCO_2 is the best index of alveolar ventilation. When the P_aCO_2 rises, the direct cause is always generalized alveolar hypoventilation. Hypoventilation causes respiratory acidosis and a fall in the pH of the blood. Alveolar hypoventilation may occur if the tidal volume is decreased (the dead-space effect) as occurs in rapid, shallow breathing. Hypoventilation may also occur if the

TABLE 31-3
Normal values for the arterial blood gases

BLOOD GAS MEASUREMENT	SYMBOL	NORMAL VALUE
Carbon dioxide tension	P_aCO_2	36–44 mmHg (average = 40)
Oxygen tension	P_aO_2	85–100 mmHg
Oxygen percent saturation	S_aO_2	97%
Hydrogen ion concentration	pH	7.35–7.45

respiratory rate is decreased as it is in narcotic or barbiturate drug overdose. The P_aCO_2 may also rise to compensate for a metabolic alkalosis. Consequently, in order to interpret the P_aCO_2 correctly, one must also consider the blood pH and bicarbonate levels to determine if a change is due to a primary respiratory condition or is compensatory for a metabolic condition.

The direct cause of a lowered P_aCO_2 is always alveolar hyperventilation. Hyperventilation causes respiratory alkalosis and a rise in the pH of the blood. Hyperventilation is common in asthma and pneumonia and represents an effort to raise the P_aO_2 at the expense of excreting excess CO_2 from the lungs. Hyperventilation may also be caused by brain injury or tumor, anxiety, or may be compensatory for metabolic acidosis. Table 31-4 summarizes the acid–base changes in compensated

TABLE 31-4
Acid–base changes in acidosis and alkalosis

ACID–BASE DISTURBANCE	pH	HCO₃⁻	P_aCO_2
Respiratory acidosis	↓	↑	↑
Respiratory alkalosis	↑	↓	↓
Metabolic acidosis	↓	↓	↓
Metabolic alkalosis	↑	↑	↑

acidosis and alkalosis. The heavy arrows indicate the primary disorder. The change in the bicarbonate level represents the kidneys' attempt to compensate for the respiratory acidosis or alkalosis, while the change in the P_aCO_2 in the metabolic disorders represent the lung's role in compensation. The purpose of the compensation is to return the blood pH to normal.

When the P_aO_2 falls below the normal value, hypoxemia is the result. P_aO_2 levels fall slightly with age, so that it is normal for persons over the age of 60 years to have a P_aO_2 as low as 70 mmHg. In severe respiratory failure, the P_aO_2 may fall to 30 to 40 mmHg. Hypoxemia resulting from respiratory disease is caused by one or more of the following mechanisms: (1) ventilation–perfusion imbalance (most common cause), (2) alveolar hypoventilation, (3) impaired diffusion, or (4) intrapulmonary anatomic shunts. Hypoxemia resulting from the first three abnormalities can be corrected by administering oxygen. However, the intrapulmonary anatomic shunt (arteriovenous shunt) cannot be corrected by oxygen therapy.

Changes in the blood gases are critical measurements in the diagnosis of respiratory or ventilatory failure which may be insidious in onset. Respiratory insufficiency exists when the P_aO_2 falls below the normal values, and respiratory failure exists when the P_aO_2 falls to 50 mmHg. The P_aCO_2 may be increased or decreased below the normal values in respiratory insufficiency or failure. Respiratory failure will be discussed in greater detail in Chap. 35.

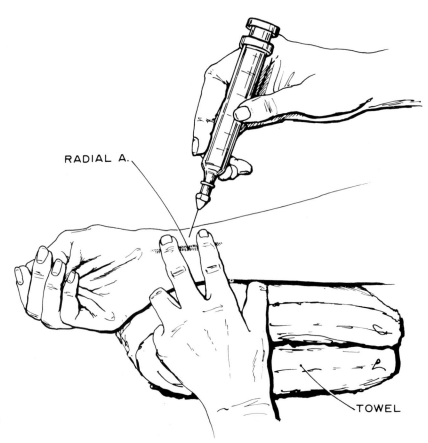

FIGURE 31-4 Radial artery puncture technique for obtaining blood for blood gases.

Some of the common changes in ventilatory function and blood gases in restrictive and obstructive patterns of pulmonary disease are summarized in Table 31-5.

QUESTIONS

Diagnostic procedures in respiratory disease—Chap. 31

Directions: Answer the following questions on a separate sheet of paper.

1 List five radiologic methods commonly used to detect pulmonary disease.

2 List four distinct features that are depicted on a routine chest x-ray.

Directions: Circle the letter which correctly answers the question.

3 Which of the following diagnostic methods is *not* used to detect pulmonary disease and adequacy of pulmonary function?
  a Blood gas measurements *b* Ventilatory function tests *c* Intravenous pyelogram *d* Fluoroscopy

Directions: Match each of the diagnostic tests in col. A to its description in col. B.

Column A
4 ____ Bronchography
5 ____ Angiography of pulmonary vessels

Column B
a Most accurate method of diagnosing pulmonary embolism
b Used to obtain informa-

6 ____ Fluoroscopy
7 ____ Perfusion lung scan
8 ____ Percutaneous needle biopsy of lung
9 ____ Bronchoscopy
10 ____ Sputum studies

tion about how various zones of the lung behave during the respiratory cycle
c Reveals the size and appearance of the tracheobronchial tree; useful in confirming the diagnosis of bronchiectasis
d Closed technique for obtaining lung biopsy specimen
e Useful technique to obtain biopsy specimen under direct visualization
f Involves the injection of albumen microspheres tagged with an isotope in a peripheral vein
g Specimen may be obtained by aspiration of gastric contents

Directions: Match each of the diagnostic procedures in col. A to the potential hazards and precautions in col. B. Letters in col. B may be used more than once.

Column A
11 ____ Fluoroscopy
12 ____ Bronchography
13 ____ Bronchoscopic biopsy
14 ____ Perfusion and ventilation scan
15 ____ Pulmonary angiography
16 ____ Lung biopsy by open and closed techniques

Column B
a Food and fluids are withheld after this exam until the gag reflex returns
b The major risk during this procedure is the development of a cardiac arrhythmia
c Safer procedure for the diagnosis of pulmonary embolism though less definitive
d Excess radiation is the chief hazard associated with this procedure
e Percussion and postural drainage should follow this procedure
f Pneumothorax and bleeding are possible complications
g Laryngospasm or edema is a possible complication following this procedure

TABLE 31-5
Changes in ventilatory function as a result of pulmonary disease

TEST	OBSTRUCTIVE PATTERN	RESTRICTIVE PATTERN
RV (residual volume)	↑	↓
FRC (functional residual capacity)	↑	↓
TLC (total lung capacity)	N or ↑	↓
VC (vital capacity)*	N or ↓	↓
FVC (forced vital capacity)	N or ↓	↓
MBC (maximum breathing capacity)	↓	N or ↓
$FEV_{1.0}$†	↓	N or ↓
FEV_1/FVC	↓ (<80%)	N or ↑ (>80%)
C (compliance)	N or ↑ (slight)	↓
P_aO_2	↓	N (↓↓ exercise)
P_aCO_2	↑	N or ↓
pH	↓ (during exacerbations)	N or ↑

Key: N = normal; ↓ = decreased or tends to decrease; ↑ = increased or tends to increase
*Useful test to monitor progress of restrictive lung disease.
†Most useful test to monitor progress of obstructive lung disease.
Source: John Crofton and Andrew Douglas, *Respiratory Diseases*, Blackwell, Oxford, England, 1969.

Directions: Answer the following questions on a separate sheet of paper.

17 Describe the role of ventilatory function tests and blood gas analysis in the diagnosis and treatment of

pulmonary disorders. Are any of these tests specifically diagnostic?

18 Explain why alveolar ventilation is a better index of effective ventilation than minute volume or tidal volume.

19 Describe the procedure for the measurement of compliance of the lungs and thoracic cage. How is compliance calculated from the measurements?

20 List three common causes of decreased lung compliance and three causes of decreased chest wall compliance.

21 Why does a patient with emphysema adopt a slow, deep pattern of respiration?

22 What breathing pattern might a patient with normal airways resistance but very stiff lungs (low compliance) adopt? Why?

23 Describe the correct technique for the collection of blood in the measurement of arterial blood gases.

24 List three causes of alveolar hyperventilation and hypoventilation.

25 List four causes of hypoxemia. Which one is not corrected by oxygen administration?

Directions: Circle T if the statement is true and F if it is false.

26   T   F   Rapid, shallow breathing results in less effective ventilation because the respiratory rate is greater than the normal rate per minute.

27   T   F   The ratio of physiologic dead space to tidal volume does *not* normally exceed 30 to 40 percent.

28   T   F   Alveolar ventilation in a 120-lb female with a tidal volume of 200 ml and a respiratory rate of 30 breaths per minute is about 6 liters/minute.

29   T   F   The work of breathing refers to the form of energy expenditure required to move the chest bellows (the amount of oxygen consumed by the respiratory muscles).

30   T   F   Elastic properties of the lungs are the result of the surface tension of fluid lining the alveoli and the elastic fibers throughout the lung.

31   T   F   The maximum breathing capacity test is a good test to measure pulmonary reserve.

32   T   F   Nonelastic resistances consist of the frictional resistance to flow in the airways.

Directions: Circle the letter preceding each item below that correctly answers each question. More than one answer may be correct.

33 The primary lung volume which measures the amount of air inhaled or exhaled with each breath is the:
a Tidal volume (V_T) b Expiratory reserve volume (ERV) c Inspiratory reserve volume (IRV) d Residual volume (RV)

34 The lung capacity which measures the maximum volume of air that can be expired after a maximum inspiratory effort is the:
a Total lung capacity (TLC) b Vital capacity (VC) c Inspiratory capacity (IC) d Functional residual capacity (FRC)

35 Which of the following combinations of lung capacities and volumes can be measured directly by the spirometer?
a V_T, TLC, RV, IC b FRC, TLC, ERV, VC c V_T, IRV, ERV, VC, IC

36 In healthy young persons, the 1-second forced expiratory volume/forced vital capacity ratio is approximately:
a 30 percent b 50 percent c 80 percent d 100 percent

37 The normal range for P_aCO_2 is:
a 22–30 mmHg b 36–44 mmHg c 50–62 mmHg d 85–100 mmHg

38 Alveolar hypoventilation can be readily diagnosed by measuring the:
a P_aO_2 b pH of the arterial blood c Respiratory rate d P_aCO_2 e Tidal volume

39 Physiologic dead space can be increased by:
a Enlargement of the anatomic dead space b Pulmonary units with high ventilation/perfusion ratios c Pulmonary units with low ventilation/perfusion ratios

40 Laboratory test results which indicate adequate compensation for a respiratory acidosis are:
a Increase in pH towards 7.4 b Decrease in the serum bicarbonate c Increase in the serum bicarbonate

Directions: Match each of the pulmonary functions in col. A to its definition in col. B.

Column A	Column B
41 _____ FVC	a The carbon dioxide tension in the arterial blood
42 _____ $FEV_{1.0}$	
43 _____ V_D/V_T	b The volume of air exchanged in the airway in one minute
44 _____ $\dot{V}_A$	
45 _____ $\dot{V}_E$	c The volume of air expired during the first second of the forced vital capacity maneuver
46 _____ P_aCO_2	
	d The proportion of tidal volume that is physiologic dead space
	e The effective ventilation per minute
	f Expiration performed as rapidly and as forcefully as possible following a maximum inspiration

47 Indicate the common changes in ventilatory function and blood gases in restrictive and obstructive patterns of pulmonary disease by filling in the blanks in Table 31-6. Use the following key: N = normal, ↓ = decreased, ↑ = increased.

TABLE 31-6
Changes in ventilatory function as a result of pulmonary disease

TEST	OBSTRUCTIVE PATTERN	RESTRICTIVE PATTERN
Residual volume		
Functional residual capacity		
Total lung capacity		
Vital capacity		
Forced vital capacity		
Maximum breathing capacity		
FEV_1		
FEV_1/FVC		
Compliance		
P_aO_2		
P_aCO_2		
pH		

BIBLIOGRAPHY

BURROWS, B., R. J. KNUDSON, and L. J. KETTEL: *Respiratory Insufficiency*, Yearbook, Chicago, 1975, pp. 25–38, 67–73.

CHERNIACK, R. M., L. CHERNIACK, and A. NAIMARK: *Respiration in Health and Disease*, 2d ed., Saunders, Philadelphia, 1972, pp. 1–51, 140–163, 263–300.

COMROE, JULIUS H., JR., et al.: *The Lung*, 2d ed., Yearbook, Chicago, 1962.

GESCHICKTER, C. F.: *The Lung in Health and Disease*, Lippincott, Philadelphia, 1973, pp. 43–62.

SHAPIRO, B. A.: *Clinical Application of Blood Gases*, Yearbook, Chicago, 1973.

WEST, J. B.: *Respiratory Physiology*, Williams & Wilkins, Baltimore, 1974.

CHAPTER 32   Cardinal Signs and Symptoms of Respiratory Disease

OBJECTIVES   **At the completion of Chap. 32, you should be able to:**

1 Describe the following cardinal signs and symptoms of respiratory disease: cough (causes, importance, and types); sputum (cause of excessive secretion, source, color, and consistency); hemoptysis (detection, cause, and importance); dyspnea (causes, classification, and significance); chest pain (type and description); digital clubbing (causes, detection, and significance); cyanosis (types, detection, causes, and importance).

2 Differentiate between hypoxemia and hypoxia.

3 List the laboratory findings associated with hypoxia.

4 List the clinical signs associated with hypoxia in the cardiovascular, respiratory, and central nervous systems.

5 Identify skin changes associated with hypoxia.

6 Differentiate between hypercapnia and hypocapnia.

Pulmonary diseases may give rise to both respiratory and general signs and symptoms. Respiratory signs and symptoms include cough, excessive or abnormal sputum, hemoptysis, dyspnea, and chest pain. General signs and symptoms include cyanosis, digital clubbing, and other manifestations related to inadequate gas exchange. The reader is referred to other textbooks for a discussion of adventitious chest sounds and systematic assessment of the respiratory status.

COUGH

Coughing is a protective reflex caused by irritation of the tracheobronchial tree. The ability to cough is an important mechanism in clearing the lower airways, and many adults normally cough a few times upon first arising to clear the trachea and pharynx of secretions which have accumulated during sleep. Coughing is also the most common symptom of respiratory disease. Any cough persisting for longer than 3 weeks should be investigated to determine the cause.

Stimuli that commonly produce a cough are mechanical, chemical, and inflammatory. Inhalation of smoke, dust, and small foreign bodies is the most common cause of cough. Smokers often have a chronic cough as a result of inhaling foreign bodies (smoke) and chronic inflammation of the airways. Mechanical stimulation from tumors either extrinsic or intrinsic to the airways are another cause of cough (the most common tumor causing cough is bronchogenic carcinoma). Any inflammatory process of the airways with or without exudate may produce a cough. Chronic bronchitis, tuberculosis, and pneumonia typically have coughing as a prominent symptom. A cough may be productive, hacking and nonproductive, brassy (as when there is pressure on the trachea), frequent, infrequent, or paroxysmal (intermittent coughing episodes).

SPUTUM

The normal adult produces about 100 ml of mucus in the respiratory tract per day. This mucus is transported to the pharynx by the normal cleansing actions of the cilia that line the airways. When excess mucus is formed, the normal process of removal may be ineffective and result in the accumulation of mucus. When this occurs, the mucous membrane is stimulated, and the mucus is coughed up as sputum. Excess mucus production may be caused by physical, chemical, or infective insults to the mucous membrane.

Whenever a patient produces sputum, it is important to observe its source, color, volume, and consistency. Sputum produced by "hawking" is most likely to have originated in the sinuses or nasal passages rather than in the lower respiratory tract. Profuse purulent sputum suggests the presence of a suppurative process such as lung abscess, while sputum production which gradually increases over a period of years suggests chronic bronchitis or bronchiectasis.

The color of sputum is also important. Yellow sputum indicates an infection. Green sputum is indicative of stagnant pus. The green color is produced by the presence of verdoperoxidase, which is liberated from polymorphonuclear leukocytes (PMNs) in the sputum. Green sputum is common in bronchiectasis because of the stagnation of sputum in dilated, infected bronchioles. Many patients with lower respiratory tract infection report having green sputum early in the morning, which becomes yellow as the day progresses. This is probably caused by the accumulation of purulent sputum during the night, with the consequent release of verdoperoxidase.

The character and consistency of sputum also yields useful information. Pink, frothy sputum is characteristic of acute pulmonary edema. Sputum may be mucoid, sticky, and grey or white in color in chronic bronchitis. A foul odor to the sputum may indicate a lung abscess or bronchiectasis.

HEMOPTYSIS

Varying amounts of blood may be mixed with sputum, or blood may comprise the entire expectorate. Hemoptysis is the term applied to the expectoration of both pure blood and blood-streaked sputum. Any process resulting in the interruption of the continuity of the pulmonary blood vessels may result in bleeding. The expectoration of pure blood is a serious symptom. It may be the first manifestation of active tuberculosis. Other common causes of hemoptysis are bronchogenic carcinoma, pulmonary infarction, and lung abscess. Blood-streaked sputum (which may be rust-colored) is a common feature of pneumococcal pneumonia. When blood or blood-streaked sputum is expectorated, it is important to determine that the source is actually the lower respiratory tract rather than the nasal passages or the gastrointestinal tract.

DYSPNEA

Dyspnea is a term used to designate awareness of difficulty in breathing and is a cardinal symptom of cardiopulmonary disease. A patient suffering from dyspnea is likely to experience shortness of breath or a sensation of suffocation. Dyspnea is by no means always an indication of disease; the normal person commonly experiences this sensation after varying degrees of physical exertion. The amount of exertion sufficient to induce dyspnea varies with age, sex, altitude, state of physical training, and emotional involvement in the task. Thus it is important to correlate dyspnea in an individual with the minimal level of activity sufficient for its induction. Dyspnea may occur (1) after moderate exertion such as climbing a flight of stairs, (2) after a short walk, (3) after light activities such as talking, bathing, or shaving, (4) at rest, and (5) while lying down (orthopnea). The key factor which seems to determine whether or not dyspnea is experienced is whether the level of ventilation or effort is appropriate to the degree of activity. The stimuli, sensory receptors, and nerve pathways by which the appropriateness is recognized have not been established with certainty.

Dyspnea is a prevalent symptom in diseases which affect the tracheobronchial tree, the lung parenchyma, and the pleural space. Dyspnea is commonly associated with pulmonary diseases in which there is increased respiratory work as a result of decreased ventilatory capacity. However, when the work of breathing is increased chronically, the patient may become accustomed to this and not experience dyspnea. Weak respiratory muscles may also result in dyspnea.

CHEST PAIN

There are many causes of chest pain, but the most characteristic pain of lung disease is that resulting from inflammation of the pleura (pleurisy). Only the parietal layer of the pleura is a source of pain, as the visceral pleura and the lung parenchyma are regarded as insensitive organs.

Typical pleurisy may develop gradually but is usually abrupt in onset. The pain occurs at the site of inflammation and is usually well localized. The pain is cutting and sharp in character, aggravated by coughing, sneezing, and deep breathing, so that the patient often adopts a pattern of rapid, shallow breathing and avoids unnecessary movement. The pain may be somewhat relieved by applying pressure (splinting) over the involved area. The most common causes of pleuritic pain are pulmonary infection or infarction, although such conditions may be present without pain.

DIGITAL CLUBBING

Digital clubbing is a peculiar change in the shape of the tips of the fingers and toes characterized by a bulbous appearance. It is a significant physical sign since it is associated with a number of serious conditions. Pulmonary disease (such as bronchogenic carcinoma, bronchiectasis, lung abscess, and pulmonary tuberculosis) is the most common cause of digital clubbing (70 to 80 percent of cases). Cardiovascular disease (such as congenital intracardiac shunting and subacute bacterial endocarditis) ranks second (10 to 15 percent of cases). Five to 10 percent of the cases of digital clubbing are associated with chronic diseases of the gastrointestinal tract, including the liver. The pathogenesis of digital clubbing is not understood. A popular hypothesis ascribes it to hypoxia, but this does not explain its presence in many entities. Clubbing often develops early in bronchogenic carcinoma and is not associated with arterial desaturation. It is curious that the chronic hypoxia of emphysema rarely seems to be associated with digital clubbing, while the chronic hypoxia of tetralogy of Fallot is often associated with severe clubbing.

It is important to detect clubbing as early as possible because of its diagnostic significance. The earliest sign is a loss of the angle between the nail and the dorsum of the terminal phalanx; this angle is normally 160°. The normal variations, early and advanced clubbing, may be seen in Fig. 32-1. In early clubbing the skin at the base of the nail may have a shiny appearance and gentle pressure on the nail root reveals a spongy feeling (floating nail). Normally the nail plate rests firmly against the bone. Early clubbing must be differentiated from the normal curved nail that is common in blacks. If one views the normal curved nail from the side, the base angle is still about 160°. In early clubbing, the base angle of the nail becomes greater than 160°. As the condition progresses, the tissue at the root of the nail becomes heaped up and the curvature of the nail becomes pronounced until the soft tissue of the digit tip becomes bulbous, producing the classic drumstick appearance.

SIGNS OF INADEQUATE GAS EXCHANGE

Cyanosis

Cyanosis is a bluish coloration of the skin and mucous membranes which develops as a result of an increase in the absolute amount of reduced hemoglobin (hemoglobin not united with oxygen). It may be a sign of respiratory insufficiency, although this is a highly unreliable indication. There are two types of cyanosis: central and peripheral. Central cyanosis resulting from insufficient oxygenation of hemoglobin in the lungs is most easily observed on the face, lips, and earlobes and under the tongue. Cyanosis is generally not detected until the absolute amount of reduced hemoglobin is 5 g% or more in a person with normal hemoglobin concentration. The normal amount of reduced hemoglobin in the capillary bed is 2.5 g%. In the person with a normal hemoglobin concentration, oxygen saturation is about 75 percent and the P_aO_2 is 50 mmHg or less when cyanosis is first detected. Anemic patients (low hemoglobin concentration) may never become cyanotic even though they have severe tissue hypoxia, because the absolute amount of

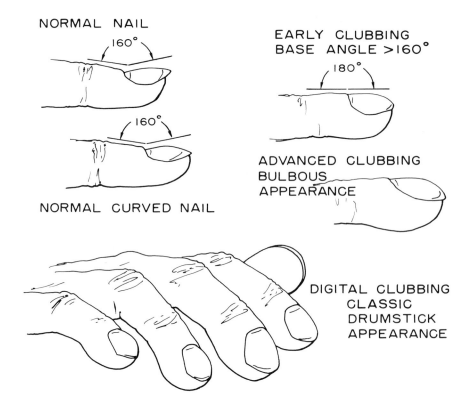

FIGURE 32-1 Digital clubbing.

reduced hemoglobin is not likely to reach 5 g%. On the other hand, a person with polycythemia (high hemoglobin concentration) can easily have 5 g% of reduced hemoglobin when there is only mild hypoxia. Other factors which make cyanosis difficult to recognize are variations in skin thickness, pigmentation, and lighting conditions.

In addition to cyanosis caused by respiratory insufficiency (central cyanosis), peripheral cyanosis occurs when severely reduced blood flow causes a great reduction in the venous saturation, thereby turning the area blue. Peripheral cyanosis may result from cardiac insufficiency, obstruction of blood flow, or vasoconstriction due to cold temperatures.

Cyanosis may also be produced by small amounts of circulating methemoglobin and by even smaller amounts of sulfhemoglobin, although these causes are uncommon. These variations in cause and the difficulty in recognizing cyanosis make it an unreliable sign of respiratory insufficiency.

Hypoxemia and hypoxia

The term "hypoxemia" refers to values of P_aO_2 which are abnormally low and is frequently associated with hypoxia, or inadequate tissue oxygenation. Hypoxemia is not necessarily accompanied by tissue hypoxia. One can have normal tissue oxygenation with hypoxemia, just as one can have a normal P_aO_2 with tissue hypoxia (because of the abnormalities of oxygen delivery and utilization by the cells, which were discussed in Chap. 30). There is a relationship, however, between the P_aO_2 and tissue hypoxia, although the precise P_aO_2 at which impairment of tissue utilization of oxygen occurs is variable. All things being equal, the more rapid the onset of hypoxemia, the more extensive the tissue abnormalities. In general, P_aO_2 values that are persistently less than 50 mmHg are associated with tissue hypoxia and acidosis (caused by anaerobic metabolism). Since hypoxia may exist with both normal and low values of P_aO_2, evaluation of blood gas measurements must always be correlated with clinical observation of the patient. Cyanosis, as has been concluded, is an unreliable sign of hypoxia because the oxygen saturation must be below 75 percent in persons with normal hemoglobin before it is detectable. Clinical signs and laboratory findings which indicate hypoxia are listed in Table 32-1.

Hypercapnia and hypocapnia

Just as ventilation is considered adequate when O_2 supply is matched with O_2 demand, so also must CO_2 elimination through the lungs be matched with CO_2 production for adequate ventilation. Because CO_2 is highly diffusible, the CO_2 tensions are equal in alveolar air and arterial blood; thus, P_aCO_2 is the direct and immediate reflection of the alveolar ventilation in relation to the metabolic rate. Adequate ventilation maintains the P_aCO_2 at about 40 mmHg. Hypercapnia is defined as a rise in the P_aCO_2 above 44 mmHg; hypocapnia occurs when the P_aCO_2 is less than 36 mmHg. The direct

cause of CO_2 retention is alveolar hypoventilation (ventilation inadequate to cope with CO_2 production). Hypercapnia is always accompanied by some degree of hypoxia when the patient is breathing room air.

The major causes of hypercapnia are obstructive airway disease, respiratory depressant drugs, weakness or paralysis of the respiratory muscles, chest trauma or abdominal surgery causing shallow respirations, and loss of lung tissue. Clinical signs associated with hypercapnia are mental confusion progressing to coma, headache (as a result of cerebral vasodilatation), asterixis or flapping tremor of the outstretched hands, and a pulse of large volume with warm, sweaty extremities (as a result of the peripheral vasodilatation caused by the hypercapnia). In chronic hypercapnia resulting from chronic pulmonary disease, the patient may become abnormally tolerant to the high P_aCO_2, so that the principal drive to respiration is hypoxia. Under these circumstances, if oxygen is administered at a high concentration, respiration is diminished, and the hypercapnia is increased.

Excessive loss of CO_2 from the lungs, hypocapnia, occurs when there is hyperventilation (ventilation in excess of metabolic need to remove CO_2). Common causes of hyperventilation were listed in Chap. 31 and include excessive mechanical ventilation, anxiety states, cerebral trauma, and as a compensatory response to

TABLE 32-1
Indicators of hypoxia

Laboratory findings	$P_aO_2 < 70$ mmHg $S_aO_2 < 90\%$ pH of blood < 7.35 $P_aCO_2 < 36$ mmHg if hyperventilation or > 44 mmHg if hypoventilation
Central nervous system	Mental confusion, bizarre behavior Restlessness; agitation Anxious facial expression; sweating Drowsiness progressing to coma when hypoxia severe
Cardiovascular	Tachycardia early; bradycardia later when heart muscle not receiving adequate oxygen Arrhythmias Rise in blood pressure followed by a drop when hypoxia remains uncorrected
Respiratory	Increased respiratory rate Dyspnea, yawning Use of accessory respiratory muscles; flared nostrils
Skin	Cyanosis of lips, oral mucosa, and nail beds

hypoxia. Signs and symptoms commonly associated with hypocapnia include frequent sighing and yawning, dizziness, palpitations, tingling and numbness in the extremities, and muscular twiches. Severe hypocapnia ($P_aCO_2 < 25$ mmHg) may cause convulsions.

QUESTIONS

Cardinal signs and symptoms of respiratory disease—Chap. 32

Directions: Match the signs and symptoms in col. B with the possible causative factor in col. A. Each letter may be used only once.

Column A

1 _____ Interruption in the continuity of the pulmonary blood vessels
2 _____ Inflammation of the pleura
3 _____ Increase in the absolute amount of reduced hemoglobin
4 _____ Physical, chemical or infectious insults to the mucous membrane of the respiratory tract
5 _____ Protective reflex initiated by irritation of the tracheobronchial tree
6 _____ Pathogenesis unknown; associated with early stage of bronchogenic carcinoma and with certain chronic respiratory, cardiovascular, and gastrointestinal diseases.
7 _____ Increased ventilatory work; must be correlated with the minimum level of activity sufficient for its induction

Column B

a Cough
b Excess sputum production
c Hemoptysis
d Dyspnea
e Digital clubbing
f Chest pain
g Cyanosis

Directions: Circle T if the statement is true and F if it is false. Correct the false statements.

8 T F Hypoxia refers to inadequate tissue oxygenation.

9 T F P_aO_2 values that are persistently less than 85 mmHg are associated with tissue hypoxia.

10 T F Cyanosis is a reliable sign of hypoxia.

11 T F Confusion, restlessness, and agitation are clinical signs that may indicate hypoxia.

12 T F Anemic patients frequently become cyanotic even with moderate degrees of hypoxemia.

13 T F The P_aCO_2 is the best index of alveolar ventilation adequacy.

14 T F Hypercapnia refers to a rise in the P_aCO_2 above 44 mmHg.

15 T F The direct cause of hypocapnia is alveolar hypoventilation.

16 T F Symptoms of headache, drowsiness, and asterixis are associated with hypercapnia.

Directions: Answer the following questions on a separate sheet of paper.

17 What is digital clubbing? Why is it important to detect?

18 How would you detect cyanosis in a black patient?

BIBLIOGRAPHY

Cough, sputum, hemoptysis

SKILLING, DAVID M.: "Cough, Hemoptysis," in C. M. MacBryde (ed.), *Signs and Symptoms* 3d ed., Lippincott, Philadelphia, 1957, pp. 321–348.

Dyspnea

BURROWS, B., R. J. KNUDSON, and L. J. KETTEL: *Respiratory Insufficiency*, Yearbook, Chicago, 1975, pp. 84–85.
CHERNIACK, R. M., L. CHERNIACK, and A. NAIMARK: *Respiration in Health and Disease*, 2d ed., Saunders, Philadelphia, 1972, pp. 180–182.
MACBRYDE, C. M. (ed.): op. cit., pp. 349–367.

Cyanosis

MACBRYDE, C. M.: op. cit., pp. 368–375.

Digital clubbing

CHERNIACK, et al.: op. cit., pp. 210–212.
MACBRYDE, C. M.: op. cit., pp. 258–272.

Hypoxemia, hypoxia, hypercapnia, hypocapnia

SHAPIRO, B. A.: *Clinical Application of Blood Gases*, Yearbook, Chicago, 1973, pp. 71–77, 89–99.

CHAPTER 33 Obstructive Patterns of Respiratory Disease

OBJECTIVES

At the completion of Chap. 33, you should be able to:

1 Describe the pattern of ventilatory dysfunction in chronic obstructive pulmonary disease (COPD).

2 Identify the criteria used to characterize chronic bronchitis, pulmonary emphysema, and asthma.

3 Define chronic bronchitis, pulmonary emphysema, and asthma in regard to symptoms, pathologic anatomy, and physiology.

4 Illustrate the interrelationships between the disease entities comprising COPD.

5 Describe the pathologic changes resulting in airway obstruction found in asthma.

6 Differentiate between the three categories of asthma.

7 Identify the major symptoms, treatment, and complications of an asthmatic attack.

8 Describe the etiology of chronic bronchitis and identify the pathologic changes found in chronic bronchitis.

9 Contrast the two morphologic patterns of emphysema.

10 Identify the process of formation and significance of blebs and bullae.

11 Outline the objectives of treatment for chronic bronchitis and emphysema.

12 Identify the pathogenesis of COPD and the morphologic types of emphysema which may result.

13 Differentiate between the pure bronchitic (blue bloater) and emphysematous (pink puffer) types of COPD in regard to onset, etiology, sputum, dyspnea, $\dot{V}/\dot{Q}$, body build, polycythemia, blood gases, lung volumes, morphologic type, and tendency to develop cor pulmonale.

14 Describe the clinical course, complications, and treatment of a patient with COPD.

15 Describe the pathologic changes that occur in bronchiectasis.

16 Describe the pathogenesis, clinical features, and treatment of bronchiectasis.

17 Describe the etiology, pathologic features, treatment, and prognosis of cystic fibrosis (mucoviscidosis).

PATTERNS OF RESPIRATORY DISEASE

Respiratory diseases have been classified on the basis of etiology, anatomic site, chronicity, and changes in structure and function. None of these classifications is entirely satisfactory. The etiologic agents are unknown in some cases, while in others the same causal agent may affect different anatomic sites and produce different pathophysiologic effects. In this chapter and the following one, respiratory diseases will be classified according to ventilatory dysfunction and will be divided into two categories: diseases which primarily produce an obstructive ventilatory disorder and those that produce a restrictive ventilatory disorder. This classification was chosen because spirometric and other tests of ventilatory function are carried out almost routinely, and most respiratory diseases affect ventilation. There are two limitations to this approach. In some respiratory disorders the ventilatory abnormality may produce a mixed pattern (e.g., chronic emphysema with superimposed pneumonia), while in other disorders affecting respiration, ventilatory function may be normal (e.g., anemia or right-to-left shunt). Pulmonary disorders which do not readily fit into obstructive or restrictive patterns of disease will be discussed separately. These are cardiovascular diseases affecting the lung, respiratory insufficiency and failure, pulmonary neoplasms, and tuberculosis. Only those disorders most commonly encountered in hospital practice will be considered.

CHRONIC OBSTRUCTIVE PULMONARY DISEASE

Chronic obstructive pulmonary disease (COPD) is a term which is often applied to a group of pulmonary diseases of long duration which are characterized by increased resistance to airflow as the main pathophysiologic feature. Chronic bronchitis, pulmonary emphysema, and bronchial asthma are the three diseases which make up the entity known as COPD. There appears to be an etiologic and sequential relationship between chronic bronchitis and emphysema which does not seem to exist between these two diseases and asthma. This is particularly true in regard to etiology, pathogenesis, and treatment as will be discussed later in this chapter.

Chronic bronchitis is a clinical disorder characterized by excessive production of mucus in the bronchi and is manifested by a chronic cough and production of sputum for a minimum of 3 months a year for at least 2 consecutive years. This definition assumes that diseases such as bronchiectasis and tuberculosis, which also cause chronic cough and sputum production, have been excluded. The sputum produced in chronic bronchitis may be mucoid or mucopurulent.

Pulmonary emphysema is an anatomic alteration of the lung parenchyma characterized by abnormal enlargement of the alveoli and alveolar ducts and destruction of the alveolar walls.

Asthma is a disease characterized by hypersensitivity of the tracheobronchial tree to various stimuli. It is manifested by periodic, reversible airway-narrowing caused by bronchospasm.

Note the different basis of the definitions of the diseases given above: chronic bronchitis is defined by clinical symptoms, pulmonary emphysema by pathologic anatomy, and asthma by clinical pathologic physiology. Although each disease may exist in its pure form, it is more usual for chronic bronchitis and emphysema to exist together in the same patient. Asthma is more easily separated from chronic bronchitis and emphysema on the basis of a history of paroxysmal attacks of wheezing beginning in childhood and associated with allergies. Occasionally, however, patients with chronic bronchitis have asthmatic features to their disease. The interrelationships among chronic bronchitis, asthma, and emphysema are illustrated in Fig. 33-1. The shaded areas represent those persons with features of more than one disease, while the unshaded areas represent each disease in the predominantly pure form. For the purpose of clarity, we will consider asthma separately from chronic bronchitis and emphysema, since the former is more easily separated from the other two diseases.

Asthma

The term "asthma" comes from the Greek word for "panting" and means attacks of shortness of breath. Although in the past this term has been used for the clinical picture of shortness of breath resulting from any cause, today it is confined to a condition of abnormal responsiveness of the air passages to certain substances.

The pathologic changes involved in airway obstruction are found in the medium-sized bronchi and bronchioles as small as 1 mm in diameter. Airway narrowing is caused by bronchospasm, mucosal edema, and hypersecretion of viscous mucus (see Fig. 33-2).

Asthma can be divided into three categories. *Extrinsic* or *allergic asthma*, found in a minority of patients, is clearly caused by a known allergen. This form generally begins in childhood in a member of a family with a history of atopic diseases including hay fever, eczema,

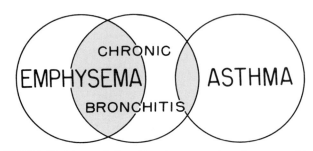

FIGURE 33-1 *Interrelationships between the disease entities comprising COPD.*

and dermatitis, as well as asthma. Allergic asthma results from the sensitization of such an individual to an allergen, usually a protein, in the form of an inhaled pollen, animal dander, mold spore, feather dust, lint, or less commonly, to a food such as milk or chocolate. Exposure to the allergen, even in minute quantities, produces an asthmatic attack. *Intrinsic* or *idiopathic asthma,* on the other hand, is characterized by the absence of clearly defined precipitating factors. Such nonspecific factors as the common cold, exercise, or emotion may trigger the asthmatic attack. The intrinsic type of asthma is more apt to develop after the age of 40, with the onset of attacks after infections of the nasal sinuses or tracheobronchial tree. The attacks become more frequent and severe as time goes on, and the condition merges into chronic bronchitis and, sometimes, emphysema. *Mixed asthma* is a form of asthma afflicting the majority of patients and is composed of components of both extrinsic and intrinsic types. Often patients with intrinsic asthma later develop the mixed type, although children who have the extrinsic type often have a complete recovery at adolescence.

The pathogenesis of asthma was discussed in Part II of this book. The clinical manifestations are easy to recognize. After exposure to the causative allergen or precipitating factor, dyspnea may begin suddenly. Patients feel as if they are suffocating and must stand or sit up and devote all their energy to breathing. On the basis of the anatomic changes which have been described, one can predict that the major difficulty is with expiration. The tracheobronchial tree widens and lengthens during inspiration, but it is difficult to force air out of the constricted, edematous, mucus-filled

bronchioles, which normally contract to a certain degree during expiration. Air is trapped distal to the obstruction, so that there is progressive hyperinflation of the lungs. Prolonged wheezing expirations are thus characteristic as the patient struggles to force the air out. It is usual for an asthmatic attack to last from a few minutes to several hours, followed by a cough which is productive of considerable whitish sputum. Treatment consists of administering bronchodilator drugs, specific long-term desensitization, avoidance of known allergens, and occasionally corticosteroid drugs. Intervals between attacks are characteristically free from respiratory difficulty. Asthma is distinguished from chronic bronchitis and emphysema by its intermittent nature and the fact that destructive emphysema rarely occurs. Occasionally, however, an asthmatic attack known as *status asthmaticus* may be sustained for days and is intractable to ordinary methods of treatment. In these cases, ventilatory function may be so impaired as to result in cyanosis and death.

Chronic bronchitis and emphysema

The main pathologic findings in chronic bronchitis are hypertrophy of the bronchial mucosal glands and an increase in the number of goblet cells, accompanied by inflammatory cell infiltration and edema of the bronchial mucosa. The resulting increased production of mucus leads to the characteristic symptoms of cough and expectoration. The chronic cough in the presence of increased bronchial secretions appears to affect the minute bronchioles to the point of destruction and dilatation of their walls. The prime etiologic factor seems to be cigarette smoking, and other forms of air pollution common to the industrial environment. Continued air pollution also predisposes the individual to recurrent infections because it slows down ciliary and phagocytic activity, causing increased mucus accumulation at the same time defense mechanisms are weakened.

Two types of emphysema are recognized in relationship to COPD. *Centrilobular emphysema* (CLE) selectively affects the respiratory bronchioles. Fenestrations develop in the walls, enlarge, become confluent, and tend to form a single space as the walls disintegrate (see Fig. 33-3). Initially, the more distal alveolar ducts and sacs and the alveoli are preserved. This disease commonly affects the upper portions of the lung more severely, but it tends to be unevenly distributed. Centrilobular emphysema is more prevalent in males than in females. It is usually associated with chronic bronchitis and is seldom found in nonsmokers.

Panlobular emphysema (PLE), or *panacinar emphysema,* is another less common morphologic pattern in which there is nearly uniform enlargement and destruction of the alveoli distal to the terminal bronchiole (see Fig. 33-3). As the disease progresses, there is gradual loss

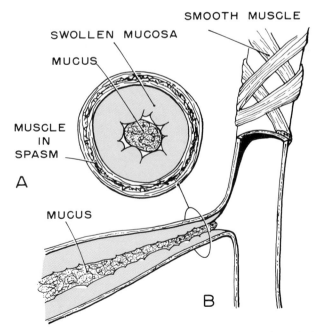

FIGURE 33-2 Factors causing expiratory obstruction in bronchial asthma: A, cross section of bronchiole occluded by muscle spasm, swollen mucosa, and mucus in lumen; B, longitudinal section of bronchiole.

of all components of the acinus until only a few strands of tissue remain, which are usually blood vessels. PLE is characteristically uniform in distribution throughout the lung, although the basal sections tend to be more severely affected. PLE, but not CLE, is associated with a small group of patients with primary emphysema. This form of emphysema is characterized by the insidious development of increased airway resistance without evidence of chronic bronchitis. In England, less than 6 percent of patients with COPD have primary emphysema, which affects females as often as males. The cause of this form of emphysema is unknown, but a familial kind associated with a deficiency of the enzyme α_1-antitrypsin has been described. It has an early onset and usually produces symptoms between the ages of 30 and 40 years.

Panlobular emphysema, although characteristic of primary emphysema, may also be associated with the emphysema of aging and with chronic bronchitis. It is believed that the deterioration of the elastic and reticular fibers of the lung with the resultant loss of elastic recoil of the lung leads to progressive generalized distention of the lung in the aging process. Senile emphysema,

however, is not true emphysema, since most of these elderly patients do not develop significant impairment of lung function. The panlobular emphysema associated with chronic bronchitis is thought to be an end stage of progressive centrilobular emphysema, since both morphologic patterns may exist in the same lung.

When the thorax of a patient who has emphysema is opened during surgery or at an autopsy, the lungs are seen to be grossly enlarged; they remain filled with air and do not collapse. They are whiter than normal and feel downy or billowy. Subpleural air-filled spaces called *blebs* and parenchymal air-filled spaces greater than 1 cm in diameter called *bullae* are commonly seen (see Fig. 33-4). There is also generalized dilatation of the air spaces. Bullae are common in both PLE and CLE but may exist in the absence of either. Bullae generally develop because of a check-valve bronchiolar obstruction (see Fig. 33-5). During inspiration, the bronchiolar lumen widens so that air is able to pass by the obstruction caused by thickening of the mucosa and excess mucus. During expiration, however, when the bronchiolar lumen normally becomes more narrow, the obstruction may prevent the egress of air. A loss of elasticity of the bronchiolar walls in emphysema may also cause premature collapse. Air is thus trapped in the affected pulmonary segment, leading to overdistention and coalescence of several alveoli. This is caused by fragmentation of the interalveolar elastic tissue and subse-

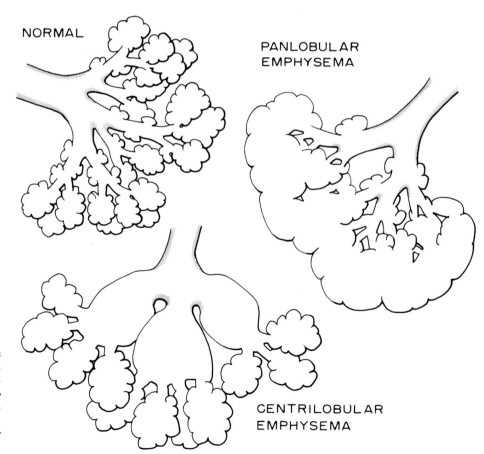

NORMAL

PANLOBULAR EMPHYSEMA

CENTRILOBULAR EMPHYSEMA

FIGURE 33-3 Morphologic types of emphysema: panlobular—entire primary lobule involved, destruction and distention distal to the respiratory bronchioles; centrilobular—destruction is central, primarily involving the respiratory bronchioles.

quent rupture of the attenuated interalveolar septae, resulting in a bulla. In emphysema there may be a single bulla or many which may or may not communicate with each other. Blebs, which are formed by ruptured alveoli, may rupture into the pleural cavity and cause a spontaneous pneumothorax (collapse of the lung). Other changes commonly seen in the COPD lung are a reduction in the capillary bed and histologic evidence of chronic bronchiolitis (involvement of the minute bronchioles).

The flow diagram in Figure 33-6 illustrates the pathogenesis of COPD and the morphologic types of emphysema which result. This diagram emphasizes the fact that while a genetic predisposition may be a factor in the development of pulmonary emphysema, and smoking and air pollution are the prime factors in the pathogenesis of the bronchitic type of emphysema, there is an interaction between the two. For example, persons with a genetic predisposition might develop emphysema if exposed to varying degrees of air pollution. Although senile dilatation of the air spaces is not considered true emphysema, it is possible that normal loss of elasticity of the lung parenchyma associated with aging is a factor in the development of true emphysema.

The clinical course of patients with COPD ranges from what is known as the "pink puffers" to the "blue bloaters." The clinical hallmark of "pink puffers" (associated with primary panlobular emphysema) is the development of dyspnea without significant cough and sputum production. Usually the dyspnea begins between the ages of 30 and 40 years and becomes increasingly severe. In advanced disease the patient may be too breathless to eat and characteristically has a thin, wasted appearance. Later on in the course of the disease, the "pink puffer" may develop secondary chronic bronchitis. The chest of the patient is barrel-shaped; the diaphragm is low and moves poorly. Polycythemia and cyanosis are rare (hence the term "pink"), and cor pulmonale (heart disease resulting from pulmonary hypertension and lung disease) rarely develops until the terminal stage. There is minimal ventilation–perfusion imbalance, so that by hyperventilating, the "pink puffer" is usually able to keep blood gases within the normal

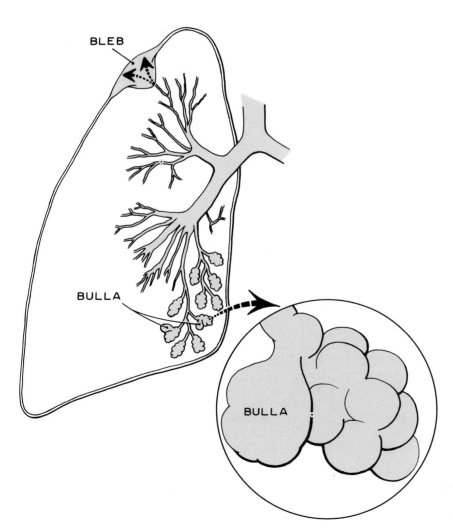

FIGURE 33-4 Pulmonary blebs and bullae.

range until late in the course of the disease. The lungs are usually greatly enlarged so that there is a large increase in total lung capacity and residual volume.

At the other extreme of the range of COPD are patients who could be described as "blue bloaters" (bronchitis with little evidence of obstructive emphysema). These patients usually have a productive cough and frequent respiratory infections which continue for years before there is noticeable functional impairment. Eventually, however, they develop dyspnea on exertion. These patients show a diminished respiratory drive; they hypoventilate and become hypoxic and hypercapnic. There is also a markedly distorted ventilation/perfusion ratio. The chronic hypoxia stimulates the kidney to produce erythropoietin, which in turn stimulates increased production of red blood cells, resulting in secondary polycythemia. Hemoglobin levels may be 20 g% or more, so that cyanosis is more readily apparent since there may easily be 5 g% of reduced hemoglobin when only a small proportion of the circulating blood hemoglobin is in the reduced form (hence the name blue bloater). As these patients are not dyspneic at rest, they appear to be comfortable. There is generally not a great weight loss, and body build is normal. The total lung capacity may be normal, and the diaphragm is in the normal position. Death usually results from cor pulmonale (which develops early) or from respiratory failure. At autopsy, emphysema is often, although not always, seen. The emphysema tends to be of the centrilobular type, although the panlobular type may also be present.

Table 33-1 contrasts the pure bronchitic ("blue

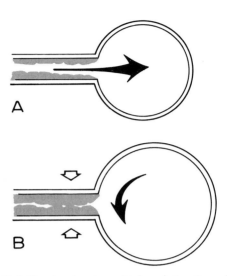

FIGURE 33-5 Check-valve bronchiolar obstruction. A, during inspiration, lumen widens enough to allow air entry. B, during expiration, premature collapse and narrowed lumen prevent egress of air which becomes trapped in the alveoli.

TABLE 33-1
Clinical types of COPD and their differentiation

FEATURE	"PINK PUFFER" (EMPHYSEMATOUS)	"BLUE BLOATER" (BRONCHITIC)
Onset	30–40 years of age	20s and 30s—cigarette cough Disability in middle age
Etiology	Unknown factors Genetic predisposition Smoking Air pollution	Unknown factors Smoking Air pollution Climate
Sputum	Minimal	Copious
Dyspnea	Relatively early dyspnea	Relatively late dyspnea
$\dot{V}/\dot{Q}$ ratio	Minimal $\dot{V}/\dot{Q}$ imbalances	Marked $\dot{V}/\dot{Q}$ imbalance
Body build	Thin, asthenic	Well-nourished
AP diameter of chest	"Barrel chest" common	Not increased
Pathologic lung anatomy	Panlobular emphysema	Centrilobular emphysema predominant
Respiratory pattern	Hyperventilation and marked dyspnea which may occur at rest	Diminished respiratory drive Hypoventilation common with resultant hypoxia and hypercapnia
Lung volumes	Low FEV_1 Increased TLC and RV	Low FEV_1 Normal TLC; moderate increase in RV
P_aCO_2	Normal or low	Elevated
S_aO_2	Normal	Much desaturation due to $\dot{V}/\dot{Q}$ imbalance
Polycythemia	Hemoglobin and hematocrit normal until late	Elevated hemoglobin and hematocrit common
Cyanosis	Rare	Common
Cor pulmonale	Rare except terminally	Frequent with many episodes

bloater") and emphysematous ("pink puffer") types of COPD. Most patients with COPD lie somewhere between these two extremes.

The typical course of COPD is a long one, beginning in the twenties and thirties with a "cigarette cough" or "morning cough" and the production of a small amount of mucoid sputum. Minor respiratory infections tend to persist longer than usual in these patients. Although there may be some decrease in exercise tolerance, it usually goes unnoticed as the patient becomes less energetic with the passage of time. Eventually episodes of acute bronchitis occur more regularly, particularly in the winter, and the patient's working capacity decreases, so that work may have to be given up sometime in the patient's fifties or sixties. In patients of the predominantly emphysematous type, the course appears to be less protracted, with no previous history of a productive cough. Severe debilitating dyspnea may develop within a few years. When hypercapnia, hypoxemia, and

cor pulmonale develop, the prognosis is poor, and death usually comes within a few years after the onset. A combination of respiratory and heart failure precipitated by pneumonia is the usual cause of death.

Therapy for the patient with chronic bronchitis and obstructive emphysema requires measures to relieve obstruction of the small airways. Although airway collapse secondary to emphysema is irreversible, many patients have some degree of bronchospasm, retention of secretions, and mucosal edema which may be relieved by the appropriate therapy. Of paramount importance is the cessation of smoking and the avoidance of other forms of air pollution or allergens which may aggravate the symptoms. Often the cessation of smoking alone

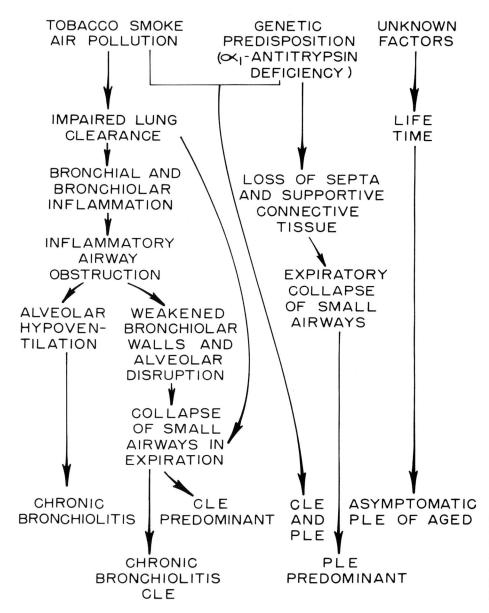

FIGURE 33-6 Pathogenesis of COPD. (Modified from Chronic Obstructive Pulmonary Disease: A Manual for Physicians, 3d ed., National Tuberculosis and Respiratory Disease Association, 1972, p. 29.)

may bring about a marked relief of symptoms and improvement of ventilation. Infection should be treated promptly and patients who are particularly susceptible to respiratory infection may be directed to use prophylactic antibiotics. The patient is instructed to seek this medication whenever dyspnea or the amount of sputum production increases. Tetracycline, ampicillin, and penicillin are usually the drugs of choice. All patients should receive influenza vaccine.

Additional measures to relieve airway obstruction include providing adequate hydration to thin bronchial secretions, administering expectorants, and administering bronchodilator drugs to relieve smooth muscle spasm. Sympathomimetic drugs such as isoproterenol, epinephrine, ephedrine, and xanthines (such as aminophylline) are commonly administered. In patients with copious secretions, percussion and postural drainage is administered to assist in the removal of obstructive secretions which may also predispose to infection. Breathing exercises may also be helpful. The patient is taught to use slow, relaxed expiration against pursed lips. This exercise prevents collapse of small bronchioles and reduces the amount of trapped air. A graduated program of physical exercise during the administration of low concentration oxygen may be helpful in improving the patient's sense of well-being. Oxygen, however, must be administered with *caution* in the later stages of

the illness when there is hypercapnia and hypoxemia. Respiratory failure may be precipitated, as these patients depend on hypoxia to stimulate breathing. The treatment of cor pulmonale and respiratory failure complications will be discussed in Chaps. 35 and 36.

Two other diseases which may result in an obstructive pattern of pulmonary dysfunction deserve mention in this chapter—bronchiectasis and cystic fibrosis.

BRONCHIECTASIS

Bronchiectasis is a condition characterized by chronic dilatation of the bronchi. Two anatomic types are commonly described. Saccular bronchiectasis consists of rounded cavitylike dilatations and is often found in children. Cylindrical bronchiectasis shows a tubular dilatation of the bronchi and is typically found in adults. Bronchiectasis develops when the bronchial walls are weakened by chronic inflammatory changes involving the mucosa and muscular coat. As seen in Fig. 33-7, purulent materials collect in these dilated areas and lead to persistent infection of the affected segment or lobe. Chronic infection causes further damage to the bronchial walls, and a vicious cycle is set up. There is no single, specific cause of bronchiectasis, as it is a disease based on an abnormal anatomic condition. Most commonly, bronchiectasis begins in childhood following a lower respiratory tract infection which develops as a complication of measles, whooping cough, or influenza. Bronchial obstruction resulting from a neoplasm or an

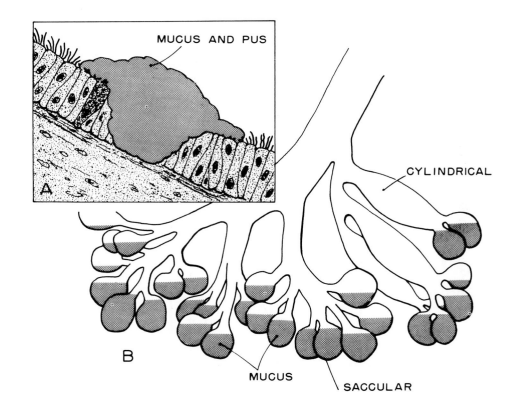

aspirated foreign body (especially if it is organic, such as a peanut) may also lead to bronchiectasis and secondary infection of the distal bronchial tree. Bronchiectasis of the upper lobes may be associated with tuberculosis, although it is frequently asymptomatic because bronchial drainage is achieved by gravity. Cystic fibrosis and Kartagener's syndrome (bronchiectasis associated with sinusitis and displacement of the heart to the right side of the thorax) are examples of congenital diseases associated with bronchiectasis.

The principle clinical feature of bronchiectasis is a chronic, loose cough productive of a large amount of mucopurulent, foul-smelling sputum. Coughing is most severe when the patient changes position. The amount of sputum varies with the stage of the disease but may be 200 ml daily in severe cases. Hemoptysis is common, usually consisting of blood streaks in the sputum. Characteristic features of advanced untreated disease are recurrent pneumonia, malnutrition, digital clubbing, cor pulmonale, and right heart failure.

The degree of functional disturbance depends on the extent of the involvement of pulmonary tissue. Bronchiectasis localized to one or two segments of the lung may cause little impairment of pulmonary function, while diffuse bronchiectasis may be associated with anastomoses between the bronchial and pulmonary circulation with resultant right-to-left shunting.

The most important feature of treatment is daily, vigorous bronchial hygiene with postural drainage which generally must be continued for the rest of the patient's life. Antibiotic therapy for the control of infection is another important aspect of therapy. Before the advent of antibiotics, bronchiectasis was much more common, and the prognosis was poor. Patients rarely lived beyond the age of 40 years. Bronchiectasis is much less common today and, except for the congenital forms of the disease, should be regarded as preventable. Timely vaccinations against childhood diseases commonly complicated by pneumonia, the vigorous antibiotic and other appropriate treatments of pneumonia, and the prompt removal of aspirated foreign bodies are all preventive measures.

CYSTIC FIBROSIS

Cystic fibrosis or mucoviscidosis is a disease of genetic origin occurring in about 1 out of 2000 births in the Caucasian race but is rarely seen in the Negro. The secretions of the exocrine glands that produce mucus and some other exocrine fluids produce abnormally viscid secretions. (The sweat and saliva are not particularly viscid but do contain abnormal amounts of salt.) The viscid secretions commonly cause obstruction of the

FIGURE 33-7 Pathologic changes in bronchiectasis. A, longitudinal section of bronchial wall—chronic infection causes damage to the bronchial walls. B, collection of purulent material in dilated bronchioles leading to persistent infection.

pancreatic and hepatic ducts and the bronchioles. The obstruction, in turn, can lead to fibrotic changes in the involved organs. A few patients may live to be adults, but survival does not generally extend beyond adolescence. Accompanying respiratory disease and complications account for over 90 percent of the deaths from this disease. The sequence of events in this disease proceed from recurrent pulmonary infections that gradually develop into bronchiectasis from retention of thick secretions, to chronic pneumonia, fibrosis, ventilation–perfusion imbalance, chronic hypoxemia, cor pulmonale, and respiratory failure. Since pulmonary dysfunction is the overriding factor in determining survival, the management of this aspect of the disease is crucial, with removal of the obstructing bronchial secretions as the most crucial aspect of treatment. Generally, aerosol therapy is used to liquefy secretions and is followed by percussion and postural drainage. Prevention of infection and its prompt treatment are also important.

QUESTIONS

Obstructive patterns of respiratory disease—Chap. 33

Directions: Answer the following questions on a separate sheet of paper.

1 What is the ventilatory functional disorder associated with COPD?

2 Describe the interrelationships between chronic bronchitis, pulmonary emphysema, and asthma.

3 Describe the symptoms of an asthmatic attack. How is it treated? What is status asthmaticus?

4 Contrast the morphologic patterns of emphysema according to anatomic changes, distribution in lung, sex prevalence, type of COPD associated with, and etiology.

5 What are the objectives of treatment for chronic bronchitis and emphysema?

6 What are the two criteria for establishing a diagnosis of chronic bronchitis? What is the period of time within which these symptoms must be manifested (months per year and consecutive years)?

7 Describe the pathologic anatomic changes in the lung parenchyma present in pulmonary emphysema.

8 What are subpleural air-filled spaces called? What is the cause?

9 What are parenchymal air-filled spaces greater than 1 cm in diameter called? What generally causes them?

10 How does the tracheobronchial tree of the asthmatic

patient respond to various stimuli? How is this manifested?

11 What anatomic changes occur in bronchiectasis? What are some possible precipitating factors and what features tend to cause persistence and progression of the disease?

12 What are the principal clinical features of bronchiectasis?

13 Identify the mode of treatment for bronchiectasis.

14 What is the most crucial aspect of treatment of cystic fibrosis?

15 Match each of the diseases in col. A with its basis for definition in col. B.

Column A	Column B
____ Chronic bronchitis	a Pathologic anatomy
____ Pulmonary emphysema	b Clinical symptoms
____ Asthma	c Pathophysiology

Directions: Circle the letter preceding each item below that correctly answers the question. More than one item may be correct.

16 Which of the following pathologic changes is associated with chronic bronchitis?
a Hypertrophy of the bronchial mucosal glands
b Destruction of alveolar walls c Increase in the number of goblet cells d Edema, scarring, and increased thickness of bronchioles e Decreased production of surfactant

17 In bronchial asthma:
a Bronchiolar smooth muscle is atrophic b Medium and small-sized bronchi are plugged with viscid mucus c The lungs are pale and emphysematous d The patient is usually free from symptoms between attacks

18 Emphysema is an anatomic entity which:
a Has one basic morphologic pattern b Causes serious respiratory insufficiency when it develops as a result of the aging process c Is characterized by increased size of the air spaces distal to the terminal bronchioles with associated parenchymal destruction d Is always related to chronic bronchitis

19 The major source of disability and death in pediatric patients with cystic fibrosis is:
a Malnutrition b Recurrent pulmonary infection c Hyponatremia resulting from the loss of salt in sweat and saliva d Chronic pancreatitis

20 Centrilobular emphysema:
a Is more common than PLE b Appears to be related to cigarette smoking c Usually affects the upper lobes more severely d Is associated with deficiency of α_1-antitrypsin

21 The pathophysiology of asthma is characterized by:
a Bronchodilatation b Alveoli filled with exudate c Loss of support of bronchiolar walls d Bronchiolar narrowing

Directions: Circle T if the statement is true and F if it is false in regard to cystic fibrosis. Correct the false statements.

22 T F Mucoviscidosis is another name for the disease.

23 T F It is a disease of genetic origin.

24 T F It is more common in Negroes than in Caucasians.

25 T F 200 ml of mucopurulent, foul-smelling sputum may be produced daily.

26 T F The exocrine glands are affected by this disease.

27 T F Digital clubbing is a characteristic feature of advanced disease.

28 T F The prognosis of cystic fibrosis is generally good.

Directions: Match the "pink puffer" and "blue bloater" types of COPD in col. B to their associated features in col. A.

Column A	Column B
29 ____ PLE	a "Pink puffer"
30 ____ CLE predominant	b "Blue bloater"
31 ____ Genetic predisposition	
32 ____ Late onset of dyspnea	
33 ____ Minimal sputum	
34 ____ Polycythemia common	
35 ____ Early cor pulmonale	
36 ____ Marked $\dot{V}/\dot{Q}$ imbalance	
37 ____ Thin, wasted appearance	
38 ____ Hypercapnia (early)	

Directions: Match the type of asthmatic condition in col. A with the appropriate descriptive features in col. B. Each item in col. B may be used more than once.

Column A	Column B
39 ____ Extrinsic asthma	a Absence of clearly defined precipitating factor
40 ____ Intrinsic asthma	b Clearly caused by a known allergen; usually develops in early childhood
41 ____ Mixed asthma	c Attacks may be associated with infection of the tracheobronchial tree or of the nasal sinuses
	d Afflicts the majority of patients
	e Exposure to the allergen precipitates an asthmatic attack

AMERICAN THORACIC SOCIETY: "Chronic Bronchitis, Asthma, and Pulmonary Emphysema: A Statement by the Committee on Diagnostic Standards for Nontuberculosis Respiratory Diseases," *American Review of Respiratory Disease,* **85**: 762–768, 1962.

CHERNIACK, R. M., L. CHERNIACK, and A. NAIMARK: *Respiration in Health and Disease,* 2d ed., Saunders, Philadelphia, 1972, pp. 303–338.

LYONS, HAROLD A.: "Obstructive Emphysema," *Hospital Medicine,* **7**: 56–75, January 1971.

NATIONAL TUBERCULOSIS AND RESPIRATORY DISEASE ASSOCIATION: *Chronic Obstructive Pulmonary Disease: A Manual for Physicians* 3d ed., New York, 1972.

ROBBINS, S. L., and MARCIA ANGELL: *Basic Pathology,* Saunders, Philadelphia, 1971, pp. 320–321, 330, 333–342.

CHAPTER 34 Restrictive Patterns of Respiratory Disease

OBJECTIVES   At the completion of Chap. 34, you should be able to:

1 State the physiologic consequences of a restricted pattern of ventilation.

2 Describe at least two extrapulmonary diseases or altered conditions causing alveolar hypoventilation. Identify the mechanism responsible for the altered conditions in the following systems or structures: central nervous system, peripheral nervous system, and muscular and chest cage.

3 List four types of fixed chest wall deformities.

4 Differentiate between kyphosis and scoliosis.

5 Identify the relationship of the four types of fixed chest wall deformities to respiratory failure.

6 State the relationship between the Pickwickian syndrome and respiratory insufficiency.

7 Describe the effect that multiple rib fractures (flail chest) has on respiration.

8 Define pleural effusion.

9 Differentiate between a pleural effusion which is a transudate and one which is an exudate.

10 Define the following terms: hydrothorax, empyema, hemothorax, and chylothorax.

11 State the possible consequences of inadequately treated empyema.

12 Define a pneumothorax.

13 List the three classes of pneumothorax according to cause and give examples of each.

14 Differentiate between an open, closed, and tension pneumothorax.

15 Describe the complications and treatment of a penetrating chest wound.

16 Explain why a pneumothorax occurs.

17 State the most common cause of idiopathic spontaneous pneumothorax in young people.

18 Differentiate between the signs and symptoms of a pneumothorax and a pleural effusion.

19 Describe the treatment for a pneumothorax and pleural effusion.

20 List several conditions that result in damage to lung alveoli and interstitium and identify the specific damage to lung tissue caused by each disorder.

21 Describe two physiologic abnormalities seen in patients with disease of the lung parenchyma.

22 Define atelectasis.

23 Differentiate between absorption and compression atelectasis on the basis of cause and mechanism involved.

24 Explain how collateral ventilation prevents absorption atelectasis.

25 Describe the importance of measures used to prevent atelectasis in predisposed individuals.

26 List four lung defense mechanisms which play a role in the prevention of atelectasis and factors which interfere with these defense mechanisms.

27 Identify the morbidity and mortality of pneumonia for susceptible population groups.

28 Describe four anatomic patterns of pneumonitis or pneumonia, the micropathologic changes, and the common infecting agent.

29 Identify and describe the four stages in the pathologic response to pneumococcal pneumonia by identifying the name of the stage, time period, and description of lung changes for each stage.

30 Describe the signs, symptoms, physical findings, treatment, and prognosis of pneumococcal pneumonia.

31 List the common complications and prognosis of pneumonias caused by gram-negative or staphylococcus organisms.

32 Describe the symptoms, treatment, complications, and prognosis of pneumonias caused by viruses or *Mycoplasma pneumoniae*.

33 Differentiate between aspiration and hypostatic pneumonia.

34 Name the three most common fungal infections in the United States.

35 Identify the most common causes of diffuse pulmonary fibrosis.

36 List the criteria used to determine whether a particular dust will cause disease of the lung parenchyma.

37 Describe the mechanism causing pulmonary fibrosis; include inorganic and organic dusts and noxious gases.

38 Describe the pulmonary manifestations of diffuse pulmonary fibrosis.

39 State the pathologic findings in respiratory distress syndrome.

40 Describe the treatment of respiratory distress syndrome.

EXTRAPULMONARY DISEASE

A restrictive ventilatory disorder is characterized by increased stiffness of the lungs or thorax or both, resulting from decreased compliance, and a reduction in all lung volumes including the vital capacity. There is an increase in the work of breathing to overcome the elastic forces of the respiratory apparatus, so that a pattern of rapid, shallow breathing is adopted. The physiologic consequences of a restricted pattern of ventilation are alveolar hypoventilation and an inability to maintain normal blood gas tensions.

There are a number of diseases which may contribute to pulmonary restriction through varying mechanisms. In this chapter, these diseases are divided into two classes: extrapulmonary disorders, including neurologic, neuromuscular, and thoracic cage disorders, and diseases of the pleura and lung parenchyma.

Neurologic and neuromuscular disorders

When one refers to extrapulmonary disorders, the term "extrapulmonary" implies that the lung tissue itself may be quite normal. The common pathophysiologic disturbance in these disorders is alveolar hypoventilation, although this is not entirely true in the case of kyphoscoliosis.

A number of disorders directly affecting the medullary respiratory center may cause alveolar hypoventilation. Carbon dioxide retention from a variety of causes may depress rather than stimulate respiration when the P_aCO_2 exceeds about 70 mmHg. A number of drugs are capable of depressing the respiratory center and thereby causing alveolar hypoventilation. For example, narcotic or barbiturate drug overdose in a suicide attempt are common causes of death due to respiratory depression and failure. Anatomic damage to the respiratory center resulting from head trauma or cerebral lesions caused by a cerebral vascular accident can also cause respiratory center depression and alveolar hypoventilation. Abnormalities of neural or neuromuscular transmission to the respiratory muscles may result in paresis or paralysis and alveolar hypoventilation. Amyotrophic lateral sclerosis, poliomyelitis, Guillain-Barré syndrome, and myasthenia gravis are all neurologic disorders which may produce ventilatory insufficiency. The muscles themselves are diseased in progressive muscular dystrophy. The severity of the respiratory involvement in any of the above diseases depends on the amount of anatomic involvement; vital capacity is reduced in proportion to the degree of paresis of the respiratory muscles. Although parenchymal lung disease is not primary, secondary infection is frequent because of ineffective coughing and limitation of respiratory excursions. Table 34-1 summarizes the extrapulmonary disorders causing alveolar hypoventilation and the mechanism responsible.

Thoracic cage disorders

There are four major types of fixed chest wall deformities which may restrict ventilation by interfering with the bellows mechanism. These are kyphoscoliosis, pectus excavatum, ankylosing spondylitis, and healed thoracoplasty.

Kyphosis is a term which refers to any posterior angulation of the spine (hunchback), and scoliosis refers to a lateral displacement of the spine. Kyphoscoliosis is, therefore, characterized by angulation of the spine both posteriorly and laterally. About 80 percent of the cases are idiopathic, while the remaining 20 percent result from the aftereffects of poliomyelitis or tuberculosis of the spine (Pott's disease). Kyphoscoliosis is quite common, with about 1 percent of the American population affected, although the defect is severe enough to pro-

TABLE 34-1
Extrapulmonary disorders causing alveolar hypoventilation

SYSTEM OR STRUCTURE	DISEASE OR ALTERED CONDITION	ALTERED MECHANISM
Neurologic (central nervous system)	$P_aCO_2 > 70$ mmHg Narcotics and barbiturates	Depression of the respiratory center
	Head trauma, CNS lesions	Direct anatomic damage to the respiratory center
	Poliomyelitis	Interruption of nerve transmission to respiratory muscles due to lower motor neuron lesion
	Amyotrophic lateral sclerosis	Interruption of nerve transmission to respiratory muscles due to upper motor neuron lesion
Neurologic (peripheral nervous system)	Guillain-Barré syndrome	Interruption of nerve transmission to respiratory muscles due to inflammation involving ganglion cells and peripheral nerves
	Myasthenia gravis	Interruption of nerve transmission to respiratory muscles due to disease involving the neuromuscular junction
Muscular	Progressive muscular dystrophy	Paresis of the respiratory muscles due to diffuse disease of the skeletal muscles
Chest cage	Kyphoscoliosis	Deformity of the chest cage causing abnormal positioning and functioning of the respiratory muscles and compression of the chest cage contents
	Closed chest wall trauma	Voluntary restriction of ventilation due to pain or paradoxical movement of the chest wall and thoracic contents in "flail chest" injury
	Pickwickian syndrome (extreme obesity)	Limitation of thoracic movement by accumulated body fat

duce cardiopulmonary symptoms in only a small proportion of these cases. Severe kyphoscoliosis is associated with marked asymmetry of the chest and leads to abnormal functioning and positioning of the respiratory muscles and to compression of the lungs.

The sequence of events which may lead to both respiratory and cardiac failure in kyphoscoliosis are shown in Fig. 34-1. In these cases, breathing entails a high work and energy cost, so that a rapid, shallow pattern is adopted. This in turn leads to alveolar hypoventilation by preferential ventilation of the anatomic dead space at the expense of alveolar ventilation. In addition, compression of the lungs by the thoracic deformity causes a small lung volume and unequal distribution of ventilation and perfusion, since both alveoli and pulmonary blood vessels are compressed. The consequent physiologic shunting leads to hypoxemia. When alveolar ventilation is also limited, the result is hypoxemia, hypercapnia, and respiratory acidosis. Compression of the pulmonary blood vessels and the acidosis also leads to pulmonary hypertension and cor pulmonale. The common cause of death from this chain of events is a combination of respiratory and heart failure.

Pectus excavatum (funnel chest) is a congenital deformity in which the lower end of the sternum is attached to the thoracic spine by fibromuscular bands, giving the lower sternal area a "caved-in" appearance. Compare this deformity with kyphoscoliosis in Fig. 34-2. Pectus excavatum, unlike severe kyphoscoliosis, rarely causes more than mild restriction of ventilation.

Thoracoplasty is a surgically induced depression of the thoracic cage which was performed for the treatment of tuberculosis in the past but is no longer common. Since this procedure is performed for an underlying lung disease, the subsequent pulmonary dysfunction is usually more closely related to the original disease than to the induced deformity.

Ankylosing spondylitis is a disease which causes symmetrical reduction in mobility of the bony thorax as a result of the ossification of the vertebral joints and ligaments. Rib fixation and increased stiffness of the chest wall cause mild ventilatory restriction which is not usually symptomatic.

Closed chest wall injury may also restrict ventilation. The most common chest wall injury is simple rib fracture. As a result of the pain and muscle splinting, there is ventilatory restriction of tidal volume, increase in respiratory rate and frequency, and voluntary inhibition of the cough reflex. Chest strapping and administration of narcotics further restrict the chest movement and depress the respiratory center and cough reflex, thus compounding the problem. Healthy young persons tend to tolerate these changes well, but in elderly persons, these changes may lead to impaired clearing of secretions, respiratory tract infection, blood gas abnormalities, and even respiratory failure. Flail chest is a major defect in chest wall continuity caused by a crushing chest injury (commonly seen in steering wheel injuries in auto accidents) with multiple rib fractures. The resulting

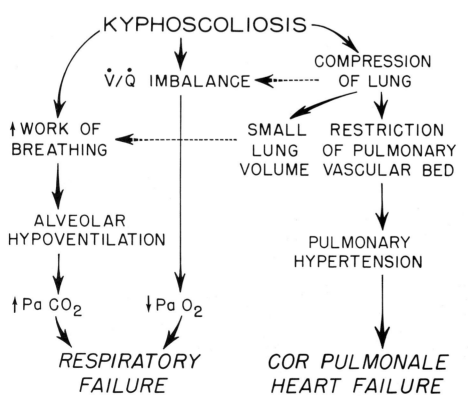

FIGURE 34-1 Pathogenesis of respiratory and heart failure in kyphoscoliosis.

instability of the chest wall causes a paradoxical movement of the chest wall accompanied by pendulum movement of the mediastinal contents during the breathing cycle. This condition may cause interference with venous return to the heart and cause dead space air to be shunted back and forth between the lungs (pendelluft) as illustrated in Fig. 34-3. The treatment for flail chest is stabilization of the chest wall and mechanical ventilation.

The Pickwickian syndrome is the term used to describe a group of clinical features found in persons who are extremely obese. These features include chronic alveolar hypoventilation, somnolence, polycythemia, hypoxemia, and hypercapnia. (The syndrome was named after the "sleepy fat boy" in Charles Dickens' *Pickwick Papers*.) The somnolence common to this syndrome can be related to the carbon dioxide retention which depresses the central nervous system; polycythemia is the compensatory response to chronic hypoxia. In persons with the Pickwickian syndrome, the accumulated body fat appears to limit thoracic movement and greatly increases the work of breathing. It is not uncommon for respiratory impairment to progress to the point of cor pulmonale and respiratory failure. It is important to note that not all extremely obese persons develop alveolar hypoventilation and blood gas abnormalities. The inconsistency of this relation is not understood. Reduction in weight generally reverses the respiratory insufficiency in those persons who exhibit it.

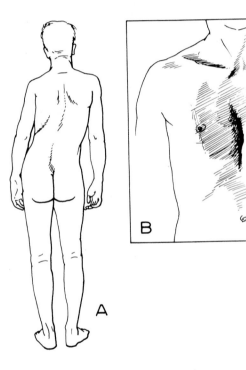

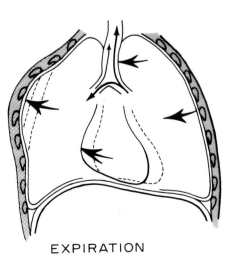

FIGURE 34-2 Thoracic deformities restricting ventilation. A, *kyphoscoliosis.* B, *pectus excavatum (funnel chest).*

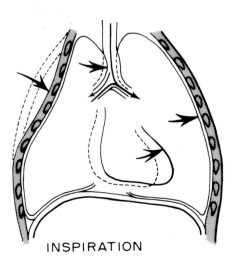

INSPIRATION

EXPIRATION

Pleural disorders

The pleura and pleural space are the site of a number of disorders which may restrict the expansion of the lungs or the alveoli or both. This reaction may result from compression of the lung as a result of the accumulation of air, fluid, blood, or purulent material in the pleural cavity. Pain resulting from inflammation or fibrosis of the pleura may also cause limitation of chest expansion.

PLEURAL EFFUSION

The parietal and visceral pleura are in close apposition to one another and are separated by a thin layer of serous fluid. This thin layer of fluid represents a balance between transudation from the pleural capillaries and reabsorption by the visceral and parietal veins and lymphatics. *Pleural effusion* is the term applied to a collection of fluid in the pleural cavity (see Fig. 34-4). Pleural effusions may be transudates or exudates. A *transudate* occurs if there is a rise in pulmonary venous pressure, as in congestive heart failure. In these cases the balance of forces favors the passage of fluid out of the vessels. Transudation may also occur if there is hypoproteinemia, as in liver and renal disease, or pressure from a tumor on the venae cavae. The accumulation of a transudate in the pleural cavity is called *hydrothorax*. The pleural fluid tends to accumulate at the base of the lungs as a result of the force of gravity. The accumulation of an *exudate* is secondary to involvement of the pleura by inflammation or malignancy and results from increased capillary permeability or impaired lymphatic absorption. An exudate is differentiated from a transudate by the protein content and specific gravity of the pleural fluid. Transudates have a specific gravity of less than 1.015 and a protein content of less than 3 percent, while exudates have a higher specific gravity and protein content because of their cellular content.

When the pleural effusion contains pus, it is termed *empyema*. Empyema is the result of extension of infection from contiguous structures and may be a complication of pneumonia, lung abscess, or perforation of a carcinoma into the pleural cavity. An empyema which is not adequately treated by drainage may have disastrous effects on the thoracic cage. The inflammatory exudate becomes organized, and fibrous adhesions weld the parietal and visceral pleura together. This condition is termed *fibrothorax* (see Fig. 34-4). If the fibrothorax is extensive, it may cause serious mechanical restriction of

FIGURE 34-3 Altered cardiopulmonary dynamics in flail chest injury. Arrows indicate the direction of motion; arrows within trachea and bronchi indicate air being shunted back and forth between lungs during respiratory cycle (pendelluft). Note the paradoxical motion of the unstable portion of the chest wall on the right side. (After B. Burrows, R. J. Knudson, and L. J. Kettel, Respiratory Insufficiency, *Yearbook, Chicago, 1975, p. 111.)*

the underlying tissue. Surgical peeling in an operation, called *decortication,* is sometimes necessary to separate the pleural membranes.

The term hemothorax is used to designate frank bleeding into the pleural cavity and does not designate a hemorrhagic pleural effusion. Trauma is the most common cause of hemothorax. The trauma may be classified as penetrating (e.g., knife wound) or nonpenetrating (e.g., fractured rib which in turn lacerates the lung or an intercostal blood vessel). The thoracic duct can also drain lymph into the pleural cavity as a result of trauma or malignancy; this condition is termed *chylothorax.*

PNEUMOTHORAX

The presence of air in the pleural cavity caused by a breach in the pleura is termed *pneumothorax*. A pneumothorax may be classified as to the cause: (1) traumatic, (2) spontaneous, or (3) therapeutic. It may also be classified according to the sequence of events which follow the breach in the pleura: (1) open, (2) closed, and (3) tension pneumothorax.

A penetrating wound to the chest is a common cause of *traumatic pneumothorax.* As the air enters the pleural space, which is normally subatmospheric in pressure, the lung collapses to a variable extent. If the communication is *open,* a massive collapse occurs until the pressure in the pleural cavity is equal to that of the atmosphere (open pneumothorax—see Fig. 34-4). The mediastinum is shifted in the direction of the collapsed lung and may shift to and fro during the respiratory cycle as air moves in and out of the pleural cavity. Emergency treatment of a penetrating chest wound consists of applying an airtight seal immediately over the wound. If the defect causing the communication between the pleural space and the atmosphere seals itself off, it is called a *closed* pneumothorax. On the other hand, if the defect remains open during inspiration and closes during expiration (check valve effect), a large volume of air may collect in the pleural space, so that pressure builds up above that of the atmosphere, causing complete collapse of the lung. This is termed *tension* pneumothorax. Tension pneumothorax is a serious emergency which must be treated immediately by aspiration of air from the pleural cavity.

Spontaneous pneumothorax is the term used to designate a sudden, unexpected pneumothorax which may occur with or without underlying pulmonary disease. Common pulmonary diseases which may cause a spontaneous pneumothorax include emphysema (rupture of blebs or bullae), pneumonia, and neoplasms. A pneumothorax occurs when there is a communication between a bronchus or alveolus and the pleural cavity, so that air gains access to the pleural cavity through the defect which may result in an open, closed, or tension pneumothorax. A spontaneous pneumothorax may occur in apparently healthy young persons usually between the ages of 20 and 40 years and is termed idiopathic spontaneous pneumothorax. The usual cause is rupture of a subpleural bleb at the surface of the lung or localized bullous disease (refer to Fig. 33-4 in Chap. 33). The etiology of such a bleb or bulla formation in otherwise healthy persons is unknown, although a familial predisposition has sometimes been reported.

A *therapeutic pneumothorax* deserves brief mention for historical reasons. Induced collapse of the lung (therapeutic pneumothorax) was a common treatment for tuberculosis until about 1960, but it is not done today. It was surmised that this procedure inhibited spread of the disease and growth of the bacteria, although there was no definite evidence to support this notion.

Both pleural effusion and pneumothorax limit function by restricting the expansion of the underlying lung. The degree of functional impairment and disability depends on the size and rapidity of development. If fluid accumulates slowly, as is usually the case in pleural effusion, a large amount of fluid may be accommodated with little apparent distress. On the other hand, the rapid decompression of a lung from a massive pneumothorax may be accompanied by the rapid development of shock. The signs and symptoms of pleural effusion and pneumothorax are summarized in Table 34-2. The presence of both conditions is confirmed by x-ray.

A first pneumothorax is treated by conservative observation if the collapse is 20 percent or less. The air is gradually absorbed through the pleural surfaces, which act as wet membranes allowing oxygen and carbon dioxide to diffuse through them. If the pneumothorax is large and dyspnea is severe, a thoracotomy tube attached to water-sealed drainage will be necessary to aid reexpansion of the lung. If bloody effusion is associated with pneumothorax, it must be removed by drainage, because clotting and organization lead to extensive pleural fibrosis. A pleural effusion is treated by needle aspiration (thoracentesis). This is particularly important if the effusion is an exudate, since fibrothorax may result. A small, noninflammatory effusion (transudate) may be resorbed into the capillaries once the cause of the effusion has been reversed.

Lung parenchymal diseases

There are a large number of diseases affecting the lung alveoli and/or interstitium either locally or diffusely which lead to respiratory impairment of varying degrees. Damage to healthy lung tissue may result from invasion by bacteria, viruses, fungi, malignant cells, and inhalation of irritating dust and fumes. Damage to the alveolar capillary endothelium from a variety of causes leads to interstitial, alveolar wall, and intraalveolar edema. Excess fibrotic tissue may be deposited as the sequela to a variety of diseases, usually inflammatory or allergenic in nature. The result is a reduction in lung compliance (stiff lungs) and interference with the gas diffusion pathway. A deficiency of surfactant, called respiratory distress syndrome, may also produce the same results.

The physiologic abnormalities seen in patients with disease of the lung parenchyma vary widely and depend, to some degree, on the extent of the pathologic process. A restrictive defect with its concomitant decrease in lung volume and a rapid, shallow breathing pattern is common. Hypoxemia is the most important blood gas abnormality and is commonly caused by a ventilation–perfusion imbalance resulting in excess wasted ventilation or wasted perfusion due to shunting. None of the physiologic abnormalities are specific, but pulmonary function tests are helpful in quantifying the degree of abnormality, guiding therapy, and assessing the results. Only selected, frequently encountered lung parenchymal diseases will be discussed in this chapter.

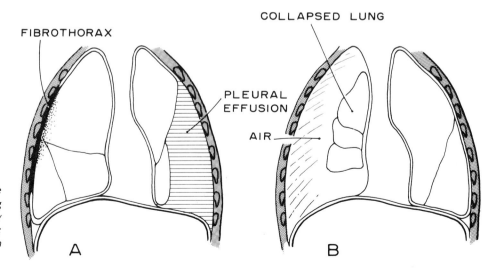

FIGURE 34-4 Disorders of the pleura: A, fibrothorax resulting from organization of inflammatory exudate and pleural effusion; B, collapse of lung due to open pneumothorax.

Atelectasis, although not a disease per se, is a condition which is associated with disease of the lung parenchyma and must be understood in order to prevent its occurrence. Atelectasis is a term meaning "imperfect expansion," and it implies that the alveoli in the affected part of the lung have become airless and collapsed. There are two major causes of collapse: absorption atelectasis secondary to bronchial or bronchiolar obstruction and atelectasis caused by compression.

In *absorption atelectasis,* obstruction of the airway prevents air from entering the alveoli distal to the obstruction. The air which is already present in the alveoli is then absorbed gradually into the bloodstream, and the alveoli collapse. (It takes more air pressure and work to reinflate an alveolus from a completely collapsed position, just as one must blow harder at the beginning when blowing up a balloon.) Absorption atelectasis may result from intrinsic or extrinsic bronchial obstruction. Intrinsic bronchial obstruction is most commonly caused by retained secretions or exudate. Extrinsic pressure on a bronchus commonly results from neoplasm, lymph node enlargement, aneurysm, or scar tissue. This discussion will be concerned with intrinsic obstruction resulting from retained secretions, since it is most .common and preventable to a large degree.

We have already discussed the physiologic defense mechanisms which act to keep the lower respiratory tract sterile. Some of these mechanisms also act to prevent atelectasis by preventing obstruction. These mechanisms include the combined action of the "ciliary escalator," which may be assisted by cough to move

TABLE 34-2
Signs and symptoms of pleural effusion and pneumothorax

PLEURAL EFFUSION	PNEUMOTHORAX
Dyspnea variable	Dyspnea (if large)
Pleuritic pain usually precedes effusion if secondary to pleuritic disease	Pleuritic pain severe
Trachea deviated away from the side of effusion	Trachea deviated away from the side of pneumothorax
Bulging of intercostal spaces (large effusion)	Tachycardia
	Cyanosis (if large)
Diminished and delayed chest movement on the involved side	Diminished and delayed chest movement on the involved side
Flat percussion note over the pleural effusion	Hyperresonant percussion note over pneumothorax
Egophony over compressed lung next to effusion (spoken syllables have a peculiar nasal or bleating quality when heard through stethoscope)	Flatness to percussion over collapsed lung
Decreased breath sounds over pleural effusion	Decreased or absent breath sounds on affected side
Decreased vocal and tactile fremitus	Decreased vocal and tactile fremitus

noxious particles and bacteria to the posterior pharynx where they are swallowed or expectorated. Another mechanism which serves to prevent atelectasis is collateral ventilation. Although a subject of debate for the past 50 years, recent experimental studies of collateral ventilation leave no doubt that air can pass from one lung acinus to another, other than by the normal airways. It is now well established that small pores, called the pores of Kohn after their discoverer in 1873, between the alveoli provide a path for collateral ventilation.

Figure 34-5 illustrates how collateral ventilation prevents absorption atelectasis in the presence of bronchiolar obstruction by a mucus plug. Also illustrated is one of the causes of ineffective ventilation and its effect. Only deep inspiration is effective in opening up the pores of Kohn and providing collateral ventilation to an adjacent obstructed alveolus. Collapse caused by the absorption of gases in the obstructed alveolus is thus prevented. (Normally gas absorption into the blood is favored because the total partial pressure of the blood gases is slightly less than atmospheric pressure because more oxygen is absorbed into the tissues than carbon dioxide is excreted.) During expiration the pores of Kohn close, and pressure builds up in the obstructed alveolus, which aids in the expulsion of the mucus plug. Even greater expiratory force may be built up if, after taking a deep breath, the glottis is closed and then suddenly opened as in the normal cough. In contrast, the pores of Kohn remain closed with shallow inspiration, so that there is no collateral ventilation to the obstructed alveolus. Pressure adequate to expel the mucus plug is thus not attained. Absorption of alveolar gases into the bloodstream continues resulting in collapse of the alveolus. As the air leaves the alveolus, it is gradually replaced by edematous fluid.

The purpose of this discussion is to emphasize the importance of coughing and deep breathing exercises and other physical activity to prevent atelectasis in predisposed individuals. This is particularly important in postoperative, bedridden, or otherwise debilitated patients, since atelectasis is the prevalent cause of morbidity in this population group. Atelectasis at the lung bases is especially common in patients whose respirations are shallow as a result of pain, weakness, or abdominal distention. Retained secretions may lead to pneumonia and more extensive atelectasis.

Prolonged atelectasis may lead to the replacement of the involved lung tissue with fibrous tissue. Adequate prevention also requires familiarity with factors which interfere with normal lung defense mechanisms. Although some of these factors were discussed previously, they are listed again in Table 34-3 for added emphasis and consideration.

Compression atelectasis results from extrinsic pressure on all or part of the lung, driving the air out and causing collapse. Common causes are pleural effusion, pneumothorax, or abdominal distention elevating the diaphragm. Compression atelectasis is much less common than absorption atelectasis.

INFECTIONS OF THE LUNG PARENCHYMA: PNEUMONIAS

Acute inflammation of the lung parenchyma, which is usually infectious in origin, is called *pneumonia* or *pneumonitis*. It is preferable to use the term "pneumonia," since the latter term has been frequently used to designate a nonspecific pulmonary inflammation of unknown etiology. Pneumonia is a common malady and affects about 1 percent of the American population annually. In 1970, the reported cases of pneumonia of all kinds numbered 2,700,000 in the United States,

accounting for 8.5 percent of 33 million hospital admissions. In spite of antibiotics, pneumonia is still a major killer and accounted for 3 percent of American deaths in 1970. The infant and young child are particularly susceptible because of poorly developed immune responses. Pneumonia is frequently the terminal event in the elderly and those debilitated by chronic diseases. Alcoholics, postoperative patients, and patients with chronic respiratory disease or virus infections are also particularly vulnerable. Infectious agents are most frequently inhaled or are already normal flora of the respiratory tract. Consequently, predisposing factors include any deficiency in the lung's defense mechanisms.

The pathologic picture depends, to some extent, on the etiologic agent. *Bacterial pneumonia* is characterized by an intra-alveolar suppurative exudate with consolidation. The infectious process may be classified on an anatomic basis. There is consolidation of an entire lobe in *lobar* pneumonia, while *lobular* or *bronchopneumonia*

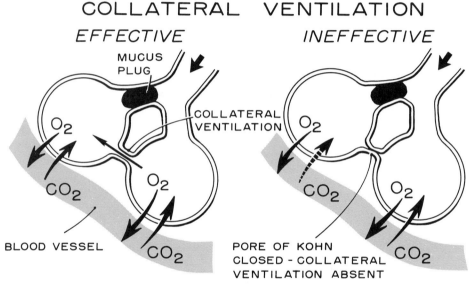

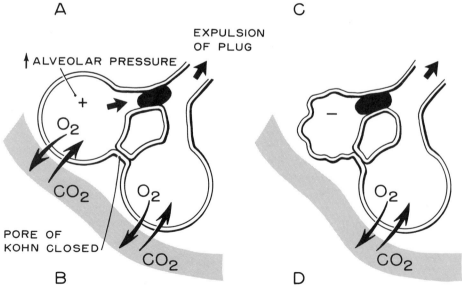

FIGURE 34-5 The role of collateral alveolar ventilation in the prevention of absorption atelectasis. Effective ventilation: A, during deep inspiration, pore of Kohn opens, and air enters adjacent obstructed alveolus; B, during expiration, the pores of Kohn close; positive pressure builds up in obstructed alveolus and aids in expulsion of mucus plug. Ineffective ventilation: C, pores of Kohn do not open during shallow inspiration, so that collateral ventilation is not provided to obstructed alveolus; D, obstructed alveolus collapses as alveolar gases are absorbed into bloodstream. (Modified from Edwin J. Kroeker, "Atelectasis," Hospital Medicine, March 1969.)

refers to a patchy distribution of infectious areas about 3 to 4 cm in diameter surrounding and involving the bronchi. *Virus* or *mycoplasma* (viruslike bacteria) pneumonias are characterized by an interstitial inflammation with accumulation of an infiltrate in the alveolar walls, although the alveolar spaces themselves are free of exudate and there is no consolidation. If the infecting agent is a *fungus* or *Mycobacterium tuberculosis,* the common pathologic pattern is a patchy distribution of granulomas which may undergo caseous necrosis with the development of cavities (see Fig. 34-6 illustrating the forms of pneumonia and the common etiologic agent).

The pattern of response also depends on the specific etiologic agent. Three organisms most commonly involved in bacterial pneumonia are the pneumococcus (accounting for more than 90 percent of the cases), *Klebsiella* or Friedländer's bacillus (1 percent), and staphylococcus (1 to 5 percent). Less commonly, hemolytic streptococcus and gram-negative organisms such as *Pseudomonas aeruginosa* and *Escherichia coli* may cause pneumonia.

Among the bacterial pneumonias, the pathogenesis of pneumococcal pneumonia has been the most extensively studied. The current concept is that the pneumococci reach the alveoli in droplets of mucus or saliva.

The lower lobes of the lungs are commonly involved because of the effect of gravity. Once established in the alveolus, the pneumococcus elicits a typical pathologic response involving four successive stages:[1]

1 Engorgement (first 4 to 12 hours)—serous exudate pours into alveloi from the dilated, leaking blood vessels.
2 Red hepatization (next 48 hours)—lung assumes a red, granular appearance (hepatization = liverlike) as red blood cells, fibrin, and polymorphonuclear leukocytes fill the alveoli.
3 Gray hepatization (3 to 8 days)—lung assumes a grayish appearance as the leukocytes and fibrin consolidate in the involved alveoli.
4 Resolution (7 to 11 days)—exudate is lysed and resorbed by macrophages restoring the tissue to its original structure.

The onset of pneumococcal pneumonia is typically sudden, with chills, fever, pleuritic pain, cough, and rust-colored sputum. Rales and a friction rub may be heard over the involved tissue because of the exudate and fibrin that are in the alveoli and may be deposited on the pleural surface. There is almost always some degree of hypoxemia as a result of the shunting of blood through the nonventilated, consolidated area of lung, and the patient may have a "dusky" appearance. Chest x-ray, white blood cell count, and sputum examination, including gross appearance, microscopic examination, and culture, may all be helpful in making the diagnosis and following the course of the pneumonia.

The general treatment of patients with pneumonia consists of the administration of antibiotic drugs effective against the specific organism, oxygen therapy for hypoxemia, and treatment of complications. Likely complications and mortality are related to the specific infecting organism. Pneumococcal pneumonia generally runs an uncomplicated course, resulting in restoration of normal tissue structure. The most likely complication is a small pleural effusion. Before the era of antibiotics there was a 20 to 40 percent mortality for pneumococcal pneumonia, but this has now been reduced to 5 to 13 percent. Death is more likely to occur in elderly, chronically ill persons. The presence of bacteremia also affects the prognosis for pneumonia. The mortality in patients with bacteremia is about double that observed in the absence of bacteremia, although transient bacteremia may occur in all patients with pneumococcal pneumonia. Demonstrable bacteremia suggests ineffective localization of the pulmonary process, and it is not surprising that the mortality is higher in this group. The consequences of bacteremia may be metastatic lesions result-

TABLE 34-3
Lung defense mechanisms preventing atelectasis

PROTECTIVE MECHANISM	FACTORS CAUSING INTERFERENCE WITH MECHANISM
Mucus and ciliary action	General dehydration causes production of viscous mucus and scant volume
	Inhalation of dry air increases viscosity of mucus so that crusting occurs
	Excess mucus production (e.g. chronic bronchitis) overwhelms ciliary escalator
	Cigarette smoke reduces or paralyzes ciliary action
	Trauma (suctioning) reduces ciliary action
	Anesthetics and atropinelike drugs reduce both mucus production and ciliary action
Cough	Pain reduces expiratory force
	Sedatives and narcotics inhibit cough initiation
	Airflow rate reduced by COPD
Collateral ventilation	Shallow breathing due to pain or sedation
	Pulmonary edema from congestion or infection
	Constant tidal volume respiration on a mechanical respirator
	Anesthetic gases and oxygen rapidly absorbed allowing less time for collateral ventilation
Pharyngeal clearing	Unconsciousness; obtundation favors aspiration of gastric contents or upper respiratory tract secretions

[1]These stages represent the temporal course in untreated pneumococcal pneumonia. With the use of antibiotics the course is now run in about 3 days.

ing in such conditions as meningitis, bacterial endocarditis, and peritonitis.

Pneumonias caused by gram-negative organisms or by staphylococcus frequently have a poor prognosis even with antibiotic therapy. These pneumonias cause extensive damage of the lung parenchyma, and complications such as lung abscess and empyema are common. The mortality is 25 to 50 percent when the infecting organism is *K. pneumoniae*, 70 percent with *P. aeruginosa*, 45 percent with *E. coli*, and 15 to 50 percent with *S. aureus*.

A large number of patients who survive *Klebsiella* (or Friedländer's) pneumonia develop a chronic pneumonia with severe progressive destruction of lung tissue that ultimately converts the patient into a respiratory cripple. A thick "red currant jelly" sputum is characteristic of this pneumonia. Most cases of *Klebsiella* pneumonia occur in middle-aged or elderly males who are chronic alcoholics or who have some other chronic disease. Pneumonia caused by *Pseudomonas* organisms is most common in hospitalized patients who are terminally ill or who have marked suppression of immunologic body defenses (e.g., a patient with leukemia or a renal transplant who is receiving large doses of immunosuppressive drugs). Other predisposing causes of gram-negative pneumonias include prior antimicrobial therapy

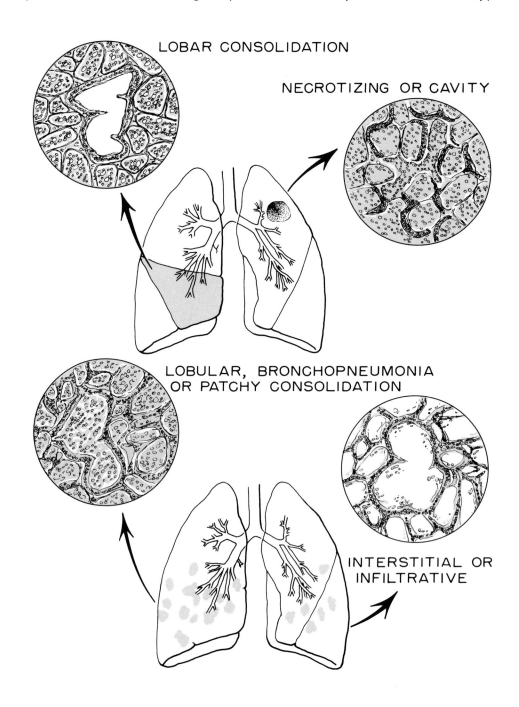

LOBAR CONSOLIDATION

NECROTIZING OR CAVITY

LOBULAR, BRONCHOPNEUMONIA
OR PATCHY CONSOLIDATION

INTERSTITIAL OR
INFILTRATIVE

which alters the normal resident flora of the respiratory tract and allows overgrowth of certain microorganisms. Contaminated ventilatory equipment is a common source of *Pseudomonas* infection. *Staphylococcus aureus* is commonly a secondary infection in hospitalized, debilitated patients and is most likely to cause a bronchopneumonia.

Viral pneumonias account for about 50 percent of all acute pneumonias and are characterized by symptoms of headache, fever, generalized aching of muscles, extreme fatigue, and a dry cough. Most of these pneumonias are mild, do not require hospitalization, and leave no permanent lung damage. Types A and B influenza virus are common infecting agents. The treatment of viral pneumonia is symptomatic and palliative, since antibiotics are not effective against viruses. Vaccination may give protection for a limited time but does not give protection against the many other types of viruses (some unidentified) which may cause respiratory infections. Viral pneumonia may set the stage for secondary invasion by bacteria, which has already been discussed. More rarely, a fatal patchy or diffuse pneumonitis may be attributed to the virus.

Pneumonia caused by *M. pneumoniae* is generally discussed with virus pneumonias even though it is a bacterium. The clinical picture of mycoplasmal pneumonia is similar to influenza virus pneumonia with evidence of interstitial pneumonitis. It is highly contagious and, unlike viral pneumonia, responds to tetracycline or erythromycin. Myoplasmal pneumonia is often referred to as primary atypical pneumonia.

Aspiration pneumonia refers to a pneumonia caused by the aspiration of gastric contents. The resultant pneumonia is partly chemical as a result of the reaction to the gastric juice and partly bacterial as a result of the organisms which may inhabit the mouth or stomach. Aspiration is most common during or following anesthesia (especially in obstetrical patients and surgical emergencies because of the lack of surgical preparation), in infants, and in any obtunded patient with depressed cough or gag reflexes. This type of pneumonia may be extremely fulminant and has a high mortality. Massive inhalation of gastric contents may lead to sudden death from obstruction, while aspiration of smaller quantities of gastric contents may lead to widespread pulmonary edema and respiratory failure. The severity of the inflammatory response depends on the pH of the aspirate more than on any other factor. Aspiration pneumonia always results when the pH of the aspirate is 2.5 or less. Abscesses, bronchiectasis, and gangrene are common

complications of aspiration pneumonia. It is important to realize that vomiting is not a prerequisite to the entrance of gastric contents into the tracheobronchial tree, as silent regurgitation may occur in obtunded patients. Proper positioning to drain oropharyngeal secretions from the mouth is most important in the care of these patients.

Hypostatic pneumonia is a pneumonia which develops frequently at the lung bases and is caused by shallow breathing and constantly remaining in the same position. Gravity causes blood to become congested in the dependent part of the lung, and infection aids the development of true pneumonia.

Fungi may be the cause of pneumonia, although this is a much less frequent cause than bacteria. A few fungi are capable of producing a chronic granulomatous suppurative lung disease which is often mistaken for tuberculosis. Many of these fungal infections are endemic to certain geographic regions. The most important fungal infections in the United States are histoplasmosis (midwest and east), coccidiodomycosis (southwest), and blastomycosis (southeast). Spores of these fungi are found in the soil and are inhaled. Spores carried into the smaller divisions of the lung are phagocytized and cause an allergic reaction. After allergy develops, the reaction becomes inflammatory, with tubercle formation, central caseation, scarring, calcification, and even cavity formation. All the pathologic changes resemble tuberculosis so closely that differentiation can only be made by identification and culture of the fungus from lung tissue. Serologic and delayed hypersensitivity skin tests are not positive until a few weeks after the initial infection and may even be negative with severe disease.

It is not unusual for fungal pneumonia to complicate the final stages of terminal diseases such as cancer or leukemia. *Candida albicans*, a yeastlike fungus frequently found in the sputum of healthy persons, may invade the pulmonary tissue under these conditions. Infections with *Candida* is termed candidiasis. Prolonged use of antibiotics may also alter the natural body flora and permit invasion of *Candida*. Amphotericin B is the drug of choice for the pulmonary fungal infections.

PULMONARY FIBROSIS

Pulmonary fibrosis is not an etiologic entity but a pathologic term which implies that there is an excessive amount of connective tissue in the lung. Fibrosis results from a method of tissue repair which may follow any disease process of the lung which produces inflammation or necrosis. The most common type of pulmonary fibrosis is localized fibrosis which follows localized damage to the lung parenchyma caused by such conditions as tuberculosis, pulmonary abscess, bronchiectasis, or unresolved pneumonias. Although less common, pulmonary fibrosis may diffusely involve the lung paren-

FIGURE 34-6 Forms of pneumonia: *lobar*—entire lobe consolidated, exudate chiefly intra-alveolar (inset), Pneumococcus and Klebsiella common infecting organisms; *necrotizing*—granuloma may undergo caseous necrosis and form cavity, fungi and tubercle bacillus common cause; *lobular*—patchy distribution, fibrinous exudate chiefly in bronchioles, Staphylococcus and Streptococcus common infecting organisms; *interstitial*—perivascular exudate and edema between the alveoli, caused by virus or mycoplasmal infection.

chyma, particularly affecting the interalveolar septa. Unlike localized fibrosis, diffuse pulmonary fibrosis is a disabling and frequently fatal disorder. Diffuse pulmonary fibrosis represents end-stage lung disease from a host of known and unknown causes. A few of the more common causes of diffuse pulmonary fibrosis are listed in Table 34-4.

The *pneumoconioses* are a group of diseases caused by the inhalation of certain inorganic and organic dusts. Some dusts, when inhaled in sufficient concentration into the lungs, produce a fibrous tissue reaction, while others are quite inert. The dust inhalation diseases are of particular interest, since exposure is usually related to certain occupations and are theoretically preventable by the institution of industrial safety standards. Only a few examples of noxious dusts or gases causing pulmonary fibrosis are listed in Table 34-4. Whether a particular dust causes disease depends on (1) the size of the particle—the most dangerous dust particle seems to be 1 to 5 μm, since larger particles never reach the alveoli; (2) the concentration and length of exposure—high concentration is usually required to overcome the action of the "ciliary escalator," and long exposure is usually required (e.g., coal miner's pneumoconiosis or "black lung" disease usually requires 20 years of exposure before there is extensive pulmonary fibrosis); (3) the

TABLE 34-4
Common causes of diffuse pulmonary fibrosis

DISEASES OF KNOWN ETIOLOGY	DISEASES OF UNKNOWN ETIOLOGY

1 Pneumoconioses (occupational inhalation of dusts)
 a Inorganic dusts:
   silica—silicosis
   coal—"black lung"
   iron—siderosis
   asbestos—asbestosis
   talc—talcosis
   beryllium—berylliosis
 b Organic dusts:
   cotton—byssinosis
   sugar cane—bagassosis
   moldy hay—"farmer's lung"
   maple bark
2 Noxious gas inhalation—nitrogen oxides (silo filler), chlorine, sulfur oxides, metal fumes
3 Drug sensitivity to diphenylhydantoin (Dilantin), busulfan (Myleran)
4 Irradiation
5 Viral pneumonias
6 Chronic pulmonary edema
	1 Hamman-Rich syndrome
	2 Sarcoidosis
	3 "Collagen diseases"—progressive systemic sclerosis
	4 Chronic interstitial pneumonia
	5 Mucoviscidosis (cystic fibrosis)

nature of the dust—certain materials [particularly the organic dusts such as cotton fiber which causes byssinosis, sugar cane (bagassosis), and moldy hay (farmer's lung)] have an unusual antigenic effect and cause an allergic alveolitis. The chemical nature of inorganic dusts also influences their capacity to produce disease. Silica dust, which causes silicosis (commonly inhaled by grinders, sandblasters, and rock quarry workers), is particularly harmful. It is thought that these dust particles regularly destroy the macrophages by which they are phagocytized, resulting in the formation of fibrotic nodules. Widespread fibrosis is produced by the coalescence of the fibrotic nodules.

The inhalation of noxious gases may be associated with certain occupations. The result is a chemical pneumonitis. Of particular interest is silo filler's disease, which is not a pneumoconiosis but is caused by the inhalation of nitrogen oxides from fermentation of the vegetation in a freshly filled silo. The severity of reaction to noxious gases depends on the concentration of gas and length of exposure. Viral pneumonias, chronic pulmonary edema, irradiation involving the chest, and certain drugs that produce a hypersensitivity reaction are other known causes of diffuse pulmonary fibrosis.

Among diseases of unknown etiology causing diffuse pulmonary fibrosis is the Hamman-Rich syndrome. This is an unusual interstitial pneumonia which may have a rapidly fatal course or a more protracted course, both with the development of severe intra-alveolar and interstitial fibrosis. Other chronic interstitial pneumonias tend to result in progressive pulmonary fibrosis. Certain systemic diseases such as sarcoidosis, collagen diseases (especially scleroderma), and mucoviscidosis also result in progressive pulmonary fibrosis.

The systemic symptoms in the group of diseases causing pulmonary fibrosis vary widely. In the early stages there may be no symptoms at all. The pulmonary symptoms, however, are strikingly similar. The primary symptom seems to be a progressive dyspnea on exertion. The common pathologic denominator is interstitial fibrosis, with the extent of fibrosis determining the effect on pulmonary function. When the fibrosis is extensive, there is a decrease in lung elasticity, total lung capacity, vital capacity, and residual volume, which all indicate restrictive lung disease. The dyspnea reflects the poor compliance and results in a concomitant increase in the work of breathing. With marked destruction of alveoli and pulmonary vessels, hypoxemia, pulmonary hypertension, cor pulmonale, and heart failure may result. Many of the cases, however, do not progress beyond mild exertional dyspnea.

RESPIRATORY DISTRESS SYNDROME

Respiratory distress syndrome is a restrictive lung disorder in which the main pathologic finding is widespread atelectasis, pulmonary edema, intense congestion, and in some cases, hyaline membranes lining the alveolar walls. The lungs are stiff and inelastic. Continued perfusion of the nonventilated atelectic areas of the lungs results in profound shunting and hypoxemia. This syndrome commonly occurs in premature infants (25 percent) and accounts for about 40 percent of premature infant deaths. The syndrome is also called *hyaline membrane disease*. One of the primary etiologic factors in respiratory distress syndrome is thought to be a deficiency of surfactant so that alveoli are more apt to collapse. The hyaline membrane which forms along the alveolar walls is a secondary development common to a variety of respiratory insufficiency states.

Adult respiratory distress syndrome results in pathologic findings similar to that found in the infant and results from a number of diverse insults. Many of the synonyms reflect the underlying causes (e.g., shock lung, aspiration pneumonia, smoke inhalation, and oxygen toxicity). It is also associated with gram-negative sepsis, overwhelming viral pneumonia, acute hemorrhagic pancreatitis, drowning, and cardiopulmonary bypass. The loss of pulmonary surfactant secondary to initial damage to the alveolar–capillary membrane is thought to be an important factor in the development of the diffuse atelectasis.

The management of respiratory distress syndrome is aimed at correcting the accompanying shock, acidosis, and hypoxemia. The use of positive end expiratory pressure (PEEP) with the volume respirator is a major advance in the treatment of this condition. PEEP helps to correct the respiratory distress syndrome by reexpanding previously atelectic areas and by reversing the flow of atelectic edema from capillaries. A device which provides continuous positive airway pressure (CPAP) without using a respirator has been developed for infants and has greatly reduced mortality. The principle is the same as PEEP in the treatment of the adult respiratory distress syndrome.

QUESTIONS

Restrictive patterns of respiratory disease—Chap. 34

Directions: Match each of the extrapulmonary disorders causing alveolar hypoventilation in col. A with its appropriate altered mechanism in col. B.

Column A
1 ____ Kyphoscoliosis
2 ____ Progressive muscular dystrophy
3 ____ P_aCO_2 70 mmHg
4 ____ Myasthenia gravis
5 ____ CNS lesion
6 ____ Amyotrophic lateral sclerosis

Column B
a Depression of the respiratory center
b Interruption of nerve transmission to respiratory muscles due to disease involving the neuromuscular junction
c Interruption of nerve transmission to respiratory muscles due to upper motor neuron lesion
d Direct anatomic damage to the respiratory center
e Paresis of the respiratory muscles due to diffuse disease of the skeletal muscles
f Deformity of the chest cage causing abnormal positioning and functioning of its respiratory muscles

Directions: Circle T if the statement is true and F if it is false. Correct the false statements.

7   T   F   In kyphoscoliosis, compression of the lungs by the thoracic deformity causes a small lung volume and unequal distribution of ventilation and perfusion.

8   T   F   Pectus excavatum refers to a lateral displacement of the spine.

9   T   F   Flail chest injury is associated with paradoxical movement of dead-space air between the airways of the right and left lungs during the respiratory cycle.

10   T   F   Ankylosing spondylitis is a disease which causes asymmetric deformity of the chest cage.

Directions: Circle the letter preceding each item below that correctly answers each question. Only one answer is correct.

11 The Pickwickian syndrome is characterized by all of the following *except*:
a Hypoxemia   b Hypercapnia   c Increased arterial pH   d Polycythemia   e Cor pulmonale

12 Patients with kyphoscoliotic lung disease would be expected to exhibit all of the following physiologic abnormalities *except*:
a Increased nonelastic work of breathing   b Increased elastic work of breathing   c Decreased lung compliance   d Decreased vital capacity

13 Alveolar hypoventilation results in all of the following abnormalities of the blood gases *except*:
a low P_aO_2 b low P_AO_2 c high P_aCO_2
d low P_ACO_2

14 Children with muscular dystrophy are most likely to exhibit which of the following abnormalities of pulmonary function?
a Obstructive ventilatory pattern   b Restrictive ventilatory pattern   c Pulmonary diffusion block   d Normal ventilatory function

Directions: Answer the following questions on a separate sheet of paper.

15 What are two physiologic alterations which occur as a consequence of a restricted pattern of ventilation?

16 List possible causes of the following types of pneumothorax: traumatic, therapeutic, and spontaneous.

17 Describe the emergency treatment of a penetrating chest wound.

18 Why does a pneumothorax occur when there is a communication between a bronchus or alveolus and the pleural cavity?

19 Describe the treatment for a large pneumothorax and a large pleural effusion.

20 What is a collection of fluid in the pleural cavity called?

21 When a transudate occurs, there is a rise in pressure so that the balance of forces favors the passage of fluid out of the vessels. What is this pressure called?

22 What is formed in the pleural cavity as the result of increased capillary permeability or impaired lymphatic absorption?

23 What is the pleural fluid called which has a specific gravity of less than 1.015 and a protein content of less than 3 percent?

24 List five general disorders which may cause damage to the lung alveoli and interstitium. State the specific damage to lung tissue that each disorder causes.

25 Contrast absorption and compression atelectasis with respect to the common cause of each and the mechanism involved.

26 Why are the pores of Kohn important in maintaining collateral ventilation? Illustrate how collateral ventilation prevents absorption atelectasis caused by bronchial obstruction by a mucus plug.

27 List in sequence the four stages describing the pathologic changes in the lung in untreated pneumococcal pneumonia (include name of stage, time period, and description of lung changes).

28 List three principles of treatment for patients with pneumonia.

29 List three criteria used to predict whether a particular dust will cause disease of the lung parenchyma. State the reason why each of these criteria is important.

30 What is thought to be the primary etiologic factor in the development of respiratory distress syndrome in the premature infant and in the adult?

31 What are the principles of treatment for adult respiratory distress syndrome?

32 List the three most important fungal infections in the United States.

33 What are two consequences of pulmonary fibrosis?

34 The manifestations of extensive diffuse pulmonary fibrosis are typical of what type of pattern of ventilatory dysfunction?

Directions: Complete the following statements by filling in the blanks.

35 Pulmonary fibrosis is characterized pathologically by _____ fibrosis.

36 Pneumonia caused by gram-negative or staphylococcus organisms cause extensive damage to the lung _____. Common complications include _____ and _____. The prognosis is generally _____.

37 The major pathologic findings in respiratory distress syndrome are _____, _____ and _____. In some cases the alveolar walls are lined with a _____ membrane.

Directions: Circle T if the statement is true and F if it is false. Correct the false statements.

38 T F Patients with Friedländer's pneumonia often develop a chronic pneumonia following the original infection.

39 T F Gram-negative pneumonias often occur in hospitalized or debilitated patients.

40 T F Viral pneumonia commonly has a poor prognosis.

41 T F Viral pneumonia is successfully treated with erythromycin.

42 T F The clinical picture of mycoplasmal pneumonia is similar to that of viral pneumonia.

43 T F Aspiration pneumonia develops at the lung bases and is caused by shallow breathing and constantly remaining in the same position.

44 T F Amphotericin B is the drug of choice for the treatment of candidiasis.

45 T F Fungal pulmonary lesions are often granulomatous and similar to lesions caused by *Mycobacterium tuberculosis*.

Directions: Match the type of pneumothorax in col. A with the correct description in col. B.

Column A
46 ___ Open
47 ___ Closed
48 ___ Tension

Column B
a Communication between pleural cavity and atmosphere sealed off
b Communication between pleural cavity and atmosphere open during inspiration and closed during expiration
c Communication between pleural cavity and atmosphere does not seal off

Directions: Match each of the anatomic patterns of pneumonia in col. A with its pathologic description or common etiologic agent in col. B. More than one letter may be used for each blank in col. A.

Column A
49 ___ Lobar consolidation
50 ___ Lobular consolidation

Column B
a Fungi or *Mycobacterium tuberculosis*
b Virus or *Mycoplasma* pneumonia

51 ____ Necrotizing or cavity formation

52 ____ Interstitial

c Pneumococcus
d Staphylococcus or streptococcus
e Perivascular exudate and edema between the alveoli
f May undergo caseous necrosis
g Exudate chiefly intra-alveolar
h Fibrinous exudate chiefly in bronchioles
i Patchy distribution of infection
j Whole lung lobe infected

Directions: Match each of the protective mechanisms in col. A with the factors causing interference with it in col. B. More than one letter may be used for each blank in col. A.

Column A

53 ____ Cough
54 ____ Mucus and ciliary action
55 ____ Collateral ventilation
56 ____ Pharyngeal clearing

Column B

a Cigarette smoke
b General dehydration
c Pain
d Shallow breathing
e Constant tidal volume breathing
f Sedatives and narcotics
g Atropinelike drugs
h Unconsciousness
i Reduction of airflow rate

Directions: Match each item in col. A with its description or cause in col. B. Items are associated with occupational diseases resulting in diffuse pulmonary fibrosis.

Column A

57 ____ Organic dusts
58 ____ Silica dust
59 ____ Farmer's lung
60 ____ Silo filler's disease
61 ____ Byssinosis
62 ____ Black lung disease

Column B

a Caused by inhalation of nitrogen oxides
b Caused by inhalation of cotton dust
c Mechanism of adverse reaction is allergic alveolitis
d Caused by moldy hay
e Mechanism of adverse reaction is production of chemical pneumonitis
f Mechanism of adverse reaction is destruction of macrophages with formation of fibrotic nodules
g Common occupational disease among rock quarry workers, grinders, and sandblasters
h Caused by inhalation of coal dust

Directions: Circle the correct answer to the following questions. More than one answer may be correct.

63 Which of the following are common causes of diffuse pulmonary fibrosis?
a Tuberculosis b Inhalation of noxious gases c Inhalation of silica dusts d Sarcoidosis e Dilantin therapy

64 Which of the following are typical signs, symptoms, and findings associated with pneumococcal pneumonia?
a "Red currant jelly" sputum b "Rusty" sputum c Dry, nonproductive cough d Decreased white blood cell count e Fever, chills, pleuritic pain f Lobar consolidation evident on chest x-ray

65 What percentage of the American population is affected by pneumonia annually?
a 1 percent b 5 percent c 10 percent d 15 percent

66 Which of the following abnormalities are commonly seen in patients with disease of the lung parenchyma?
a A restrictive pattern of pulmonary dysfunction
b An obstructive pattern of pulmonary dysfunction
c Rapid, shallow breathing pattern d Slow, deep breathing pattern e Decrease in lung volume
f Hypercapnia g Hypoxemia

Directions: Circle the one best answer to the following questions.

67 Inadequately treated empyema may result in which of the following conditions?
a Hydrothorax b Chylothorax c Hemothorax d Fibrothorax

68 Which of the following statements is the best description of a pneumothorax?
a Air within the pleural cavity b Cohesion and positive intrapleural pressure c A pathologic lesion of the lung d Accumulation of fluid in the pleural cavity

69 The most common cause of idiopathic spontaneous pneumothorax in healthy young adults is:
a Bulging of the intercostal spaces b Rupture of a subpleural bleb or localized bullous disease c Lesions of the parietal pleura d Diffuse emphysematous disease of the lungs

70 Which of the following signs and symptoms would best differentiate between a pleural effusion and a pneumothorax?
a Moderate dyspnea b Diminished and delayed chest movement on the involved side c Decreased vocal fremitus over the involved area d Diminished or absent breath sounds on the affected side
e Egophony over lung above effusion (bleating sound heard by stethoscope when patient speaks)

71 A patient with pneumonia is having severe pain in the right lateral chest accompanying respiratory movements. This is because the:
a Inflamed lung is painful b Visceral pleura is in-

flamed and sensitive to pain *c* Parietal pleura is inflamed and sensitive to pain *d* Patient has an intercostal peripheral neuritis

72 Nosocomial (arising from hospitalization) infections associated with respirators, resusitation equipment, and humidifiers are especially likely to be caused by: *a* Klebsiella pneumoniae *b* Staphylococcus aureus *c* Fungi *d* Pseudomonas organisms

73 The normal respiratory tract is sterile:
a Below the oropharynx *b* Below the larynx
c Below the mainstem bronchi *d* Below the terminal bronchioles *e* Nowhere

74 The usual course of pneumococcal lobar pneumonia terminates with:
a Diffuse pulmonary fibrosis *b* Organization of the inflammatory exudate *c* Complete resolution of the pulmonary inflammation *d* Abscess formation and empyema

BIBLIOGRAPHY

Chest wall abnormalities and injuries

Burrows, B., R. J. Knudson, and L. J. Kettel: *Respiratory Insufficiency*, Yearbook, Chicago, 1975, pp. 110–112.

Fishman, Fred P.: "Chronic Cor Pulmonale," *Hospital Practice*, May, 1971, pp. 101–117.

Geiger, J. R.: "Diagnosis of Chest Injuries," *Hospital Medicine*, 7: 109, October, 1971.

Harlan, D. E., and J. M. Mattloff: "Initial Management of Rib Fractures and their Complications," *Hospital Medicine*, 9: 71, March, 1973.

Pleural disorders

Adler, Richard H.: "Spontaneous Pneumothorax," *Hospital Medicine*, 1: 2, May 1965.

Baum, Gerald L.: "Diseases of the Pleura," *Hospital Medicine*, 5: 6, October 1969.

Cherniack, R. M., L. Cherniack, and A. Naimark: *Respiration in Health and Disease*, 2d ed., Saunders, Philadelphia, 1972, pp. 392–407.

Scharer, Lawrence: "Pleurisy, Pleural Effusions, and Empyema," in C. W. Holman and C. Muschenheim (eds.), *Bronchopulmonary Diseases and Related Disorders*, Harper & Row, New York, 1972, vol. 1, pp. 766–783.

Atelectasis

Kroeker, Edwin J.: "Atelectasis," *Hospital Medicine*, 5: 67, March 1969.

Robbins, S. and M. Angell: *Basic Pathology*, Saunders, Philadelphia, 1971, pp. 321–322.

Spencer, H.: *Pathology of the Lung*, 2d ed., Pergamon, New York, 1968, p. 43.

Pneumonia

Cherniack, et al.: op. cit., pp. 339–352.

Cole, R. B.: *Essentials of Respiratory Diseases*, Medcom, New York, 1975.

"Deaths from 69 Selected Causes by Age, Color, and Sex: U.S.A. 1970," *Vital Statistics of the U.S., 1970, Vol. II, Mortality*, U.S. Department of Health, Education, and Welfare, Public Health Service, 1974.

Geschickter, Charles F.: *The Lung in Health and Disease*, Lippincott, Philadelphia, 1973, pp. 144–134.

Hook, Edward W.: "The Pneumonias and Viral Respiratory Infections," in Holman and Muschenheim, op cit., pp. 279–340.

Reimann, Hobart A. (ed.): *Acute Respiratory Tract Diseases*, Medcom, New York, 1975.

"Respiratory Diseases: Task Force on Problems, Research Approaches, Needs," Publication No. (NIH) 732. Department of Health, Education, and Welfare, October 1972, p. 118.

Robbins and Angell: op. cit., pp. 334–338.

Sandritter, W., and W. B. Wartman: *Color Atlas and Textbook of Tissue and Cellular Pathology*, 4th ed., Yearbook, Chicago, 1973, pp. 74–97.

Pulmonary fungal infections

American Lung Association: *Introduction to Lung Diseases*, 5th ed., 1973, pp. 49–58.

Cherniack, et al.: op. cit., pp. 357–360.

Cole: op. cit., pp. 190–195.

Geschickter: op. cit., pp. 152–159.

Pulmonary fibrosis and pneumoconioses

American Lung Association: op. cit., pp. 87–104.

Cherniack, et al.: op. cit., pp. 357–360.

Cox, Paul M.: *Synopsis of Clinical Pulmonary Disease*, Mosby, St. Louis, 1974, pp. 142–145.

Dickie, Helen Aird: "Dust Inhalation Diseases," in Holman and Muschenheim, op. cit., pp. 449–467.

Robbins and Angell: op. cit., pp. 327–330.

Robin, Eugene D.: "Restrictive and Diffusional Disorders of the Lung," in M. Wintrobe, et al. (eds.), *Harrison's Principles of Internal Medicine*, 6th ed., McGraw-Hill, New York, 1970, pp. 1269–1307.

Respiratory distress syndrome

Ashbaugh, D. G., and T. L. Petty: "Positive End-Expiratory Pressure," *Journal of Thoracic and Cardiovascular Surgery*, 65: 165, 1973.

Burrows, et al.: op. cit., pp. 157–158.

Cherniack, et al.: op. cit., pp. 360–366.

Gracey, D. R.: "Adult Respiratory Distress Syndrome," *Heart & Lung*, 4: 280, March–April 1975.

Northway, W. H., and W. J. R. Daily: in Holman and Muschenheim, op. cit., pp. 210–217.

CHAPTER 35 Respiratory Insufficiency and Respiratory Failure

RESPIRATORY INSUFFICIENCY

Respiratory insufficiency may be defined as an impairment of the normal ability to oxygenate the arterial blood or to eliminate carbon dioxide, resulting in an inability to maintain normal arterial blood gases under conditions of increased demand, namely, exercise. An increased breathing effort to maintain adequate ventilation and oxygenation at rest may also be obvious. Respiratory insufficiency may be associated with any of the broad categories of diseases previously discussed—restrictive and obstructive disorders and diseases affecting the neuromuscular system or the chest wall. The most common cause of respiratory insufficiency, however, is chronic obstructive pulmonary disease. In the initial stages of the underlying disease, blood gas disturbances are corrected by an increase in ventilation and, possibly, by some redistribution of ventilation and perfusion. However, if the disease progresses, or if it is complicated by superimposed pulmonary infection, these compensatory mechanisms become inadequate and serious abnormalities of the blood gases are present at rest, which indicates that respiratory insufficiency has progressed to respiratory failure.

Respiratory failure

Respiratory failure is numerically defined as having a P_aO_2 of 50 mmHg or less or a P_aCO_2 of 50 mmHg or greater. A numerical definition has been established for this entity because the line between respiratory insufficiency and respiratory failure is very subtle, and clinical observations alone are very unreliable. In the beginning chapters of this section it was noted that cyanosis is a very unreliable index of oxygenation, since it is influenced by hemoglobin concentration, the state of the peripheral circulation, and the observer's perception and interpretation of skin color. Clinical observation of alveolar ventilation has been shown to be quite inaccurate. The cardiovascular, neurologic, and respiratory signs of hypoxia and hypercapnia discussed in Chap. 32 are most easily recognized when the onset of respiratory failure is acute. Patients with chronic respiratory insufficiency, however, may be able to tolerate a significant degree of hypoxemia and hypercapnia. Only when the condition progresses to coma with slow or gasping respirations is the diagnosis of respiratory failure clinically obvious. Clinical observations, a high degree of suspicion, and final confirmation by blood gas determinations must all be utilized in diagnosing respiratory failure. Respiratory failure should be suspected in the patient with progressive neuromuscular disease, in narcotic overdose, shock, severe burns, and in all patients showing symptomatic exacerbations of chronic lung disease.

There are two primary causes of respiratory failure and two broadly classified types. One of the causes of respiratory failure is alveolar hypoventilation, which is most commonly traceable to chronic airway obstruction or restriction. It can also result from neuromuscular disease, drugs which depress the respiratory center, or high-flow oxygen therapy in patients with chronic lung disease. The second primary cause of respiratory failure is ventilation–perfusion imbalance which increases either the physiologic dead space or the physiologic shunt (venous admixture). Other less common causes of respiratory failure are impaired diffusion of gases caused by an increase in the anatomic distance which the gas must travel from the alveolar space to the lumen of the pulmonary capillary. The most common cause of impaired diffusion is pulmonary edema which may be cardiogenic. Pulmonary fibrosis may be associated with some impairment in diffusion of gases, but ventilation–perfusion imbalance is of much more importance in causing abnormal blood gases. A true anatomic right-to-left shunt is uncommon and therefore is a less important cause of blood gas abnormalities. The two types of respiratory failure are (1) hypoxemia without hypercapnia (decreased P_aO_2, normal or low P_aCO_2) and (2) hypoxemia with hypercapnia (decreased P_aO_2, increased P_aCO_2).

Although the terminology is confused in the literature, when both hypoxemia and hypercapnia are present, the condition is often referred to as ventilatory failure. Others may refer to the first condition as hypoxemic respiratory failure and to the second condition as hypercapnic respiratory failure. The importance of distinguishing between these two types of respiratory failure lies mainly in determining the use of oxygen as therapy. In the absence of hypercapnia, high concentrations of oxygen may be given for a limited period of time without danger of harming the patient. However, when there is significant hypercapnia, there is great danger in administering high concentrations of oxygen,

since this will reduce the hypoxic respiratory drive and may aggravate hypoventilation and carbon dioxide retention. The common causes and principles of treatment for these two types of respiratory failure are discussed in the following paragraphs.

Hypoxemic respiratory failure (hypoxemia without hypercapnia)

Hypoxemia with a normal or low P_aCO_2 is always caused by disease of the lung itself and is associated with those conditions affecting the alveolar wall and interstitium, resulting in a restrictive pattern of ventilation. Hypoxemic respiratory failure is also associated with diseases affecting the pulmonary vascular bed, which will be discussed in Chap. 36. Common disorders producing this condition include pneumonia, diffuse lung diseases causing pulmonary fibrosis, pulmonary edema, atelectasis, pulmonary emboli, and respiratory distress syndrome or oxygen toxicity (causing atelectasis).

Hypoxemia in these patients results, in part, from diffusion abnormalities (interference with the diffusion path as in pulmonary edema, fibrosis, or reduction of the diffusion surface as in atelectasis) but is mainly the result of ventilation–perfusion imbalance (shunt effect caused by the perfusion of unventilated atelectic areas or ventilation of underperfused areas, as when there is destruction of the pulmonary vascular bed).

Mild hypoxemia which is exercise-induced is more common in disorders resulting in hypoxemic respiratory failure, although the hypoxemia may become quite severe in lobar pneumonia or massive atelectasis. When a patient is breathing room air, hyperventilation to improve oxygenation has little effect on the hypoxemia and may cause a reduction of the P_aCO_2, since its excretion is directly related to ventilation. The sigmoid shape of the oxyhemoglobin curve (see Fig. 30-13) explains why hyperventilation causes little improvement in oxygenation. In fact, if there is significant respiratory alkalosis ($P_aCO_2 = 20$ to 25 mmHg) produced by hyperventilation combined with significant hypoxia, cerebral oxygenation may become impaired because the oxyhemoglobin curve is shifted to the left as a result of the high pH and the oxygen that is delivered to the cells is reluctant to dissociate from hemoglobin.

Oxygenation or hypoxemic respiratory failure may progress to hypercapnic respiratory failure if the hypoxemia becomes severe enough to cause hypoxia, circulatory failure, and metabolic acidosis, which in turn results in depression of the respiratory center and the respiratory system.

Hypercapnic respiratory failure (hypoxemia with hypercapnia)

Alveolar hypoventilation is the main cause of respiratory failure associated with hypoxemia and hypercapnia. Hypercapnic respiratory failure is the most common type of respiratory failure. Patients with this type of respiratory failure may be divided into two groups—those with essentially normal lungs and those with intrinsic lung disease. Carbon dioxide retention in the first group results from generalized alveolar hypoventilation caused by abnormalities in respiratory control, abnormalities in the neuromuscular events required to maintain ventilation, or abnormalities of the chest wall (as occurs in narcotic overdose, myasthenia gravis, and extreme obesity). Respiratory failure is often overlooked in this group of patients. The second group of patients with hypercapnic respiratory failure is composed of those with chronic obstructive pulmonary disease. In these patients, alterations in the mechanical and gas exchange characteristics of the lung lead to inadequate elimination of carbon dioxide (alveolar hypoventilation) even though minute ventilation may be normal or increased. A reduction of the $\dot{V}/\dot{Q}$ ratio (shunting) also contributes to the hypoxemia and hypercapnia in chronic bronchitis. A rise in the P_aCO_2 can usually be prevented by hyperventilation in an acute asthmatic attack, but hypercapnia may develop in a sustained attack (status asthmaticus).

Treatment of respiratory failure

The priorities in the management of respiratory failure vary according to the etiology, but the primary aims of treatment are the same in all cases, that is, to treat the cause of the respiratory failure and at the same time ensure adequate ventilation and clear airways.

Since the most life-threatening feature of respiratory

failure is the impairment of gas exchange, the first goal of therapy is to ensure that hypoxemia, acidosis, and hypercapnia do not reach hazardous levels. A P_aO_2 of 40 mmHg or a pH of 7.2 or less is poorly tolerated by adults and can result in cerebral, kidney, and cardiac impairment and the development of cardiac arrhythmias. A P_aCO_2 of 60 mmHg which has developed slowly in a patient with COPD is usually well tolerated, whereas rapid development to this level is not well tolerated. A P_aCO_2 of 70 mmHg or more is usually poorly tolerated in any patient and causes central nervous system depression and coma.

Oxygen may be delivered at a concentration of 40 to 60 percent to a patient with hypoxemia and a normal or low P_aCO_2 (mask or catheter at 8 liters/minute with adequate humidification) in order to achieve a rapid correction of the hypoxemia. However, this concentration should not be continued for more than a few hours, as it has a direct toxic effect on alveolar cells, causing decreased pulmonary compliance. Prolonged administration of oxygen at high concentrations also causes atelectasis.

Hypoxemia with hypercapnia is always treated with low graduated oxygen therapy beginning with a venti-mask which delivers 24 percent oxygen. The concentration is increased to 28 percent oxygen if necessary to maintain a P_aO_2 of 50 mmHg or more. Careful monitoring of blood gases is utilized at all times to ensure that the oxygen therapy does not cause a deterioration in the patient's respiratory status. In the patient with COPD, attempts are made to achieve P_aO_2 values which are normal for the patient (e.g., 50 to 70 mmHg) and not those normal for the healthy adult (85 to 100 mmHg). When it is not possible to achieve P_aO_2 values of 50 mmHg, artificial ventilation with a respirator may be required.

The approach to the problem of retained lung secretions includes measures to liquefy and remove them. Liquefaction is best achieved by adequate hydration of the patient. Drugs such as potassium iodide taken orally or aerosol delivery of water may also help in the mobilization of sputum. Secretions are best removed by encouraging the patient to cough or assisting the patient's efforts by percussion, vibration, and postural drainage. When the patient is too depressed or weak to cough, secretions may be removed by aspiration via an endotracheal tube or bronchoscopy. If these methods fail, tracheostomy may be necessary.

If bronchospasm is present in respiratory failure, bronchodilatory or corticosteroid drugs may be used. Respiratory infection, which is a common cause of hypoxemic respiratory failure, is treated with the appropriate antibiotics.

Finally, a thorough search is made for other factors which may have induced the respiratory failure, such as pulmonary embolism and left ventricular failure. Table 35-1 lists the priorities and aims of treatment of hypercapnic respiratory failure. A number of excellent books

TABLE 35-1
Priorities and principles of the treatment of hypercapnic respiratory failure

PRIORITY	PROBLEM	TREATMENT
1	Retained secretions (ineffective cough)	Adequate hydration, expectorants, aerosols Supervised coughing Catheter aspiration (deep suction) Bronchoscopic suction Endotracheal tube aspiration Tracheostomy
2	Hypoxemia	Graduated oxygen therapy with frequent monitoring of blood gases to direct therapy
3	Hypercapnia	Respiratory stimulants (drug overdose) Avoidance of sedation Artificial ventilation via endotracheal tube or tracheostomy
4	Respiratory infection	Antibiotics
5	Bronchospasm	Bronchodilatory drugs (isoproteranol by inhalation therapy; intravenous, oral, or rectal aminophylline; corticosteroid drugs
6	Cardiac failure	Diuretics Digoxin (with caution if given at all)

Source: J. Crofton and A. Douglas, *Respiratory Diseases*, Blackwell, Oxford, England, 1969, pp. 342–346.

dealing with the management of respiratory failure are suggested in the references for those who wish to gain more extensive knowledge of this subject.

QUESTIONS

Respiratory insufficiency and respiratory failure—Chap. 35

Directions: Answer the following questions on a separate sheet of paper.

1 What is the relationship between respiratory insufficiency and the maintenance of normal arterial blood gases?

2 What is the most common cause of respiratory insufficiency?

3 List the two types of respiratory failure based on blood gas changes.

4 Explain why high concentrations of oxygen must not be administered in hypercapnic respiratory failure.

5 What level of P_aO_2 or P_aCO_2 would not be well tolerated in most adults?

6 List at least three measures used to treat the problem of retained secretions and pulmonary infection in hypercapnic respiratory failure.

7 What is the primary goal and first priority in the treatment of respiratory failure?

Directions: Circle T if the statement is true and F if it is false. Correct false statements.

8 T F The clinical signs of respiratory failure are most easily detected in a patient who has chronic respiratory insufficiency which has progressed to respiratory failure.

9 T F Cyanosis is the most reliable index of respiratory failure.

10 T F Acute respiratory failure may be manifested by cardiovascular and neurologic signs and symptoms.

11 T F Hypoxemia with a normal or low P_aCO_2 is associated with conditions affecting the alveolar wall and interstitium of the lung.

12 T F Hypoventilation may cause the P_aCO_2 to fall below normal, since its excretion is directly related to ventilation.

13 T F Hyperventilation when breathing room air fails to correct hypoxemia.

14 T F Cerebral oxygenation may become impaired when significant hypocapnia is combined with hypoxemia.

15 T F Impaired cerebral oxygenation can be explained by the shift of the oxyhemoglobin dissociation curve to the left as a result of respiratory alkalosis.

Directions: Circle the letter next to each item which correctly answers the following questions. More than one choice may be correct.

16 Ventilation failure is numerically defined as:
a $P_aO_2 = 80$ mmHg, $P_aCO_2 = 60$ mmHg
b $P_aO_2 = 70$ mmHg, $P_aCO_2 = 35$ mmHg
c $P_aO_2 \geq 60$ mmHg, $P_aCO_2 \geq 40$ mmHg
d $P_aO_2 \leq 50$ mmHg, $P_aCO_2 \geq 50$ mmHg

17 Which of the following best describes the primary causes of respiratory failure?
a Hypersensitivity of the tracheobronchial tree to various stimuli b Ventilation–perfusion imbalance which increases physiologic shunt or dead space c Alveolar hypoventilation associated with obstructive or restrictive disease d Impaired diffusion due to alveolar–capillary block

18 The major cause of hypoxemia with hypercapnia is:
a Alveolar hypoventilation b Alveolar hyperventilation c Neither a nor b d Both a and b

19 Treatment of patients with hypoxemia with hypercapnia includes:
a Oxygen delivered at a concentration of 40 to 60 percent in order to achieve a rapid correction of hypoxemia b Low graduated oxygen therapy beginning with a ventimask which delivers 24 percent oxygen concentration c Careful monitoring of blood gases d Achievement of a P_aO_2 of 90–100 mmHg for all these patients

20 Tissue hypoxia may occur even when the P_aO_2 is normal if:
a Severe anemia is present b Cardiac output is low c The oxyhemoglobin curve is shifted to the left d Local vasoconstriction is present

BIBLIOGRAPHY

Burrows, B., R. J. Knudson, and L. J. Kettel: *Respiratory Insufficiency*, Yearbook, Chicago, 1975, pp. 91–96.

Cherniack, R. M., L. Cherniack, and A. Naimark: *Respiration in Health and Disease*, Saunders, Philadelphia, 1972, pp. 427–437.

Cole, R. B.: *Essentials of Respiratory Disease*, Medcom, New York, 1975, pp. 103–107.

National Tuberculosis and Respiratory Disease Association: *Chronic Obstructive Pulmonary Disease: A Manual for Physicians*, 3d ed., New York, 1972, pp. 97–104.

SMITH, JAMES P.: "Respiratory Failure and its Management," in C. W. Holman and C. Muschenheim, *Bronchopulmonary Diseases and Related Disorders,* Harper & Row, New York, 1972, vol. 2, pp. 694–728.

Additional references on respiratory failure

BENDIXEN, H. H., et al.: *Respiratory Care,* Mosby, St. Louis, 1965.

CREWS, E. R., and LEOPOLDO LAPUERTA: *A Manual of Respiratory Failure,* Thomas, Springfield, Ill., 1972.

CHAPTER 36 Cardiovascular Disease and the Lung

Chronic lung disease is an increasingly frequent cause of heart disease, and conversely, heart disease with decompensation or vascular disease may cause changes in the structure and function of the lung. The basis of this close interrelationship relates to the functional position of the lungs in the circulation (refer to Fig. 30-4). This chapter discusses pulmonary embolism, pulmonary edema, and cor pulmonale, all diseases demonstrating the close relationship between the heart and the lungs.

PULMONARY EMBOLISM

Pulmonary embolism occurs when an embolus, usually a blood clot which breaks free from its attachment in a vein of the lower limbs, circulates through the blood vessels and the right side of the heart to become lodged in the main pulmonary artery or one of its branches. Pulmonary infarction is the term used to describe a local focus of necrosis resulting from the vascular obstruction (see Fig. 36-1).

The true incidence of pulmonary embolism cannot be determined because of the difficulty of the clinical diagnosis, but it is an important cause of morbidity and mortality in a hospital population and is said to account for 5 percent of sudden deaths. Pulmonary embolism has been described in over 50 percent of consecutive autopsies in some studies, suggesting that many cases are clinically undetected.

Three basic factors are related to the development of venous thrombosis and subsequent pulmonary embolism: (1) venous stasis or slowing of the blood flow, (2) injury to the vein wall, and (3) hypercoagulability. Several diseases and activities seem to increase the risk of forming a thrombus, and patients in these states should be watched closely to detect any evidence of the formation of a thrombus. The risk of thrombus formation is increased by pregnancy, the use of oral contraceptive drugs, obesity, heart failure, varicose veins, abdominal infection, cancer, sickle cell anemia, and any prolonged inactivity such as plane, train, or bus rides. Many of these conditions are common in hospitalized patients. Venous thrombosis and pulmonary embolism occur predominantly in bedridden patients. The single most important condition predisposing to venous thrombosis is congestive heart failure; the postoperative state is the next in importance. The most common site for a blood clot to form is in the deep veins of the legs (90 percent), although clots may form in the pelvic veins and in the right side of the heart. Emboli of nonthrombotic origin are uncommon but include obstruction caused by air, fat, malignant cells, amniotic fluid, parasites, vegetations, and foreign material.

The signs and symptoms of a pulmonary embolus are extremely variable, depending on the size of the clot or clots. The clinical picture may range from no signs at all to sudden and almost immediate death caused by a massive "saddle embolus" at the bifurcation of the main pulmonary artery, resulting in blockage of the entire outflow of the right ventricle. In a patient with the signs

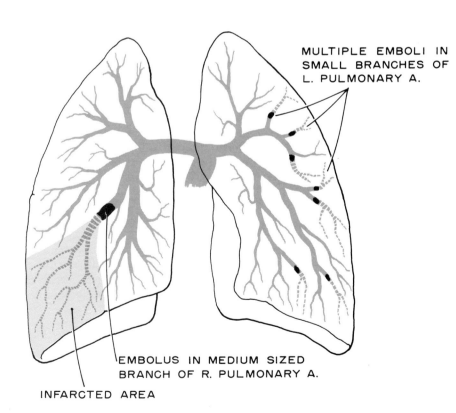

MULTIPLE EMBOLI IN
SMALL BRANCHES OF
L. PULMONARY A.

EMBOLUS IN MEDIUM SIZED
BRANCH OF R. PULMONARY A.

INFARCTED AREA

FIGURE 36-1 Pulmonary embolism and infarction.

of thrombophlebitis in leg veins, the classic syndrome associated with a *moderate-sized pulmonary embolus* consists of chest pain of sudden onset, dyspnea, cough, rapid respiratory rate, fever, and occasionally hemoptysis. The pain is usually pleuritic, and a pleural friction rub may be heard on auscultation. *Massive pulmonary embolism* may result in a sudden, shocklike state with tachycardia, hypotension, cyanosis, stupor, or syncope. Death usually follows within a few minutes. Frequently, however, the symptoms of pulmonary embolism are subtle, such as unexplained fever or worsening of a preexisting cardiac or cardiopulmonary condition. These subtle symptoms are apt to be associated with *recurrent small, multiple pulmonary emboli*. They may go unnoticed until right ventricular hypertrophy and failure direct attention to the pulmonary vascular disease.

The effect of pulmonary embolism is to produce an area of lung which is ventilated but underperfused, thus increasing physiologic dead-space ventilation. Reflex bronchoconstriction occurs in the affected area and is thought to result from the release of histamine or serotonin from the clot. Reflex bronchoconstriction is considered to be compensatory in the occluded area, as it reduces the unevenness of ventilation and perfusion. In adjacent areas, however, reflex bronchospasm may result in considerable hypoxemia. If the pulmonary vascular bed is sufficiently reduced by a large embolus or by recurrent multiple emboli, pulmonary hypertension may result. It is estimated that two-thirds of the vascular bed must be obliterated before this happens.

A localized area of ischemic necrosis (infarction) is an uncommon complication of pulmonary embolism because of the lung's dual blood supply. Pulmonary infarction is usually associated with occlusion of a medium-sized lobar or lobular artery and insufficient collateral flow from the bronchial circulation (see Fig. 36-1). A pleural friction rub and a small pleural effusion are common signs.

There are few diagnostic tests which specifically distinguish a pulmonary infarction from a pulmonary infiltrate. Radioactive lung perfusion scans will be abnormal in either case or in the presence of emphysema. The chest x-ray may be normal, or the presence of a pleural effusion may occur in both cases. Physiologic tests and serum enzymes are likewise of little value in distinguishing an infarction from pneumonia. In addition, the signs and symptoms of pneumonia may be very similar to pulmonary embolism. The most reliable method of diagnosis is pulmonary angiography.

Objectives in treatment of pulmonary embolism are to prevent initial or recurrent embolism, to relieve symptoms resulting from the embolus, and surgical removal of a massive embolus. In high-risk patients, the effectiveness of oral anticoagulants in preventing pulmonary embolism has been clearly shown. "Low-dose heparin" (3000 to 5000 units every 8 to 12 hours subcutaneously) has also been effective in preliminary studies and may prove to be a valuable prophylactic

agent. Treatment of an acute pulmonary embolism includes general cardiopulmonary support with oxygen, digitalization, intensive care monitoring, elastic stockings, and the administration of aqueous heparin in full doses of 20,000 to 40,000 units per day by continuous infusion or divided doses. Surgical embolectomy is considered only when the embolus is massive, since the mortality from this kind of surgery is about 50 percent. Other surgical measures to prevent recurrent pulmonary emboli from the lower extremities include ligation of the inferior vena cava or the insertion of a filtering device or screen in the inferior vena cava.

PULMONARY EDEMA

Pulmonary edema is an excessive accumulation of serous or serosanguinous fluid in the alveoli. If the edema is acute and extensive, death may rapidly ensue. Pulmonary edema may be precipitated by an increase of hydrostatic pressure within the pulmonary capillaries, a decrease in the colloid osmotic pressure as in nephritis, or damage to the capillary walls. Damage to the capillary walls may result from the inhalation of noxious gases, inflammation as in pneumonia, or from local interference with oxygenation. The most common cause of pulmonary edema is left ventricular failure resulting from arteriosclerotic heart disease or mitral stenosis (mitral valve obstruction). If the left side of the heart fails while the right side continues to pump blood, the pulmonary capillary pressure rises until pulmonary edema results. Blood plasma is poured out into the alveoli faster than coughing or the lymphatics of the lung can clear it. This interferes with diffusion of oxygen, and the consequent tissue hypoxia further increases the tendency to edema. Asphyxia may result unless measures are taken to reverse the pulmonary edema. Emergency treatment for acute pulmonary edema includes measures to reduce pulmonary hydrostatic pressure, such as placing the patient in Fowler's position with the feet dependent; rotating tourniquets; or phlebotomy (removal of about a pint of blood). Other measures include the administration of diuretics, oxygen, and digitalis to improve myocardial contractility.

In the presence of chronic passive congestion of the lungs, structural changes in the lung, namely pulmonary fibrosis, may result. These changes enable the lung to function for a time with the increased hydrostatic pressure without the development of pulmonary edema. The balance, however, is precarious, and the patient may have attacks of dyspnea at night (paroxysmal nocturnal dyspnea) due to the increase in pulmonary hydrostatic pressure which results from a horizontal position.

COR PULMONALE

Cor pulmonale is the condition in which hypertrophy and dilatation of the right ventricle, with or without right heart failure, develop as a result of disease affecting the structure or function of the lung or its vasculature. Implied in this definition is the provision that neither disease of the left side of the heart nor congenital heart disease is responsible for its pathogenesis.

The prerequisite for the development of cor pulmonale is pulmonary hypertension. Pulmonary hypertension, in turn, increases the work load of the right ventricle, causing it to hypertrophy and eventually fail. Because the pulmonary circulation is a low-pressure, low-resistance circulation under normal circumstances, cardiac output can increase many times (as happens during exercise) without a significant increase in pulmonary artery pressure. The critical point in the sequence leading to pulmonary hypertension seems to be an increase in pulmonary vascular resistance through the small muscular arteries and arterioles. The increase in vascular resistance may be anatomic or vasomotor in origin. The cross-sectional area of the pulmonary vascular bed may be reduced by a number of pathologic processes. Reduction can occur as a result of a loss of capillaries, as in chronic bronchitis/emphysema; the internal diameter may be occluded by pulmonary emboli; external pressure may reduce the diameter, as occurs in pulmonary fibrosis or high alveolar pressures in obstructive lung diseases; and the various forms of pulmonary fibrosis may reduce the distensibility. When about two-thirds or three-fourths of the vascular bed is destroyed, pulmonary arterial hypertension occurs even at rest.

Anatomic alterations in the pulmonary vascular bed are only one cause of pulmonary hypertension. Another important condition resulting in pulmonary hypertension is pulmonary arteriolar vasoconstriction. Pulmonary vasoconstriction occurs in response to a number of stimuli but the most important ones are hypoxemia (results in alveolar hypoxia) and hypercapnia (which causes acidosis and evokes pulmonary vasoconstriction). Hypoxemia, hypercapnia, and acidosis, three conditions important in the pathogenesis of pulmonary hypertension and cor pulmonale, are present in a number of different pulmonary diseases as a result of generalized alveolar hypoventilation or as a consequence of ventilation–perfusion abnormalities.

It is evident from the above discussion that any pulmonary disease that affects ventilatory mechanics, gas exchange, or the pulmonary vascular bed may result in cor pulmonale. Since this is true of most all pulmonary diseases, a list of the causes of cor pulmonale includes all possible types of pulmonary disease. This list also includes extrapulmonary disease such as kyphoscoliosis, the Pickwickian syndrome, and others which affect ventilatory mechanics. The development of cor pulmonale simply means that the primary disease was sufficiently advanced to impair cardiac function. Right heart failure is often the terminal event in these diseases. The etiology and pathogenesis of cor pulmonale is illustrated in Fig. 36-2.

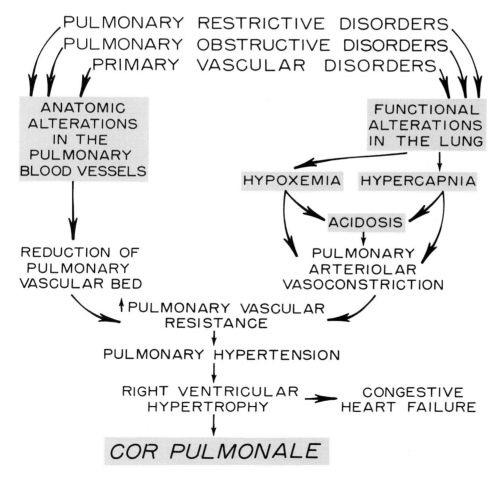

FIGURE 36-2 Etiology and pathogenesis of cor pulmonale.

The most common cause of cor pulmonale in the United States is chronic obstructive pulmonary disease, which accounts for about 75 percent of the cases. A second important cause is recurrent multiple pulmonary emboli. The exact incidence of cor pulmonale is unknown, but one study in Cleveland, Ohio, during 1941–1947, using the criteria of postmortem ventricular wall thickness, found an incidence of 7.1 percent of all patients with cardiac disease (most patients being over the age of 50).

The treatment of cor pulmonale is directed toward improvement of the underlying pulmonary disorder and correction of the accompanying hypoxemia. In the event of right ventricular failure, digitalis is seldom used, as it may produce toxicity in patients who have fluctuating serum electrolytes and blood gases.

QUESTIONS

Cardiovascular disease and the lung—Chap. 36

Directions: Answer the following questions on a separate sheet of paper.

1 List three factors which directly relate to the development of venous thrombosis.

2 What disease is the most common cause of cor pulmonale in the United States?

3 List four conditions that may precipitate pulmonary edema.

4 What is paroxysmal nocturnal dyspnea?

5 Define cor pulmonale.

6 What is the relationship between left-sided heart failure and pulmonary edema? Is this condition the most frequent cause of pulmonary edema?

7 List three objectives in the treatment of pulmonary embolism.

8 What are the two goals in treatment of cor pulmonale?

9 Describe two mechanisms that can lead to increased pulmonary vascular resistance.

Directions: Circle the letter next to each item which correctly answers the following questions. More than one choice may be correct.

10 The classical signs and symptoms associated with a moderate-sized pulmonary embolism are:
a Dyspnea *b* Rapid respiratory rate *c* Pleuristic chest pain *d* Unconsciousness and death within minutes *e* Hemoptysis (occasionally)

11 Which of the following types of pulmonary embolism is most frequent?

a Massive occlusion at bifurcation of main pulmonary artery *b* Moderate-sized occlusion of lobar or lobular pulmonary artery *c* Occlusion of small pulmonary vessels as a result of recurrent, multiple emboli

12 Which of the following are effects of pulmonary embolism?
a Pulmonary infarction *b* $\dot{V}/\dot{Q}$ imbalance resulting in increased dead space *c* $\dot{V}/\dot{Q}$ imbalance resulting in increased shunting *d* Reflex bronchoconstriction

13 The most reliable method of diagnosing a pulmonary embolism is:
a Chest x-ray *b* Perfusion lung scan with albumin tagged with radioactive isotope *c* Pulmonary angiography *d* Physical examination

14 The usual treatment of an *acute* pulmonary embolism includes:
a Oral anticoagulants in low dosage *b* Intense care monitoring *c* General cardiopulmonary support with oxygen *d* Elastic stockings *e* Surgical embolectomy

15 What is the approximate mortality for surgical removal of a massive pulmonary embolus?
a 1 percent *b* 10 percent *c* 50 percent

16 Emergency treatment of acute pulmonary edema might include:
a Placing the patient in a high Fowler's position with the feet dependent *b* Placing the patient in a horizontal position with the feet elevated *c* Rotating tourniquets *d* Rapid infusion of intravenous solutions

17 A pulmonary embolism usually occurs when a thrombus from a leg vein breaks off and:
a Circulates through the left ventricle and lodges in the main pulmonary artery or its branches *b* Circulates through the right ventricle of the heart and lodges in the pulmonary vein *c* Circulates through the right side of the heart and lodges in the main pulmonary artery or its branches

18 The most likely location for the formation of a blood clot causing a pulmonary embolism is:
a A deep vein in the legs *b* In the left ventricle *c* An artery in the legs *d* In the right ventricle

19 Which of the following conditions is associated with an increased risk of pulmonary embolism?
a Carcinoma of the small bowel *b* Postoperative bedridden patients *c* Thrombophlebitis *d* Congestive heart failure

Directions: Determine which are the first and second most important conditions predisposing a patient to venous thrombosis by writing 1 beside the first choice, and 2 beside the second.

20 ____ Thrombophlebitis
____ Postoperative bedridden patients
____ Congestive heart failure
____ Carcinoma of the small bowel

Directions: Circle T if the statement is true with respect to pulmonary infarction and F if it is false.

21 T F It is a localized area of ischemic necrosis.

22 T F It is an infrequent complication of pulmonary embolism as a result of the lung's dual blood supply.

23 T F It is frequently associated with a small pleural effusion.

24 T F It is easily differentiated from pneumonia by chest x-ray.

Directions: Complete the following statements by filling in the blanks.

25 A freely circulating blood clot which lodges in a blood vessel causing an obstruction is called a(n) _____ _____.

26 Pulmonary embolism is the cause of sudden death in hospitalized patients in at least _____ percent of the cases.

27 A prerequisite for the development of cor pulmonale is an increased pulmonary vascular resistance leading to _____ _____.

BIBLIOGRAPHY

Pulmonary embolism

Burrows, B., R. J. Knudson, and L. J. Kettel: *Respiratory Insufficiency*, Yearbook, Chicago, 1975, pp. 151–155.

Cherniack, R. M., L. Cherniack, and A. Naimark: *Respiration in Health and Disease*, 2d ed., Saunders, Philadelphia, 1972, pp. 375–383.

Cole, R. B.: *Essentials of Respiratory Diseases*, Medcom, New York, 1975, pp. 251–260.

Fitzmaurice, J. B., and A. A. Sasahara: "Current Concepts of Pulmonary Embolism: Implications for Nursing Practice," *Heart & Lung*, **3**: 209, March–April, 1974.

Genton, Edward, and Ray Pryor: "Acute Pulmonary Embolism," *Hospital Medicine*, **9**: 9, April 1973.

Pulmonary edema

Cherniack, et al.: op. cit., pp. 386–391.

Geschickter, C. F.: *The Lung in Health and Disease*, Lippincott, Philadelphia, 1973, pp. 99–103.

Cor pulmonale

Burrows, et al.: op. cit., pp. 86–90.

Robin, Eugene, and Ralph Gaudio: "Cor Pulmonale," *Disease-a-Month*, May 1970.

CHAPTER 37 Pulmonary Malignant Neoplasms

OBJECTIVES **At the completion of Chap. 37, you should be able to:**

1 List three factors that appear to account for the increase in bronchogenic carcinoma.

2 Describe the relationship between cigarette smoking and the development of bronchogenic carcinoma.

3 Identify one possible reason why bronchogenic carcinoma is more common in the lowest socioeconomic classes.

4 Identify at least one example of an important industrial hazard associated with an increased incidence of bronchogenic carcinoma.

5 Describe the four histologic types of bronchogenic carcinoma with respect to anatomic site, frequency, sex, association with smoking, mode of spread, and general prognosis.

6 Define the carcinoid syndrome.

7 Identify one reason why the lung is a common site for cancer metastasis.

8 List the manifestations of bronchogenic carcinoma.

9 Name and describe briefly the diagnostic tests used in the diagnosis of lung cancer and identify the significant findings expected with each technique.

10 State the objectives for the treatment of lung cancer.

11 State the general prognosis for patients with lung cancer.

Over 90 percent of primary lung tumors are malignant, and about 95 percent of these malignant tumors are bronchogenic carcinoma. This is the disease that is meant whenever reference is made to "lung cancer," since the majority of primary malignant tumors of the lower respiratory tract are epithelial in nature and arise from the mucosa of the bronchial tree.

Although once considered a rare form of malignancy, the incidence of lung cancer among males in the large cities of the industrialized countries has risen to epidemic proportions in the decades since 1930. Some of the alarming statistics were cited in the introduction to this section.

BRONCHOGENIC CARCINOMA

Although the exact etiology of bronchogenic carcinoma is unknown, three factors appear to account for the increase in incidence—smoking, industrial hazards, and air pollution. Of these factors, smoking appears to play the major role. Massive statistical evidence indicates that there is a relationship between heavy cigarette smoking and the development of lung cancer. Three prospective studies, one involving nearly 200,000 men aged 50 to 69, followed for 44 months revealed that the death rate from cancer of the lung per 100,000 was 3.4 in the male nonsmoker; 59.3 in those who smoked 10 to 20 cigarettes daily; and 217.3 in those who smoke 40 or more cigarettes daily. Those who give up smoking permanently are much less likely to develop carcinoma after an abstinence of 5 years. The risk in pipe smokers or cigar smokers is only slightly greater than in nonsmokers. Mortality from lung cancer is related to atmospheric pollution, but its effect is small compared to that of cigarette smoking. The death rate from cancer of the lung is twice as high in cities as in rural areas. Statistical evidence also shows that the disease is more common in the lowest socioeconomic classes and decreases in the higher classes. This may be partly explained by the fact that the lowest social classes are more apt to live near their jobs, where the atmosphere may be more polluted.

A carinogen (cancer-producing material) which has been found in polluted air (and also in cigarette smoke) is 3,4-benzpyrene. The nicotine in cigarette smoke is not a carcinogen.

In certain instances, bronchogenic carcinoma appears to be an occupational disease. Of the various industrial hazards, the most important is undoubtedly asbestos, which is widely used in the construction industry. The risk of lung cancer in asbestos workers is about 10 times greater than in the general population. There is also increased risk in those who work with uranium, chromate, arsenic (insectiside used in agriculture), iron, and iron oxides.

In many tissues, chronic inflammatory changes are known to precede cancer. Evidence supports the view that chronic inflammation of the bronchial mucosa from inhaled irritants may be of greater importance than the carcinogenic affect of any one substance. Another factor which has not received much attention is the close correspondence between the increase in the number of motor vehicles and the incidence of lung cancer.

These facts suggest that although smoking clearly plays a major part in the increasing incidence of lung cancer, there are many indications that it is by no means the only factor. Chronic infection, air pollution from motor vehicles and industry, occupational exposure to carcinogens, and perhaps other unknown factors may (either alone or in combination) predispose to cancer of the lung.

Primary lung cancer can be classified in terms of its anatomic location and on the basis of histologic type. The approximate anatomic distribution is illustrated in Fig. 37-1. About 50 percent of the lesions arise centrally about the hilus and the first few orders of bronchi; the others have a more peripheral origin in the terminal bronchioles. Bronchogenic carcinoma may be classified into the following histologic types (approximate frequencies are listed in parentheses): (1) squamous cell or epidermoid carcinoma (45 to 60 percent); (2) anaplastic or undifferentiated carcinoma (20 to 30 percent) (includes the oat cell, small cell, and large cell varieties); (3) adenocarcinoma (10 to 15 percent); and (4) bronchiolar-alveolar cell carcinoma (1 to 2 percent).

Squamous cell carcinoma is the most common histologic type of bronchogenic carcinoma and arises from the surface of the bronchial epithelium. Squamous cell carcinoma is usually centrally located about the hilus and is almost always associated with cigarette smoking. The tumor is seldom more than a few centimeters in diameter, and it tends to spread by direct extension to the hilar lymph nodes, chest wall, and mediastinum. Squamous cell carcinoma often presents with manifestations of cough and hemoptysis as a result of irritation or ulceration and pneumonia and abscess formation from the obstruction and secondary infection. The life expectancy in this type of tumor is greater than in the anaplastic variety, since it tends to metastasize locally and somewhat later.

Anaplastic carcinomas are the second most common histologic type. They are undifferentiated cell types, since no squamous or adenomatous pattern can be defined. Metastasis occurs early, chiefly via the lymphatics, so that the prognosis in this type of cancer is very poor. Death usually occurs within a few months after discovery. The oat cell variety of anaplastic carcinoma is the most common and generally is centrally located about the mainstem bronchi. This type of cancer is also related to heavy cigarette smoking.

Adenocarcinoma, as the name implies, shows a cellular organization like bronchial glands that may contain mucus. The majority of these tumors arise in the peripheral segmental bronchi and are sometimes associated with focal lung scars and chronic interstitial fibrosis. These lesions often spread via the bloodstream and remain clinically silent until distant hematogenous metastases occur. There is no clear correlation between this type of bronchogenic carcinoma and smoking. Unlike the squamous and oat cell varieties which are much more common in men, both sexes are affected about equally.

Bronchiolar-alveolar cell carcinoma is a rare type of malignant lung tumor which arises from either the alveolar or possibly from the bronchiolar epithelium. This type of lung cancer does not seem to be related to smoking and is equally distributed between the sexes. In contrast to anaplastic and squamous carcinomas which have a peak incidence between the ages of 50 to 60 and are located centrally, bronchiolar-alveolar cell carcinoma is almost always located in the peripheral portions of the lung and occurs in patients of all ages. The onset is generally insidious, with signs resembling pneumonia. Grossly this neoplasm resembles in some cases the uniform consolidation of lobar pneumonia. Microscopically, groups of alveoli are lined with clear

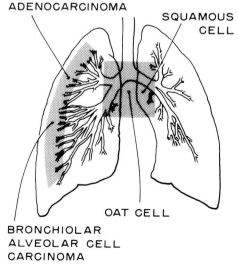

ADENOCARCINOMA

SQUAMOUS CELL

OAT CELL

BRONCHIOLAR ALVEOLAR CELL CARCINOMA

FIGURE 37-1 Anatomic distribution of lung cancer (50 percent is located centrally, while the other 50 percent is peripheral).

mucus-secreting cells, and there is abundant expectoration of mucoid sputum. The prognosis is poor unless surgical removal of the diseased lobe is performed early.

OTHER FORMS OF LUNG CANCER

Other rare types of primary lung cancer include sarcomas (affecting less than 1 percent of the population) and bronchial adenomas. Bronchial adenomas are a group of small tumors arising in the lower trachea or major bronchi, the most important being the bronchial carcinoid and the rarer cylindroma. The carcinoid affects adults of either sex under the age of 40 years. Some of these tumors secrete serotonin, 5-hydroxy-tryptophan and other biologically active substances which give rise to a symptom complex known as the *carcinoid syndrome*. Symptoms include hypotension, flushing, bronchoconstriction, cyanosis, anxiety, and tremulousness. Carcinoid tumors follow a relatively benign course, and surgical resection is usually successful.[1]

Finally, it should be remembered that the lung is affected by metastatic cancer much more often than by a primary malignant neoplasm. The lung is a common site for secondary deposits of cancer originating from other organs because bloodborne microscopic tumor emboli are likely to become enmeshed in the pulmonary capillary bed. Lymphborne tumors from the lower half of the body and abdominal cavity may also be arrested as they pass through the thoracic duct. The most common neoplasms giving rise to pulmonary metastasis are carcinoma of the breast, gastrointestinal tract, female genital tract, and kidneys, melanomas, and male genital cancer.

MANIFESTATIONS OF BRONCHOGENIC CARCINOMA

Bronchogenic carcinoma imitates a variety of other pulmonary diseases and has no typical mode of onset. It often masquerades as a pneumonitis which fails to resolve. Cough is a common symptom which is often ignored by the patient or attributed to smoking or bronchitis. When bronchial carcinoma develops in a patient with chronic bronchitis, cough often becomes more frequent or the volume of sputum may increase. Hemoptysis is another common sign. Initial symptoms of localized wheeze and mild dyspnea may result from varying degrees of bronchial obstruction. Chest pain may appear in various forms but is commonly experienced as an ache or discomfort caused by neoplastic

[1]Carcinoid tumors are more common in the gastrointestinal tract than in the lungs. Although usually benign, they can be malignant.

spread to the mediastinum. Pleuritic pain may occur when there is secondary involvement of the pleura resulting from neoplastic spread or pneumonia. Rapid development of digital clubbing is an important sign, since it is often associated with bronchogenic carcinoma. General symptoms such as anorexia, fatigue, and weight loss are late symptoms. Symptoms of intrathoracic or extrathoracic spread may also be present when the patient is first seen by the physician. Local extension of the tumor to the mediastinal structures may produce hoarseness as a result of involvement of the recurrent laryngeal nerve, dysphagia from involvement of the esophagus, and paralysis of the hemidiaphragm from involvement of the phrenic nerve. Symptoms of extrathoracic spread depend on the site of metastasis. Structures commonly involved are the scalene lymph nodes (especially in peripheral lung tumors), adrenals (50 percent), liver (30 percent), brain (20 percent), bone (20 percent), and kidneys (15 percent). The oat cell tumors are known to produce virtually any of the polypeptide hormones such as parathormone, ACTH, or ADH, so that the patient may show features which resemble hyperparathyroidism, Cushing's syndrome, or fluid retention with hyponatremia.

THE DIAGNOSIS AND TREATMENT OF LUNG CANCER

The main tools in the diagnosis of lung cancer are radiology, bronchoscopy, and cytology. A solitary, circumscribed nodule or "coin lesion" on the chest x-ray is of particular importance and may be the earliest indication of bronchogenic carcinoma, although it may occur in many other conditions. Bronchoscopy with biopsy is the most successful technique in the diagnosis of squamous cell carcinoma, which is generally located centrally. Scalene node biopsy is most successful in the diagnosis of those cancers which are inaccessible to bronchoscopy. Cytologic examination of the sputum, bronchial brushings, and examination of the pleural fluid also play an important role in the diagnosis of lung cancer.

The treatment of lung cancer consists of surgical resection and palliative treatment such as chemotherapy and irradiation. The general prognosis is poor. The average survival time after diagnosis is 5 to 14 months. About one-third of the cases are inoperable at the time of diagnosis. Of the remaining patients who undergo exploratory thoracotomy, about one-third are found to be unresectable. The 5-year survival of the remaining resectable group is only about 20 percent. This results in an overall 5-year survival of all patients of about 5 percent.

On the basis of present knowledge, the only practical means of treating lung cancer is to prevent it by advising people not to smoke cigarettes or live in an atmosphere polluted by industry. Protective measures must also be taken for those who work with asbestos, uranium, chrome, and other carcinogenic materials. Men over the age of 40 should have routine chest x-rays for earlier detection of lung malignancy.

Pulmonary malignant neoplasms—Chap. 37

Directions: Answer the following questions on a separate sheet of paper.

1 What is the carcinoid syndrome and what type of tumor causes it?

2 What are some common signs and symptoms of bronchogenic carcinoma and why is it difficult to diagnose on the basis of these signs and symptoms?

3 List three major diagnostic tools used for the detection of lung cancer and describe the significant findings of each technique.

Directions: Match each histologic type of bronchogenic carcinoma in col. A with its characteristics in col. B.

Column A	Column B
4 _____ Squamous or epidermoid	a Least common of all types
5 _____ Anaplastic (oat cell)	b Most common type
6 _____ Adenocarcinoma	c Spreads chiefly by direct extension to hilar lymph nodes
7 _____ Bronchiolar-alveolar cell	d Spreads chiefly via lymphatics
	e Spreads chiefly via bloodstream
	f Spreads directly through airways
	g Mucus-producing tumor cells
	h Associated with heavy cigarette smoking
	i Not associated with smoking
	j Located centrally about hilus and first few orders of bronchi
	k Located in peripheral part of lung
	l Both sexes affected equally
	m Undifferentiated cell type
	n Poorest prognosis
	o May secrete hormones

Directions: Circle T if the statement is true and F if it is false. Correct the false statements.

8 T F Three factors which appear to account for the increase in lung cancer over recent decades are cigarette smoking, industrial hazards, and air pollution.

9 T F Statistical evidence indicates a negative relationship between heavy cigarette smoking and bronchogenic carcinoma.

10 T F Of the industrial hazards, the most common material responsible for increasing the risk of developing lung cancer is uranium.

11 T F Primary malignant neoplasms of the lung are more common than secondary metastasis to the lung from another primary site.

12 T F About 95 percent of primary malignant neoplasms of the lung are bronchogenic carcinoma.

13 T F About 50 percent of malignant bronchogenic tumors are centrally located about the hilus and first few orders of bronchi.

Directions: Circle the letter next to each item which correctly answers the following questions. More than one item may be correct.

14 The lung is a common site for secondary metastasis because:
a Bloodborne tumor emboli are likely to become enmeshed in the capillary beds of the lungs b It is anatomically close to the abdominal organs c All the lymph of the body passes through the thoracic duct and may transport lymphborne tumor cells to the lungs

15 The overall survival rate for patients with primary lung cancer is about:
a 75 percent b 50 percent c 10 percent
d 5 percent

16 Methods of treatment for lung cancer include:
a Irradiation b Lung scan c Surgical resection
d Chemotherapy

BIBLIOGRAPHY

AUERBACH, OSCAR, E. C. HAMMOND, and L. GARFINKEL: "Bronchial Carcinoma in Relation to Smoking," in Robert F. Johnston (ed.), *Pulmonary Care,* Grune & Stratton, New York, 1973, pp. 231–242.

BURNEY, L. E.: "Smoking and Lung Cancer: A Statement of the Public Health Service," *J.A.M.A.,* **171**: 1829, 1957.

CROFTON, JOHN, and ANDREW DOUGLAS: *Respiratory Diseases,* Blackwell, Oxford, England, 1969, pp. 482–488, 517–564.

"The Health Consequences of Smoking: A Report to the Surgeon General: 1971," Washington: U.S. Department of Health, Education, and Welfare, Public Health Service.

O'DONNEL, W. M., R. H. MANN, and J. L. CROSH: "Asbestos, an Extrinsic Factor in the Pathogenesis of Bronchogenic Carcinoma and Mesothelioma," *Cancer (N.Y.),* **19**: 1143, 1966.

Pool, John L., G. F. Gray, and C. W. Holman: "Tumors of the Lung and Trachea," in C. W. Holman and C. Muschenheim (eds.), *Bronchopulmonary Diseases and Related Disorders*, Harper & Row, New York, 1972, pp. 785–821.

Robbins, S. L. and M. Angell: *Basic Pathology,* Saunders, Philadelphia, 1971, pp. 352–359.

Selikoff, I. J., et al.: "Asbestosis and Neoplasia" (editorial), *American Journal of Medicine,* **42**: 487, 1967.

Spencer, H.: *Pathology of the Lung,* 2d ed., Pergamon, New York, 1968, pp. 778–869.

Weiss, William: "Smoking and Pulmonary Disease," in Robert F. Johnson, op. cit., pp. 221–231.

CHAPTER 38 Pulmonary Tuberculosis

OBJECTIVES   **At the completion of Chap. 38, you should be able to:**

1 List the characteristics of mycobacterum tuberculosis.

2 Differentiate between the staining and culture methods used to detect the tubercle bacillus.

3 Identify the most common mode of transmission and site of implantation of the tubercle bacillus.

4 Describe the inflammatory process at the site of infection (the Ghon complex) that is evoked by the tubercle bacillus.

5 Describe caseous necrosis as to appearance and responses that occur as the result of its formation.

6 Differentiate between the lymphohematogenous and hematogenous dissemination of mycobacterial tuberculosis.

7 List the typical pathologic findings of pulmonary tuberculosis on a roentgenographic examination.

8 Describe a hypersensitivity reaction in the host of the tubercle bacillus.

9 Describe the technique used in tuberculin skin testing with respect to injection site, peak of reaction, interpretation and recording of the result, and significance of the reaction.

10 Identify the signs and symptoms that are associated with tuberculosis as it develops.

11 List the antimicrobial drugs used in the treatment and preventive therapy for tuberculosis with respect to usual dosage and minimum duration of therapy.

12 Explain the risk associated with isoniazid therapy.

13 List at least three groups that should be placed on preventive therapy against tuberculosis.

14 State the rationale that was used to develop a classification system for tuberculosis.

15 State the risk factors that must be examined when considering a person's susceptibility to tuberculosis.

16 Explain the rationale for the public health efforts to control tuberculosis in the United States.

The incidence of and mortality from tuberculosis in the United States have been declining. However, in recent years this trend has begun to plateau. In 1974, data indicated that there were approximately 30,000 new cases and 3600 deaths, which corresponds to 14.3 new cases and 1.8 deaths per 100,000 population. The incidence of infections has also declined, particularly for susceptible groups, such as young children.

DEFINITION

Tuberculosis is an infectious disease caused by *Mycobacterium tuberculosis*. The aerobic, acid-fast rods include both pathogenic and saprophytic organisms. There are several pathogenic mycobacteria, but only the bovine and human strains are pathogenic to humans. The tubercle bacillus is $0.3 \times 2-4$ μm, which is smaller than a red blood cell.

BACTERIOLOGIC STUDIES

Microscopic examination of stained specimens may be done on sputum specimens, catheterized urine, cerebrospinal fluid, and gastric contents. However, bacteriologic examination of the sputum is the most important study in the etiologic diagnosis of tuberculosis. The Ziehl-Neelsen method is used for staining bacilli. The slide is flooded with steaming carbofuchsin, then decolorized with acid-alcohol. It is then counterstained with methylene blue or brilliant green. The best accepted method of staining is the auramine-rhodamine technique of fluorescent staining. This solution, once attached to the mycobacteria, resists acid-alcohol decolorization. The clinician is provided with an estimate of the number of acid-fast bacilli detected on the slide. The microscopic examination provides the clinician with a preliminary indication of the diagnosis if the specimen is positive. It does not rule out an infection with disease if the specimen is negative.

The most accurate diagnostic method is the culture technique. The mycobacteria are slow-growing and require complex media to grow. The microorganism takes 2 or more weeks at 36 to 37°C to grow. Mature colonies are cream-colored or buff, and a warty, cauliflower appearance is very characteristic. As few as 10 bacteria per milliliter of digested, concentrated material can be detected on the culture media. The mycobacterial growth that is observed on the culture media should be quantified as to the number of colonies that are present.

PATHOGENESIS

The majority of tuberculosis infections result from the inhalation of the tubercle bacillus. The infecting particle is usually disseminated to an individual from a patient infected with active disease. The gastrointestinal tract is the usual portal of entry for the bovine strain, which is spread by contaminated milk. However, in the United States, with widespread pasteurization of milk and detection of diseased cattle, bovine tuberculosis is extremely rare.

The most common site of implantation of the tubercle bacillus is on the alveolar surface of the lung parenchyma—in the lower part of the upper lobe or upper part of the lower lobe. The reaction evoked by the tubercle bacillus is described as an inflammatory process. Polymorphonuclear leukocytes appear on the scene and phagocytize the bacteria but do not kill the organism. After the first few days, replacement of leukocytes by macrophages occurs. The involved alveoli are consolidated, and acute pneumonia develops. This cellular pneumonia may resolve itself so that no residue remains, or the process may continue, whereby the bacteria continue to be phagocytized or to multiply within the cells. There is also lymphatic drainage of the bacilli into the regional lymph nodes. The infiltrating macrophages elongate and partially fuse together to form the epitheloid cell tubercle. Surrounding the tubercle are lymphocytes. This reaction usually takes 10 to 20 days. Necrosis of the central portion of the lesion results in a relatively solid, cheesy appearance called caseous necrosis. The area of caseous necrosis and surrounding granulation tissue of epitheloid cells and fibroblasts evoke different responses. The granulation tissue may become more fibrous, forming collagenous scar tissue resulting in a capsule surrounding the tubercle. The primary lesion in the lung is called the Ghon focus, and the combination of regional lymph node involvement and the primary lesion is termed the Ghon complex. This calcified Ghon complex may be seen on a routine chest x-ray of healthy individuals.

Another response which may occur at the site of the necrotic area is liquefaction, with the liquid material sloughing into a connecting bronchus and producing a cavity. The tubercular material sloughed from the walls of the cavity enters the tracheobronchial tree. The process may be repeated in other parts of the lung, or bacilli may be carried to the larynx, middle ear, or gut.

Even without therapy, small cavities close and leave a fibrous scar. As inflammation subsides, the bronchial lumen may be narrowed and closed by scarring near the broncho-cavity junction. The caseous material may thicken and be unable to flow through the communicating channel. The cavity therefore fills with this material, and the lesion becomes similar to the unsloughed encapsulated lesion. It may remain in a quiescent stage for long periods or reestablish its bronchial communication and be the site of active inflammation.

The disease may spread through the lymphatics or blood vessels. The organisms that pass through the lymph nodes reach the bloodstream in small numbers which may initiate occasional lesions in various organs. This is referred to as lymphohematogenous dissemination, which is usually self-limited. The other type of hematogenous dissemination is an acute phenomenon and usually gives rise to miliary tuberculosis. This occurs when a necrotic focus erodes a blood vessel, allowing large numbers of organisms to enter the vascular system and be disseminated to organs in the body.

The roentgenographic examination often suggests the presence of tuberculosis, but it is almost impossible to make a diagnosis on this basis alone because almost all the manifestations of tuberculosis can be mimicked by other diseases.

There are pathologic features of tuberculosis. The earliest manifestation of tuberculous involvement of the lung is usually a parenchymal lymph node complex. In adults, the apical and posterior segments of the upper lobe or the superior segments of the lower lobe are the usual sites where lesions occur. Lesions may appear dense and homogenous. Also, there may be evidence of cavity formation and scattered disease which is often bilateral.

HYPERSENSITIVITY REACTION

The pathogenicity of the bacillus does not arise from any intrinsic toxicity but from its capacity to induce a hypersensitive reaction in the host. Tuberculoproteins derived from the bacillus appear to induce this reaction. The tissue responses of inflammation and necrosis are the results of a cellular (delayed) hypersensitivity response of the host to the tubercle bacillus. The development of a tuberculosis hypersensitivity reaction usually occurs 3 to 10 weeks from the onset of infection. As stated previously (see Chap. 5), individuals who have been exposed to the tubercle bacillus develop sensitized T-lymphocytes. If an individual has lymphocytes sensitized to tuberculoprotein and if purified protein derivative (PPD) tuberculin is injected into the skin, the sensitized lymphocytes interact with the extract and attract macrophages to the area.

Tuberculin skin testing

The standard technique (Mantoux) is the intracutaneous injection of 0.1 ml of tuberculin (PPD) into the ventral surface of the forearm. The injection is made with a short, bluntly beveled needle with a tuberculin syringe. The injection should be beneath the surface of the skin. A wheal should be produced when the prescribed amount is accurately injected.

Other types of tests for tuberculosis include the jet-gun test and the multiple puncture tests. The jet-gun test is a method of administering large numbers of tuberculin tests rapidly and painlessly. The testing material is administered intradermally by high pressure without a needle. Multiple puncture tests are rapidly administered by devices that pierce the skin at several points simultaneously. However, the Mantoux test is the method of choice and the standard of comparison for other types of tests.

The skin reaction requires 48 to 72 hours to reach its peak after the injection. The reaction should be read during that time period. The reaction must be recorded as the diameter of induration in millimeters. The measurement should be made transversely to the long axis of the forearm. Only *induration,* not erythema alone, is significant. Induration may be determined by inspection and by palpation by stroking the area with a finger. The interpretation of the skin test includes:

Positive reactions measure 10 mm or more of the induration. This reaction reflects sensitivity resulting from infection with the bacillus.

Doubtful reactions measure 5 to 9 mm of induration. This reaction can result from cross-sensitivity to atypical mycobacteria. The test should be repeated.

Negative reactions measure 0 to 4 mm of induration. No repetition of the test is usually necessary.

It is important to emphasize that a positive reaction to the tuberculin test indicates the presence of infection but does not necessarily signify clinical disease. However, this test is an important diagnostic tool in the evaluation of an individual patient. It is also very useful in determining the prevalence of tuberculous infection in individual members of the population.

CLINICAL MANIFESTATIONS

In the early stages of tuberculosis there are usually no specific signs or symptoms. Tuberculosis can be diagnosed only by tuberculin testing, roentgenogram examination, and bacteriologic studies. As the disease progresses and there is more destruction of lung tissue, there may be an increase in sputum production and coughing. Chest pain is usually not a symptom and hemoptysis is usually associated with more advanced cases. Some patients present with productive cough, fatigue, weakness, night sweats, and weight loss, which are similar to the signs and symptoms of acute bronchitis and pneumonia.

TREATMENT

The treatment of tuberculosis consists primarily of the prolonged administration of antimicrobial drugs. These drugs can also be used to prevent disease in an infected individual.

Every tuberculosis patient with clinical disease should receive a minimum of two drugs which are used to prevent emergence of drug resistant strains. The drug of first choice is isoniazid (INH) with ethambutal (EMB) or rifampin. The usual adult dosage of INH is 5 to 10 mg/kg body weight or 300 mg/day; EMB, 25 mg/kg for 60 days, then 15 mg/kg; rifampin, 600 mg once daily. Side effects of ethambutal include retrobulbar neuritis with a decrease in visual acuity. Monthly tests of visual acuity are recommended in order to detect this condition. Serious side effects to INH are rare. The most serious complication is hepatitis. The risk of hepatitis is very low in persons under 20 years of age and reaches a peak among persons over 50 years of age. Mild hepatic dysfunction, as evidenced by elevation of serum aminotransferase activity, occurs in 10 to 20 percent of persons taking INH. The minimum duration of the combined therapy is 18 months after sputum conversion to negative cultures. An additional year of INH alone is also necessary.

Isoniazid is also used for preventive therapy in a dosage of 300 mg/day for adults for a 1-year period. At present, no other drug has been demonstrated to be effective for preventive therapy.

Priorities must be established for determining which groups should be placed on preventive therapy. The following groups are recommended for preventive therapy:

1 Household members and other close associates of persons who have been recently diagnosed as having tuberculosis.

2 Positive tuberculin skin test reactor with findings on chest x-ray that are consistent with nonprogressive tuberculous disease.

3 Newly infected persons. This would apply to persons who had a tuberculin skin test conversion within the past 2 years.

4 Positive tuberculin in special clinical situations. The following situations increase the risk of developing tuberculosis: (a) therapy with corticosteroids, (b) immunosuppressive therapy, (c) certain hematologic and reticuloendothelial diseases, (d) diabetes mellitus, and (e) silicosis.

5 Positive tuberculin reactors who are under 35 years of age.

CLASSIFICATION

The American Lung Association has developed a classification system of tuberculosis which is based on the broad host–parasite relationships as described by exposure history, infection, and disease. This system applies to both children and adults. The basic classifications are divided into four categories which include the following:

0 No tuberculosis, not infected
  Negative tuberculin
  No history of exposure

I Tuberculosis exposure with no evidence of infection
  History of exposure
  Negative tuberculin

II Tuberculous infection without disease
  Positive tuberculin test
  Negative bacteriologic studies
  No roentgenographic findings compatible with tuberculosis
  No symptoms due to tuberculosis

III Tuberculosis infected with disease
  The current status of the patient's tuberculosis shall be described by:
    Location of the disease
    Bacteriologic status
    Chemotherapy status
    Roentgenogram findings
    Tuberculin skin test

Terms such as active and inactive that were previously used to describe the status of clinical activity are not included. Bacteriologic status and chemotherapy status are now used to indicate clinical condition.

EPIDEMIOLOGY

In the United States, it is estimated that 10 percent of the population, or approximately 20 million people, are infected. An adult tuberculin reactor with an abnormal chest x-ray consistent with tuberculosis has a 5 to 10 percent chance of developing clinical evidence of tuberculosis over the ensuing 10-year period. More than 80 percent of the reported new cases of tuberculosis are in persons over 25 years of age, the majority of whom were infected in the past. In general, 2 or 3 percent of the newly infected population will contract (develop) pulmonary tuberculosis.

When considering a person's susceptibility to tuberculosis, two risk factors must be examined. One is the risk of acquiring the infection and the other is of developing clinical disease after infection has occurred. The risk of acquiring the infection and developing clinical disease is dependent on the following factors: infection in the population, crowding, socially disadvantaged populations, and inadequacy of medical care. Black and Indian populations have a higher rate of tuberculosis infection than do white populations.

PREVENTION AND CONTROL

Public health measures are designed for early detection of cases and sources of infection. Preventive therapy of tuberculosis with antimicrobial drugs is an effective tool in the control of the disease. It is a preventive health measure that benefits not only the infected individual but the community as well. Therefore, populations that are at risk of developing tuberculosis must be identified, and priorities for setting up treatment programs must take into account the risk of therapy versus the benefit to the individual.

Tuberculosis eradication involves a combination of effective chemotherapy, prompt contact identification and follow-up, and chemoprophylactic therapy of high-risk population groups.

QUESTIONS

Pulmonary tuberculosis—Chap. 38

Directions: Circle the letter next to each item which correctly answers the following questions. More than one item may be correct.

1 Mycobacterium tuberculosis is described as a(n):
 a Nonpathogenic organism *b* Acid-fast rod
 c Aerobic bacillus

2 Which of the following is the most accurate diagnostic method used for the detection of the tubercle bacilli?
 a Ziehl-Neelsen method *b* Auramine-rhodamine technique *c* Culture technique

3 Of the four possible portals of entry into the body by the tubercle bacillus, which one is responsible for the majority of tuberculosis infections in the United States?
 a Respiratory tract *b* Lymphoid tissue of the oropharynx *c* Gut *d* Skin

4 The most common site of implantation of the tubercle bacillus is on the alveolar surface of the lung parenchyma in the:
 a Lower part of the upper lobe *b* Upper part of the lower lobe *c* Both *a* and *b* *d* Neither *a* nor *b*

5 The tissue lesion or tubercle produced by the causative agent *Mycobacterium tuberculosis* usually results in:
 a Hyperplasia of epithelial tissue with many mature cells *b* Dilatation and erosion of a pulmonary artery *c* Bacilli surrounded by lymphocytes and fibroblasts *d* Erosion of the epithelial lining of the mainstem bronchus

6 Which one of the following is the earliest reaction to the tubercle bacillus?
 a Cavity *b* Fibrosis *c* Calcification
 d Caseous necrosis

7 The development of caseous necrosis in tuberculosis occurs as a result of which of the following?
 a Immunity *b* Hypersensitivity

8 The period from the onset of infection with tuberculosis bacilli to the development of a tuberculin hypersensitivity reaction is usually:
 a 4 to 6 months *b* 3 to 10 weeks *c* 2 to 4 days
 d 8 to 12 hours

9 A tuberculin skin test detects which one of the following?

 a A humoral sensitivity reaction to the tubercle bacillus *b* Tuberculosis, infected with disease *c* Caseous necrosis *d* Cellular (delayed) immunologic sensitivity to the tubercle bacillus

10 A negative tuberculin skin test usually indicates that an individual:
 a Is immune to tuberculosis *b* Has been treated for tuberculosis with drugs *c* Has not been exposed to *Mycobacterium tuberculosis* *d* Has not been exposed to the tubercle bacillus or, if recently exposed, has not developed a tuberculin hypersensitivity reaction

11 Which of the following indicates a positive tuberculin test?
 a Formation of a vesicle followed by a pustule
 b A region of 10 mm of erythema around the injection site *c* An area of 10 mm of induration *d* An area of 5 mm of induration with erythema

12 The signs and symptoms that may be present in the more advanced stages of pulmonary tuberculosis include:
 a Chest pain *b* Hemoptysis *c* Increase in sputum production and cough *d* Low-grade fever

13 A 30-year-old male factory worker was diagnosed with pulmonary tuberculosis. His treatment included prolonged administration of antituberculosis drugs—isoniazid (INH) and rifampin. The usual adult dosage of INH is ___ mg/day and ___ mg of rifampin daily.
 a 100; 300 *b* 200; 400 *c* 300; 600 *d* 500; 800

14 Which of the following groups should be considered for preventive therapy with isoniazid?
 a Positive tuberculin reactors who are receiving adrenocorticoid therapy *b* Positive tuberculin reactors over 35 years of age *c* Casual contacts of persons who have been recently diagnosed with tuberculosis *d* Persons who are newly infected as demonstrated by a tuberculin skin test conversion within the past 2 years

Directions: Circle T if the statement is true and F if it is false. Correct the false statements.

15 T F Antimicrobial drugs such as ethambutal and rifampin are usually administered with isoniazid in an attempt to prevent the emergence of drug-resistant strains of *M. tuberculosis*.

16 T F The risk of developing hepatitis in persons receiving isonizid drug therapy is greatest in persons under 20 years of age.

17   T   F   The American Lung Association classification system of tuberculosis is based on the status of clinical activity of the disease (i.e., active and inactive).

18   T   F   It is estimated that 10 percent of the population in the United States, or approximately 20 million people, are infected with tuberculosis.

Directions: Answer the following questions on a separate sheet of paper.

19 Describe the two risk factors that must be examined when considering a person's susceptibility to tuberculosis.

20 What are the primary public health measures for prevention and control of tuberculosis in the United States?

BIBLIOGRAPHY

AMERICAN LUNG ASSOCIATION: *Diagnostic Standards and Classification of Tuberculosis and other Mycobacterial Diseases*, 13th ed., New York, 1974.

BAUM, G. L., and P. B. BARLOW: "Tuberculosis Patients, Old Myths, New Realities," in R. F. Johnston (ed.), *Pulmonary Care*, Grune & Stratton, New York, 1973, pp. 181–193.

CROFTON, J., and A. DOUGLAS: *Respiratory Diseases*, Blackwell, Oxford, England, 1969, pp. 163–195.

JAWETZ, E., J. MELNICK, and E. ADELBERG: *Review of Medical Microbiology*, 11th ed., Lange Medical Publications, Los Altos, Calif., 1974, pp. 200–206.

NOBLE, JOHN: "Isoniazid Prophylaxis Re-examined," *The New England Journal of Medicine*, **285**: 687, 1971.

ROBBINS, S. L. and M. ANGELL: *Basic Pathology*, Saunders, Philadelphia, 1971, pp. 411–418.

U.S. DEPARTMENT OF HEALTH, EDUCATION, AND WELFARE: *Morbidity and Mortality*, Public Health Service, Center for Disease Control, Atlanta, February 22, 1975.

WEG, JOHN: *Treatment and Control of Tuberculosis*, American Lung Association, New York, 1972.

WIDMANN, F. K.: *Goodale's Clinical Interpretation of Laboratory Tests*, 7th ed., Davis, Philadelphia, 1973.

PART VII Normal Renal Function and Renal Pathophysiology

LORRAINE M. WILSON

It has only been within recent years that the role of the kidney as a vital organ has begun to be appreciated and understood. The concept of the kidney as an organ of urine excretion is no longer adequate. Indeed, the kidney as master chemist of the body has the unique role of regulating the fluid, electrolyte, and acid-base balance of the internal environment. Its excretory function is only incidental to its regulatory function.

This new understanding gained from intensive research in normal renal physiology, pathophysiology, and effective methods of treatment has resulted in an appreciation of the impact of renal disease on the health of the nation.

The National Kidney Foundation reports that over 8 million Americans suffer with kidney-related diseases and it is the fourth greatest health problem in the nation today. They also estimate that 3.3 million persons have unrecognized and undiagnosed infection of the urinary tract. Most of these persons do not develop renal failure but there is a relationship between urinary infection and chronic pyelonephritis, one of the major causes of death due to renal failure. The financial impact of kidney-related diseases on the national economy is in excess of 3.6 billion dollars annually. This figure includes wages lost, medical services, drug costs, and insurance disbursements.*

Deaths directly related to kidney disease have been estimated to be about 55,000 annually.† This estimate

*State Health Planning Advisory Council and Office of Health and Medical Affairs, *Management of Renal Disease in Michigan, A Statement of Public Policy*, State Health Planning Advisory Council, Lansing, Michigan, November, 1973.

†"Report to the Congress: Treatment of Chronic Kidney Failure: Dialysis, Transplant, Costs, and the Need for More Vigorous Efforts," Department of Health, Education, and Welfare, GAO Report no. MWD-75-53, Washington, D.C., June 24, 1975.

is conservative since it does not take into account cases in which renal disease was a contributing cause of death. For example, many patients dying of diabetes, hypertension, or septicemia may have significant renal involvement which is not reported. It should be noted that deaths directly attributed to renal disease exceed those due to diabetes, stroke, rheumatic heart disease, and hypertensive disease through the age of 34 years. In fact, kidney disease continues to be a significant factor throughout the productive years.

Although much more knowledge of the etiology of the major renal diseases (notably chronic glomerulonephritis and pyelonephritis) is needed before effective prevention is possible, much progress has been made in prolonging the lives of persons with end-stage renal failure. These two methods of treatment are chronic dialysis and renal transplantation.

As of May 1, 1976 the National Transplant Registry reports that 15,701 renal transplants have been performed, of which approximately 12,500 have been performed during the past five years.‡ In addition, over 10,000 persons with end-stage renal disease are being kept alive by hemodialysis. Since 1973 the Federal government has taken the responsibility of paying for this expensive treatment under the Medicare program. Medicare's first year cost was 240 million dollars. Yet, little more than half of the actual treatable patients with end-stage renal disease are actually being treated. One of the reasons for this management-delivery gap is because the body of scientific, technical, and clinical knowledge in nephrology has mushroomed during the past decade and health care personnel outside of the medical centers have not kept pace with this expanding body of knowledge.§

This section is concerned with the problem of renal failure. The first three chapters discuss normal renal structure and function, methods of detecting renal disease, and the etiology and pathophysiology of chronic renal disease. The consequences of renal failure and its treatment are discussed in Chaps. 4 and 5. Acute renal failure is discussed in Chap. 6.

‡Report of the American College of Surgeons/National Institutes of Health, Organ Transplant Registry, 55 East Erie St., Chicago, Ill., May 1, 1976.
§Department of Health, Education, and Welfare, loc. cit.

OBJECTIVES

At the completion of Part VII you should be able to:

1 Describe normal renal structure and function and the effects of disordered renal function as a disease process.

2 Describe the consequence of renal failure and the principles of its treatment.

CHAPTER 39 Normal Renal Function

OBJECTIVES   **At the completion of Chap. 39 you should be able to:**

1 Identify the anatomic structures of the urinary tract.

2 Describe and recognize the importance of the location of the kidney in relation to other anatomic structures in close proximity.

3 Identify the structures that enter and leave the kidney.

4 Describe the gross anatomy of the kidney.

5 Trace the blood route supplying and draining the kidney.

6 Describe the special features of renal blood flow including total blood received, its distribution, and autoregulation.

7 Give one example of a possible complication of variations in the renal blood supply.

8 Identify the component parts of the nephron.

9 Name, locate, and describe the function of the various types of cells of the renal corpuscle.

10 Identify and describe the components of the juxtaglomerular apparatus.

11 Describe the function of the juxtaglomerular apparatus in relation to renal blood flow.

12 Describe the renin-angiotensin system.

13 Describe glomerular filtration including the forces involved, its measurement, and normal values for men and women.

14 Differentiate between reabsorption and secretion in the nephron.

15 Distinguish two types of transport mechanisms in the nephron.

16 Identify three classes of substances and the major components of each which are filtered by the glomerulus.

17 Describe tubular regulation of filtered substances in each component part of the nephron.

18 Describe the role of the kidneys in acid-base regulation.

19 Identify three hormones which influence tubular secretion or reabsorption and the substances influenced.

20 List seven major functions of the kidney (four excretory and three nonexcretory).

21 Define the concept of *osmolality*.

22 Name the single factor that influences osmotic activity.

23 List the four colligative properties of solutions.

24 Illustrate how each of these colligative properties is affected by the addition of particles to water.

25 Differentiate between two methods of measuring the concentration of body fluids (osmometer and urinometer).

26 Write the formula used to calculate the osmotic concentration (osmolality) of a solution, and given appropriate values, calculate the plasma osmolality.

27 Distinguish between osmolality and osmolarity.

28 Describe reabsorption of glomerular filtrate in the proximal tubule.

29 Differentiate between the cortical and juxtamedullary nephrons (number and anatomic features).

30 Define the *vasa recta*.

31 Explain the two basic processes involved in the countercurrent mechanism.

32 Describe the concentration gradient of the filtrate as it moves from the glomerulus to the end of the collecting duct.

33 Explain the anatomic relations which allow a concentration gradient to become established and maintained in the kidney.

34 Explain how the chloride pump (active chloride transport) is involved in countercurrent multiplication of concentration.

35 Describe how the vasa recta act as a countercurrent exchange system.

36 Describe the effect of antidiuretic hormone (ADH) on the distal tubule, collecting ducts, and the vasa recta.

37 Describe the recirculation of urea and its contribution to the osmotic concentration of the interstitial fluid.

38 Explain the role of ADH in maintaining a constant volume and osmolality of the plasma.

ANATOMY OF THE KIDNEYS AND URINARY TRACT

The kidneys perform the vital function of regulating the volume and chemical composition of the blood (and the internal environment) by selective excretion of solutes and water. If both kidneys were to fail to perform this function for any reason, death would follow within 3 or 4 weeks. This vital function of the kidney is accomplished within the organ by filtration of the blood plasma through the glomerulus followed by reabsorption of the appropriate amounts of solute and water along the renal tubules. Excess solutes and water are excreted as urine through the urinary collecting system to the outside of the body. This chapter will review the gross and microscopic anatomy of the kidney and discuss its physiologic functions.

The urinary tract

The urinary tract consists of the kidneys, which constantly manufacture urine, and the various tubes and reservoirs necessary to carry urine to the outside of the body (Fig. 39-1).

The kidneys are bean-shaped organs situated on either side of the vertebral column. The right kidney is slightly lower than the left because it is pushed down by the liver. Its upper pole lies on the level of the twelfth rib. The upper pole of the left kidney lies at about the level of the eleventh rib.

The two ureters are tubes about 10 to 12 in long extending from the kidneys to the bladder. Their only function is to convey urine to the bladder.

The bladder is a collapsible muscular bag located behind the symphysis pubis. There are three openings in the bladder, two from the ureters and one into the urethra. The bladder has two functions: (1) it serves as a reservoir for urine before it leaves the body, and (2) aided by the urethra, it expels urine from the body.

The urethra is a small, dilatable tube leading from the bladder to the outside of the body. It is about 1½ in long in the female and about 8 in long in the male. The opening to the outside of the body is called the urinary meatus.

Anatomic relations of the kidney

The kidneys lie at the back of the upper abdomen behind the peritoneum, in front of the last two ribs and three major muscles—the transversus abdominus, quadratus lumborum, and psoas major (Fig. 39-2). They are kept in position by a heavy cushion of fat. The adrenal glands are situated over the upper pole of each kidney.

The kidneys are well protected from direct trauma—

posteriorly by the ribs and overlying muscles, and anteriorly by a thick cushion of intestines. When they are injured, it is almost always as a result of a force acting upon the twelfth rib, which rotates inwards and squeezes the kidney between itself and the bodies of the lumbar vertebrae. This excellent protection from direct injury also accounts for their difficult position for palpation and surgical access. The normal-sized left kidney is not generally palpable on physical examination because the upper two-thirds of the anterior surface is overlaid by the spleen. The lower pole of the normal-sized right kidney, however, may be bimanually palpated in many persons. Gross enlargement or displacement of either kidney may be detected by palpation, though this is more easily accomplished on the right.

Gross structure of the kidney

In the adult each kidney is 12 to 13 cm long, 6 cm wide, and weighs from 120 to 150 g. The size does not vary appreciably with body build. A difference of more than 1.5 cm in the length of a particular kidney or a change in its shape is significant since the majority of renal diseases are manifested by structural changes of the organ.

The anterior and posterior surfaces, upper and lower poles, and lateral margin of the kidney have a convex contour while the medial margin is concave due to the presence of the hilus (Fig. 39-3A). Several structures

enter or leave the kidney through the hilus including the renal artery, renal vein, nerves, and lymphatics. The kidney is encased in a thin, fibrous, glistening capsule, which is loosely adherent to the underlying tissue and can be easily stripped from the surface.

A longitudinal section of the kidney reveals two distinct regions, the outer cortex and inner medulla (Fig. 39-3B). The medulla is divided into triangular wedges called pyramids. The pyramids are interspersed with cortical material called the columns of Bertin. Pyramids have a striated appearance because they are made up of segments of the tubules and collecting ducts of the nephron. The papilla (apex) of each pyramid forms the papillary ducts of Bellini, which in turn are created by the terminal fusion of many collecting ducts. Each papillary duct is thrust into a cup-shaped terminal extension of the renal pelvis called a minor calyx (Gk. *kalyx,* cup). Several minor calyces unite to form major calyces, which in turn unite to form the pelvis of the kidney. The renal pelvis is the main reservoir for the renal collecting system. The ureter connects the renal pelvis to the urinary bladder.

Knowledge of renal anatomy is basic to understanding urine formation. Urine formation begins in the cortex and continues as the material flows through the tubules and collecting ducts. The formed urine then flows into the papillary ducts of Bellini, enters the minor calyces, major calyces, renal pelvis, and finally exits the kidney via the ureter to the urinary bladder. The walls of the calyces, pelvis, and ureter contain smooth muscle, which contracts rhythmically and helps to propel urine along its course by peristalsis.

Gross vascular supply of the kidney

The renal arteries arise from the abdominal aorta at approximately the level of the second lumbar vertebra. Because the aorta is to the left of the midline, the right renal artery is longer than the left (Fig. 39-2). Each renal artery branches as it enters the hilus of each kidney.

The renal veins which drain each kidney empty into the inferior vena cava which lies to the right of the midline. Consequently, the left renal vein is about twice as long as the right. Because of these anatomic features, the transplant surgeon generally prefers the left kidney from the donor, which is rotated and placed in the right pelvis of the recipient. Few technical difficulties are encountered with a short renal artery which is anastomosed with the internal iliac (hypogastric) artery. The renal vein, however, must be longer since it is implanted directly into the external iliac vein (Fig. 43-8).

As the renal artery enters the hilus, it breaks down into the *interlobar* arteries which pass between the pyramids to form the *arcuate* branches, which arch over the bases of the pyramids (Fig. 39-4).

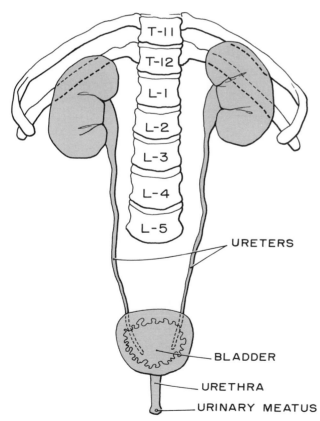

FIGURE 39-1 The urinary tract, anatomic relations.

The arcuate arteries give rise to the *interlobular arterioles*, which form a parallel array in the cortex. These interlobular arterioles give rise to *afferent arterioles*.

The afferent arterioles terminate in capillary tufts called the *glomeruli*. The capillary tufts, or glomeruli, converge into *efferent arterioles* which in turn subdivide into a portal network of capillaries surrounding the tubules, sometimes called the *peritubular capillaries* (not shown). The blood passing through this portal network drains into a venous network to the interlobular, arcuate, interlobar, and renal veins to reach the inferior vena cava.

SPECIAL FEATURES OF RENAL BLOOD FLOW

The kidneys are perfused with about 1200 ml of blood per minute—a volume equal to 20 to 25 percent of the cardiac output (5000 ml/minute). This fact is quite remarkable when one considers that the combined weight of the kidneys is less than 1 percent of the total body weight.

More than 90 percent of the blood perfusing the kidney is distributed to the cortex, while the remainder is distributed to the medulla (the physiologic significance of this for urine concentration will be discussed later).

Another special feature of renal blood flow is autoregulation of blood flow through the kidney. The afferent arterioles have an intrinsic capacity to vary their resistance in response to changes in arterial blood pressure thus keeping renal blood flow and glomerular filtration constant. It is effective over an arterial pressure range of 80 to 180 mmHg. The result is the prevention of large changes in solute and water excretion. Autoregulation, however, can be overpowered in certain circumstances even in the autoregulatory range. Renal nerves may cause vasoconstriction in states of emergency and shunt blood away from the kidney to the heart, brain, or skeletal muscles at the expense of the kidney. Disturbances in autoregulation and the distribution of intrarenal blood flow may be important in the pathogenesis of acute oliguric renal failure (see Chap. 44).

VARIATIONS IN RENAL VASCULAR SUPPLY

There are cases in which multiple arteries or veins supply the kidneys (Fig. 39-5). Anomalies of the renal arteries are far more common than those of the veins. In fact, about 25 percent or more of the population have more than one renal artery supplying a kidney. These additional arteries usually originate as small, multiple branches from the aorta and supply the poles of the kidney. An arteriogram of the renal blood supply is essential in the donor before kidney transplantation is attempted because of the possibility of these variations, which may present technical difficulties for the surgeon.

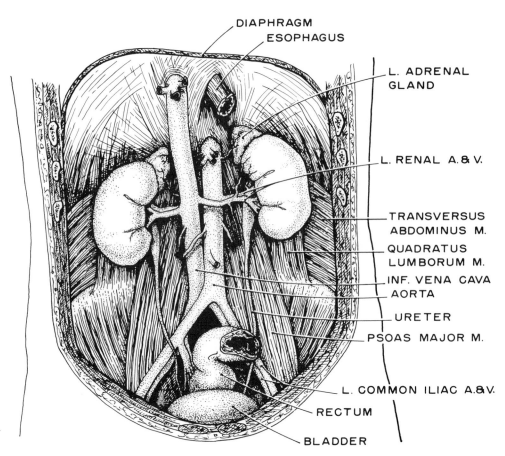

DIAPHRAGM
ESOPHAGUS
L. ADRENAL GLAND
L. RENAL A. & V.
TRANSVERSUS ABDOMINUS M.
QUADRATUS LUMBORUM M.
INF. VENA CAVA
AORTA
URETER
PSOAS MAJOR M.
L. COMMON ILIAC A. & V.
RECTUM
BLADDER

FIGURE 39-2 The kidneys, anatomic relations.

THE NEPHRON

The functional work unit of the kidney is called the nephron. There are about 1 million nephrons in each kidney, basically similar in structure and function. Thus the work of the kidneys may be considered to be the sum total of the function of all the nephrons put together. Each nephron consists of *Bowman's capsule,* which surrounds the glomerular capillary tuft, the *proximal convoluted tubule,* the *loop of Henle,* and the *distal convoluted tubule,* which empties into the *collecting ducts* (Fig. 39-6). A normal person can survive, albeit with difficulty, with less than 20,000 nephrons, or 1 percent of the total nephron mass. Thus, it is possible to donate one kidney for transplantation without endangering life.

THE RENAL CORPUSCLE

The renal corpuscle consists of Bowman's capsule and the glomerular capillary tuft. The term glomerulus is often used interchangeably with renal corpuscle, though it properly refers only to the capillary tuft.

Bowman's capsule is a specialized invagination of the proximal tubule (Fig. 39-7). There is a urine-containing space between the capillary tuft and Bowman's capsule called *Bowman's space,* or the *capsular space.*

Bowman's capsule is lined with epithelial cells. *Parietal epithelial cells* are flat and form the outermost part of the capsule; the much larger *visceral epithelial cells*

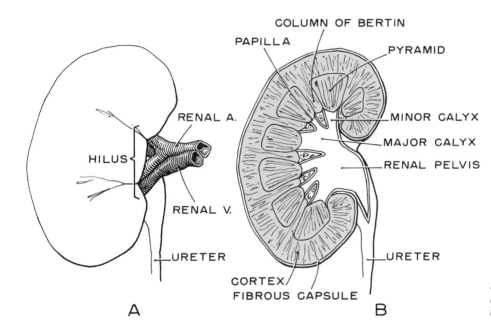

FIGURE 39-3 Gross structure of the kidney. A. anterior surface; B. longitudinal section.

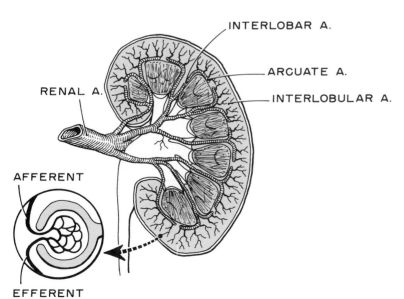

FIGURE 39-4 Vascular supply to the kidney. Approximately 90 percent of the blood is distributed to the cortex and 10 percent to the medulla. Inset depicts the glomerular capillary tuft with afferent and efferent arterioles.

form the innermost part of the capsule and line the outer side of the capillary tuft. Foot processes, or *podocytes,* form extensions of the visceral epithelial cells which come in contact with the basement membrane at intervals, leaving many areas free of epithelial cell contact. The area between the foot processes, usually referred to as the *slit pore,* has an average width of about 400 Å (angstrom units).

The *basement membrane* forms the middle layer of the capillary wall, sandwiched between the epithelial cells on one side and the endothelial cells on the other. The capillary basement membrane is continuous with that of the tubule. No pores are visible in the basement membrane, although it behaves as if it had pores about 70 to 100 Å in diameter.

Endothelial cells form the innermost layer of the capillary tuft. Unlike the epithelial cells, the endothelial cells are in continuous contact with the basement membrane. However, there are numerous windowlike openings called fenestrations which are about 600 Å in diameter. The endothelial cells are continuous with the endothelial lining of the afferent and efferent arterioles.

The endothelial cells, basement membrane, and visceral epithelial cells are the three layers which make up the *glomerular filtration membrane.* The function of the glomerular filtration membrane is to allow ultra-filtration of the blood. In separating the formed elements of the blood and the large protein molecules from the rest of the plasma, it delivers the plasma as primary urine to the urinary space of Bowman's capsule. The mechanism involved in the filtration process is not fully understood. Recent evidence seems to indicate that the structural basis for the relative impermeability of the glomerular capillary may be the slit pores or the gelatinous basement membrane. A small amount of albumin, molecules of which have a diameter slightly less than that of the smallest "pores," enters the filtrate but is reab-sorbed in the proximal tubule. Larger protein molecules and blood cells do not normally appear in the filtrate and urine.

The *mesangial cells* are endothelial cells which form a continuous network between the capillary loops of the glomerulus and are thought to function as a supporting network. Mesangial cells are not part of the filtration membrane.

THE JUXTAGLOMERULAR APPARATUS

In each nephron the first part of the distal tubule rises from the medulla so that it is situated in the angle between the afferent and efferent arteriole of the glomerulus of that nephron (Fig. 39-7). At this point the *juxtaglomerular cells* within the wall of the afferent arteriole contain secretory granules which are believed to secrete renin. Renin is an enzyme important in the regulation of blood pressure. The distal tubular cells come into intimate contact with the granular cells and are called the *macula densa* because of their prominent nuclei. This specialized group of cells (including some connective tissue cells) near the vascular pole of each glomerulus is known as the juxtaglomerular (JG) apparatus and is believed to regulate renin release.

There are two important theories concerning the regulation of renin release. According to one theory, the juxtaglomerular cells function as baroreceptors (pressure sensors) sensitive to blood flow through the afferent arteriole. A decrease in arterial pressure stimulates increased granularity of the juxtaglomerular cells and increased renin secretion. According to the other theory, the macula densa cells of the distal tubule act as chemoreceptors sensitive to the sodium concentration of the tubular fluid. A decreased sodium concentration in the distal tubule influences the juxtaglomerular cells (in close apposition to the macula densa) to increase renin output. There is also evidence that the sympathetic nervous system and the catecholamines influence renin secretion. It is probable that both the baroreceptor and macula densa theories are valid, and the juxtaglomerular apparatus may be a site for the integration of several diverse inputs.

FIGURE 39-5 Anomalies in renal vasculature. About 25 percent of the population have multiple renal arteries supplying a kidney, A; multiple renal veins, B. (Modified from Frank H. Netter, Ciba Collections of Medical Illustrations: Kidneys, Ureters, and Urinary Bladder, *Ciba Pharmaceutical Co., Summit, N.J., 1973, vol. 6.)*

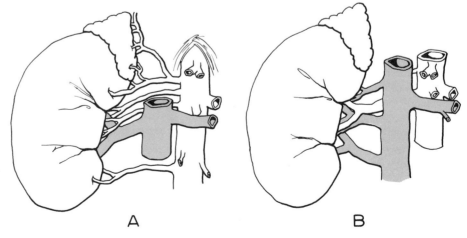

A   B

The release of renin from the kidney results in the conversion of angiotensinogen (a glycoprotein made in the liver) to angiotensin I. Angiotensin I is changed to angiotensin II by a converting enzyme found in the pulmonary capillary bed. Angiotensin II increases blood pressure by causing vasoconstriction of peripheral arterioles and stimulating secretion of aldosterone. Elevated aldosterone levels stimulate sodium reabsorption in the distal tubules and collecting ducts. Increased sodium reabsorption causes increased water reabsorption, and thus plasma volume is increased. This increased plasma volume contributes to blood pressure elevation which in turn facilitates the reduction of renal ischemia. The schema for the renin-angiotensin mechanism is outlined in Fig. 39-8.

BASIC RENAL PHYSIOLOGY

The primary function of the kidney is to maintain within normal limits the volume and composition of the extracellular fluid. The composition and volume of the extracellular fluid is controlled by glomerular filtration, tubular reabsorption, and secretion. The following discussion will be concerned with these processes.*

*It may be helpful for the reader to read the summary of renal functions in Table 39-1 at the end of this chapter before proceeding.

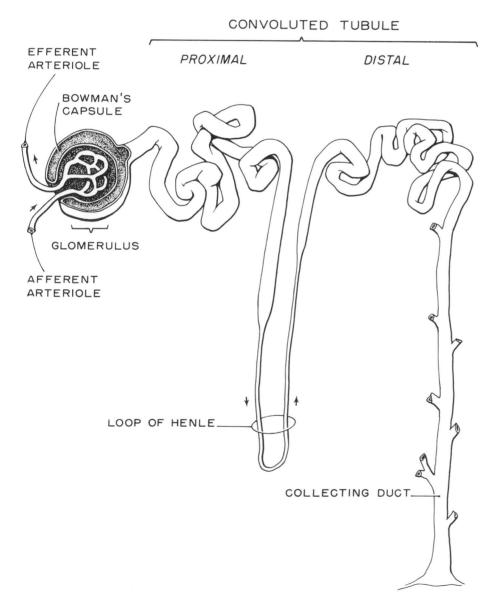

FIGURE 39-6 The nephron.

Glomerular ultrafiltration

Urine formation begins with glomerular filtration of plasma. Renal blood flow (RBF) is equal to about 25 percent of the cardiac output, or 1200 ml/minute. Assuming a normal hematocrit of 45 percent, renal plasma flow (RPF) is equal to 660 ml/minute ($0.55 \times 1200 = 660$). Approximately one-fifth of the plasma or 125 ml/minute passes through the glomerulus into Bowman's capsule. This is called the glomerular filtration rate (GFR). Filtration at the glomerulus is termed glomerular ultrafiltration because the primary filtrate has the same composition as plasma with the exception of the absence of proteins. Blood cells and large molecules such as proteins are effectively restrained by the filtration membrane "pores" while water and crystalloids (solutes of small molecular dimensions) are readily filtered. Calculation reveals that 173 liters of fluid is filtered through the glomerulus in one day—an astonishing amount in organs whose combined weight is about 10 oz! As the filtrate travels through the tubules, various substances are added or subtracted from it so that eventually only about 1.5 liters/day is excreted as urine.

The forces that account for this high glomerular filtration rate are entirely passive since metabolic energy is not expended by the kidney for the process of filtration. The filtration force is a result of the pressure gradient between the glomerular capillary and Bowman's capsule. The hydrostatic pressure of the blood in the glomerular capillaries favors filtration, and this force is opposed by the hydrostatic pressure of the filtrate in Bowman's

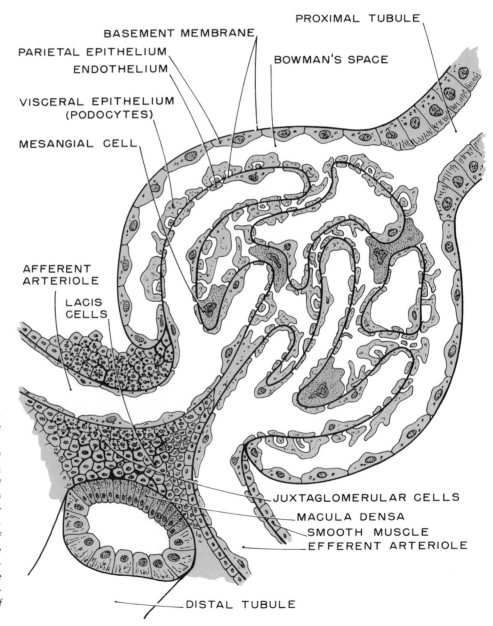

PROXIMAL TUBULE
BASEMENT MEMBRANE
PARIETAL EPITHELIUM
ENDOTHELIUM
BOWMAN'S SPACE
VISCERAL EPITHELIUM
(PODOCYTES)
MESANGIAL CELL
AFFERENT
ARTERIOLE
LACIS
CELLS
JUXTAGLOMERULAR CELLS
MACULA DENSA
SMOOTH MUSCLE
EFFERENT ARTERIOLE
DISTAL TUBULE

FIGURE 39-7 The renal corpuscle. The glomerular capillary filter consists of three layers of cells—the endothelium, basement membrane, and visceral epithelium containing podocytes or foot processes. Mesangial cells (between the capillaries) form a supporting network for the glomerular tuft. The juxtaglomerular apparatus consists of a specialized group of cells (the macula densa and juxtaglomerular cells) near the vascular pole of the glomerulus and is important in the regulation of blood pressure.

capsule and the colloid osmotic pressure (COP) of the blood. The COP in Bowman's capsule is essentially zero. Although never measured in human beings, the glomerular capillary pressure was estimated by R. F. Pitts to be about 50 mmHg and intracapsular pressure to be about 10 mmHg. These estimates are based on actual recent measurements in rats. Colloid osmotic pressure of the blood is about 30 mmHg. Net glomerular filtration pressure is thus about 10 mmHg. The glomerular filtration is influenced not only by these physical forces, but by the permeability of the capillary walls. The balance of forces involved in glomerular ultrafiltration is summarized below:

$$\text{GFR} = \begin{matrix}\text{filtration}\\\text{permeability}\\\text{factor}\end{matrix}$$
$$\times \left[\begin{matrix}\text{intracapillary}\\\text{hydrostatic}\\\text{pressure}\end{matrix} - \left(\begin{matrix}\text{intracapsular}\\\text{hydrostatic}\\\text{pressure}\end{matrix} + \begin{matrix}\text{colloid}\\\text{osmotic}\\\text{pressure}\end{matrix} \right) \right]$$

Net filtration pressure = 10 mmHg
$$= 50 - (10 + 30) \text{ mmHg}$$

The most accurate way to measure the GFR is to use a substance which is freely filtered at the glomerulus and is neither secreted nor reabsorbed by the tubules. Inulin is a substance which satisfies these criteria. The clearance of a substance is the volume of plasma from which that substance is completely cleared by the kidneys per unit time. The rate of the clearance of inulin is exactly equal to the GFR. This is measured by the administration of inulin at a constant intravenous drip rate to ensure constant plasma concentration level. Measurement of inulin concentration in plasma (p_{in}) in milligrams per hundred milliliters (mg/100 ml), in urine (U_{in}) in milligrams per hundred milliliters and of the volume of urine (V) in milliliters per minute (ml/minute) will permit calculation of inulin clearance (C_{in}) in milliliters per minute. The result must be corrected for body surface area estimated by using a normogram which relates height and weight to body surface area. Example: if a person is passing urine at the rate of 4.2 ml/minute, the inulin concentration in the urine specimen is 600 mg/100 ml, and the plasma inulin concentration is constant at 25 mg/100 ml, then

$$\text{GFR} = C_{in} = \frac{(U_{in})\ 600 \text{ mg/100 ml} \times (V)\ 4.2 \text{ ml/minute}}{(P_{in})\ 25 \text{ mg/100 ml}}$$
$$= 100 \text{ ml/minute}$$

The calculated GFR of 100 ml/minute would then be normalized by correcting it to the standard normal body

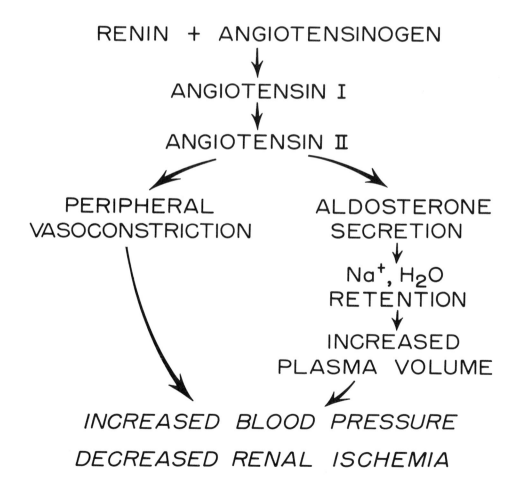

RENIN + ANGIOTENSINOGEN

↓

ANGIOTENSIN I

↓

ANGIOTENSIN II

PERIPHERAL VASOCONSTRICTION   ALDOSTERONE SECRETION

↓

Na⁺, H₂O RETENTION

↓

INCREASED PLASMA VOLUME

INCREASED BLOOD PRESSURE

DECREASED RENAL ISCHEMIA

FIGURE 39-8 Schema for the renin-angiotensin system.

surface area of 1.73 m². This correction makes it possible to compare function in persons of varying physical stature. The GFR of normal young men averages 125 ± 15 ml/minute/1.73 m², and that for normal young women is 110 ± 15 ml/minute/1.73 m².

Tubular reabsorption and secretion

Three classes of substances are filtered at the glomerulus (Fig. 39-9). These are electrolytes, nonelectrolytes, and water. Some of the most important electrolytes are sodium (Na^+), potassium (K^+), calcium (Ca^{2+}), magnesium (Mg^{2+}), bicarbonate (HCO_3^-), chloride (Cl^-), and phosphate (HPO_4^{2-}). Important nonelectrolytes are glucose, amino acids, and the metabolic end products of protein metabolism: urea, uric acid, and creatinine.

The second step in urine formation after filtration is the selective reabsorption of filtered substances. Most of the substances filtered are reabsorbed through minute "pores" in the tubule where they pass back into the peritubular capillaries which surround the tubule. In addition, some substances are secreted from the surrounding peritubular blood vessels into the tubule.

Reabsorption and secretion take place by both active and passive transport mechanisms. A mechanism is active if it transports a substance against an electrochemical gradient; i.e., against a gradient of electrical potential, chemical potential, or both. Work is performed directly on the substance reabsorbed or secreted by the tubular cells, and energy is expended in the process. A transport mechanism is passive if the sub-

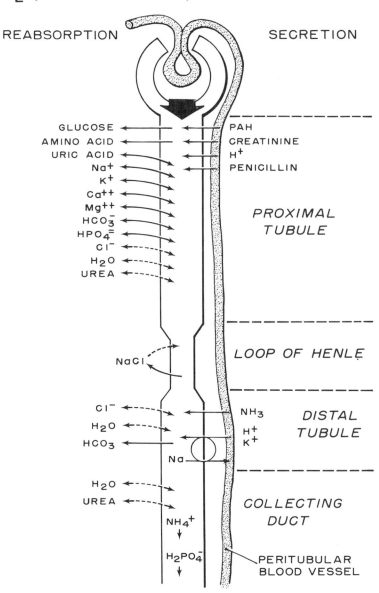

FILTRATION
H₂O, ELECTROLYTES, NONELECTROLYTES

REABSORPTION   SECRETION

GLUCOSE   PAH
AMINO ACID   CREATININE
URIC ACID   H⁺
Na⁺   PENICILLIN
K⁺
Ca⁺⁺
Mg⁺⁺   PROXIMAL
HCO₃⁻   TUBULE
HPO₄⁼
Cl⁻
H₂O
UREA

NaCl   LOOP OF HENLE

Cl⁻   NH₃   DISTAL
H₂O   H⁺   TUBULE
HCO₃   K⁺
                   Na

H₂O
UREA   COLLECTING
                    DUCT
NH₄⁺

H₂PO₄⁻   PERITUBULAR
                   BLOOD VESSEL

FIGURE 39-9 Tubular reabsorption and secretion along the glomerular nephron. Solid arrows indicate active transport, and broken arrows indicate passive transport.

stance being reabsorbed or secreted moves down an electrochemical gradient. No energy is directly expended in moving the substance.

Along the proximal tubule glucose and amino acids are completely reabsorbed by active transport. Almost all of the potassium and uric acid are actively reabsorbed, and both are secreted into the distal tubule. At least two-thirds of the filtered sodium is actively reabsorbed in the proximal tubule. Reabsorption of sodium continues in the loop of Henle, distal tubule, and collecting ducts so that less than 1 percent of the filtered load is excreted in the urine. Most of the calcium and phosphate is reabsorbed in the proximal tubule by active transport. Water, chloride, and urea are reabsorbed in the proximal tubule by passive transport. As large numbers of positively charged sodium ions leave the tubular lumen, negatively charged chloride ions must follow for reasons of electrical neutrality. The exit of a large number of ions and nonelectrolytes from the proximal tubular fluid leaves it osmotically dilute, and as a result, water diffuses out of the tubule into the peritubular blood. Urea then diffuses passively down a concentration gradient established by the reabsorption of water. Hydrogen ion (H^+), organic acids such as para-amino-hippurate (PAH) and penicillin, and creatinine (an organic base) are all actively secreted in the proximal tubule. About 90 percent of the bicarbonate is reabsorbed in the proximal tubule indirectly by Na^+-H^+ exchange. When H^+ is secreted into the tubular lumen (in exchange for Na^+), it combines with the HCO_3^- present in the glomerular filtrate to give carbonic acid (H_2CO_3). The H_2CO_3 dissociates to water and carbon dioxide (CO_2). Both CO_2 and H_2O diffuse out of the tubular lumen into the tubular cell. In the tubular cell, carbonic anhydrase catalyzes the reaction of CO_2 and H_2O to form H_2CO_3 once again. The dissociation of H_2CO_3 produces HCO_3^- and H^+. The H^+ is resecreted, and the HCO_3^- passes into the peritubular blood along with Na^+.

In the loop of Henle, Cl^- is actively transported out of the ascending limb followed passively by Na^+. NaCl then diffuses passively into the descending limb. This process is important for urine concentration and will be discussed later in this chapter.

The selective process of secretion and reabsorption is completed in the distal tubule and collecting ducts. Two important functions of the distal tubule are the final regulation of water balance and acid-base balance. If the cells are to function normally, the pH of the extracellular fluid must be maintained within the narrow range of 7.35 to 7.45. Several biological mechanisms working in coordination contribute toward maintaining the pH within normal limits. The principal blood buffer is the bicarbonate–carbonic acid system given by the equation:

$$CO_2 + H_2O \underset{\substack{\text{carbonic} \\ \text{anhydrase}}}{\rightleftharpoons} H_2CO_3 \rightleftharpoons H^+ + HCO_3^-$$

The blood pH is given by the Henderson-Hasselbalch equation:

$$pH = pK + \log \frac{HCO_3^- \text{ (kidneys)}}{H_2CO_3 \text{ (lungs)}}$$

where pK is the dissociation constant of carbonic acid. The lungs eliminate CO_2 which is produced when H^+ is buffered by HCO_3^- (left shift of the reaction above) and thus play an important role stabilizing the pH. The role of the kidneys in maintaining acid-base balance is the reabsorption of most of the filtered HCO_3^-. When considering disturbances in acid-base balance, it is often helpful to keep in mind that the serum pH is largely a function of the HCO_3^-/H_2CO_3 ratio and that the numerator is largely regulated by renal mechanisms, while pulmonary mechanisms regulate the denominator (through control of CO_2 elimination). A change in the numerator or denominator is followed by a unidirectional change in the other. This change is known as compensation and serves to protect the pH.

In addition to reabsorbing and conserving most of the HCO_3^-, the kidneys also eliminate excess H^+. About 60 meq of acids other than H_2CO_3 are produced in the body each day. Since these acids cannot be eliminated by the lungs they are called *fixed acids*. These acids are eliminated in the tubular fluid, so that it is possible for the urine to achieve a pH as low as 4.5 (a hydrogen-ion gradient that is 800 times that in the plasma). All along the tubule, H^+ is secreted into the tubular fluid. The H^+ may then be excreted by combination with filtered dibasic phosphate (HPO_4^{2-}) or with ammonia (NH_3). Thus H^+ is excreted as the titratable monobasic acid salt (NaH_2PO_4) or as ammonium ion (NH_4^+). NH_3 diffuses readily into the tubular lumen, but after combination with H^+ to form the charged particle NH_4^+, it is unable to diffuse back into the tubular cell. Because the minimum urine pH that can be achieved is 4.5, the amount of free H^+ that can be excreted is limited. Therefore the ammonium mechanism (and the phosphate mechanism) is very important in eliminating an acid load, since NH_4^+ does not affect the urine pH. The buffering of H^+ by NH_3 or HPO_4^{2-} also has the effect of adding a *new* HCO_3^- to the plasma for every H^+ excreted into the urine. The H^+ that is secreted is derived from H_2CO_3 in the tubular cell leaving HCO_3^- behind in equimolar amounts. In contrast, when HCO_3^- is reabsorbed from the tubular fluid by the mechanism previously described in this discussion, HCO_3^- is merely conserved, since one H^+ is returned to the plasma for each one that is secreted into the tubular fluid. Therefore the regeneration of HCO_3^- (i.e., the de novo synthesis) by the buffering mechanism is very important in preventing acidosis.

Both uric acid and potassium are secreted into the distal tubule, as already mentioned. Normally about 5 percent of the filtered potassium load is excreted in the urine. Water reabsorption is also completed in the distal tubule and collecting ducts.

Several hormones regulate the tubular reabsorption and secretion of solutes and water. Water reabsorption depends on the presence of antidiuretic hormone (ADH). Aldosterone influences Na^+ reabsorption and K^+ secretion. Increased aldosterone causes increased Na^+

reabsorption and increased K^+ secretion. A decrease in aldosterone has the opposite effect. Another hormone of the parathyroid glands, parathormone, regulates Ca^{2+} and HPO_4^{2-} reabsorption along the tubule. Increased parathormone results in increased reabsorption of Ca^{2+} and increased HPO_4^{2-} excretion. A decrease in parathormone has the opposite effect.

Figure 39-9 summarizes the major function of each part of the nephron. It is by means of this selective reabsorption and secretion along the tubule that the kidney is able to regulate the internal body environment in a very precise manner. The following discussion will examine in greater detail the role of the kidney in water metabolism.

Regulation of water balance

The total solute concentration of body fluids is remarkably constant in the normal person despite wide fluctuation in water and solute intake and excretion. It is through the production of urine much more concentrated or dilute than the plasma from which it is derived that the concentration of the plasma and body fluids is maintained within narrow limits. When a large volume of fluids is ingested causing dilution of body fluids, the urine becomes dilute, and the excess water is rapidly excreted. Conversely, under conditions of water deprivation or excess solute intake causing the body fluids to become concentrated, the urine becomes highly concentrated so that solute is lost in excess of water. The water retained tends to return the body fluids to a normal solute concentration.

Before proceeding to describe the processes involved

in the regulation of body fluid balance, it is necessary for you to understand the concept of *osmolality*. This is a term used to express the concentration of body fluids.

OSMOTIC CONCENTRATION

Osmotic concentration (osmolality) refers to the number of particles dissolved in a solution. When a solute is added to water, the effective concentration (activity) of water is lowered relative to that of pure water. Osmotic activity is influenced only by the relative number of solute and solvent particles and is ideally independent of the nature of the solute. Solute particles differing in mass, shape, and charge have the same effect on the osmotic activity of the solvent provided they are equal in number. Thus six sodium and chloride ions which are completely dissociated have the same effect on the osmotic activity as six glucose molecules in one kilogram of water even though they are quite different in mass, shape, and charge (Fig. 39-10).

Colligative properties of solutions

The addition of solute particles to a solvent is manifested as lowering of vapor pressure and freezing point and raising of the boiling point and osmotic pressure of the solvent. These phenomena are referred to as the colligative properties of solutions. All of these properties depend on osmotic concentration.

Figure 39-11 illustrates the four colligative properties of solutions. The first two colligative properties are vapor pressure lowering and boiling point elevation. When particles are added to water, it is more difficult for the water to escape from the surface since the effective concentration of water is decreased. Consequently, pure water boils at 100°C while a solution of glucose and water boils at a temperature greater than 100°C.

When solute particles are added to water, the osmotic pressure is increased, which is a third colligative prop-

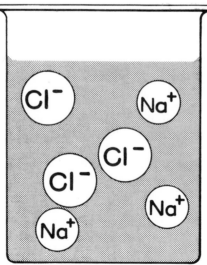

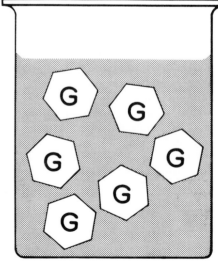

FIGURE 39-10 Osmotic concentration equals the number of particles per kilogram of water. It does not depend on the mass, shape, or charge of the particles in an ideal solution.

6 PARTICLES
NaCl/KgH₂O

6 PARTICLES
GLUCOSE/KgH₂O

erty of a solution. In the diagram in Fig. 39-11 note that there are two glucose molecules in the left compartment and six in the right compartment separated by a semi-permeable membrane. The pores in the membrane are too small to allow glucose to diffuse readily. Water, a smaller molecule, diffuses easily from the area of low osmotic concentration in the left-hand compartment to the area of higher osmotic concentration in the right-hand compartment. This process is called *osmosis*. Actually, water is moving from an area of higher water concentration (in the left compartment) to an area of lower water concentration (in the right compartment). Osmosis is thus only a special case of diffusion.

The diffusion of water from the left to the right compartment continues until osmotic equilibrium is achieved, with the result that the fluid level is elevated in the right compartment. The force driving the water through the semipermeable membrane is called *osmotic pressure*. To prevent the water from diffusing into the right-hand compartment, it would be necessary to apply physical pressure over the solution in the right-hand compartment which would be equal to the higher potential of water in the left compartment. It is common usage to speak of the osmotic pressure of a solution though it is virtually never measured. Several other properties of solutions vary in exact proportion to the osmotic pressure and are more easily measured (e.g., depression of the freezing point and vapor pressure

lowering). In fact, even the use of the term osmotic pressure is rather loose since it is commonly expressed in terms of concentration rather than pressure (see later).

The principle of osmosis is basic to the movement of water between compartments in the body. This principle is also applied in dialysis by putting high concentrations of glucose in the dialysis bath to facilitate removal of excess fluid from the body which has accumulated when the kidneys are not functioning adequately.

The fourth colligative property of a solution is the freezing point depression. Particles added to water cause the solution to freeze at a lower temperature than that of pure water which freezes at 0°C.

Measurement of osmotic concentration

There are two common methods of measuring the osmotic concentration of body fluids. Measuring the freezing point depression by the *osmometer* is a true measure of osmotic concentration but is complex and must be carried out in a laboratory.*It is based on the

*More recently a device to measure osmotic concentration based on vapor pressure lowering has been used in some laboratories. This method is more rapid and less complicated to use than the osmometer.

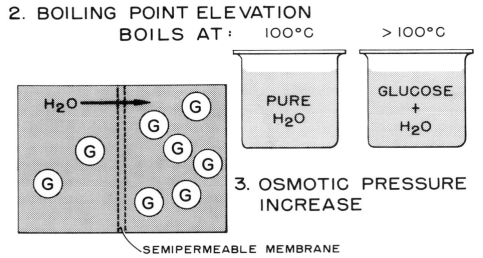

I. VAPOR PRESSURE LOWERING
2. BOILING POINT ELEVATION
BOILS AT: 100°C   > 100°C

3. OSMOTIC PRESSURE INCREASE

SEMIPERMEABLE MEMBRANE

4. FREEZING POINT DEPRESSION
FREEZES AT: 0°C   < 0°C

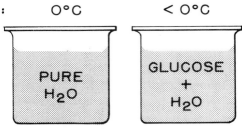

FIGURE 39-11 Colligative properties of solutions.

principle that the freezing point of a solution consisting of one gram-molecular weight (or mole, mol) of any nondissociated substance dissolved in one kilogram of water will be −1.86°C.* Such a solution is called an osmolal solution, and it contains one osmol of solute particles (i.e., the number of particles to lower the freezing point of water by 1.86°C). The change in temperature is called the molal freezing point constant (K_f) and is equal to one osmol.

In the absence of dissociation, each molecule of solute behaves as a single particle. Therefore, since molecular size has no effect on colligative properties, one gram-mole of albumin (mol wt 70,000) affects the freezing point of water to the same degree as one gram-mole of glucose (mol wt 180). If dissociation occurs as with sodium chloride, for example, and two ions are formed, each molecule has the effect of two particles. In this case, then, one osmol is one-half the molecular weight.

In order to calculate the osmotic concentration (osmolality) of a solution, it is only necessary to measure the lowering of the freezing point below that of pure water (ΔT). This number is then divided by K_f, the molal freezing point constant

$$\text{Osmolality} = \frac{\Delta T}{K_f}$$

For example, blood plasma freezes at −0.53°C. When this number is divided by −1.86 (K_f), the calculated concentration is 285 mOsm (1 milliosmol = 0.001 osmol)

$$\text{Plasma concentration} = \frac{-0.53°C}{-1.86°C} \times 1000$$
$$= 285 \text{ mOsm}$$

*One mole of any element or molecular compound contains the same number of particles (Avogadro's number: 6.02×10^{23} molecules/mol).

In the healthy person, plasma concentration is 285 ± 10 mOsm/kg H_2O.

The second method of estimating concentration of body fluids is to measure the specific gravity with the urinometer (see photographs of the urinometer and osmometer in Fig. 39-12). Specific gravity is not a true measure of concentration, but because of its simplicity, it is commonly used in the clinical unit. What is actually being measured is the density (which depends on the *weight* of the solute particles) and not the concentration (which depends on the *number* of solute particles). However, estimating the concentration of urine by measuring specific gravity is fairly accurate provided the urine has normal constituents. In Chap. 40 the correlation between the osmolal and specific gravity measurements will be discussed.

Osmolality vs. osmolarity

In the literature and in practice you will observe that the term osmolarity is frequently used in place of or interchangeably with the term osmolality when speaking of the concentrations of intravenous solutions or body fluids. This interchange often causes confusion. Osmolality is an expression of concentration *in terms of one thousand grams of water*. Accordingly, neither temperature nor space taken up by the solids present in the solution has any bearing on the osmolality figure, and a direct comparison can be made of various body fluids with different water or solids content. On the other hand, such a comparison is not possible when concentration is expressed *in terms of one liter of solution* (i.e., osmolarity). The amount of water in one liter of solution is a function both of its temperature and the space occupied by the solids in solution. Inasmuch as colligative properties are determined only by the ratio of solute to solvent particles, the osmolarity of various body fluids is not directly comparable. The difference between osmolality and osmolarity is apparent in the diagram in Fig. 39-13. To make up a one-osmol solution, one gram-mole of solute particles is added to a beaker with exactly

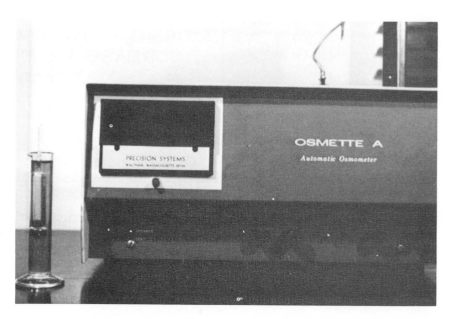

FIGURE 39-12 Osmometer and urinometer. The osmometer measures the freezing point depression of a solution which is used to calculate osmolality. The urinometer (left) does not actually measure osmotic concentration but the density of a solution.

one thousand grams of water. The volume of the solution is thus greater than 1 liter. The one-osmolar solution is made by first adding one gram-mole of solute particles to the beaker and then sufficient water to reach the one-liter mark. Thus the volume of the solute is included in the solution. It is obvious that the concentrations of the two solutions are not equal. The difference between osmolality and osmolarity is negligible in the range of concentration and temperature of body fluids. It is, however, important to use osmolal units of concentration in the accurate preparation of intravenous solutions.

It is the function of the kidneys to keep the concentration of the body fluids constant at 285 mOsm. How this is accomplished will be explored in the following pages.

ISOOSMOTIC REABSORPTION IN THE PROXIMAL TUBULE

When the glomerular filtrate first enters the proximal tubule, it has the same concentration as the plasma, 285 mOsm. It is therefore called isoosmotic. Along the proximal tubule as much as 80 percent of the filtrate is reabsorbed into the peritubular capillaries.* This reab-

*Reported values of filtrate reabsorption in the proximal tubule vary from two-thirds to seven-eighths depending on the source (see R. F. Pitts, p. 109; see "References" at the end of Part VII).

sorption is isoosmotic since both water and solutes are reabsorbed in the same proportion as they exist in the filtrate. So at the end of the proximal tubule the concentration of the filtrate is still 285 mOsm, and about 20 percent of the filtrate still remains (Fig. 39-14). Even though the flow has been significantly reduced (from 125 to about 25 ml/minute), urine excretion directly out of the proximal tubule would be about 1500 ml/hour. At this rate of urine excretion, death would occur within a few hours from dehydration, since a loss of 12 to 14 percent of the body weight in water is fatal. The next step in the process of urine formation is to greatly reduce the volume of the filtrate before it is expelled as urine.

COUNTERCURRENT MECHANISM

In the kidney there are two types of nephrons—the cortical and the juxtamedullary (next to the medulla), illustrated in Fig. 39-15. The juxtamedullary nephron has a much longer loop of Henle than the cortical nephron, and its peritubular blood supply is in the form of hair-

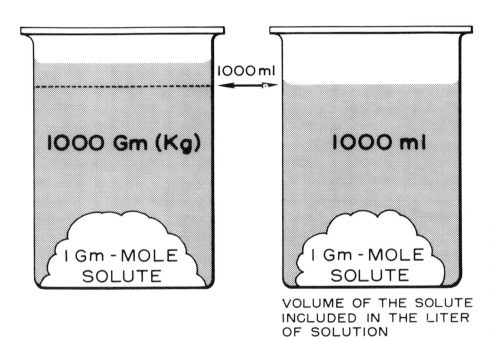

VOLUME OF THE SOLUTE
INCLUDED IN THE LITER
OF SOLUTION

FIGURE 39-13 Osmolality vs. osmolarity. Osmolality is an expression of concentration in terms of 1000 g of water. Osmolarity is concentration expressed in terms of 100 ml of solution. Osmolality is approximately equal to osmolarity for dilute solutions when the volume occupied by the solute is very small.

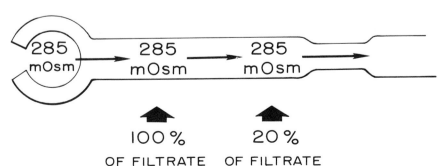

FIGURE 39-14 Eighty percent isoosmotic reabsorption of the glomerular filtrate in the proximal tubule.

pin loops which dip down beside the loop of Henle. These blood vessels are called the *vasa recta*. These anatomic features of the juxtamedullary nephrons largely account for the concentration of urine. In fact, the longer the hairpin loop, the greater the concentrating ability of the animal. The kangaroo rat, a desert rodent, has unusually long loops and can excrete urine with an osmolality of about 6000 mOsm. In the human, about one out of seven nephrons are juxtamedullary with long loops, and the maximum concentration of urine is about 1400 mOsm.

The countercurrent mechanism, which is responsible for the conservation of water by the kidney actually involves two basic processes: (1) the countercurrent multiplier of concentration in the loop of Henle and (2) the countercurrent exchanger in the vasa recta which is also in the form of a hairpin loop. The main function of the loop of Henle is to make the interstitial fluid in the medulla hyperosmotic and the tubular fluid which emerges from it into the distal tubule hypoosmotic; these changes permit the concentration of the final urine to be modified over a wide range. The main function of the vasa recta is to prevent the dissipation of the osmotic gradient in the medullary interstitial fluid which has been built up by the loop of Henle. Along the nephron, the fundamental processes involved in the production of a concentrated or dilute urine are the active reabsorption of chloride in the ascending limb of Henle and the variable permeability to the passive diffusion of water and urea along their concentration gradients.

First, let us examine the overall relationships during the production of a concentrated urine (Fig. 39-16). Beginning at the glomerulus where filtration starts, the filtrate is isoosmotic with the plasma at 285 mOsm. By the end of the proximal tubule 80 percent of the filtrate has been reabsorbed, although the concentration is still 285 mOsm. As the filtrate moves down the descending limb of Henle, the concentration of the filtrate reaches a maximum at the tip of the loop. Then

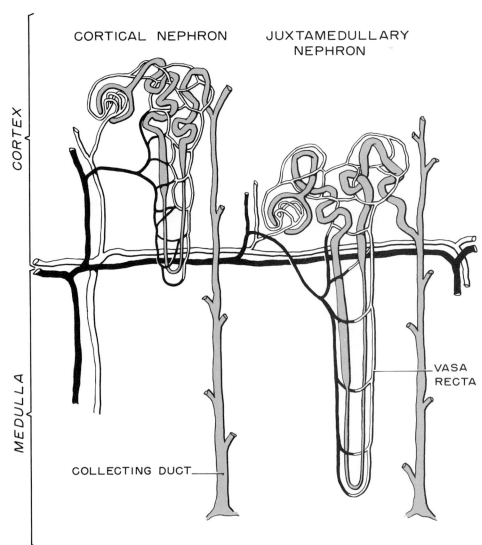

FIGURE 39-15 Cortical and juxtaglomerular nephrons with vasa recta.

as the filtrate moves up the ascending limb, the concentration becomes more and more dilute until it is hypoosmotic at the top of the limb. As the filtrate proceeds along the distal tubule, it becomes more concentrated until it is isoosmotic with the blood plasma at the top of the collecting duct. As the filtrate moves down the collecting duct, it again becomes increasingly concentrated. At the end of the collecting duct about 99 percent of the water has been reabsorbed, and about 1 percent of the filtrate is excreted as urine.

Note on the diagram that there is also a concentration gradient in the interstitial fluid increasing from the cortex to the medulla. The vasa recta which dip down beside the loop of Henle also have a concentration gradient which increases going down the descending limb and decreases moving up the ascending limb, though the decrease is much less than in the ascending limb of Henle. Note also that the limbs of the loop of Henle form parallel columns and that the filtrate flow is in opposite directions. This is known as countercurrent

flow and allows the loop of Henle to function as a countercurrent multiplier building up the concentration gradient in the interstitium. (The principle of countercurrent multiplication is reviewed in Fig. 39-17.) The entire process may now be described in greater detail.

The operation of the countercurrent multiplier in the loop of Henle is initiated by the active transport of chloride out of the ascending limb. This causes sodium to passively follow down the potential gradient created by the active chloride transport. Water, however, cannot passively follow the sodium chloride transport since the ascending limb is impermeable to water (indicated by the heavy lines in Fig. 39-16). Consequently, the filtrate becomes hypoosmotic as the top of the ascending limb is approached. The interstitial fluid becomes more con-

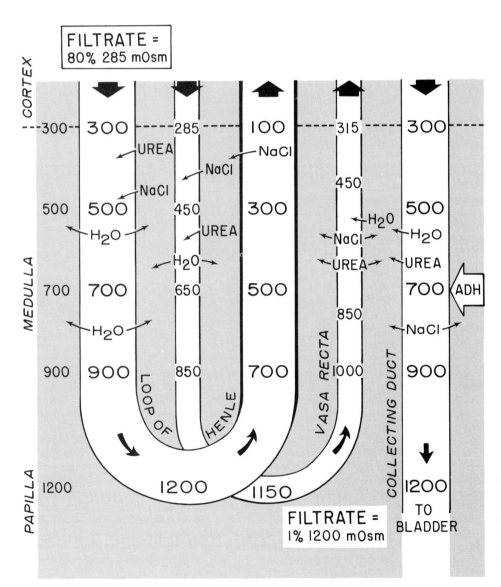

FIGURE 39-16 The countercurrent mechanism. See text for explanation. (Modified from Frank H. Netter, Ciba Collections of Medical Illustrations, Kidneys, Ureters, and Urinary Bladder, *Ciba Pharmaceutical Co., Summit, N.J., 1973, vol. 6.*)

centrated, setting up an osmotic gradient between the interstitial fluid and the descending limb of Henle. Water flows out of the descending limb and sodium chloride passively enters, causing the filtrate to become increasingly concentrated. As this process continues, a concentration gradient increasing from cortex to medulla is established in both the descending limb of Henle and in the interstitium until a steady state is reached.

The vasa recta, which dip down beside the loop of Henle, act as a countercurrent exchanger by passive diffusion (active transport is not involved). The blood in the vasa recta is in osmotic equilibrium with the interstitial fluid. As blood flows through the descending limb of the vasa recta, sodium chloride passively moves in and water moves out, causing the blood to become increasingly concentrated as it approaches the tip of the loop. In the ascending limb of the vasa recta, opposite events occur. Sodium passively diffuses out into the interstitium while water is reabsorbed into the blood vessel and returned to the general circulation. The fact that the blood flow through the vasa recta is sluggish allows it to act as an efficient exchanger (recall that the medulla only receives 10 percent of the blood supply to the kid-

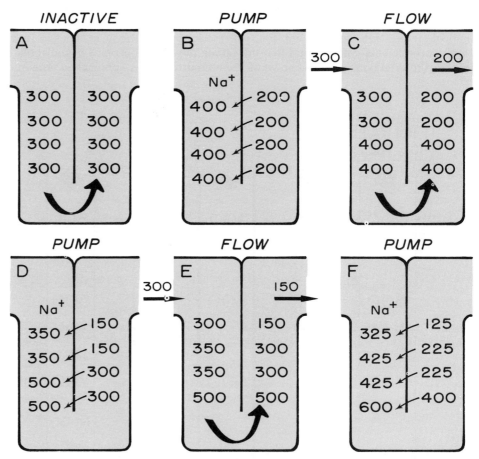

FIGURE 39-17 *The principle of countercurrent multiplication of concentration is based on the assumption that at any level along the loop of Henle a gradient of 200 mOsm can be achieved between the limbs by active transport of chloride and passive diffusion of sodium ions. The changes in concentration along the loop are illustrated in a series of discontinuous steps. Step A, Multiplier not active, filtrate enters at 300 mOsm. Step B, Flow stopped, ion pump activated generating a horizontal gradient of 200 mOsm between the limbs. Step C, Flow started, more filtrate enters at 300 mOsm pushing some fluid around the tip from descending to ascending limb. Some fluid is ejected. Step D, Flow stopped, ion pump activated generating another gradient of 200 mOsm between the limbs. Step E, More filtrate enters at 300 mOsm pushing filtrate around the tip from descending to ascending limb. Step F, Flow stopped, ion pump activated generating another gradient of 200 mOsm between the limbs. Note that the concentration of the filtrate at the tip of the loop is now 600 mOsm, and there is a longitudinal gradient of 275 mOsm whereas the ion pump was only able to generate a horizontal gradient of 200 mOsm. Continuation of this process further increases the longitudinal gradient. (Modified from R. F. Pitts,* Physiology of the Kidney and Body Fluids, *3d ed.,* Year Book Medical Publishers Inc., Chicago, 1974.)

ney). If the blood flow were very rapid, the sodium chloride which entered the descending limb would be washed away. Thus the vasa recta acting as a countercurrent exchanger prevents the disssipation of the concentration gradient in the interstitium built up by the loop of Henle acting as a countercurrent multiplier of concentration.

Along the distal tubule sodium (chloride) is actively reabsorbed. Under conditions of antidiuresis the hypoosmotic filtrate at the beginning of the distal tubule becomes isoosmotic by the time it reaches the top of the collecting duct. The final concentration of urine takes place in the distal tubule and collecting ducts under the control of antidiuretic hormone (ADH). The distal tubule and collecting ducts are permeable to water in the presence of ADH. Water then diffuses out into the interstitium in response to the osmotic gradient in the medulla. The water then enters the ascending limb of the vasa recta and is returned to the general circulation. The final urine produced is low in volume and high in osmotic concentration.

In contrast, under conditions of diuresis and the absence of ADH, the distal tubule and collecting ducts are virtually impermeable to water. Sodium (chloride) is

actively reabsorbed from the distal tubule and collecting ducts, but water does not diffuse out to maintain osmotic equilibrium. Since sodium is reabsorbed and water is left behind, a large volume of dilute urine is produced.

Urea also diffuses out of the collecting ducts into the interstitial fluid where it contributes to the high osmotic concentration in the medulla. Some of the urea also enters the descending limb of the loop of Henle and the vasa recta and is recirculated. The effect is to trap urea in the medullary interstitium. A person on a low protein diet is unable to concentrate urine as well as a person on a normal or high protein diet since urea is the end product of protein metabolism.

ADH MECHANISM FOR THE REGULATION OF PLASMA OSMOLALITY

The ADH mechanism is important in maintaining the volume and osmolality of the extracellular fluid (ECF) at

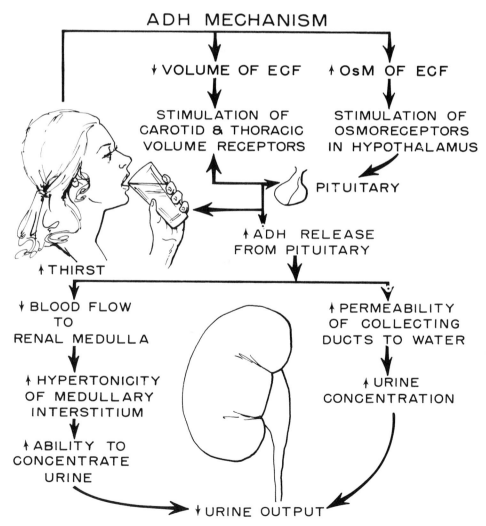

FIGURE 39-18 ADH mechanism for the regulation of plasma osmolality.

a constant level by controlling the final volume and osmolality of the urine.

Changes in plasma volume or osmolality from the ideal constant of 285 mOsm control the release of ADH. ADH is produced in the supraoptic nuclei of the hypothalamus and descends along nerve fibers to the posterior pituitary where it is stored for subsequent release. ADH release is controlled by a feedback mechanism with two pathways (Fig. 39-18).

ADH release is increased by an increase in the plasma osmolality or a decrease in the plasma volume. Osmoreceptor cells located in the hypothalamus are sensitive to the concentration of the circulating blood, and pressure-sensing cells in the left atria are sensitive to blood volume. These sensors stimulate the release of ADH. Increased osmolality and/or decreased volume of the ECF, for example, may be caused by factors such as water deprivation, fluid loss from vomiting, diarrhea, hemorrhage, burns, sweating, or displacement of fluid as in ascites.

The subjective feeling of thirst which drives one to ingest water is also stimulated by a decrease in volume and/or an increase in ECF osmolality, the adaptive significance of both being self-evident in the illustration. The centers which mediate thirst are also located in the hypothalamus close to those areas which produce ADH. Increased thirst in the person who has suddenly lost 800 ml of blood due to hemorrhage (decrease in ECF) or in the person who has just eaten a candy bar (increase in the osmolality of ECF due to more glucose particles in the blood) is explained by this mechanism.

In the kidney, ADH indirectly augments the key events which occur in the loop of Henle by two interrelated mechanisms: (1) blood flow through the vasa recta of the medulla is diminished in the presence of ADH, thus minimizing solute depletion of the interstitium which in turn becomes more hyperosmotic, and (2) ADH increases the permeability of the collecting ducts and distal tubules so that more water diffuses out to equilibrate with the hyperosmotic interstitial fluid. Both mechanisms operate to produce a concentrated urine and thus reduce the volume of excretion.

Conversely, low plasma osmolality and/or volume expansion from increased water intake inhibits ADH release. The final volume of urine excreted is increased and more osmotically dilute.

Even in extreme cases of a huge volume of fluid ingestion or of a very limited fluid intake, normal human beings have amazing flexibility in maintaining the osmolality of the ECF at a constant 285 mOsm. To accomplish this we are able to excrete urine as dilute as 40 mOsm or as concentrated as 1200 to 1400 mOsm. As will be shown later, the patient with renal insufficiency loses this great flexibility.

Functions of the kidney

The major functions of the kidneys are summarized in Table 39-1 which emphasizes their regulatory role in the body. Vander summarized the function of the kidneys in a poignant manner when he said, "This regulatory role is obviously quite different from the popular conception of the kidneys as glorified garbage-disposal units which rid the body of assorted wastes and poisons."* The kidneys do excrete certain foreign chemicals (drugs, etc.), hormones, and other metabolites, but their most important function is maintaining the volume and composition of the ECF within normal limits. This is accomplished, of course, by varying the excretion of water and solutes, and the high filtration rate allows great precision in this function. Renin and erythropoietin production and vitamin D metabolism are all important nonexcretory functions. Excessive renin secretion may be important in the etiology of some forms of hypertension and will be discussed in Chap. 41. Deficiency of erythropoietin and vitamin D activation is believed to be important in the etiology of anemia and bone disease in uremia and will be discussed in Chap. 42.

*A. J. Vander, *Renal Physiology*, p. 4 (see Part VII References).

TABLE 39-1
Major functions of the kidney

EXCRETORY	NONEXCRETORY
Maintain plasma osmolality near 285 mOsm by varying the excretion of water	Produce renin—important in the regulation of blood pressure
Maintain the plasma concentration of each individual electrolyte within normal range	Produce erythropoietin—important factor in stimulating red blood cell production by the bone marrow
Maintain the plasma pH near 7.4 by eliminating excess H^+ and regenerating HCO_3^-	Metabolize vitamin D to its active form
Excrete the nitrogenous end products of protein metabolism; chiefly, urea, uric acid, and creatinine	

QUESTIONS

Normal renal function—Chap. 39

Directions: Label Figs. 39-19 to 39-22 with the appropriate term from each group.

1 Fig. 39-19. The urinary tract.

Urinary meatus	Ureter
Bladder	Right kidney
Urethra	Left kidney

2 Fig. 39-20. Posterior abdominal wall, vertebrae, ribs.

Eleventh rib	Psoas major muscle
Twelfth rib	Transversus abdominus muscle

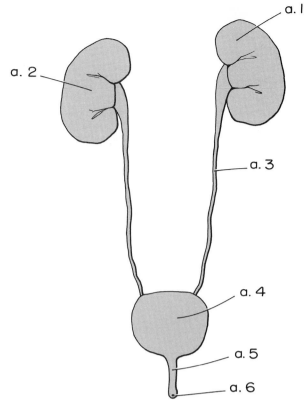

FIGURE 39-19 *The urinary tract.*

3 Fig. 39-21. Cross section of the kidney.

Pyramid	Minor calyces
Ureter	Major calyx
Renal pelvis	Fibrous capsule
Papilla	Medulla
Cortex	Column of Bertin

4 Fig. 39-22. The nephron.

Proximal convoluted tubule	Bowman's capsule
	Macula densa
Distal convoluted tubule	Juxtaglomerular cells
	Afferent arteriole
Collecting duct	Efferent arteriole
Loop of Henle	Glomerular capillary tuft

5 Draw the kidneys on the diagram in Fig. 39-20 in the appropriate relationship to the ribs and vertebrae.

6 Trace the formation and transit of urine from the renal cortex to the bladder by lettering the following structures in sequence.

Ureter	Bladder
Renal pelvis	Minor calcyces
Collecting ducts	Distal convoluted tubule
Bowman's capsule	Major calyces
Proximal convoluted tubule	Papillary ducts of Bellini

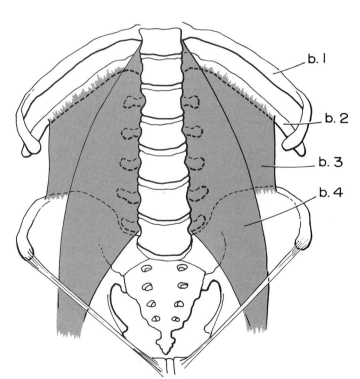

FIGURE 39-20 *Posterior abdominal wall, vertebrae, ribs.*

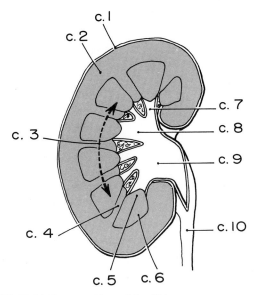

FIGURE 39-21 Cross section of the kidney.

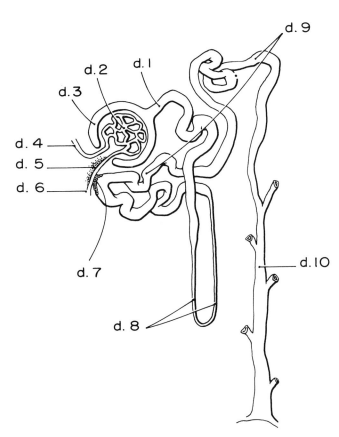

FIGURE 39-22 The nephron.

7 This list contains the names of blood vessels supplying and draining the kidneys. Letter this list in the correct sequence beginning with the blood vessel supplying the kidney.

Renal vein   Interlobular arterioles
Afferent arterioles   Interlobar arteries
Abdominal aorta   Arcuate veins
Arcuate arteries   Renal artery
Inferior vena cava   Peritubular capillaries
Interlobar veins   (portal network)
Glomerular capillaries   Interlobular veins
Efferent arterioles

Directions: Answer the following questions on a separate sheet of paper.

8 Why is it especially important to obtain a renal arteriogram in a healthy individual who is supplying a donor kidney for transplantation?

9 Explain how the juxtaglomerular cells and macula densa cells help to control blood pressure.

10 Why is a heavy blow over the twelfth rib particularly dangerous to the kidney?

Directions: Match the type of renal corpuscular cell in col. A with its proper description in col. B by placing the correct letter in the blank.

Column A
11 ___ Parietal epithelium
12 ___ Visceral epithelium
13 ___ Podocytes
14 ___ Endothelial cells
15 ___ Basement membrane
16 ___ Mesangial cells

Column B
a Network between capillary loops of the glomerulus
b Extensions of visceral cells contacting basement membrane
c Layer that separates epithelial from endothelial cells
d Flat cells, outermost part of capsule
e Innermost layer of capillary tuft containing fenestrations
f Large cells which line the outside of the capillary tuft

Directions: Circle the letter preceding each item below that correctly answers the questions. Only one answer is correct.

17 The glomerular filtration membrane is composed of all of the following cell layers *except:*
a Endothelial cells b Basement membrane
c Visceral epithelium d Mesangial cells

18 Which of the following structures of the glomerular filtration membrane is least effective in preventing entry of protein molecules into the filtrate?
a Fenestrations in the endothelial cell layer b Slit pores between visceral epithelial cells c Basement membrane d Long pores in the mesangial cells

19 Pole-to-pole length of the normal-sized kidney is:
a 6 to 7 cm b 9 to 10 cm c 12 to 13 cm
d 16 to 19 cm

20 The normal-sized _____ kidney is not generally palpable during physical examination.
a Right   *b* Left

21 The minimal number of nephrons needed to sustain life is about:
a 2 million   *b* 1 million   *c* 200,000   *d* 20,000

22 The substance which *directly* causes peripheral vasoconstriction and increased aldosterone secretion is:
a Angiotensinogen   *b* Renin   *c* Angiotension II
d Angiotensin I

23 What percentage of the cardiac output is normally delivered to the kidneys?
a 90 percent   *b* 50 percent   *c* 25 percent
d 10 percent

24 The cortex/medulla ratio of blood distribution in the kidney is normally about:
a 9:1   *b* 1:9   *c* 1:1   *d* 1:3

25 The adaptive value of autoregulation of blood flow by the kidney is:
a To increase total renal blood flow in response to hypotensive shock   *b* To decrease cortical blood flow in response to hypotensive shock   *c* To increase sodium and water retention in severe cases of hypertension   *d* To increase medullary blood flow in cases of dehydration shock   *e* To prevent changes in solute and water excretion in response to fluctuations in arterial pressure

Directions: Answer the following questions on a separate sheet of paper.

26 Why is glomerular filtration called ultrafiltration?

27 How is net filtration pressure derived?

28 Define and give the normal numerical value of the GFR for men and women.

29 What kind of substance must be used to measure the GFR and why?

30 During an inulin clearance test the following values were obtained from a patient: concentration of inulin in plasma 25 mg/100 ml and in urine 500 mg/100 ml; urine volume 2 ml/minute. Calculate this patient's GFR ignoring body surface area. Is it within normal range?

31 What are the two most important functions of the distal tubule and collecting ducts?

32 Explain how the kidneys and lungs work together in the regulation of acid-base balance in the body.

33 How does phosphate excretion and ammonia secretion contribute to the excretion of acid by the kidney?

34 List the seven major functions of the kidney.

35 How are the four colligative properties of a solution affected by the addition of particles to water?

36 What does the osmometer measure? the urinometer?

Which is the most accurate in estimating concentration and why?

37 Write the formula to calculate plasma osmotic concentration from the freezing point. Given that plasma freezes at −0.53°C, calculate the concentration of plasma in milliosmols.

38 Draw a cortical and juxtamedullary nephron illustrating their position in relationship to the cortex and medulla.

39 What are the vasa recta and what do they do?

40 What is the purpose of the countercurrent mechanism? What are the two basic processes involved?

Directions: Circle the letter preceding each item below that correctly answers the questions. (Only one answer is correct; exceptions noted.)

41 The forces that determine the glomerular filtrate are:
a Hydrostatic pressure of the blood in the glomerulus
b Plasma protein concentration   *c* Hydrostatic pressure of the fluid in Bowman's capsule   *d* All of the above

42 Tubular secretion involves the movement of substances:
a From the peritubular capillaries into the tubular lumen   *b* From the tubular lumen into the peritubular capillaries   *c* From the glomerular capillaries into the tubular lumen   *d* From the tubular lumen into the bladder

43 Normal renal plasma flow is about:
a 1200 ml/minute   *b* 660 ml/minute
c 125 ml/minute   *d* 1 ml/minute

44 The fraction of plasma filtered by the glomerulus (filtration fraction) is:
a 100 percent   *b* 50 percent   *c* 20 percent
d 1 percent

45 The type of tubular transport involving the movement of a substance up a chemical or electrical gradient is called:
a Osmosis   *b* Passive diffusion   *c* Active
d Hydrostatic

46 Substance normally filtered by the glomerulus include all of the following *except*:
a Electrolytes   *b* Water   *c* Nonelectrolytes
d Blood cells

47 The proportion of glomerular filtrate reabsorbed in the proximal tubule is about:
a 20 percent   *b* 50 percent   *c* 80 percent
d 99 percent

48 The osmolality of a solution depends on:
a Density of particles   *b* Size of particles   *c* Elec-

trical charge of the particles   d Number of particles
e All of these

49 The ascending limb of the loop of Henle:
a Actively transports sodium   b Is permeable to
water   c Is hyperosmotic   d Actively transports
chloride   e Actively transports water

50 The medullary interstitial fluid in health is:
a Always hypoosmotic   b Always hyperosmotic
c Hyperosmotic during antidiuresis only   d Hypoosmotic during diuresis and hyperosmotic during
antidiuresis

51 All of the following factors are important in the formation of a concentrated urine *except*:
a Presence of a long loop of Henle   b Presence of
ADH   c Intact chloride pump in the ascending limb
of Henle   d Increase in medullary blood flow in the
vasa recta   e Diffusion of urea into the medullary
interstitium

52 Which of the following stimulate increased ADH
release? (More than one answer is correct.)
a Increase in ECF volume   b Decrease in ECF volume
c Increase in the osmolality of the ECF   d Decrease
in the osmolality of the ECF

53 ADH exerts all of the following effects on the kidney
except (more than one answer is correct):
a Increases blood flow in the vasa recta   b Decreases blood flow in the vasa recta   c Increases
permeability of distal tubule and collecting ducts to
water   d Decreases isoosmotic reabsorption in the
proximal tubule

54 Under conditions of severe water deprivation in
human beings, maximum urine osmolality is greater
than plasma osmolality by a factor of about:
a 10   b 5   c 3   d 2

55 Which of the following osmolalities represents the
maximum urine dilution ability in human beings
under conditions of excess water ingestion?
a 40 mOsm   b 100 mOsm   c 285 mOsm
d 1400 mOsm

*Directions: Match the appropriate osmotic concentration in col.
B with each region of the nephron or interstitium in col. A:*

Column A		Column B
56 _____	Bowman's space	a Hypoosmotic
57 _____	Ascending limb of Henle	b Isoosmotic
58 _____	Descending limb of Henle	c Hyperosmotic

59 _____	Proximal tubule	d Isoosmotic or
60 _____	Distal tubule	hypoosmotic
61 _____	Collecting duct	
62 _____	Medullary interstitium	
63 _____	Cortical interstitium	

*Directions: Answer questions 64 to 73 in relation to the fol-
lowing list of substances.*

a Sodium	g Amino acids	l Renin
b Potassium	h Creatinine	m Ammonia
c Calcium	i Chloride	n Uric acid
d Phosphate	j Urea	o Hydrogen ion
e Glucose	k Bicarbonate	p Water
f Urine		

64 Check the substances in this list which are filtered
by the glomerulus.

65 Which two substances are 100 percent reabsorbed in
the proximal tubule?

66 Which two substances are regulated by parathyroid
hormone?

67 Which three substances are passively reabsorbed in
the proximal tubule?

68 Which substance is actively transported out of the
ascending limb of Henle?

69 Which three substances are end products of protein
metabolism?

70 Which two substances are regulated by aldosterone?

71 Which two substances are secreted into the distal
tubule in exchange for sodium reabsorption?

72 Which substance is secreted into the distal tubule,
unites with H^+, and is unable to diffuse out of the
tubule?

73 Which substance when reabsorbed is most important
as a blood buffer?

*Directions: Match the correct estimated pressures in col. B to
the proper glomerular filtration forces in col. A.*

Column A		Column B
74 _____	Glomerular hydrostatic pressure	a 50 mmHg
75 _____	Colloid osmotic pressure	b 30 mmHg
76 _____	Net filtration pressure	c 10 mmHg
77 _____	Hydrostatic pressure in Bow-man's capsule	

*Directions: Select the one correct answer to the following
questions.*

78 The ratio of juxtaglomerular nephrons to cortical
nephrons in the human kidney is about:
a 1:1   b 1:3   c 1:7   d 1:15

79 Osmolality is solute concentration:
a Per 1000 g (kg) of water   b Per 1000 ml of solution

CHAPTER 40 Diagnostic Procedures in Renal Disease

OBJECTIVES At the completion of Chap. 40 you should be able to:

1 Describe the significance of proteinuria as a pathological condition.

2 Illustrate some of the advantages and disadvantages of the dipstick test for proteinuria.

3 Describe the diurnal pattern of urine pH.

4 List the points to consider when testing the pH of the urine.

5 Describe the factors contributing to the formation of urinary tract calculi.

6 Discuss the prevention of urinary tract calculi.

7 Explain the significance of hematuria.

8 List the steps for measuring specific gravity with a urinometer.

9 Describe the relationship between specific gravity and osmolality of the urine.

10 Describe the creatinine clearance test and its relationship to the glomerular filtration rate.

11 Give the normal value for serum creatinine and blood urea nitrogen levels and discuss the significance of an elevation of each.

12 Discuss the effects of aging on the glomerular filtration rate.

13 Describe two tests used to estimate renal plasma flow and proximal tubule function.

14 Explain the significance of the concentration and dilution tests as tests of distal tubule function.

15 Describe the test used in the diagnosis of renal tubular acidosis.

16 Discuss the value of a sodium conservation test in renal disease.

17 List four types of morphological renal investigations.

18 List the normal constituents of the urine sediment.

19 List the most common abnormal constituents of the urine and their significance.

20 Describe how casts are formed in the kidney (source of constituents, shape).

21 Differentiate between the various types of casts (hyaline, cellular, granular, fatty, and broad granular).

22 Describe the significance of bacteriuria.

23 Discuss the proper procedure of urine collection for bacteriologic study.

24 Differentiate between an intravenous and a retrograde pyelogram.

25 Describe the procedure, precautions, and indications for a renal arteriogram.

26 Describe the procedure, precautions, and indications for a renal biopsy.

BIOCHEMICAL METHODS

It will be the purpose of this chapter to discuss some of the commonly performed diagnostic tests for the detection of renal disease and evaluation of renal function. These tests are divided into methods which are predominantly biochemical or morphological. These diagnostic tests are especially important in the detection of renal disease since many serious renal diseases do not produce symptoms until renal function is significantly impaired.

Chemical examination of the urine

Chemical testing of the urine has been greatly simplified by the introduction of impregnated paper strips which detect substances such as glucose, acetone, bilirubin, protein, and blood. The pH of the urine can also be measured using a dipstick test. Of particular importance in renal disease is the detection of protein or blood in the urine, the measurement of osmolality or specific gravity, and microscopic examination of the urine (to be considered in "Morphological Methods").

PROTEINURIA

Normal healthy adults excrete very small amounts of protein in the urine—up to 150 mg/day—which consists mainly of albumin and Tamm-Horsfall protein. The latter is secreted by the distal tubule. Proteinuria in amounts greater than 150 mg/day is considered pathological.

Because it is easy to use, the dipstick test (Albustix, Combistix) is the most commonly used test for proteinuria. The end of the stick is dipped in urine, removed immediately, and the excess urine shaken off by tapping the stick on the side of the container. The result is then read by comparison with the color chart on the label. Grading is from 0 to 4+, and the corresponding amounts of protein are trace (less than 30 mg/100 ml urine; 1+ (30 mg/100 ml urine); 2+ (100 mg/100 ml urine); 3+ (300 mg/100 ml urine); and 4+ (1 g/100 ml urine). While the dipstick test is generally accurate, there are a number of pitfalls and difficulties in interpretation. Early morning samples are normally more concentrated and should preferably be tested for protein. A "trace" response found in an early morning specimen is probably within normal limits, less than 150 mg/day. On the other hand, if the urine specimen is collected later in the day and is more dilute (e.g., specific gravity 1.006), a trace response might in fact indicate significant proteinuria. A common cause of a false positive in females is contamination of the urine with vaginal secretions. A simple test for pro-

tein should be done on all routine urine examinations for purposes of screening. More accurate quantitative tests for protein may be carried out in the laboratory on a 24-hour specimen.

Persistent proteinuria almost always indicates renal disease, especially involving the glomerulus. The direct cause of proteinuria is always an increase in glomerular permeability. Recall that the glomerulus is composed of three layers (endothelium, basement membrane, and epithelium) which have a series of "pores" of varying sizes. Normally, only a small amount of albumin (the smallest protein molecule in the serum) is filtered at the glomerulus, and most of this is reabsorbed in the tubules. Albuminuria is very common in the various types of glomerulonephritis. Heavy proteinuria refers to the passage of ≥3.5 g per day and is the laboratory definition of the nephrotic syndrome (to be discussed later). Some patients with the nephrotic syndrome may pass as much as 20 or 30 g of protein per day. Moderate proteinuria is associated with a broad spectrum of renal diseases, and minimal proteinuria (less than 1 g/day) is more apt to be associated with renal diseases such as chronic pyelonephritis with less glomerular involvement.

HEMATURIA

The dipstick test for occult blood is an excellent screening test for hematuria. Whenever it is positive, a microscopic examination of the urine should be made. Hematuria is a common finding in a number of renal diseases and pathological processes in the lower urinary tract. The dipstick test can easily be used by patients to follow the course of hematuria during their treatment.

HYDROGEN-ION CONCENTRATION (pH)

In the healthy adult, the pH of the urine ranges widely from 4.5 to 8.0, but the average pooled specimen is quite acidic at 6.0 because of acidic metabolites produced by the normal breakdown of body tissues and nutrients. The usual diurnal pattern consists of a rise in pH after a meal (alkaline tide) followed by a gradual fall until the next meal ingestion, while during normal sleeping hours pH reaches its minimum (nocturnal acid tide due to hypoventilation during sleep). A diet high in animal protein tends to produce an acid urine while a predominantly vegetable diet tends to produce an alkaline urine.

A persistently acid urine may occur in respiratory or metabolic acidosis and in pyrexia (fever). A persistently alkaline urine is suggestive of urinary tract infection with urea-splitting organisms. For example, in *Proteus* infections, the urine pH is consistently at a pH of 8 or higher. Persistently alkaline urine also occurs in renal tubular acidosis (a renal disease in which there is inability to conserve bicarbonate), in potassium depletion, and in Fanconi syndrome (a renal disease in which ammonia excretion is defective).

Although random pH readings are of little diagnostic value, they are helpful in the management of certain clinical conditions in which the pH of the urine should be kept persistently high or low by diet or drugs. Alkaline urine is desirable in the treatment of patients with calculi which form in acid urine, and acid urine is desirable in patients with calculi which form in alkaline urine or who have urinary tract infections (Table 40-1).

Common stones formed in acid urine are composed of calcium oxalate, uric acid crystals, or cystine. Hyperuricemia leading to uric acid crystallization is a particular hazard in patients who are receiving cytotoxic drugs for cancer or leukemia. Uric acid is formed principally as an end product of nucleoprotein metabolism. With increasing proliferation and destruction of cells there is a proportional increase in uric acid because of degradation of cellular nucleoproteins. The physician may order the administration of sodium bicarbonate or citrate to alkalinize the urine. It is important to encourage a high fluid intake in these patients, especially before bedtime when the urine normally becomes more acid, to prevent crystallization of uric acid in the renal tubules and interstitium and consequent obstruction. Some foods which help alkalinize the urine are milk, vegetables, and fruits (except prunes, plums, and cranberries).

Common stones formed in alkaline urine are composed of calcium phosphate or magnesium ammonium phosphate (triple-phosphate stones). Calcium phosphate or oxalate is often present in triple-phosphate stones.

Triple-phosphate stones are often associated with urinary tract infections, especially with urea-splitting organisms. These stones occasionally grow to occupy the entire pelvicalyceal system. Such a stone is referred to as a "staghorn" calculus because of its shape, and it must be removed surgically. Since 90 percent of all calculi contain calcium, hypercalciuria is an important predisposing cause. Hypercalciuria is associated with hyperparathyroidism, renal tubular acidosis, and prolonged immobilization. All are associated with mobilization of calcium salts from bone. Meat, bread, protein foods, cranberry juice, plums, and prunes tend to produce an acid urine and thus help prevent the formation of these stones. The physician may order a drug such as Mandelamine to acidify the urine for persistent urinary tract infections. Probably the most important factor in the prevention of all stones regardless of composition is a high fluid intake.

The pH of the urine may be tested using Squibb Nitrazine paper or a dipstick test. The following points should be kept in mind while performing this test: (1) only fresh urine should be used (when urine is allowed to stand, urea breaks down to ammonia and the pH becomes more alkaline); (2) the test strip should be removed promptly after being dipped in the urine to avoid washing out the test reagent; and (3) the color comparison with the standard should be made immediately in good light (daylight is preferable and fluorescent light should be avoided).

SPECIFIC GRAVITY

The measurement of specific gravity is commonly performed in the clinical unit to determine the concentration of urine. It is measured by the flotation of a hydrometer or urinometer in a cylinder of urine (Fig. 40-1).

The proper procedure for measuring the specific gravity of urine is as follows:

1 Check the accuracy of the urinometer against distilled water to read 1.000 at its calibration temperature. Most urinometers are calibrated at a temperature of 16°C (60.8°F). This is necessary since the density of water changes with temperature.
2 Fill the cylinder about three-quarters full of well-mixed urine. A uniform solution is necessary since solute concentration is being measured.
3 Give the urinometer a gentle spin as it is plunged into the urine to avoid errors of surface tension at the stem and to prevent it from adhering to the sides of the cylinder.
4 Read from top to bottom. The urinometer is calibrated in units of 0.001 starting with 1.000 at the top and progressing downward to 1.060. The correct reading is at the level of the bottom of the meniscus which should be read at eye level.
5 Correct the specific gravity reading if the temperature

TABLE 40-1
Factors contributing to the formation of urinary tract calculi and their prevention

URINARY STONE CONTENT	PREDISPOSING FACTORS	URINE pH DESIRED (THERAPY)*
	Acid urine	Alkaline urine (pH > 6)
Calcium oxalate	Hypercalciuria	Vegetables, milk, fruit (except plums, prunes, cranberries)
Uric acid crystals	Chemotherapy, gout	Sodium bicarbonate or citrate
Cystine	Aminoaciduria	
	Alkaline urine	Acid urine
Triple-phosphate	Urinary tract infection	Meat, breads, protein foods, cranberry juice, prunes, plums
Calcium phosphate	Hypercalciuria	
	Prolonged immobility	Mandelamine

*High fluid intake is the most important preventive measure against all calculi.

of the specimen deviates from the calibration temperature of the urinometer. Use a thermometer to determine the actual temperature of the urine. Add 0.001 to the reading for every 3°C (5.4°F) above the calibration temperature and subtract 0.001 for each 3°C below. For example, if a urinometer calibrated at 16°C is placed in a freshly voided urine specimen with a temperature of 31°C (88°F) and shows a reading of 1.015, then 0.005 is added to the reading

$$(31°C - 16°C) = 15°C \times \frac{0.001}{3°C} = 0.005$$

The true specific gravity corrected for temperature is 1.020.

Although specific gravity is simple and convenient to measure, it is important to realize that density is being measured. The density depends on the weight as well as on the number of the solute particles in solution. The kidney's capacity to concentrate, however, is related to the concentration of particles in solution (i.e., osmolality) and not to their weight. True concentration, osmolality, is measured by freezing point depression or vapor pressure lowering, though this is more expensive and time-consuming.

Fortunately, when urine contains only normal constituents (mainly NaCl), the correlation between specific gravity and osmolality is sufficiently close to use specific gravity as a clinical guide to the osmolality of the urine. The relationship between specific gravity and the osmolality of urine is shown in Fig. 40-2. When the urine contains normal constituents (middle line), a specific gravity of 1.010 corresponds to the osmolality of the blood at 285 mOsm. When given large amounts of water, the healthy person can excrete urine with a minimum specific gravity of 1.001 (about 40 mOsm). When deprived of fluid, maximum specific gravity is about 1.040 (1300 mOsm). If the urine should contain glucose or protein (dense particles), the specific gravity will be greater at a fixed osmolality than in normal urine (shifted toward the pure glucose curve); and conversely, if the

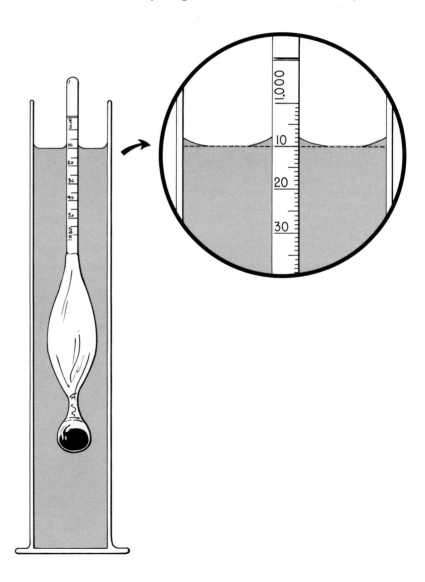

FIGURE 40-1 Urinometer with scale featured.

urine contains much urea (a less dense molecule), the specific gravity will be lower. For example, at a concentration of 400 mOsm the specific gravity of urine with normal constituents would be about 1.013. At the same osmolality, if the urine contained a large amount of protein or glucose, the specific gravity would be about 1.030; if it contained a large amount of urea, the specific gravity would be about 1.007. These facts must be taken into consideration when the specific gravity measurement is used to estimate the ability of the kidneys to concentrate urine.

In chronic renal disease, the kidney loses first the ability to concentrate urine. Later, the ability to dilute urine is lost as well so that the specific gravity of urine becomes fixed near 1.010 (the specific gravity of the plasma). This generally occurs when 80 percent of the nephron mass has been destroyed.

Glomerular filtration rate (GFR)

One of the most important indices of renal function is the glomerular filtration rate (GFR). The GFR gives information about the amount of functioning renal tissue. As noted previously, the most accurate way to measure GFR is by means of the inulin clearance test. However, this test is infrequently used in the clinical unit because it involves an intravenous infusion at a constant rate and timed collections of urine by catheterization. The endogenous creatinine clearance test is much more simple to carry

CREATININE CLEARANCE TEST

Creatinine is an end product of muscle metabolism which is liberated from the muscles at virtually a constant rate and excreted in the urine at the same rate. The plasma (serum) level is therefore nearly constant and ranges from 0.7 to 1.5 mg% (higher value in males than in females because of their greater muscle mass). Creatinine is excreted in the urine by filtration at the glomerulus, but it is not reabsorbed by the tubules. A small amount, however, is secreted by the tubules especially when serum creatinine levels are high. In spite of the fact that a small amount is secreted, the creatinine clearance test is a convenient test to estimate the GFR in the clinical unit. To perform the creatinine clearance test, it is only necessary to collect a 24-hour urine specimen and a blood specimen during that 24-

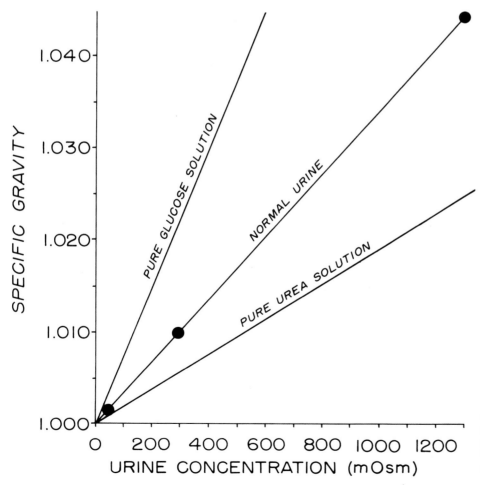

FIGURE 40-2 Relationship between specific gravity and osmolality of the urine. (Modified from H. E. De Wardner, The Kidney, 4th ed., Longman, Inc., New York, 1973.)

hour period (Fig. 40-3). Creatinine clearance is then calculated using the clearance formula

$$C_{cr} = \frac{U_{cr}V}{P_{cr}}$$

Creatinine clearance is a fairly good index of GFR although it is not a true measurement since it is secreted by the tubules to some extent. The slight secretion of creatinine tends to cause an overestimation of the GFR. On the other hand, plasma creatinine is overestimated because of the difficulties inherent in the laboratory determination. Luckily, these two errors are of nearly the same magnitude and cancel each other out so that creatinine clearance approximates GFR.

In chronic renal disease, the GFR is decreased below the normal value of 125 ml/minute. GFR also decreases with advancing age. After the age of 30, it decreases at the rate of about 1 ml/minute/year.

PLASMA CREATININE AND BLOOD UREA NITROGEN

The plasma creatinine and blood urea nitrogen (BUN) concentrations are also used as guides to the glomerular filtration rate. The normal BUN concentration is about 10 to 20 mg%, and plasma creatinine concentration is 0.7 to 1.5 mg%. Both of these substances are nitrogenous end products of protein metabolism normally excreted in the urine. When the GFR decreases as in renal insufficiency, the plasma levels of creatinine and BUN rise. This condition is called *azotemia* (nitrogenous

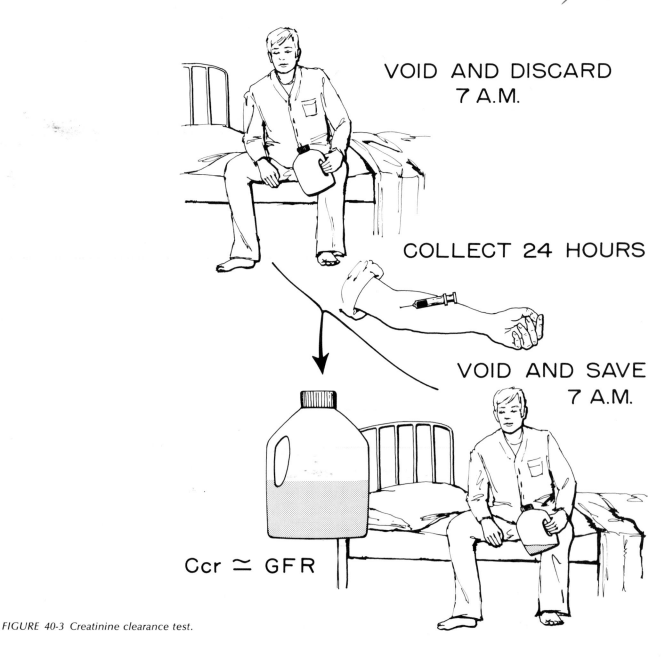

VOID AND DISCARD
7 A.M.

COLLECT 24 HOURS

VOID AND SAVE
7 A.M.

$Ccr \simeq GFR$

FIGURE 40-3 Creatinine clearance test.

substances in the blood). Plasma creatinine as an index of GFR is more accurate than the BUN since its production rate is mainly a function of the size of the muscle mass, which changes very little. The BUN, however, is affected by the amount of protein in the diet and the catabolism of body protein. The relationship of a rising plasma creatinine and BUN level to a decreasing GFR will be discussed in Chap. 41.

Tubular function tests

A number of tests are carried out to evaluate the function and integrity of the renal tubules. The function of the tubules, of course, is selective reabsorption of the contents of the tubular fluid and secretion of substances into the tubular lumen which are either circulating in the peritubular capillaries or are formed by the tubular cell. These processes are under the control of a wide variety of hormones, gas pressures, and plasma electrolyte concentrations. Common tests of proximal tubular function include the phenolsulfonphthalein (PSP) and para-aminohippurate (PAH) excretion tests. Distal tubular function tests include tests of concentration, dilution, acidification, and sodium conservation.

PSP EXCRETION TEST

Phenolsulfonphthalein is a remarkably nontoxic dye which is eliminated primarily by secretion into the proximal tubule. Binding of PSP to plasma proteins is so high that only about 4 percent is excreted by glomerular filtration. With the usual 6-mg intravenous dose the plasma level of the dye is only about one-fifth of the tubular capacity to excrete PSP. The excretion rate of PSP is therefore usually limited by the rate of delivery to the tubules via the renal plasma flow and, in severely

impaired kidneys, by proximal tubular function. The 15-minute PSP test is most commonly performed (Fig. 40-4).

Thirty minutes before the PSP dye is given, the patient is asked to drink two or three glasses of water to ensure sufficient bladder urine for urination. Exactly 1 ml (6 mg) of PSP is injected intravenously using a tuberculin syringe for accuracy. Exactly 15 minutes after the dye is given, the patient is asked to completely empty the bladder. All of the urine is then placed in a 1-liter volumetric flask; 5 ml of 10% NaOH is added, and enough water to bring the volume up to 1 liter. A test tube of the pink, diluted specimen is then compared with the appropriate standards or by the use of a colorimeter. The person with normal renal function should excrete a minimum of 28 percent of the dye in 15 minutes.

The primary value of the PSP excretion test is in the detection of functional impairment early in the course of renal disease. Many physicians no longer perform this test and consider the creatinine clearance test alone to be an adequate assessment of renal function. The analysis of the PSP test is so simple that it can be performed without the aid of a clinical laboratory, so it might be useful in situations where these facilities are not available.

PAH EXCRETION TEST

Para-aminohippurate is a substance which is both filtered by the glomerulus and secreted by the proximal tubule. When given in low concentrations to human subjects,

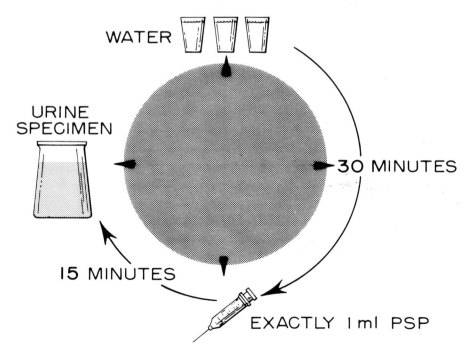

FIGURE 40-4 Fifteen-minute PSP excretion test. Twenty-eight percent or more of the dye is normally excreted in 15 minutes.

$< 7 = $ acid
$> 7 = $ basic
$7 = $ neutral

about 92 percent is cleared in one circulation through the kidneys. It is therefore, a fairly accurate measure of renal plasma flow. If the plasma concentration is further increased until secretory capacity is exceeded, the secretory capacity of the proximal tubule can be calculated from the filtered load and urinary excretion. This test is most commonly used in research.

CONCENTRATION AND DILUTION TESTS

The measurement of urine specific gravity after water restriction is a sensitive measure of the ability of the renal tubules to reabsorb water and produce a concentrated urine. Renal function is considered normal if an early morning urine specimen has a specific gravity of 1.025 or greater. When concentrating ability is doubtful, a more elaborate concentration test may be carried out. The Fishberg concentration test is commonly used. To ensure accuracy of results, the person must be on a normal diet (normal salt, protein, and fluid intake) and must not be taking diuretics prior to the administration of the test. The patient is instructed to eat a normal evening meal at 6 P.M. and not to take food or fluids until the test is completed the next morning. Urine specimens are collected the next morning at 6, 7, and 8 A.M. At least one of these specimens should have a specific gravity of 1.025 (800 mOsm) or greater (Fig. 40-5A).

The urinary dilution test is performed by having the patient drink 1 liter of water within a 30-minute period. Urine specimens are then collected over the next 3 hours. At least one of these specimens should have a specific gravity of 1.003 (80 mOsm) or less (Fig. 40-5B). The urinary dilution test is much less useful than the concentration test since nonspecific factors such as nausea or emotions may interfere with a water diuresis even in normal subjects. Diluting ability may be defective in adrenal insufficiency, hepatic disease, and cardiac failure. The ability to dilute urine is lost late in most renal diseases, while concentrating ability is lost early. Neither the concentration nor the dilution tests should be carried out on azotemic patients since dehydration and water intoxication could result.

URINE ACIDIFICATION TEST

The urine acidification test is designed to measure the maximum acid-excreting capacity of the kidney and is specific for the diagnosis of renal tubular acidosis.

In the 5-day test, 2 days of control urine collections are made. The patient is then given ammonium chloride (about 12 g/day in the adult) for the next 3 days. The ammonium chloride is metabolized to urea and hydrogen chloride, producing an acidosis in the patient. The urinary pH is determined daily, and on the fifth day ammonium and titratable acids are also measured. Normally the kidney excretes the acid load and the urine pH

is 5.3 or less (Fig. 40-6). In renal tubular acidosis a hydrogen-ion gradient between the tubular lumen and the plasma cannot be maintained, and a low urine pH is not achieved. Many patients with chronic renal failure can achieve a urine pH of 5.3, but excretion of ammonium and titratable acids is impaired.

SODIUM CONSERVATION TEST

The healthy person can produce urine that is virtually sodium-free under conditions of dietary restriction of sodium. In renal disease the ability to conserve sodium may be lost, and some patients suffer sodium depletion. If a patient is losing more sodium than is ingested, the result is a contraction of the plasma volume, a decrease in the GFR, and an accelerated course toward final renal failure. A salt-losing nephritis is more common in patients who have chronic pyelonephritis or polycystic disease. Both diseases primarily involve the renal tubules. Many patients in renal failure oscillate between states of sodium retention and depletion so that their daily intake of sodium must be defined within very narrow limits.

The sodium conservation test is sometimes used to determine how much sodium is needed in the diet of a patient with a salt-losing nephritis. The patient eats a low sodium diet (10 meq or 500 mg). Sodium excretion in the urine normally falls to equal sodium intake within a week. In salt-losing nephritis, a large amount of sodium continues to be lost in the urine in spite of the restricted intake. Additional sodium may be added to the diet when the magnitude of the deficit is determined. For example, a patient who is excreting 50 meq of sodium in urine on a 10-meq sodium diet should be allowed an additional 40 meq of sodium in the diet, or 50 meq.

MORPHOLOGICAL METHODS

Diagnostic methods in renal disease which are primarily morphological include microscopic and bacteriologic examination of the urine, renal radiology, and renal biopsy. These methods will be discussed briefly.

Microscopic examination of the urine

Microscopic examination of the urine is carried out on a freshly collected, centrifuged specimen, the deposit from which is suspended in 0.5 ml urine. In health, the urine contains a small number of cells and other elements derived from the entire length of the genitourinary tract—casts, epithelial cells from the lining of the urinary tract and vagina (females), spermatozoa (males), mucus threads, and no more than one or two red blood cells and three or four white blood cells per high-power field.

FIGURE 40-5 Urine concentration and dilution tests. See text for explanation.

The most common abnormal constituents of the urine are red blood cells (RBCs), white blood cells (WBCs), bacteria, and casts. All casts arise in the kidney and are thought to be "moldings" of renal tubules. Thus, they indicate conditions exclusively within the kidneys and, for this reason, are of great diagnostic value. Casts consist of a mucoprotein matrix, the Tamm-Horsfall mucoprotein, in which cells or debris are embedded and in which a variety of serum and renal proteins may be absorbed. The Tamm-Horsfall protein is secreted by the distal tubule cells. As it passes down the tubule, it dehydrates and takes on the shape of the tubule.

Hyaline casts consist of this protein and appear as clear cylinders. Cellular elements may be incorporated into hyaline casts (cellular casts) at the time of their formation. In this way, various types of casts are formed, depending on the cell type embedded in the cast (Fig. 40-7). Normally there is not enough protein in the renal tubules to provide more than an occasional cast.

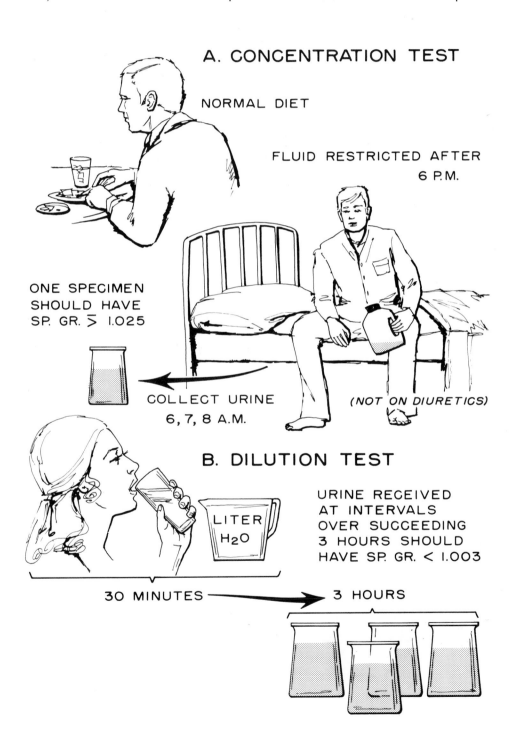

A. CONCENTRATION TEST

NORMAL DIET

FLUID RESTRICTED AFTER 6 P.M.

ONE SPECIMEN SHOULD HAVE SP. GR. ≥ 1.025

COLLECT URINE 6, 7, 8 A.M.

(NOT ON DIURETICS)

B. DILUTION TEST

LITER H₂O

URINE RECEIVED AT INTERVALS OVER SUCCEEDING 3 HOURS SHOULD HAVE SP. GR. < 1.003

30 MINUTES → 3 HOURS

Cylindruria (excessive excretion of casts in the urine) usually means increased proteinuria or renal excretion of cells or both, and indicates renal disease.

Casts are classified according to shape or constituents. Cellular casts may contain RBCs, WBCs, bacteria, or tubular epithelial cells, or may be mixed. Red blood cells and *red cell casts* are seen in active glomerulonephritis.

White cell casts are often seen in pyelonephritis. Oval fat bodies and *fatty casts* are common in the nephrotic syndrome. Oval fat bodies are the remains of degenerated fat-filled tubular cells. *Granular casts* or *waxy casts* represent stages in the degeneration of a cellular cast, and the progression is from coarse, to fine, and, finally, to waxy. *Broad, granular casts* are a typical finding in end-stage kidney disease. They are granular because of dead cells and broad because they are formed in the collecting ducts due to decreased urinary flow. These broad, granular casts are sometimes called *renal failure casts*.

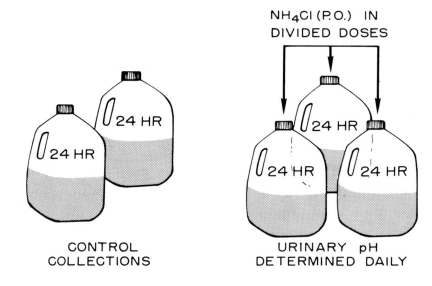

NH₄Cl (P.O.) IN
DIVIDED DOSES

CONTROL
COLLECTIONS

URINARY pH
DETERMINED DAILY

pH: NORMAL • 4.5 - 5.3
RENAL TUBULAR ACIDOSIS • > 5.3

FIGURE 40-6 Urine acidification test.

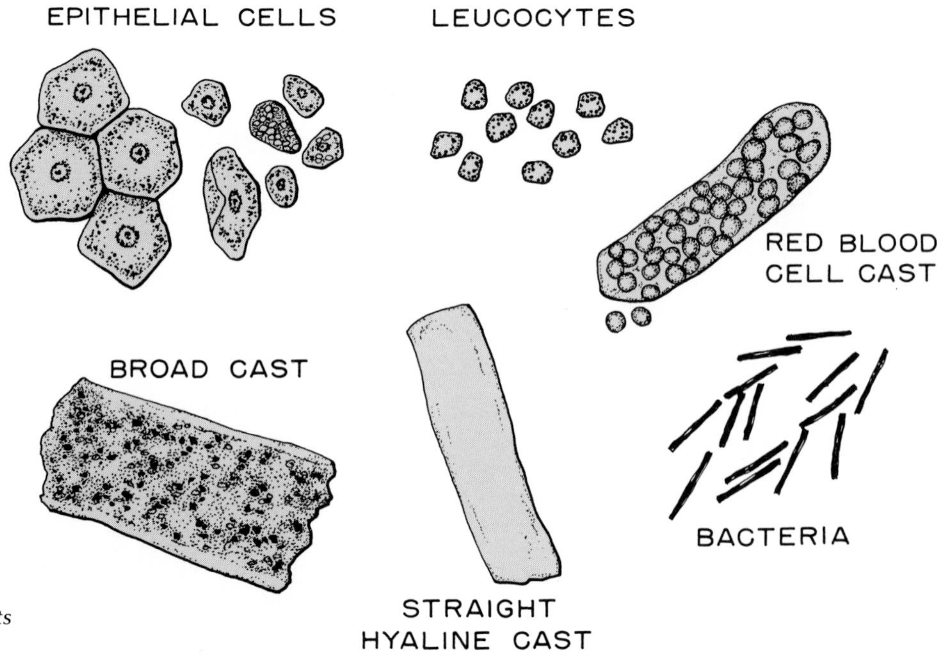

EPITHELIAL CELLS   LEUCOCYTES

RED BLOOD
CELL CAST

BROAD CAST

BACTERIA

STRAIGHT
HYALINE CAST

FIGURE 40-7 Some formed elements in the urine sediment.

Bacteriologic examination of the urine

Bacterial counts may be carried out by inoculating the surface of a nutrient agar plate using a calibrated loop which delivers 0.001 ml of urine (Fig. 40-8). The agar plate is then incubated for 24 hours at 37°C, and colonies are counted. Counts of 100 or more colonies (10^5 organisms per milliliter of urine) constitute a significant degree of bacteriuria. The bacteria may be subcultured for identification and for an antibiotic sensitivity test. This procedure is commonly referred to as "C & S," or the culture and sensitivity test. The results of this test are a useful guide in the choice of an antibiotic for the most effective treatment.

In order for a bacteriologic study of the urine to have validity, the specimen must be free of contaminating bacteria from the urethra, external genitalia, and perineum. Proper techniques and precautions are therefore important in the collection of urine specimens. Collection of the urine by catheterization into a sterile container is the best way to ensure that the specimen is uncontaminated. Catheterization, however, is avoided if possible, because of the danger of introducing bacteria into the urinary tract. A "sterile-voided" specimen is generally considered adequate for a bacteriologic study. Men, and particularly women, are instructed to wash the area around the urinary meatus with soap and water. A midstream specimen is then collected in a clean or sterile specimen container. The urine is examined within 30 minutes, or a preservative is added and it is refrigerated at 4°C. Refrigeration prevents the growth of bacteria, and the preservative prevents the deterioration of casts and cells.

Radiologic examinations

A number of radiologic procedures are available to evaluate the urinary system. The intravenous pyelogram and renal arteriogram are most common and will be described.

INTRAVENOUS PYELOGRAM (IVP)

The usual procedure for performing the IVP includes a flat plate (plain film) of the abdomen followed by intravenous injection of contrast medium. The contrast medium circulates via the bloodstream and heart to the kidneys where it is excreted. After injection, a film is taken every minute for the first 5 minutes for the purpose of visualizing the cortex of the kidney. The cortex is thinned in glomerulonephritis and has a moth-eaten appearance in pyelonephritis and ischemia. Adequacy of the filling of the calyces is evaluated by examination of the 3- and 5-minute films. Another film is taken at 15 minutes, which makes the calyces, pelvis, and ureters visible. Cysts, lesions, and obstructions cause a distortion of these structures. A final film is taken at 45 minutes which makes the bladder visible. If the patient is severely azotemic (BUN > 70 mg%), an IVP is not usually done since this indicates that the GFR is very low. Consequently, the dye will not be excreted, and the pyelogram will be difficult to visualize.

Sometimes a retrograde pyelogram is done by passing a catheter up the ureter and injecting contrast medium directly into the kidney. The main indications for this procedure are urologic—e.g., further investigation of a nonfunctioning kidney or on occasions when visualization of the IVP is not clear. This procedure is avoided if at all possible since it involves anesthesia, and there is a very real danger of infection.

The standard IVP serves many purposes. It can establish the presence and position of the kidneys and evaluate their size and shape. The effect of different disease states on the kidney's ability to concentrate and excrete the dye can also be evaluated. The diagram in Fig. 40-9 shows some typical abnormalities revealed by the IVP.

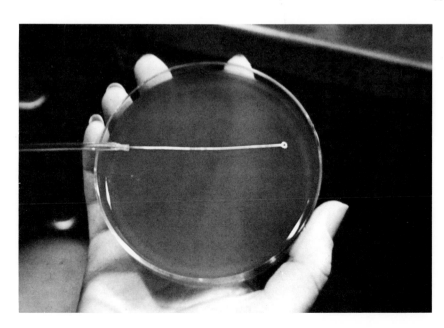

FIGURE 40-8 Inoculation of the surface of a blood agar plate by means of a calibrated loop. The plate is incubated for 24 hours at 37°C. Significant bacteriuria is 10^5 (100,000) or more organisms per milliliter of urine.

The small, atrophic kidney may be due to unilateral renal ischemia or unilateral chronic pyelonephritis (Fig. 40-9A). Distortion of the renal pelvis with *clubbing of* the calyces is a common finding in chronic pyelonephritis (Fig. 40-9B). Note also the irregular shape and the greatly thinned cortex.

RENAL ARTERIOGRAM

The renal blood vessels may be visualized in an arteriogram. The usual procedure is to introduce a catheter via the femoral artery and abdominal aorta to the level of the renal artery. Contrast medium is injected at this level and then flows into the renal artery and its accessory branches (Fig. 40-10).

Indications for this procedure are (1) to visualize renal artery stenosis which may cause some cases of hypertension, (2) to visualize the blood vessels of a neoplasm, (3) to visualize the blood supply of the cortex, which, for example, may have a patchy appearance in chronic pyelonephritis, and (4) to ascertain the structure of the renal blood supply of the donor before renal transplantation. Figure 40-11 is an arteriogram showing marked narrowing of the right renal artery.

Angiography is not done without discomfort and some hazard. The patient usually experiences an intense burning sensation for a few seconds as the solution enters the blood vessel. Prior to injection, the patient is usually tested for iodide sensitivity to avoid an anaphylactic response. Other complications following arteriogram include thrombus or embolus formation, and local inflammation or hematoma at the site of entry. Although these complications are rare, vital signs are checked every 15 minutes until stable and then every 4 hours for 24 hours. Peripheral pulses are also checked for diminished strength to detect occlusion of blood flow due to a thrombus.

Renal biopsy

Renal biopsy is one of the most important diagnostic techniques developed during the past few decades. It has resulted in considerable advancement of knowledge of the natural history of renal disease. The main indication for renal biopsy is for the diagnosis of diffuse renal disease and for following its progress.

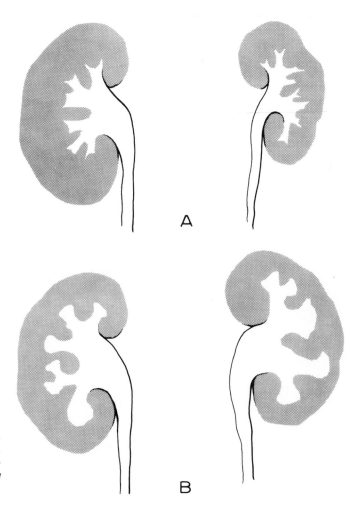

FIGURE 40-9 Diagram of abnormalities viewed on the intravenous pyelogram (IVP). A. Small, atrophic kidney due to unilateral renal ischemia. B. Clubbing of the calyces, irregularity of contour, and thinning of cortical substance may be found in chronic pyelonephritis.

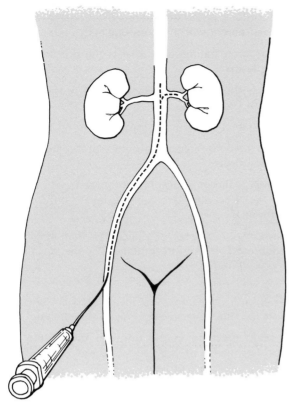

FIGURE 40-10 Transfemoral approach in renal angiography.

The most common renal biopsy procedure is the percutaneous, or blind, procedure. The patient lies prone with sandbags under the abdomen to fix the kidney against the back (Fig. 40-12). Local anesthesia is used. The usual site for the biopsy is over the right renal angle just below the twelfth rib. The site is located by x-ray reference. A biopsy needle is used to obtain a specimen of renal tissue. The tissue is examined, after appropriate preparation, by light microscopy, electron microscopy, and immunofluorescent microscopy. Figure 40-13 illustrates the appearance of a normal renal biopsy by light microscopy.

Renal biopsy should only be performed by a skilled nephrologist. The procedure is dangerous in patients who are uncooperative or who have a coagulative disorder or a solitary kidney. The most common complications are intrarenal and perirenal bleeding. Serious bleeding with gross hematuria occurs in about 5 percent and mortality in about 0.17 percent. Arteriovenous fistula is the second most common complication.

Immediately after a biopsy, pressure is applied over the biopsy site for 10 minutes with 4 by 4 in sponges, and the patient is kept in a prone position for 30 minutes. A pressure dressing is then applied to the biopsy site. The dressing from above and the sandbag from below provide pressure on the kidney and aid in the prevention of extrarenal bleeding. Lying on the sandbag is usually

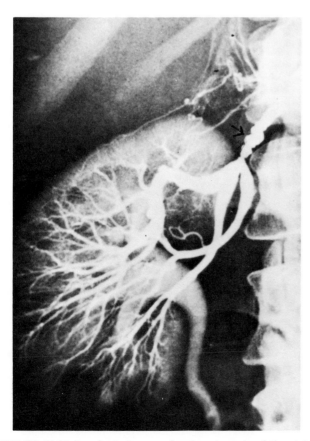

FIGURE 40-11 Renal arteriogram showing stenosis of the right renal artery.

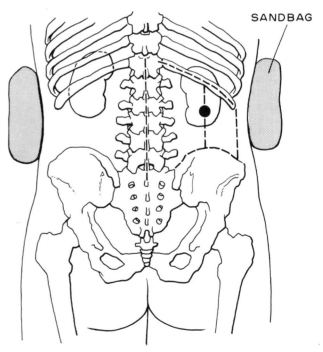

SANDBAG

FIGURE 40-12 Percutaneous renal biopsy. Site is located by x-ray reference; patient lies prone with sandbag under abdomen to fix kidney against back. Vital signs are monitored.

uncomfortable but immobilizes the kidney in the antero-posterior plane and is a necessary measure to ensure hemostasis. The patient should be kept in bed and as quiet as possible for the next 24 hours and should be instructed not to cough or sneeze. During this period frequent observations of the vital signs, abdomen, and urine should be made. The patient is kept on bed rest as long as hematuria occurs.

QUESTIONS

Diagnostic procedures in renal disease—Chap. 40

Directions: Answer the following questions on a separate sheet of paper.

1 Contrast the amount of protein a healthy adult and a person with the nephrotic syndrome might excrete in a day. Explain the significance.

2 What is always the *direct* cause of proteinuria regardless of the underlying disease process?

3 Explain why only fresh urine should be used for measuring pH.

4 Hyperuricemia leading to uric acid crystallization in the renal tubules is a particular hazard for patients receiving cytotoxic drugs. Why?

5 What are the most common factors predisposing towards formation of calculi in alkaline urine? Explain.

6 What is the most important *preventive* measure against all calculi?

7 What are the five important points that must be con-

sidered in obtaining an accurate specific gravity measurement with the urinometer?

8 What is creatinine, and what is the normal range in the plasma?

9 Why is the creatinine clearance test not a true measure of GFR?

10 What effect does increasing age have on the GFR?

11 What test most accurately measures effective renal plasma flow?

12 Which is the most accurate index of renal function—the BUN or plasma creatinine level? Why? What is azotemia?

13 Give two examples of difficulties that may be encountered in the interpretation of the dipstick test for proteinuria.

Directions: Fill in the blanks with the correct words or numbers or circle the letter to the correct answers as indicated.

14 Protein excreted in the urine of the healthy adult consists mainly of _____ and _____-_____ protein.

15 The average pooled daily urine specimen has a pH of about _____.

16 After a meal, one expects a (a) rise or (b) fall in the urine pH. This is referred to as the _____ tide.

17 During normal sleeping hours the urine pH reaches its (a) maximum or (b) minimum due to (c) hypoventilation or (d) hyperventilation during sleep. This is referred to as the _____ _____ tide.

18 When the urine contains normal constituents, a specific gravity of 1.010 corresponds to the normal osmolality of the blood at _____ mOsm.

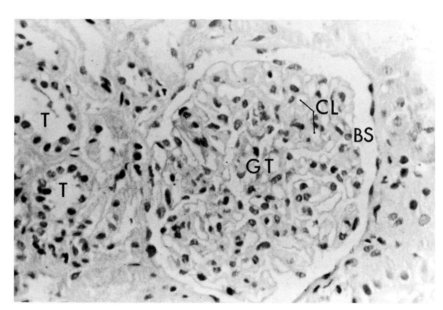

FIGURE 40-13 Light microscopy of normal renal biopsy section. BS = Bowman's space; GT = glomerular tuft; CL = capillary lumen; T = tubule.

19 When given large amounts of water, the healthy human being can dilute urine to a minimum specific gravity of about _____ (40 mOsm). Under conditions of water deprivation a normal person can excrete a concentrated urine with a maximum specific gravity of about _____ (1300 mOsm). What is the purpose of this great flexibility?

20 In the 15-minute PSP test the kidneys normally excrete _____ percent of the dye in the urine.

21 After about 14 hours of water deprivation, the urine of a person with normally functioning kidneys has a specific gravity of _____ or greater. After a water load (1 liter in 30 minutes) the specific gravity should be _____ or less within the next 3 hours.

22 The _____ _____ test is specific for the diagnosis of renal tubular acidosis (RTA). The urine pH should be _____ or less in the 5-day test.

23 The _____ _____ test is used to determine the proper dietary intake of sodium, especially in a patient with "salt-losing" nephritis. A negative sodium balance is most frequently found in patients with renal disorders primarily involving the (a) tubules or (b) glomerulus.

Directions: Circle the letter preceding each item which correctly answers the questions. Only one answer is correct; exceptions will be noted.

24 The normal pH range of the urine is:
a 7.0–14.0   b 6.0–12.0   c 4.5–8.0   d 3.0–6.0

25 The most clinically useful test for the measurement of the glomerular filtration rate is:
a Urea clearance   b Uric acid clearance
c Creatinine clearance   d PSP excretion

26 Which of the following foods tend to produce an acidic urine? (More than one answer may be correct.)
a Meat   b Vegetables   c Cranberry juice, prunes
d Milk

27 The following data was obtained from a creatinine clearance test on a patient: 24-hour urine volume = 1440 ml; urine creatinine level = 50 mg/100 ml; plasma creatinine level = 2 mg/100 ml. Calculate the creatinine clearance (uncorrected for body surface area).
a 100 ml/minute   b 1440 ml/minute
c 25 ml/minute   d 36,000 ml/minute

28 At the usual rate of decrease with aging, the GFR in a 90-year-old man would be about:
a 25 percent of normal   b 50 percent of normal
c 75 percent of normal   d 100 percent of normal

Directions: Answer the following questions on a separate sheet of paper.

29 Name the most common abnormal constituents of the urine sediment.

30 When is bacteriuria significant? (List proper conditions of urine collection and significant bacterial count.)

31 Differentiate between an intravenous pyelogram (IVP) and a retrograde pyelogram. State the purpose of each.

32 List four indications for performing a renal arteriogram.

33 Why is it not worthwhile to do an IVP if the patient is severly azotemic (BUN level greater than 70 mg%)?

34 Outline a plan of care for a patient following a renal arteriogram.

35 Outline a plan of care for a patient during and after a renal biopsy. What observations should be made?

Directions: Fill in the blanks with the correct words.

36 Four types of morphological renal investigations are (a) _____ examination of the urine sediment; (b) _____ study of the urine; (c) renal _____, a method which reveals the shape, size, and position of the kidneys; and (d) renal _____, a method which reveals the microscopic structure of the kidney.

37 Hyaline casts are made up of coagulated _____ _____ protein secreted by the _____ tubule.

38 Excessive excretion of casts in the urine is called _____ and usually means that there is an increased glomerular permeability to _____.

39 A _____ and _____ test is sometimes done to determine the best choice of an antibiotic for treating a urinary tract infection.

40 An abnormality seen on the IVP which is diagnostic of chronic pyelonephritis is _____ of the calyces.

Directions: Circle the letter preceding each item which correctly answer each question. Only one answer is correct.

41 Casts are classified according to:
a Number of particles   b Shape and constituents
c Number of bacteria

42 Long-standing renal ischemia usually results in _____ of the kidney.
a Atrophy   b Hypertrophy

43 Significant hematuria revealed by microscopic examination of the urine sediment would be more than _____ RBCs per high-power field.
a 100,000   b 5000 to 9000   c 1 to 2

44 Which of these statements with respect to renal biopsy is false?
a Death occurs in 1 percent of the cases. b The procedure is dangerous in patients who are uncooperative. c Postbiopsy hematuria occurs in 5 percent of the cases. d During the procedure the patient lies in a prone position on a sandbag.

Directions: Match the renal disease in col. B to the type of cast most frequently seen in the urine sediment in col. A.

Column A

45 _____ Broad, granular casts

46 _____ Red blood cell casts

47 _____ Leukocyte casts

48 _____ Fatty casts and oval fat bodies

Column B

a Pyelonephritis

b Nephrotic syndrome

c Advanced renal disease

d Active glomerulonephritis

CHAPTER 41 Chronic Renal Failure

OBJECTIVES

At the completion of Chap. 41 you should be able to:

1 Differentiate between acute and chronic renal failure.

2 List the three primary structures involved in the kidney in chronic renal disease.

3 Describe the three stages in the natural history of progressive renal failure.

4 Explain why nocturia and polyuria are often early symptoms of chronic renal failure.

5 Describe anatomic changes in chronic renal disease which may alter renal function.

6 Describe the intact nephron hypothesis and give the supporting evidence for this theory.

7 Explain why the original cause of end-stage renal disease may be difficult to determine.

8 List the four leading causes of end-stage renal disease.

9 Name the most common infecting organism in urinary tract infections and say how it may reach the kidney.

10 Describe the urinary tract defense mechanisms against infection.

11 Describe nine factors which may predispose to urinary tract infection and chronic pyelonephritis.

12 Differentiate between symptomatic and asymptomatic bacteriuria as a cause of chronic pyelonephritis.

13 Compare the sex distribution, clinical features, and gross and microscopic changes in the kidney in acute and chronic pyelonephritis.

14 Explain the principles of treatment of acute pyelonephritis.

15 Delineate controversial issues concerning the etiology of chronic pyelonephritis.

16 Define the meaning of the term *glomerulonephritis*.

17 Explain why confusion exists in the classification and separation of the various types of glomerulonephritis.

18 Distinguish between diffuse, focal, and local glomerulonephritis.

19 Discuss the distinguishing features and the natural history of the broad clinical forms of diffuse glomerulonephritis.

20 Describe a classical case of acute poststreptococcal glomerulonephritis (age group commonly affected, specific organisms involved, presenting features, treatment, and prognosis).

21 Describe the sequence of events that results in glomerular injury following an antigen-antibody reaction along the basement membrane.

22 Describe the pathogenetic basis of the hypertension, edema, hematuria, albuminuria, and urinary casts in acute poststreptococcal glomerulonephritis.

23 Differentiate between the two distinct immune mechanisms involved in diffuse glomerulonephritis.

24 Describe the significance of epithelial crescent formation.

25 Describe the gross and microscopic changes in end-stage kidney disease.

26 Describe four histologic types of glomerulonephritis associated with the nephrotic syndrome (population affected, morphology, treatment, prognosis).

27 Describe the nephrotic syndrome (clincial features, physiological disturbances, causes, treatment).

28 Describe the relationship between hypertension and chronic renal failure.

29 Distinguish between benign and malignant essential hypertension (rate of progress, target organs, clinical signs and symptoms, arterial lesions).

30 Define *nephrosclerosis.*

31 Explain the importance of the early diagnosis of renal artery stenosis.

32 Discuss the relationship of connective tissue disorders to renal disease.

33 Relate the histologic changes in lupus nephritis to prognosis and compare the histologic changes with those seen in primary glomerulonephritis.

34 Describe polyarteritis nodosa and scleroderma (pathogenesis, population affected, renal lesions).

35 Compare renal tubular acidosis and polycystic disease of the kidneys (heredity, forms of the disease and population affected, renal lesions or pathophysiology, clinical features, treatment, prognosis).

36 Describe diabetic nephropathy.

37 Explain the importance of gout, hyperparathyroidism, and amyloidosis to renal failure.

38 List three reasons why the kidney is vulnerable to the hazards of drug or chemical toxicity.

39 Describe the characteristic renal changes and presenting clinical features that may result from chronic analgesic abuse with phenacetin.

40 Describe the pathogenesis of lead nephropathy.

The purpose of this chapter is to give you an overview of the course of deterioration in progressive renal failure, its general pathophysiology, and various causes.

Renal failure is usually divided into two broad categories—chronic and acute. Chronic renal failure is a progressive, slow development of renal failure, usually over a period of years, as contrasted with acute renal failure, which develops over a period of days or a few weeks. In both cases the kidneys lose their ability to maintain the volume and composition of the body fluids under conditions of normal dietary intake. Although the terminal functional disability is similar in both types of renal failure, acute renal failure has some unique features and will be discussed separately in Chap. 44.

Chronic renal failure follows a great number of conditions which devastate the nephron mass of the kidney. The majority of these conditions involve diffuse, bilateral disease of the renal parenchyma, although obstructive lesions of the urinary tract may also lead to chronic renal failure. In the beginning, some renal diseases primarily involve the glomerulus (glomerulonephritis), while others primarily involve the renal tubules (pyelonephritis or polycystic kidney disease) or may interfere with blood perfusion to the renal parenchyma (nephrosclerosis). In all cases, however, if the disease process is progressive, the entire nephron is destroyed and is replaced by scar tissue. The individual features of the various parenchymal renal diseases will be discussed later in this chapter.

Despite the diversity of causes, the clinical features of chronic renal failure are remarkably similar, for progressive renal failure may be explained simply as a deficiency in the total number of functioning nephrons, and a fairly fixed combination of disturbances is inevitable.

OVERVIEW: CLINICAL COURSE OF CHRONIC RENAL FAILURE

An overview of the general course of chronic renal failure may be obtained by looking at the relationship of the creatinine clearance and glomerular filtration rate (GFR) (as a percentage of normal) to the serum creatinine and the blood urea nitrogen (BUN) levels as the nephron mass is progressively destroyed by chronic renal disease (Fig. 41-1).

The general course of progressive renal failure may be divided into three stages (designated as I, II, and III in Fig. 41-1). The first stage is called decreased renal reserve. During this stage the serum creatinine and BUN levels are normal, and the patient is asymptomatic. Impairment of renal function may only be detected by imposition of severe demands on the kidney, such as a prolonged urine concentration test, or by careful testing of the GFR.

The second stage in the progression is called renal insufficiency, when more than 75 percent of the functioning tissue has been destroyed (GFR is 25 percent of normal). At this point the BUN level is just beginning to rise above the normal range. The rise in BUN concentration is variable depending on the dietary intake of protein (compare the BUN graphs for a low and normal protein intake). Serum creatinine level also begins to rise above normal during this stage. The azotemia is generally mild unless, for example, the patient is stressed by infection, heart failure, or dehydration. It is also during the stage of renal insufficiency that the symptoms of nocturia and polyuria (caused by impaired concentrating ability) begin to appear. These symptoms occur in response to stress and sudden changes in food or fluid intake. The patient usually takes little note of these

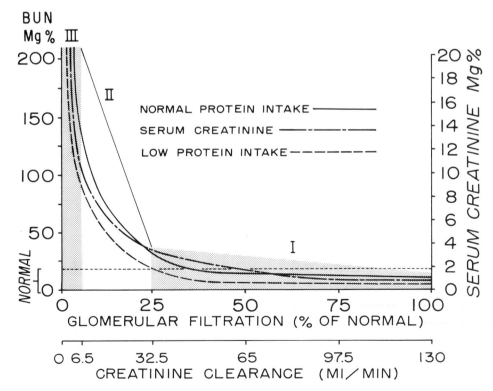

FIGURE 41-1 The relationship of the blood urea nitrogen (BUN) and serum creatinine levels to the glomerular filtration rate during the three stages of progressive renal failure. Note that a low protein diet delays azotemia.

symptoms, so that they are revealed only by careful questioning. *Nocturia* (urinating at night) is defined as persistent symptoms of a nocturnal output of 700 ml or having to get up more than once to void during the night. Nocturia is due to the loss of the normal diurnal pattern of concentrating urine to a greater degree at night. The ratio of day to night urine is normally 3 or 4:1. Of course, nocturia may occasionally occur in response to anxiety or to a high fluid intake, especially of tea, coffee, or beer taken just before retiring. *Polyuria means a persistent increase in the volume of urine.* Normal urine output is about 1500 ml/day and varies considerably with fluid intake. The polyuria of renal insufficiency is usually greater in diseases which primarily affect the tubules though it is generally moderate and rarely exceeds 3 liters/day.

The third and final stage of progressive renal failure is called *end-stage renal failure or uremia.* End-stage renal failure occurs when about 90 percent of the nephron mass has been destroyed, or only about 200,000 nephrons remain intact. The GFR is 10 percent of normal, and the creatinine clearance may be 5 to 10 ml/minute or even less. At this point, the serum creatinine and BUN levels rise very sharply in response to small decrements in the GFR. During end-stage renal failure the patient begins to suffer severe symptoms as the kidneys are no longer able to maintain fluid and electrolyte homeostasis in the body. The urine becomes isoosmotic with the plasma at a fixed specific gravity of 1.010. The patient usually becomes oliguric (urine output less than 500 ml/day) because of glomerular failure even though the renal tubules may have been initially affected by the disease process. The complex of biochemical changes and symptoms which is called the uremic syndrome affects every system in the body and will be discussed in detail in Chap. 42. In end-stage renal failure, unless the patient receives treatment in the form of dialysis or renal transplantation, death will surely follow.

Although the clinical course of chronic renal disease has been divided into three stages, in practice there are no sharp divisions between the stages. The hyperbolic shape of the graph of azotemia plotted against GFR reflects this continuous but slowly accelerating course.

General pathophysiology of chronic renal failure

Two theoretical approaches are generally offered to account for the impaired function of the kidneys in chronic renal failure. The traditional point of view is that all of the nephron units are diseased to varying degrees and that specific parts of the nephron concerned with particular functions may be destroyed or their structure altered. For example, organic lesions of the medulla disrupting the anatomic arrangement of the loop of Henle and vasa recta or the chloride pump in the ascending limb would interfere with countercurrent multiplication and exchange. The second approach, known as the *Bricker hypothesis or the "intact nephron" hypothesis,* maintains that nephrons, when diseased, are totally destroyed. The remaining intact nephrons behave normally. Uremia results when the total number of nephrons is so reduced that fluid and electrolyte balance can no longer be maintained. The intact nephron hypothesis is most useful in explaining the orderly pattern of functional adaptation in progressive renal disease, i.e., the ability to maintain a balance of body water and electrolytes in spite of a marked decrease in the GFR.

The sequence of events in the general pathophysiology of progressive renal failure may be outlined in terms of the intact nephron hypothesis. As chronic renal disease advances the amount of solute which must be excreted by the kidney in order to maintain body homeostasis does not change although there is a progressive reduction in the number of nephrons performing this function. Two important adaptations occur in the kidney in response to the threat of fluid and electrolyte imbalance. The remaining nephrons hypertrophy in an attempt to carry on the entire workload of the kidneys (Fig. 41-2). There is an increase in filtration rate, solute load, and tubular reabsorption in each individual nephron even though the GFR for the entire nephron mass of the kidneys is decreased below normal. This adaptive mechanism is successful in maintaining body fluid and electrolyte balance down to very low levels of renal function. Finally, when about 75 percent of the nephron mass is destroyed, the filtration rate and solute load per nephron is so high that glomerular-tubular balance (balance between increased filtration and increased tubular reabsorption) can no longer be maintained (note that six out of the eight nephrons are destroyed in Fig. 41-2). There is a loss of flexibility in both the excretion and conservation of individual solutes and water. Modest dietary changes may upset the precarious balance, since the lower the GFR (which means fewer nephrons), the greater must be the change in excretion rate per nephron. Loss of the ability to concentrate or dilute causes the specific gravity of urine to become fixed at 1.010 or 285 mOsm (the concentration of plasma) and accounts for the symptoms of polyuria and nocturia. For example, a person on a normal diet excretes about 600 mOsm of solute each day. If that person is incapable of concentrating urine from the normal plasma osmolality of 285 mOsm, then there is an obligatory loss of 2 liters of water with the 600 mOsm solute excretion (285 mOsm/liter) regardless of water intake. In response to the same solute load and water deprivation, the normal person could concentrate urine to about 4 times the plasma concentration and thus excrete a small volume of concentrated urine. As the GFR progresses toward zero, it becomes increasingly important to regulate intake of water and solutes very precisely to accommodate the decreased flexibility in renal function.

The intact nephron hypothesis is supported by several experimental observations. Dr. Neal Bricker and his associates have shown that in patients with naturally occurring pyelonephritis and in dogs with experimental destruction of the kidney, the surviving nephrons hypertrophy and become more active than normal. It is also known that when one kidney is removed in the healthy person, the remaining kidney undergoes hypertrophy, and the function of this kidney approaches that formerly possessed by both.

It has also been demonstrated that normal kidneys under conditions of an increased solute load behave in a similar manner as the kidney in progressive renal failure, giving further support to the intact nephron hypothesis. The experimental data in Fig. 41-3 illustrates that with progressive increases in solute load, the ability to concentrate the urine under conditions of water deprivation (upper curve) or to dilute the urine under conditions of high water intake (lower curve) is progressively lost. Both curves approach the specific gravity of 1.010 until the urine is isoosmotic with the plasma at 285 mOsm so that a fixed specific gravity exists.

The above experimental conditions could be induced in a normal person by giving mannitol (an osmotic diuretic). The number 10 on the x-axis is arbitrarily chosen to show that the kidneys are excreting 10 times the usual solute load. At this point each normal nephron is undergoing an osmotic diuresis with an obligatory loss of water. The kidney has lost its flexibility to either concentrate or dilute the urine from the plasma osmolality of 285 mOsm.

Similar events probably occur in the patient with progressive renal failure. The patient with 90 percent destruction of nephron mass is at the same point on the graph as the normal person with an induced solute load that is 10 times normal. The remaining 10 percent of the nephrons are forced to excrete 10 times the normal solute load and therefore lose their flexibility; they are unable to compensate properly by the usual changes in tubular reabsorption for excesses or deficiencies of sodium or water.

CAUSES OF CHRONIC RENAL FAILURE

Chronic renal failure is a clinical state of progressive, irreversible renal damage arising from many different causes. The most common causes of chronic renal failure may be divided into eight classes listed in Table 41-1. No attempt is made to be all-inclusive, and only selected examples are listed under each class. These diseases will be discussed in this chapter but not necessarily in the same order in which they appear in the

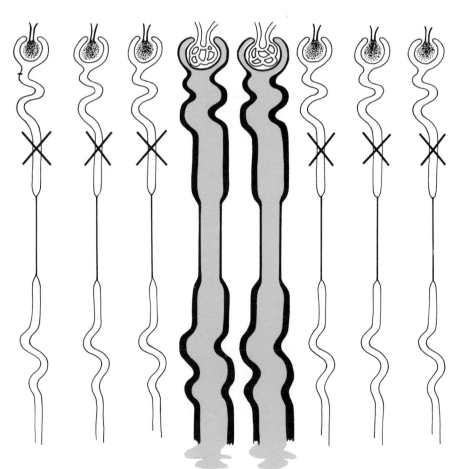

FIGURE 41-2 Diagram illustrating the intact nephron hypothesis. As chronic renal disease advances and nephrons are progressively destroyed, the remaining intact nephrons hypertrophy in an attempt to carry on the entire workload of the kidney. Solute load per nephron is increased, resulting in osmotic diuresis, i.e., rise in urine flow and reduction in concentration. (Modified from Frank H. Netter, Ciba Collection of Medical Illustrations: Kidneys, Ureters, and Urinary Bladder, Ciba Pharmaceutical Co., Summit, N.J., 1973, vol. 6.)

table. It should be emphasized that while the early stages of renal disease may be quite variable, the end stages are remarkably similar, and in many cases the original cause cannot be identified. According to the 1975 report of the American College of Surgeons/National Institutes of Health Organ Transplant Registry, the leading causes of end-stage renal disease (in transplant recipients) are glomerulonephritis (56.0 percent), pyelonephritis (13.1 percent), polycystic disease (5.4 percent), and hypertensive nephrosclerosis (4.9 percent).* There is also great variation in the rate of progression of these chronic renal diseases. The course terminating in end-stage renal disease may vary from 2 or 3 months to 30 or 40 years.

Urinary tract infections and pyelonephritis

Urinary tract infection is a very common condition and usually implies pyelonephritis or cystitis. Cystitis is an infection of the bladder, and pyelonephritis is an infection involving the renal pelvis and interstitium. Pyelonephritis may be acute or chronic. While both cystitis and acute pyelonephritis are usually benign, they may

---

*Figures may overrepresent glomerulonephritis and underrepresent pyelonephritis since patients with pyelonephritis may have been rejected more often as unsuitable for transplant. In the United States in 1964, the Committee on Chronic Dialysis ("Gottschalk Report") reported the following distribution of primary renal diseases: nephritis and nephrosis (45 percent), infections of the kidney (36 percent), and polycystic disease (15 percent). In a 1967 report by Hood in Sweden the diseases responsible for death in uremia were nonobstructive pyelonephritis (includes patients with papillary necrosis in which analgesic abuse may have played a role), 42 percent; chronic glomerulonephritis, 21 percent; diabetic renal disease, 18 percent; obstructive pyelonephritis, 7 percent; polycystic kidney, 5 percent; and malignant hypertension, 3 percent. From M. B. Strauss and L. G. Welt, *Diseases of the Kidney*, 2d ed., Little, Brown, Boston, 1971, p. 235.

lead to chronic pyelonephritis and renal failure. Obstruction of the urinary tract is an important predisposing factor in recurrent or chronic infections. Chronic pyelonephritis is the second leading cause of end-stage renal disease and is theoretically preventable by the control of urinary tract infections. It is unfortunate, however, that many chronic urinary tract infections involving the kidney may be silent and asymptomatic until irreversible renal damage occurs.

ETIOLOGY AND PATHOGENESIS

The most common infecting organism of the urinary tract is *Escherichia coli*, which accounts for more than 80 percent of the cases. *E. coli* is a normal inhabitant of the colon. Other infecting organisms often include the *Proteus, Klebsiella, Pseudomonas, Enterococcus,* and *Staphylococcus* groups. In most cases the organisms gain access to the bladder via the urethra. The infection, beginning as a cystitis, may remain confined to the bladder or may ascend via the ureter to the kidney. Organisms may also reach the kidney via the bloodstream or lymphatics, but this is believed to be uncommon. The bladder and upper urethra are normally sterile, although bacteria are present in the lower urethra. The normal urinary tract can decontaminate itself of bacteria before they have a chance to invade the mucosa by the flushing action of urine flow. Other defense mechanisms include the antibacterial effect of the urethral mucosa, the bactericidal properties of prostatic fluid in the male, and the phagocytic properties of the bladder epithelium. In spite of these defenses, many urinary infections do occur and are believed to be related to certain predisposing factors listed in Table 41-2.

Obstruction of the urinary outflow proximal to the bladder can result in the accumulation of fluid under pressure in the renal pelvis and ureter. This alone is enough to cause severe atrophy of the renal parenchyma. It is a condition called *hydronephrosis*. In addition, obstruction below the level of the bladder is often

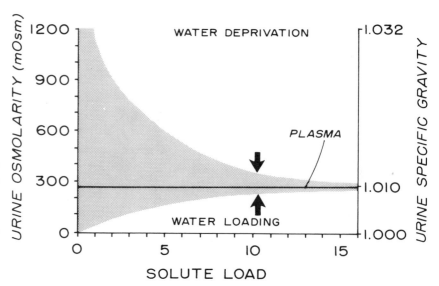

FIGURE 41-3 The response of normal kidneys to an increasing solute load under conditions of water loading and deprivation. Ability to concentrate or dilute the urine is progressively lost as the solute load increases. Urine specific gravity becomes fixed near 1.010 (285 mOsm). (Modified from A. Gordon, and M. H. Maxwell, "Reversible Uremia," Hospital Medicine, Jan., 1967.)

associated with vesicoureteral reflux (see later) and infection of the kidney. Common causes of obstruction are renal or ureteral scarring, calculi, neoplasms, prostatic hypertrophy (common in males over 60 years), congenital anomalies of the bladder neck and urethra, and urethral stricture.

Females have a much higher incidence of urinary tract infections and pyelonephritis than males, presumably because of a shorter urethra and its proximity to the anus and consequent fecal contamination. Epidemiologic studies have shown that significant bacteriuria (10^5 organisms per ml urine) exists in 1 to 4 percent of schoolgirls, 5 to 10 percent of women of childbearing age, and about 25 percent of women greater than 60 years of age. Only a few of these persons have clinical symptoms of urinary tract infection, and the relationship of significant bacteriuria to the development of chronic pyelonephritis is not known. Infection in the male is rare, and when it occurs, it is usually related to obstruction.

It has been known for some time that hydroureter and hydronephrosis, most marked on the right, always occurs during pregnancy and persists for some time afterwards. The dilatation is attributed partly to muscular relaxation caused by the high progesterone levels and partly to obstruction of the ureters by the enlarged uterus. About 5 to 7 percent of these women have asymptomatic bacteriuria, and if untreated, 40 to 50 percent develop acute pyelonephritis.

Normally all the urine contained in the bladder is expelled through the urethra during micturation. Vesico-

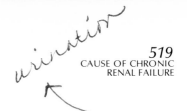

ureteral reflux is the backflow of urine up the ureters as well as out the urethra during micturation. Vesicoureteral reflux has been demonstrated in a high proportion of patients, especially children with recurrent urinary tract infections, and appears to be the mechanism by which organisms ascend to the kidney.

Urethral and ureteric catheterization and cystoscopy are common forms of instrumentation whereby infection is introduced into the bladder or kidney. About 2 percent of simple, single bladder catheterizations result in infection. There is a 98 percent incidence of infection within 48 hours when an indwelling catheter is placed unless meticulous attention is directed to keeping a closed drainage system. Even when the system is closed, the urine is only sterile for about 5 to 7 days. These facts indicate that catheterization is a procedure to be avoided if possible.

Neurogenic bladder, common in patients with spinal cord injury, is frequently associated with urinary retention and infection. The use of catheters and urinary drainage are additional predisposing factors. These patients often die because of renal complications due to chronic infection.

Chronic phenacetin abuse alone may cause chronic interstitial nephritis (see "Analgesic Abuse" later in this chapter), but it also predisposes to chronic pyelonephritis. Various underlying renal diseases increase susceptibility to infection and pyelonephritis. Finally, metabolic disturbances such as diabetes, gout, and renal stones are often complicated by renal infection.

It is not known with certainty what proportion of the cases of chronic bacterial pyelonephritis can be explained on the basis of these predisposing factors. It is clear, however, that infection beginning in the lower urinary tract can ascend to the kidney. Various studies have shown that the renal medulla has unique characteristics which favor the survival of bacteria. This increased susceptibility to infection is apparently due to the high ammonia content and hyperosmolality which interfere with host defense mechanisms such as leukocyte migration, phagocytosis, and complement activity. In addition, some bacteria when in a hyperosmotic

TABLE 41-1 *causes of CRF*
Classification of the causes of chronic renal failure

DISEASE CLASSIFICATION	DISEASE
Infections	Chronic pyelonephritis
Inflammatory diseases	Glomerulonephritis
Hypertensive vascular disease	Benign nephrosclerosis Malignant nephrosclerosis Renal artery stenosis
Connective tissue disorders	Systemic lupus erythematosis Polyarteritis nodosa Progressive systemic sclerosis
Congenital and hereditary disorders	Polycystic kidney disease Renal tubular acidosis
Metabolic disorders	Diabetes mellitus Gout Hyperparathyroidism Amyloidosis
Toxic nephropathy	Analgesic abuse Lead nephropathy
Obstructive nephropathy	Upper urinary tract—calculi, neoplasms, retroperitoneal fibrosis Lower urinary tract—prostatic hypertrophy, urethral structure, congenital anomalies of the bladder, neck, and urethra

TABLE 41-2
Predisposing factors in the development of urinary tract infections and chronic pyelonephritis

Obstruction of urinary outflow
Sex, age
Pregnancy
Vesicoureteral reflux
Instrumentation (especially indwelling catheters)
Neurogenic bladder
Chronic analgesic abuse (phenacetin)
Renal disease
Metabolic disturbances (diabetes, gout, urinary calculi)

environment enter a spherocyte or protoplast form (bacteria with defective cell walls) in which they become resistant to antibiotics and can revert later to the parent form.

ACUTE PYELONEPHRITIS

The clinical features of acute pyelonephritis are usually quite characteristic. The patient is a woman in about 90 percent of the cases. There is an abrupt onset of fever, chills, malaise, back pain, tenderness to palpation over the costovertebral area, leukocytosis, pyuria, and bacteriuria. These symptoms are often preceded by dysuria, urgency, and frequency indicating that the infection began in the lower urinary tract. The finding of leukocyte casts indicates that the infection is in the kidney.

Figure 41-4 illustrates the gross and microscopic appearance of the kidney in acute pyelonephritis. The kidney is swollen with multiple, small abscesses on the surface. On the cross section, abscesses appear as yellowish gray streaks in the pyramids and cortex. Microscopically, numerous polymorphonuclear leukocytes (PMNs) are found within the tubules (arrow) and in the interstitium surrounding the tubules. Segments of the tubules are destroyed, and this leukocytic material is flushed out into the urine as casts.

E. coli is the most common infecting organism in acute, uncomplicated pyelonephritis. Of these patients 90 percent respond to antibiotic therapy, while the remaining 10 percent may have acute recurrent infections or persistent asymptomatic bacteriuria. When acute pyelonephritis is complicated by obstruction, recurrent or persistent bacteriuria occurs in 50 to 80 percent of patients within 2 years. It is not known with certainty how many of these patients will develop significant renal damage or how long the process might take. Treatment is directed towards appropriate antibacterial

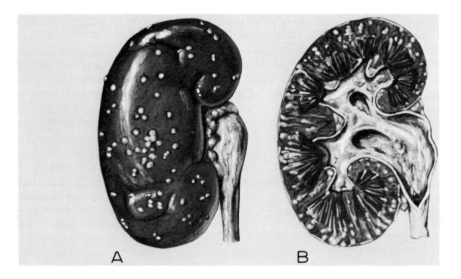

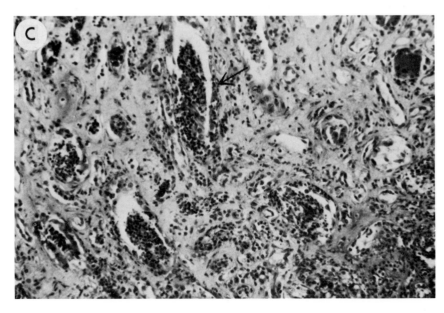

FIGURE 41-4 Gross and microscopic appearance of the kidney in acute pyelonephritis. A. The kidney is swollen with multiple abscesses on the surface. B. Abscesses appear as yellowish gray streaks on the cross section. C. Histologically, many PMNs appear in the interstitium and within the tubules. (Art by Judy Simon, Dept. of Medical and Biological Illustrations, University of Michigan.)

therapy, correction of predisposing factors, and careful long-term follow-up with urine cultures at intervals to ensure that the urine is sterile.

CHRONIC PYELONEPHRITIS

There are many controversial issues among the authorities concerning the etiology of chronic pyelonephritis, since about one-half the patients have no recallable history of urinary tract infection, and more than one-half of patients with established chronic pyelonephritis have negative urine cultures. Nevertheless, many believe that it develops from inadequately treated or recurrent pyelonephritis. Explanations given to account for the above facts are that recurrent infection may be sub-clinical, and bacteria (which can convert to the proto-plast form) may only be expelled into the urine inter-mittently. Evidence against bacterial infection as a cause include the fact that the sex incidence of chronic pyelo-nephritis is about equal although acute urinary tract infection is probably 10 times more frequent in females. Furthermore, bacterial infection is a common complica-tion of other renal diseases, and nonbacterial agents such as phenacetin produce similar lesions.

In contrast to acute pyelonephritis, the clinical fea-tures of chronic pyelonephritis are quite vague. The diagnosis is often made when the patient presents with symptoms of chronic renal insufficiency or hypertension, or proteinuria may be discovered in a routine examina-tion. In some cases there is a documented history of urinary tract infections dating from childhood. In other cases careful questioning may reveal a history of vague symptoms of dysuria, frequency, and sometimes loin pain. Many patients are asymptomatic until the disease is advanced. Typical findings in chronic pyelonephritis include intermittent bacteriuria and white blood cells or white cell casts in the urine. Proteinuria is usually minimal. Because chronic pyelonephritis is chiefly a medullary interstitial disease, the concentrating ability of the kidney is affected early in its course before there is a significant decrease in the glomerular filtration rate. Consequently, polyuria, nocturia, and urine with a low specific gravity are prominent early symptoms. In addi-tion, many patients have a tendency to lose salt in the urine. About one-half the cases may develop hyper-tension. Azotemia is common in the course of chronic pyelonephritis, although advancement to renal failure is usually very slowly progressive.

The IVP reveals clubbing of the calyces, a thinned cortex, and small, irregular-shaped kidneys which are usually asymmetric (see Fig. 40-9B). Figure 41-5 illustrates the pathological changes in chronic pyelonephritis. The surface of the kidney is coarsely granular with U-shaped depressions (Fig. 41-5A); subcapsular scars; and a dilated, fibrosed pelvis; and calyces are seen on the cross section (Fig. 41-5B). Microscopic examination of tissue sections reveals characteristic parenchymal changes: Many chronic inflammatory cells consisting of plasma cells and lymphocytes (dark-staining dots) are scattered throughout the interstitium. The three glomeruli are intact while surrounded by many tubules which are small and atrophied or dilated. There is an

area of interstitial fibrosis near the glomerulus (arrow, Fig. 41-5C). Large areas of thyroidization (having the appearance of thyroid gland tissue) are seen, consisting of dilated tubules lined with flattened epithelial cells and filled with glassy-appearing casts (Fig. 41-5D).

Glomerulonephritis

Most deaths from renal failure are due to chronic glomerulonephritis. This disease also accounts for the greatest number of patients who enter chronic dialysis and transplant programs.

Glomerulonephritis is a bilateral inflammatory disease of the kidneys which begins in the glomerulus and is manifested by proteinuria and/or hematuria. Although the lesions are primarily glomerular, entire nephrons may eventually be destroyed, leading to chronic renal failure. The original disease described by Richard Bright in 1827 (called Bright's disease) is now known to be a collection of many diseases of different etiologies (most of which are unknown), although immune responses seem to be implicated in several forms of glomerulo-nephritis.

In recent years, knowledge of the pathological changes in renal disease has been greatly expanded by renal biopsy studies using light, immunofluorescent, and electron microscopy. As knowledge has expanded, new categories have emerged based on a greater ability to define the nature of renal lesions. Numerous attempts have been made to separate and classify the various types of glomerulonephritis by relating histologic and clinical features. Unfortunately, the various categories are not exclusive. This overlap is understandable since the kidney only has a limited number of morphological and functional responses. To add to this confusion, many systemic and metabolic disorders (when there is renal involvement) may have changes in the glomeruli which are indistinguishable from primary glomerulo-nephritis.

Table 41-3 lists the various ways in which glomerulo-nephritis is described and classified. This table will serve as a guide for the discussion in the remainder of this chapter and should be read before proceeding. It will be helpful for the reader to remember that the gen-eral term *glomerulonephritis* (GN) is generally used to refer to a number of primary renal diseases pre-dominantly affecting the glomeruli, but it is also used to refer to glomerular lesions which may or may not be the result of primary renal disease. For example, the renal lesion in systemic lupus erythematosis may be referred to as proliferative glomerulonephritis. The following discussion will focus on primary renal diseases which cause glomerulonephritis although references will be made to systemic diseases causing similar lesions in the kidney. Systemic diseases causing renal injury will be considered in more detail later in the chapter.

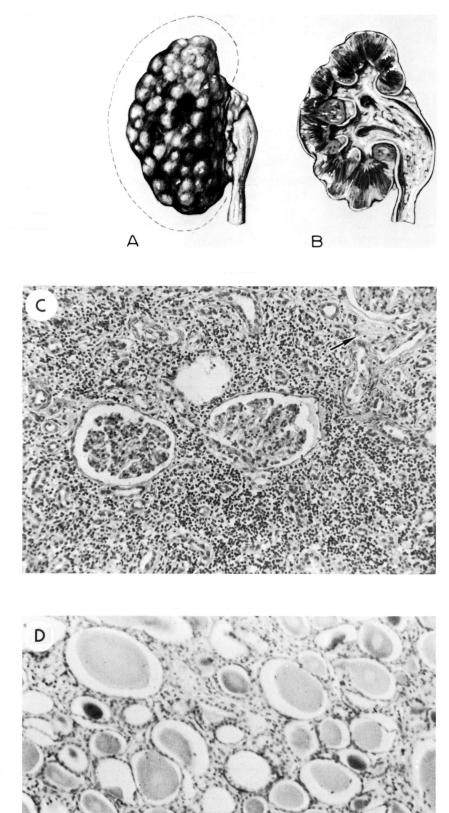

FIGURE 41-5 Gross and microscopic appearance of the kidney in chronic pyelonephritis. A. Coarsely granular surface with U-shaped depressions. B. Thinning of the cortex, subcapsular scars, dilated, fibrosed pelvis and calyces. C. Chronic inflammatory cells throughout interstitium, small, atrophied tubules, and an area of interstitial fibrosis (arrow). D. Thyroid-gland appearance due to dilated tubules containing glassy-looking casts. (Art by Judy Simon, Dept. of Medical and Biological Illustrations, University of Michigan.)

TABLE 41-3
Various classifications of glomerulonephritis

CLASSIFICATION	DESCRIPTION
1 Distribution	
a Diffuse	Involves all the glomeruli; most common form results in chronic renal failure (CRF).
b Focal	Only a proportion of the glomeruli are abnormal.
c Local	Only a part of the glomerular tuft is abnormal, such as a single capillary loop.
2 Broad clinical forms of diffuse glomerulonephritis	
a Acute (AGN)	Classic, benign disorder which is nearly always preceded by a streptococcal infection and associated with immune-complex deposition in the glomerular basement membrane (GBM) and proliferative cellular changes.
b Subacute (RPGN)	Rapidly progressive form of glomerulonephritis characterized by intense cellular proliferative changes that destroy the glomeruli and result in death from uremia within a few months from the onset.
c Chronic (CGN)	Slowly progressive glomerulonephritis leading to sclerosing and obliterative changes in the glomeruli; small, contracted kidneys; and death from uremia; entire course varies from 2 to 40 years.
3 Pathogenetic immune mechanism and immunofluorescent pattern	
a Immune-complex, granular	Antibody (Ab) to either exogenous or endogenous nonglomerular antigens (Ag) is involved in the formation of circulating Ab-Ag complexes which are passively trapped in the GBM. Complement fixation and the release of immunologic mediators results in glomerular injury; deposit is along epithelial surface and reveals a lumpy or granular pattern on immunofluorescent microscopy; associated with poststreptococcal GN, idiopathic membranous GN, and the GN of serum sickness, subacute bacterial endocarditis, malaria, and anaphylactoid purpura.
b Nephrotoxic (anti-GBM), linear	Antibodies form which react with the patient's own GBM as the antigen (anti-GBM or anti-kidney antibodies). True autoimmune disease in contrast to immune-complex GN in which the GBM is like an innocent bystander; immune deposits are subendothelial and result in a ribbonlike linear pattern on immunofluorescence; associated with RPGN and Goodpasture's syndrome.
4 Histologic pattern	
a Minimal change	Also referred to as lipoid nephrosis or foot-process disease; glomeruli appear normal or nearly normal on light microscopy, while electron microscopy reveals fusion of the foot processes; only major form of GN without evidence of immunopathology; commonly presents as the nephrotic syndrome in children of 1 to 5 years; responds well to corticosteroid therapy; prognosis excellent.
b Proliferative	Deposition of immunoglobulin, complement, and fibrin leads to proliferation of endothelial, mesangial, and epithelial cells; latter leads to crescent formation which may encircle and obliterate the glomerular tuft—ominous sign; common in RPGN and advanced CGN.
c Membranous	Epimembranous deposit of immune material along GBM causing the GBM to thicken, but there is little or no inflammation or cellular proliferation, though the capillary lumen may eventually be obliterated; most common lesion in adults with the nephrotic syndrome; responds poorly to corticosteroid and immunosuppressive therapy; generally poor prognosis and slow progression to renal failure; membranous changes are also common in systemic nephritic diseases such as diabetes mellitus and systemic lupus erythematosis (SLE).
d Membranoproliferative	Also referred to as mesangiocapillary, lobular, or hypocomplementemic GN; immune complex material deposited between the GBM and endothelium causing GBM thickening and proliferation of the mesangial cells giving the glomerulus a lobular or "wipe-loop" appearance on light microscopy; characterized by low serum complement level, hematuria, and the nephrotic syndrome; responds poorly to therapy, generally progresses slowly to renal failure.
e Focal	Proliferative or sclerosing lesions which occur at random throughout the kidneys (focal as opposed to diffuse) and often only affect part of the glomerular tuft (local); occurs during at least part of the course of SBE, SLE, polyarteritis nodosa, Goodpasture's syndrome, and purpura; idiopathic focal GN sometimes appears in children; prognosis good.

TABLE 41-3—(Continued on next page)

TABLE 41-3—(Continued)
Various classifications of glomerulonephritis

CLASSIFICATION	DESCRIPTION
5 Clinical syndromes	
a Acute nephritic syndrome	Acute nephritis of sudden onset usually associated with poststreptococcal GN but can occur in many other renal diseases and as an acute exacerbation of CGN.
b Nephrotic syndrome	Clinical complex characterized by massive proteinuria (>3.5 g/day), hypoalbuminemia, edema, and hyperlipidemia. Occurs in many primary renal and systemic diseases; 50 percent of patients with CGN have it at least once.
c Persistent, asymptomatic urine abnormalities	"Latent" stage in CGN characterized by minimal proteinuria and/or hematuria but without symptoms; glomerular function relatively stable or may show slow progression ("silent azotemia").
d Uremic syndrome	Symptomatic end-stage renal failure.

Key: GBM, glomerular basement membrane; GN, glomerulonephritis; CRF, chronic renal failure; CGN, chronic glomerulonephritis; SLE, systemic lupus erythematosis; SBE, subacute bacterial endocarditis; RPGN, rapidly progressive or subacute glomerulonephritis.

ACUTE GLOMERULONEPHRITIS

The classic case of acute glomerulonephritis follows a streptococcal infection of the throat or sometimes of the skin after a latent period of 1 to 2 weeks. The responsible organism is usually a type 12 or 4, group A, β-hemolytic streptococcus, and rarely others. However, the streptococcus itself does not cause the renal damage by infection. It is believed that antibodies are directed against a specific antigen which is a constituent of the specific streptococcal plasma membrane. An antigen-antibody complex is formed in the blood and circulates to the glomerulus, where it is mechanically trapped in the basement membrane. Complement is fixed, resulting in injury and inflammation which attracts polymorphonuclear leukocytes (PMNs) and platelets to the damaged site. Phagocytosis and release of lysosomal enzymes also damage the endothelium and glomerular basement membrane (GBM). As a response to injury there is proliferation of endothelial cells, then of mesangial cells, and later epithelial cells may increase as well. The resulting increased porosity of the glomerular capillary permits the escape of proteins and blood cells into the forming urine causing proteinuria and hematuria. It is presumably these antigen-antibody-complement complexes which appear as subepithelial nodules (or epimembranous humps) on electron microscopy and as a granular, "lumpy-bumpy" pattern on immunofluorescent microscopy; by light microscopy the glomeruli appear swollen and hypercellular with invasion of PMNs (Fig. 41-6).

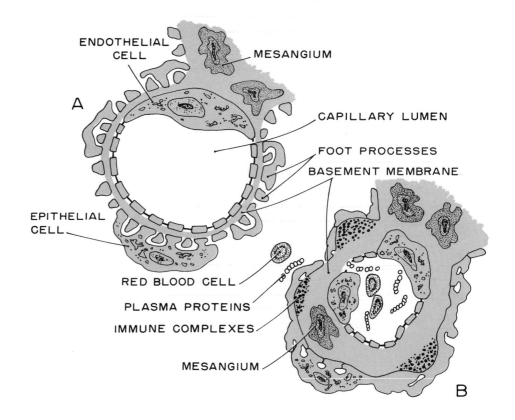

Acute poststreptococcal glomerulonephritis (APSGN) most frequently affects children between the ages of 3 and 7 years, though adolescents and young adults are also affected. The ratio of male to female is about 2:1.

The common presenting features of APSGN include hematuria, proteinuria, oliguria, edema, and hypertension. Common symptoms associated with the onset are fatigue, anorexia, and sometimes fever, headache, nausea, and vomiting. Elevation of the antistreptolysin O (ASO) titer may indicate the presence of antibodies to streptococcal organisms. Serum complement levels may be low due to depletion. This common finding gives further support to the hypothesis that the disease has an immune basis.

The major physiological distrubances in APSGN are depicted on the diagram in Fig. 41-7. The GFR is usually depressed (though renal plasma flow is generally nor-

mal). Consequently, the excretion of water, sodium, and nitrogenous substances may be decreased, resulting in edema and azotemia. Increased aldosterone may also play a role in sodium and water retention. Facial edema, particularly periorbital edema, is extremely common in the morning though it may become more apparent in the lower extremities as the day progresses. The degree of edema usually depends on the severity of the glomerular inflammation, whether there is concomitant congestive heart failure, or how soon dietary salt is restricted.

Hypertension almost always occurs, though the rise in

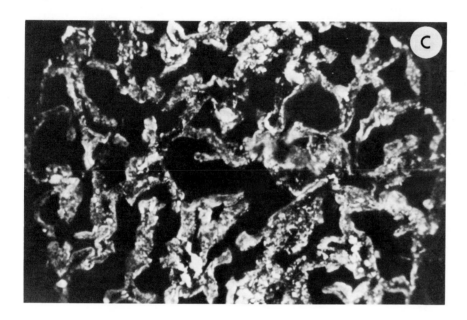

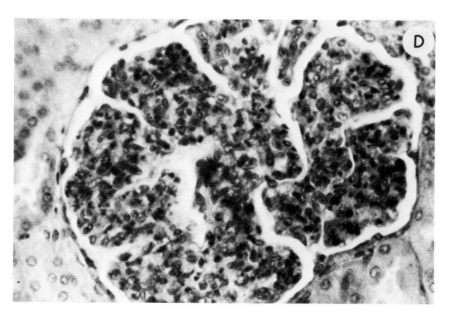

FIGURE 41-6 Acute poststreptococcal glomerulonephritis. A. Diagram of electron microscopy (EM) appearance of a single capillary loop of the glomerular tuft. B. Diagram of EM appearance of subepithelial deposits of immune complex, thickened basement membrane, cellular proliferation, and damage to capillary. C. Photomicrograph of immunofluorescent preparation showing lumpy pattern of immunoglobulin and complement deposits along glomerular capillary walls in circulating immune-complex disease. D. Light microscopy slide from kidney of a patient with APSGN showing infiltration with PMNs and hypercellularity which crowds the glomerulus filling Bowman's space. (Modified from Frank H. Netter, Ciba Collection of Medical Illustrations: Kidneys, Ureters, and Urinary Bladder, Ciba Pharmaceutical Co., Summit, N.J., 1973, vol. 6.) (Immunoflorescent micrograph courtesy of Michael J. Deegan.)

blood pressure may only be moderate. Whether the hypertension results from an expansion of the extracellular fluid (ECF) volume or from vasopasm is not clear.

Damage to the glomerular capillary tuft results in hematuria and albuminuria, as previously described. The urine may be grossly bloody or coffee-colored. Microscopic examination of the sediment reveals cylindruria (many casts), red blood cells (RBCs), and red cell casts. The latter establish the glomerular origin of the bleeding. The loss of protein is usually not great enough to cause hypoalbuminemia, and the nephrotic syndrome rarely occurs in APSGN. The urine specific gravity is usually high despite azotemia, a combination rarely occurring in renal diseases other than APSGN. This finding is explained by the fact that tubular function has been affected very little by the acute disease.

The usual treatment of APSGN is penicillin to eradicate any residual streptococcal infection, bed rest during the acute phase, sodium restriction in the presence of edema or signs of heart failure, and antihypertensive drugs if indicated. Corticosteroid drugs have no known beneficial effect in APSGN. Symptoms usually subside within days although microscopic hematuria and proteinuria may persist for months. It is estimated that more than 90 percent of children have a complete recovery. The prognosis is less favorable for adults (30 to 50 percent). Death occurs in 2 to 5 percent of all patients during the acute phase. In the remainder of patients, the disease may advance to a rapidly progressive glomerulonephritis (RPGN) or a more slowly progressive chronic glomerulonephritis (CGN). In RPGN, death in uremia usually occurs within a few months, while the entire course may vary from 2 to 40 years in CGN.

The natural history of the various forms of diffuse glomerulonephritis is depicted in the diagram in Fig. 41-8. Contrary to popular belief, only a small percentage of the cases of RPGN and CGN have their origin in APSGN. The precipitating factors are usually unknown.

Although APSGN has been more clearly defined, it should be noted that an acute nephritic syndrome may be associated with many other diseases affecting the

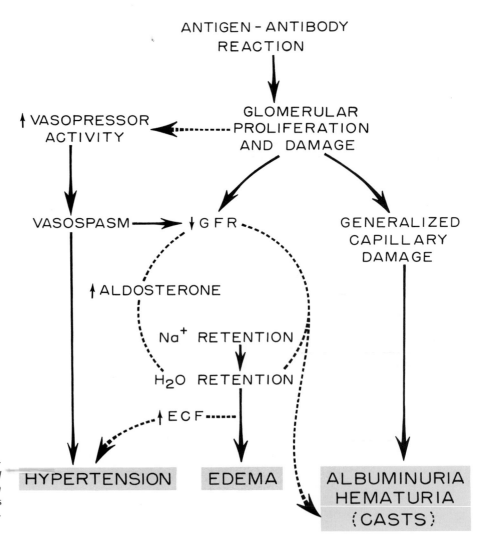

FIGURE 41-7 The major disturbances in acute poststreptococcal glomerulonephritis. (Modified from A. G. White, Clinical Disturbances of Renal Function, Saunders, Philadelphia, 1961.)

kidney [e.g., subacute bacterial endocarditis (SBE), malaria, anaphylactoid purpura, and the collagen diseases]. An acute nephritic syndrome may also occur during the course of CGN (Table 41-3).

RAPIDLY PROGRESSIVE GLOMERULONEPHRITIS (sub acute GN)

Rapidly progressive glomerulonephritis (formerly called subacute) is a term used to designate a fulminant renal disease with characteristic clinical and morphological features. There is hematuria, proteinuria, and rapidly progressive azotemia resulting in death within 2 years. At autopsy, the salient features are widespread epithelial crescent formation and diffuse glomerular involvement. Goodpasture's syndrome is a good example of this type of disease. Though a rare disease, it is most common in young men. The onset may be insidious or acute and is associated with lung hemorrhage and hemoptysis. There is usually no preceding illness to suggest the origin of the autoimmune antibodies against the glomerular basement membrane which develop in the patient's blood. Subendothelial immune-complex material is seen with electron microscopy, and a linear pattern of immunofluorescence suggests that a nephrotoxic immune mechanism is involved in the pathogenesis (Fig. 41-9). Immunoglobulin deposits have also been found along the basement membrane in the lung alveoli. There is no known treatment for this condition. The patient may be kept alive by hemodialysis but may die of lung hemorrhage.

CHRONIC GLOMERULONEPHRITIS (C G N)

Chronic glomerulonephritis (CGN) is characterized by slow, progressive destruction of the glomeruli from long-standing glomerulonephritis. In most instances, CGN has no known relationship to APSGN and RPGN but appears to represent de novo disease. The onset tends to be insidious, and it is usually discovered late in its course when symptoms of renal insufficiency appear. According to the stage of the disease there may be polyuria or oliguria, proteinuria of varying degrees, hypertension, progressive azotemia, and death in uremia.

In advanced CGN the kidneys are grossly contracted, sometimes weighing as little as 50 g, and the surface is granular. These changes are due to the loss of nephrons and ischemia. Microscopically, most of the glomeruli are altered. There may be a mixture of membranous and proliferative changes and epithelial crescent formation. Eventually there is atrophy of the tubules, interstitial fibrosis, and thickening of the arterial walls. When marked damage to all structures has occurred, the organ is called an "end-stage kidney," and it may be difficult to determine whether the original lesion was glomerular, interstitial due to chronic pyelonephritis, or vascular (Fig. 41-10).

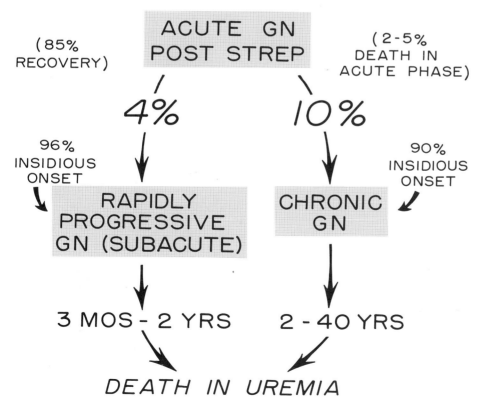

FIGURE 41-8 Natural history of the various forms of diffuse glomerulonephritis.

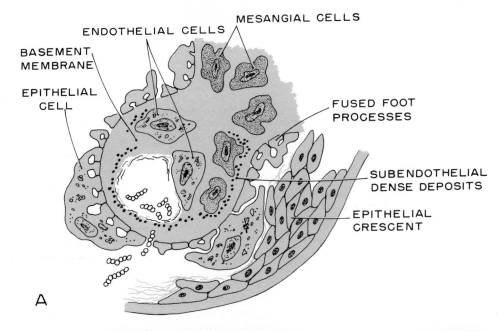

ENDOTHELIAL CELLS
MESANGIAL CELLS
BASEMENT MEMBRANE
EPITHELIAL CELL
FUSED FOOT PROCESSES
SUBENDOTHELIAL DENSE DEPOSITS
EPITHELIAL CRESCENT

A

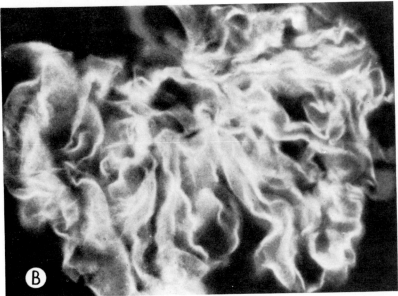

B

FIGURE 41-9 *Rapidly progressive glomeru-lonephritis.* A. *Cross section of a single capillary loop showing subendothelial dense deposits and glomerular damage.* B. *Photomicrograph of immunofluorescent preparation showing linear pattern of im-mune deposit typical of anti-GBM disease.* C. *Light microscopy slide from a patient with rapidly progressive glomerulonephritis showing large fibroepithelial crescent (arrow) crowding a lobulated glomerular tuft. (Diagram modified from Frank H. Netter, Ciba Collection of Medical Illustra-tions: Kidneys, Ureters, and Urinary Blad-der, Ciba Pharmaceutical Co., Summit, N.J., 1973, vol. 6.) (Immunofluorescent slide from A. J. Fish, A. F. Michael, and R. A. Good, in M. B. Strauss and L. G. Welt (eds.),* Diseases of the Kidney, *2d ed., Little, Brown, Boston, 1971.)*

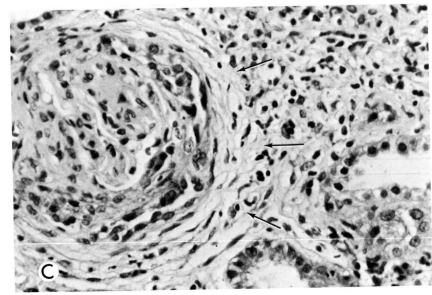

C

Although many patients with CGN have persistent, asymptomatic proteinuria throughout the course of the disease, about 50 percent develop the nephrotic syndrome. The nephrotic syndrome is a clinical state in which there is massive proteinuria (>3.5 g/day), hypoalbuminemia, edema, and hyperlipidemia. Usually the BUN level is normal.

According to Robson's review of over 1400 cases, several varieties of primary glomerulonephritis account for 78 percent of the nephrotic syndrome in adults and 93 percent in children. In 22 percent of the adults the condition was due to a systemic disorder (chiefly diabetes, amyloidosis, and renal vein thrombosis) in which the kidney was secondarily involved or to an abnormal response to drugs or other allergens.

There are four histologic entities found in the nephrotic syndrome included in the general category of glomerulonephritis. These are minimal change, membranous change, proliferative change, and mixed membranous and proliferative change glomerulonephritis (described in Table 41-3). Focal glomerulonephritis is a less frequent cause of the nephrotic syndrome.

1 Minimal change glomerulonephritis (GN) is the typical lesion of the nephrotic syndrome in childhood (69 percent) and accounts for 18 percent of adult cases. The older term for this disease is lipoid nephrosis. It is also called *foot-process disease* since the normally discrete foot processes (podocytes) of the epithelial cells appear to be fused together on electron microscopy (Fig. 41-11). Minimal change GN is the only major form of glomerulonephritis in which immune pathogenetic mechanisms do not appear to be involved. It is generally treated successfully with corticosteroids. In a minority of patients who do not respond to steroid therapy, the disease can sometimes be suppressed by immunosuppressive drugs such as cyclophosphamide (Cytoxin) or azathioprine (Imuran). The small proportion of patients who do not recover generally follow a long, remitting-relapsing course ending in uremia.

2 Membranous change GN accounts for 25 percent of the cases of nephrotic syndrome in adults and only 2 percent in children. About 95 percent of these patients develop azotemia and die in uremia in 10 to 20 years. The predominant histologic change is thickening of the basement membrane visible by both electron microscopy and light microscopy.

3 Proliferative and membranoproliferative change GN account for the remaining 35 percent of the adult nephrotic syndrome cases and for 22 percent in children. Proliferative change GN is characterized by hypercellularity of the glomerular cells, while there is both hypercellularity and basement membrane thickening in membranoproliferative change GN. Response to therapy is generally poor in these histologic types of GN, and there is progressive renal failure.

The major physiological disturbances leading to edema in the nephrotic syndrome are depicted in Fig. 41-12. The initial event in most cases is an antigen-antibody reaction at the glomerulus resulting in increased GBM permeability, massive proteinuria, and hypoalbuminemia. Patients with the nephrotic syndrome commonly pass 5 to 15 g protein per 24 hours. Hypoalbuminemia, by decreasing colloid osmotic pressure (COP), favors the transudation of fluid out of the vascular compartment into the interstitium. This serves as a fairly direct mechanism for the production of edema. In addition, the hypovolemia results in a decrease of renal plasma flow (RPF) and GFR activating the renin-angiotensin mechanism. The hypovolemia also activates volume receptors in the left atria. The result is increased aldosterone and ADH production. Salt and water are retained by the kidneys, further aggravating the edema. By repetition of this chain of events, massive edema (anasarca) may occur. The amount of protein lost, however, does not correlate precisely with the severity of

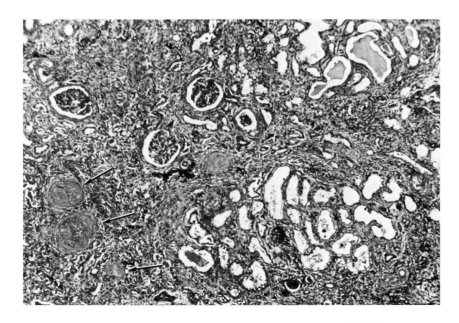

FIGURE 41-10 End-stage kidney (light microscopy) from a patient with chronic pyelonephritis showing marked distortion of the renal architecture. There is interstitial fibrosis, several glomeruli are completely hyalinized (arrow) while three are spared. There is marked tubular distortion and atrophy and casts appear in several tubules.

the edema since people vary in the rate of protein synthesis to replace that which is lost. The cause of the hyperlipidemia which often accompanies the nephrotic syndrome is obscure. Serum cholesterol, phospholipids, and triglycerides are all usually increased. Note that the mechanism of neophrotic edema differs from that of APSGN.

Treatment of the nephrotic syndrome consists of corticosteroid and immunosuppressive drugs directed toward the nature of the lesion; high protein and salt-restricted diet; diuretics; sometimes intravenous infusion of albumin; and restricted activity during the acute phase. It is also important to isolate patients from sources of infection. Patients with the nephrotic syndrome are highly susceptible to infection, and in pre-antibiotic days often died of empyema, pneumonia, or peritonitis. Long-term management is important since many patients follow a course of repeated exacerbations and remissions over a period of years, but with advancing glomerular hyalinization, proteinuria usually diminishes as azotemia progresses.

Hypertensive nephrosclerosis

Hypertension and chronic renal failure are closely related. Hypertension may be the primary disease and cause damage to the kidneys, and conversely, severe chronic renal disease may cause hypertension or contribute to its maintenance through the mechanism of sodium retention and the vasopressor effects of the renin-angiotensin system. Sometimes it is difficult for the nephrologist to determine which was primary.

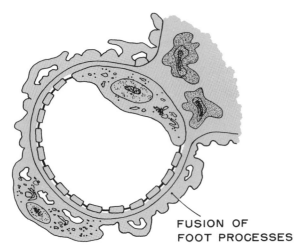

FUSION OF
FOOT PROCESSES

FIGURE 41-11 Schema of glomerular loop showing fusion of foot processes in minimal change glomerulonephritis. (Modified from Frank H. Netter, Ciba Collection of Medical Illustrations: Kidneys, Ureters, and Urinary Bladder, Ciba Pharmaceutical Co., Summit, N.J., 1973, vol. 6.)

Nephrosclerosis (hardening of the kidneys) refers to the pathological changes in the renal blood vessels as a result of hypertension. It is one of the leading causes of chronic renal failure.

ESSENTIAL HYPERTENSION AND THE KIDNEYS

Hypertension is defined as a sustained elevation of blood pressure above the accepted normals of 90 mmHg diastolic or 140 mmHg systolic. According to this definition, about 5 percent of the United States population has hypertension. However, as many as 25 percent of individuals may have this disorder by the age of 50 years. The cause of hypertension is unknown in about 90 percent of the cases and is termed *essential hypertension* (unknown etiology and pathogenesis). The onset of essential hypertension is usually between the ages of 20 and 50 years, and it is more frequent in blacks and females. Essential hypertension is classified as *benign* and *malignant*. Benign hypertension is slowly progressive while malignant hypertension is a clinical state in which there is rapid acceleration in the course of the hypertensive disease resulting in severe organ damage.

The rate of progression of benign essential hypertension is variable, but it generally runs a slowly progressive course over a period of 20 to 30 years. Long-standing hypertension produces structural changes in the arterioles throughout the body characterized by fibrosis and hyalinization (sclerosis) of the blood vessel walls. The chief target organs of this condition are the heart, brain, and kidneys. The usual cause of death is myocardial infarction, congestive heart failure, or cerebral vascular accident. If essential hypertension remains benign, only about 1 percent of patients are likely to suffer renal damage sufficient to die of uremia. Proteinuria and mild azotemia may exist for years without symptoms, and most patients who die of uremia do so as a result of the hypertension entering the malignant phase. This occurs in less than 10 percent of the cases of essential hypertension.

Malignant hypertension implies severe hypertension with the diastolic blood pressure greater than 120 to 130 mmHg, grade IV retinopathy,* and renal excretory dysfunction ranging from proteinuria, to hematuria, to azotemia. Malignant hypertension may occur at any time during the course of benign hypertension but usually occurs after many years. Occasionally it occurs de novo especially in black males in their third and fourth decades.

In the kidney, renal arteriosclerosis due to long-standing hypertension results in the disorder called *benign nephrosclerosis*. This disorder is the direct result of ischemia due to the narrowed lumen of the intrarenal blood vessels. The kidney may be reduced in size, usually symmetrically, and has a granular pitted surface. Histologically, the essential lesion is sclerosis of the small arteries and arterioles which is most marked

---

*Grade IV retinopathy refers to the most severe changes in the retina due to hypertension. These changes may be viewed with the ophthalmoscope and consist of vascular sclerosis, exudates, hemorrhages, and papilledema.

in the afferent arterioles. The closure of the arteries and arterioles leads to destruction of the glomeruli and atrophy of the tubules, so that entire nephrons are destroyed.

Malignant nephrosclerosis is a term used to designate the structural renal changes often associated with the malignant phase of essential hypertension.* The kidneys may be of normal size, with minimal granularity and some petechiae from rupture of arterioles, or they may be shrunken and scarred. Histologically, there are three types of lesions: (1) proliferative endarteritis, (2) fibrinoid necrosis of arteriolar walls, and (3) fibrinoid necrosis of glomerular tufts. At first there is marked thickening of the intima of the interlobular arteries caused by proliferation of the endothelial cells. These changes produce an appearance often referred to as "onion skin." The narrowed lumina produce ischemia of the afferent arterioles and the release of renin, and the blood pressure rises still further. Focal necrosis then occurs in the walls of the afferent arterioles, and as the

*Although these gross and microscopic renal lesions are characteristic of the malignant phase of essential hypertension, they are not specific and may be superimposed upon a variety of diseases associated with hypertension (e.g., chronic pyelonephritis, chronic glomerulonephritis, polyarteritis nodosa).

necrosed areas contain fibrin, the change is called *fibrinoid necrosis*. Fibrinoid necrosis of the glomerular tufts is probably an extension of the fibrinoid necrosis of the feeding afferent arterioles. If the blood pressure remains elevated, these localized changes become widespread, with the formation of thrombi, glomerular hemorrhage, infarction of entire nephrons, and rapid death of all renal cells. Figure 41-13 illustrates some of the above lesions.

RENAL ARTERY STENOSIS

The renal artery may be occluded by atherosclerotic plaques or fibrodysplasia causing hypertension which is often of the rapidly progressive type. Atherosclerosis is found chiefly in older men and usually involves the proximal one-third of the renal artery near the aorta. Fibrodysplasia is characterized by excesses in fibrous connective tissue within the layers of the blood vessel and is most apt to occur in middle and distal thirds of

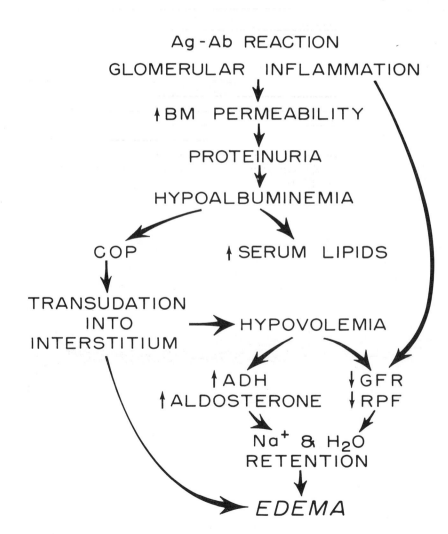

FIGURE 41-12 Pathogenesis of nephrotic edema. (Modified from F. E. Schreiner, "The Nephrotic Syndrome," in M. B. Strauss and L. G. Welt (eds.) Diseases of the Kidney, 2d ed., Little, Brown, Boston, 1971.)

the renal artery and sometimes involves segmental branches. There are several histologic types of fibrodysplasia, and the disorder is most common in women between the ages of 20 and 50 years.

Renal artery stenosis may be unilateral or bilateral. If the caliber of the artery is reduced by 70 percent or more, renal ischemia occurs. The renal ischemia activates the renin-angiotensin system, and hypertension follows. Though uncommon (about 5 to 7 percent of hypertension cases), renal artery stenosis is important because surgical correction may alleviate or markedly ameliorate the hypertensive state.

Unilateral renal artery stenosis not only causes ischemic atrophy of the involved kidney but may eventually cause hypertensive nephrosclerosis of the contralateral kidney. The pathogenetic mechanism is depicted in Fig. 41-14. If the contralateral kidney has developed significant nephrosclerosis from the renin-induced hypertension, the function of the ischemic kidney may even be the better of the two, since the stenosed renal artery protects the occluded kidney from the full effects of the systemic hypertension.

An intravenous pyelogram suggests unilateral renal artery stenosis when it shows a smaller kidney on the affected side (at least 1.5 cm shorter than the other), when there is delayed appearance of the contrast medium or reduced concentration on the affected side, and when late films show an increased density of contrast material. Selective renal arteriography gives further evidence. An elevated plasma renin measurement implies that a renal artery stenosis is significant. The test can be extended to determine the renin concentration from each renal vein in order to discover the source of an elevated renin level.

Tests used

*Contralateral.
on the opposite side*

Elevated plasma renin levels suggest that surgery would be beneficial. Surgical treatment consists of revascularization of the ischemic kidney, often by means of a saphenous vein bypass graft. The increased perfusion suppresses the increased renin secretion, and the hypertension is cured in more than one-half of the cases. Most of the remaining cases are improved by the surgery, allowing easier medical control of the hypertension.

Connective tissue disorders *(Collagen diseases)*

The connective tissue diseases (collagen diseases) are systemic diseases whose manifestations are mainly attributable to the soft tissues of the body (see Part XI). They are of particular interest in nephrology because of the high incidence of renal involvement. About two-thirds of patients with systemic lupus erythematosis (SLE) and progressive systemic sclerosis (scleroderma) have clinical evidence of renal involvement. The incidence is about 80 percent for patients with polyarteritis nodosa. Death from renal failure is common in these patients. In addition, death in uremia occurs in one in four patients with rheumatoid arthritis (to be discussed in "Amyloidosis" later).

SYSTEMIC LUPUS ERYTHEMATOSIS

Systemic lupus erythematosis is a disease that predominantly affects women, who account for 90 percent of the cases. The age of onset is usually between 20 and 40 years. The blood usually gives a positive test for antinuclear factor and LE (lupus erythematosis) cells, especially during the active phase of the disease. Many different tissues and organs may be involved, but renal involvement is the most significant in terms of outcome.

Lupus nephritis is caused by circulating immune complexes which become trapped in the glomerular basement membrane and cause damage. The mechanism is

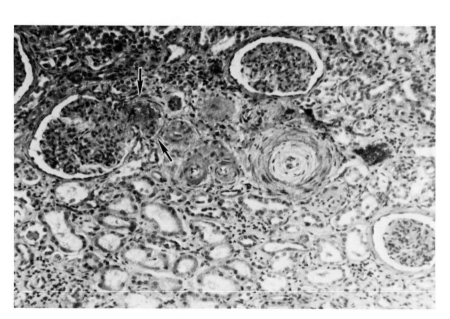

FIGURE 41-13 Malignant nephrosclerosis. Light microscopy slide showing several hyalinized arterioles (center field), dilated tubules with atrophied lining cells (lower center), and an area of fibrinoid necrosis (arrow).

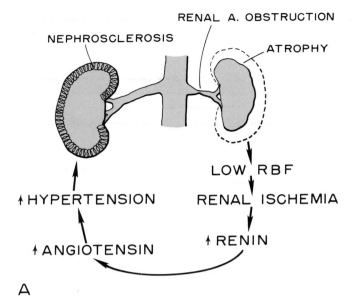

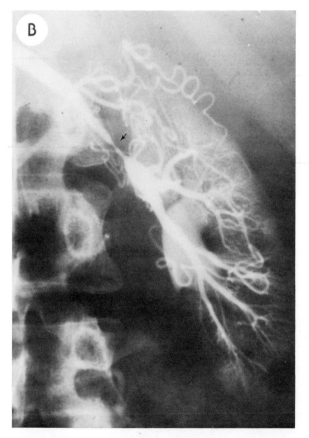

FIGURE 41-14 A. Pathogenesis of nephrosclerosis in the contra-lateral kidney in renal artery stenosis. B. Renal arteriogram show-ing renal artery stenosis due to fibrodysplasia. (Arteriogram from James C. Stanley and William F. Fry, "Renovascular Hyperten-sion Secondary to Arterial Fibrodysplasia in Adults," Archives of Surgery, **110**: 922, 1975. Copyright © 1975, American Medical Association.)

similar to that in APSGN except that the source of the antigen is the body's own DNA rather than the strep-tococcal plasma membrane. In the case of SLE the body produces antibody against its own DNA. The clinical picture may be of an acute glomerulonephritis or of the nephrotic syndrome. Although the basic cause is thought to be the same in each case, focal, membranous, and proliferative changes in the glomeruli may all be seen. The earliest change often involves only part of the glomerular tuft (local), or only scattered glomeruli may be involved (focal). Focal and local glomerulonephritis respond quite well to corticosteroid drugs, and there may be a complete remission. The prognosis is poor for those who develop diffuse membranous or proliferative changes, and these patients often die of renal failure (Fig. 41-15).

POLYARTERITIS NODOSA

Polyarteritis nodosa is an inflammatory and necrotizing disease involving the medium-sized and small arteries throughout the body. Males are more commonly af-fected than females, and the peak incidence is in the seventh decade. Although the exact etiology and patho-genesis are unknown, there is evidence to suggest some form of hypersensitivity mechanism. In many cases the onset is associated with a sensitivity reaction to drugs.

Renal lesions are of two types. If the medium-sized vessels within the kidney are affected, areas of renal infarction develop. If the disease is confined to the arterioles, the renal histology is that of severe, focal, proliferative glomerulonephritis and fibrinoid necrotic changes with epithelial crescents.

Polyarteritis nodosa is treated with corticosteroid drugs, which are more effective during the early course of the disease. The prognosis is generally poor. Death results from uremia or hypertension secondary to the arteritis following a slowly progressive course or one characterized by exacerbations and remissions.

PROGRESSIVE SYSTEMIC SCLEROSIS (scleroderma)

Progressive systemic sclerosis or scleroderma is an un-common, systemic disease characterized by diffuse sclerosis of the skin and other organs. Females are affected more often than males. The onset is usually between the ages of 20 and 50 years. As in SLE, a variety of antibodies may be found in the serum suggesting that immune mechanisms may be involved in the pathogenesis.

The interlobar arteries typically show changes re-sembling hypertensive nephrosclerosis. Progressive renal impairment may develop slowly over a period of years. In a few cases, hypertension and uremia may follow a malignant course with the development of end-stage renal failure within weeks.

Congenital and hereditary disorders

Renal tubular acidosis and polycystic disease of the kidneys are hereditary disorders primarily affecting the renal tubules which may terminate in renal failure, though this is more common in polycyctic disease. Both diseases have an infantile and an adult form, whose manifestations may be quite distinct.

POLYCYSTIC KIDNEY DISEASE (PCKD)

Polycystic kidney disease (PCKD) is characterized by bilateral, multiple, expanding cysts which gradually encroach upon and destroy the normal renal parenchyma by compression. The kidney may be enlarged (sometimes as large as a football) and filled with grapelike clusters of cysts (Fig. 41-16). The cysts are filled with clear or hemorrhagic fluid.

The rare infantile form of the disease appears to be inherited as an autosomal recessive trait. The cysts are closed, blind pouches into which the glomerular filtrate flows. The course of the disease is rapidly progressive, usually resulting in death before the age of 2 years.

In contrast, adult polycystic disease is much more common (about 1 per 500 population); it is an autosomal dominant trait; the cysts communicate with the tubules; and the course is slowly progressive with symptoms of renal insufficiency usually occurring during the fourth decade. Flank pain, hematuria, polyuria, proteinuria, and palpably enlarged, "knobby" kidneys are often the presenting signs and symptoms. Hypertension and urinary tract infections are frequent complications. While this disease is ultimately fatal, some persons may complete a normal life span and die of nonrenal causes. Adult

PCKD is an important disease because of its frequency (third leading cause of end-stage renal failure) and because it is potentially eradicable by genetic counseling.

RENAL TUBULAR ACIDOSIS (RTA)

Primary renal tubular acidosis (RTA) is a clinical disorder in which there is systemic acidosis due to the inability to excrete an appropriately acid urine. RTA may stem from disease of the proximal tubule in which there is defective bicarbonate reabsorption or from disease of the distal tubule in which there is a transport defect for hydrogen ion, resulting in an inability to develop an adequate pH gradient between the blood and urine.

The classic distal RTA in the adult is believed to be transmitted through autosomal dominant heredity. Twice as many females as males are afflicted. The first symptoms generally appear during adolescence or young adulthood. These include bone pain due to osteomalacia, renal colic due to nephrocalcinosis or calculi, and weakness due to hypokalemia. These changes may be explained as a consequence of the tubular defect. The transport defect of H^+ in the distal tubule results in reduced urine titratable acidity and ammonia. Not all the filtered HCO_3^- is reabsorbed. The missing anion is replaced by Cl^-, giving a hyperchloremic acidosis. There is also increased loss of K^+ and Na^+ in the urine. The sustained acidosis due to H^+ retention (or HCO_3^- loss) results in mobilization of Ca^{2+} salts from the bone and hypercalciuria. Bone resorption is manifested as osteomalacia in adults and as rickets in children. Calcium salts may precipitate diffusely in the renal parenchyma (nephrocalcinosis) or within the collecting system (calculi). Renal failure is secondary to these complications. The condition is diagnosed by the urine acidification test described in Chap. 40. Proximal tubule RTA, however, cannot be diagnosed by this test, since these patients can acidify their urine when given an acid load.

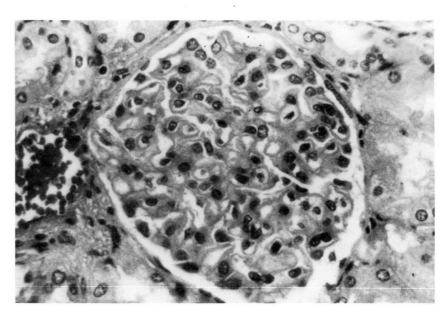

FIGURE 41-15 Glomerulus from a patient with membranous lupus nephritis. Capillary walls (basement membrane) are uniformly thickened, but there is no increase in cellularity. Note the wire-loop appearance. Note the RBCs in the lumen of the tubule (left center).

The infantile form of RTA occurs during the first 18 months of life and commonly presents as a "failure to thrive." It is not believed to be hereditary. The clincial picture is one of thirst, polyuria, anorexia and vomiting, rickets, and sometimes nephrocalcinosis.

RTA is treated by alkali therapy—sodium bicarbonate or citrate in divided doses. The infant responds well to this therapy, and the condition is usually completely reversed. In some adults the calcium deposits are re-absorbed after prolonged alkali therapy while in others the nephrocalcinosis is permanent. The prognosis depends on the extent of renal damage prior to treatment.

Metabolic disorders

Metabolic disorders which may lead to chronic renal failure include diabetes mellitus, gout, primary hyper-parathyroidism, and amyloidosis.

DIABETES MELLITUS

Renal involvement is very common is diabetes. In some of the more recent investigations, over 50 percent of all patients (juvenile- and adult-onset) who had this disease for 20 years were found to be in renal failure.*

Common renal lesions include nephrosclerosis due to lesions of the arterioles, pyelonephritis and necrosis of the renal papilla, and glomerulosclerosis. Glomerulo-sclerosis is the most characteristic lesion and may be diffuse or nodular. Nodular glomerulosclerosis is also known as the *Kimmelstiel-Wilson lesion* and is virtually pathognomonic of diabetes (Fig. 41-17). Both lesions are due to increased deposit of mesangial matrix.† In the

---

*Renal failure is the most common cause of death in juvenile-onset diabetes.

†The mesangial matrix is a spongy network of basement membrane–like trabeculae at the center of the glomerular lobule surrounding the mesangial cells. It merges with the capillary basement membrane.

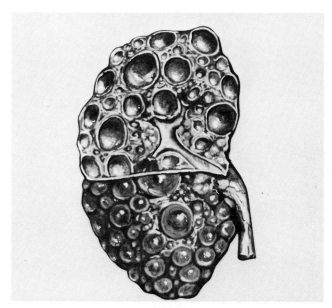

FIGURE 41-16 Polycystic kidney. (Art by Judy Simon, Dept. of Medical and Biological Illustrations, University of Michigan.)

diffuse type, the matrix is more diffusely distributed in each glomerulus and is less discrete. There is more thickening of the peripheral basement membrane. In the nodular type the matrix is deposited within the core of the capillary lobule, giving the appearance of a nodule. Initially the capillary lumina are patent, but they are gradually obliterated as the disease progresses.

Diabetic retinopathy, characterized by microaneurysms around the macula, precedes nearly all cases of diabetic glomerulosclerosis. Proteinuria, hypertension, and an increased incidence of pyelonephritis often precede end-stage renal failure.

GOUT

Gout is a metabolic disease characterized by hyperuricemia (increased plasma uric acid concentrations). There are two forms of the disease. Primary gout is a hereditary disorder of deranged uric acid metabolism affecting males in 95 percent of the cases. Secondary gout may arise either from increased uric acid production in such conditions as leukemia, polycythemia vera, or multiple myeloma, or from decreased uric acid excretion as in chronic renal failure. The source of the increased uric acid in the myeloproliferative disorders is the massive breakdown of cells (which contain nucleoproteins).

The major lesions of gout are principally due to the deposition and crystallization of urates in the fluids and tissues of the body. The joints and kidneys are the prime targets. In chronic gout, deposit of urate crystals in the renal interstitium causes interstitial nephritis and nephrosclerosis. Approximately 20 percent of these patients eventually develop renal failure. Acute renal failure may develop secondary to complete obstruction of renal tubules by uric acid during cytotoxic drug therapy for malignant disease (discussed in Chap. 40).

HYPERPARATHYROIDISM

Primary hyperparathyroidism, resulting in hypersecretion of parathormone, is a relatively rare disease which can result in nephrocalcinosis and subsequent renal failure. The usual cause is adenoma of the parathyroid glands. Secondary hyperparathyroidism is a very common complication of chronic renal failure. Whether the disease is primary or secondary, the manifestations are similar. These will be discussed in detail in Chap. 42.

AMYLOIDOSIS

Amyloidosis is a metabolic disease in which amyloid, an insoluble, waxy glycoprotein, is deposited in the various soft tissues of the body, where it can produce pressure and cause atrophy of the contiguous cells. In primary or congenital amyloidosis, amyloid is more often found in the tongue, heart, gastrointestinal tract, and peripheral nerves than in the kidneys. Secondary amyloidosis is frequently associated with chronic infectious disease, such as tuberculosis, chronic rheumatoid arthritis (25 percent), and multiple myeloma (10 to 20 percent), and with paraplegic patients (40 percent). The kidneys are frequently involved in secondary amyloidosis. The nephrotic syndrome and death from renal failure are common in these patients.

Toxic nephropathy

The kidney is especially vulnerable to the toxic effects of drugs and chemicals for the following reasons: (1) it receives 25 percent of the cardiac output, so it may readily be exposed to large amounts of a chemical; (2) the hyperosmotic interstitium allows chemicals to be concentrated in a relatively hypovascular region; and (3) the kidney is an obligatory excretory route for most drugs, so that renal insufficiency results in drug accumulation and increased concentration in the tubular fluid. The most frequently encountered nephrotoxins result in acute renal failure and will be discussed in Chap. 44. Chronic renal failure may result from analgesic abuse and exposure to lead.

ANALGESIC ABUSE (PHENACETIN NEPHRITIS)

It is now generally accepted that chronic abuse of analgesics can cause renal injury. The responsible ingredient is believed to be phenacetin, a constituent of the common APC tablet (aspirin, phenacetin, and caffeine) and many other over-the-counter preparations. The American tablet contains 150 mg phenacetin. The amount sufficient to induce renal failure is not known with certainty. Gault defines *abuse* as the ingestion of five tablets per day for 3 years, the minimum time-dose to induce a nephrotoxic response. Neurotic individuals or those with chronic headaches are most likely to be analgesic abusers. The highest incidence of this disease is in the Scandinavian countries and in Australia.

The characteristic renal lesion is papillary necrosis and interstitial nephritis. The papillary tips may slough off completely and be excreted in the urine. Since the distal tubule bears the brunt of the disease, urine concentration and acidification tend to be severely impaired, and a salt-losing state may also develop. Common clinical features are hematuria (in cases of papillary necrosis), renal colic (flank pain), and urinary tract infection, including chronic pyelonephritis. Frequently the disease progresses insidiously so that the patient may have advanced chronic renal failure and hypertension at the time of diagnosis.

LEAD NEPHROPATHY

Exposure to lead occurs in a number of occupations and may be ingested in illicitly distilled whisky. Lead intoxication is still a problem in the United States, although not as great as when lead-based paints were used. Lead is chiefly incorporated into the bone and gradually released over a period of years. Lead is also incorporated into renal tubular cells. The basic renal lesion is interstitial nephritis and slowly progressive renal failure.

QUESTIONS

Chronic renal failure—Chap. 41

Directions: Answer the following questions on a separate sheet of paper.

1 What is the major difference between acute and chronic renal failure and what happens to the function of the kidneys in both categories?

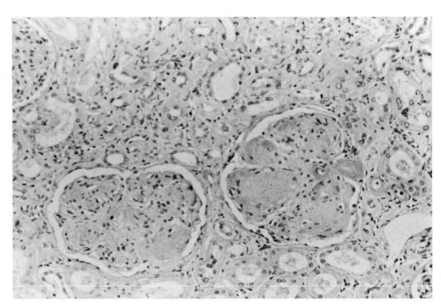

FIGURE 41-17 Diabetic nephropathy (light microscopy) showing the typical nodular lesion in the two central glomeruli. Nodular appearance is due to the deposit of mesangial matrix within the core of the peripheral capillary lobules. Initially the capillary lumina are patent but are gradually obliterated as the disease progresses. Note also the thickening of the basement membrane of the tubules in the lower central field.

2 List the four leading causes of end-stage renal disease and the primary renal structures involved in each case.

3 Name in order the three stages in the natural history of progressive renal failure. What percentage of nephrons have been destroyed in each case?

4 From the list below, indicate whether the laboratory value would be normal, rising just above normal, or rising very sharply.

	BUN	PLASMA CREATININE
First-stage renal failure		
Second-stage renal failure		
Third-stage renal failure		

5 What happens to the creatinine clearance in progressive renal failure?

6 What is the difference between polyuria and oliguria? Define *nocturia*.

7 Explain why the symptoms in question 6 occur as more and more functioning nephrons are destroyed in chronic renal failure. Explain how renal lesions could cause these symptoms.

8 Explain how the normal kidney responds to an increasing solute load, how this condition might be induced, and how this evidence supports the intact nephron hypothesis.

9 What happens to the remaining functioning nephrons in progressive renal failure (size, filtration rate, tubular reabsorption, solute load)?

10 Explain why the original cause of chronic renal failure may be difficult to identify in some cases?

11 Differentiate between symptomatic and asymptomatic bacteriuria as a cause of chronic pyelonephritis.

12 Why is long-term follow-up important in acute pyelonephritis?

13 Why is it often difficult to diagnose chronic pyelonephritis?

14 Recite the arguments for and against the bacterial etiology of chronic pyelonephritis.

15 What is the difference between the typical gross appearance of the kidneys in acute and chronic pyelonephritis?

Directions: Circle the letter preceding each item which correctly answers the questions. Only one answer is correct; exceptions noted.

16 Which of the following best describes nocturia?
a A decrease in the volume of urine   *b* Loss of the normal diurnal pattern of concentrating urine to a greater degree at night   *c* Both *a* and *b*   *d* Neither *a* nor *b*

17 The earliest symptoms of chronic renal failure are which of the following? (More than one answer is correct.)
a Pruritis   *b* Oliguria   *c* Polyuria   *d* Nocturia

18 The most common infecting organism in urinary tract infections is:
a Proteus vulgaris   *b* Klebsiella pneumoniae   *c* Staphylococcus aureus   *d* Escherichia coli

19 Defense mechanisms present in males but lacking in females which may account for their greater resistance to urinary tract infections include which of the following? (More than one answer may be correct.)
a Phagocytic capacity of the bladder epithelium   *b* bactericidal properties of prostatic fluid   *c* Long entry pathway for bacteria   *d* Short urethra

20 A simple, single urethral catheterization leads to urinary tract infection in approximately what percentage of cases?
a 2 percent   *b* 20 percent   *c* 50 percent   *d* 98 percent

21 Conditions interfering with host defense mechanisms in the renal medulla include which of the following? (More than one answer may be correct.)
a High ammonia content   *b* Hypertonicity   *c* Poor blood supply   *d* High glucose content

22 The salt-losing tendency in early chronic renal failure and especially in chronic pyelonephritis is due to:
a Obligatory sodium wastage to preserve acid-base balance   *b* Defective sodium reabsorption   *c* An osmotic diuresis in each functioning nephron   *d* Decreased aldosterone production

23 Factors predisposing to urinary tract infection include:
a Indwelling catheter drainage   *b* Urethral stricture   *c* High progesterone levels in pregnancy   *d* Vesicoureteral reflux   *e* All of these

24 The most important cause of chronic renal failure from a preventive or remediable point of view is probably:
a Chronic pyelonephritis   *b* Chronic glomerulonephritis

Directions: Circle T if the statement is true and F if it is false.

25   T   F   Typical findings in chronic pyelonephritis are intermittent bacteriuria, white blood cells, or white cell casts in the urine.

26   T   F   Absence of bacteriuria rules out chronic pyelonephritis.

27   T   F   In chronic pyelonephritis, the concentrating ability of the kidney is often diminished before there is a significant decrease in GFR.

Directions: Fill in the blanks with the correct words.

28 In acute pyelonephritis, _____ (inflammatory cells) are usually found throughout the cortex and medulla and segments of the _____ are destroyed. Whereas in chronic pyelonephritis, in the interstitium there are many _____ and _____ cells.

29 Label Fig. 41-18 by matching the letters with the renal histologic findings from the list below.
_____ Normal tubule
_____ Area of interstitial fibrosis
_____ Hypertrophied tubule with atrophy of epithelial cells
_____ Atrophied tubule containing cast
_____ Inflammatory cells (PMNs)

Directions: Answer the following questions on a separate sheet of paper.

30 Define the term *glomerulonephritis.*

31 Why does confusion exist in the classification and separation of the various types of glomerulonephritis?

32 Name three types of glomerulonephritis based on clinical classification. What is the prognosis of each type, generally speaking? Describe their natural history and relationship.

33 Describe the classic case of acute poststreptococcal glomerulonephritis with respect to common age group affected, causative organisms, signs and symptoms, major physiological disturbances, pathogenetic mechanisms involved, and treatment.

34 What is the nephrotic syndrome? Why does the patient become edematous? What diseases is it commonly associated with? General principles of treatment?

35 Explain the importance of early diagnosis of unilateral renal artery stenosis. Explain the mechanism resulting in damage to the contralateral kidney (illustrate).

36 List three reasons why the kidney is especially vulnerable to the toxic effect of drugs or chemicals.

Directions: Match the descriptions in col. B to the terms in col. A which refer to the distribution of glomerular lesions.

Column A	Column B
37 _____ Diffuse	a Only a portion of the glomeruli are involved.
38 _____ Local	b Part of the glomerulus is involved.
39 _____ Focal	c All of the glomeruli are affected.

Directions: Match the descriptive characteristics in col. B to the appropriate pathogenic immune mechanism in col. A.

Column A	Column B
40 _____ Circulating immune complex	a Associated with Goodpasture's syndrome.
41 _____ Anti-GBM	b Associated with APSGN and SLE.
	c Immunoglobulin is deposited subepithelially.
	d Immunoglobulin is deposited subendothelially.
	e Autoimmune mechanism.
	f Linear or ribbonlike pattern of deposit on immunofluorescent biopsy slide.
	g Ag-Ab complexes are mechanically trapped in the filtration membrane.
	h Results in more serious injury to the glomerulus.

Directions: Match the appropriate description in col. B to the histologic type of glomerulonephritis in col. A. (Letters may be used more than once.)

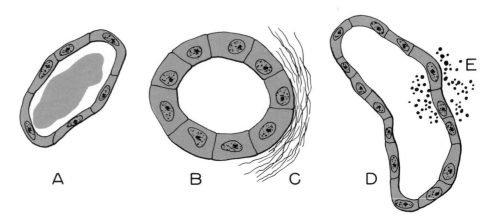

Column A | Column B

42 ＿＿ Minimal change GN
43 ＿＿ Membranous GN
44 ＿＿ Proliferative GN

a Primary change in the glomerulus is an increase in endothelial, mesangial, or epithelial cells.
b Predominant change is thickening of the basement membrane.
c Only morphological change is fusion of the foot processes.
d Most common lesion in children associated with the nephrotic syndrome.
e Nephrotic patients with these lesions often progress to renal failure.

Directions: Match the descriptive phrases in col. B with the terms in col. A to which they apply. (Letters may be used more than once.)

Column A | Column B

45 ＿＿ Polycystic kidney disease (adult form)
46 ＿＿ Polycystic kidney disease (infantile form)
47 ＿＿ RTA (adult form)
48 ＿＿ RTA (child form)
49 ＿＿ Kimmelsteil-Wilson disease
50 ＿＿ Gout
51 ＿＿ Hyperparathyroidism
52 ＿＿ Amyloidosis

a Characteristic lesion of diabetic nephropathy.
b Hereditary disorder.
c Commonly presents as "failure to thrive."
d Nephrocalcinosis is a common complication.
e Deposits in kidney common in rheumatoid arthritis, paraplegia, and multiple myeloma.
f Cysts communicate with tubules.
g Cysts are closed.
h Urate crystals may be deposited in the renal tubules or interstitium.
i Treated with sodium bicarbonate or sodium citrate.
j Urine acidification test may aid in diagnosis.

Directions: Circle the letter preceding each item which correctly answers the questions. Only one answer is correct; exceptions noted.

53 Which of the following antibodies is most significant in the pathogenesis of the glomerulonephritis of systemic lupus erythematosis?
a Anti-RNA b Anti-GBM c Anti-DNA
d Antikidney

54 Which statement is false with respect to immune-complex glomerulonephritis?
a Ag-Ab complexes form in the blood and circulate to the glomerulus. b PMNs produce glomerular injury

FIGURE 41-18 Histologic findings in chronic pyelonephritis.

by the release of lysosomal enzymes. c Immunofluorescent studies show a pattern of granular deposits. d The major glomerular injury is caused by streptococcal renal infection.

55 Which of the following findings is uncommon in APSGN?
a Decreased serum complement b Ability to produce concentrated urine c Massive proteinuria (nephrotic syndrome) d Red cell casts

56 Which of the following types of glomerulonephritis (GN) associated with the nephrotic syndrome does not show evidence of an immune pathogenetic mechanism?
a Idiopathic membranous GN b Minimal lesion GN (lipoid nephrosis) c Membranoproliferative GN d Proliferative GN of systemic lupus erythematosis

57 Mortality from minimal change GN is primarily due to:
a Infection b Toxic effects of corticosteroid drugs c Acute renal failure d Chronic renal failure

58 Which of the following statements is false concerning the histologic changes in the end-stage kidney of chronic glomerulonephritis?
a Only the glomeruli are involved in the pathological destruction. b Destructive lesions involving the glomeruli, renal tubules, and vasculature are all present. c Some glomeruli are completely hyalinized. d Epithelial crescents are frequently seen.

59 The characteristic lesion in benign nephrosclerosis is:
a Fibrinoid necrosis, glomerular hemorrhage
b Nodular glomerulosclerosis c Hyalinized thickening of the arteriolar walls with narrowing of lumina
d Widespread infarction of entire nephrons

60 The leading cause of death in systemic lupus erythematosis is:
a Infection b Renal disease c Hemorrhage
d Neurologic lesions

61 Which of the following commonly precedes diabetic glomerulosclerosis?
a Hyperlipidemia b Hypertension c Retinopathy
d Increased insulin requirement

62 Which statements are true concerning scleroderma?
a Renal changes resemble those of hypertensive nephrosclerosis. b Immunopathic mechanisms may be involved in causation. c Incidence is higher in females. d All are correct.

63 Which statements are true concerning polyarteritis nodosa? (More than one answer may be correct.)
a Most frequently affects young adult females. b Arterial lesions in the kidney are common. c Other renal lesions include proliferative GN and tubular atrophy.

64 Chronic abuse of which of the following drugs may result in papillary necrosis?
a Ethyl alcohol b Aspirin c Phenacetin
d Caffeine

Directions: Circle T if the statement is true and F if false. Correct the false statements.

65   T   F   Surgical correction of renal artery stenosis or removal of the ischemic kidney always results in cure of the hypertension.

66   T   F   About one-third of all patients with SLE, PN, and scleroderma have clinical evidence of renal disease.

67   T   F   SLE patients with focal and local glomerular lesions respond well to corticosteroid therapy and the prognosis is good.

68   T   F   The most frequent cause of death in juvenile-onset diabetes is uremia.

69   T   F   Hypoproteinemia is important in the pathogenesis of edema in APSGN.

70   T   F   The kidney is larger than normal with multiple petechiae on the surface in advanced chronic renal failure.

71   T   F   Polyuria and "salt wasting" are common clinical features of analgesic nephropathy.

72   T   F   Chronic renal failure may cause hypertension.

73   T   F   Widespread epithelial crescent formation signifies remission and a good prognosis in chronic renal failure.

74   T   F   Immunopathic mechanisms are probably involved in the pathogenesis of most of the connective tissue disorders.

CHAPTER 42 The Uremic Syndrome

OBJECTIVES **At the completion of Chap. 42 you should be able to:**

1 Define the *uremic syndrome.*

2 Relate the decrease in GFR to the development of the uremic syndrome.

3 Distinguish between two groups of clinical symptoms present in the uremic syndrome.

4 Describe the events that lead to the development of metabolic acidosis in the uremic syndrome.

5 Explain why the total NH_4^+ excretion is decreased in renal failure.

6 Explain why the acidosis of chronic renal failure usually stabilizes at a moderate level.

7 List three symptoms common in the uremic patient which may be associated with renal acidosis.

8 Describe Kussmaul respirations.

9 Discuss the development of potassium imbalances in chronic renal failure.

10 Explain why systemic acidosis contributes to hyperkalemia.

11 Describe the most serious complication of hyperkalemia.

12 Differentiate between early renal insufficiency and terminal renal failure in relation to the ability of the kidney to regulate sodium.

13 Explain what condition may result in renal failure when magnesium is not excreted.

14 Explain why uremic patients may have attacks of gouty arthritis.

15 Explain the meaning of a constant finding of the urine specific gravity at 1.010.

16 Describe how uremia usually affects sexual and reproductive function.

17 Describe cardiovascular, respiratory, and hematologic manifestations of the uremic syndrome.

18 List some of the factors that predispose the uremic patient to infection.

19 Describe changes in skin coloration in the uremic patient for Caucasian and dark-skinned patients.

20 Describe hair and nail changes associated with renal failure.

21 Describe "uremic frost."

22 Explain why the uremic patient often complains of itching.

23 Describe the gastrointestinal manifestations of uremia.

24 Give the rationale for dietary restriction of protein in the uremic patient.

25 Explain how protein, fat, and carbohydrate metabolism is altered in the uremic patient.

26 Describe muscular and central nervous system disturbances associated with the uremic syndrome.

27 Describe peripheral neuropathy and the stages in its development.

28 Describe renal osteodystrophy and the types of bone disorders present in this disorder.

29 Discuss the pathogenesis of secondary hyperparathyroidism and the bone disorders associated with terminal renal failure.

30 Explain the significance of the calcium-phosphate cross product.

31 List some common sites of calcium salts deposition in metastatic soft-tissue calcification.

32 Give the etiology of "uremic red eye."

Each of the principal kidney diseases that lead to chronic progressive renal failure has unique features which relate to etiology, pathogenesis, and morphology. These differences were discussed in Chap. 41. It was also pointed out that these diseases produce kidneys which may have many morphological features in common. This is particularly true when the terminal stage of chronic renal disease is reached, when it may be difficult to determine the etiology of the chronic renal failure by examination of the end-stage kidney.

You also learned in Chap. 41 that, from a functional point of view, regardless of the cause there is a common sequence of changes in renal function due to the progressive destruction of nephrons. The rate of destruction can vary greatly, with quiescent periods and exacerbations, and the duration from beginning to end may vary from months to as long as 40 years. However, once the GFR begins to fall and the BUN and creatinine levels rise, there is a tendency toward rapid progression to end-stage renal failure. Because of these common functional patterns, it is possible to consider the events in the pathophysiology of chronic renal failure as a single phenomenon rather than discuss the changes in function on a disease-by-disease basis.

MANIFESTATIONS OF THE UREMIC SYNDROME

The common sequence of changes has this effect on the patient: When the GFR falls to 5 to 10 percent of normal and progresses towards zero, the patient develops what is called the uremic syndrome. The *uremic syndrome* is a symptom complex that results from or is associated with retention of nitrogenous metabolites because of renal failure. In advanced uremia, some functions of virtually every organ system in the body may become abnormal.

Two groups of clinical symptoms are present in the uremic syndrome. First, symptoms referrable to deranged regulatory and excretory functions are prominent: fluid volume and electrolyte abnormalities, acid-base imbalance, retention of nitrogenous and other metabolites, and anemia due to renal secretory deficiency. A second group of clinical features includes a constellation of cardiovascular, neuromuscular, gastrointestinal, and other abnormalities. Surprisingly little is known about the basis of these multiple-system abnormalities, though diligent research is now being conducted to uncover these mysteries. Table 42-1 lists some of the common manifestations of the uremic syndrome which will be discussed in this chapter.

Biochemical disturbances

METABOLIC ACIDOSIS $\angle 40-60$ meq/day of H^+

Renal failure is characterized by a wide variety of biochemical disturbances. One of the constant abnormalities exhibited by the uremic patient is metabolic acidosis. On a normal diet, the kidney has to excrete 40 to 60 meq/day of H^+ in order to prevent acidosis. In renal failure, impaired ability of the kidney to excrete H^+ results in a systemic acidosis with a decrease in the plasma pH and HCO_3^- concentration. The HCO_3^- level decreases because it is used up in buffering H^+. NH_4^+ excretion is the kidney's most important mechanism for the excretion of H^+ and the regeneration of HCO_3^- (since it allows de novo addition of new HCO_3^- rather than just reabsorption of the filtered HCO_3^- to the extracellular fluid). Total NH_4^+ excretion is decreased in renal failure due to the diminished number of nephrons. Phosphate excretion provides another mechanism for the excretion of H^+ as titratable acid (i.e., phosphate-buffered H^+). The rate of phosphate excretion, however, is determined by the need to maintain phosphate balance rather than acid-base balance. Phosphate tends to be retained in renal failure due to the diminished nephron mass and to factors related to calcium metabolism which will be discussed later. The retention of sulfate and other organic anions also contributes to the depletion of HCO_3^-.

The serum bicarbonate level usually stabilizes at about 18 to 20 meq/liter (moderate acidosis) and rarely progresses below this level. The most likely explanation for this lack of progression in the presence of a positive hydrogen-ion balance is that hydrogen ion is being buffered by calcium carbonate from the bone.

It is possible that the symptoms of anorexia, nausea, and lethargy that are common in the uremic patient may be due in part to the acidosis. One symptom which is undoubtedly due to acidosis is Kussmaul respirations, though this symptom may be less prominent in chronic acidosis. *Kussmaul respirations* are deep, sighing respirations which occur because of the need to increase carbon dioxide excretion and thus reduce the severity of the acidosis.

POTASSIUM IMBALANCES

Potassium imbalance is one of the very serious disturbances which may occur in renal failure because only a very narrow plasma concentration range is compatible with life (normal = 3.5 to 5 meq/liter). About 80 percent of the normal intake of 60 to 80 meq/day is excreted in the urine. Hypokalemia may be associated with the polyuria of early chronic renal failure particularly in tubular diseases such as chronic pyelonephritis. However, as the patient becomes oliguric in end-stage renal failure, hyperkalemia invariably develops.

The systemic acidosis also contributes to the hyperkalemia by causing K^+ to shift from the cells to the extracellular fluid. The major life-threatening effect of hyperkalemia is its influence on the electrical conduction of the heart. Fatal arrhythmias of cardiac standstill may occur when serum K^+ levels reach 7 to 8 meq/liter.

TABLE 42-1
Manifestations of the uremic syndrome

Biochemical	Metabolic acidosis (serum HCO_3^- 18–20 meq/liter)		Ammoniacal odor to breath
	Azotemia ($\downarrow$ GFR $\rightarrow$ $\uparrow$ BUN, $\uparrow$ creatinine)		Metallic taste, dry mouth
	Hyperkalemia		Stomatitis, parotitis
	Sodium retention or wasting		Gastritis, enteritis
	Hypermagnesemia		GI bleeding
	Hyperuricemia		Diarrhea
Genitourinary	Polyuria $\rightarrow$ oliguria $\rightarrow$ anuria	Intermediate metabolism	Protein—intolerance, abnormal synthesis
	Nocturia, reversal of diurnal rhythm		Carbohydrate—hyperglycemia, $\downarrow$ insulin need
	Fixed urine sp. gr. 1.010		
	Proteinuria; casts		Fat—$\uparrow$ triglycerides
	Loss of libido, amenorrhea, impotency, sterility	Neuromuscular	Easy fatigability
Cardiovascular	Hypertension		Muscle wasting, weakness
	Hypertensive retinopathy, encephalopathy		Central nervous system
			Decreased mental acuity
	Circulatory overload		Poor concentration
	Edema		Apathy
	Congestive heart failure		Lethargy/restlessness, insomnia
	Pericarditis (friction rub)		Mental confusion
Respiratory	Kussmaul breathing, dyspnea		Coma
	Pulmonary edema		Muscle twitching, asterixis, convulsions
	Pneumonitis		Peripheral neuropathy
Hematologic	Anemia $\rightarrow$ fatigue		Slowed nerve conduction, restless leg syndrome
	Hemolysis		
	Bleeding tendency		Sensory changes in the extremities—paresthesias
	$\downarrow$ Resistance to infection (urinary tract infection, pneumonia, septicemia)		Motor changes—foot drop $\rightarrow$ paraplegia
Cutaneous	Pallor, pigmentation		
	Hair and nail changes (nails brittle, thin, ridged, alternating red and light bands associated with protein wasting)	Calcium and skeletal disorders	Hyperphosphatemia, hypocalcemia
			Secondary hyperparathyroidism
	Pruritis		Renal osteodystrophy
	Uremic "frost"		Pathological fractures (demineralization of bones)
	Dry skin		
	Bruises		Calcium salts deposited in soft tissue (around joints, blood bessels)
Gastrointestinal	Anorexia, nausea, vomiting $\rightarrow$ weight loss		Conjunctivitis (uremic red eye)

SODIUM IMBALANCES

In most normal persons, there is great flexibility in the kidney's ability to vary excretion of sodium in response to a variable intake. Salt excretion may vary from nearly zero to as much as 20 g/day. Patients with chronic renal failure lose this great flexibility and may be "poised on a razor's edge" with respect to the ability to vary salt output. In early renal insufficiency when there is polyuria, there may be salt wasting because of the increased solute load of each intact nephron. The osmotic diuresis results in obligatory salt losses. This salt-losing tendency is more common in chronic pyelonephritis and polycystic kidneys, which primarily affect the tubules.

When oliguria supervenes in terminal renal failure, the patient is more likely to retain sodium. The retention of sodium and water may result in circulatory overload, edema, hypertension, and congestive heart failure. The development of congestive heart failure secondary to the hypertension and the increased aldosterone levels present in uremic patients may also play a major role in sodium retention.

HYPERMAGNESEMIA

Like potassium, magnesium is chiefly an intercellular cation and is excreted chiefly by the kidneys. The ability to excrete magnesium is reduced in the uremic patient. However, hypermagnesemia is generally not a serious problem since intake of magnesium is usually reduced due to anorexia, reduced protein intake, and decreased absorption from the gastrointestinal tract. A sudden load of magnesium from the ingestion of laxatives such as milk of magnesia or magnesium citrate may cause death.

AZOTEMIA

As has been previously discussed, a sharp rise in the plasma urea and creatinine levels generally signals the onset of terminal renal failure and accompanies uremic symptoms. There is much evidence, however, that urea itself is not responsible for the symptoms and metabolic defects found in uremia. Some of the substances found in the blood of uremic patients which might act as toxins are the guanidines. Some of these compounds act as potent enzyme inhibitors. It is more likely that a combination of factors such as the acidosis and other electrolyte disturbances, hormonal disturbances, and retained "toxins" produce the metabolic defects and the multiple-system involvement.

HYPERURICEMIA

We have alluded to the intimate association of gout and the kidney in Chap. 41. A rise in serum uric acid concentration and the formation of obstructive crystals in the kidney can cause chronic or acute renal failure. On the other hand, the serum uric acid level generally rises early in the course of chronic renal failure due to excretory impairment of the kidneys. The kidneys normally account for about 75 percent of the excreted uric acid. A rise in serum uric acid concentration above the normal 4 to 6 mg% may or may not be associated with symptoms. It is not uncommon, however, for uremic patients to have attacks of gouty arthritis due to the deposition of urate salts in the joints and soft tissues.

Genitourinary disturbances (Ꮞ‌Ꮜ)

Urinary symptoms in uremia are intimately associated with water metabolism. We have already discussed these findings in previous chapters. Polyuria due to osmotic diuresis gradually gives way to oliguria and even anuria as the nephron mass is gradually destroyed. Nocturia and a reversal of the normal diurnal pattern of urine excretion, resulting in a relatively constant rate of urine formation throughout the day and night, is another important symptom due to the osmotic diuresis. A constant urine specific gravity near 1.010 in the uremic patient reflects the loss of the ability to concentrate or dilute the urine from that of the plasma concentration. These changes make the uremic patient vulnerable to acute changes in water balance. Diarrhea or vomiting may quickly cause dehydration (with subsequent hypovolemia, decreased GFR, and further deterioration of renal function), and excess water intake may cause circulatory overload, edema, and congestive heart failure.

As the nephron mass and the GFR decrease, proteinuria, which may have been prominent earlier in the chronic renal disease, may become insignificant or may disappear altogether. Broad, granular casts may occasionally be found in the urine sediment and are characteristic of advanced renal failure.

The young uremic female ceases to menstruate, and the male is generally impotent and sterile when the GFR falls to 5 ml/minute. Both sexes experience a loss of libido as the uremia becomes more severe. Sexual and reproductive function may return after renal transplantation or a regular hemodialysis program. Most physicians, however, advise women not to become pregnant when there is advanced renal insufficiency.

Cardiovascular abnormalities

Hypertension and congestive heart failure often accompany the uremic syndrome. The combination of hypertension, anemia, and circulatory overload due to sodium and water retention all contribute to the increased propensity for congestive heart failure. Other side effects of severe hypertension include retinopathy and encephalopathy. The symptoms of these disorders are the same as in nonuremic patients.

A fibrinous pericarditis is clinically evident in about one-half the patients presenting with severe uremia. The patient may complain of pain on deep inspiration or when lying down, but about two-thirds of the patients are asymptomatic. A "to-and-fro" friction rub may be heard over the precordium with auscultation. Occasionally the patient with uremic pericarditis may develop a massive hemorrhagic effusion and cardiac tamponade. In the event of this emergency, prompt aspiration of the fluid by the physician may be lifesaving.

Respiratory changes

The deep, sighing (Kussmaul) respirations of severe acidosis have already been mentioned. However, the patient with moderate acidosis of chronic renal insufficiency is more apt to complain of dyspnea on exertion, and the increased depth of breathing is overlooked except by an experienced observer.

Other respiratory complications of renal failure are the "uremic lung" and pneumonitis. Chest x-ray of the uremic lung reveals a bilateral butterfly-shaped infiltration of the lungs (Fig. 42-1). It is actually pulmonary edema and is inevitably associated with fluid overload due to sodium and water retention and/or left ventricular failure. Bilateral infection causing a pneumonitis may be superimposed on the chronically wet lung. Pulmonary congestion disappears with the reduction of body fluids by salt restriction and hemodialysis.

Hematologic problems

A characteristically normochromic, normocytic anemia is an inevitable feature of the uremic syndrome. Usually the hematocrit falls to the 20 to 30 percent range and

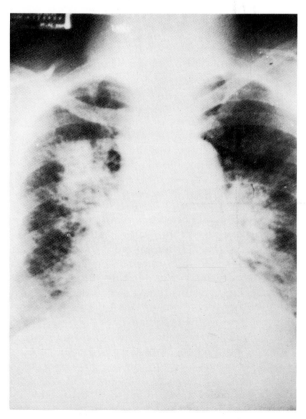

FIGURE 42-1 *Uremic lung, showing marked central distribution of pulmonary edema. (From George L. Bailey,* Hemodialysis, *Academic, New York, 1972.)*

parallels the degree of azotemia. The primary cause of the anemia is bone marrow suppression due to the deficient or absent production of erythropoietin by the failing kidneys. A second factor contributing to the anemia is that the life span of the red blood cell (RBC) in a patient with renal failure is about one-half that of the normal person. The increased hemolysis of red blood cells (RBCs) appears to be due to the abnormal chemical environment in the plasma and not to a defect in the cells themselves. In addition to the deficient erythropoiesis and hemolytic tendency, blood loss in the gastrointestinal tract may further aggravate the anemia. The bleeding tendency of uremia is apparently due to a qualitative defect in the platelets and consequently results in defective adhesion. Inhibition of certain coagulation factors may also play a role.

Pallor due to persistent anemia is characteristic of the anemic patient. The anemia undoubtedly contributes to the symptoms of fatigue. Dyspnea on exertion may be experienced when the hemoglobin is 8 g% or less. Bruising, nosebleeds, and GI bleeding may be manifestations of the coagulation defect.

Infection is a fairly common complication of patients with advanced renal insufficiency. Poor nutrition, pulmonary edema, and the use of cannulas and indwelling catheters may be predisposing factors to the increased susceptibility to infection. The use of large doses of corticosteroid and other immunosuppressive drugs following renal transplant to suppress tissue rejection makes these patients unusually susceptible to severe infection which may result in death.

Cutaneous changes

The accumulation of urinary pigments (principally urochrome) combined with anemia in advanced renal insufficiency gives the skin of the Caucasian person a peculiar waxy, yellow cast. In the brown-skinned person, this is observed as a yellowish brown coloration, and in the black-skinned person as an ashen-gray color with yellow tones, particularly on the palmar and plantar surfaces. The skin may be dry and scaly, and the hair may be brittle and may change color. The nails may be thin, brittle, ridged, and show alternating light and reddish bands. These nail changes are characteristic of chronic protein wasting (Muercke's lines). Pruritis is common in the uremic patient and is considered to be a manifestation of increased parathyroid gland function and deposition of calcium in the skin. When the BUN level is very high, fine, white crystals of urea may appear on areas of the skin where there is heavy perspiration. This is called "uremic frost." Uremic frost is not ordinarily seen when good hygienic care is given to the skin. Multiple bruises caused by minor trauma are often seen on the skin of the uremic patient due to increased capillary fragility.

Gastrointestinal signs and symptoms

The gastrointestinal manifestations of uremia can cause the patient great distress. Anorexia, nausea, and vomiting are very common in uremia and are often the first symptoms of disease. They are responsible, in part, for the extensive loss of weight in chronic renal failure. The entire GI tract itself becomes affected in uremia. Patients often complain of a metallic taste in the mouth, and there may be an odor of ammonia to the breath. The mouth may become inflamed and ulcerated (stomatitis), and the tongue may be dry and coated. Occasionally parotitis (inflammation of the parotid gland) occurs. The normal flora of the mouth contains organisms (tooth calculus bacteria) which can split urea in the saliva to produce ammonia. This accounts for the uriniferous odor to the breath and altered sense of taste, and predisposes the tissue to inflammation and infection. Mucosal ulcerations may occur in the stomach and the small or large intestine, and may result in profuse bleeding. The effect of GI hemorrhage is extremely serious, as the fall in blood pressure lowers the GFR even further, and the digestion of the blood causes a precipitous rise in the BUN level. Diarrhea occurs at times and may cause serious dehydration.

Intermediate metabolism abnormalities

Abnormalities of intermediate metabolism are characteristic of the uremic syndrome though the physiological mechanisms are poorly understood, as they are in other body systems.

PROTEIN

Whatever other elements are responsible for uremic symptoms, the breakdown products of protein metabolism are of prime importance. The dietary restriction of protein generally relieves somewhat the symptoms of lassitude, nausea, and anorexia, though it does not improve the GFR. The patient tends to decrease protein intake voluntarily as azotemia progresses, since the appetite for protein foods generally is lost. Another reason for protein restriction in uremia is because H^+, K^+, and phosphates are derived chiefly from protein foods and must be restricted to prevent accumulation in the blood. There is evidence of abnormal protein synthesis in uremia manifested by elevation or depression of selected amino acids. The significance of this phenomenon is not known.

CARBOHYDRATES AND FATS

Defective carbohydrate metabolism is commonly associated with uremia. Fasting blood sugar levels are elevated in more than 50 percent of uremic patients but not usually over 200 mg%. Insensitivity of the peripheral tissues to insulin is the possible cause. On the other hand, insulin-dependent diabetics who develop uremia may improve their carbohydrate metabolism and require a lower dosage of insulin, in apparent contradiction to the glucose intolerance of nondiabetics. A possible explanation is an elevated serum insulin level due to a prolonged half-life (the kidney normally inactivates insulin) in uremia. Carbohydrate metabolism generally becomes normal with regular hemodialysis.

Abnormal fat metabolism is manifested by high serum triglyceride levels in the uremic patient, even in patients who are regularly dialyzed.

Neuromuscular abnormalities

Involvement of the neuromuscular system is a nearly universal complication of uremia. Both the central and peripheral nervous system are involved with diverse consequences. The muscles may be involved partly through the peripheral neuropathy and partly through the muscle wasting.

CENTRAL NERVOUS SYSTEM

The degree of cerebral disturbance roughly parallels the degree of azotemia. Early symptoms are decreased mental acuity and ability to concentrate, apathy, and lethargy. The patient complains of feeling weak and tired and may be unable to perform a normal day's work without frequent rest periods. Lethargy may alternate with periods of restlessness and insomnia. The untreated patient will eventually become confused and comatose. If convulsions occur, they are usually associated with hypertensive encephalopathy. Neuromuscular irritability is reflected by involuntary jerking and twitching of muscles. Asterixis (flapping tremor of the hands) may sometimes be present and is a manifestation of cerebral toxicity. The physical sign is induced by having the patient raise both arms with forearms fixed and fingers extended; this will result in alterations of flexion and extension at the wrist (flapping tremor).

PERIPHERAL NEUROPATHY

Affliction of the peripheral nervous system follows a characteristic course. The earliest sign of peripheral neuropathy is the slowing of nerve conduction. The "restless leg syndrome" may sometimes be an early symptom. The patient may describe this symptom as a peculiar feeling which is relieved by walking or moving the legs. The second stage in the development of peripheral neuropathy is the advent of sensory changes in the extremities. The patient experiences burning pain, numbness, or tingling (paresthesias) of the toes and feet, which progresses up the leg in a stockinglike fashion. Later, paresthesias may occur in the fingers and hands. Finally, motor nerves are involved. Motor involvement usually begins as a "foot drop" and may progress to paraplegia.

Hemodialysis may halt the progress of peripheral neuropathy, but once these changes occur, they are

poorly reversible (sensory) or irreversible (motor). Therefore, hemodialysis (or transplant) should be started before clinical signs and symptoms occur.

547
MANIFESTATIONS OF THE
UREMIC SYNDROME

Calcium and skeletal disorders (renal osteodystrophy)

If a patient with chronic renal failure survives long
enough, calcium and phosphate imbalances with skeletal
involvement are inevitable. The skeletal disorders called
renal osteodystrophy consist of three lesions.

Osteomalacia is the most common bone disorder
and is seen in about 60 percent of all patients with
chronic renal failure. It consists of defective mineralization of bone. It is caused by a deficiency of 1,25-di-
hydroxycholecalciferol [1,25(OH)$_2$D$_3$], the most active
form of vitamin D metabolized by the kidneys. The
deficiency of the most active form of vitamin D leads to
severely impaired absorption of calcium from the gut.
In the bone, osteoblasts continue to manufacture
osteoid tissue (the framework on which calcium salts are
laid down to produce bone) but the low serum calcium
level and ineffective action of vitamin D on the bone do
not allow mineralization. Osteoid tissue eventually
replaces normal bone, producing osteomalacia in adults
and rickets in children. Osteoid is structurally weak and

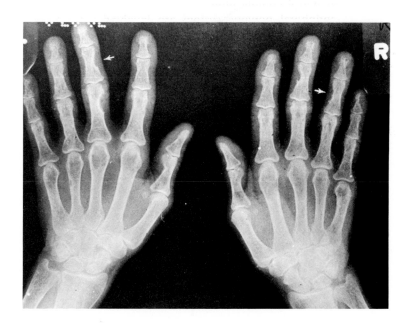

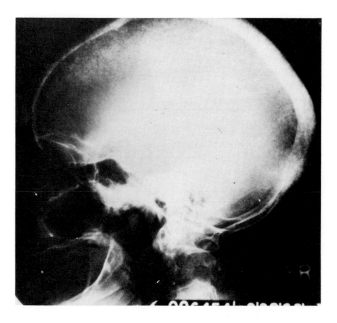

FIGURE 42-2 *Renal osteodystrophy. A. Subperiosteal resorption
is present in all phalanges but is seen best on the middle phalanx
of both the right and left hands (arrows) producing a jagged appearance. B. Skull x-ray shows spotty demineralization of bone
producing a "moth-eaten" appearance. (Courtesy of D. E.
Schteingart.)*

may fracture or deform under stress. On x-ray, osteomalacia presents as a generalized decrease in bone density, especially of the hands, skull, ribs, and spine.

Osteitis fibrosa, occurring in over 30 percent of patients, is characterized by osteoclastic resorption of bone and replacement by fibrous tissue. The bone demineralization may be localized and may present as cystlike lesions (osteitis fibrosa cystica) or may appear as a generalized decrease in bone density on the x-ray. Osteitis fibrosa is caused by the increased levels of parathormone (secondary hyperparathyroidism) in chronic renal failure. The classic x-ray appearance of osteitis fibrosa is often seen in the fingers as subperiosteal bone resorption and in the skull as a patchy loss of bone density (Fig. 42-2).

Osteosclerosis is the third, less common bone disorder and is often manifested as a banded or striped appearance of the vertebrae ("rugger-jersey spine") on x-ray due to alternate bands of decreased and increased bone density.

Any of the above lesions may occur alone but a combination is more common. Hemodialysis alone does not prevent renal osteodystrophy. Only within the past few years has research uncovered some of the complex relationships in the pathogenesis of renal osteodystrophy so that effective treatment is possible. The principal factors are decreased renal function, secondary hyperparathyroidism, and vitamin D deficiency and/or resistance.

PATHOGENESIS OF RENAL OSTEODYSTROPHY

The sequence of events leading to secondary hyperparathyroidism and renal osteodystrophy is most easily followed in Fig. 42-3.

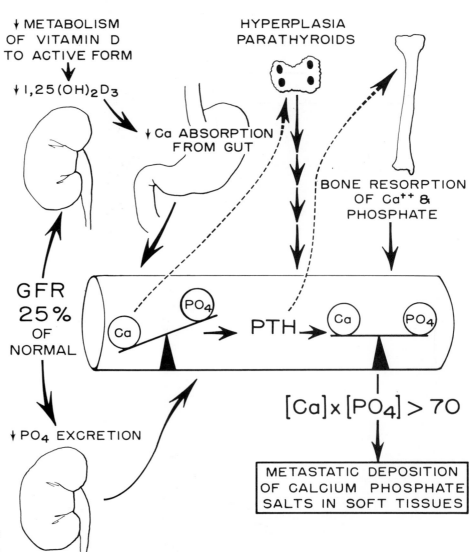

FIGURE 42-3 Pathogenesis of renal osteodystrophy. (See text for explanation.)

Normally the serum calcium and phosphate are in equilibrium with solid-phase calcium and phosphate in the bones. The absorption from the gut, excretion by the kidneys, deposition and resorption from the bone of these minerals is primarily controlled by parathormone (PTH) and vitamin D. Moreover, serum calcium and phosphate levels have a reciprocal relationship, i.e., when serum calcium levels go up, serum phosphate levels go down and vice versa. This interrelationship serves the purpose of keeping the serum calcium-phosphate cross product constant so that precipitation of calcium phosphate does not occur in the vascular system. For example, the normal serum calcium level is 9.0 to 11.0 mg%, and the normal phosphate level is 3.0 to 4.5 mg%. The normal cross-product value in mg% of calcium and phosphate is thus: 3 to 4.5 × 9 to 11 = 27.0 to 49.5. Precipitation of calcium phosphate salts in the soft tissues is believed to occur when their cross product exceeds 60 to 70 mg%.

As renal disease advances, calcium-phosphate interrelationships become progressively disrupted. When the GFR falls to about 25 percent of normal, phosphate is retained by the kidneys. Phosphate retention causes the depression of serum calcium levels. The azotemic state also interferes with vitamin D activation by the kidney, which is necessary for the absorption of calcium from the gut. Both of these factors tend to cause hypocalcemia. Hypocalcemia stimulates the parathyroid glands to put out more parathormone. PTH causes bone resorption of calcium and phosphate, increased excretion of phosphate, and activation of vitamin D by the kidneys. Serum calcium and phosphate levels thus tend to be restored to normal. As the GFR continues to decrease, however, the low serum calcium and high phosphate levels continue to stimulate parathyroid activity more and more. The parathyroid glands may show hyperplasia of the secretory cells with apparent independence of physiological controls. The result is increasing demineralization of the bony skeleton. A rise in the serum alkaline phosphatase level is evidence that this process is occurring. The calcium-phosphate cross product may become exceedingly high, resulting in the precipitation of calcium phosphate salts in the soft tissues of the body.

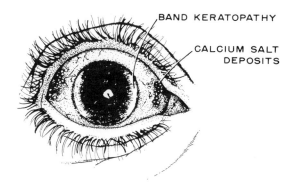

BAND KERATOPATHY

CALCIUM SALT DEPOSITS

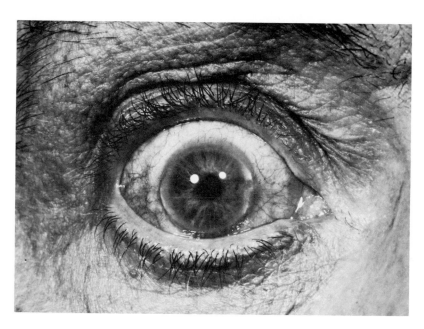

FIGURE 42-4 Band keratopathy due to deposit of calcium salts in the eye. Conjunctival deposits of calcium salts are also present. Diagram of abnormalities seen in photograph. (Photograph from M. H. Maxwell and C. R. Kleeman (eds.), Clinical Disorders of Fluid and Electrolyte Metabolism, 2d ed., McGraw-Hill, New York, 1972.)

Common sites for the deposition of calcium salts are in and around joints, resulting in painful arthritis; in the kidney (nephrocalcinosis), resulting in obstruction; in the blood vessels, which may have the appearance of an arteriogram on the x-ray; and in the eyes. The deposition of calcium salts in the conjunctiva and cornea of the eye is called *band keratopathy*. Band keratopathy appears as grayish or whitish granular opacities in the form of a crescent on the nasal or temporal side of the limbus (where cornea and sclera meet at colored and white part of eye) (Fig. 42-4). Precipitation of calcium phosphate salts occurs on the surface of the eye because here the pH is high and favors precipitation. These depositions can be seen with the naked eye but are most easily outlined by slit lamp examination. The conjunctival deposits sometimes cause intense irritation with redness and watering of the eyes ("uremic red eye").

This completes the description of the syndrome which is called uremia. Not all components are present in every patient, and the dominant features may vary from one patient to another. The prevention and treatment of these complications will be considered in Chap. 43.

QUESTIONS

The uremic syndrome—Chap. 42

Directions: Answer the following questions on a separate sheet of paper.

1 What is meant by the uremic syndrome?

2 What are the two groups of clinical symptoms present in the uremic syndrome?

3 Explain why total NH_4^+ excretion is decreased in renal failure.

4 Why does the acidosis of chronic renal failure generally stabilize at a moderate level when there is a positive H^+ balance? What relationship might the acidosis of renal failure have to the bone pathology?

5 Why is salt wasting associated with polyuria in early renal insufficiency?

6 Name two common laxatives which, if administered to the uremic patient, might result in death.

7 Explain the meaning of a constant finding of urine specific gravity at 1.010.

8 How is sexual and reproductive function affected in terminal renal failure? (Explain how it affects males and females.)

9 Name four factors which contribute to the development of an infection in the uremic patient.

10 Describe skin color changes in the uremic patient who is Caucasian, brown-skinned, or black-skinned.

11 Illustrate the mechanisms by which GI bleeding, vomiting, or diarrhea could cause the deterioration of renal function. (Draw flow diagrams.)

12 List several changes you might expect to observe in the mental, emotional, neuromuscular statuses and rest patterns of a patient who is developing uremia.

13 List the stages in the development of peripheral neuropathy and the signs and symptoms you would expect to observe in the patient with renal failure.

14 Illustrate the appearance of the phalanges seen on x-ray when there is subperiosteal bone resorption in renal osteodystrophy.

15 Draw a flow diagram of the pathogenesis of secondary hyperparathyroidism and list several examples of the consequences of this condition.

16 A uremic patient has a serum phosphate level of 8 mg% and a calcium level of 10 mg%. Would you expect metastatic calcification in the soft tissues of the body? Explain.

17 What is "band keratopathy"? Illustrate. What causes "uremic red eye"?

Directions: Circle the letter preceding each item that correctly answers each question. Only ONE answer is correct; exceptions will be noted.

18 In renal failure there is an impaired ability to excrete H^+. This results in:
a Respiratory acidosis b Metabolic acidosis
c Respiratory alkalosis d Metabolic alkalosis

19 Which of the following describes the plasma pH and bicarbonate levels in the condition in question 18?
a Increase in pH and decrease in HCO_3^- b Decrease in pH and increase in HCO_3^- c Decrease in both pH and HCO_3^- d Increase in both pH and HCO_3^-

20 Which of the following mechanisms is most important for the excretion of H^+ by the kidney?
a Excretion of H^+ as NH_4^+ by combination with NH_3
b Excretion of H^+ as acid phosphate

21 Hypokalemia associated with polyuria is most apt to be associated with:
a Acute renal failure b Acute pyelonephritis
c Chronic pyelonephritis

22 As the patient becomes oliguric in end-stage renal failure, which of the following K^+ disturbances usually develops?
a Hypokalemia b Hyperkalemia

23 Metabolic acidosis contributes to hyperkalemia by which of the following mechanisms?
a K^+ (cells) → extracellular fluid b Mg^{2+} (cells) → extracellular fluid c K^+ (extracellular fluid) → cells d Mg^{2+} (extracellular fluid) → cells

24 Fatal arrhythmias and cardiac arrest are most apt to occur when serum K$^+$ levels reach:
a 3.5 to 4.5 meq/liter *b* 4.5 to 5.5 meq/liter
c 6.5 to 7.5 meq/liter

25 When oliguria occurs in terminal renal failure, the patient is likely to do which of the following? (More than one answer may be correct.)
a Increase salt-losing tendency *b* Retain sodium
c Increase circulatory overload *d* Increase aldosterone secretion

26 Symptoms of gouty arthritis experienced by some uremic patients are most likely caused by serum elevations of:
a Urea *b* Creatinine *c* Uric acid *d* Bicarbonate

27 Which of the following factors contribute to the development of congestive heart failure in uremic patients? (More than one answer may be correct.)
a Anemia *b* Hypertension *c* Excess sodium and water intake *d* Circulatory overload

28 Which statements are true related to the anemia in the uremic patient? (More than one answer may be correct; correct false statements.)
a Due to excess hemolysis *b* Due to iron deficiency *c* Normochromic, normocytic *d* Due to excess production of erythropoietin *e* When severe may cause symptoms of fatigue, dyspnea, and pallor

29 What is the mechanism of the bleeding tendency in uremia? (More than one answer may be correct.)
a Defective platelet adhesion *b* Severe thrombocytopenia *c* Inhibition of some of the circulating coagulation factors

30 Symptoms of uremia generally begin when the GFR falls to which of the following ranges of normal?
a 80 to 90 percent *b* 50 to 60 percent
c 30 to 40 percent *d* 4 to 10 percent

Directions: Circle T if the statement is true and F if false. Correct false statements.

31 T F Anorexia, nausea, and lethargy are common symptoms in the uremic patient and may be due, in part, to metabolic acidosis.

32 T F Kussmaul respirations are shallow respirations which occur because of the need to decrease CO_2 excretion by the lungs.

33 T F The symptoms of anorexia, nausea, and lassitude are often relieved by the dietary restriction of protein.

34 T F Dietary protein restriction causes a marked improvement of the GFR.

35 T F Dietary protein restriction helps reduce K$^+$, H$^+$, and phosphate intake.

36 T F There is no evidence of abnormal protein synthesis in uremia.

37 T F Hypoglycemia is the usual manifestation of abnormal carbohydrate metabolism in uremia.

38 T F Insulin-dependent diabetics who become uremic often require lower dosages of insulin.

39 T F Elevation of serum triglycerides in uremia is related to abnormal fat metabolism in uremia.

Directions: Fill in the blanks with the correct words.

40 Organisms normally in the mouth split _____ producing _____ which contributes to the uriniferous odor to the breath, inflammation and ulceration of the mucus membranes, predisposition to _____, and altered taste sensation common in the uremic patient.

41 Three types of bone lesions seen in renal osteodystrophy are (a) _____ due to hyperparathyroidism; (b) _____ due to vitamin D deficiency; (c) _____ which gives a banded (rugger-jersey) appearance to the spine due to alternating areas of bone demineralization and sclerosis.

Draw arrows from the abnormalities found in uremia in col. A to the most likely complication resulting from that abnormality in col. B. (More than one arrow from each condition may be drawn from left to right.)

Column A	Column B
42 Pericarditis	*a* Pneumonia
	b Retinopathy
43 Circulatory overload	*c* Cardiac tamponade
	d Pulmonary edema
44 Hypertension	*e* Encephalopathy

Directions: Match the following integumentary manifestations of the uremic syndrome in col. B with the probable causative factor in col. A.

Column A	Column B
45 ____ Urochrome	*a* Bruises
46 ____ Anemia	*b* Yellow cast
47 ____ Urea	*c* Pruritis
48 ____ Proteinuria	*d* Fine, white crystal deposits in areas of increased perspiration
49 ____ Calcium deposits in skin	*e* Brittle, ridged nails with alternating light and red bands
50 ____ Capillary fragility	*f* Pallor

CHAPTER 43 The Treatment of Chronic Renal Failure

OBJECTIVES

At the completion of Chap. 43 you should be able to:

1 Describe the two stages in the treatment of chronic renal failure.

2 Describe the principles of dietary regulation in the management of chronic renal failure.

3 Illustrate how fluid allowance is determined in the uremic patient.

4 List common complications encountered in uremia.

5 Describe prevention and treatment measures for the above complications.

6 List two reasons why the treatment of advanced renal insufficiency has been changed in recent years.

7 Describe the modalities of treatment the uremic patient may choose and how they are related to each other.

8 Identify the criteria for transition from conservative methods of treatment of the uremic patient to more definitive therapy.

9 Define *dialysis*.

10 Describe the two major techniques and the basic principles of dialysis (diffusion; osmotic and hydrostatic pressure gradients).

11 Identify the three basic types of hemodialyzers.

12 Describe a hemodialysis system in operation.

13 Differentiate between an external and an internal arteriovenous shunt.

14 Compare the efficiency of hemodialysis and peritoneal dialysis.

15 Describe the placement of a transplanted kidney.

16 Identify the most important antigens involved in renal transplantation.

17 Describe the major complications of renal transplantation.

18 Compare hemodialysis and renal transplantation as methods of treatment in end-stage renal disease.

The treatment of chronic renal failure may be divided into two stages. The first stage consists of conservative measures which are designed to temper or delay the progressive deterioration of renal function. Conservative measures are begun when the patient becomes azotemic. The physician makes every effort to determine the primary cause of the renal failure and search out any reversible factors such as infection, obstruction, or malignant hypertension which may be the immediate cause of the renal failure. Treatment of reversible factors may stabilize and prevent any further deterioration of renal function. The second stage of treatment begins when conservative measures are no longer effective. Terminal renal failure exists at this point [glomerular filtration rate (GFR) usually less than 2 ml/minute] and the only effective treatment is either intermittent dialysis or renal transplantation.

CONSERVATIVE MANAGEMENT

The basic principles of conservative management are quite simple and are based on an understanding of the range of excretion that can be achieved by the failing kidney. Dietary regulation of individual solutes and fluid is then adjusted to the limitations. In addition, therapy is directed towards prevention and treatment of complications as they occur.

Dietary regulation of protein, potassium, sodium, and fluids

Dietary regulation is of primary importance in the treatment of chronic renal failure. It is customary to restrict the protein intake of the azotemic patient though there is controversy about how severe this restriction should be. The restriction of protein not only reduces the BUN level, and perhaps other poorly defined toxic products of protein metabolism, but also reduces the intake of potassium, phosphate, and hydrogen-ion production which stem from protein. Though the GFR is not improved, uremic symptoms such as nausea, vomiting, and fatigue may be ameliorated. One suggested predialysis schedule based on the GFR is as follows:

GFR	PROTEIN RESTRICTION
10 ml/minute	40 g
5 ml/minute	25 to 30 g
3 ml/minute or less	20 g

Not only is the amount of protein important but also the quality. It is possible to maintain nitrogen balance even on a 20-g protein diet provided the protein is of the highest biological value (i.e., contains all the essential amino acids, as do milk and eggs) and adequate calories are supplied in the form of fats and carbohydrates to prevent the breakdown of body protein to satisfy caloric requirements. However, acceptability may be a problem with a protein diet less than 40 g/day, and dietary treatment does not seem to be too successful once the GFR has fallen below 4 to 5 ml/minute.

Hyperkalemia generally becomes a problem in advanced renal failure, and it becomes necessary also to restrict dietary intake of potassium. Care must be taken not to administer foods or drugs which are high in potassium. These include salt substitutes (which contain ammonium chloride and potassium chloride), expectorants, potassium citrate, and foods such as soups, dates, bananas, and pure fruit juices. Inadvertent administration of food or drugs high in potassium might cause a serious hyperkalemia.

The dietary regulation of sodium is very important in renal failure. The optimal sodium intake must be determined individually for each patient in order to maintain good hydration. An intake that is too liberal can lead to fluid retention, peripheral edema, pulmonary edema, hypertension, and congestive heart failure. Sodium retention is generally a problem in glomerular disease and in advanced renal failure. On the other hand, if sodium is restricted to the point of negative sodium balance, then hypovolemia, decreased GFR, and a deterioration of renal function would ensue. Sodium depletion is more common in tubular disease and may be precipitated by vomiting or diarrhea. It is therefore important for the physician to determine the optimum sodium intake for each patient. The sodium conservation test and a careful observation of the daily weight, signs of edema, and other complications may all be helpful.

The intake of fluids requires careful regulation in advanced renal failure as the patient's thirst is an unreliable guide to the state of hydration. Daily weight is the critical parameter to follow in addition to *accurate* intake and output records. An intake that is too liberal may result in circulatory overload, edema, and water intoxication, and less than optimal intake will result in dehydration, hypotension, and a deterioration in renal function. The general rule for allowed fluid intake is: intake = urine output during last 24 hours + 500 ml. The 500 ml represents insensible losses. For example, if the patient's urine output during the past 24 hours was 400 ml, then the total intake per day should be 500 + 400 ml = 900 ml. Anephritic patients are allowed 800 ml/day, and patients on dialysis are given sufficient fluid to allow a 2- to 3-pound weight gain between treatments. Obviously, both sodium and fluid intake must both be manipulated to achieve fluid balance.

Prevention and treatment of complications

The second category of conservative measures used in the treatment of renal failure are those directed towards the prevention and treatment of complications.

HYPERTENSION

It is generally agreed that renal function deteriorates more rapidly if severe hypertension develops. In addition, extrarenal complications such as retinopathy and encephalopathy may develop. Hypertension can be brought under control most effectively by a combination of a low sodium diet and a hypotensive drug. Methyldopa (Aldomet) is generally the drug of choice for mild cases of hypertension (diastolic pressure below 115 mmHg), and guanthidine (Ismelin) may be used for more severe cases. Great care is taken to lower the blood pressure gradually so that the patient does not become hypotensive with the consequent lowering of GFR and further deterioration of renal function. Hypertension in the majority of uremic patients is due to fluid overload and is most effectively restored to normal by regulation of sodium and fluid intake and intermittent dialysis.

HYPERKALEMIA

One of the most serious complications in the uremic patient is the development of hyperkalemia. When serum K^+ reaches a level of about 7 meq/liter, serious arrhythmias and cardiac arrest may occur. In addition, hypocalcemia, hyponatremia, and acidosis enhance the deleterious effects of hyperkalemia. For this reason, the patient may be put on a cardiac monitor to detect the effect of the hyperkalemia (and the effects of all the other ions) on cardiac conduction.

Acute hyperkalemia may be treated by the administration of intravenous glucose and insulin which drives K^+ into the cells, or by the careful intravenous administration of 10% calcium gluconate with continuous ECG monitoring if the patient is hypotensive with widening of the QRS complex. The effect of these measures is only temporary and subsequent correction of the hyperkalemia must be made with dialysis. When it is not possible to lower K^+ by dialysis, the cation exchange resin, Kayexalate, may be used. Each gram of the resin binds one milliequivalent of K^+. Kayexalate may be given by mouth or by rectal installation. When given rectally, 50 to 100 g is mixed in 200 to 300 ml water. To facilitate the K^+ exchange 25 to 30 ml of 70% sorbitol (a poorly absorbed, osmotically active alcohol which has a laxative effect) is added. Needless to say, orange juice (high K^+ content) should not be given to disguise the taste when Kayexalate is administered orally!

ANEMIA

The anemia of renal failure is unresponsive to hematinics except erythropoietin, which is not commercially available. Patients can usually function quite well with hematocrits of 18 to 20 percent. Blood transfusions are kept to a minimum since they further suppress an already depressed red blood cell (RBC) production. Blood transfusions can also induce sensitivity to a large number of leukocyte antigens which increases the risk of tissue rejection in the event of renal transplantation. Limiting blood transfusions also reduces the incidence of pulmonary edema and hepatitis.

ACIDOSIS

The mild chronic metabolic acidosis of the uremic patient usually stabilizes at a plasma bicarbonate level of 16 to 20 meq/liter. It does not usually progress beyond this point, since H^+ production is balanced by bone buffering. The renal acidosis is not usually treated unless the plasma HCO_3^- falls below 15 meq/liter, when symptoms of acidosis may appear. Severe acidosis may be precipitated by the superimposition of an acute acidosis on the mild chronic acidosis. This might occur, for example, in the event of profuse diarrhea with its HCO_3^- loss. When severe acidosis is corrected by the parenteral administration of $NaHCO_3$, it is important to be aware of the hazard involved. Overcorrection of blood pH may precipitate tetany, convulsions, and death. Remember that chronic renal failure patients are usually hypocalcemic. A mild degree of induced alkalosis may reduce the ionized fraction of serum Ca^{2+} (usually in an acidic environment) to the point of severe hypocalcemia. The most logical mode of treatment, finally, is dialysis.

RENAL OSTEODYSTROPHY

One of the most crucial therapeutic measures used to prevent the development of secondary hyperparathyroidism and its consequences is a low phosphate diet along with the administration of gels which bind phosphate in the bowel. The prevention and correction of hyperphosphatemia prevents the sequents of events leading to calcium and bone disorders discussed in Chap. 42. A low protein diet is also low in phosphate. The usual agents chosen as phosphate binders are aluminum antacid gels (Amphojel or Basojel) administered in tablet or liquid form. *Most other antacids contain magnesium and should not be given.* These antacids form an insoluble aluminum phosphate in the bowel which is subsequently excreted in the stool. Phosphate-binding gels should be taken *with* meals. The greatest problem is obtaining the cooperation of the patient in carrying out the treatment regimen.*

If severe skeletal involvement occurs for the lack of or in spite of preventive therapy with antacid gels, subtotal parathyroidectomy or vitamin D therapy may be indicated. Severe bone demineralization, hypercalcemia, and/or intractable pruritis are considered indications for parathyroidectomy. When the predominant lesion is osteomalacia, the nephrologist may begin vitamin D therapy with great care. This treatment may be quite hazardous. Not only may calcium absorption be increased, but it may in fact lead to progressive soft-tissue calcification when bone resorption and hyperphosphatemia continue unabated.

Other methods used to prevent renal osteodystrophy include increasing calcium intake to 1.2 to 1.5 g/day by diet or by calcium supplement (only after the serum phosphate level is lowered to normal) and keeping the concentration of calcium in the dialysate between 6.5 and 7.0 meq/liter.

HYPERURICEMIA

Allopurinol is usually the drug of choice for treating the hyperuricemia of advanced renal disease. This drug reduces uric acid levels by blocking the biosynthesis of some part of the total uric acid produced by the body.

---

*Recent experimental evidence with uremic dogs reveals that a secondary hyperparathyroidism was prevented by the early administration of a low phosphate diet (N. S. Bricker, *New England Journal of Medicine*, **286**: 1093, 1972). Treatment should begin early when the GFR is 20 to 30 ml/minute. In addition, bread sticks impregnated with a dehydrated aluminum oxide gel may soon be commercially available and provide a more palatable form of phosphate binder. (From a lecture on "Renal Osteodystrophy" by Edwardo Slatopolsky at North Central Dialysis and Transplant Society Symposium, Dearborn, Michigan, June 12, 1976.)

Colchicine (anti-inflammatory drug for gout) may be given for the relief of symptoms of gouty arthritis.

PERIPHERAL NEUROPATHY

Usually, symptomatic peripheral neuropathy does not occur until renal failure is far advanced. There is no known treatment for these changes except dialysis which stops its progression. Therefore, the development of sensory neuritis is a signal that dialysis should not be delayed any longer. Motor neuropathy may be irreversible.

PROMPT TREATMENT OF INFECTION

Patients with chronic renal failure have an increased susceptibility to infection, particularly urinary tract infection. Since infection of any sort may accentuate the catabolic process and impair adequate nutrition and fluid and electrolyte balance, infections should be treated promptly to prevent further deterioration of renal function.

CAUTIOUS DRUG ADMINISTRATION

Since many drugs are excreted by the kidney, caution must be exercised in their administration to the uremic patient. The half-life of drugs excreted by the kidney is greatly prolonged in uremia so that toxic serum levels may occur. The dosages of these drugs must therefore be reduced. The choice of antibiotics (nonnephrotoxic) and their dosages are made by the nephrologist with consideration of these facts. Particular caution is necessary when digitalis drugs are ordered for the treatment of intrinsic cardiac disease in the uremic patient. In fact, *cautious drug administration to the uremic patient should be the rule.*

In progressive renal failure, conservative therapeutic measures finally become inadequate. Hemodialysis and/ or renal transplantation are then the only means of preserving life. Continuation of many of the conservative measures may be necessary, particularly with hemodialysis.

DIALYSIS AND RENAL TRANSPLANTATION

The treatment of end-stage renal failure has been transformed by the development of techniques for dialysis and renal transplantation during the past 15 years. In the past, these patients were doomed to die when all conservative methods failed. Now, their lives may be prolonged many years with maintenance dialysis or renal transplantation.

There is an intimate relationship between these two techniques, and advances in both have closely paralleled each other. For example, the uremic patient may choose to undergo renal transplantation with a related or cadaver donor rather than be maintained on chronic intermittent dialysis. Nevertheless, dialysis will undoubtedly play an important role in the treatment. Dialysis may be used to maintain the patient in an optimum clinical state until the donor kidney is available. In the case of a cadaver renal transplant, the patient may have to wait many months. There are several choices of treatment depending on the resources available. The initial treatment will be carried out in the medical center hemodialysis unit. The patient may then undergo home dialysis training to permit self-administration of the procedure at home until the donor kidney is available; or more commonly treatment may be given in a satellite (out-of-hospital) or mobile hemodialysis unit near the individual's home. Dialysis may sustain the renal transplant patient through periods of postoperative oliguria, and it provides an alternative other than death if the transplanted kidney should fail due to rejection or other complications. Both renal transplantation and chronic maintenance dialysis offer about the same prognosis of longevity. There are problems unique to both modes of treatment. Renal transplantation, if successful, probably offers a better quality of life because it is less restrictive. There are usually no dietary restrictions, and it is not necessary to commit large blocks of time several times each week for performing dialysis.

Preparation of the patient

It is important that the patient be prepared for the transition from conservative management to more definitive therapy long before the need arises for maintenance dialysis or renal transplantation. Not only does this give the patient hope, but it allows time for indoctrination of the patient in preparation for the treatment and makes it possible for the treatment to start at the proper time.

Originally, extremely rigid criteria were used to select patients for either renal transplantation or maintenance dialysis, especially because of limited facilities and the high cost of treatment. The increase in facilities, financial support by the federal government, improvements in techniques, and success in treating some children, older people, diabetics, and patients with systemic lupus erythematosis are all factors which have helped to liberalize the criteria so that a greater number of patients can be helped.

When to begin treatment

There are no clear-cut guidelines in terms of measurable blood levels of creatinine or BUN to determine when definitive therapy should begin. Most nephrologists' decisions are based on the well-being of the patient, who is followed very closely as an outpatient. Therapy is generally begun when the patient is no longer able to work full-time, develops peripheral neuropathy, or shows other signs of clinical deterioration. The serum creatinine level is generally above 6 mg% in males (4 mg% in females), and the GFR is below 4 ml/minute. In no case should the patient be allowed to become bedridden or so sick that usual activities are impossible.

Sometimes, in spite of being carefully followed, the patient may rapidly deteriorate over a period of a few days. This rapid deterioration is usually in response to an infectious disease. Sometimes one or two peritoneal dialyses will restabilize the patient. If this is not successful, then intermittent hemodialysis may be initiated. If a decision for a renal transplant has been made, then this may be done on an elective basis at a later date.

Dialysis

Dialysis refers to the diffusion of solutes and water through a passive, porous membrane from one fluid compartment to another. Hemodialysis and peritoneal dialysis are the two major techniques used in dialysis and the basic principles involved are the same for both—diffusion of solutes and water from the plasma to the dialysis solution in response to a concentration or pressure gradient.

Figure 43-1 illustrates the basic principles of diffusion and osmotic and hydrostatic pressure gradients involved in dialysis. Given a semipermeable membrane with the patient's blood on one side and a solution of known composition on the other side (the dialysate or dialysis "bath"), substances to which the membrane is permeable will move from where their concentration is high to where it is low. If the blood potassium level is high and the potassium level in the dialysis bath is low (round dots), the net movement of potassium will be out of the blood into the dialysis bath (long arrows indicate direc-

tion of net diffusion). The black squares represent solutes which are in higher concentration in the dialysate (e.g., bicarbonate) so that net diffusion is from the bath solution to the blood. Ultrafiltration is achieved by mechanically increasing the hydrostatic pressure in the blood compartment and by adding glucose to the dialysis bath. The resulting osmotic and hydrostatic pressure gradients cause a net movement of water from the blood to the dialysis bath. The positive pressure in the blood compartment also speeds up the diffusion of both solutes and water. Note that protein, blood cells, and bacteria are too large to pass through the pores in the dialysis membrane.

By using a dialysis solution which contains the important electrolytes in concentrations which are normal for healthy individuals, the concentration of these electrolytes can be corrected in the blood of the patient with renal failure. The basic practical problems in dialysis are to bring enough blood into contact with enough dialysis solution across a semipermeable membrane of adequate area. This may be accomplished inside the patient's body using the peritoneum as the semipermeable membrane (peritoneal dialysis) or outside the body using an "artificial kidney" and cellophane or Cuprophane as the semipermeable membrane (hemodialysis).

HEMODIALYSIS

An artificial kidney machine, or hemodialyzer, consists simply of a semipermeable membrane (cellophane or Cuprophane) with blood on one side and dialysis fluid on the other. Three basic types of dialyzers have been developed. The *coil dialyzer* consists of two cellophane coils arranged in parallel supported by a rigid mesh screen. Blood is pumped through the inside of the coil, and dialysis fluid is bubbled up around the outside of

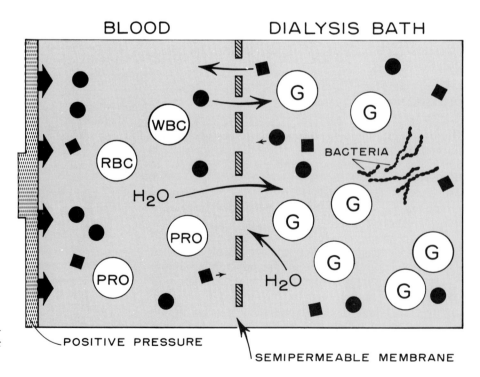

FIGURE 43-1 Basic principles of diffusion and osmosic and hydrostatic pressures involved in dialysis.

the coil and is recirculated (Fig. 43-2). The *parallel plate dialyzer* consists of two cellophane sheets sandwiched between two rigid supports to form an envelope. Two or more envelopes are arranged in parallel. Blood flows between the membrane layers and dialysis fluid may flow in the same direction as the blood or in the opposite direction (countercurrent) shown in Fig. 43-3. The *hollow fiber* or *capillary dialyzer* consists of thousands of tiny capillary fibers arranged in parallel (Fig. 43-4). Each fiber has a wall thickness of 30 μm, an inside diameter of 200 μm, and is 21-cm long (for comparative purposes, a red blood cell has a diameter of 7 μm). Blood flows

down the center of these tiny tubes, and dialysis fluid bathes the outside. The flow of the dialysis fluid is opposite to that of the blood (countercurrent). This dialyzer is very small and compact because of the large surface area provided by the many capillary tubes.

Figure 43-5 is a diagrammatic representation of a hemodialysis system using a hollow fiber dialyzer.

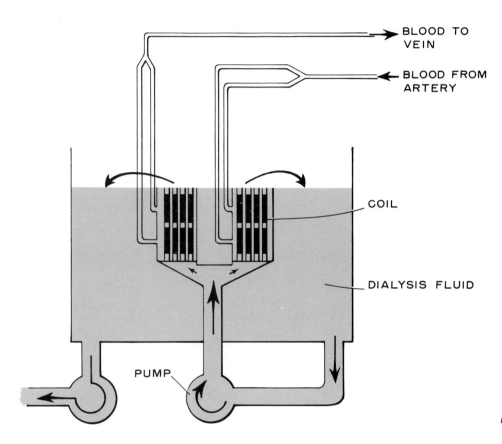

FIGURE 43-2 Coil dialyzer.

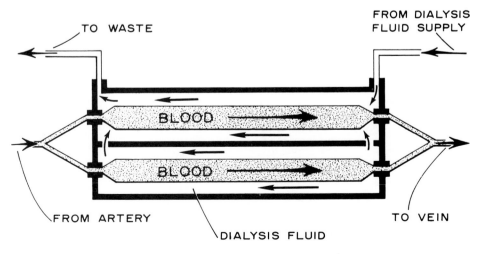

FIGURE 43-3 Parallel plate dialyzer.

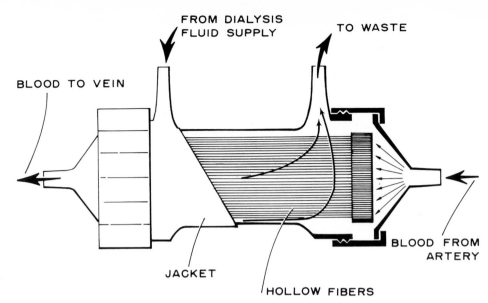

FIGURE 43-4 Hollow fiber or capillary dialyzer.

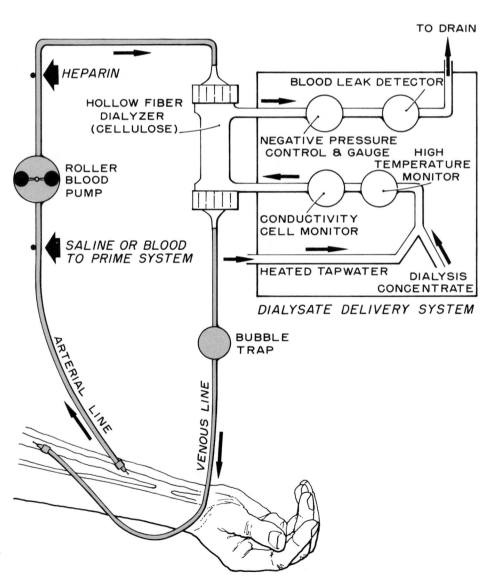

FIGURE 43-5 Diagram of a hemodialysis system using hollow fiber dialyzer.

A dialysis system consists of two circuits, one for the blood and one for the dialysis fluid. When the system is in operation, blood flows from the patient through plastic tubing (arterial line), through the hollow fibers of the dialyzer, and back to the patient through the venous line. The dialysis fluid forms the second circuit. Tap water is filtered and heated to body temperature and is then mixed with a concentrate by a proportioning pump to make the dialysate or bath. The bath is then delivered to the dialyzer, where it flows on the outside of the hollow fibers before exiting to a drain. Equilibrium between the blood and the dialysate takes place across the dialyzing membrane by the processes of diffusion, osmosis, and ultrafiltration described in Fig. 43-1.

The composition of the dialysis bath is designed to approximate the ionic composition of normal blood, modified slightly to correct the common fluid and electrolyte disorders which accompany renal failure. The usual components are Na^+, K^+, Ca^{2+}, Mg^{2+}, Cl^-, acetate, and glucose. Urea, creatinine, uric acid, and phosphate diffuse readily from the blood to the dialysis fluid since they are not present in the dialysis fluid. Sodium acetate and glucose which are in higher concentration in the dialysis bath diffuse into the blood. The purpose of adding the acetate is to correct the uremic patient's acidosis. Acetate is metabolized into bicarbonate in the patient's body. Glucose is added to the dialysis bath to provide an osmotic gradient and thus facilitate the removal of water from the patient (ultrafiltration). Water diffuses from the patient's blood (lower osmolality or higher water concentration) to the dialyzing fluid (higher osmolality or lower water concentration*). In hemodialysis, ultrafiltration is achieved mainly by effecting a hydrostatic pressure difference between the blood and dialysis fluid. The hydrostatic pressure gradient is achieved by increasing the positive pressure within the dialyzer blood compartment by increasing resistance to venous outflow (not shown) or by exerting a vacuum effect in the dialysis fluid compartment by manipulating the negative pressure control. The hydrostatic pressure gradient across the dialyzing membrane also increases the diffusion rate of the solutes.

The blood circuit of the dialysis system is initially primed with saline or blood before connection to the circulation of the patient. The blood pressure of the patient may be adequate to propel the blood through the extracorporeal circuit, or a blood pump may be used to assist the flow (about 200 ml/minute is a desirable flow rate). Heparin is continuously delivered to the arterial line by a slow infusion pump to prevent clotting. A clot and bubble trap in the venous line prevents air or blood clots from returning to the patient. To ensure patient safety, monitors with alarms for various parameters are included in modern hemodialyzers. A con-

*Some glucose does diffuse from the dialysis bath into the blood, but, since water diffuses much more rapidly than glucose, the major shift will be that of water from blood to bath.

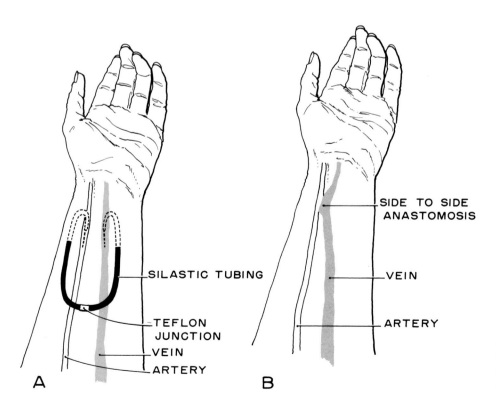

A

SILASTIC TUBING

TEFLON
JUNCTION

VEIN

ARTERY

B

SIDE TO SIDE
ANASTOMOSIS

VEIN

ARTERY

FIGURE 43-6 Access to the circulation. External AV shunt or cannula system (A) and internal AV fistula (B).

ductivity cell monitors the chemical composition of the dialysis fluid. Dialysis fluid at body temperature increases the rate of diffusion, but a temperature that is too high would cause hemolysis of red blood cells, with possible death to the patient. Any tear in the dialysis membrane causing either a minor or a massive leak is detected by a photocell in the dialysate outflow.

Maintenance hemodialysis is usually performed 3 times a week, and the length of a single treatment varies from 4 to 6 hours depending on the type of dialysis system used and the condition of the patient.

ACCESS TO THE BLOODSTREAM

In order to perform long-term intermittent dialysis, reliable access to the circulation is necessary. Blood must exit and return to the patient at the rate of about 200 ml/minute. The major access techniques that can provide flow rates of this magnitude are the internal *arteriovenous (AV) fistula* and the external *AV cannula* or *shunt* (Fig. 43-6). Other techniques include bovine vein graphs and direct cannulation.

The external AV shunt is created by placing Teflon cannula tips in an artery (usually the radial or posterior tibial) and a nearby vein. The cannula tips are then connected by silicone rubber tubing and a Teflon bridge to complete the shunt. At the time of dialysis, the external shunt tubing is separated, and connection is made to the dialyzer. Blood then flows from the arterial line,

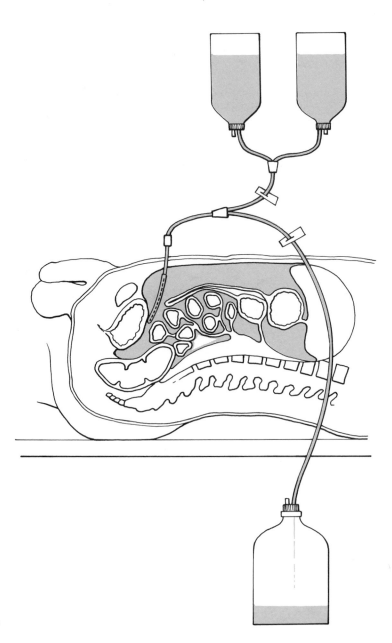

FIGURE 43-7 Peritoneal dialysis.

through the dialyzer, and then back to the vein. The cannula system was devised by Scribner in 1960 and made chronic intermittent dialysis possible for the first time. The main problem with the external shunt is a short life span due to clotting and infection (average life = 9 months).

More recently, use has been made of the AV fistula constructed by anastomosing an artery directly to a vein (usually the radial artery and cephalic vein at the wrist). Blood is shunted from the artery to the vein causing the vein to enlarge ("ripening") after a few weeks. Venipuncture with large-bore needles becomes easy and gives access to rapidly flowing blood under arterial pressure. Connection with the dialysis system is made by placing one needle distally (arterial line) and the other needle proximally (venous line) in the arterialized vein. The internal fistula circumvents the problems of infection, clotting, and possible hemorrhage associated with the cannula. The average life of a fistula is about 4 years. The main problems are painful venipuncture, formation of aneurysms, achieving hemostasis postdialysis, and ischemia of the hand (steal syndrome).

PERITONEAL DIALYSIS

Peritoneal dialysis accomplishes the same functions and operates on the same principles of diffusion and osmosis as hemodialysis. In this instance, however, the peritoneum is the semipermeable membrane. A catheter is placed in the peritoneal cavity by paracentesis (Fig. 43-7). In the adult, 2 liters of sterile dialysis solution are allowed to run into the peritoneal cavity through the catheter (10 to 20 minutes). Equilibrium between the dialysis fluid and the highly vascular semipermeable peritoneal membrane takes place. This is called "dwell time" and is generally 30 to 45 minutes. The fluid is then

allowed to drain by gravity into a closed, sterile collecting system. The cycle is repeated successively over a period of 1 to 2 days. The main advantage of this method of dialysis is its simplicity (it does not require highly skilled personnel or sophisticated equipment), and it does not require access to the bloodstream. On the other hand, peritoneal dialysis requires about 6 times longer than hemodialysis to achieve the same results. In addition, the procedure is often painful (especially when high glucose concentrations are used to achieve ultrafiltration), and repeated treatments may lead to peritonitis.

RENAL TRANSPLANTATION

A successful renal transplant is the preferred method of treatment for patients in end-stage renal failure, although some patients may elect to perform intermittent dialysis in their own home after being taught the procedure by a "home-training nurse."

The first successful renal transplant was performed on identical twins in 1954 by Murray, Merrill, and Harrison in Boston, Massachusetts. Since that time over 25,000 renal transplants have been performed in the world, of which more than 15,000 have been in the United States.

The surgical technique involved in renal transplantation is relatively simple and is generally performed by a surgeon with a background in urologic, vascular, or general surgery. It is the standard procedure to rotate the donor kidney and place it in the contralateral iliac

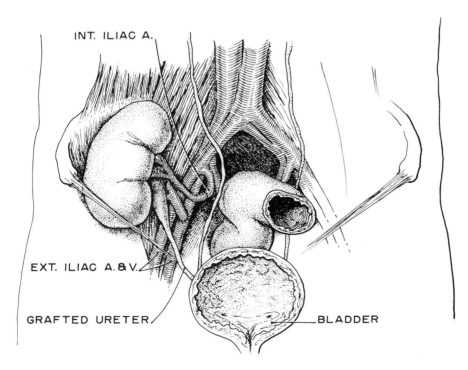

INT. ILIAC A.

EXT. ILIAC A. & V.

GRAFTED URETER

BLADDER

FIGURE 43-8 Renal transplantation.

fossa of the recipient. The ureter then lies anterior to the renal vessels and is more readily anastomosed or implanted into the recipient bladder. The renal artery is anastomosed end-to-end to the internal iliac artery, while the renal vein is anastomosed to the external or common iliac vein (Fig. 43-8).

The major limiting factor in this procedure is the body's immunologic response that leads to rejection of the transplanted kidney. Rejection may occur by two processes: cell-mediated and humoral-mediated rejection. Cell-mediated rejection involves T-lymphocytes produced in response to antigens in the donor kidney which are recognized as foreign cells. These lymphocytes invade the foreign donor kidney and contribute to its destruction. Humoral-mediated rejection involves the production of antibodies against antigens in the donor kidney which the recipient's plasma cells recognize as foreign. Rejection can occur within hours or several years after a transplant.

The most important antigens from the point of view of transplantation are those of the ABO blood groups and the human leukocyte antigens (HLA). As far as the ABO system is concerned, the same rules apply as with blood transfusions. An O kidney can be transplanted into any recipient while an A kidney can only be given to an A or an AB recipient.

The HLA system is more complex, and there are about 15 different leukocyte antigens. Each person has two pairs of these antigens, one inherited from each parent. The two genes responsible for each pair of antigens are located on the same chromosome. Because of this pattern of inheritance, one out of four siblings may have identical HLA antigens. In general, the closer the genetic similarity between donor and recipient, the greater the chance of a successful transplant. When the donor and recipient are identical twins or HLA-identical siblings, some 90 percent of the graphs are functioning at the end of 2 years. The next best choice for a donor is a non-identical-HLA sibling, then a parent, and finally an unrelated person (source of cadaver kidneys). Tissue typing is a technique which has been developed in recent years to predict the outcome of a particular match of antigens between donor and recipient.

The survival of the transplanted kidney depends on minimizing the body's defense mechanisms. Common drugs used to suppress the immune response are azothioprine (Immuran) and prednisone. These drugs make the patient more susceptible to infection. Consequently, overwhelming infection is also a major complication in a renal transplant recipient.

Table 43-1 is a comparison of hemodialysis and renal transplantation as methods of treatment in end-stage renal failure.

QUESTIONS

The treatment of chronic renal failure—Chap. 43

Directions: Answer the following questions on a separate sheet of paper.

TABLE 43-1
Comparison of renal transplantation and hemodialysis

	RENAL TRANSPLANT	HEMODIALYSIS
One-year survival, %†	80	95
Five-year survival, %†	60	75
One-year graft survival, %*		
Sibling	76.5	
Parent	69.2	
Cadaver	54.2	
Five-year graft survival, %*		
Sibling	60.8	
Parent	42.0	
Cadaver	35.2	
Cost	$10,000–$30,000	$30,000/year (medical center)
		$20,000/year (satellite unit)
		$5,000–$8,000/year (home)
Activity restriction	None	Some
General well-being	Complete	Incomplete
Generalized infection	Yes	No
Localized infection	No	Yes
Diet restriction	No	Yes
Renal osteodystrophy	No	Yes
Neuropathy	No	Yes
Rehabilitation	Yes	Yes

*"Year of Transplant, 1969," from "12th Report of the Human Transplant Registry," *Journal of the American Medical Association,* **233**: 787, 1975.
†D. J. Brundage, *Nursing Management of Renal Problems,* Mosby, St. Louis, 1976, p. 81.

1 When are conservative measures of treatment begun for the patient with chronic renal failure? What are the basic principles of conservative treatment?

2 When conservative therapeutic measures are no longer adequate in the treatment of the uremic patient, what are the alternatives for the patient?

3 Describe the principles of dietary regulation of protein, carbohydrate, sodium, and potassium in the treatment of the patient with terminal renal failure.

4 Mr. Walker, who is oliguric and in uremia, has a total urine output of 500 ml during the past 24 hours. What should his approximate fluid intake be for the next day?

5 What are the two modalities of treatment for the end-stage renal failure patient and how are they related?

6 Define *dialysis*.

7 Differentiate between the two common methods for providing access to the bloodstream for hemodialysis.

Directions: Match the uremic complication in col. A with the common therapies for the prevention or treatment of the condition in col. B. Conditions may have more than one treatment.

Column A	Column B
8 ____ Hyperkalemia	a Cardiac monitor
9 ____ Hyperparathy-roidism	b Kayexalate
	c Colchicine
10 ____ Hypertension	d IV glucose + insulin
11 ____ Osteomalacia	e Methyldopa
12 ____ Hyperuricemia	f Allopurinol
13 ____ Peripheral neuropathy	g Amphojel or Basojel
	h Vitamin D
14 ____ Gouty arthritis	i IV calcium gluconate
	j Progress halted only by dialysis
	k Sodium restriction

Directions: Circle the letter preceding each item that correctly answers each question. Only ONE answer is correct; exceptions will be noted.

15 The anemia of end-stage renal failure:
a Is readily corrected by the administration of iron *b* Is treated by weekly blood transfusions *c* Is intractable and generally not treated except when severe *d* Is treated by injections of vitamin B$_{12}$

16 The IV administration of sodium bicarbonate to correct the systemic acidosis in renal failure may result in which of the following complications?
a Tetany and convulsions *b* Hypermagnesemia *c* Azotemia *d* Renal osteodystrophy

17 Antacids for the uremic patient are properly administered:
a One hour before meals *b* During meals *c* One hour after meals *d* Ad lib by patient for gastric distress

18 Which of the following findings in a patient with renal insufficiency would indicate that dialysis treatment should be initiated? (More than one answer may be correct.)
a BUN 60 mg% *b* K$^+$ 6.3 meq/liter *c* Unable to carry on usual job as telephone operator *d* Burning sensation on soles of feet

19 Peritoneal dialysis removes waste products from the blood because of all of the following principles *except:*
a Water moves across the semipermeable membrane by osmosis. *b* The peritoneal surface acts as a semipermeable membrane. *c* Red blood cells are removed by ultrafiltration. *d* Na$^+$ and K$^+$ are removed by diffusion.

20 The objectives of hemodialysis are all of the following *except:*
a Removal of excess extracellular and intracellular fluid *b* Diffusion of K$^+$ out of the blood *c* Stimulation of urine production by the osmotic pressure gradient *d* Diffusion of urea out of the blood

21 The most compact of the basic types of hemodialyzers is the:
a Coil dialyzer *b* Parallel plate dialyzer *c* Hollow fiber dialyzer

22 All of the following substances may leave the blood and enter the dialyzing fluid *except:*
a Albumin *b* Urea *c* Magnesium *d* Potassium

23 In hemodialysis, blood is pumped through a _____ _____ tubing bathed in a dialysis fluid which is similar to plasma in composition.
a Permeable *b* Semipermeable *c* Osmotic *d* Ultrafiltrate

24 The purpose of adding sodium acetate to the dialyzing fluid is to:
a Correct the hyperuricemia *b* Decrease the incidence of peripheral neuropathy *c* Alleviate the pruritis *d* Provide bicarbonate to the body to correct acidosis *e* Increase the osmolality of the dialyzing solution to provide for ultrafiltration

25 The flow of blood through an artificially created internal AV fistula causes the vein to enlarge and is referred to as which of the following? What is the purpose of this procedure? State in words.
a Fistulation *b* Ripening *c* Ultrafiltration *d* Cannulation

26 Which drug is used to prevent clotting of blood during extracorporeal circulation?
a Protamine *b* Heparin *c* Warfarin sodium (Coumadin) *d* Fibrinogen

27 The most common cause of failure of a renal transplant is:
a Obstruction of the ureterovesicular anastomasis

b Infection of the transplanted kidney *c* Immunologic rejection of the transplanted kidney *d* Recurrence of the patient's original kidney disease

28 Which of the statements are true concerning the procedure for renal transplantation? (More than one answer may be correct.)
a The left kidney of the donor is rotated and placed in the right iliac fossa of the recipient. *b* The left kidney of the donor is rotated and placed in the left iliac fossa of the recipient. *c* The left kidney of the donor is placed in the left upper abdominal cavity of the recipient, and the renal artery anastomosed to the recipient's renal artery. *d* The renal vein is anastomosed to the common iliac vein. *e* The renal artery is anastomosed to the internal iliac artery. *f* The ureter of the transplanted kidney is implanted into the colon.

29 The most important antigens from the point of view of renal transplant are which of the following? (More than one answer may be correct.)
a ABO blood group *b* Leukocytes *c* Hemoglobin *d* Thrombocytes

30 In general, a donor kidney from which of the following persons would most likely be successful?
a Parent *b* Sister *c* Cadaver *d* Cousin

31 The advantage of kidney transplant is:
a Generally eliminates the need for dialysis *b* Side effects easily treated with corticosteroids *c* No danger to the donor *d* Minimal danger of postoperative infections

CHAPTER 44   Acute Renal Failure

OBJECTIVES   **At the completion of Chap. 44 you should be able to:**

1 Define *acute renal failure*.

2 List the two major causes of acute renal failure.

3 Describe the common clinical situations leading to acute ischemic renal failure.

4 Discuss three examples of acute nephrotoxic injury to the kidneys.

5 List two other causes of acute renal failure that are not the two major causes.

6 Describe two types of histologic lesions commonly observed in acute tubular necrosis.

7 Describe the prognosis for each of these two lesions.

8 Describe the general prognosis, extent of acute damage, and residual effects on the kidney in acute cortical necrosis.

9 Describe the clinical course of acute renal failure (three stages and characteristics).

10 Differentiate between prerenal azotemia, postrenal obstruction, and acute tubular necrosis (etiology, laboratory tests, treatment, prognosis).

11 Describe the complications of acute tubular necrosis (principles of management, mortality rates).

CAUSES OF ACUTE RENAL FAILURE

Acute renal failure may be defined as the sudden cessation of renal function, usually manifested by a fall in urine output to less than 400 ml/day. Acute renal failure may result from a wide variety of diseases, drugs, surgical procedures, and trauma. There are two broad categories of causes of acute renal failure: (1) renal ischemia and (2) nephrotoxic injury.

Renal ischemia

Common clinical situations leading to acute ischemic renal failure are major surgical procedures, septic abortion, postpartum hemorrhage, extensive burns, the release of hemoglobin due to hemolysis in mismatched blood transfusions, myoglobinemia especially from massive crush injuries, and acute pancreatitis. In short, any clinical situation associated with severe trauma, infection, dehydration, hemorrhage, and shock may lead to

acute renal failure. The *common denominators* resulting in ischemic renal injury are shock and anoxia.* Any of the above insults are commonly referred to as *prerenal causes* of acute renal failure.

Nephrotoxic injury

Acute nephrotoxic injury to the kidneys is most frequently related to ingestion of bichloride of mercury, ethylene glycol (antifreeze), and carbon tetrachloride. The inhalation of fumes from carbon tetrachloride, a common ingredient of spot remover and other cleaning fluids, accompanied by the ingestion of ethyl alcohol, is particularly dangerous due to the chemical reaction between these two compounds. A potent toxin is formed

---

*The mechanism by which ischemia leads to renal damage and oliguria is poorly understood. Total renal blood flow (RBF) is reduced to about 30 percent of normal, which would not produce oliguria and uremia in a patient with chronic renal failure. It is believed that there is increased vascular resistance and redistribution of RBF from the cortex to the medulla.

which is nephrotoxic. The above set of circumstances (alcohol ingestion at a party and removing a clothing stain with spot remover) has resulted in acute renal failure in a number of innocent persons. For the same reasons, hobbyists using organic solvents and glues should work in well-ventilated rooms and refrain from drinking alcohol at the same time. Less frequent causes of nephrotoxic injury are mushroom poisoning, sulfonamides, certain antibiotics, and a wide variety of other drugs and chemicals.

Other causes

Other causes of acute renal failure which do not fit into either of the above categories are mechanical postrenal obstruction and acute-on-chronic renal failure. Patients with chronic renal failure from any of the causes previously discussed may easily be thrown into acute renal failure by relatively minor upsets such as vomiting, diarrhea, or infections. Patients with acute glomerulonephritis or acute pyelonephritis may also develop acute renal failure. Patients with previous renal disease will not be considered in this discussion.

ACUTE TUBULAR NECROSIS

The term *acute tubular necrosis* (ATN) is commonly applied to both nephrotoxic and ischemic renal injuries, although it does not reflect the nature and severity of the observed tubular changes. Two types of histologic lesions are commonly observed in ATN: (1) *necrosis of the tubular epithelium* leaving the *basement membrane intact,* commonly resulting from the ingestion of nephrotoxic chemicals, and (2) *necrosis of the tubular epithelium and the basement membrane* commonly associated with renal ischemia.

The severity of tubular damage in ATN due to nephrotoxins is highly variable, and the prognosis varies accordingly. There may be necrosis of the proximal tubule epithelium with complete healing in 3 or 4 weeks. Bichloride of mercury and carbon tetrachloride commonly produce this type of lesion. The prognosis is generally good with conservative management or supportive dialysis. In contrast, other poisons such as glycols may produce irreversible renal failure with infarction of the entire nephron, termed *acute cortical necrosis.* The prognosis in this case is very poor. Calcification commonly occurs in the area of cortical necrosis if the patient is fortunate enough to survive.

Tubular damage due to renal ischemic causes is also highly variable. It depends on the extent and period of time in which the decreased renal blood flow and ischemia exists. There may be patchy or widespread destruction of the tubular epithelium and basement membrane or cortical necrosis. Many cases of acute cortical necrosis have followed complications of pregnancy, particularly premature separation of the placenta, postpartum hemorrhage, eclampsia, and septic abortion. When the basement membrane is disrupted, epithelial regeneration occurs in a random, haphazard manner, frequently leading to obstruction of the nephron at the site of necrosis. The prognosis depends on the extent of this type of change.

CLINICAL COURSE OF ACUTE RENAL FAILURE

The clinical course of acute renal failure may be divided into three stages: oliguria, diuresis, and recovery.

Oliguric stage

The clinical picture is often dominated by the surgical, medical, or obstetrical calamity causing the acute renal failure. Oliguria is usually present within 24 to 48 hours after the initial injury, though this symptom may not occur until several days after exposure to nephrotoxic chemicals. Azotemia accompanies the oliguria.

It is critically important to recognize the onset of oliguria, determine the cause, and begin treatment of any reversible causes. Oliguria due to acute-on-chronic renal failure is usually evident from the history. Bladder retention of urine and postrenal obstruction must be ruled out, especially if the cause of the renal failure is not apparent. The presence of anuria or periods of anuria alternating with periods of normal urine flow suggests obstruction. Postrenal obstruction, if left uncorrected, may result in ATN. Finally, prerenal oliguria must be distinguished from ATN.

PRERENAL OLIGURIA VERSUS ATN

Prerenal oliguria and azotemia is physiologic and potentially reversible. It results from shock, decreased plasma volume, and consequent decrease in renal blood flow and GFR. Prerenal oliguria may result from any of the prerenal causes of acute renal failure previously discussed. If left uncorrected, prerenal oliguria may progress to ATN. Serial determinations of the urine output, BUN level, creatinine level, and electrolytes should therefore be made following any major surgery, trauma, serious infection, or obstetrical complication.

A few simple tests are helpful in distinguishing prerenal oliguria from true acute renal failure. In prerenal oliguria, when there is not yet any damage to the renal parenchyma, the oliguric urine is concentrated. The urine/plasma osmolality ratio is greater than 2:1 in prerenal oliguria and progresses to 1:1 (specific gravity 1.010) in established acute tubular necrosis. The urine/plasma urea concentration ratio is generally greater than 20:1 in prerenal oliguria and less than 10:1 in established ATN.

Correction of circulatory insufficiency and the resulting decreased renal perfusion is very important in preventing the progression of prerenal oliguria to ATN.

Blood transfusion to replace any losses and hydration with intravenous fluids may be successful in restoring circulation. A trial of mannitol or furosemide may be successful in the induction of diuresis.

In established ATN, the period of oliguria may last no longer than a day, or it may last as long as 6 weeks. The average duration of the oliguria is from 7 to 10 days. During the oliguric phase, the usual rise in BUN level is 25 to 30 mg%/day, and creatinine rises at the rate of about 2.5 mg%/day. The retention of fluids, electrolytes, and nitrogenous substances causes the rapid development of uremic symptoms.

Diuretic stage

The diuretic stage of acute renal failure begins when the urine output increases to more than 400 ml/day. This stage generally lasts 2 or 3 weeks. Daily urine output rarely exceeds 4 liters, provided the patient is not over-hydrated. The high urine volume of the diuretic phase is due partly to the osmotic diuresis produced by the high blood urea concentration and partly to the impaired ability of the recovering tubules to conserve filtered salts and water. During the diuretic phase patients may develop deficits of potassium, sodium, and water. If the urinary losses are not replaced, death may complicate the diuresis. During the early diuretic stage, the BUN level may continue to rise largely because urea clearance does not keep up with endogenous urea production. As the diuresis continues, however, the azotemia gradually disappears, and there is great clinical improvement.

Recovery stage

The recovery stage of acute renal failure lasts up to a year, during which time the anemia and concentrating ability of the kidneys gradually improves. Some patients, however, are left with a permanent reduction in the GFR.

Even though damage to tubular epithelium is theoretically reversible, the development of ATN is a dangerous condition with a serious prognosis. The mortality rate is still about 50 percent (down from a previous rate of about 90 percent two decades ago) in spite of the most careful management of fluid and electrolyte balance and the aid of dialysis. About two-thirds die during the oliguric stage, and about one-third during the diuretic stage. The mortality rate is related to the causal background of the associated illnesses leading up to the acute episode. Mortality is about 70 percent in cases following surgery, crush injuries, and other major trauma and about 25 percent following incompatible blood transfusions and carbon tetrachloride poisoning.

TREATMENT OF ESTABLISHED ACUTE TUBULAR NECROSIS

After ATN is established, the primary consideration in management is the maintenance of fluid and electrolyte balance. The same principles of conservative management which were discussed in the treatment of chronic renal failure also apply to acute renal failure. The early use of hemodialysis to prevent severe fluid and electrolyte imbalance and uremic symptoms has undoubtedly reduced the mortality. Careful attention to fluid and electrolyte balance is necessary not only during the oliguric stage but also during the diuretic stage, when severe sodium and potassium depletion may occur. The most frequent complication in acute renal failure resulting in death is infection. It is the contributing cause of death in about 70 percent of patients and the primary cause in about 30 percent. Not only is the uremic patient more susceptible to infection, but once it is established, it is difficult to control. The presence of infection may go unrecognized due to the lack of the usual symptom of fever since hypothermia is common in renal failure. Once infection is identified, it should be treated with nonnephrotoxic antibiotics.

QUESTIONS

Acute renal failure—Chap. 44

Directions: Answer the following questions on a separate sheet of paper.

1 Why is it particularly hazardous to use organic solvents (containing CCl_4) and drink an alcoholic beverage at the same time?

2 List the two major causes of acute renal failure based on the mechanisms of renal injury.

3 What is meant by acute-on-chronic renal failure? Precipitating causes?

4 What is the difference between the two types of histologic lesions commonly observed in ATN? Common etiology?

5 What is acute cortical necrosis? List the common causes, complications, and prognosis.

6 What is the most common complication resulting in death in acute renal failure?

Directions: Circle the letter preceding each item that correctly answers the question. Only ONE answer is correct; exceptions will be noted.

7 Acute renal failure usually refers to the sudden cessation of renal function resulting in urine output less than:
 a 800 ml/day   *b* 1200 ml/day   *c* 400 ml/day

8 In ATN, proximal tubular epithelial damage associated

with CCl₄ or HgCl₂ poisoning (mild exposure) usually results in:

a Irreversible renal failure with infarction of the entire nephron *b* Complete healing of the lesion in 3 to 4 weeks

9 Acute tubular necrosis may result from which of the following? (More than one answer may be correct.)

a Exposure to nephrotoxic chemicals *b* Obstruction of the ureteropelvic junction *c* Hyperkalemia *d* Massive crush injuries *e* Excessive sodium restriction *f* Prolonged shock

10 Which of the following will not cause necrosis of the tubular epithelial cells?

a CCl₄ *b* Severe acute renal ischemia *c* Transfusion reactions *d* Mercuric ions *e* Diodrast (x-ray contrast medium)

11 Which of the following statements is true concerning the treatment and differentiation of prerenal azotemia and established ATN? (More than one answer may be correct.)

a Oliguric urine is concentrated in established ATN. *b* The urine/plasma osmolality ratio is greater than 2:1 in prerenal azotemia. *c* The urine/plasma urea concentration is less than 10:1 in established ATN. *d* The correction of circulatory insufficiency by blood and IV administration of fluids may prevent the progress of prerenal azotemia to ATN. *e* The administration of IV mannitol will correct established ATN.

Directions: Match the stage in the clinical course of acute renal failure in col. B to the statement which applies to it best in col. A.

Column A	Column B
12 ＿＿ Azotemia gradually subsides in this stage.	*a* Oliguric stage
13 ＿＿ Concentrating ability of the kidneys gradually improves during this stage (may last up to 1 year).	*b* Diuretic stage
14 ＿＿ BUN may rise 25 to 30 mg%/ day during this stage.	*c* Recovery stage
15 ＿＿ Average duration is 7 to 10 days.	
16 ＿＿ Most deaths occur during this stage.	
17 ＿＿ Most common complications during this stage are hyperkalemia, pulmonary edema, and cardiac failure.	
18 ＿＿ About one-third of the deaths occur during this stage.	

REFERENCES

AVIOLI, PAUL F.: "Vitamin D Metabolism in Uremia," *The Kidney,* vol. 8, no. 1, 1975.

BAILEY, GEORGE L.: "Uremia as a Total Body Disease," in G. L. Bailey (ed.), *Hemodialysis,* Academic, New York, 1972.

BERLYNE, G. M.: *A Course in Renal Disease,* 3d ed., Blackwell, Oxford, 1971, chaps. 3 and 4.

———: "Renal Involvement in the Collagen Diseases," in D. A. K. Black (ed.), *Renal Disease,* 3d ed., Blackwell, London, 1972, pp. 559–585.

BLACK, D. A. K.: "Immunosuppressive Therapy in Glomerulonephritis," *The Kidney,* vol. 4, no. 6, 1971.

BRICKER, N. S., et al.: "The Kidney in Chronic Renal Disease," in M. H. Maxwell and C. R. Kleeman (eds.), *Clinical Disorders of Fluid and Electrolyte Metabolism,* 2d ed., McGraw-Hill, New York, 1972, pp. 697–723.

———: "On the Functional Transformations in the Residual Nephrons with Advancing Disease," *Pediatric Clinics of North America,* **18**: 595, 1971.

———: "On the Meaning of the Intact Nephron Hypothesis," *American Journal of Medicine,* **46**: 1, 1969.

———: "Renal Function in Chronic Renal Disease," *Medicine,* **44**: 263, 1965.

BROWN, J., et al.: "Diabetes Mellitus: Current Concepts and Vascular Lesions (Renal and Retinal)," *Annals of Internal Medicine,* **68**: 643, 1968.

BRUNDAGE, D. J.: *Nursing Management of Renal Problems,* Mosby, St. Louis, 1976, pp. 83–127.

CAMERON, J. S.: "Natural History of Glomerulonephritis," in D. A. K. Black (ed.), *Renal Disease,* 3d ed., Blackwell, London, 1972, pp. 295–331.

CARTER, N. W.: "Regulation of Acid-Base Balance in Renal Disease," *The Kidney,* vol. 6, no. 2, 1973.

CASTELLAN, GILBERT W.: *Physical Chemistry,* Addison-Wesley, Reading, Mass., 1964, pp. 250–266.

CHURG, J. and H. DOLGER: "Diabetic Renal Disease," in M. B. Strauss and L. G. Welt (eds.), *Diseases of the Kidney,* Little, Brown, Boston, 1971, pp. 873–885.

COLTON, ROGER S. and WARD L. EMMERSON: "Uric Acid, Gout, and the Kidney," *Medical Clinics of North America,* **50**: 1031–1041, 1966.

COUPLAND, R. E.: "Anatomy of the Human Kidney," in D. A. K. Black (ed.), *Renal Disease,* Blackwell, Oxford, 1972, pp. 1–18.

DALGAARD, O. Z.: "Polycystic Disease of the Kidney," in M. B. Strauss and L. G. Welt (eds.), *Diseases of the Kidney,* 2d ed., Little, Brown, Boston, 1971, pp. 1223–1253.

DE WARDNER, H. E.: *The Kidney,* 4th ed., Longman, New York, 1973, pp. 5, 55, 68, 101, 118–132, 266–272, 322–325.

DIXON, FRANK J.: "Glomerulonephritis and Immunopathology," *Hospital Practice,* November, 1967.

DOUGLAS, A. P. and D. S. KERR: *A Short Textbook of Kidney Disease,* Pitman, London, 1968, pp. 34–36, 84–86, 156–206.

EPSTEIN, F. H.: "Acute Glomerulonephritis," *Hospital Medicine,* November, 1968.

EPSTEIN, F. H.: "Glomerulonephritis," in *Harrison's Principles of Internal Medicine*, 7th ed., McGraw-Hill, New York, 1974, pp. 1388–1400.

FINKELBERG, C. and C. M. KUNIN: "Clinical Evaluation of Closed Urinary Drainage Systems," *Journal of the American Medical Association*, **207**: 1657, 1969.

FISH, A. J., A. F. MICHAEL, and R. A. GOOD: "Pathogenesis of Glomerulonephritis," in M. B. Strauss and L. G. Welt (eds.), *Diseases of the Kidney*, 2d ed., Little, Brown, Boston, 1971, pp. 373–395.

FRANKLIN, S. S. and M. H. MAXWELL: "Acute Renal Failure," in M. H. Maxwell and C. R. Kleeman (eds.), *Clinical Disorders of Fluid and Electrolyte Metabolism*, 2d ed., McGraw-Hill, New York, 1972, pp. 727–759.

FREEDMAN, L. R.: "Urinary Tract Infection, Pyelonephritis, and Other Forms of Chronic Interstitial Nephritis," in M. B. Strauss and L. G. Welt (eds.), *Diseases of the Kidney*, 2d ed., Little, Brown, Boston, 1971, pp. 667–713.

GAULT, M. H., et al.: "Syndrome Associated with the Abuse of Analgesics," *Annals of Internal Medicine*, **68**: 906–925, 1968.

GOLDEN, A. and J. F. MAHER: *The Kidney—Structure and Function*, Williams & Wilkins, Baltimore, 1971, pp. 69–87, 145–165, 176–189.

GORDON, ARTHUR and M. H. MAXWELL: "Reversible Uremia," in *Hospital Medicine*, January, 1969, pp. 11–18.

GUTCH, C. F. and MARTHA STONER: *Review of Hemodialysis for Nurses*, Mosby, St. Louis, 1971.

HEPINSTALL, R. H.: "Pathology of Acute Glomerulonephritis," in M. B. Strauss and L. G. Welt (eds.), *Diseases of the Kidney*, Little, Brown, Boston, 1971, pp. 405–452.

KOUNTZ, S. L., et al.: "Complications of Renal Transplantation," *The Kidney*, vol. 5, no. 5, 1972.

KUNIN, CALVIN M.: *Detection, Prevention, and Management of Urinary Tract Infections*, 2d ed., Lea & Febiger, Philadelphia, 1974, pp. 1–41, 127–128, 144–155.

LANGLEY, L. L., I. R. TELFORD, and J. B. CHRISTENSEN, *Dynamic Anatomy and Physiology*, 4th ed., McGraw-Hill, New York, 1974, pp. 667–692.

LINDEMAN, ROBERT D.: "Percutaneous Renal Biopsy," *The Kidney*, vol. 7, no. 2, 1974.

LUKE, R. G.: "Acute Renal Failure," *Hospital Medicine*, May, 1970, pp. 62–75.

MAXWELL, M. and C. R. KLEEMAN, *Clinical Disorders of Fluid and Electrolyte Metabolism*, 2d ed., McGraw-Hill, New York, 1972, pp. 215–233, 246–250, 697–703.

MERRILL, JOHN P.: "Uremia," *New England Journal of Medicine*, **282**: 953–961, 1014–1024, 1968.

METHANY, N. M. and W. D. SNIVELY, *Nurses' Handbook of Fluid Balance*, 2d ed., Lippincott, Philadelphia, 1974, pp. 71–73, 110.

MILNE, MALCOLM D.: "Renal Tubular Dysfunction," in M. B. Strauss and L. G. Welt (eds.), *Diseases of the Kidney*, 2d ed., Little, Brown, Boston, 1971, pp. 1114–1116, 1071–1127.

NETTER, FRANK H.: *Ciba Collection of Medical Illustrations: Kidneys, Ureters, and Urinary Bladder*, Ciba Pharmaceutical Co., Summit, N.J., 1973.

OLSSON, OLLIE: "Renal Radiography," in M. B. Strauss and L. G. Welt (eds.), *Diseases of the Kidney*, 2d ed., Little, Brown, Boston, 1971, pp. 139–196.

PAPPER, S.: *Clinical Nephrology*, Little, Brown, Boston, pp. 20–23, 85–120, 159–197, 227–245, 359–387.

——— and C. A. VAAMONDE: "Nephrosclerosis," in M. B. Strauss and L. G. Welt (eds.), *Diseases of the Kidney*, 2d ed., Little, Brown, Boston, 1971, pp. 735–760.

PITTS, ROBERT F.: *Physiology of the Kidney and Body Fluids*, 3d ed., Year Book, Chicago, 1974, pp. 1, 3–10, 40–41, 71–96, 124–168, 198–239.

RAPPAPORT, F. T. and J. DAUSSET (eds.): *Human Transplantation*, Grune & Stratton, New York, 1968.

REED, G. M. and VINCENT F. SHEPPARD: *Regulation of Fluid and Electrolyte Balance*, Saunders, Philadelphia, 1971.

RELMAN, A. S.: "Pyelonephritis," in D. A. K. Black (ed.), *Renal Disease*, 3d ed., Blackwell, London, 1972, pp. 399–415.

RELMAN, A. S. and N. G. LEVINSKY: "Clinical Examination of Renal Function," in M. B. Strauss and L. G. Welt (eds.), *Diseases of the Kidney*, 2d ed., Little, Brown, Boston, 1971, pp. 87–96, 116–120, 121–125.

ROBBINS, S. L. and M. ANGELL: *Basic Pathology*, Saunders, Philadelphia, 1971, pp. 196–198, 374–376, 385–398.

ROSS, E. J.: "Chronic Renal Failure," in D. A. K. Black (ed.), *Renal Disease*, 3d ed., Blackwell, London, 1972, pp. 463–495.

ROBSON, J. S.: "The Nephrotic Syndrome," in D. A. K. Black (ed.), *Renal Disease*, 3d ed., Blackwell, London, 1972, pp. 331–359.

SCHREINER, G. E.: "Toxic Nephropathy," *American Journal of Medicine*, **38**: 409, 1965.

———: "The Nephrotic Syndrome," in M. B. Strauss and L. G. Welt (eds.), *Diseases of the Kidney*, 2d ed., Little, Brown, Boston, 1971, pp. 503–607.

———: "Renal Biopsy," in M. B. Strauss and L. G. Welt (eds.), *Diseases of the Kidney*, 2d ed., Little, Brown, Boston, 1971, pp. 197–207.

SELDIN, D. W., et al.: "Consequences of Renal Failure and Their Management," in M. B. Strauss and L. G. Welt (eds.), *Diseases of the Kidney*, 2d ed., Little, Brown, Boston, 1971, pp. 211–272.

SHERMAN, JAMES H.: "Osmosis," unpublished manuscript (Associate Professor of Physiology, Assistant Director of Allied Health Education, University of Michigan, Ann Arbor, Michigan).

SMITH, JR., L. H. and H. E. WILLIAMS: "Kidney Stones," in M. B. Strauss and L. G. Welt (eds.), *Diseases of the Kidney*, 2d ed., Little, Brown, Boston, 1971, pp. 973–992.

THEIL, G: "Membranous Glomerulopathy," *The Kidney*, vol. 5, no. 6, 1972.

VANDER, ARTHUR J.: *Renal Physiology,* McGraw-Hill, New York, 1975, pp. 1–9, 36–59, 75–78.

WARHOL, B. A., et al.: "Osmolality," *Archives of Internal Medicine,* **116**: 743, 1965.

WEINER, M. W. and F. H. EPSTEIN: "Signs and Symptoms of Electrolyte Disorders," in M. H. Maxwell and C. R. Kleeman (eds.), *Clinical Disorders of Fluid and Electrolyte Metabolism,* 2d ed., McGraw-Hill, New York, 1972, pp. 629–661.

WELLER, JOHN M. and JAMES A. GREENE: *Examination of the Urine,* Meredith Publishing Co., New York, 1966.

WELT, L. G. (ed.): "Symposium on Uremia," *American Journal of Medicine,* **44**: 653–802, 1968.

WILSON, L. M. and R. E. EASTERLING: *Fistula or Cannula? Hemodialysis Blood Access Systems,* University of Michigan Renal Disease Control Program, 1975.

WINTER, C. C. and M. R. BARKER: *Urologic Diseases,* 3d ed., Mosby, St. Louis, 1972, p. 205.

WOODS, J. W. and T. F. WILLIAMS: "Hypertension Due to Renal Vascular Disease, Renal Infarction, Renal Cortical Necrosis," in M. B. Strauss and L. G. Welt (eds.), *Diseases of the Kidney,* 2d ed., Little, Brown, Boston, 1971, pp. 772–774.

PART VIII Neurologic Disorders

MARIE TRAVA KING
MARY CARTER LOMBARDO

Disorders of the nervous system cause a staggering number of problems in the United States today. Statistics from the National Institutes of Health estimate that approximately 12 percent of the deaths in the United States are directly caused by a neurological disorder. This statistic does not include the chronic neurological conditions that contribute to the cause of death, thereby significantly underestimating the magnitude of the problem. An excess of 19 billion dollars is spent annually in the care of persons with neurological disorders.*

More than 200 clinical syndromes associated with dysfunction, disease, and injury of the nervous system are recognized. The clinical manifestations of disease involving the nervous system are perhaps the most complex and intriguing in all of medicine. Signs and symptoms of these diseases vary in type and range from relatively simple, objective, and easily elicited signs to complex and highly individualized signs.

Only a small number of neurological disorders are presented in this section. Basic concepts and the principles and practices of care and treatment can be applied to all patients experiencing symptoms of a neurological disorder.

*National Institutes of Neurological Diseases and Stroke, *Neurological and Sensory Disabilities: Estimated Numbers and Cost*, Bethesda, Maryland, National Institutes of Health, U.S. Department of Health, Education, and Welfare Bulletin 1973, no. (NIH) 73-152.

OBJECTIVES

At the completion of Part VIII, you should be able to:

1 Describe the normal structure and function of the central and peripheral nervous system and relate this to the elicited signs and symptoms of neurological disorders.

2 Identify the etiology, pathogenesis, and treatment principles for selected neurological disorders.

CHAPTER 45 The Nervous System

OBJECTIVES   **At the completion of Chap. 45 you should be able to:**

1 Review the major components of the central nervous system.

2 Review the structure of the neuron.

3 Identify each unit of a neuron with a particular function.

4 Distinguish between two different nerve cell processes.

5 Identify the relationships of one neuron to another.

6 Distinguish between nerves and tracts.

7 Explain the normal physiology of conduction of an impulse in the neuron.

8 Discuss whether nerve cells regenerate.

9 Name, in addition to the neuron, the major cell types in the nervous system.

10 List the structures that constitute the central nervous system and the peripheral nervous system.

11 Describe the function of the thalamus.

12 Differentiate between the functions of the somatic (cerebrospinal) and the autonomic (visceral) nervous systems.

13 List and describe the function of the subdivisions of the autonomic nervous system.

14 Trace the major pathways from the periphery to the higher centers in the brain for pain, temperature, conscious knowledge of position sense and vibration, information to discriminate size and shape, and touch sensation.

15 Identify for the corticospinal tracts (pyramidal) the origin of the nerve fibers, the pathway from the higher centers of the brain to the periphery, and the type of impulses carried.

CENTRAL NERVOUS SYSTEM

The nervous system is a complicated, functional component of the human body. It is composed of approximately 100 billion neurons and 1 trillion glial cells. Its anatomic variability is a major reason that contributes to its complexity. Sensory organs are continually providing input to the brain, which in turn integrates this information and initiates the body's reaction. Sensory information can be utilized immediately or stored and recalled at a future time when it will help determine the body's response.

Nervous control is always exerted on a muscle or gland by effector, or motor, nerves. Muscles are made to shorten (contract) or lengthen (relax), and glands are stimulated to secrete or cease secretion. Neural control is transmitted from the brain and spinal cord by either the spinal nerves or the cranial nerves (except cranial nerves I and II).

In the evolution of the central nervous system (CNS) almost nothing has been discarded. Rather, the new (higher) centers have been superimposed on lower centers. This process is referred to as *encephalization*. The spinal cord was functionally developed before the evolution of the brain. All basic reflexes are contained within the spinal cord, with the brain acting to modify and facilitate. These basic reflexes can still occur if the brain is removed.

Best and Taylor identify five levels of neural control:

1 Segmental—which is a reflex control.
2 Reticular—involving the reticular formation of the brainstem. Selective facilitation and inhibition modify the segmental reflexes.
3 Level of unconscious control (respiration, body temperature, water balance)—mechanisms of brainstem and diencephalon are involved.
4 Level of voluntary control (skeletal muscles and principal sensory systems). Included are components that contribute to normal movement such as cerebral cortex, basal ganglia, thalamus, and corticopontine cerebellar pathways.
5 Cortical level where neural activity is not measurable in an empirical manner because it is not necessarily translated into movement or secretion; thinking cannot be measured empirically. We only know someone is thinking who tells us that.

Neuroglia

The term *neuroglia* refers to the supportive tissue of the brain or spinal cord, which is composed of specialized connective tissue cells with many protoplasmic processes. These cells are called astrocytes, oligodendroglia, and microglia.

The largest of the glia cells are the astrocytes. The two types of astrocytes are the fibrous and protoplasmic astrocytes. Oligodendroglia cells appear to function in the formation of myelin in the central nervous system.

Neuron

The basic anatomic and functional unit of the nervous system is the neuron, or nerve cell. The neurons consist of cylindrical processes connected to a large central mass which is referred to as the *cell body*. Neurons have at least two processes: an axon and one or more dendrites.

There is a great variation in the size and shape of the cell bodies and their axon lengths. The cell body, or perikaryon, is classically depicted as polyhedral in shape with a large, vesicular, well-defined nucleus.

The cytoplasm of the neuron contains clumps of a chromaphilic substance called Nissl granules or bodies which is the endoplasmic reticulum of the nerve cell. Specialized structures of the nerve cell are neurofibrils, which are delicate, homogeneous strands consisting of neurofilaments and microtubules. Other cell parts that have been demonstrated are Golgi apparatus, mitochondria, lysosomes, and inclusions (Fig. 45-1).

Almost all nerve cell bodies are within the central nervous system. The relatively few outside the central nervous system are usually in clustered groups called *ganglia*.

The *axon*, or nerve fiber, is a single, long process which extends from the cell body. It leaves the cell at the axon hillock, an area of the cell free of Nissl granules. The axon may extend a minute distance, as between two neurons within the spinal cord, or 2 to 3 ft to skeletal muscles.

Dendrites receive the stimuli that initiate conduction and, in turn, conduct or transmit impulses to the cell body. They contain Nissl substance and some neurofibrils.

It is thought that the nerve impulse, or action potential, is generated along the length of the axon's membrane. The potential change occurs at the point of stimulation where the potential inside the cell changes as permeability of the cell membrane is altered. Positive ions from adjacent areas flow inward. The potential difference between the two sides of the membrane is reduced. The resting potential becomes less negative; the permeability increases, and sodium moves in. Polarity reversal occurs, and the outside becomes negative.

An axon often has one or more branches called *collaterals*. Near the end the collaterals branch into divisions called axon terminals which conduct impulses from the neuron to the cell contacted by the axon terminal.

The point or junction between two nerve cells where an impulse from one fiber is connected to another is called a *synapse*. Neurons that conduct information toward synapses are referred to as presynaptic neurons and those neurons conducting information away are postsynaptic neurons (Fig. 45-2).

There are many terminal fibrils of the presynaptic neuron in contact with the dendrites or cell body of the postsynaptic neuron. These terminal fibrils are called synaptic knobs. These synaptic knobs contain many mitochondria and vesicles. Transmitter substances such

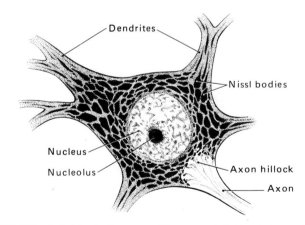

FIGURE 45-1 A typical neuron. Also present but not shown in this drawing are neurofibrils, mitochondria, a Golgi body, and various amounts of fat droplets and pigment granules. (From L. L. Langley, I. R. Telford, and J. B. Christensen, Dynamic Anatomy and Physiology, *4th ed., McGraw-Hill, New York, 1974, p. 210.)*

as acetylcholine (Ach) and norepinephrine are contained within these vesicles. There is a space, the synaptic cleft, between the knob and the postsynaptic neuron. A sequence of events occurs whereby the molecules of transmitter substance are emptied into the synaptic cleft. Receptor sites are located in the postsynaptic membrane. These receptors bind the transmitter (Ach) to a specific site in the receptor which produces the response of the postganglionic neuron. There is also a substance that inactivates the transmitter in order to prevent repetitive postganglionic responses (Fig. 45-3).

There are specific presynaptic neurons that appear to liberate an inhibitory transmitter which raises the threshold of excitation of the postsynaptic neuron. Evidence indicates that the inhibitory transmitter is γ-aminobutyric acid (GABA). GABA appears to cause hyperpolarization by increasing the postsynaptic neuron membrane permeability for potassium and chloride. This causes potassium to diffuse out of the neuron and more chloride to move in. The inside of the membrane becomes more negative in reference to the outside.

Impulses generally move along a neuron in only one direction. A resting neuron has a membrane potential of 70 millivolts (mV), and this remains stationary until the cell is stimulated. When the neuron is stimulated, a generator current is evoked in the receptor. When this reaches threshold magnitude, an action potential results, and the neuron has discharged or fired. A single neuron may polarize but not fire. Other impulses are sent rapidly so they overlap (summation) and fire—called temporal facilitation.

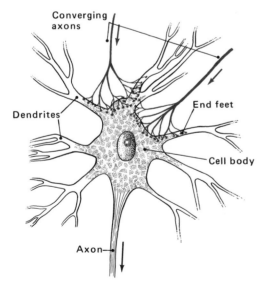

FIGURE 45-2 Synapsis upon a neuron cell body. The arrangement shown is convergence: two presynaptic neurons impinge upon a single postsynaptic neuron. (From L. L. Langley, I. R. Telford, and J. B. Christensen, Dynamic Anatomy and Physiology, 4th ed., McGraw-Hill, New York, 1974, p. 219.)

Regeneration

Nerve cells generally do not have centrosomes and, therefore, are incapable of mitosis and do not reproduce. When a cell body dies, it is not replaced. After birth neurons are not produced by multiplication or differentiation of primordial cells. Adult nerve cells are never seen in mitosis.

However, injuries (called lesions) to the nervous system often do improve with time. There are several theories that may clarify how this process seems to occur (J. Brobeck, 1973):

1 The neurons are temporarily incapacitated—but not destroyed. If the pathology interfering with their metabolism is short-lived, they will recover function normally. Situations that may be responsible for inactivating neurons are anoxia, anesthetics, hypnotics, acidosis, hypothermia, and pressure.

2 A lesion may destroy one component of a system, and the remaining one may be temporarily affected. An example is spinal shock (loss of spinal reflexes), which originally results in areflexia below the lesion. Even though the higher centers are permanently removed (transection of spinal cord), spinal neurons eventually recover the ability to respond to reflex stimuli.

3 Intact neurons may assume the functions of those that were destroyed. However, this is at present a controversial issue.

4 Redundant systems may have innervated a particular part or may be responsible for a particular function. As recovery occurs, one of the backup systems may assume control of the situation.

A nerve cell may recover (with or without structural change), or it may die, depending on the intensity and duration of the offending agent. If the nerve cell dies immediately, 6 to 12 hours are necessary before microscopic changes occur. Loss of function can occur without morphological change being evident.

Initially, there is edema and Nissl disintegration, with the nucleus being displaced to the periphery of the cell. Hyperchromatism occurs, and the nuclear structure loses its clarity. The proximal processes stand out distinctly. Vacuolation and disintegration of cytoplasmic and nuclear membrane indicate a dead cell ready for dissolution and phagocytosis.

If the offending agent produces a chronic pathology, the cell atrophies and hyperchromatism occurs in the cytoplasm and nucleus. Acute and chronic nerve cell involvement are accompanied by glial and blood vessel alterations.

FIGURE 45-3 Electron micrograph of a synapse. The two rounded areas at the bottom are terminal knots of axons. Their synaptic vesicles hold the transmitter substance. When the nerve impulse reaches the terminal knob, the vesicles release the substance into the cleft between the knob and an adjacent dendrite (center of micrograph). (From L. L. Langley, I. R. Telford, and J. B. Christensen, Dynamic Anatomy and Physiology, 4th ed., McGraw-Hill, New York, 1974, p. 220.)

At about age 20, and with increasing age, in the normal population there is shrinkage and dissolution of cell bodies and consequent degeneration of axons. Lost neurons are replaced by glia, chiefly astrocytes.

If an axon is severed, the neuron may generate a new one. However, the neurilemma is necessary for this regeneration. Since neurilemma is present only on peripheral axons, the axons contained in the brain and spinal cord are not capable of regenerating.

AXONAL REACTION

Wallerian degeneration refers to the phenomenon that occurs when an axon of a peripheral neuron is severed; the part separated from the cell body degenerates. The nerve cell can also undergo retrograde changes (swelling, Nissl breakup, loss of angularity). There is a maximum reaction in 12 days as the cytoplasm assumes a ground-glass appearance with a few remaining Nissl granules at the periphery. The cell body (if not destroyed) will undergo restoration and return to a normal appearance. If the cell body is destroyed, the entire neuron dies. If not, the neural process (axon) will grow back into the empty neurilemma, at the rate of approximately 2.5 mm/day.

STRUCTURES OF THE NERVOUS SYSTEM

The nervous system consists of structures and cells so correlated and integrated that they function as a single unit. The basic mechanisms of the nervous system are divided as follows:

1 Central nervous system
    a Brain
    b Spinal cord
2 Peripheral nervous system
    a Afferent system
    b Efferent system
    c Somatic nervous system
    d Autonomic nervous system
        (1) Sympathetic nervous system
        (2) Parasympathetic nervous system

The central nervous system is actually a single, continuous structure divided into the brain and spinal cord.

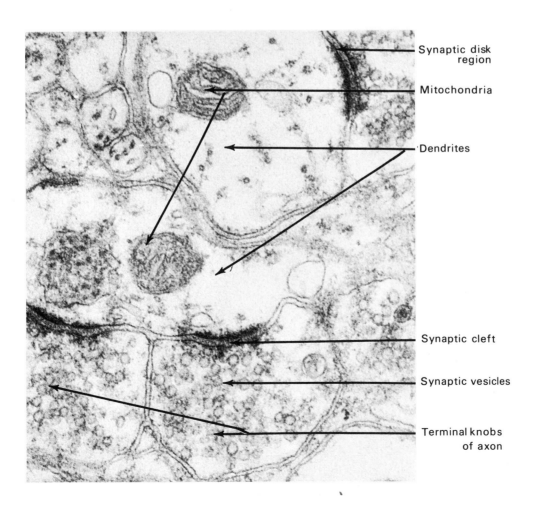

Synaptic disk region

Mitochondria

Dendrites

Synaptic cleft

Synaptic vesicles

Terminal knobs of axon

Spinal cord

The spinal cord is elongated and nearly cylindrical, 1 cm in diameter and 42 to 45 cm in length. Its position varies with the movement of the spinal column. For example, it is drawn upward when the spinal column is flexed. The cord is enclosed in the vertebral column and surrounded by cerebral spinal fluid and meninges. It is anchored in the dura by paired longitudinal ligaments.

The spinal cord consists of two major divisions—the central gray matter and the peripheral white regions. The gray matter contains cell bodies and dendrites of interneurons, efferent neurons, and the entering fibers of afferent neurons. The white matter contains nerve axons which transmit action potentials between various levels of the spinal cord or between the brain and spinal cord. This region has a whitish appearance due to the myelin content of the fibers. The gray matter is composed of nonmyelinated fibers; the white matter, of myelinated fibers. The fibers can be divided into bundles of nerve processes which are referred to as *pathways* or as *tracts*. These tracts can be composed of processes conveying information from the spinal cord to the brain and from the brain to the spinal cord.

The efferent nerves are motor fibers that originate in the anterior horn of the cord. The afferent nerves are sensory fibers and originate in the posterior root ganglion. Immediately outside of the cord these two nerves join to form the spinal nerve.

Each spinal cord segment has four nerves attached to it. The two anterior or ventral roots carry axons to innervate muscles (motor axons). The two posterior or dorsal roots carry sensory information into the cord (Figs. 45-4 and 45-5).

Brainstem

The brainstem connects the spinal cord with the higher brain centers. It is composed of the medulla oblongata, pons, and mesencephalon (midbrain). The cerebellum is attached to the medulla and pons with the fourth ventricle intervening.

Diencephalon

The diencephalon and midbrain lie centrally within the brain between the cerebrum and the pons. The thalamic portion of the diencephalon is subdivided into an epithalamus, thalamus, hypothalamus, and subthalamus. The thalamus is the end station for sensory impulses, all of which synapse there with the exception of the olfactory. In lower forms of life without a cortex, the thalamus is the highest center for sensation. The thalamus correlates all sensory impulses (except olfactory) and relates them to the cortex. It is also involved in crude sensation.

If the cortex is removed, there is a dull awareness of pain or sensation, but the area sending the sensation can not be well localized.

Cerebrum

The cerebrum is the largest portion of the human brain and is located in the upper portion of the cranial cavity. The cortex of the cerebrum is marked by a series of grooves called sulci, or fissures, which divide it into two hemispheres. Prominent fissures include the central fissure (of Rolando), the lateral fissure (of Sylvius), and the parietooccipital fissure. These indentations subdivide each cerebral hemisphere into four lobes—frontal, parietal, temporal, and occipital. The cerebral cortex consists of a thin surface layer of the cerebrum.

Cerebellum

The cerebellum is the second largest portion of the brain. It is located above the medulla and is covered dorsally by the cerebral hemispheres. The cerebellum is separated from the cerebrum by the tentorium cerebelli. The tentorium is a fold of dura mater which serves as a frame of reference for designating locations within the cranium (Fig. 45-6).

Peripheral nervous system

The peripheral nervous system, as mentioned previously, is divided into the autonomic and somatic systems. It consists of 31 pairs of spinal nerves—8 cervical, 12 thoracic, 5 lumbar, 5 sacral and 1 coccygeal. There are also 12 pairs of cranial nerves. All the spinal nerves transmit both motor and sensory impulses mainly to body walls and limbs. The cranial nerves may transmit only motor, only sensory, or both motor and sensory im-

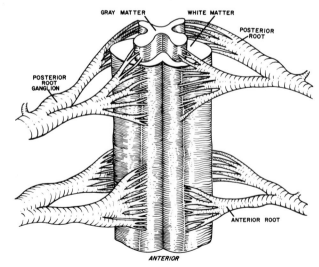

FIGURE 45-4 A view of the anterior aspect of the spinal cord showing the segmental nature of the spinal cord roots. (From B. Curtis, S. Jacobson, and E. Marcus, An Introduction to the Neurosciences, *Saunders, Philadelphia, 1972, p. 11.*)

pulses. The peripheral nervous system is primarily composed of nerve fibers, but it also has cerebrospinal and autonomic ganglia. The cell bodies of all primary sensory neurons are found in the cerebrospinal ganglia located on the dorsal roots of the spinal nerves. Cell bodies or ganglia for special senses (eye, ear, and nose) are found within the particular organ.

The somatic, or motor, portion of the peripheral nervous system innervates skeletal muscle and is chiefly concerned with movement.

The autonomic division is further subdivided into sympathetic and parasympathetic components. The sympathetic division leaves the central nervous system from the thoracic and lumbar regions of the spinal cord, and the parasympathetic from the brain and sacral portion of the spinal cord. Both sets innervate smooth muscle, cardiac muscle, and glands. The autonomic nervous system is mainly concerned with regulation of internal glands. In general, the autonomic nervous system tends to regulate activity of structures not under voluntary control and functions below the level of consciousness.

The differences between the autonomic and somatic nervous systems are summarized below:

1 Autonomic nerves outside the central nervous system synapse once in ganglia.
   a The fiber before the synapse is called the preganglionic (from origin to synapse).
   b The fiber after the synapse is called the postganglionic (from synapse to gland, muscle, etc.).
2 The structures innervated are different—autonomic nerves end at smooth or cardiac muscle or gland; somatic nerves end at skeletal muscle.
3 If the somatic (or skeletal) nerve is destroyed, the muscle innervated will atrophy. Skeletal muscles must be innervated in order to function.
4 Structures innervated by the autonomic nervous system have some intrinsic activity. For example, the heart beats automatically without nerves. The nerves regulate the heart rate.
5 The somatic nervous system always leads to excitation of the effector organ; the autonomic nervous system can lead to excitation or inhibition of the effector organ.

Selected tracts of the spinal cord

ASCENDING SPINOTHALAMIC

The *lateral spinothalamic* tract carries pain and temperature sensation from the cord to the thalamus. The fibers are very small; those for pain are nonmyelinated; temperature fibers may be either myelinated or nonmyelinated. The fibers enter the posterior root of the spinal cord, and they bifurcate and ascend or descend a few segments before entering and synapsing in the posterior horn and cross over to the contralateral side. This information is then relayed to the thalamus, where it is integrated and transmitted to the primary somesthethic cortex.

Posterior columns of the spinothalamic tract carry the modalities of conscious position sense and vibration, information to discriminate size and shape, and touch sensation. Their axons enter the posterior root, synapse in the medulla, and cross to opposite side in the medulla.

CORTICOSPINAL TRACTS

The corticospinal tracts (pyramidal) are descending tracts that carry impulses for voluntary movement. Pyramidal tract is a more accurate term because all fibers do not end in the spinal cord; some end in the nuclei of motor-cranial nerves and in the reticular formation. These fibers originate in the precentral cortex (specifically, from the motor and premotor cortex of the frontal lobe). The fibers join in the internal capsule and continue through the brainstem. In the medulla the majority decussate and travel in the lateral and posterior region of white matter of the spinal cord, forming the lateral corticospinal tract. About 15 percent of the original pyramidal tract fibers continue uncrossed to form the *anterior corticospinal tract*. It generally does not extend below the cervical level; it occasionally is completely absent. Axons leaving the tract are thought to cross at the midline of the cord before synapsing with the anterior horn cells. The *lateral*

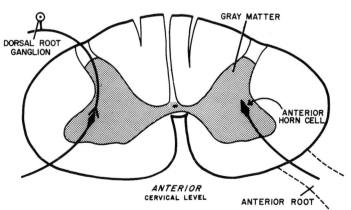

FIGURE 45-5 A cross section of the spinal cord showing the synaptic connection between a sensory root entering the spinal cord through the posterior root and a motor fiber leaving via the anterior root. This particular section is from the neck region. (From B. Curtis, S. Jacobson, and E. Marcus, An Introduction to the Neurosciences, Saunders, Philadelphia, 1972, p. 11.)

corticospinal tract is the major tract for voluntary muscle control. These axons synapse with anterior horn cells. Almost one-half of these fibers end in the cervical area.

EXTRAPYRAMIDAL TRACTS

These tracts descend from nuclei in the brainstem. Current knowledge does not attribute specific function to them so they are together called extrapyramidal tracts. They are concerned with the integration of movement.

SPINOCEREBELLAR TRACTS

These tracts are two pathways from the posterior roots to the cerebellum. They are clinically indistinguishable, and both carry information regarding unconscious position sense.

The *posterior spinocerebellar tract* is made up of large axons whose cell bodies are in the posterior and medial gray matter above the level of T4 and up to C7. This tract enters the cerebellum, uncrossed, by way of the inferior cerebellar peduncle.

The *anterior spinocerebellar tract* originates in the sacral lumbar areas. The fibers synapse in the gray matter upon entry and then cross the cord. They enter the cerebellum by the superior cerebellar peduncle, crossing again as they enter.

Intersegmental tracts are tracts that connect segments of the cord to each other.

QUESTIONS

The nervous system—Chap. 45

Directions: Circle the T for true and the F for false. Correct the false statements.

1   T   F   The nervous system consists of two major cell types, the neurons, their processes, and supporting connective tissue.

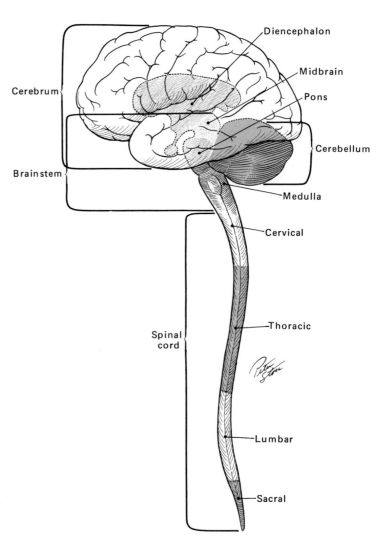

FIGURE 45-6 Lateral view of the central nervous system. (From L. L. Langley, I. R. Telford, and J. B. Christensen, Dynamic Anatomy and Physiology, 4th ed., McGraw-Hill, New York, 1974, p. 228.)

2 T F The nervous system is a communication system which directs and integrates all body activity.

3 T F Dendrites conduct impulses away from the cell body.

4 T F GABA decreases the excitability of neurons.

5 T F Nerve cells are not mitotic; they do not reproduce.

6 T F The thalamus is a crude receptor for sensory phenomena, including olfactory.

7 T F The central nervous system includes the brain, spinal cord, and peripheral nerves.

8 T F All spinothalamic fibers cross in the white matter of the spinal cord.

9 T F Nerve fibers for pain ascend in the posterior gray root of the spinal cord.

10 T F The direction of a nerve impulse can be reversed.

Directions: Circle the letter preceding each item below that correctly answers each question. More than one answer may be correct.

11 The processes of the neuron are:
  a Cytoplasm *b* Axon and one or more dendrites *c* Cell body and one or more axons

12 The point at which an electrical activity from one neuron influences the excitability of another neuron is the:
  a Sensory receptor *b* Effector *c* Synapse *d* Cell body

13 The nerve cell has a resting potential because its membrane is selectively permeable to different ions. The *most* important ion species in the maintenance of resting membrane potential and production of action potential are:
  a Calcium and phosphorus *b* Magnesium and calcium *c* Phosphorus and sodium *d* Sodium and potassium

14 Which of the following appears to function in myelin formation in the central nervous system?
  a Fibroblasts *b* Granulation tissue *c* Collagen *d* Oligodendroglia

15 The gray matter of the spinal cord consists primarily of:
  a Cell bodies and dendrites of interneurons
  b Nerve axons which transmit action potentials
  c Both *a* and *b* *d* Neither *a* nor *b*

16 Cells of the sympathetic division of the autonomic nervous system leave the nervous system from which of the following areas?

  a Ventral gray matter of the spinal cord *b* Lateral gray matter of the spinal cord *c* Medulla *d* Thalamus

17 The thin surface layer of the cerebrum is referred to as the:
  a Cortex *b* Midbrain *c* Pons *d* Sulcus

18 After leaving the spinal cord which of the following join to form the spinal nerve?
  a Efferent nerves that originate in the anterior horn of the cord *b* Afferent nerves that originate in the posterior root ganglion *c* Both *a* and *b* *d* Neither *a* nor *b*

19 Loss of voluntary muscular activity on the left side of the body occurs as a result of injury to which one of the following?
  a Neurons of the spinocerebellar tract in the right hemisphere of the cerebellum *b* Lower motor neurons in the ventral horn on the left side of the cord *c* Neurons of the corticospinal tract in the left hemisphere of the cerebrum *d* Neurons of the corticospinal tract in the right hemisphere of the cerebrum

20 If the _____ root of a spinal nerve were severed, impulses could not be conducted to the particular muscle cells supplied by the axon in that root.
  a Posterior *b* Anterior

21 Which of the following structures is *not* included in the central nervous system?
  a Cerebellum *b* Glia cells *c* Spinal cord *d* Basal ganglia *e* Ganglia of the sympathetic chain

22 Which of the following are characteristic of the autonomic nervous system?
  a It controls involuntary activities. *b* If the nerve is destroyed, the muscle innervated will atrophy. *c* It lies outside the spinal cord. *d* It always leads to excitation of the effector organ.

23 When a nerve cell is acutely injured by an offending agent, which of the following changes can occur if the nerve cell dies immediately?
  a Cell atrophies and hyperchromatism occurs in the cytoplasm. *b* Microscopic changes occur within 6 to 12 hours. *c* Edema occurs along with Nissl disintegration. *d* Vacuolation and disintegration of cytoplasmic and nuclear membrane.

24 Regeneration of nerve fibers will occur if the cell body is intact and the fiber has:
  a A myelin sheath *b* An axon *c* A dendrite *d* A neurilemma

25 Which of the following tracts of the spinal cord carry impulses for sense and vibration and touch sensation?
  a Posterior columns of spinothalamic *b* Lateral spinothalamic *c* Corticospinal *d* Spinocerebellar

26 Voluntary movement nerve fibers:
   a Decussate in the medulla   *b* Enter the posterior
   root of the spinal cord   *c* Originate in the precentral
   cortex   *d* Travel in the lateral and posterior region of
   white matter of the spinal cord

27 What is the resting potential of nervous tissue?
   a 25 mV   *b* 50 mV   *c* 70 mV   *d* 90 mV

28 A neuron can secrete only one neurotransmitter substance. If the neuron is excitatory (versus inhibitory),
   it will secrete:
   a γ-Aminobutyric acid (GABA)   *b* Acetylcholine
   c Both *a* and *b*   *d* Neither *a* nor *b*

CHAPTER 46 The Neurologic Examination: Evaluation of the Neurologic Patient

At the completion of Chap. 46 you should be able to:

1 List the six major areas of the neurologic examination.

2 Explain the purpose of history taking during a neurologic examination.

3 State the function of the cerebellum.

4 Describe at least one function of each lobe (frontal, parietal, temporal, occipital) of the cerebral cortex.

5 Locate the structures of the brain that regulate vital-organ functions (such as heartbeat and respiration) and other body functions (such as hearing and other sensory impulses).

6 Describe the 12 cranial nerves by identifying their function and know how to test each one.

7 Differentiate between normal and abnormal responses to each test for the cranial nerves.

8 Describe the neurologic diseases usually associated with cranial nerve responses.

9 Distinguish between upper and lower motor neurons as to origin and their pathways for eliciting a muscle response.

10 Describe a reflex arc.

11 Describe the procedures for eliciting deep tendon and superficial reflexes.

12 State an example of a deep tendon and a superficial reflex.

13 List four areas that are investigated when examining the sensory nervous system.

14 Describe the effects of a lesion in the lateral spinothalamic tract and the corticospinal tract.

Neurology is a discipline that is concerned with diseases and disorders of the nervous system. This system is a complex and vital network which allows the individual to cope and adapt to environmental stresses. Diseases of the nervous system may develop insidiously (e.g., in multiple sclerosis) or acutely, with sudden interference in normal functioning (e.g., in ruptured aneurysm). Regardless of the cause, the professional health practitioner is dealing with a patient who must adapt to a new method of functioning, whether it is temporary or permanent.

The neurological examination is an essential segment of the diagnostic evaluation of the patient with a neurological disorder. The neurological examination yields valuable information concerning the particular neurological deficit. This information is used to order special diagnostic tests which will confirm the examiner's suspicions in an attempt to establish the diagnosis.

In order for the neurological examination to yield the necessary information, it is important whenever possible, to gain the patient's cooperation. During the process of examination the patient may be asked to do something that may appear to be senseless or likely to make him or her look ridiculous. During the neurologic examination reassurance to the patient that this examination is a vital part of the diagnostic process must be given. Patient education prior to testing should accomplish the following goals: (1) establish the patient's confidence in the person performing the examination; (2) explain what to expect, such as whether the examination will be painful, whether the examiners will say when to expect pain; (3) describe the type of treatment that will be received during the examination; and (4) answer questions as accurately as possible.

THE NEUROLOGICAL EXAMINATION

Evaluation of the patient with a neurological disorder begins with a systematic method of viewing the nervous system. The neurological examination is an integral part of a complete physical examination because of the close relationship of the results with symptoms of medical disease states (e.g., diabetes mellitus, hypertension, thyroid disorders). Therefore, a complete medical evaluation is necessary even when the patient's symptoms suggest a neurological problem. An explanation of the above information to the patient may relieve concerns about the diagnostic procedures that seem to have no relationship to the diseased condition.

The neurological examination focuses on why the patient seeks medical attention. It is important that this information be elicited and recorded in the patient's own words; it should not include diagnostic terms. Important information includes past medical history, a review of systems, social history, and family history. The patient may be asked specifically about dizziness, headaches, visual disturbances, bowel or bladder dysfunction, weakness, numbness, and pain. The examiner observes the patient's behavior, attitude, personal appearance, ability to relate information, and ability to concentrate. This part of the examination provides the examiner with valuable information concerning the patient which will help establish or localize the disease process. In some instances, the physical examination can be negative, and diagnosis is made on history alone, such as in the conditions of migraine or trigeminal neuralgia.

The actual examination of the nervous system is organized into functional segments which include tests of mental status, language abilities, the cranial nerves, motor function, reflexes, and sensory function. The results from each segment are correlated with information gained from the medical history, leading to an accurate localization of the disease process.

Examination of mental status

This portion of the examination evaluates the patient's ability to reason, abstract, plan ahead, and make judgments. Changes in behavior and personality may be associated with organic brain dysfunction and, therefore, these changes need to be elicited from the patient or the patient's family. In evaluating the patient's mental status the examiner must be cognizant of socioeconomic, ethnic, and educational status. The patient is observed for level of consciousness, which may range from alert to comatose. Awareness of time, place, and person is also elicited from the patient. For example, general knowledge and intellect may be evaluated by asking the patient to name five countries or five major rivers. The patient's ability to remember past events may be difficult to assess. This may be accomplished by asking the patient questions concerning his or her own past. Recent memory may be assessed by asking the patient to repeat at least six digits. Normal individuals have the ability to remember and repeat seven digits forward and four backward. Important information is obtained by evaluating the patient's ability to produce abstract thoughts and generalizations from concrete statements. Asking the patient to interpret a common saying (e.g., "A rolling stone gathers no moss") is frequently the method used.

Cerebral functions

The frontal lobe predominantly functions in conceptualizing, abstracting, and forming judgments. Lesions of the frontal lobe are frequently accompanied by impaired judgment and reasoning and slovenly attention to dress and personal grooming.

Functioning as the highest integrative and coordinating center for perception and interpretation of sensory phenomena is the parietal cortex. Patients with disorders affecting the parietal lobes have difficulty understanding receptive communications.

Memories are thought to be stored in temporal areas, with recent memory located in the hippocampus (part of the limbic system, which is located along the medial portion of the cerebral cortex). Disorders affecting the temporal lobes frequently affect recent memory but leave memory of past events intact (Fig. 46-1).

Language and speech examination

One of the most important functions of the dominant hemisphere is speech. The left hemisphere is dominant for speech in right-handed individuals and in the majority of left-handed persons. In approximately 20 percent of left-handed individuals the right hemisphere is dominant for speech. There are three speech disorders of neurological origin—dysarthria, dysphonia, and aphasia.

Dysarthria is a defect in articulation, enumeration, and rhythm of speech related to a weakness in the muscles involved in speech. This abnormality is usually detected in ordinary conversation with the patient but may be confirmed by asking for repetition of a difficult word or phrase, such as "methodist episcopal." The causes for this weakness can be amyotrophic lateral sclerosis, pseudobulbar palsy, and myasthenia gravis.

Dysphonia is a disorder of vocalization giving a hoarse quality to the voice. Confirmation of this problem can be made by asking the patient to say "E," which should result in hoarseness or a rough quality to the voice, and by indirect laryngoscopy. This problem has many non-neurologic causes. The neurologic causes of dysphonia are injury to the recurrent laryngeal nerve and tumors of the brainstem.

Aphasia is a general term meaning the loss of ability to comprehend, elaborate, or express speech concepts. Motor aphasia is the loss of the ability to express one's thoughts in speech or writing and sensory aphasia is the loss of the ability to comprehend spoken or written language. Evaluation can be done by directing the patient to perform certain tasks by written or verbal orders, such as, "Fold this paper, write your name." The most common cause of aphasia is a cerebrovascular disorder involving the middle cerebral artery, which supplies the speech and language center.

Examination of the cranial nerves

There are 12 pairs of cranial nerves arising from the undersurface of the brain through small foramina. The cranial nerves are numbered according to the order in which they emerge from front to rear (Fig. 46-2).

The cranial nerves are composed of afferent or efferent fibers, and some are of both types, which are referred to as mixed fibers. The cell bodies of the afferent fibers are located in ganglia outside the brainstem while the cell bodies of the efferent fibers are located in various nuclei of the brainstem.

The cranial nerves are not examined in sequence but are examined according to function. The method of examination of the cranial nerves and some pathophysiologic implications will be discussed.

OLFACTORY NERVE (CRANIAL NERVE I)

The olfactory nerve conveys smells to the brain for appreciation. With the patient's eyes closed and one nostril occluded at a time, mildly aromatic substances such as vanilla, cologne, and cloves are offered for identification. The patient is requested to indicate the moment of first

detection of the odor and, if possible, to identify the substance. Perception of the odor is more important than correct identification of the substance.

Nasal disorders, e.g., sinusitis, allergies, and upper respiratory infections, are the most common causes of loss of smell. The neurologic causes include tumor in the olfactory groove (olfactory groove and meningioma). Anosmia may also occur after meningitis, subarachnoid hemorrhage, or head injury involving the nerve fibers as they pass through the cribriform plate.

OPTIC NERVE (CRANIAL NERVE II)

The optic nerve transmits impulses from the retina to the optic chiasm and then through visual pathways to the occipital cortex for recognition and interpretation. Examination of this nerve involves testing visual acuity either by using a Snellen or a Jaeger test or, if these are not available, by asking the patient to read various sizes of newspaper print. Reduction of visual acuity is generally caused by diseases involving the eye, the optic nerve, or the optic chiasm. Visual field examinations give the examiner information concerning the optic nerve and visual pathways from the eye to the occipital cortex. For general purposes as part of a neurological examination, visual fields are examined by confrontation. The patient is asked to cover one eye with the examiner sitting directly in front with the eye opposite to the patient's shut eye closed; a pencil or finger is brought into the field of vision from four quadrants and should be seen by both people. This method provides a gross screening device. For a more thorough evaluation a perimeter and target screen is used.

The optic disc is visualized by use of the ophthalmoscope. Neurologically the two most significant findings

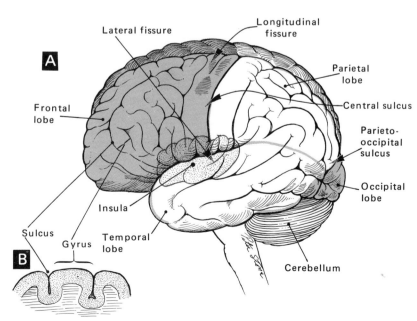

FIGURE 46-1 A. *Lateral view of the cerebrum. Note the line that demarcates the parietal and temporal lobes. B. A portion of the cortex in cross section. (From L. L. Langley, I. R. Telford, and J. B. Christensen,* Dynamic Anatomy and Physiology, *4th ed., McGraw-Hill, New York, 1974, p. 229.)*

are papilledema and optic atrophy. Changes in the disc occur with tumors, infections, and trauma. Other changes visualized are exudates, hemorrhages, and arteriovenous abnormalities associated with diabetes and hypertension.

OCULOMOTOR, TROCHLEAR, AND ABDUCENS NERVE (CRANIAL NERVES III, IV, AND VI)

These three nerves are examined together since they act conjugately to control the extraocular muscles (EOM). In addition, the oculomotor nerve elevates the upper eyelid and innervates the constrictor muscle, which alters the pupil size. The innervation of the EOM is examined by asking the patient to follow a moving finger or pencil with eyes turning upward, downward, medially, and laterally. Weakness in muscles becomes evident when an eye cannot move in a certain direction. Pupils are examined in subdued light and should be round and ap-

proximately equal in size, although unequal pupils are found in approximately 20 to 25 percent of the population. However, the difference is rarely greater than 1 mm. Both pupils should react to light directly and consensually.

The nuclei of the oculomotor nerves and the trochlear nerve are located in the midbrain. The nuclei of the abducens nerve lie beneath the floor of the fourth ventricle in the lower pons and are very close to fibers from the facial nerve nucleus.

Myasthenia gravis is an important cause of weakness of the extraocular muscles causing weakness in more than one muscle and ptosis (see Chap. 49). Horner's syndrome consists of ptosis of the lid, constriction of the pupil, and absence of sweating on the same side of the face. This can be due to vascular lesions in the brainstem, cervical spinal cord injuries and tumors, and trauma affecting the sympathetic fibers in the neck, and can be a temporary side effect of cerebral angiography.

Nystagmus, rapid oscillations of the eye as it gazes laterally, is an important neurological sign. It is seen normally on extreme lateral gaze. Neurological causes include multiple sclerosis, lesions of one cerebellar

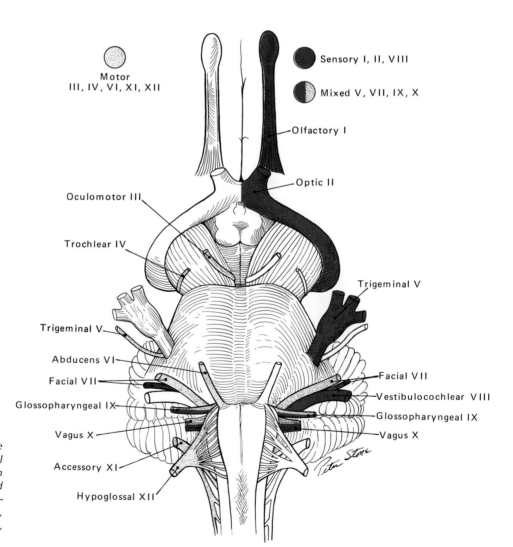

Motor
III, IV, VI, XI, XII

Sensory I, II, VIII

Mixed V, VII, IX, X

Olfactory I

Optic II

Oculomotor III

Trochlear IV

Trigeminal V

Trigeminal V

Abducens VI

Facial VII

Facial VII

Glossopharyngeal IX

Vestibulocochlear VIII

Vagus X

Glossopharyngeal IX

Vagus X

Accessory XI

Hypoglossal XII

FIGURE 46-2 Emergence of the cranial nerves from the ventral surface of the brainstem. (From L. L. Langley, I. R. Telford, and J. B. Christensen, Dynamic Anatomy and Physiology, 4th ed., McGraw-Hill, New York, 1974, p. 250.)

hemisphere, or tumor of one side of the brain. Non-neurologic causes include the use of barbiturates and tranquilizers.

TRIGEMINAL NERVE (CRANIAL NERVE V)

The trigeminal nerve carries both motor and sensory fibers. It supplies innervation to the temporal and masseter muscles, which are the muscles of mastication. Examination of the motor division of this nerve is accomplished by asking the patient to clench the teeth and move the jaw from side to side while the examiner palpates the muscles and judges the strength of contraction.

The sensory fibers of the trigeminal nerve are divided into three main branches—ophthalmic, maxillary, and mandibular (Fig. 46-3). In order to evaluate areas of sensory loss each area is tested by asking the patient to respond to a touch with a piece of cotton. The corneal reflex is tested in each eye—a wisp of cotton with a fine point is touched to the cornea causing the patient to blink.

Tumors of the posterior fossa cause loss of corneal reflex and facial numbness as an early sign. The most notable disorder affecting the trigeminal nerve is trigeminal neuralgia, or tic douloureux, causing brief, excruciating pain along the maxillary or mandibular divisions of the trigeminal nerve. Myasthenia gravis and amyotrophic lateral sclerosis cause weakness and fatigue of the muscles of mastication causing chewing to be difficult and at times impossible.

FACIAL NERVE (CRANIAL NERVE VII)

This nerve has both sensory and motor function. It carries sensory fibers which mediate taste perception from the anterior tongue and motor fibers which innervate all the muscles necessary for the varied facial expressions individuals are capable of—including smiling, frowning, grimacing, etc.

The motor division of the facial nerve is evaluated by asking the patient to perform various facial movements and observing the patient talk. Weakness of the facial muscle would evidence itself by flattening of the nasolabial fold, drooping of one side of the mouth, and sagging of the lower eyelid. The sense of taste is evaluated by asking the patient to identify sweet, sour, bitter, and salty substances that are applied to the tongue.

Since the nucleus of the facial nerve lies in the lateral portion of the lower pons, a lesion in the area of the

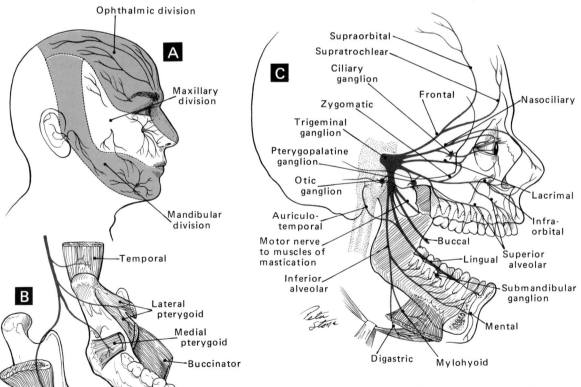

FIGURE 46-3 A. *Distribution of sensory fibers to the skin by the three branches of the trigeminal nerve.* B. *Distribution of the cheif motor fibers to muscles of mastication.* C. *Distribution of terminal branches. (From L. L. Langley, I. R. Telford, and J. B. Christensen,* Dynamic Anatomy and Physiology, *4th ed., McGraw-Hill, New York, 1974, p. 254.)*

brainstem will often cause facial nerve dysfunction. Since the facial nerve enters the temporal bone and is in close proximity to the middle ear, it is subject to trauma from fractures of the base of the skull and the temporal bone; from surgical procedures; and from diseases of the ear. Other disorders that may result in facial nerve weakness include myasthenia gravis and Guillain-Barré syndrome. Bell's palsy is the most common type of nerve paralysis.

ACOUSTIC NERVE (CRANIAL NERVE VIII)

The acoustic nerve functions to maintain balance and to transmit impulses which allow the individual to hear. Maintenance of balance is the function of the vestibular division, while the cochlear division mediates hearing. The acoustic nerve cochlear division can be tested by observing the patient's ability to hear a whisper from a distance of 2 ft. Another method of testing is by using the tuning fork, which will distinguish between conductive hearing loss and sensorineural loss. There are two commonly used hearing tests which are referred to as the Weber and Rinne tests. In the Weber test, a vibrating tuning fork is placed on the mastoid process; when the patient indicates that the vibration is no longer audible, the tuning fork is placed next to the ear. If the patient again hears the vibration, then air conduction (AC) is better than bone conduction (BC), which is normally the case. The Rinne test is often done by placing the vibrating tuning fork on the top of a patient's head or on the forehead. The patient is asked where the sound is loudest. Normally the individual will hear best on the occluded side. In conductive loss the sound is referred to the diseased ear, while in sensorineural loss, it is not heard on the affected side. If an abnormality is detected, a complete audiometric evaluation is recommended.

Acute dysfunction of the vestibular division of the acoustic nerve is manifested by vertigo, nausea, vomiting, and ataxia. The cold caloric test is used to screen for problems which may be performed with the patient upright. Five ml of ice water is injected into the ear. The normal response to this stimulus is nystagmus of both eyes, vertigo, nausea, and vomiting. Little or no reaction to this stimulus indicates an abnormality of the vestibular nerve. Ménière's disease involves a dilation of the endolymphatic channels in the cochlea with eventual atrophy of the hearing mechanism resulting in vertigo, tinnitus, and hearing loss in the affected ear.

The acoustic nerve leaves the brainstem and travels along a similar path as the facial nerve. Like the facial nerve it is subject to damage from fractures of the base of the skull and the temporal bone. Vascular occlusions and tumors of the brainstem are other causes of damage to the acoustic nerve.

THE GLOSSOPHARYNGEAL AND VAGUS NERVES (CRANIAL NERVES IX AND X)

These two nerves are closely related anatomically and functionally and are evaluated together. The glosso-pharyngeal nerve has a sensory division which carries taste from the posterior portion of the tongue, innervates the carotid sinus and the carotid bodies, and supplies sensation to the pharynx. The motor division innervates the posterior wall of the pharynx. The vagus nerve innervates all the thoracic and abdominal viscera and conveys impulses from the walls of the intestines, the heart, and the lungs. It is not possible clinically to examine all of these functions; therefore, evaluation of the vagus nerve is directed toward evaluating the motor function of the palate, pharynx, and larynx.

The first step in evaluation of the glossopharyngeal and vagus nerves is inspection of the soft palate. The soft palate should be symmetrical and should not deviate to either side. When the patient says "ah," the soft palate should rise symmetrically. To induce a gag reflex the posterior wall of the pharynx is touched, causing elevation of the palate and constriction of the pharyngeal muscles. The patient's swallowing reflex is tested by observing the reaction to drinking a glass of water. Observations are made of difficulty in swallowing or regurgitation of fluid through the nose, which would indicate weakness of the soft palate and an inability to close off the nasopharynx when swallowing. Indirect laryngoscopy is done when the patient's complaint is a voice disturbance or hoarseness. The vocal cords can be observed for paresis or lesions. Bilateral lesions may cause great difficulty in swallowing and in the ability to mobilize secretions.

The glossopharyngeal and the vagus nerves leave the skull through the jugular foramen with the internal jugular vein. Therefore trauma or a tumor in close proximity to this area would affect these structures. The recurrent laryngeal nerve, a branch of the vagus which supplies the larynx, is susceptible to injury during surgery of the neck because of its close proximity to the thyroid gland. Amyotrophic lateral sclerosis and myasthenia gravis frequently cause weakness in the muscles innervated by the glossopharyngeal and the vagus nerve.

SPINAL ACCESSORY NERVE (CRANIAL NERVE XI)

The spinal accessory nerve is a motor nerve innervating the sternocleidomastoid muscle and the upper portion of the trapezius muscle. These muscles act to flex the neck; the sternocleidomastoid muscle acts to rotate the head from side to side, and the trapezius rotates the scapula when the arm is raised.

The function of the spinal accessory nerve is evaluated by observing the muscles for atrophy and assessing their strength. It is examined by asking the patient to turn the head toward one shoulder and to resist attempts of the examiner to move the head in the opposite direction. The strength of the sternocleidomastoid muscle on the opposite side is evaluated by repeating the test on the opposite side. The trapezius muscle is evaluated by asking the patient to shrug the shoulders while the examiner attempts to push downward. The patient is then asked to elevate both arms to a vertical position. A patient with weakness in the trapezius muscle will not be able to perform this action.

The spinal accessory nerve lies in close proximity to the glossopharyngeal and the vagus nerves. Tumors affecting these frequently affect this nerve. The cell bodies of the spinal accessory nerve lie in the upper part of the spinal cord at levels C1 through C5 and receive innervation from both cerebral hemispheres. A unilateral lesion causes little or no dysfunction in the two muscles innervated by this nerve. The most common cause for spinal accessory nerve dysfunction is neck trauma.

HYPOGLOSSAL NERVE (CRANIAL NERVE XII)

The hypoglossal nerve innervates the musculature of the tongue. Normal functioning of the tongue is essential for normal speech and swallowing. Slight bilateral weakness will be evident by difficulty in enunciating consonants and difficulty in swallowing. Severe bilateral weakness causes extreme difficulty with speech and swallowing.

The tongue is examined for asymmetry, deviation to one side, and the presence of fasciculations. This examination is done first inside the mouth with the tongue at rest and then with the tongue protruded. Strength of the muscle is evaluated by asking the patient to push out a cheek with the tongue while the examiner opposes the effort with fingers on the patient's cheek.

The nuclei of the hypoglossal nerves lie within the medulla beneath the floor of the fourth ventricle and receive innervation from both cerebral hemispheres.

Injuries to the neck may cause unilateral weakness of the tongue with atrophy and fasciculations. Tumors at the base of the posterior fossa near the foramen magnum may cause ipsilateral paralysis of the tongue. Bilateral weakness can be due to amyotrophic lateral sclerosis and myasthenia gravis.

Examination of motor function

Motor performance is dependent upon an intact muscle, a functioning neuromuscular junction, and intact cranial and spinal nerve tracts. In order to understand how the nervous system functions to coordinate muscle activity, it is important first to be able to distinguish between the upper and the lower motor neuron.

The *upper motor neuron* originates in the cerebral cortex and projects downward, one part (the corticobulbar tract) ending in the brainstem and the other (the corticospinal tract) crossing in the lower medulla and descending into the spinal cord. The cranial nerve nuclei

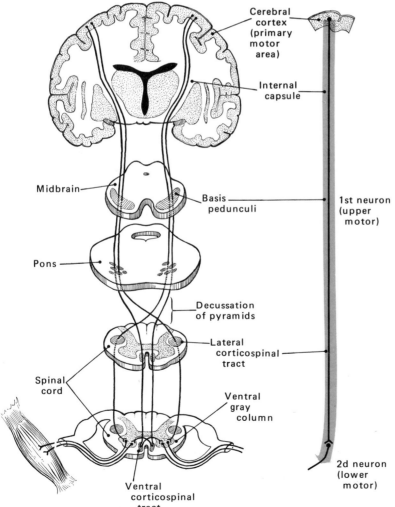

FIGURE 46-4 Pyramidal motor pathways, the corticospinal tracts. The tracts originate in pyramidal cells of the cortex. Fibers that cross at the medulla form the lateral corticospinal tracts, while the remaining fibers form the ventral corticospinal tracts. The basis pedunculi are part of the cerebral peduncles. (From L. L. Langley, I. R. Telford, and J. B. Christensen, Dynamic Anatomy and Physiology, 4th ed., McGraw-Hill, New York, 1974, p. 286.)

serve as the end point for the corticobulbar tracts. The corticospinal tracts terminate in the region of the anterior horn of the spinal cord from the cervical to the sacral areas. Those corticospinal fibers that travel through the medullary pyramids constitute the pyramidal tracts. Nerve fibers in the corticospinal tract mediate voluntary movement, particularly fine, discrete, conscious movement (Fig. 46-4).

The *lower motor neuron* includes the motor cells of the cranial nerve nuclei and their axons as well as the anterior horn cells of the spinal cord and their axons. The motor fibers leave through the anterior, or motor, root of the spinal column and innervate the muscles.

Lesions involving the upper motor neuron and the lower motor neuron produce characteristic changes in muscle response. Awareness of the differences in muscle weakness will help locate the neurologic lesion.

Certain observations are made of the musculature during this phase of the neurologic examination. These include observations of the way the patient walks and stands. These activities require adequate muscle strength, coordination, plus vestibular function and vision. Abnormalities in strength and coordination can be accentuated by asking the patient to walk heel to toe (tandem walking). This test will often reveal a lack of coordination. Coordination is further tested by requesting the patient to follow through on simple rapid movements (placing a hand on a knee quickly). An additional test is to ask the patient to place the heel of one foot on the opposite knee and to slide it down the front of the leg.

Major muscle groups should be observed for any evidence of muscle wasting, fasciculations, or contractures. Muscle strength is tested by comparing muscles of one side to those on the other as the patient resists the examiner's movements. Age, sex, and the physical condition of the patient must be considered when evaluating these tests. Muscle tone, which is the resistance detected by the examiner when a joint is moved through passive range of motion, is frequently altered in nervous system disorders. Upper motor neuron disorders increase the tone, while lower motor neuron disorders decrease muscle tone. The patient is observed for any evidence of involuntary movements; these include tremors, chorea, athetosis, dystonia, hemiballism, and tic.

Tremors are involuntary, rhythmic, tremulous movements that may be more pronounced at rest (resting tremor) or as the patient reaches for an object (intention tremor). Tremors are the result of lesions of the cerebellar pathways (Bates, 1974).

Involuntary movements of the face, extremities, or trunk that are rapid, irregular, jerky, and purposeless are known as chorea. These occur in diseases of the basal ganglia and are present in two particular disorders: Huntington's chorea and Sydenham's chorea.

Athetosis, frequently seen in cerebral palsy, is infrequent, slow, twisting, irregular motions, especially of the face and hand. Dystonia is a movement disorder in which parts of the body are held in abnormal positions for varying periods of time. Some of these movements include extreme pronation or supination or forced head or trunk rotation, sometimes combined with powerful flexion or extension at various joints. These abnormal movements may be seen with Wilson's disease, after injection of phenothiazine, and with virus infections of the brain (Simpson and Magee, 1973).

Hemiballism, a rare disorder of movement, is due to cerebrovascular occlusions involving the subthalamic nucleus. The movements are unilateral, affecting the side opposite the occlusion, and involve violent, flinging movements at the proximal joint. These movements are continuous in the early stage but diminish in intensity after a few weeks.

Tics are repetitive twitching of muscles, frequently in the face and around the eye and mouth. The cause is in most cases benign.

Evaluation of reflexes

A deep tendon reflex is elicited by a brisk tap with a reflex hammer over a partially stretched tendon. The impulse then travels along afferent fibers to the spinal cord, where it synapses with a motor neuron or anterior horn cell. After it synapses, the impulse is transmitted down the motor neuron to the anterior nerve root through the spinal nerve and then the peripheral nerve. After being transmitted across the neuromuscular junction, the muscle is stimulated to contract. In simplest form this is the reflex arc (Fig. 46-5).

Different deep tendon reflexes commonly tested are the biceps reflex, the triceps reflex, the brachioradialis reflex, the patellar reflex, and the achilles reflex. The response to reflexes is graded on a scale of 0 to +4 (see Table 46-1).

It is important to compare sides when evaluating reflex responses.

Superficial reflexes are tested by stroking the skin with a firm object such as the end of a reflex hammer or applicator, causing the muscles to contract. These reflexes include abdominal, cremasteric, plantar, and gluteal. Abdominal and cremasteric reflexes may be ab-

TABLE 46-1
Grading of reflexes

GRADE	SIGNIFICANCE
+4	Very brisk, suggestive of disease of the upper motor neuron, frequently associated with clonus (rhythmic oscillations between flexion and extension)
+3	Brisker than average but not necessarily indicative of disease
+2	Average/normal
+1	Somewhat diminished
0	No response

Source: Modified from B. Bates, *A Guide to Physical Examination*, Lippincott, Philadelphia, 1974.

sent in both upper and lower motor neuron disorders. The plantar reflex is elicited by stroking the lateral aspect of the sole from the heel to the ball and curving medially across the ball of the foot. The normal response to this stimulus is flexion of the toes. An abnormal response, dorsiflexion of the great toe with fanning of the other toes, is known as the Babinski reflex and indicates upper motor neuron disease (Fig. 46-6). This reflex may be present normally in children under the age of 2 years.

Sensory evaluation

The sensory system plays a vital role in conveying to the central nervous system information concerning the environment. When examining the sensory system the fol- lowing four areas are investigated: (1) superficial tactile sensation including pain, temperature, and touch; (2) proprioceptive sense, which is motion or position sense; (3) vibratory sense; and (4) cortical sensory functions. Patterns of sensory loss may lead to a diagnosis of lesions of the cerebral hemisphere, the brainstem, the spinal cord, the nerve root, and single or multiple peripheral nerves.

Perceptions of pain and temperature are carried by nerve fibers to the dorsal root ganglia where the nuclei

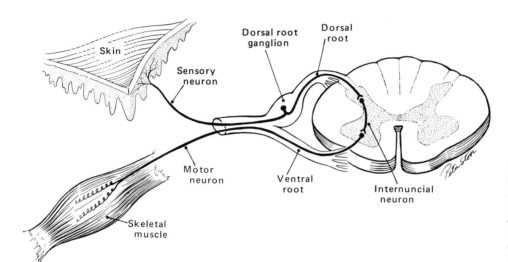

FIGURE 46-5 Components of a simple reflex: a sensory, an internuncial, and a motor neuron. (From L. L. Langley, I. R. Telford, and J. B. Christensen, Dynamic Anatomy and Physiology, 4th ed., McGraw-Hill, New York, 1974, p. 280.)

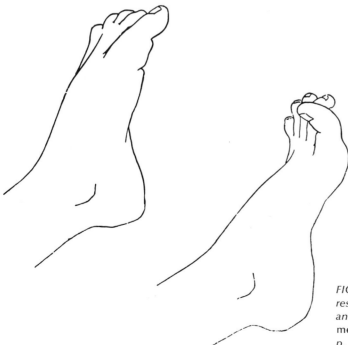

FIGURE 46-6 The Babinski response. Upper, the normal adult response to stimulation of the foot. Lower, the normal infant and abnormal adult response. (From E. D. Gardner, Fundamentals of Neurology, 6th ed., Saunders, Philadelphia, 1975, p. 215.)

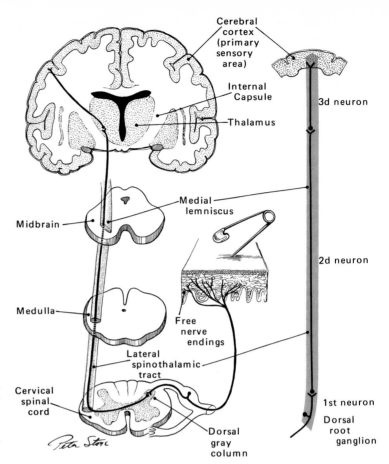

FIGURE 46-7 The central pathway for impulses perceived as pain, the lateral spinothalamic tract. Note that the fibers cross upon entering the spinal cord. (From L. L. Langley, I. R. Telford, and J. B. Christensen, Dynamic Anatomy and Physiology, 4th ed., McGraw-Hill, New York, 1974, p. 271.)

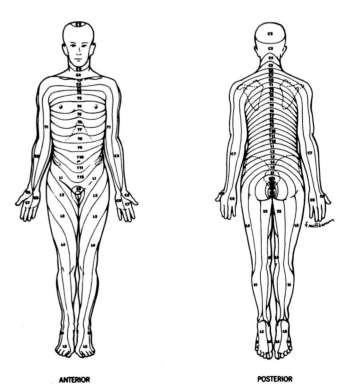

FIGURE 46-8 Arrangement of the dermatomes. (From J. Simpson and K. Magee, Clinical Evaluation of the Nervous System, Little, Brown, Boston, 1973, p. 77.)

of these nerve fibers are located. After synapsing in the dorsal horn they cross over the midline and enter the opposite lateral spinothalamic tract. This tract ascends through the entire length of the spinal cord, medulla, pons, and midbrain and terminates in the thalamus. The thalamus, acting as a relay station, transmits the impulse to the sensory cortex for interpretation. Simple touch sensation is transmitted by the ventral spinothalamic tract. A lesion involving the lateral spinothalamic tract will result in loss of pain and temperature sensation on the opposite side of the body below the level of the lesion. Lesions of the nerve roots and of peripheral nerves impair the perception of touch (Fig. 46-7).

Fibers conducting the sensation of position, vibration sense, and touch sensations requiring a high degree of localization, like stereognosis, graphesthesia, and two-point discrimination, enter the spinal column and pass into the dorsal column system. Traveling upward to the lower medulla where they synapse and cross over, the fibers ascend as the medial lemniscus, terminating in the thalamus. The fine distinction and perception of these sensations is made in parietal cortex.

The pattern of the dermatomes is shown in Fig. 46-8. Theoretically, a lesion in the dorsal root produces loss of sensation in the area supplied by the root. However, there is considerable overlap of nerve supply, which frequently confuses the clinical picture.

Sensory testing is done with the patient's eyes closed, using a wisp of cotton to test for touch, a safety pin to test for superficial pain, and test tubes filled with hot and cold water, respectively, to test for temperature.

Proprioception, position, and motion sense is first evaluated in distal joints. If proprioception is normal in the distal joints, then it is not necessary to test the proximal joint. A distal phalanx of one of the patient's fingers is grasped, slowly moved upward or downward, and the patient is asked to indicate the movement of the phalanx. The Romberg test evaluates the position sense for the legs and trunk: the normal individual should be able to stand with feet together and eyes closed without swaying markedly or losing balance. Frequently patients with abnormality in the proprioceptive pathway can maintain their balance with eyes open since the visual orientation serves to keep them balanced. The patient with a cerebellar disorder, on the other hand, sways and loses balance with eyes open as well as closed.

QUESTIONS

The neurologic examination: evaluation of the neurologic patient—Chap. 46

Directions: Answer the following questions on a separate sheet of paper.

1 What is the purpose of history taking during a neurological examination?

2 List the six major areas of the neurological examination.

Directions: Mark T for true and F for false. Correct the false statements.

3 T F The highest integrative and coordination center for perception and interpretation of sensory input is the frontal lobe.

4 T F The neurologic examination of the mental status evaluates the patient's ability to reason, make abstract thoughts, plan ahead, make judgments.

5. T F The right hemisphere is dominant for speech in right-handed individuals and in the majority of left-handed persons.

6 T F Dysarthria is a defect in articulation, enunciation, and rhythm of speech related to a weakness in the muscles involved in speech.

Directions: Match the respective functions in col. B to the appropriate location of its cerebral control in col. A.

Column A

7 _____ Medulla (brainstem)
8 _____ Frontal lobe
9 _____ Precentral gyrus of frontal lobe (strip along central fissure in posterior part frontal lobe)
10 _____ Occipital lobe
11 _____ Temporal lobe
12 _____ Parietal lobe (strip along central fissure)
13 _____ Cerebellum
14 _____ Thalamus

Column B

a Hearing
b Balance, coordination
c Relay center for sensory impulses
d Voluntary muscle movements
e Vital organ functions—heartbeat, respiration
f Reception of fine sensory stimuli
g Sight
h Intellect, memory, thought

Directions: Select the letter which best answers the question. More than one answer may be correct.

15 During a cranial nerve examination which of the following *may* be abnormal if there is damage to the medulla?
a Pupillary reflex b Gag reflex c Corneal reflex
d Patient's ability to shrug shoulders

16 During a cranial nerve exam, Mr. B demonstrates the ability to smile without any apparent impairment but indicates that he is unable to chew. Where do you suspect the problem to be?
a Abducent (VI) b Facial (VII) c Trigeminal (V)
d Acoustic (VIII) e Trochlear (IV)

17 Which of the following cranial nerves is responsible for vision?
a Olfactory (I) b Optic (II) c Oculomotor (III)
d Facial (VII)

18 Mrs. Jones presents with a dilated left pupil, left ptosis (drooping of the eyelid), and the inability to look up, down, or medially with her left eye. These signs indicate a problem with:
a Right optic nerve b Left optic nerve c Left oculomotor nerve d Left trochlear nerve e Left abducent nerve

19 On neurological examination it was observed that a positive Babinski reflex was demonstrated. Which of the following best describes this reflex?
a Extension of the leg when the patellar tendon is struck b Tremor of the foot following brisk, forcible dorsiflexion c Dorsiflexion of the great toe when the sole is stroked d Flexion of the forearm when the biceps tendon is tapped

20 Mr. J. has an extensive tumor of the cerebellum. In view of the functions of this organ, which symptom would you expect to observe?
a Absence of the knee jerk and other reflexes
b Inability to execute smooth, precise movements
c Inability to respond to verbal commands d All of the above

21 Reflex activity of the central nervous system:
a Requires at least two nerve cells b Is a simple process in higher mammals c Requires more than three nerve cells to become activated d Is a mechanical process

22 In the patellar reflex, efferent impulses originate from cell bodies located in the:
a White matter of the spinal cord b Ventral gray column of the spinal cord c Dorsal root spinal ganglion d Ventral root spinal ganglion

23 A lesion in the corticospinal tract may cause:
a Problems with visual acuity b Weakness with decreased reflexes c Weakness with increased reflexes d Problems with auditory reflexes

24 A lesion in the lateral spinothalamic tract may cause:
a Weakness with increased reflexes b Problems of perception of pain and temperature c Problems of perception of movement of joint d Problems with integration of movement

Directions: Match the correct procedure in col. B associated with its corresponding cranial nerve in col. A.

Column A	Column B
25 ____ Optic (II)	a Occlude one nostril with digital compression; have patient indicate when odor is first detected and identify substance, if possible.
26 ____ Trigeminal (V)	
27 ____ Facial (VII)	
28 ____ Acoustic (VIII)	
29 ____ Oculomotor (III)	
30 ____ Glossopharyngeal (IX)	b Have patient say "ah" in order to note phonation and symmetry of the soft palate.
31 ____ Vagus (X)	c Test positional sense.
32 ____ Spinal accessory XI)	d Cover one eye and bring finger into visual field.
33 ____ Olfactory (I)	e Test gag reflex.

f Have patient raise eyebrows, frown, close eyes, and tightly close eyes; observe symmetry.

g Test for conductive versus sensorineural hearing loss.

h Ask patient to shrug shoulders and turn head with and without resistance.

i Have patient clench teeth; palpate masseters for tension.

j Check for ptosis of lids and note equality of pupils.

Directions: Match the cranial nerves in col. A with responses indicating pathology of the respective cranial nerves from col. B.

Column A	Column B
34 ____ Trigeminal (V)	a Dilatation of the pupil, decreased reaction to light
35 ____ Glossopharyngeal, vagus (IX, X)	b Loss of corneal reflex when cotton wisp is touched to cornea
36 ____ Oculomotor (III)	c Absence of gag reflex when tongue blade is touched to posterior pharynx
37 ____ Spinal accessory (XI)	d Inability to "shrug" the shoulders

e Deviation of protruding tongue toward the weak side (muscle atrophy also present on the paralyzed side)

Directions: Answer the following question on a separate sheet of paper.

38 List the four areas that are investigated when examining the sensory system.

CHAPTER 47 Cerebrovascular Disease

OBJECTIVES

At the completion of Chap. 47 you should be able to:

1 Explain the importance of vascular disease as compared with other diseases of the nervous system.

2 Describe the historical significance of cerebrovascular disease.

3 State the approximate percentage of the total body weight comprised by the brain and the percentage of the total body oxygen supply utilized by the brain.

4 State how long the brain can survive without oxygen.

5 Describe the arterial blood supply to the brain.

6 Identify the major arteries that form the circle of Willis.

7 Describe the extrinsic (extracranial) factors and the intrinsic (intracranial) factors thought responsible for cerebral circulatory control.

8 Explain the significance of the mortality and morbidity effects of cerebrovascular accidents (stroke) in the United States.

9 List and describe the three types of strokes according to the chronological pattern of their clinical progression and regression of their signs and symptoms.

10 Identify for cerebral arteriosclerosis the characteristic degenerative process, arteries affected, progressive changes, and related diseases and conditions.

11 Describe the association of cerebral thrombosis with arteriosclerosis, etiology, onset, incidence of cerebral vascular accidents, age group most often affected, and prognosis.

12 Describe transient ischemic attacks (TIA) by identifying the frequency of occurrence, associated symptoms, and prognosis.

13 Identify for cerebral embolism the etiology, incidence, age group most often affected, signs and symptoms, and prognosis.

14 Identify for cerebral hemorrhage the etiology, pathogenesis, incidence of cerebral vascular accidents, onset, neurologic findings, clinical features, age group affected according to vessel involved, and prognosis.

15 Describe for a saccular (berry) aneurysm the most common site of occurrence, signs and symptoms, treatment, and prognosis.

16 Describe the major clinical features associated with arterial insufficiency to the brain from the internal carotid artery; vertebral-basilar system; anterior, middle, and posterior cerebral arteries.

17 Explain for arteriography, computerized axial tomography, brain scans, EEG, and EMI scanner the purpose and technique of each procedure.

18 List four critical factors that must be considered in an acute care situation for cerebrovascular accidents (CVAs).

19 Describe the effectiveness of treatment modalities such as vasodilators, anticoagulants, and platelet antiaggregants in the treatment of CVAs.

20 Explain the primary goal of surgical intervention for stroke patients.

21 Describe the procedure and prognosis of these surgical treatments of stroke patients: carotid endarterectomy, revascularization, evacuation of blood clots, and aneurysmal surgery.

22 List the preventive (for risk factors associated with the development of a CVA) treatment for cerebral vascular accidents.

Vascular disease of the nervous system is the most commonly occurring neurologic disease. Cerebrovascular disease (or apoplexy, as it is called in Europe) was first described pathologically by Morgagni in the eighteenth century (1761). He described two forms: a nonsanguineous type which caused cerebral softening with arterial changes; and a sanguineous form with arterial occlusion and venous regurgitation. The symptoms were assumed to arise on the basis of local etiology, and studies in that direction continued until the twentieth century. Early in the twentieth century, isolated investigators noted that extracranial factors might be significant in the causation of cerebrovascular pathology. However, these investigators were generally ignored. The practice of embalming with the carotid arteries left intact did not help pursuit in this direction.

In 1927, carotid arteriography was introduced by E. Moniz (in Lisbon). In 1951, Fisher emphasized the importance of internal carotid occlusion as a cause for cerebral ischemia. Refinement of angiographic techniques and discovery of other valuable diagnostic tools has revolutionized care in certain stroke victims.

The brain accounts for approximately 2 percent of the body's total weight. In a resting state the brain receives one-sixth of the cardiac output; it uses 20 percent of the body's oxygen. When cerebral ischemia occurs, neurons begin to undergo metabolic alterations. Within a period of 3 to 10 minutes the neurons may become totally inactive. Oxygen deprivation leading to loss of function is followed by destruction of the neuron.

When an isolated artery is stenosed, blood flow to the brain continues until the lumen of that vessel is narrowed by 80 percent. Successive stenosis, however, will be significant when the flow is decreased by a lesser amount. For example, if one carotid is occluded, a 50 percent decrease in flow through the other will produce neurological deficits.

CEREBRAL CIRCULATION

The arterial blood to the brain is supplied by the two internal carotid arteries (anteriorly) and the two vertebral arteries (posteriorly). They arise from the aortic arch. On the right, the brachiocephalic trunk (innominate) artery divides into the right common carotid, which supplies the head, and the right subclavian artery, which supplies the arm. On the left side, the left common carotid and left subclavian arteries each arise directly from the aortic arch.

In general, the cerebral arteries are either conducting or penetrating. The conducting arteries (carotid, middle and anterior cerebral, vertebral, basilar, posterior cerebral, and their branches) form an extensive network over the surface of the brain. The penetrating arteries are nutrient vessels which are derived from the conducting arteries. These vessels enter the brain at right angles (Fig. 47-1).

Circulation to the two hemispheres is generally symmetrical, with each side retaining its own separate blood supply. However, anomalies of the classical distribution are very common and generally insignificant. When a problem arises, these anomalies can cause confusion when an attempt is made to correlate clinical findings with pathophysiological phenomena.

Collateral circulation is developed when normal flow to a part is decreased. Most cerebral collateral circulation between major arteries is via the circle of Willis. It has been estimated that anomalies in the circle of Willis occur in nearly one-half of the population. The brain also has collateral circulation sites that function only when other routes are impaired, such as between external and internal carotid arteries via the ophthalmic artery. Theoretically, these communicating channels are capable of providing an adequate blood supply to all areas of the brain. Practically, this is often not the case. A major vessel occlusion in one person will produce either no symptoms or a transient neurological deficit; in another the same occlusion site may cause a major loss of function. These differences would seem to be related to the state of the individual's collateral circulation.

The normal brain has the ability to regulate its own blood supply. "Normal" needs to be emphasized here, because pathological states are capable of altering or even abolishing this autoregulatory mechanism. Exactly how this mechanism functions has not been proven. McHenry has arbitrarily divided factors that control cerebral circulation into extrinsic or extracranial and intrinsic or intracranial:

EXTRINSIC (EXTRACRANIAL) FACTORS	INTRINSIC (INTRACRANIAL) FACTORS
1 Systemic blood pressure	1 Cerebral autoregulatory mechanisms related to cerebral perfusion pressure
2 Cardiovascular function	2 Cerebral blood vessels
3 Blood viscosity	3 Intracranial or cerebro-spinal fluid pressure

The extrinsic factors regulating cerebral blood flow (CBF) are related primarily to the cardiovascular system.

If systemic mean blood pressure (BP) drops below 60 mmHg, the brain's autoregulatory mechanism becomes less effectual. The brain will initially attempt to compensate by extracting more oxygen from the available blood, but if the BP continues to drop until CBF is decreased to 30 ml/100 g of tissue per minute, signs of cerebral ischemia will appear.

Cardiac arrythmias can change cardiac output. If cardiac output is decreased by more than one-third, there is often a fall in CBF.

The significance of blood viscosity is demonstrated by the fact that CBF may increase by as much as 30 percent with anemia; in polycythemia it may decrease by 50 percent.

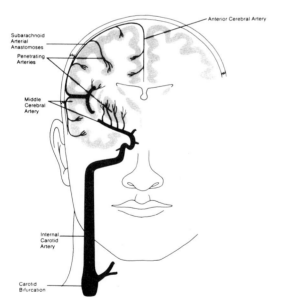

FIGURE 47-1 On the left is shown the course of the internal artery from the carotid bifurcation to its continuation as the middle cerebral artery. The penetrating lenticulostriate arteries arise from the first portion of the middle cerebral artery to supply the basal ganglia and internal capsule. The middle cerebral artery continues to course over the cerebral hemisphere sending short and deep penetrating arteries into the brain. The penetrating arteries are end arteries. The subarachnoid arterial anastomoses, which supply collateral circulation, are shown between the middle and anterior cerebral arteries. (From Smith, Kline, and French, Essentials of Stroke and Diagnostic Management, rev., 1973.)

The intrinsic factors as noted above are three in number. McHenry calls the cerebral perfusion pressure the "driving force in cerebral circulation." It is the pressure difference between the cerebral arteries and veins. The CBF will remain constant (750 ml/minute) due to autoregulation even when systemic BP fluctuates. The range whereby this mechanism can be effective is 150 to 60 mmHg for the systemic BP. When systemic BP falls, there is a compensatory decrease in cerebral vascular resistance. An elevation of BP results in an increase in cerebral vascular resistance.

The cerebral blood vessels are considered the most important factor relating to cerebrovascular resistance.

Recent microcirculatory studies have identified a myogenic response. This hypothesis proposes that parenchymal tissue of arterioles releases a vasodilating metabolite in response to their oxygen needs and thereby exerts control on arterial smooth muscle tone.

$$\text{Decrease perfusion pressure} \rightarrow \text{decrease CBF}$$

$$= \text{increase accumulation of metabolites} \rightarrow \text{vasodilation with restoration of blood flow toward normal}$$

The third intrinisic factor regulating CBF is the intracranial pressure (ICP). An increase in ICP will increase cerebrovascular resistance. CBF does not decrease until ICP has increased to 450 mm water (normal range 60 to 180 mm water).

Three metabolic factors considered very important (Guyton, 1972) are:

1 CO_2 concentration. High CO_2 tension is a potent vasodilator, possibly due to accumulation of CO_2 in vasomotor centers. In normal subjects CO_2 inhalations have produced up to 75 percent increase in CBF (raising PCO_2 by 9 mmHg will raise CBF by 75 percent).
2 H^+ concentration. An increase in H^+ yields an increase in blood flow.
3 O_2 concentration. Low O_2 tension is a powerful vasodilator; high O_2 concentration is a moderate vasoconstrictor.

CEREBRAL VASCULAR ACCIDENTS

Cerebral vascular disease, or stroke, is, in general terms, a disturbance in cerebral circulation. It is a focal neurological disorder. It may be secondary to a pathologic process within a cerebral blood vessel.

The pathologic process may encompass one of these phenomena:

1 Circulatory failure due to hypotension
2 Change in vessel lumen size
3 Altered permeability of vascular wall
4 Change in quality of the blood

Pathological processes within the blood vessel may include:

1 Thrombosis
2 Embolus
3 Rupture of vessel wall
4 Basic vascular disease such as atherosclerosis, arteritis, trauma, aneurysm, and developmental malformations

Stroke is responsible for 200,000 deaths in the United States each year. It is the third most frequent cause of death in the country. One-half million Americans each year suffer a new, acute cerebral vascular accident (CVA). There are an estimated 2 million people in the United States today with neurological deficit that is a result of stroke. About 50 percent of all adult neurological hospital admissions are due to vascular disease.

The major causes of stroke in order of importance are:

Atherosclerosis (thrombosis)

Embolism

Hypertensive intracerebral hemorrhage

Ruptured saccular (berry) aneurysm

Stroke is generally accompanied by one or more associated medical problems:

Hypertension

Cardiac disease

Elevated blood cholesterol level

Diabetes mellitus

Peripheral vascular disease

The severity of the stroke process is variable. Some infarcts are found on autopsy when cause of death was unrelated. (Of all adults examined postmortem 80 to 90 percent have significant atheromatous disease.) In others the stroke is sudden and dramatic with the patient literally being "struck down." In this latter form, hemiplegia and unconsciousness may both be evident.

Strokes may be categorized according to etiology or on the basis of their course. According to course, or temporal profile (which is defined as the chronological pattern of clinical progression and regression of signs and symptoms), strokes may be divided into three types:

1 Transient ischemic attacks (TIAs). These are focal neurological deficits that develop suddenly and disappear within a few minutes to hours.
2 Progressive (stroke in evolution). Evolution of stroke is gradual though acute.
3 Completed stroke. Deficits are maximal at onset with little improvement.

Major clinical features associated with arterial insufficiency to the brain (points of bifurcation or angulation are most vulnerable) may be focal and temporary, or the dysfunction may be permanent with actual tissue death and neurological deficit. There is difficulty in attempting to establish a close correlation between symptomatology associated with a particular vessel and actual clinical manifestations any particular patient has because:

1 There is variability of collateral circulation between individuals with regard to the circle of Willis (Fig. 47-2). Total occlusion of a carotid artery may give no symptoms if the left anterior cerebral and left middle cerebral arteries receive adequate blood from the anterior communicating artery. If this blood supply is not adequate, symptoms may include confusion, contralateral monoparesis or hemiparesis, and incontinence.
2 Leptomeningeal anastomoses are significant over the cerebral cortex between the anterior, middle, and posterior cerebral arteries. There are also anastomoses between the anterior cerebral arteries of the two hemispheres across the corpus callosum.
3 Each of the cerebral arteries has a central area to supply with blood and a peripheral supply area, or border area, which it may share with another artery. Anastomoses exist between external and internal carotid arteries, as around the orbit, with blood from external carotid vessels going to the ophthalmic artery.
4 Various systemic and metabolic factors are of significance in determining symptoms that a particular pathology will produce. A stenosed vessel may produce no symptoms as long as systemic blood pressure is 190/110, but should it be reduced to 120/70, variable symptoms will result depending on the location of the stenotic area. Hyponatremia and hyperthermia are metabolic factors that facilitate development of neurological deficits.

When identifying symptoms associated with particular blood vessels, it is important to recognize that symptoms may not apply to every patient with the particular involvement.

*FIGURE 47-2 The circle of Willis and some common anatomical variations. The anomalies are indicated by arrows. A. Normal circle of Willis. B. Reduplication of the anterior communicating artery. C. Stringlike anterior cerebral artery. D. Stringlike posterior cerebral artery. E. Embryonic derivation of posterior cerebral artery from the internal carotid artery. (Modified from B. J. Alpers, R. G. Berry, and R. M. Paddison, "Anatomical Studies of the Circle of Willis in Normal Brain," Archives of Neurology and Psychiatry, **81**: 409, 1959.)*

Major clinical features associated with arterial insufficiency to the brain may be associated with the following signs and symptoms:

1 Vertebral-basilar.
  a Weakness in one to four extremities.
  b Increased tendon reflexes.
  c Ataxia.
  d Bilateral Babinski sign.
  e Cerebellar signs.
  f Dysphagia.
  g Dysarthria.
  h Syncope, stupor, coma, dizziness, memory disturbances.
  i Visual disturbances (diplopia, nystagmus, ptosis, paralysis of single eye movements).
  j Numbness of face.

2 Internal carotid artery—most common location of lesion is the bifurcation of the common carotid into the internal and external carotid. Branches of the internal carotid are the *ophthalmic, posterior communicating, anterior choroidal, anterior cerebral,* and *middle cerebral.* Variable syndromes may develop. The pattern depends on the amount of collateral circulation.

  a *Monocular blindness,* episodic and called *amaurosis fugax,* on the side of involved carotid; it is due to retinal artery insufficiency. Sensory and motor symptoms involve contralateral extremities due to middle cerebral artery insufficiency.
  b Area between anterior and middle cerebral arteries and predominantly middle: symptoms will initially develop in upper extremities (weak, numb hand) then may involve the face—weak, supranuclear-type weakness. If in the dominant hemisphere, expressive aphasia (Broca's motor-speech area involved).
  c Possibly partial Horner's syndrome (slight ptosis and miosis) on side opposite the paresis (probably due to hypothalamic damage).
3 Anterior cerebral artery—confusion is the primary symptom.
  a Contralateral weakness greater in leg. Proximal arm may also be involved. Voluntary movement of that leg impaired.

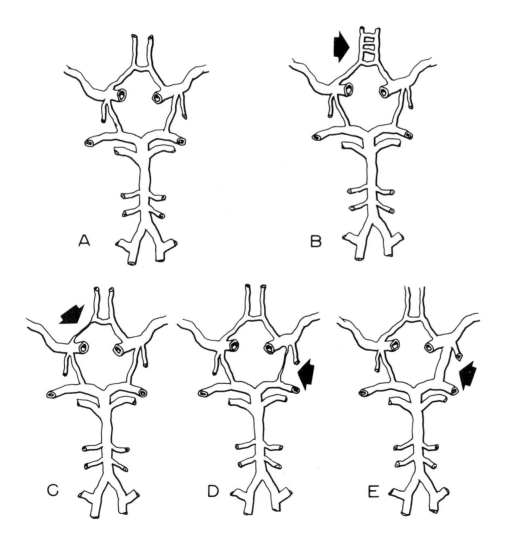

b Contralateral sensory deficits.

c Dementia, grasp, pathologic reflexes (frontal lobe dysfunction).

d Bilateral infarction may cause akinetic mutism.

4 Posterior cerebral artery (in lobe of midbrain or thalamus).

   a Coma.

   b Contralateral hemiparesis.

   c Visual aphasia or word blindness (alexia).

   d Third cranial nerve palsy—hemianopsia, choreoathetosis.

5 Middle cerebral artery.

   a Contralateral monoparesis or hemiparesis (usually affecting arm).

   b Occasional contralateral hemianopsia (blindness).

   c Global aphasia (if *dominant* hemisphere is involved)—disturbance of all functions involving speech and communication.

   d Dysphasia.

Thrombosis

Thrombosis (thrombo-occlusive disease) is the most common cause of stroke. It accounts for about 40 percent of all pathologically verified strokes.

The *atherosclerotic process* is characterized by yellow, fatty plaques which involve the intima of large and medium-sized arteries. The intima of the cerebral artery becomes thin and fibrous, with loss of muscle cells. The internal elastic lamina is split and frayed, and sclerotic material partly fills the lumen of the vessel.

The plaques show a tendency to form at branchings and curves. The connective tissue is exposed from loss of intima. Platelets adhere to this exposed, roughened surface. They release an enzyme, adenosine diphosphate, which initiates the coagulation mechanism. This fibrinoplatelet plug may break off and embolize, or it may remain in place and eventually cause complete occlusion of the artery. It is rare for cerebral arteries to be significantly affected beyond their first major branchings (Fig. 47-3).

Cerebral thrombosis is a disease of older age groups. In one study the peak age was 60 to 69 years, with only 8 percent occurring before the age of 50. Hypertension and/or diabetes appear to be important etiological factors, and one of these is found in two-thirds of clients who have CVA (Mancall, 1975).

The onset or progression of symptoms tends to occur during sleep or soon after arising (60 percent of cases according to one source). Maximum intensity is generally realized within 48 hours. Progression is generally stepwise (series of sudden changes) rather than smooth. Postural hypotension is more common in patients with cerebrovascular disease than in normal controls, possibly due to interference with the baroreceptor reflex. The pressor response to Valsalva maneuver is often ab-

sent in the aged with arteriosclerosis. Recumbency even for a night's rest can decrease sympathetic activity and lower blood pressure in the elderly. Additional factors, such as sedation or prolonged rest, can seriously compromise their precarious position.

Transient ischemic attacks (called cerebral angina) are characteristic, if not pathognomonic, of thrombosis.

About 80 percent of thrombotic victims suffer TIAs before their major stroke. TIAs rarely precede embolic or intracerebral hemorrhagic.

The nature of TIAs is not clearly understood. Possible explanations for its pathogenesis include (a) hypoperfusion, possibly due to vasospasm, (b) microembolization, and (c) hypotension.

Anoxic encephalopathy may occur with cerebral thrombosis. Symptoms and the clinical picture are dependent on the location. The brain distal to the clot becomes swollen. There may be discoloration, with the appearance being muddy-looking. There is a loss of demarcation between the gray and white matter. As time passes, nerve cells disintegrate and are replaced by glia.

Pathologically the infarcted area may be classified as either red infarct or anemic (white) infarct. With a red

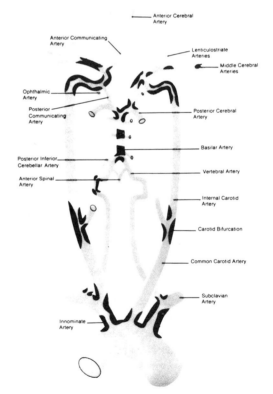

FIGURE 47-3 Extracranial and intracranial arteries supplying blood to the brain. The circle of Willis and its principal branches are also shown. The sites of atherosclerosis of the cerebral blood vessels are designated, the main locations being the carotid bifurcation and takeoff of the branches from the aorta, innominate, and subclavian arteries. These are the sites that are amenable to surgery. (From Smith, Kline, and French, Essentials of Stroke and Diagnostic Management, rev., 1973.)

infarct there is hemorrhage or blood flow into the necrotic area. This is usually seen with an occluded vein. The anemic infarct is arterial and does not have blood flowing into it.

Embolism

Cerebral embolism is the second most common cause of stroke. Its incidence is estimated in a range from 3 to 25 percent of all strokes. With refinements in diagnostic methods the upper level of the range is being increasingly realized. These patients are younger than those with thrombosis. Most cerebral emboli originate from a thrombus in the heart, so this problem is essentially a manifestation of heart disease. Less frequently the embolus originates from an atheromatous plaque in the carotid sinus or internal carotid artery. Any area of the brain may be involved, but generally the embolus will lodge at a narrow area. The middle cerebral artery, especially the upper division, is the most frequent site of cerebral emboli.

Symptoms may occur at any time, and they are rapidly progressive. Symptoms of small emboli may be contrasted with those of TIAs in that the latter tend to recur with the same clinical picture each time [same vessel(s) involved]. With numerous small emboli (as from a chronic atrial fibrillation) the pattern would vary with each episode depending upon which vessels were involved.

In general, there is a greater amount of tissue death with emboli than with more gradually occurring situations because anastomotic vessels do not have time to dilate and thus compensate. Within the cranium, nerve cells and their processes and oligodendroglia are most vulnerable. Astrocytes are more resistant, and microglia and capillaries survive longest under hypoxic conditions.

Cerebral hemorrhage is the third most frequent cause of CVA, accounting for one-tenth of all cases. Ruptured cerebral arteries are the usual source of intracranial bleeding. Extravasation of blood occurs in the brain and/or subarachnoid space. Adjacent tissue may be displaced and compressed. Massive hemorrhages have a tendency to track along tissue planes, separating rather than destroying nerve tissue (Norman et al.). Blood, though, is particularly irritating to brain tissue, as it hemolyzes and breaks down into its pigments. Phagocytosis occurs around the outer rim, producing an orange-brown area of hemosiderin-filled macrophages. The mass, which is originally soft and resembles red currant jelly, will eventually decrease in size and within 2 to 6 months only an orange-stained cleft may remain at the hemorrhage site. This mass represents dead cells that for an unknown reason have not undergone phagocytosis and have absorbed calcium and iron onto their surfaces. Histologically, the brain adjacent to the clot may be swollen and necrotic. Some nerve cells and glia disappear from it. Numerous petechial hemorrhages are visible in the adjacent brain tissue.

With cerebral hemorrhage hypertension is usually present. Other causes commonly associated are rupture of saccular aneurysm and hemorrhage associated with bleeding disorders. If an aneurysm is involved, 85 percent develop in the anterior portion of the circle of Willis.

Neurological findings are dependent upon the site and severity of the hemorrhage. The vessel involved is usually a penetrating artery. The most common site is the putamen and adjacent internal capsule.

The onset is abrupt and evolution rather rapid and steady, lasting minutes, hours, and occasionally days. The average patient takes 1 to 24 hours to reach the peak. The speed of bleeding determines the time involved.

Frequently the clinical features include severe headache, nuchal rigidity, vomiting, stupor, coma, and convulsions. Cerebrospinal fluid is bloody in 90 percent of the cases (when hemorrhage is small and away from the ventricles, it may be clear). Of these patients 70 to 75 percent die in 1 to 30 days, generally on the basis of hemorrhage extending into the ventricular system, temporal lobe herniation and midbrain compression, or seepage into vital centers.

With smaller hemorrhages these people do well since brain has been pushed aside and possibly not destroyed. As reabsorption of the clot occurs, functions can return. Rebleeding from the same site is unlikely.

When cerebral hemorrhage occurs on the basis of a ruptured aneurysm, it is usually in the 35- to 65-year age group, and 20 percent have more than one aneurysm. As noted earlier, most are located in the circle of Willis.

Saccular (or berry) aneurysms can be smaller than a pin's head or 2 to 3 cm in diameter. They are frequently the size of a pea and arise at or close to points of divisions of an artery. These aneurysms are thin-walled (covered only by intima) blisters protruding from the artery at a point where a local weakness exists. They gradually enlarge, and rupture can occur. They may be asymptomatic until they rupture. Generally, rupture occurs during activity. The usual clinical picture includes sudden, violent headache, "like something snapped in my head"; collapse; brief unconsciousness and confusion; no warning symptoms; few, if any, lateralizing signs. An outstanding feature of aneurysms is their tendency to rebleed (Fig. 47-4).

Diagnosis

A thorough history and physical examination should be done on all patients with cerebrovascular disease. An inadequate history is probably the most frequent cause of diagnostic error. Often neither the patient nor the family can recall when initial symptoms started (Thorn, 1977). The specific type of stroke should be determined. Contributory diseases need to be identified and treated.

Two significant phenomena that are characteristic of all varieties of stroke are (1) the temporal profile: suddenness of evolution, especially, marks the event as vascular, along with the findings of some degree of improvement following stabilization; (2) focal or lateralizing neurological signs. Hemiplegia is the classic sign of stroke and is found in lesions involving the cerebral hemispheres or brainstem.

ANGIOGRAPHY

With the clinical diagnosis of cerebrovascular pathology, arteriography is essential to demonstrate the cause and site. Practically all intracranial vascular areas, from the aorta on up, may be visualized. Special magnification, subtraction, and stereoscopic techniques have increased the diagnostic and localizing capabilities of these studies. The medium used is less toxic and irritating than in the past.

Some practitioners favor waiting 8 days following a hemorrhage before angiography to avoid aggravating a fresh infarct. A combination of carotid and vertebral angiography will demonstrate aneurysms in 85 percent of cases.

Many practitioners now avoid direct punctures into the carotid artery, which may result in a disruption of plaque formation and consequent emboli. Also extravasation in this area can result in respiratory difficulty. Instead, femoral, brachial, axillary, or subclavian arteries are utilized.

Computerized axial tomography (CAT), where it is available, is proving a valuable diagnostic tool for demonstrating hematomas, infarcts, and hemorrhage. It it totally reliable in diagnosing lesions 1.5 cm or more in diameter.

Brain scans are good as a screening device, and if the lesion has damaged the blood-brain barrier, the isotope may localize in the area. It is best for lesions near the surface. Scans are safe and can be repeated as desired.

Electroencephalograms (EEG) may assist in localization. The delta waves would be slower over the affected area.

The EMI scanner is a rotating x-ray tube with a recording device, a small, computer digital readout system, and an oscilloscope with a Polaroid camera. It depends on the difference in densities between x-rays absorbed by normal and damaged tissue. This method is safe, rapid, and seems accurate.

Treatment

In the acute care situation the critical factors to be considered are

1 Stabilization of vital signs which entails (a) maintaining a patent airway (frequent and deep suctioning, O_2, tracheotomy, respiratory assistance if brainstem is involved), and (b) blood pressure control on an individualized basis. This entails correcting hypotension as well as hypertension.
2 Detection and correction of cardiac arrhythmias.

3 Bladder care. The trend is to avoid indwelling catheters.
4 Proper positioning is stressed immediately. The patient should be turned every hour and passive range of motion (ROM) exercises instituted every 2 hours. Within a few days full ROM to a total of 50 times per day is recommended. This is necessary to avoid pressure areas and contractures (especially at shoulder, elbow, and ankle).

Current treatment of cerebrovascular disease remains to be clarified. There is no single method of treatment that has been consistently useful. Several modes of therapy seem useful, but survivorship has not increased.

CONSERVATIVE TREATMENT

Vasodilators have increased cerebral blood flow (CBF) experimentally but have not proven beneficial in human strokes. Effective dilators of vessels in other areas of the body have little or no effect on cerebral vessels, especially when used orally (nicotinic acid, tolazoline, papaverine, etc.). Based on a few clinical trials the following have been suggested as useful: histamine, aminophylline, acetazolamide, intraarterial papaverine.

The use of vasodilators may also exert an adverse effect on CBF by lowering systemic BP and thereby decreasing intracerebral anastomotic flow.

Anticoagulants exert no beneficial effect on established strokes or on those in active evolution. They may be of value in TIAs since they seem to decrease the frequency and severity of the attacks. The hazards of long-term use must be evaluated in all cases. In three, separate, randomized trials of anticoagulant therapy for TIAs the results showed (1) no decrease in total mortality, (2) a small decrease in number of strokes and related deaths, and (3) decrease in frequency of TIAs (Kuller 1974).

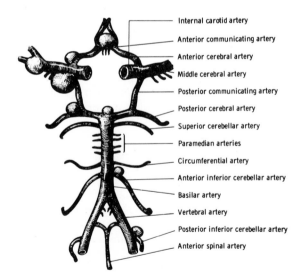

FIGURE 47-4 *The common sites of saccular (berry) aneurysms. Each is drawn in direct proportion to the frequency at that site. (From F. McDowell, in P. B. Beeson, and W. McDermott (eds.), Textbook of Medicine, 14th ed., Saunders, Philadelphia, 1975, p. 663.)*

Platelet antiaggregants have not had long-term clinical trials as yet. Aspirin and sulfinpyrazone are used to inhibit the platelet aggregation-release reaction which occurs after ulceration of an atheroma.

SURGICAL THERAPY

Several surgical procedures are now being utilized in stroke clients. The proper selection of the individual who would most benefit from surgery remains a most difficult task. Improving cerebral blood flow is the primary goal of surgical intervention.

One of the first successful reconstructions of an internal carotid artery (*Carotid endarterectomy*) was reported in 1954 by C. Rab et al. (St. Mary's Hospital, London, England). With this procedure the carotid artery in the neck is exposed. The vessel is incised at the site of stenosis, and the clot and plaque material are removed (Fig. 47-5). DeBakey has reported the success of carotid endarterectomy for cerebral vascular insufficiency in a 19-year follow-up study.

In the 1960s with the use of stereoscopic microscopes and microsuturing techniques patent anastomoses were successfully performed through the *revascularization procedure*. Normal CBF is 50 ml/(100 g·minute). The brain can adapt to lesser amounts and still carry out its metabolic activity up to a point. A critical level of CBF is defined as 15 to 18 ml/(100 g·minute). Many people can no longer maintain normal electrical activity at this level. Other groups have reported a reduction of blood supply by 20 percent or more on the involved side as good physiological grounds for microsurgical cerebral revascularization. It is assumed that increasing regional blood flow to areas that are being compromised would benefit properly selected cases. Revascularization procedures are being done to this end. Various vessels can be utilized. Commonly, the superficial temporal artery is anastomosed to a superficial cortical artery. In another procedure (the subclavian–external carotid bypass graft) a segment of the saphenous vein is anastomosed to the subclavian artery and the proximal end of the external carotid. Revascularization is primarily a prophylactic procedure and is most likely to benefit clients with TIAs or who are early in the course of a thrombosis-in-evolution. Clients manifesting fixed neurological deficits can expect no benefit from these procedures and are not considered appropriate candidates.

Evacuation of blood clots is seldom beneficial in the acute stage of stroke. Exceptions to this are surface lesions where the client is conscious and some cerebellar hemorrhages where surgical evacuation of the clot has lead to improvement.

Surgical intervention in the case of *aneurysms* is directed toward prevention of a recurrence of the hemorrhage. Ligation of the common carotid artery in the neck is the most conservative treatment of aneurysm.

Intracranial procedures such as clipping or ligating the neck of the aneurysm necessitates major neurosurgical intervention. Aneurysms can also be painted with a physiological glue which provide an elastic cap and keep them from rupturing.

Various *shunt* procedures may be done (ventriculoatrial shunt) if obstructive hydrocephalus is an overriding concern.

Occasionally *decompression craniotomies* are recommended to reduce increased intracranial pressure.

Vascular surgery for *stroke* is a debatable area. Some feel that a stroke is generally due to small intracranial vessel involvement and is not amenable to surgery. For those favoring surgery, removing the emboli or its source and improving CBF are of primary concern. Clients need to be carefully selected for surgery since the surgery is hazardous, and mortality rate is high.

In the 1960s, using stereoscopic operating microscopes and microsuturing techniques, patent anastomoses were successfully performed. Revascularization procedures are most likely to benefit clients with TIAs and prevent disastrous stroke. Patients with severe fixed deficits or with embolic etiology are not considered appropriate candidates for surgery.

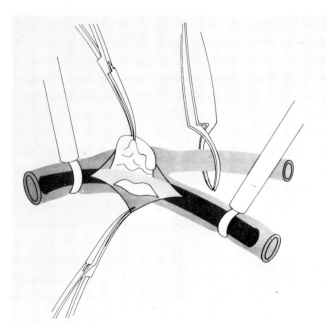

FIGURE 47-5 Diagram of a carotid endarerectomy. A bypass tube is used during the removal of an atherosclerotic lesion at the carotid bifurcation. (From Smith, Kline, and French, Essentials of Stroke and Diagnostic Management, rev., 1973.)

PREVENTATIVE MEASURES

In a 24-year follow-up study by the American Heart Association involving 5184 men and women (ages 30 to 62 years at entry into study), 345 had suffered strokes; 60 percent of these had suffered thrombosis [called atherothrombotic brain infarction (ABI) in this work]. Unlike other manifestations of atherosclerosis, ABI occurs equally among men and women. The most important risk factor identified was *hypertension,* which was even more dangerous when coupled with other factors such as: diabetes, left ventricular hypertrophy identified by ECG, elevated blood cholesterol level, cigarette smoking, and cardiac impairments.

This study cites the control of blood pressure as the key to ABI prevention (American Heart Association, 1977).

Several other general preventative measures can be identified:

1 Decrease in salt intake—beginning in early life with salt-free or low salt baby food.
2 Especially with the elderly, extreme care to maintain blood pressure during surgical procedures.
3 Increased activity—daily walking part of a fitness program.
4 Decrease weight if overweight.
5 Avoid oversedation and prolonged bed rest especially with elderly.
6 Stop smoking cigarettes.

QUESTIONS

Cerebrovascular disease—Chap. 47

Directions: Circle the letter preceding each item below that correctly answers each question. More than one answer may be correct.

1 Which of the following is the most commonly occurring neurologic disease?
  a Tumors of the nervous system   *b* Vascular disorders of the nervous system   *c* Spinal cord diseases   *d* Epilepsy

2 Which of the following statements is (are) true concerning the pathogenesis of cerebrovascular disease as it has historically been defined?
  a Early investigators have considered extracranial factors significant in the causation of cerebrovascular pathology.   *b* Symptoms were assumed to be on the basis of local etiology.   *c* Internal carotid occlusion was identified as a cause for cerebral ischemia.   *d* Two forms of the disease were identified: a nonsanguineous type and a sanguineous form.

3 Death of brain cells due to a lack of oxygen occurs in approximately _____ minutes.
  a 15 minutes   *b* 10 minutes   *c* 4 minutes   *d* 1 minute

4 The major arterial blood vessels that supply blood to the circle of Willis are which of the following arteries?
  a External carotid   *b* Internal carotid   *c* Ophthalmic   *d* Basilar-vertebral system

Directions: Answer the following questions on a separate sheet of paper.

5 Describe the arterial blood supply to the brain.

6 Briefly describe the three extrinsic (extracranial) factors and the three intrinsic (intracranial) factors which are thought responsible for cerebral circulatory control.

7 Cerebrovascular accident (stroke) is responsible for how many deaths in the United States each year? Approximately how many people in the United States have a neurologic deficit that is a result of a stroke?

8 List and describe the three types of stroke according to the chronological pattern of clinical progression and regression of signs and symptoms.

Directions: Circle the letter preceding each item below that correctly answers each question. More than one answer may be correct.

9 Which of the following cerebral arteries are most likely to form fatty plaques?
  a Ophthalmic   *b* Basilar   *c* Carotids   *d* Vertebral

10 Cerebral emboli can be composed of which of the following?
  a Blood clot (especially with underlying heart or vascular disease)   *b* Fatty tissue   *c* Tumor cells   *d* Bacteria clumps (often from heart disease)

11 Major sites of origin of cerebral emboli causing a stroke include all of the following *except:*
  a Mural thrombi in the left atrium associated with atrial fibrillation   *b* Mural thrombi overlying ventricular infarcts   *c* Thrombi formed in rheumatic valve disease   *d* Thrombi formed on arteriosclerotic plaques in the aortic arch and carotid arteries   *e* Thrombi formed in the deep leg veins

Directions: Circle the T for true and the F for false. Correct the false statements.

12   T   F   Cerebral thrombosis usually has a gradual onset, whereas cerebral embolism usually has a sudden onset.

13   T   F   In cerebral vascular disorders the signs and symptoms the patient experiences depend upon which vessel is involved and the amount of collateral circulation in the affected area.

14   T   F   In order for a cerebral vascular disorder to be referred to as a transient ischemic attack (TIA) there must be evidence of cerebral tissue necrosis.

15   T   F   Cerebral thrombosis is a disease of the older age groups.

Directions: Select the letter that best answers each question. More than one answer may be correct.

16 Mr. B., a 60-year-old male was admitted to the general hospital. On admission his physical findings indicated a temperature of 99.8°F, pulse of 90, respirations 20 per minute, and a blood pressure of 250/140 mmHg. Lumbar puncture disclosed that the spinal fluid contained red blood cells and was under increased pressure. Shortly after admission, he became comatose. He was diagnosed as having a cerebral hemorrhage. Which of the following symptoms would likely indi-

cate a hemorrhage in the area of the brain involving the posterior cerebral artery and the thalamus?
a Contralateral hemiplegia or hemiparesis b Ipsilateral numbness and sensory loss on the face
c Dementia d Tremor

17 The predisposing factors that probably contributed to Mr. B.'s intracerebral hemorrhage include all of the following *except:*
a History of preexisting hypertension b Weakness of the vascular wall c Sudden rise in blood pressure
d Greatly reduced blood viscosity

18 Miss K., a 32-year-old woman with a history of rheumatic heart disease complicated by mitral stenosis and atrial fibrillation was admitted to the hospital with a high fever, changing heart murmurs, large tender spleen, and the *abrupt* onset of a right hemiplegia and aphasia which persisted for 48 hours. The *most likely* type of neurologic deficit which transpired is:
a Embolic b Transient ischemic attack
c Thrombosis d None of the above

19 Mr. G., aged 67, was referred to the neurologist by the public health nurse after experiencing several transient ischemic attacks. Symptoms experienced during these attacks included falling due to weakness of extremities, dizziness, and loss of equilibrium; double vision, and difficulty with speech. The most likely site of arterial occlusion is:
a Internal carotid artery b Basilar-vertebral arteries
c Radial artery d Anterior cerebral artery

20 Mr. K., a 75-year-old man with a history of mild diabetes mellitus and a previous myocardial infarction, was admitted to the hospital with a mild left hemiparesis which evolved slowly over several hours with no other neurologic deficit. This deficit improved slightly after several days in the hospital but did not entirely clear. The most likely diagnosis is:
a Subarachnoid hemorrhage b Wallenberg's syndrome (lateral medullary syndrome) on the right side of the medulla c Transient ischemic attack involving the right middle cerebral artery
d Cerebral thrombosis involving the right middle cerebral artery

21 A subarachnoid hemorrhage is most frequently associated with:
a Mycotic aneurysms b Severe hypertension
c "Berry" aneurysms d Atherosclerotic aneurysms

22 Characteristics of transient ischemic attacks (TIA) include which one of the following?
a Evidence of lasting damage to the brain after an attack b Similar to epileptic attacks in the duration of neurologic dysfunction c Return to "normal" after an attack d Hemiparesis

23 Mr. O., a 50-year-old male, was admitted to a local general hospital convulsing and unconscious. His temperature was 99°F rectally, pulse rate 98 beats per minute, and respirations 20 per minute, and blood pressure 240/140 mmHg. Twenty-four hours after admission, Mr. O. regained consciousness. His right

arm and right leg were paralyzed, and he was unable to speak. The hemorrhage responsible for his symptoms probably occurred from rupture of a branch of the:
a Anterior cerebellar artery b Posterior cerebral artery c Middle cerebral artery d Vertebral artery

24 Berry aneurysms:
a Occur most often at the bifurcation of arteries
b Commonly occur on or near the circle of Willis
c Are usually not discovered until they bleed
d Cause subdural hemorrhage when they rupture

25 A cerebral infarction in the distribution of the middle cerebral artery would be likely to cause all of these symptoms *except:*
a Contralateral hemiplegia b Aphasia c Ipsilateral Horner's syndrome d Homonymous hemianopsia (loss of vision in half of the visual field)

26 A patient is admitted to the hospital with a diagnosis of mild CVA. The patient demonstrated left-sided weakness of upper and lower extremities. With left-sided weakness of upper and lower extremities, the patient likely has a lesion located in the:
a Left cerebral hemisphere b Right cerebral hemisphere c Brainstem d Medulla

27 Which of the following diagnostic studies are used to visualize the intracranial vascular areas?
a Brain scan b Arteriography c Tomography (CAT)

28 Which of the following diagnostic procedures is able to demonstrate hematomas, infarcts, and hemorrhage?
a Brain scan b Arteriography c Tomography (CAT)

Directions: Answer the following questions on a separate sheet of paper.

29 For the acute period of a stroke, describe four critical factors in the patients treatment.

30 Describe the effectiveness of vasodilators, anticoagulants, and platelet antiaggregants in the treatment of CVA.

31 State the primary goal of surgical intervention for stroke patients.

32 Describe a surgical procedure used to increase collateral blood flow to the brain.

33 What is the major purpose of clipping the neck of a berry aneurysm located on the anterior communicating artery of the brain?

34 What are the principles of prevention and therapy after neurologic deficit?

CHAPTER 48 Epilepsy

OBJECTIVES **At the completion of Chap. 48 you should be able to:**

1 Define *epilepsy*.

2 Compare the incidence of epilepsy in the general population and in the offspring of epileptics.

3 List at least three conditions that may cause seizures.

4 Name the areas of the brain associated with lesions that are likely to be epileptogenic.

5 Describe the factors that may play an instrumental role in precipitating seizures.

6 Describe the metabolic changes that can occur during and immediately following a seizure.

7 Differentiate between the expected clinical manifestations in grand mal, petit mal, psychomotor, and Jacksonian seizures.

8 Define *status epilepticus*.

9 Identify for an electroencephalograph the changes associated with activity and the layers of the brain responsible for electrical activity, and give an interpretation of the tracing.

10 Identify the drugs used to control the treatment of grand mal, petit mal, psychomotor, and Jacksonian seizures.

11 Discuss the medical and surgical treatment modalities for epilepsy.

Epilepsy is the second most common neurological problem found in adults. Epilepsy may be defined as excessive, uncontrolled, synchronous, paroxysmal, local discharges of a group of cerebral neurons, usually in the cortex. For spread, surrounding neurons need to be activated and involved in similar abnormal activity. In a broad sense any phenomenon involving abnormal motor, sensory, or psychic activity that has an abrupt onset, short course, and is followed by a return to normal can be representative of a seizure (Harvey, Johns, 1976).

It has been estimated that 3 to 5 percent of the population have at least one seizure in their lifetime, and 0.5 percent have recurring seizures, called epilepsy (Niedermeyer, 1974).

Relatives of epileptic patients exhibit abnormal brain wave patterns 6 times more frequently than normal control groups. The incidence of epilepsy is 1:200 for the general population in the United States. For offspring of an epileptic the incidence is 1:20, or 10 times as frequent.

The incidence of epilepsy is highest in the first 4 years of life and after the age of 60.

It is often difficult to determine the prevalence of epilepsy, because many epileptics do not reveal their condition. Historically, this may be due to society's demeaning view of epilepsy in the occupational, educational, and social spheres. These social factors are often as complicated as the clinical manifestations for the patient.

PATHOLOGY

There are at least fifty conditions that may cause seizures. These conditions include such things as cerebral vascular disease, cerebral atrophy, meningitis, diabetic acidosis, and acute alcoholism. If the cause of the seizure is unknown, it is referred to as *idiopathic epilepsy*.

Following insults to the brain such as injury, seizures

may be induced in 1 to 50 percent of the cases depending on the severity of the injury. The normal equilibrium involving excitatory and inhibitory impulses may be disturbed, resulting in loss of inhibitory elements and permitting excessive neuronal discharges.

Lesions in the midbrain, thalamus, and cerebral cortex are likely to be epileptogenic, because these areas are the most sensitive in the brain; whereas, lesions in the cerebellum and brainstem do not generally elicit seizures.

Present knowledge is insufficient to explain why many abnormal cortical discharges do not evoke a seizure; or, conversely, why other abnormal discharges do evoke a seizure.

An established epileptogenic focus can create a secondary or "mirror" focus in the contralateral hemisphere. If this should occur, the seizure may persist even when the primary site is obliterated (Fig. 48-1).

When a discharging focus is governed by another lesion and the responsible lesion is removed, the seizure activity will cease in the discharging focus.

Biochemical studies have not clarified exact mechanisms involved, but several factors have emerged which may play an instrumental role in precipitating seizure. Current literature refers to the possibility of "epileptic neurons" that have lower thresholds for firing abnormal discharges (Thorn, 1977). A deafferented neuron has been identified in some focal lesions. Deafferented neurons are hypersensitive and in a chronic state of depolarization. Their cytoplasmic membranes exhibit increased permeability making them susceptible to activation by various factors (hypoxia, hyperthermia) and circumstances (repeated sensory stimuli) (Harvey, Johns, 1976). Electrolyte distribution is altered with seizure activity. The intracellular potassium content of neurons is decreased and replaced by sodium with seizure activity. Edema may precipitate seizures. Cell membrane permeability, hyperventilation, and pH all seem to play a role in seizure activity and precipitation. Their exact role is not clear.

There are metabolic changes that occur during and immediately following a seizure that are in part the result of increased energy needs from the neuronal hyper-activity. Metabolic needs are drastically increased during convulsions; the electrical discharges of motor nerve cells may be increased to 1000 per second. Cerebral blood flow is increased, as is tissue respiration and glycolysis. Acetylcholine appears in cerebral spinal fluid (CSF) during and following seizures. Glutamic acid may be depleted during seizure activity.

There is generally no gross change found at autopsy. Histopathologic evidence supports the hypothesis that the lesion is neurochemical rather than structural. There is no consistent pathological factor that has been identified. Focal abnormalities in the metabolism of potassium and acetylcholine are found to be present between seizures. Seizure foci seem especially sensitive to acetylcholine, a facilitatory transmitter. They are slow to bind and remove the acetylcholine.

SEIZURES

The following are clinical manifestations of different kinds of seizures:

Petit mal is characterized by short lapses of consciousness, rarely lasting over a few seconds. For example, there may be a brief pause in conversation or a vacant look or rapid blinking of the eyes. The patient may have one or two seizures a month or several a day. Petit mal occurs almost exclusively in children; the onset is rarely after 20 years of age. Petit mal will usually disappear after puberty or be replaced by generalized seizures.

Grand mal is the classic seizure of epilepsy and the most frequent form. It is characterized by an aura followed by a loss of consciousness and tonic-clonic spasms. The aura is a sensory indication of an impending seizure. This may consist of a momentary visual, gustatory, auditory, or olfactory sensation. The seizure starts

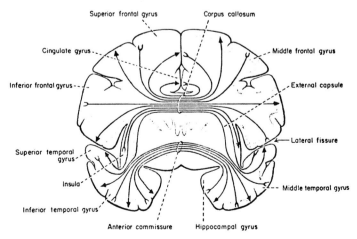

FIGURE 48-1 Possible anatomic pathways for the development of "mirror foci" in the opposite hemisphere. Coronal section of the brain at the level of the anterior commissure illustrating connections through corpus callosum and the anterior commissure. (From E. C. Crosby, T. Humphrey, and E. W. Lauer, Correlative Anatomy of the Nervous System, Macmillan, New York, copyright © 1962 by Macmillan Publishing Co., Inc., 1962.)

with a rapid loss of consciousness, a cry may be expressed due to the thoracic or abnormal spasms causing forced expiration, and then may follow loss of upright position, tonic then clonic movements, and bladder and/or bowel incontinence, along with other autonomic dysfunctions. In the *tonic phase,* muscles contract and body position may be distorted. This phase lasts for a few seconds. The *clonic phase* involves opposing muscle groups contracting and relaxing, giving a jerking movement. The contractions gradually decrease in number, but not in strength. The tongue may be bitten, which occurs in approximately one-half the cases (spasms of jaw and tongue). Following the seizure the patient relaxes and may remain unconscious for a few minutes to even as long as one-half hour. The patient regaining consciousness may appear confused, stuporous or dull. Generally, there is no recollection of the seizure.

Jacksonian motor seizures are characterized by a focal onset thought to be caused by a lesion in the contralateral motor cortex. This seizure generally starts with either a tonic spasm or a clonic rhythmic twitching of the fingers of one hand, face on one side, etc. This disorder then spreads in a progressive *march.* For example, from face, to neck, hand, forearm, arm, trunk, and leg, or on one side of the body. In some instances there is progression to the opposite hemisphere with a loss of consciousness. It is extremely important to observe where the seizure begins, as this may offer a clue as to location of the lesion. This involvement may be sensory. The patient complains of transient abnormal sensations that begin as focal phenomena and then progressively march to involve one side of the body.

Psychomotor (temporal lobe) epilepsy is characterized by transient mental disturbances and automatic movements (clapping hands, smacking lips, chewing motions) which generally last over a minute. The patients have a clouded, "dreamy" feeling of unreality.

The patient is usually conscious during the attack but may not recall what has happened. Other behavior associated with psychomotor epilepsy includes sudden recollection of past events, hallucinations (visual or olfactory are common), forgetfulness, word finding difficulty, personality changes, antisocial behavior, and inappropriate moodiness. In the postictal period this patient may enter a "fugue state" in which complex and organized activities may be performed which are not remembered (amnesia).

These attacks may be precipitated by music, blinking lights, and other stimuli. They may occur at any age but primarily occur in adults. Temporal lobe epilepsy (psychomotor) is associated with small focal lesions in the anterior temporal lobe, especially in the hippocampal (uncinate) gyrus. Psychomotor seizures can also be caused by lesions outside the temporal lobe (in the insula, orbital cortex, anterior olfactory centers, and diencephalon).

STATUS EPILEPTICUS

Status epilepticus refers to a state in which there is a succession (two or more) of generalized seizures with no recovery of consciousness between them. Exhaustion and acidosis may prove fatal if unrelieved.

Status is not a common phenomenon. Treatment consists of intravenous anticonvulsant medication and diazepam (Valium). Cardiopulmonary support systems may also be warranted.

ELECTROENCEPHALOGRAM (EEG)

The electrical activity of the cortex is of very low voltage. It is amplified and recorded by an electroencephalograph. The record is called an EEG.

Brain waves are individualized and vary with activity (e.g., intense mental activity = low amplitude, high frequency; slow-wave sleep = low frequency, amplitude increased). Spikes indicate an irritative focus. Brain waves are slowed with hypoxia, anesthesia, sedatives, low CO_2, deep sleep, relaxation. Brain waves are increased with increased CO_2 levels, sensory stimulation, light anesthesia, convulsive drugs (Medrol).

The superficial layers of cortex are responsible for electrical activity as recorded on EEGs. Masses of dendrites forming a dense network are thought to be the source. The cerebellum has a similar network, and a similar pattern can be recorded from that area.

EEGs should be used in conjunction with careful clinical evaluations. EEG is a physiological recording and does not distinguish one entity from another (for example, a tumor cannot be distinguished from a thrombosis by EEG). Ten percent of patients with seizures have normal EEGs. Also, an abnormal record does not mean a person has epilepsy. In fact, even in the case of diagnosed epileptics most seizure activity is nonclinical.

EEG is one test and not a panacea. Caution should be employed in the interpretation of EEG tracings. For example, scalp electrodes frequently may not perceive the electrical activity from the inferior aspect of the frontal and temporal and occipital lobes.

Certain activating techniques such as hyperventilation, sleep, and visual stimulation are used to initiate abnormal electrical activity in some patients.

In grand mal seizures EEG abnormalities are dependent upon the frequency and duration of the seizures. With frequent seizures, 75 to 80 percent of patients show abnormality; with infrequent seizures (four or five over several years' time) 20 to 30 percent show abnormal EEG (Fig. 48-2).

TREATMENT

The primary mode of management for the epileptic patient is drug therapy to prevent the occurrence of seizures. Approximately 70 to 80 percent of patients benefit from anticonvulsant drugs. Medications are often used in combination because one alone rarely gives effective control. Combined they tend to potentiate each other, and lower doses are possible, thus minimizing side effects. Dosages are individualized for each drug. The following are examples of some drugs used in the treatment of epilepsy.

Phenytoin (Dilantin)
Therapeutic uses: The drug of choice for grand mal, Jacksonian, psychomotor seizures.
Side effects: Nystagmus, ataxia, slurred speech, blurred vision, diplopia, vertigo, hypersensitivity, mental confusion, gingival hyperplasia, hirsutism, rash.

Phenobarbital
Therapeutic uses: Exerts a prophylactic influence against most types of seizures (except petit mal); also useful in status epilepticus.
Side effects: Sedation, nystagmus, ataxia, irritability, and hyperactivity in children; confusion in the elderly.

Primidone (Mysoline)
Therapeutic uses: Related to phenobarbital. Frequently used in grand mal, Jacksonian, and psychomotor seizures.
Side effects: Sedation, vertigo, dizziness, ataxia, nausea, diplopia, nystagmus.

Mephenytoin (Mesantoin)
Therapeutic uses: Primarily used in grand mal and psychomotor seizures.
Side effects: Similar chemical structure to phenytoin, but demethylated effect may produce rash, fever, agranulocytosis, and aplastic anemia. Monthly blood counts are necessary.

Ethotoin (Peganone)
Therapeutic uses: Less potent than phenytoin. Therapeutic uses are the same. Usually used in combination with other drugs.
Side effects: Similar to phenytoin but gingival hyperplasia and hirsutism are less common.

Phenacemide (Phenurone)
Therapeutic uses: Primarily used in psychomotor seizures and those not responsive to other drugs.
Side effects: *Very* toxic and close surveillance is essential with its use. Hepatic damage, bone marrow depression, and personality changes (toxic psychosis).

Acetazolamide (Diamox)
Therapeutic uses: Used in conjunction with anticonvulsive medication and appears to decrease frequency and severity of the seizure.
Side effects: Drowsiness, anorexia, paresthesias.

Ethosuximide (Zarontin)
Therapeutic uses: Primary drug for petit mal seizure.
Side effects: Drowsiness, dizziness, headache, anorexia, nausea, photophobia, blood dyscrasia.

Trimethadione (Tridione)
Therapeutic uses: Used in petit mal seizures when patient cannot tolerate ethosuximide.
Side effects: Sedation, visual aberrations, nephrotoxic, hepatoxic, aplastic anemia.

Diazepam (Valium)
Therapeutic uses: Given I.V. in the treatment of status epilepticus.

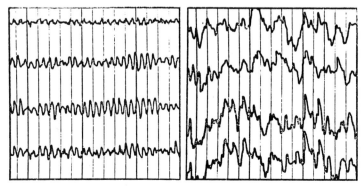

FIGURE 48-2 Electroencephalogram. On the left is the normal pattern. On the right is an EEG taken during an attack of epilepsy. (From Frank Elliott, Clinical Neurology, 2d ed., Saunders, Philadelphia, 1971.)

Side effects: Sedation, cardiovascular and respiratory depression.

Clonazepam (Clonopin)

Therapeutic uses: Relatively new drug used in all type seizures when the patient is unresponsive to other drugs, especially for the petit mal variant, akinetic and myoclonic seizures.

Side effects: Respiratory depression, drowsiness, ataxia, behavioral changes.

Carbamazepine (Tegretol)

Therapeutic uses: Major motor and psychomotor seizures unresponsive to other drugs.

Side effects: Paresthesias of extremities, skin rash.
Toxicity: fatal bone marrow depression, obstructive jaundice, urinary retention, water intoxication.

Surgical treatment is a debatable issue. It is restricted to focal epilepsy if the area is not indispensable (as the speech center is). It should be considered only after drug therapy is not effectual.

Indications for surgery include

1 Focal lesion identified by EEG and compatible with clinical manifestations.
2 Area accessible and dispensable.
3 Patient a good candidate for rehabilitation (normal IQ, motivated).

QUESTIONS

Epilepsy—Chap. 48

Directions: Answer the following questions on a separate sheet of paper.

1 Define *epilepsy*.
2 (a) What is the incidence of epilepsy in the general population of the United States? (b) for the offspring of epileptics?

3 What are three conditions that may cause seizures?

4 List the areas of the brain associated with lesions that are likely to be epileptogenic.

5 Describe the factors that may play an instrumental role in precipitating seizures.

6 Describe the metabolic changes that can occur during and immediately following a seizure.

7 Define *status epilepticus*.

Directions: Select the letter which best answers the question. More than one answer may be correct.

8 Which of the following statements concerning epilepsy are true?
a The single most important factor in diagnosing epilepsy is careful observation and reporting of a seizure. b The majority of patients can be brought under reasonable control. c There are characteristic disease inheritance patterns. d Epileptics may have difficulty in obtaining employment.

9 Psychomotor seizures are usually characterized by:
a Inappropriate behavior b A disturbance in the temporal lobe c Most common occurrence in children d Temporary loss of consciousness

10 Uncontrollable tonic, then clonic muscular spasms with loss of consciousness is characteristic of which of the following types of seizures?
a Jacksonian b Petit mal c Grand mal d Psychomotor

11 A seizure involving a momentary loss of consciousness often characterized by a blank stare and a facial twitch is referred to as:
a Jacksonian b Grand mal c Psychomotor d Petit mal

12 Which of the following interventions are of primary importance when one encounters a patient having a seizure?
a Insert a tongue blade b Observe the seizure to determine progression of muscular involvement c Restrain the patient to limit outward movement of arms and legs d Establish an open airway by maintaining the patient in a side-lying position.

13 Which of the following are likely indications for the surgical treatment of an epileptic patient?
a Focal lesion identified by EEG and compatible with clinical manifestation b Area accessible and dispensable c Drug therapy is not an effective modality of treatment d High motivation for a rehabilitation program

Directions: Match the type of drug in col. A with the associated therapeutic uses and side effects in col. B.

Column A	Column B
14 ____ Phenytoin	a Hepatic damage, bone marrow depression, toxic psychosis.
15 ____ Ethosuximide	
16 ____ Phenacemide	
17 ____ Carbamazepine	b Drug of choice for grand mal, Jacksonian and psychomotor seizures.
18 ____ Mephenytoin	
19 ____ Primidone	c Primary drug for petit mal seizures.
	d Sedation, vertigo, dizziness, ataxia, nausea, diplopia, nystagmus.
	e Fatal bone marrow depression, obstructive jaundice and water intoxication are signs of toxicity.
	f Similar to phenytoin, but demethylated effect may produce rash, fever, aplastic anemia.

CHAPTER 49 Degenerative Diseases of the Nervous System

Degenerative diseases of the nervous system have been traditionally referred to as diseases with a progressively downhill course whose etiology and pathology were generally unknown. Parkinson's syndrome (paralysis agitans, shaking palsy), multiple sclerosis, and myasthenia gravis are three entities grouped under this heading. Parkinson's syndrome commonly affects older adults and the site of pathology is believed to be the basal ganglia and extrapyramidal nerve tracts. Multiple sclerosis is one of the most common neurological disorders involving young people, and the primary pathological change is demyelinization of the nerve fibers in the central nervous system. Myasthenia gravis is actually a disease involving the neuromuscular junction, with the chief symptom of muscular weakness. These common neurological disorders and related entities will be discussed in this chapter.

ANATOMY OF THE BASAL GANGLIA

Specific delineation of the extrapyramidal system is not universally agreed upon, but there is basic concurrence that the basal ganglia and the extrapyramidal portions of the cerebral cortex are important constituents (Figs. 49-1 to 49-3).

The main cortical components arise from the posterior section of the frontal lobe. The cerebellum and other parts of the reticular formation are also part of this anatomic-physiologic unit. The whole system appears to work as a unit, making the attribution of specific functions to a prescribed, localized area very difficult.

The basal ganglia are found in each cerebral hemisphere in paired groups. They consist of neuronal cell bodies of motor control neurons. They are formed from the central gray matter of the telencephalon. The basal ganglia are the *caudate, lenticular,* and *amygdaloid nuclei,* and the *claustrum.* The caudate nucleus is the most medial of the basal ganglia and is shaped like a comma with an extended tail (Fig. 49-2). The amygdaloid nucleus lies as a knob of gray matter at the tip of the tail of the caudate. The lenticular nucleus is a lens-shaped body extending from the head of the caudate nucleus. It is further divided into the *putamen* and *globus pallidus,* or palladium. The claustrum is a thin plate of gray matter just beneath the cortex near the insula (not shown in the figure). The *internal capsule* lies in close association with the basal ganglia and consists of a band of nerve fibers passing from the spinal cord and brainstem to the cortex as well as fibers passing from the cortex to lower centers. The caudate and lenticular nucleus along with the adjacent part of the internal capsule are sometimes referred to as the *corpus striatum.* In the upper part of the midbrain lie three nuclear masses which are intimately related to the corpus striatum. These are the *red nucleus,* the *substantia nigra,* and the *subthalamic nucleus,* or *corpus Luysii.* These nuclei are considered as part of the basal ganglia system, since they are connected to the basal ganglia by important neuronal pathways. There are also neuronal connections between the cerebral cortex and the corpus striatum and between that and the reticular formation of the brainstem.

The basal ganglia are believed to function as important centers of coordination, especially in the control of automatic associated movements. The corpus striatum (caudate nucleus and putamen) are believed to be responsible for the control of the initiation and inhibition of gross intentional body movements that are unconsciously performed in the normal person. They also provide muscle tone so that exact movements can be performed, e.g., fine hand work requires the coordinated effort of the entire arm and trunk, or the hand is unable to perform. The globus pallidus is a more primitive structure. Many nonpyramidal pathways converge in this area. The claustrum is included, but details regarding its physiology are lacking. The exact function of the amygdala is unknown although it may be related to vegetative activities.

A feedback system seems to operate via circular pathways from the motor cortex to the basal ganglia, thalamus, and the motor cortex. Motor signals from the cerebral cortex to the pons and cerebellum are also circuitous, with the return to the cortex being through the ventrolateral nucleus of the thalamus through which signals from the basal ganglia also pass. Because of the proximity of these circuits it is hypothesized that basal ganglia and cerebellum feedback signals could be integrated in this area.

Broadly speaking, the basal ganglia are involved in two general activities: control of the body's motor tone

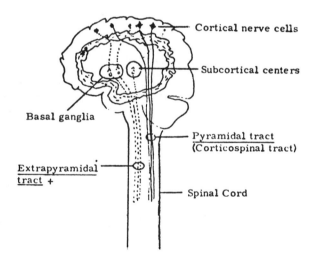

FIGURE 49-1 Simplified diagram of pyramidal and extrapyramidal systems. (From Medical Notes on Parkinsonism and Pseudoparkinsonism, PI 99–14 rev., April, 1972, Burroughs Wellcome Co., Research Triangle Park, North Carolina, 27709.)
*The basal ganglia include all subcortical motor nuclei of the forebrain and are collectively known as the striatum, the globus pallidus (pallidum), subthalamic nucleus, substantia nigra, and red nucleus.
†Posture and the performance of well coordinated movements result from an integration of information received from both the cortex and extrapyramidal systems. The cortex initiates movement while the extrapyramidal system exerts the necessary facilitation or inhibition needed for the production of purposeful, coordinated, controlled movements. Disruption of this influence results in abnormal, uncontrolled movements.
+Extra pyramidal tract: (a) Reticulospinal, (b) Vestibulospinal, (c) Tectospinal, (d) Rubrospinal.

and gross intentional movements. The general effect of basal ganglia excitation is of inhibitory signals to the bulboreticular facilitatory areas and of excitatory signals to the bulboreticular inhibitory areas. When the basal ganglia are not functioning adequately, the facilitatory areas become overactive; the inhibitory areas become underactive. This results in rigidity throughout the body. The patient with an extrapyramidal disorder has great difficulty maintaining equilibrium while standing and posture while sitting. It is difficult to change from a horizontal to a sitting position, to roll from a supine to a prone position, and to walk, since control of the center of gravity is lacking. The righting reflex, the vestibular reflex, and proprioception are all disturbed. If the spinal cord is transected at the level of the mesencephalon, a decerebrate rigidity occurs, indicating that the major effect of the basal ganglia is inhibition. The tremor (abnormal movements) observed in extrapyramidal disorders is a result of excess neural activity in one area of the brain from unopposed activity in another area. This characteristic is called the *release phenomenon* and is a common occurrence with tissue destruction in the nervous system (a lesion in A removes the regulatory control that A exerted over B, and consequently B becomes overactive).

Both the corpus striatum and the motor cortex are instrumental in the control of gross intentional movements that are normally unconscious. The control is accomplished through two pathways: globus pallidus through the thalamus to the cortex and downward via corticospinal and extracorticospinal pathways into the spinal cord; and downward through the globus pallidus and substantia nigra to the reticular formation and reticulospinal tracts to the cord. The globus pallidus seems to provide the background muscle tone necessary for performing exacting movements (especially with the

hands). Stimulation of the globus pallidus will stop a movement at any point and keep it locked at that point as long as the stimulation is continued.

EXTRAPYRAMIDAL SYNDROMES

Extrapyramidal syndromes are disorders concerned with movement which result from lesions involving those parts of the brain other than the corticospinal pathways, principally the basal ganglia. There is more data available concerning the clinical aspects of extrapyramidal dysfunction than about its pathophysiologic basis. Even the anatomy of this area escapes precise measurement. Often a patient is seen with an obvious neurological deficit based on pathologic changes in the basal ganglia, brainstem, and cerebrum, but the functional impairment may far exceed the anatomic changes that are evident. Again, when there is widespread destruction of very similar areas, the patient may escape relatively unscathed. Neurochemical changes are hypothesized to account for some of these discrepancies.

Tremor

The tremor is an involuntary movement which results from an excess of neuronal activity in one area that is a result of unopposed activity in another area. This release phenomenon is a common occurrence with nervous system pathology. The tremor is most marked peripherally. It may be suppressed by will or with vigorous activity. In general, there is alternating contractions of the flexor and extensor muscle groups so that movement is at right angles to the axis of the limb. The tremor of Parkinsonism occurs at rest and temporarily disappears during voluntary activity. In contrast, a tremor due to cerebellar deficiency is an intention tremor and is increased with purposeful activity.

Chorea

Chorea is a type of involuntary movement particularly involving the limbs, face, trunk, and head. The movements are brief, rapid, and explosive, resembling fragments of purposive movements following one another in a disorderly fashion. In the face the movements are always bilateral. Raising the eyebrows, frowning, smiling, and bizarre movements of the mouth may occur. In severe cases there may be considerable dysarthria so that speech and mastication are affected. The involuntary movements in the limbs may make walking and purposeful movement of the hands difficult. Movement and environmental stimuli aggravate the symptoms, while the movements may disappear during sleep.

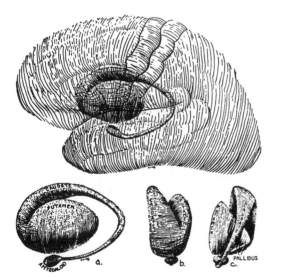

FIGURE 49-2 Upper, Phantom of the corpus striatum within the cerebral hemisphere. A, Lateral aspect; B, ventral aspect; C, caudal aspect. Copyright © W. J. Krieg, Department of Biostructure, Northwestern Medical School, Chicago, Illinois.

The pathology in chorea probably involves extensive areas of the nervous system but most importantly where there is diffuse and widespread damage (as in Huntington's chorea) includes the corpus striatum. Conversely, there are many documented cases of striatum pathology that occur with vascular softenings (area distal to the infarct becomes soft and spongy) that show no clinical evidence of chorea. Another view suggests that chorea may be the result of increased receptor site response to normal dopamine levels. The striatal dopamine content is normal in Huntington's chorea. Cerebrospinal fluid levels of homovanillic acid (the major catabolic product of dopamine) are also normal. Its normal level suggests that dopamine turnover is not increased. This would support the hypothesis that the pathophysiology in chorea is in some manner related to an increased (or altered) response of striatal dopamine receptors. This hypersensitivity hypothesis is supported by biochemical and pharmacological data. Exogenous L-dopa can cause an increase or exacerbation of chorea; neuroleptic drugs can decrease or ameliorate the abnormal movements, supposedly by competing with dopamine at the receptor sites.

Athetosis

Athetosis is marked by involuntary movements combined with instability of posture. It is evidenced by slow, rhythmic, writhing, wormlike movements that usually occur in the peripheral parts of the upper extremities (especially the fingers and hands). The face, neck, and feet may be affected. The involved muscles are spastic, and voluntary activity is impaired. Voluntary activity and emotional stimuli cause an exaggeration of the abnormal movements. Coordinated activity is not possible in the affected muscle groups.

The globus pallidus and possibly the corpus striatum are involved in the pathology of athetosis. The cerebral cortex also demonstrates lesions. Normal feedback circuits are interrupted, and the detoured impulses result in abnormal movement.

Dystonia

Dystonia may be considered as a variant of athetosis. Dystonia is a kind of frozen athetosis characterized by bizarre or grotesque postures of the limbs or trunk from excessive muscular tone in certain muscle groups. Voluntary movement is seriously impaired. The pathophysiologic basis for dystonia is poorly understood.

Hemiballismus

Hemiballismus is the involuntary, violent movement of a large body area (entire leg, shoulder, pelvic girdle). It usually involves only one side of the body. Attempting a normal activity may invoke a ballistic movement instead. This syndrome is believed to be due to extensive lesions of the subthalamic nuclei usually secondary to an infarct. Death occurs in 4 to 6 weeks in 60 percent of patients and is generally the result of exhaustion, pneumonia, or congestive heart failure. The recent use of neuroleptics (dopamine antagonists) such as haloperidol and chlorpromazine has improved the survival rate. This has raised the question of the possible role of increased presynaptic synthesis and release of dopamine (Klawans, 1976).

Parkinson's syndrome

Parkinson's disease, or paralysis agitans, is considered to be the most common neurological disorder of the aging. It affects about 1 million persons in the United

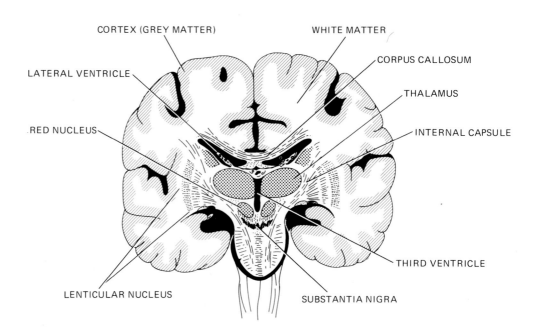

States with 50,000 new cases occurring every year. One percent of the population over the age of 50 years is affected. The majority of cases are considered *idiopathic*. Other cases are related to epidemic encephalitis (von Economo's disease, which was common from 1918 to 1926), but today there are only a few cases remaining. This type is called *postencephalitic parkinsonism*. *Drug-induced parkinsonism* is an increasingly common cause of parkinsonism in young and middle-aged patients. The phenothiazines and *Rauwolfia* (antipsychotic drugs) have been most often implicated; generally, parkinsonism is a consequence of prolonged ingestion of a high dose.

CLINICAL MANIFESTATIONS

Regardless of etiology, parkinsonism is characterized by chronic, progressive (but varyingly so) motor dysfunction. The hallmarks of the condition are rigidity, resting tremor, and poverty of movement.

The rigidity may be isolated to one muscle or joint or may be widespread and bilateral. It decreases muscle power and speed and is a major factor in the associated deformities of parkinsonism. Passive movement of an extremity meets with a plastic, dead-feeling resistance that has been likened to bending a lead pipe and is therefore called *lead-pipe rigidity*. Since both flexor and extensor muscles are tightly contracted (increased tonus), impairment of reciprocal inhibitory muscle groups is indicated. The rigidity is different than the spasticity in pyramidal tract pathology. Sometimes there is a series of "catches" during passive motion, called *cogwheel rigidity*. The sudden loss of resistance seen in a spastic extremity, however, is absent.

The tremor associated with Parkinson's disease occurs at rest and is referred to as a *rest tremor*. Extrapyramidal lesions typically produce tremors that are exaggerated with rest and decreased with voluntary movements and sleep. It is due to regular, alternating, contractions (four to six per second) of antagonistic muscles. If the head and limbs are affected, the tremor is *coarse*. The hand movements are described as "*pill-rolling*," brought about by the rhythmic movement of the thumb and first two fingers. One or both hands may be involved, and it is a very common initial symptom.

The basis for the tremor is not clear. Electromyogram tracings show rhythmic bursts of motor discharges. Two theories that have been proposed to explain the tremor are as follows: (1) Degeneration of the substantia nigra is invariably found in Parkinson's disease and the globus pallidus is often involved. These changes result in a loss of inhibitory influence, and control nuclei in the reticular substance of the brainstem are free to oscillate. (2) Loss of inhibitory influences in the lower basal ganglia causes increased feedback in the globus pallidus-thalamus-cortical circuit, and this results in

oscillation. To further complicate the possible basic explanation concerning the tremor, not all patients have it. In addition, if hemiplegia should incidentally occur in these patients, the tremor disappears on the paralyzed side.

In addition to the slowness resulting from rigidity, difficulty is experienced in initiating new movements and in performing ballistic actions; this is called *bradykinesia*. It may be seen in the patient's difficulty in rising from a chair, in starting to walk, speak, or write. Speech is slow and often slurred. Writing is small and cramped and becomes even smaller as the person continues (*micrographia*). Bradykinesia is an impairment of voluntary movements. Involuntary movements are also affected: there is a loss of associated movements (*akinesia*). For example, the patient does not swing the arms while walking; the face is expressionless and the voice unmodulated. The patient must consciously perform certain actions that are normally unconscious. This requires much expenditure of energy and effort.

Gait disturbances reflect increasing impairment of postural and righting reflexes. When pushed, the patient is unable to stop quickly but continues to move in the direction pushed (propulsion, retropulsion, lateropulsion). Poor balance is almost pathognomonic. The gait is slow and shuffling with short steps (*festinating*) to remain upright (the person is bent forward and hurries along trying to keep up with the body's center of gravity to prevent falling).

Certain autonomic manifestations appear in Parkinson's syndrome, but little is known about their precise pathophysiology. There is *hyperhidrosis*, or excessive perspiration. The skin has an oily quality with a tendency toward seborrheic dermatitis. The latter is believed to be a result of hypothalamus dysfunction and the release of excess sebotropic hormone. Drooling is probably from decreased swallowing as a reflection of bradykinesia. The volume of saliva is not increased. Constipation is an almost universal symptom of Parkinson's syndrome due to gastrointestinal hypomotility. Neurogenic bladder dysfunction is a fairly frequent complaint and is aggravated by anticholinergic drugs and prostatic hypertrophy.

DIAGNOSIS

No specific laboratory data is significant so that the diagnosis of Parkinson's syndrome is based on clinical findings. The major neurological findings are listed in Table 49-1.

PATHOLOGY

The pathologic changes in Parkinson's syndrome are not yet fully understood, although the basal ganglia appear to be involved. There is a decrease or loss of pigment in the substantia nigra along with a degeneration of a sig-

FIGURE 49-3 Coronal section of the brain showing the thalamus, basal ganglia, lateral and third ventricles, and internal capsule. (From Esta Carini and Guy Owens, Neurological and Neurosurgical Nursing, *6th ed., Mosby, St. Louis, 1974, p. 19.)*

nificant number of neurons with reactive gliosis [some of the cells have eosinophilic intracytoplasmic inclusions called Lewy bodies (Robbins, 1974)]. There is also a depletion of dopamine in the corpus striatum which appears to be proportional to the cell loss in the substantia nigra. Levodopa (L-dopa), which is transformed to dopamine within neuronal cells, causes improvement by replenishing stores toward normal levels. The dopamine neuron hypothesis offers an explanation of Parkinson's syndrome from a pharmacologic point of view but does not explain how dopamine is depleted and cells destroyed.

TREATMENT

Dopamine given orally does not cross the blood-brain barrier and is metabolized before it can reach the basal ganglia. L-Dopa, a metabolic precursor of dopamine that will cross the blood-brain barrier, relieves symptoms in about two-thirds of patients with Parkinson's syndrome (Guyton, 1972). Its main effects are produced by its decarboxylation to dopamine. Since L-Dopa is largely decarboxylated in the gastrointestinal tract and liver, only

TABLE 49-1
Major neurological findings in Parkinson's syndrome

NEUROLOGICAL FINDING	COMMENT
1 Hyperactive glabellar (blink) reflex	Exaggerated sensitivity to finger tapping over glabella (between eyebrows) causing the patient to blink with each tap. It takes effort for a normal person to blink. Early sign of Parkinson's syndrome.
2 Palmomental reflex	Palm of hand stroked by thumb causes ipsilateral response in mentalis muscle with resulting wrinkling of the skin of the chin. If the Parkinson's disease is unilateral, the response may only be found on the affected side. Palmomental reflex negative in normal persons.
3 Masklike facies	Wide-eyed, unblinking, staring expression. Blinks 2 to 3 times per minute. Normal blinking 12 to 20 times per minute.
4 Rest tremor	Pill-rolling movement of hands characteristic. Tremor decreased with voluntary movement and during sleep.
5 Cogwheel rigidity	Motion interrupted by "catches."
6 Postural abnormalities	Kyphosis, stooped posture, shuffling gait with short steps (festinating gait).
7 Micrographia, monotone	Small handwriting; expressionless speech.

small amounts reach the basal ganglia. Consequently, large doses are necessary to achieve results. Another preparation now available (Carbidopa, Sinemet) combines L-Dopa with a decarboxylase inhibitor that will not cross the blood-brain barrier. This results in less breakdown of the drug in peripheral tissue so that side effects are greatly reduced and more of the drug is available to the basal ganglia.

L-dopa therapy is begun in small doses and gradually increased until parkinsonian symptoms are obliterated or drug side effects appear (0.5 to 8 g daily in two or more divided doses with food). If the patient is taking L-dopa without an inhibitor, it is most important that the patient avoid taking pyridoxine (vitamin B_6) since it is a coenzyme for dopa decarboxylase and will enhance its activity, converting L-dopa to dopamine in peripheral tissues so that less is available to cross the blood-brain barrier. Vitamin B_6 can actually negate the therapeutic effect of L-dopa. Alcohol can antagonize the effects of L-dopa. Obesity may cause dose regulation to be a problem since L-dopa is absorbed into fat deposits and released erratically. An increase in dietary protein can aggravate parkinsonian symptoms since amino acids and L-dopa compete for absorption through intestinal epithelium and when crossing the blood-brain barrier.

Other adjuncts to treatment include anticholinergic drugs (Artane), physical and occupational therapy, and a positive attitude of encouragement. Stereotaxic surgery was introduced as a treatment in 1946 but is now reserved for unilateral cases that are normotensive and relatively young. It is not generally done unless L-dopa therapy is not effective.

DEMYELINATING DISEASES

There are a large number of neurological disorders termed demyelinating diseases because their common pathological feature is focal areas of destruction involving the myelin sheath of nerve fibers in the central nervous system. The axon often suffers damage as well, but destruction of myelin is the primary change. Multiple sclerosis is the primary demyelinating disease and will be the focus of the discussion.

Acute disseminated encephalomyelitis

Acute disseminated encephalomyelitis (postvaccinial or postinfectious), although rare, is another demyelinating disorder that deserves mention because it is essentially preventable. This is an acute encephalitic or myelitic process of variable course characterized by symptoms indicating damage to the white matter of the brain or spinal cord. The pathological findings consist of numerous circumscribed areas of perivascular demyelinization. About 1 week following measles and 10 days to 2 weeks following vaccination for rabies or smallpox, there is a rapid development of neurological symptoms consisting of headache, drowsiness, stupor, ocular palsies, and often a transverse cord lesion causing a flaccid paralysis of all four limbs. Variations in severity are common. Postvaccination encephalomyelitis may occur with an incidence of about 1 in 1000 and 1 in 4000 persons vaccinated (Thorn, 1977) and is presumably due to sensitization of brain tissue contained in the vaccine. The same condition may follow vaccination for smallpox with an incidence of 1 in 5000 vaccinated. It is more common in the primary vaccination. The mortality rate is 30 to 50 percent, and patients who recover are frequently left with some disability, such as paraplegia and epilepsy. Postinfectious encephalomyelitis following a viral infection, especially the measles, occurs in about 1 in 1000 cases. The mortality rate is 10 to 20 percent, and about 50 percent of those who survive are left with some neurologic damage (Thorn, 1977).

The use of killed duck embryo vaccine which is free of nerve tissue for rabies, the selective use of smallpox vaccine, and vaccination for measles has greatly reduced the risk and incidence of encephalomyelitis in the United States.

Multiple sclerosis

Multiple sclerosis is one of the most common neurological disorders affecting young people. It is characterized by the widespread occurrence of patches of myelin destruction followed by gliosis in the white matter of the nervous system. The hard, yellow plaques found on autopsy are responsible for it being so named. The characteristic course of the disease consists of a series of isolated attacks affecting different parts of the central nervous system. Each attack subsequently shows some degree of remission, but the overall picture is one of deterioration.

ETIOLOGY AND PATHOLOGY

The fundamental nature of the disturbance which leads to multiple sclerosis is unknown and is consequently the subject of much speculation. The illness is more common in temperate climates (northern Europe and northern United States) with an incidence of 30 to 80 per 100,000 population, and it is rare in the tropics. In Japan it is uncommon at any latitude. There is also a slightly higher familial incidence of the disease. It is about 8 times more common in immediate relatives (Thorn, 1977). It most commonly presents in young people from the age of 20 to 45 years. All of these data suggest an infectious etiology (probably viral) contracted early in life which becomes activated somewhat later, in early adulthood. Its mechanism of action may be that of an autoimmune reaction attacking myelin.

The notion of precipitating factors is viewed by many statisticians as having occurred by pure chance, and the average patient is apt to develop new symptoms every 2 to 3 years (Silberberg, 1970). Several events which are considered precipitating factors include pregnancy, excessive fatigue, stress, infection, and injury.

Necropsy examination shows that the lesions are most prominent in the pyramidal tracts and posterior columns of the cord, around the ventricles of the brain, in the

optic nerves, in the pons and medulla, especially involving the cerebellar peduncles (Peery and Miller, 1971). In the acute phase the area is edematous, and infiltrated with lymphocytes and plasma cells. This is most apparent around the veins. Macrophages remove the areas of degenerating myelin and as the acute phase subsides, there is a reactive gliosis. The end result is a shrunken area of sclerosis. The axon cylinders and cell bodies are not directly affected although the scar is capable of damaging the underlying axon fiber. The symptoms of multiple sclerosis due to the demyelinization are irreversible although there may be a substantial return of function when the edema subsides which may obscure the underlying deficit.

CLINICAL FEATURES

The greatly varied location of the lesions and the unpredictable occurrence of remissions and exacerbations makes an orderly discussion of signs and symptoms impossible. Any combination of the following signs and symptoms may coexist:

(1) *Sensory disorders* Paresthesias (numbness, tingling, "dead" feeling, "pins and needles") may vary in degree from one day to the next. If there is a lesion of the posterior columns of the cervical cord, flexion of the neck causes shocklike sensations to run down the cord (*Lhermitte's sign*). Proprioceptive disorders often give rise to a sensory ataxia and incoordination of the arms. Vibration sense is often diminished at the ankles. Since sensory disorders cannot be demonstrated objectively, these symptoms may be thought hysterical.

(2) *Visual complaints* Optic neuritis which causes increasingly blurred vision in one eye which may progress to complete uniocular blindness during a period of a few hours to 3 days is the initial disorder in 40 forty percent of patients. There is often pain on movement of the affected eye. Diplopia and scotomas (blind spots) are also reported. The symptoms generally subside when the acute exacerbation has ended.

(3) *Spastic weakness of the limbs* Weakness of a limb on one side of the body or an asymmetric distribution in all four limbs is a very common complaint. The patient may complain of tiredness and heaviness in one leg and noticeably drags that foot and has poor control. The patient may complain that the leg jumps spontaneously, especially when in bed. More profound spasticity is accompanied by painful spasm of the muscles. The tendon reflexes may be hyperactive and abdominal reflexes absent; the plantar responses are extensor.

(4) *Cerebellar signs* Nystagmus and cerebellar ataxia is another common syndrome and indicates involvement of the cerebellar and corticospinal tracts. Cere-

bellar ataxia is manifested by uncoordinated voluntary movements, intention tremors, balance disturbances, and dysarthria (scanning speech with words broken into syllables with pauses between syllables). The nystagmus (rapid oscillation of the eyeball horizontally or vertically) indicates cellebellar or brainstem involvement.

(5) *Bladder dysfunction*   Lesions in the corticospinal tracts often cause disorder of sphincter control; hesitancy, urgency, and frequency are common. Acute retention and incontinence also occur.

(6) *Disorders of mood*   Many patients develop *euphoria,* an unrealistic feeling of well-being. This is believed to be due to involvement of the white matter of the frontal lobes. Other signs of cerebral impairment may include loss of memory.

DIAGNOSIS, PROGNOSIS, AND TREATMENT

The diagnosis is usually made on a clear history of relapses and remissions and signs of multiple lesions in the central nervous system. Many times it is impossible to confirm the diagnosis until the patient is followed for several years. The colloidal gold test on the cerebrospinal fluid is positive (in the absence of a positive serology) in many cases and is supportive evidence. In about 60 percent of the cases of established multiple sclerosis the gamma globulin level in the cerebrospinal fluid is elevated, but this test is not helpful in establishing an early diagnosis. One test which is helpful in determining the presence of active demyelinization is the basic protein assay (BPA) of the spinal fluid. The level of BPA drops rapidly once the acute exacerbation is over (Cohen, Herndon, McKhann).

The progression of multiple sclerosis is extremely variable. The classic picture is of intermittent relapses followed by more or less complete remissions. The remissions are usually less complete with each ensuing attack so that within 10 to 20 years the patient is physically disabled. In a few cases the patient may become severely disabled within a couple of years.

Since the cause of the disease is not known, there is no specific therapy. During an acute relapse the patient should rest in bed, although prolonged bed rest is to be avoided. During acute relapses, vitamin B_{12} and corticosteroid drugs may be given, but evaluation of this treatment is difficult because of the episodic nature of the disease. Physical therapy is the most valuable process in which the patient should be involved. It tends to increase comfort and build morale. Gait retraining, muscle stretching, and strengthening may all be necessary.

MYASTHENIA GRAVIS

The name *myasthenia gravis* means grave muscle weakness. It is the only neuromuscular disease that incorporates both rapid fatigue of voluntary muscle and prolonged recovery time (may actually take 10 to 20 times longer than normal). Mortality rates in the past have been as high as 90 percent. The death rate has been drastically reduced since medications and respiratory care units have become available.

The clinical syndrome was first described in 1600. In the late 1800s myasthenia gravis was distinguished from muscle weakness due to true bulbar palsy. In the 1920s, a physician with myasthenia gravis noticed an improvement after taking ephedrine for menstrual cramps. Finally in 1934, another physician from England (Mary Walker) noted the similarity of symptoms in myasthenia gravis and curare poisoning. She used the curare antagonist physostigmine for myasthenia gravis and observed marked improvement.

The incidence of myasthenia gravis in the United States is 1 in 10,000. It is more common in women under the age of 40 years, and the age group most affected is 30 to 40 years old (Robbins, 1976, p. 1426); after the age of 40 men are more prone than women to develop myasthenia gravis.

Pathophysiology

Skeletal or striated muscles are innervated by large, myelinated nerves that originate in the anterior horn cell of the spinal cord and the brainstem. They send their axons out in the spinal or cranial nerves to the periphery. Individual nerves branch many times and are capable of stimulating up to 2000 skeletal muscle fibers. The junction where a nerve interacts with a muscle is generally at a midpoint section of the muscle so that the action potential travels in both directions. The *end plate* refers to a nerve ending which branches to form several nerve terminals on the muscle but is outside the muscle fiber plasma membrane (Fig. 49-4). The entire unit is insulated by Schwann cells. The point where a nerve terminal in-

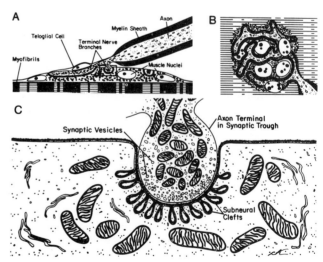

FIGURE 49-4 Muscle and nerve-muscle junction. Schematic representations of the motor end plate as seen by light and electron microscopy. A. End plate as seen in histological sections in the long axis of the muscle fiber. B. As seen in surface view with the light microscope. C. As seen in an electron micrograph of an area such as that in the rectangle in A. (From B. Curtis, S. Jacobson, and E. Marcus, An Introduction to the Neurosciences, Saunders, Philadelphia, 1972, p. 115.)

vaginates the muscle membrane is called the *synaptic gutter* or *trough*. The *synaptic cleft* refers to the space between the end-plate terminal and the fiber membrane. It is filled with a gelatinous substance through which extracellular fluid may diffuse. In the bottom of the gutter, the muscle membrane forms folds called *subneural clefts* or *secondary synaptic clefts*. These clefts increase surface area where physiochemical processes can occur.

The mitochondria in the axon terminals supply the energy necessary for the synthesis of acetylcholine (Ach) which is synthesized in the cytoplasm of the terminal but rapidly absorbed into *synaptic vesicles*. The Ach (the excitatory transmitter) is released from vesicles in the nerve ending. Approximately 300,000 vesicles are in the terminals of a single end plate. Ach diffuses across the neuromuscular cleft and interacts with a receptor substance present only on the sarcolemmal membrane of the motor end plate.

The subneural clefts in the gutter contain the enzyme acetylcholinesterase, which is capable of inactivating Ach within 2 to 3 seconds, but this is sufficient time for the Ach to excite the muscle fiber. The nerve impulse (action potential) causes calcium ions to move into membranes of the terminal (from extracellular fluid). Calcium ion causes the release of Ach from its vesicles. If there is insufficient calcium ion or excess magnesium, the release of Ach is decreased. The local end-plate potential is the result of sodium flowing in (because Ach increases permeability for sodium) causing a rise in membrane potential to 50 to 75 mV.

In myasthenia gravis myoneural conduction is impaired, and end-plate potentials are too weak to adequately stimulate muscle fibers. The number of folds in the synaptic gutter is decreased resulting in less surface area where the neurochemical reactions can occur. The synaptic cleft is widened. Antibodies that attack muscle fibers have been found in serums of many of these patients. It has been suggested that end-plate potentials in these patients are greatly reduced. Some evidence has been gathered suggesting that the motor end plates of some patients are abnormally thin and blanched.

The muscles appear normal macroscopically. If atrophy is evident, it is on the basis of disuse. Microscopically, some cases of lymphocytic infiltrates are found within the muscle and other organs.

Recent evidence is pointing toward a receptor disorder, making myasthenia gravis a muscle defect. By using snake venom to bind Ach receptor sites, the number of sites has been decreased, and symptoms of myasthenia gravis have been produced on that basis alone. Muscle biopsies on ten myasthenia gravis patients showed that all of them had marked reduction (70 to 80 percent below normal controls) in the number of Ach receptors per neuromuscular junction (Drachman, 1976). Autoimmune mechanisms may be instrumental in blocking or damaging Ach receptors. Antireceptor antibodies have been found in serums of myasthenia gravis patients. Whether this is a primary or secondary consequence of receptor damage caused by an unknown primary agent will be of great value in determining the exact pathogenisis of myasthenia gravis. Figure 49-5 illustrates some possible defects in myasthenia gravis.

Clinical manifestations

As mentioned previously, it is currently hypothesized that myasthenia gravis is an autoimmune disorder involving a neuromuscular conduction blockage. It most frequently presents as an insidious, progressive disease. However, it may remain localized to a specific group of muscles. Because the course is so variable from one patient to another, prognosis is difficult to determine. Table 49-2 divides myasthenia gravis into two groups—those with ocular myasthenia and those with generalized myasthenia. Generalized myasthenia may be mild, moderate, or severe, and the onset may be slow or rapid.

In 90 percent of patients the initial symptoms involve the ocular muscles, causing ptosis and diplopia. The diagnosis can be established by attention to the levator palpebrae muscles of the eyelids. If the disease remains confined to the eye muscles, the course is very mild, and there is no mortality.

The facial, laryngeal, and pharyngeal muscles are also frequently involved in myasthenia gravis. This may result in regurgitation through the nose when swallowing is attempted (palatal muscles); abnormal, nasal speech; and failure of the mouth to close—called the "hanging jaw" sign.

Respiratory muscle involvement is evidenced by a weak cough, eventual attacks of dyspnea, and inability to clear the tracheobronchial tree of mucus. The shoulder and pelvic girdles may become involved in advanced cases; there may be generalized weakness of any of the skeletal muscles.

POSSIBLE DEFECTS IN MYASTHENIA GRAVIS

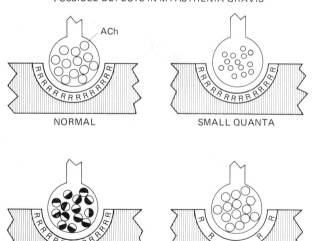

FIGURE 49-5 *Possible defects in myasthenia gravis. Schematic representations of neuromuscular junctions. Circles within nerve endings indicate Ach-containing vesicles. R represents Ach receptors. (From D. B. Drachman, I. Kao, and A. Pesbronk, et al., "Myasthenia Gravis as a Receptor Disorder," Annals of the New York Academy of Sciences, **274**: 226–234, May 28, 1976.)*

Generally, symptoms of myasthenia gravis are relieved by rest and anticholinesterase agents. Symptoms are aggravated or exacerbated by (1) alterations in hormonal balance, such as during pregnancy, fluctuations in the menstrual cycle, or disturbances in thyroid function, (2) concurrent illness, especially upper respiratory tract infections and those associated with diarrhea or fever, (3) emotional upsets—most patients experience more muscular weakness when they are upset, (4) alcohol (especially with tonic water which contains quinine, a drug promoting muscle weakness) and other drugs. Lithium carbonate aggravates symptoms once a myasthenia gravis attack has begun (*Nurses' Drug Alert*, 1977). Table 49-3 lists some of the drugs that are contraindicated or must be used with caution in patients with myasthenia gravis.

TABLE 49-2
Clinical classification of myasthenia gravis

Group I   Ocular myasthenia
Involvement of ocular muscles only, with ptosis and diplopia. Very mild, no mortality.

Group II   Generalized myasthenia

A Mild generalized
Slow onset, frequently ocular, gradually spreading to skeletal and bulbar muscles. Respiratory system not involved. Response to drug therapy good. Low mortality rate.

B Moderate generalized
Gradual onset with frequent ocular presentation, progressing to more severe generalized involvement of the skeletal and bulbar muscles. Dysarthria, dysphagia, and poor mastication more prevalent than in mild, generalized myasthenia gravis. Respiratory muscles not involved. Response to drug therapy less satisfactory and the patient's activities restricted, but mortality rate low.

C Severe generalized
  1 Acute fulminating
      Rapid onset of severe bulbar and skeletal muscle weakness with early involvement of respiratory muscles. Progression of disease usually complete within 6 months. Percentage of thymomas highest in this group. Response to drugs poor, incidence of myasthenic, cholinergic, and mixed crises high. Mortality rate high.
  2 Late severe
      Severe myasthenia gravis develops at least 2 years after onset of group I or group II symptoms. Progression of myasthenia gravis may be either gradual or sudden. Second highest percentage of thymomas. Response to drug therapy and prognosis poor.

Source: Professional Information Committee of the National Medical Advisory Board, *Myasthenia Gravis: A Manual for Nurses*, Myasthenia Gravis Foundation, Inc., New York, 1975.

Diagnosis

A diagnosis can be made by a suspicious clinician on the basis of the patient's history and the physical exam. One must keep in mind that there *is* such a disease, affecting a small number of people. Many patients have been

TABLE 49-3
Drugs that are contraindicated or must be used with caution in myasthenia gravis

DRUG GROUP	DRUG NAME
ACTH and corticosteroids	
Anesthetics	Chloroform
	Ether
	Halothane (Fluothane)
	Procaine, IV (Adrocaine)
Antiarrhythmics	Procainamide (Pronestyl)
	Quinidine
Antibiotics	Bacitracin
	Colistimethate (Coly-Mycin M)
	Colistin (Coly-Mycin S)
	Gentamicin (Garamycin)
	Kanamycin (Kantrex)
	Neomycin (Mycrifradin, Neobiotic)
	Novobiocin (Albamycin)
	Polymyxin B (Aerosporin)
	Streptomycin
	Vancomycin (Vancocin)
Anticonvulsants	Magnesium sulfate
Antimalarials	Quinine
Antipsychotics	Chlorpromazine
Barbiturates and other sedative-hypnotics	
Cathartics	
Diuretics	Carbonic anhydrase inhibitors
	Chlorthalidone (Hygroton)
	Ethacrynic acid (Edecrin)
	Furosemide (Lasix)
	Metolazone (Zaroxolyn)
	Quinethazone (Hydromox)
	Thiazides
Morphine and other narcotic analgesics	
Muscle relaxants	Decamethonium (Syncurine)
	Dimethyltubocurarine (Metubine)
	Gallamine (Flaxedil)
	Hexafluorenium (Mylaxen)
	Orphenadrine (Norflex)
	Pancuronium (Pavulon)
	Succinylcholine
	Tubocurarine
Thyroid preparations	
Tranquilizers	

Source: R. Wang and S. Lamid, "Restoring Strength in Myasthenia Gravis," *Drug Therapy*, January, 1976, p. 124.

bluntly told to see a psychiatrist. Asking the subject to perform a repetitive action until tiredness is evident can help establish a diagnosis. The diagnosis is confirmed by the *Tensilon test*. Endrophonium chloride (Tensilon), a cholinesterase inhibitor drug, is given intravenously. In myasthenia patients, there is a marked improvement of muscle strength within 30 seconds. When a positive result is obtained, it is important to make a differential diagnosis between true myasthenia gravis and myasthenic syndrome. Patients with *myasthenic syndrome* have the same symptoms as those with true myasthenia gravis, but the cause is related to other pathological processes such as diabetes, thyroid abnormalities, and widespread malignancies. The age of onset of the two conditions is an important distinguishing factor. Patients with true myasthenia are usually young; those with myasthenic syndrome are generally older. Symptoms in the myasthenic syndrome usually disappear if the basic pathology can be controlled.

Abnormalities of the thymus gland occur in myasthenia gravis. Even when too small to be radiologically observable, 80 percent of patients have histologically abnormal thymus glands, and 10 percent of that number have thymomas (Wang, 1976). Electromyography reveals no denervation, but there is a characteristic falling off in the amplitude of motor-unit potential with continued use (Elliott, 1971).

Treatment

If the patient survives for 10 years, the disease usually remains benign, and death from myasthenia gravis itself would be rare. These patients must learn to live within the limits prescribed by their disease. They need 10 hours of sleep at night to awaken refreshed, and they need to alternate work and rest periods. They must avoid precipitating factors and must take their medications on time.

Medical treatment with anticholinesterase drugs is the treatment of choice. Neostigmine inactivates or destroys cholinesterase so the Ach is not destroyed immediately. The effect is restoration to almost normal muscular activity, at least 80 to 90 percent of former strength and endurance. Besides neostigmine (Prostigmin), pyridostigmine (Mestinon), and ambenonium (Mytelase), there are other synthetic analogues of the drug originally used, physiostigmine (Eserine). Disagreeable side effects in the gastrointestinal tract (cramping, diarrhea) are called *muscarinic side effects*. It is important that the patient realize that these symptoms can mean there has been too much medication on a particular day, that the next dose must be decreased accordingly to avoid a cholinergic crisis (see below). Since neostigmine is the most apt to cause muscarinic effects, it may be prescribed initially so that the patient is made aware of exactly what this side effect is like.

Pyridostigmine is available in a timespan and is often used at bedtime so the patient can sleep through the night without being awakened to take medication.

The routine use of belladonna or atropine to neutralize muscarinic side effects is not recommended and could result in a dangerous overdose. Adrenocorticotropic hormone (ACTH) and prednisone have been used since 1966 with some degree of success, but there is doubt regarding their long-term effect.

Thymectomy in selected patients seems to bring about an earlier and more complete remission than might otherwise be expected. Young women with increasing disability and within the first 5 years after the onset seem to get the most benefit.

Crisis in myasthenia gravis

When unable to swallow, clear secretions, or breathe adequately without artificial assistance, the myasthenic patient is in crisis. There are two types of crisis: (1) *myasthenic crisis*, a condition in which there is a need for more anticholinesterase drugs; (2) *cholinergic crisis*, a condition due to an excess of anticholinesterase drugs. In either situation, artificial respiration and an adequate airway must be maintained. Tensilon (2 to 5 mg) is given intravenously as a test to differentiate between the types of crisis. The drug produces a temporary improvement in myasthenic crisis and no improvement or worsening of symptoms in cholinergic crisis.

If in myasthenic crisis, the patient is maintained on the respirator. Anticholinesterase drugs are withheld since they increase respiratory secretions and may precipitate a cholinergic crisis. Medicines are restarted gradually, and often the dosage can be lowered following a crisis.

In a cholinergic crisis the patient may have taken an excess of medication by mistake or because there had been a spontaneous remission. Many that develop this type of crisis are called "brittle myasthenics." They are difficult to control with medication and have a narrowed therapeutic range between underdose and overdose. Their response to drugs is often only partial. In cholinergic crisis the patient is maintained on artificial ventilation, anticholinergic drugs are withheld, and 1 mg of atropine may be given intravenously and repeated if necessary. When atropine is given, the patient must be carefully observed since respiratory secretions can thicken, making suctioning difficult, or a mucus plug can occlude a bronchus, causing atelectasis.

QUESTIONS

Degenerative diseases of the nervous system—Chap. 49

Directions: Answer the following questions on a separate sheet of paper.

1 Name and outline the components of the basal ganglia. What is their function?

2 Name the sites in the brain that are affected in Parkinson's disease. How are these areas of the brain affected? Where are these areas located in the brain?

3 Name the type of nerve tract that is involved in Parkinson's disease. What is the general function of this nerve tract?

4 Define *Parkinson's syndrome* and name three types of the disease.

5 Name the chemical substance that is believed to be involved in Parkinson's disease. What is the problem concerning this substance?

6 Name and briefly describe five movement disorders of the extrapyramidal motor tracts.

7 Name two drugs known to cause extrapyramidal dysfunction and parkinsonian signs and symptoms.

8 Name several neurological findings (including two reflexes) common in patients with Parkinson's disease.

9 What serious demyelinating disorder may follow the measles or vaccination for smallpox or rabies. How can this be prevented?

10 Describe the pathology in multiple sclerosis. What are the most likely symptoms which would cause you to suspect this disease in a patient?

Directions: Circle the letter preceding each item that correctly answers the question. Only ONE answer is correct. Exceptions will be noted.

11 The chief symptoms of Parkinson's disease are:
a Rigidity, aphasia, oculogyric crisis b Hemiplegia, drooling, and tremor c Tremor, rigidity, and weakness d All of the above

12 The basal ganglia are:
a Masses of white matter embedded deep inside the cerebrum b Paired structures found in each hemisphere c Six distinct structures all independent of the others d Cortical structures related to vegetative activities and having a steadying influence on muscle

13 The preferred treatment of Parkinson's disease is:
a Medical treatment with L-dopa b Surgical treatment of the older patient with bilateral disease c Anticholinergic drugs d Medical treatment with dopamine

14 Symptoms of Parkinson's disease include which of the following? (More than one answer may be correct.)
a Masklike face b Intention tremor c Bradykinesia d Choreiform movements

15 The probable site of pathology in athetosis:
a Neuromuscular junction b Cranial nerve V c Globus pallidus d Motor cortex

16 In multiple sclerosis:
a Convulsions occur in about one-half the cases. b Visual loss is generally unilateral. c Headaches and aphasia are not unusual. d Euphoria is an uncommon disturbance.

17 A patient who receives L-dopa with a decarboxylase inhibitor should avoid taking large doses of which of the following B vitamins?
a Thiamine (B₁) b Pyridoxine (B₆) c Cyanocobalamin (B₁₂) d Does not have to be concerned about ingestion of any of the B vitamins

18 Multiple sclerosis is:
a Usually inherited b Most common in tropical areas c Often a familial disease d Most common in the 20 to 40 age group

19 Which of the following statements is true about myasthenia gravis?
a Ptosis of the eyelids is an uncommon symptom. b By nature it is an acute disease common in cold climates. c It is characterized by acetylcholine deficiency at the junction of a motor nerve and skeletal muscle. d There is experimental evidence that the parathyroid glands are involved in some way with myasthenia gravis.

20 The only manifestations of myasthenia gravis are:
a Rigidity and tremor b Flaccid and/or spastic paralysis of voluntary muscle c Rapid fatigue of skeletal muscle and prolonged time for recovery of power d Rapid fatigue of smooth muscle and prolonged time for recovery of power

21 Myasthenia gravis is often associated with pathologies of the:
a Heart b Thyroid c Thymus d Liver

22 Your client has demonstrated a positive Tensilon test. What symptoms would indicate this result?
a Muscarinic effect on smooth muscle b Immediate decrease in muscle strength c Difficulty in keeping eyes open (ptosis) d Immediate increase in muscle strength

23 Anticholinesterase drugs are used to treat myasthenia gravis. The most common side effects of these medications involve:
a Central nervous system b Skeletal muscle c GI tract d Respiratory system

24 Which of the following is NOT used in treatment of myasthenia gravis?
a Neostigmine b Pyridostigmine c Ambenonium d Endrophonium

25 When a patient with myasthenia gravis is in crisis, the first consideration is to:
a Identify the type of crisis (cholinergic versus myasthenic) b Control the hemorrhage c Establish an adequate airway d Restore electrolyte balance

CHAPTER 50 Central Nervous System Injury

INCREASED INTRACRANIAL PRESSURE

Increased intracranial pressure is defined as an increase in the pressure exerted within the cranial cavity. Normally the cranial cavity is occupied by brain tissue, blood, and cerebrospinal fluid. Each portion occupies a particular volume giving a normal intracranial pressure of 50 to 200 mm water or 4 to 15 mmHg. Intracranial pressure is normally influenced by everyday activities to rise temporarily to levels much higher than normal. A few of these activities are deep abdominal breathing, coughing, and straining. Temporary increases in intracranial pressure present no difficulty, but sustained pressure has a detrimental effect on living brain tissue.

The brain, cerebral blood, and cerebrospinal fluid occupy a relatively closed space. Any increase in any one content encroaches on the space available for the other. Increased intracranial pressure not only is seen after head injury but has many additional causes of which nurses should be aware.

A brain tumor is an added mass of tissue occupying the cranial cavity. Any blockage to the flow of cerebrospinal fluid would allow a backup to occur in the ventricles, increasing the space occupied by the cerebrospinal fluid and decreasing the space available for brain tissue and blood. A tumor that obstructs the jugular vein, and, therefore, venous drainage from the head, would also lead to increased intracranial pressure.

Cerebral edema is perhaps the most common cause of increased intracranial pressure and has many causes itself. These include an increase in intracellular fluid, hypoxia, fluid and electrolyte imbalances, cerebral ischemia, meningitis, and, of course, injury. There are many causes, but the effects are basically the same.

Intracranial pressure generally increases gradually. After head injury edema formation may take 36 to 48 hours to reach its maximum (Schwartz, 1974). Like other systems within the body, the brain has mechanisms to compensate for gradual increases in intracranial pressure. But there is a limit to the brain's capacity to compensate when intracranial pressure is allowed to increase to or above the level of systemic arterial pressure. With the increase in intracranial pressure, circulation within the brain ceases (Schwartz, 1974). Relief of the pressure must be accomplished within 4 to 6 minutes, or brain death ensues.

The compensatory mechanism includes the shunting of cerebrospinal fluid from the cerebral subarachnoid space to the spinal subarachnoid space, thereby decreasing the volume occupied by the cerebrospinal fluid. A decrease in cerebral blood flow will frequently occur in response to physiological changes.

CENTRAL NERVOUS SYSTEM INJURY

Introduction to head injuries

The brain is protected from injury by the hair, skin, and bones that surround it. Without this protection, the delicate brain which makes us what we are would be very susceptible to injury and destruction. Moreover, a neuron once destroyed does not regenerate. Head injury can have catastrophic implications for an individual. Some problems are caused directly by the injury, and many others occur secondary to the injury. It is these effects that the medical team work to prevent and to detect early in order to avoid the sequence of events that lead to mental and physical deficit and even death.

Just above the skull lies the *galea aponeurotica,* a freely moveable, dense, fibrous tissue which aids in absorbing the force from external trauma. Between the galea and the skin is a fatty layer and a deep membranous layer which contains large vessels. Awareness of this fact is important because when severed, these vessels constrict poorly and may cause significant blood loss in a patient with a scalp laceration. Directly beneath the galea is the subaponeurotic space in which are found the *emissary* and *diploic veins.* These vessels may carry infection from the scalp to deep within the skull, which underscores the extreme importance of thorough cleansing and debridement of the scalp whenever the galea has been torn (Schwartz, 1974).

In the adult, the skull is a rigid compartment allowing for no expansion of intracranial contents. The bone is actually composed of two walls which are separated by cancellous bone. This structure provides for greater strength and insulation with less weight. The inner table contains grooves in which lie the anterior, middle, and posterior meningeal arteries. When fracture of the skull involves tearing of one of these arteries, the resultant arterial bleeding, which accumulates in the epidural space, may lead to a fatal outcome unless it is detected and treated immediately. This constitutes one of the true neurosurgical emergencies, demanding immediate surgical intervention (Schwartz, 1974).

Covering the brain for added protection are the meninges. The three layers of the meninges are the *dura mater,* the *arachnoid,* and the *pia mater.* Each has a separate function and differs from the other two in structure (Figs. 50-1 and 50-2).

The *dura* is the tough, semitranslucent, inelastic outer membrane. It functions to (1) protect the brain and (2) enclose the venous sinuses, and forms partitions within the skull. It is closely attached to the interior surface of the skull. Perhaps, when one reviews the problems that arise when a tear in the dura is not completely repaired and made airtight, its most important function is protection. There may be expansion of the fracture instead of healing and a chronic leakage of cerebrospinal fluid which may lead to the development of meningocerebral cicatrix causing focal epilepsy. There are instances when the dura is left open, and these include situations when it is necessary to decompress the bulging brain (e.g., with cerebral edema), to provide for drainage of cerebrospinal fluid, and after exploratory trepaning for inspection and evacuation of clots.

The dura has a rich blood supply. The middle and

FIGURE 50-1 Meninges. A. Extensions of the dura mater in the cranial cavity, sagittal view. B. The dura and arachnoid sheathe the spinal nerves at their origin. The dentate ligament separates dorsal from ventral roots and adheres to the dura. C. A vertical section through a portion of the calvaria (cranium) and cortex. (From L. L. Langley, I. R. Telford, and J. B. Christensen, Dynamic Anatomy and Physiology, 4th ed., McGraw-Hill, New York, 1974, p. 238.)

posterior areas are supplied by the middle meningeal artery, which branches off the internal carotid and vertebral arteries. The anterior and ethmoid vessels are also branches of the internal carotid and supply the anterior fossa. A branch of the occipital artery, the posterior meningeal, supplies blood to the posterior fossa.

Lying close to the dura but not attached to it is the fine, fibrous, elastic membrane known as the *arachnoid*. This membrane, because it is not attached, allows bleeding between the dura and the arachnoid (the subdural space) to spread feely, limited only by the barriers of the falx cerebri and tentorium. The cerebral veins passing through this space have little support except that provided by the dura and the archnoid and are therefore susceptible to injury and rupture in head (cerebral) trauma.

Between the arachnoid and the pia mater (which lies directly beneath the arachnoid) is the *subarachnoid space*. This space widens and deepens in places and allows for the circulation of cerebrospinal fluid. In the superior sagittal and transverse sinuses, the arachnoid forms villus projections (the Pacchionian bodies) which serve as a pathway for cerebrospinal fluid to empty into the venous system.

The *pia mater* is a very delicate membrane which is richly supplied with minute blood vessels. As the pia dips into all the sulci and conformations of the gyri, it helps form the choroid plexuses of the lateral, third, and fourth ventricles.

The brain damage seen in head trauma can be caused in two different ways: (1) by the immediate effects of the trauma on the functioning brain and (2) by the later effects of the brain cells responding to the trauma.

Immediate neurological damage is caused by an object or piece of bone penetrating and lacerating the brain tissue, the effects of force or energy transmitted to the brain, and, lastly, the effects of acceleration-deceleration on the brain, which is confined in a rigid compartment.

The degree of damage caused by these problems can be dependent upon the force applied—the greater the force, the greater the damage. There are two kinds of forces applied in two ways, causing two different effects. First, there is local injury, which is caused by a sharp object with low velocity and little force. Disruption of neurological functioning occurs in a localized area and is caused by the object or fragments of bone penetrating the dura at the point of impact. Second, there is generalized injury, which is more commonly seen in blunt trauma to the head and after automobile accidents. The damage occurs as the energy or force is transmitted to the brain. Much of the energy or force is absorbed by the protective layers of hair, scalp, and skull, but with violent trauma this is not enough to protect the brain. The remaining energy is transmitted to the brain as this energy passes through the brain tissue causing damage and disruption along the way as delicate tissues are sub-

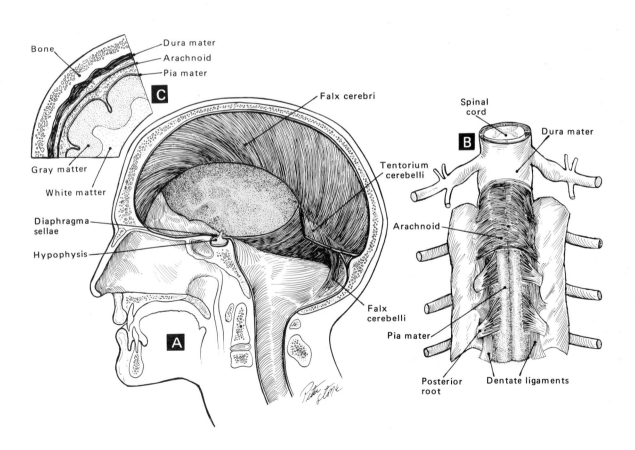

lose its ability to autoregulate the available circulating blood volume, causing ischemia to certain areas within the brain.

jected to the force (Schwartz, 1974, p. 1634). If the head is moving and is suddenly and violently stopped, as in an automobile accident, damage is caused not only by local injury to tissue but also by acceleration and deceleration (Schwartz, 1974, p. 1635). The force of acceleration and deceleration causes the contents within the rigid skull to move, thereby forcing the brain against the inner surface of the skull on the side opposite the impact. This is also called *contrecoup* injury. As has been noted before, there are areas within the cranial vault which are rough, and as the brain moves across these areas (e.g., sphenoid ridge), it tears and lacerates the tissues. The damage is intensified when trauma also causes rotation of the skull. The area of the brain most likely to receive the greatest amount of damage includes the anterior portion of the frontal and temporal lobes, the posterior sections of the occipital lobes, and the upper portion of the midbrain (Schwartz, 1974, p. 1635).

The secondary effects of the trauma, which cause severe neurological alterations, are due to the tissue response to the injury. Whenever tissue is injured, it responds in a predictable way—there is alteration in intracellular and extracellular fluid content, extravasation of blood, increased blood supply to the area, and mobilization of cells to repair and to remove cellular debris.

The neurons, the functional cells within the brain, are dependent from minute to minute on a constant supply of nutrients in the form of glucose and oxygen and are very susceptible to metabolic injury when supplies are cut off. As a result of injury the cerebral circulation may

EPIDURAL HEMATOMA

Epidural hematoma is a serious sequela to head injury and carries a mortality rate of approximately 50 percent (Schwartz, 1974). Epidural hematoma occurs most frequently in the parietotemporal area from a tear in the middle meningeal artery (Fig. 50-3). Although epidural hematomas are found in the frontal and occipital areas, hematomas in these areas are frequently not suspected and produce poorly localizing signs (Beeson and McDermott, 1975). When not associated with additional brain injuries, early treatment of epidural hematoma is generally followed by recovery with little or no neurological deficit.

The typical patient with epidural hematoma gives a history of a head injury followed by a short period of unconsciousness. After this short period of unconsciousness a lucid period follows. It is important to state here that this lucid interval is not pathognomonic of epidural hematoma. First, the lucid interval may go unobserved, especially if it is short in duration. Second, the patient with additional serious brain injury may remain stuporous (Beeson and McDermott, 1975).

An expanding hematoma in the temporal area causes the temporal lobe to be forced downward and inward. This pressure causes the medial portion of the lobe (the uncus and part of the hippocampal gyrus) to herniate under the edge of the tentorium. The effects of this are what cause the neurological signs observed by the medical team (Fig. 50-4).

The pressure of the herniation of the uncus on the arterial circulation to the reticular formation of the

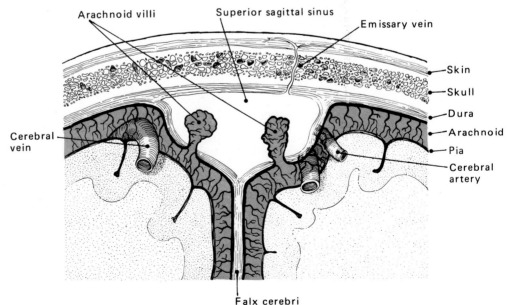

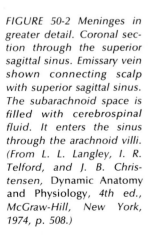

FIGURE 50-2 Meninges in greater detail. Coronal section through the superior sagittal sinus. Emissary vein shown connecting scalp with superior sagittal sinus. The subarachnoid space is filled with cerebrospinal fluid. It enters the sinus through the arachnoid villi. (From L. L. Langley, I. R. Telford, and J. B. Christensen, Dynamic Anatomy and Physiology, 4th ed., McGraw-Hill, New York, 1974, p. 508.)

medulla causes unconsciousness. Also located in this area are the nuclei to the third cranial nerve (oculomotor). Compression of this nerve produces dilation of the pupil and ptosis of the eyelid. Compression of the corticospinal pathways ascending in this area causes weakness in motor responses contralaterally (i.e., side opposite the hematoma); brisk or hyperactive reflexes; and a positive Babinski sign (Sodeman and Sodeman, 1974).

As the developing hematoma enlarges, it pushes the entire brain toward the opposite side, causing severe intracranial pressure. Late signs of increased intracranial pressure develop, including decerebrate rigidity and disturbances in vital signs and respiratory functioning.

Diagnosis of epidural hemorrhage is made by clinical signs and symptoms as well as by carotid arteriogram and echoencephalogram. Treatment is surgical evacuation of the hematoma and control of the bleeding from the lacerated middle meningeal artery. Surgical intervention must be accomplished early and before serious compression of brain tissue causes brain damage. Mortality remains high, about 80 percent, even when diagnosis and treatment are accomplished early because of the associated severe brain trauma and sequelae (Cohen, Freidan, and Samuels, 1977).

SUBDURAL HEMATOMA

While an epidural hematoma is generally arterial in origin, a subdural hematoma is venous (Fig. 50-3). It is caused by rupture of the veins in the subdural space. Subdural hematomas are divided into types which differ in symptomatology and prognosis—acute, subacute, and chronic.

Acute subdural hematoma

Acute subdural hematomas are those that cause serious and significant neurological symptoms within 24 to 48 hours after injury. Frequently associated with serious brain trauma, these hematomas are associated with a high mortality rate (Schwartz, 1974).

Progressive neurological deficit is due to the compression of brain tissue with herniation of the brainstem into the foramen magnum, leading to compression of the

brainstem. This quickly leads to cessation of respiration and loss of control of pulse and blood pressure.

Diagnosis is made by carotid arteriogram and echoencephalogram or CAT (computerized axial tomography). Acute subdural hematoma should always be considered a possibility in patients who have suffered severe neurological trauma showing signs of a deteriorating neurological status. Since more than one-half of these hematomas are bilateral, it is extremely important to consider the type of injury incurred and to use appropriate diagnostic measures (e.g., bilateral arteriograms) to rule out the possibility of bilateral hematomas (Schwartz, 1974; Cohen et al., 1977).

Treatment consists mainly of removing the hematoma, decompression by removal of areas of skull and portions of the frontal or temporal lobes if necessary and relaxation of the compressing dura. Even with prompt diagnosis and surgical intervention, mortality rates are 80 to 90 percent, most related to the severe brain trauma and major organ failure that accompanies severe trauma (Beeson and McDermott, 1975).

Subacute subdural hematoma

Subacute subdural hematoma is that which causes significant neurological deficit more than 48 hours but less than 2 weeks after injury (Schwartz, 1974). Again, like the acute subdural hematoma, it is caused by venous bleeding into the subdural space.

The typical clinical history of a patient with a subacute subdural hematoma is of head trauma causing unconsciousness but subsequent gradual improvement in neurological status. After a period of time the patient demonstrates signs of deteriorating neurological status. The level of consciousness begins to decrease gradually over a period of hours. As the intracranial pressure increases due to the accumulating hematoma, the patient may become difficult to arouse and nonresponsive to verbal and painful stimuli. As with acute subdural hematoma, the shift of intracranial contents and the increasing

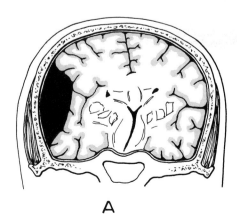

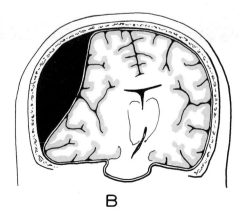

A   B

FIGURE 50-3 A. *Subdural hematoma, usually a result of laceration of the subdural veins. B. Epidural hematoma in the temporal fossa, usually a result of laceration of the middle meningeal artery.*

intracranial pressure due to the accumulation of blood will lead to herniation of the uncus. This, of course, will give rise to third nerve compression and its associated clinical signs—ptosis of the eyelid and dilation of the pupil.

Treatment, like the treatment of acute subdural hematoma, is early and prompt removal of the clot. This can be accomplished with different means dependent upon the clinical condition of the patient. Since many of these clots are bilateral, as in the acute subdural hematoma, measures should ensure that both subdural spaces have been evaluated and, if indicated, surgically explored (Schwartz, 1974).

Chronic subdural hematoma

Chronic subdural hematoma presents a very interesting clinical history. The cerebral trauma responsible for this problem may be trivial or even nonexistent or forgotten.

The onset of symptoms is usually delayed for weeks, months, and possibly years after the initial injury.

The initial trauma ruptures one of the veins traversing the subdural space. Slow bleeding thus occurs into the subdural space. Within 7 to 10 days after bleeding has occurred, the blood is surrounded by a fibrous membrane. Breakdown of blood cells within the hematoma occurs as an osmotic pressure gradient is built up, pulling fluid into the hematoma. It is this increase in the size of the hematoma that may cause further bleeding by tearing the surrounding membrane or vessels, increasing the size and pressure of the hematoma (Schwartz, 1974). If allowed to follow its natural course, the contents within the subdural hematoma undergo characteristic changes (see Table 50-1).

Chronic subdural hematoma has frequently been nicknamed the "imitator" because the signs and symptoms are generally nonspecific, nonlocalizing, and could be caused by many different disease processes. Some patients complain of a headache. The most typical signs and symptoms include progressive alteration in level of consciousness including apathy, lethargy, and decreased attention span, and decreased ability to use higher cognitive skills. Hemianopsia, hemiparesis, and pupillary

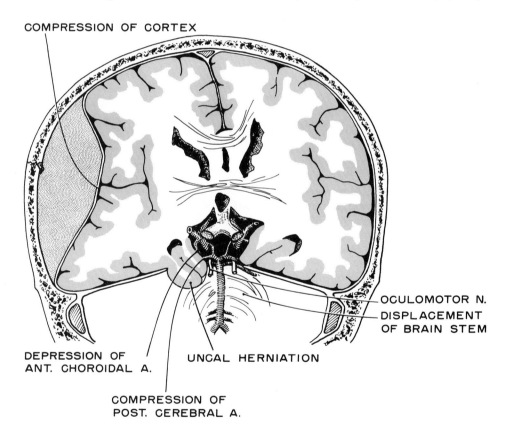

COMPRESSION OF CORTEX

OCULOMOTOR N.
DISPLACEMENT
OF BRAIN STEM

DEPRESSION OF
ANT. CHOROIDAL A.

UNCAL HERNIATION

COMPRESSION OF
POST. CEREBRAL A.

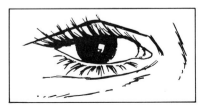

abnormalities are observed in less· than 50 percent of cases. The spinal fluid is rarely helpful in confirming a diagnosis and may be nonspecifically abnormal with increased protein content and xanthochromia, or may contain a few red blood cells, the pressure is generally normal. When aphasia is present, it is usually an *anomic* type (a fluent aphasia with repetition and comprehension) (Schwartz, 1974; Beeson and McDermott, 1975; Cohen et al., 1977).

Diagnosis is best made by arteriography. CAT may demonstrate a hematoma, thereby preventing the necessity of the arteriogram, although a negative CAT does not necessarily rule out the diagnosis of subdural hematoma.

Small hematomas will resolve spontaneously if allowed to follow their natural history. In patients with small hematomas with no neurological signs who can be closely followed, this is probably the best medical course. But for the patient with progressive neurological deficit and debilitating symptoms, the best course of treatment is surgical removal, since the greatest danger in chronic subdural hematoma is that in acting like an enlarging mass, it may cause herniation of the temporal uncus and death (Schwartz, 1974; Cohen et al., 1977).

SPINAL CORD INJURY

Most spinal cord injuries occur during sports activities such as diving and skiing, and during automobile accidents. Many of those affected are young males under the age of 30. The common mechanism of cord injury is flexion-extension and rotation.

The vertebral column is constructed with a circumferential bony ring which provides ideal protection for low-velocity penetrating injuries and contusions, but the intervertebral articulations are weak points for flexion, extension, or rotational stress. According to Schwartz, dislocation and fractures that do not break the vertebral

ring allow the vertebrae above and below the area of injury to act as a fulcrum for another vertebra and its attached soft tissue to concuss, stretch, contuse, or disrupt the spinal cord.

The stresses of flexion, extension, and rotation, along with the relative weakness of the articulations of the vertebrae cause fractures and dislocations to occur most commonly at points where a relatively mobile portion of the vertebral column meets a relatively fixed segment, namely, between the lower cervical area and the upper thoracic segment; between the lower thoracic and upper lumbar segments; and between the lower lumbar segment and the sacrum (Schwartz, 1974).

Most of the damage in spinal cord injury occurs at the time of injury. Secondary cord injury occurs from movement of the unstable vertebral column; the injury that occurs is a movement of the spinal cord against sharp fragments of bone projecting into the canal, and continued compression of the spinal cord.

The primary changes occcurring after spinal cord injury include small hemorrhages in the gray matter that occur as spinal cord blood flow falls and hypoxia ensues, followed by edema. Hypoxia of the gray matter stimulates the release of catecholamines which contribute to the hemorrhage and necrosis and cause further spinal cord dysfunction. This mechanism is still under investigation but has stimulated researchers to suggest cooling of the injured segment, norepinephrine blocking agents, and steroids as possible therapeutic measures to prevent additional damage (Beeson and McDermott, 1975; Schwartz, 1974).

When the spinal cord is completely severed, two functional disasters are immediately evident: (1) all voluntary activity in the body parts innervated by the spinal seg-

FIGURE 50-4 Mechanisms of signs and symptoms of an expanding intracranial hematoma over the parietotemporal region. The expanding hematoma compresses the cortex, pushing the brain to the opposite side and displacing the brainstem, cranial nerves, and vessels. The extreme medial portion of the temporal lobe (uncus) becomes herniated under the edge of the tentorium cerebelli. Compression of the oculomotor nerve by the herniated uncus may lead to ipsilateral pupil dilatation, ptosis, and eventual pupil fixation. Compression of the cerebral cortex and/or distortion of the brainstem will result in depression of consciousness. In the latter structure the reticular activating system is involved. The arterial supply and venous return to the brainstem may be compromised due to pressure. Interference with the cardiorespiratory centers will be evidenced by irregularity or slowing of the pulse, elevation of the blood pressure, and abnormalities of respiratory rate, depth, and rhythm. Pressure on the corticospinal and associated pathways may result in a contralateral Babinski's sign and contralateral weakness or paralysis.

TABLE 50-1
Stages in the natural history of nonlethal subdural hematoma

STAGE	DESCRIPTION
Stage I	Dark blood spreads widely over the brain surface beneath the dura.
Stage II	Blood congeals; becomes darker, thicker, and "jellylike" (2 to 4 days).
Stage III	Clot breaks down and after about 2 weeks has color and consistency of crankcase oil.
Stage IV	Organization begins with formation of encasing membrane; an outer thick, tough one derived from dura and a thin inner one from arachnoid. The contained fluid becomes xanthochromic.
Stage V	Organization is completed. Clot may become calcified or even ossified (or may resorb).

Source: Modified from F. E. Jackson, "The Pathophysiology of Head Injuries," *Ciba Clinical Symposium,* **28,** 1976.

ments is permanently lost, and (2) all sensation, which depends upon the integrity of the ascending spinal pathways, is lost. A third occurrence is immediate spinal areflexia, frequently called *spinal shock.*

Spinal shock

Spinal shock is a temporary condition of decreased excitability of neurons above the level of the transection. The period of spinal shock may extend over a period of many months. Under normal conditions axons descending from the supraspinal portions of the nervous system deliver low-frequency impulses to the neurons. This serves to maintain the neuron in a state of excitability ready to respond to a higher frequency impulse. When this "background tone" (Mountcastle, 1968) is removed by transection, the resting excitability of the spinal cord is greatly reduced, resulting in spinal shock.

Spinal shock is not due to any form of irritation at the site of the transection nor is it due to the drop in blood pressure that follows transection. The phenomenon of spinal shock is confined to the region above the level of the transection.

Spinal shock may occur in partial transection of the cord. Studies reported by Mountcastle have shown that it is the reticulospinal and the vestibulospinal tracts whose severance produces the phenomenon of spinal shock.

Transection of the spinal cord produces widespread alterations in visceral functions. Immediately after transection of the spinal cord there is complete atony of the smooth muscle of the bladder wall. At the same time there is an increase in constrictor tone of the sphincter muscle, probably due to loss of an inhibitory influence. With recovery of somatic reflexes, which may occur in 25 to 30 days after cord section, tone returns to the bladder muscles and reflex emptying of the bladder occurs. This is produced by simultaneous contraction of the smooth muscle walls and, to a certain extent, relaxation of tone of the sphincter. After reflex emptying of the bladder, a considerable residual volume is left. Cutaneous stimulation to abdomen, perineum, or lower extremities greatly facilitates reflex emptying.

In the intestinal tract it appears as if digestion and absorption proceed normally. Great difficulty is encountered in the evacuation of feces from the lower bowel and rectum. Normally the presence of fecal matter in the lower bowel and rectum passively stretching the walls produces active contraction and peristalsis; this combined with inhibitory relaxation of the sphincter causes defecation. This mechanism is depressed during spinal shock. The sphincter ani muscles relax only slightly in response to passive dilation, and, therefore, retention of fecal material occurs. With the recovery of reflex excitability, reflex evacuation of the bowel occurs. It is facilitated by tactile stimulus of the skin areas of the sacral segments and/or by manual dilation of the sphincter ani muscle.

Reflex actions upon the peripheral vessels and organs innervated by the autonomic nervous system are profoundly affected by spinal shock. Transection of the spinal cord causes an immediate and profound fall in arterial pressure. This is the result of elimination of the bulbar vasoconstrictor mechanism; when spinal nerves are separated from the medullary centers, the important coordination between the state of the blood vessels and subsidiary centers in the spinal cord is lacking. In the individual with an intact spinal cord, the spinal centers are regarded as subordinated to the higher vasoconstrictor center in the medulla. The hypotension persists for some time after transection. Spinal neurons innervating peripheral effectors concerned with body temperature control are permanently severed from the descending influences of the thermoregulatory center.

The duration of spinal shock varies greatly from one individual to another. In general the reappearance of any reflex which has been completely abolished by cord injury is a sign of recovery from spinal shock and cord activity (Mountcastle, 1968; Frohlich, 1972; Sodeman and Sodeman, 1974).

Cervical spine injury

Forced flexion injury to the cervical spine compresses the vertebral bodies, dislocates a vertebra forward on the one below, and interlocks the articular facets. Compression of the spinal cord is caused by displaced fragments of bone or a prolapsed intervertebral disc. In a flexion injury a prolapsed intervertebral disc does not occur except in conjunction with a fracture dislocation.

Direct pressure or injury to the anterior spinal artery or injury to the radicular or vertebral artery in the intravertebral foramen occludes circulation through these arteries, leading to ischemic injury.

Hyperextension injuries to the cervical spine buckle the ligamentum flavium forward, pinching the cord. Such injury can damage several centimeters of the cord. The effects of such an injury leave the upper limbs weaker than the lower limbs and variable loss of sensation, with sparing of touch, position, and vibration sense. Hematomyelia (bleeding into the central cord) may complicate the injury.

Cervical spinal cord injuries above the level of C3 are usually fatal. Injuries at C4 may be fatal and are usually associated with respiratory embarassment due to lack of innervation to the diaphragm and the respiratory muscles. As a general rule, cervical spinal cord injury causes quadriplegia; patients with a C5 injury may have partial function of shoulder and elbow; with a C6 injury partial function of the wrist in addition to the shoulder and elbow may return; in a C7 and C8 injury, shoulder, wrist, elbow, and hand function may return with some weakness in the hand.

Thoracic-lumbar spinal cord injury

The usual mechanism for thoracic-lumbar spinal cord injury is hyperextension. A hyperextension injury causes compression of one or more of the vertebral bodies, generally in the region of T12 and L3. A heavy, direct blow is needed to fracture the midthoracic vertebral bodies unless they have been previously softened by osteoporosis or neoplasm.

Damage to the cord at the thoracic-lumbar region generally causes paraplegia. Initially the paralysis is a flaccid paralysis which is usually followed by spastic paralysis (Schwartz, 1974; Beeson and McDermott, 1975.)

Treatment of spinal cord injuries

The first and foremost rule in treatment of spinal cord injury is stabilization of the vertebral column. The presence of foreign bodies adjacent to or in the spinal cord allows for additional damage from body movements. Therefore, patients with spinal cord injuries are moved carefully, keeping the body in alignment.

The primary treatment for cervical injury is reduction and stabilization of the fracture, most effectively obtained by skeletal traction with tongs or wires inserted in the skull to achieve and maintain reduction. Stabilization is achieved by anatomic reduction and by tension of the spinal ligaments and soft tissue of the cervical area. Slight extension of the neck gives tension to the anterior spinal ligament.

Reduction of fracture dislocations of the thoracic and lumbar spines are no longer recommended. At present, treatment consists of bed rest until pain subsides. Single compression fractures of the body of the vertebra, with flexion angulation of the spine without spinal cord deficit, may be treated by positioning on a Foster frame, utilizing extension to stretch the anterior spinal ligament and expand the vertebral body.

A controversial therapy is decompression of the spinal cord. There are two schools of thought on early surgical decompression of the spinal cord. Some neurosurgeons believe that severe injury of the cord can rarely be reversed. The damage that occurs with spinal cord injury occurs early in the injury and surgical intervention at this time seriously jeopardizes the patient's life with little or no chance of improving functioning postoperatively. Improvement in return of function occurs gradually in a period of up to 2 years postinjury. Therefore, taking the chance with surgery is not warranted. Another school of thought believes that the edema and swelling of the spinal cord that occurs postinjury increase the neurological deficit. Therefore, laminectomy with decompression is always of some potential value. All surgeons agree that patients showing progressive deficit of neurological function and those with open fractures benefit from surgical decompression.

QUESTIONS

Central nervous system injury—Chap. 50

Directions: Answer the following questions on a separate sheet of paper.

1 What is normal intracranial pressure in mmHg? What causes increased intracranial pressure and why is it dangerous?

2 Explain the mechanisms which account for the following signs and symptoms of intracranial hematoma: hemiparesis, seizures, mental dysfunction, depression of consciousness, changes in vital signs (increased systolic blood pressure, bradycardia), decerebrate rigidity, dilated ipsilateral pupil.

3 What are the two general mechanisms which account for brain damage in head trauma?

4 What is a contrecoup injury? What areas of the brain are most likely to be injured in a deceleration automobile accident?

5 List the three most common sites of spinal cord injury.

6 What is the first and foremost rule in the treatment of spinal cord injury?

7 Contrast the mechanisms for posttraumatic epidural and subdural hematomas.

Directions: Circle the letter preceding each item that correctly answers each question. Only ONE answer is correct. Exceptions will be noted.

8 Infection from a scalp wound may be transmitted to the brain tissue via the:
a Emissary and diploic veins *b* Middle meningeal artery *c* Cerebral veins of the subdural space *d* Carotid artery

9 Brain injury can cause which of the following changes? (More than one answer may be correct.)
a Increased intracranial pressure *b* Hypoxia *c* Hypercarbia *d* Hyperthermia

10 Billy, a 10-year-old boy, was hit by a baseball over the temporal area while playing sandlot baseball in the afternoon. Because of a short period of "dizziness," Billy sat on the bench for the next inning and resumed playing the game. Following dinner at 6 P.M., Billy vomited, complained of a headache, lay down on the sofa, and appeared to be slightly confused. His mother took him to the emergency room of the local hospital. One might suspect which of the following types of brain hemorrhage?
a Subdural *b* Subarachnoid *c* Subperiosteal *d* Epidural

11 If the condition suspected in question 10 is correct, what other neurologic signs and symptoms would Billy be expected to develop if his case is untreated? (More than one answer may be correct.)
a Ptosis of the contralateral eyelid *b* Dilatation of the ipsilateral pupil *c* Positive Babinski sign *d* Ipsilateral hemiparesis *e* Decrease in blood pressure

12 If the suspected diagnosis in question 10 is correct, therapy should consist of:
a Conservative observation for the next 24 hours prior to craniotomy *b* A spinal tap with the removal of cerebrospinal fluid to relieve the increased intracranial pressure *c* Immediate surgical removal of

the hematoma and interruption of the arterial bleeding   d Administration of a stimulant to improve mental alertness   e Administration of hypertonic urea to relieve cerebral edema with craniotomy planned within the next 3 days

13 Following a motorcycle accident, which of the following changes in the neurologic status of a patient would be most significant in indicating damage involving the central nervous system?
a Localization of headaches   b Change from alertness to increasing lethargy   c Pain and edema located near the eye   d Increase in pulse and respiratory rate

14 Which of the following statements are true concerning chronic subdural hematoma? (More than one answer may be correct.)
a Usually a result of trivial injury   b Develops very slowly   c Can be diagnosed by arteriogram   d Develops very rapidly

15 Which of the following mechanisms best explains the sign of ipsilateral pupil dilatation in the case of intracranial hematoma? (More than one answer may be correct.)
a Hemorrhage from the anterior cerebral artery   b Herniation of the uncus into the tentorial ring compressing the third cranial nerve.   c Hemorrhage from the middle cerebral artery   d Traction of the oculomotor nerve against the posterior cerebral artery

16 A young male with a head injury reveals a rise in temperature together with a slowing of his pulse and respirations. Which of the following would probably be responsible for his symptoms?
a Injury to the cortical motor speech area   b Organization of the clot   c Injury to the vital centers within the medulla   d Lesion in the occipital lobe

17 A subdural hematoma which causes the development of significant signs and symptoms within 24 to 48 hours is classified as:
a Acute   b Subacute   c Chronic

18 An injury causing unilateral transection of the spinal cord causes which of the following changes below the level of the injury?
a Contralateral loss of vibration sense and ipsilateral loss of tactile sensation   b Contralateral loss of vibration sense and tactile discrimination and a contralateral increase in touch threshold   c An ipsilateral loss of the vibration sense and tactile discrimination and a contralateral increase in the touch threshold

d An ipsilateral loss of the vibration sense and tactile discrimination and an ipsilateral increase in the touch threshold

19 Which of the following changes is expected immediately following transection of the spinal cord?
a A general increase in skeletal muscle tone   b A period of spinal shock lasting approximately 2 days   c Retention of urine and feces   d Hypotension

Directions: Match the meningeal structure in col. A with the appropriate statement from col. B.

Column A	Column B
20 ____ Dura mater	a Fine, fibrous middle layer of the meninges
21 ____ Arachnoid	b Inner meningeal layer closely applied to the brain and spinal cord
22 ____ Pia mater	c Encloses the venous sinuses and separates the brain into compartments
	d Circulation of cerebrospinal fluid in a space directly under this layer
	e Middle and posterior portions supplied by the middle meningeal artery

Directions: Circle T if the statement is true and F if it is false. Correct the false statements.

23   T   F   An epidural hematoma is described as a hemorrhage between the dura and the arachnoid.

24   T   F   Paraplegia may be caused by a bilateral lesion at C5.

25   T   F   A bilateral lesion in the middle or lower thoracic cord causes paraplegia.

26   T   F   Cervical spinal cord injuries above the level of C3 are generally fatal.

27   T   F   A quadraplegic with a C6 injury might be expected to have partial function of the shoulder, elbow, and wrist.

28   T   F   The initial treatment of all serious spinal cord injuries consists of laminectomy with decompression.

29   T   F   An ipsilateral lesion of the spinal cord at C5 would cause hemiplegia.

30   T   F   Spinal shock is a temporary condition of decreased excitability of neurons above the level of the cord transection and may last up to 2 years.

CHAPTER 51 Central Nervous System Tumors

OBJECTIVES | **At the completion of Chap. 51 you should be able to:**

1 Explain why the diagnosis of brain tumors may be difficult.

2 Identify the most common brain tumors in adults and children.

3 Identify three types of glial cells and describe their functions.

4 Identify the characteristics of astrocytomas and glioblastomas (common locations, prognosis).

5 Discuss the pathology, growth characteristics, common symptomatology, and treatment of meningiomas.

6 Identify three types of pituitary tumors and the characteristics of each.

7 Describe neurilemmomas (pathology, symptoms, treatment, and sequelae).

8 Identify the two most common locations of the primary site of metastatic brain tumors.

9 Identify three types of cerebral blood vessel tumors and their common locations.

10 Identify several brain tumors of congenital origin and their common locations.

11 Describe the effects of adnexal tumors.

12 Describe the pathophysiology of focal disturbances and increased intracranial pressure in brain tumors.

13 Describe the mechanism causing cerebral edema.

14 Explain how the body compensates for intracranial pressure and describe the effects of untreated intracranial pressure.

15 Identify three of the classic clinical manifestations of brain tumor (pathogenesis, significance).

16 Define *papilledema, amaurosis fugax, hemianopsia, quadrantanopsia, hypotonia.*

17 Describe some localizing symptoms for tumors of the frontal, occipital, temporal, and parietal lobes, the cerebellum, ventricles, and hypothalamus.

18 Describe noninvasive and invasive techniques for the diagnosis of brain tumors.

19 Compare brain and spinal cord tumors with respect to frequency and malignancy.

20 List the common locations of spinal cord tumors and common lesions associated with each.

21 List several disorders of movement seen in cerebellar tumors.

22 Describe the signs and symptoms of spinal cord compression at various levels.

BRAIN TUMORS

Intracranial tumors include space-occupying lesions both benign and malignant that develop in the brain, meninges, and skull. Because brain tumors present with diverse and confusing symptomatology, diagnosis can be difficult. Brain tumors can occur at any age; they are not uncommon in children under 10 but are most commonly found in adults during the fifth and sixth decade.

There are many classifications of brain tumors. Perhaps the one easiest to understand is the Kernahan and Sayre classification based on naming the tumor for the cells present in the adult nervous system, in vascular tissue, and in developmental defects combined with a malignancy grading of I to IV (IV being the most malignant) (see Table 51-1).

Certain tumors occur more frequently in a particular age group. During infancy and childhood, posterior fossa tumors are far more frequent than supratentorial lesions (middle or anterior fossa), which are more common in adults. The brain tumor of a child is likely to be a malignant astrocytoma of the cerebellum of grade I or II. In the middle-aged or elderly individual the most common brain tumor is a glioblastoma multiforme—this is the most malignant glioma, characterized by a rapid growth rate of the tumor.

Gliomas

Gliomas account for approximately 40 to 50 percent of brain tumors. Gliomas are classified based on embryological origin. In the adult the neuroglia cell of the central nervous system provides for the repair, support, and protection of the delicate nerve cells. Gliomas consist of connective tissue and supporting cells. The neuroglia possess the potential to continue to divide throughout life. Glial cells congregate to form dense cicatrical scars in regions of the brain where neurons disappear due to injury or disease (Mountcastle, 1968).

There are three types of glial cells—*microglia, oligodendroglia,* and *astrocytes.* Of these the microglia are of mesodermal embryologic origin and therefore are generally not classified as true glial cells. The microglia enter the nervous system through the vascular system and function as phagocytes—clearing away the debris and combating infection.

The oligodendroglia and the astrocytes are true neuroglia and like neurons arise from the ectoderm. Oligodendroglia are involved in myelin formation. The function of astrocytes is still under investigation; evidence shows that they might play some role in impulse conduction and synaptic transmission of neurons and may serve as conduits between blood vessels and neurons (Sodeman and Sodeman, 1974; Mountcastle, 1968).

Astrocytomas infiltrate the brain and are frequently associated with cysts of various sizes. Although they infiltrate the brain tissue, the effect on brain functioning is minimal early in the illness. Generally, astrocytomas are nonmalignant although they may undergo a malignant change to a glioblastoma—a highly malignant astrocytoma. These tumors are generally slow-growing. Because of this the patient frequently does not seek medical attention for several years, until debilitating symptoms occur—for instance, epileptic seizures or headaches. At the time of surgery complete excision is generally not possible because of the invasive nature of the tumor.

The glioblastoma multiforme is the most malignant of the gliomas. These tumors have a very rapid growth rate, and complete surgical excision is impossible. Life expectancy is usually about 12 months. This tumor may occur anywhere but most commonly involves the cerebral hemisphere and often spreads to the opposite side via the corpus callosum.

The oligodendroglioma is similar to the astrocytoma but is composed of oligodendroglia cells. It is relatively avascular and is prone to calcification.

Ependymoma is a malignant tumor arising from within the walls of the ventricle. In children the most common site is the fourth ventricle. These tumors invade the surrounding tissue and obstruct the ventricles. Death usually occurs in 3 years or less.

TABLE 51-1
Brain tumors

TUMOR	PERCENT
Gliomas	40–50
Astrocytoma grade I	5–10
Astrocytoma grade II	2–5
Astrocytoma grades III and IV	20–30
(glioblastoma multiforme)	
Medulloblastoma	3–5
Oligodendroglioma	1–4
Ependymoma grades I–IV	1–3
Meningioma	12–20
Pituitary tumors	5–15
Neurilemmomas (mainly cranial nerve VIII)	3–10
Metastatic tumors	5–10
Blood vessel tumors	
Arteriovenous malformations	
Hemangioblastomas	
Endotheliomas	0.5–1
Tumors of developmental defects	2–3
Dermoids, epidermoids, teratomas,	
chordomas, paraphyseal cysts,	
craniopharyngiomas	3–8
Pinealomas	0.5–0.8
Miscellaneous	
Sarcomas, papillomas of the choroid plexus,	
lipomas, unclassified, etc.	1–3

Source: S. I. Schwartz (ed.), *Principles of Surgery,* 2d ed., McGraw-Hill, New York, 1974, p. 1646.

Meningeal Tumors

The meningioma is the most important tumor arising from the meninges, the mesothelial lining cells, and the connective tissue cells of the arachnoid and the dura. The majority of these tumors are benign, encapsulated, and do not infiltrate adjacent tissue but rather compress the underlying structures. These tumors are often quite vascular and will therefore take up radioactive isotopes during a brain scan. Complete surgical excision is possible, especially if the tumor is not in a "critical area" and diagnosis is made early. Because of the slow growth of this tumor, symptoms may be overlooked and the diagnosis missed completely. Symptoms include idiopathic epilepsy, hemiparesis, and aphasia.

Pituitary tumors

Pituitary tumors arise from the chromophobe, eosinophil, or basophil cells of the anterior pituitary. These tumors cause headache, bitemporal hemianopsia (due to pressure on the optic chiasm), and signs of abnormal secretion of hormones from the anterior pituitary. Figure 51-1 illustrates the various visual field defects common when lesions involve the optic tract.

Chromophobe tumors are nonfunctioning tumors which compress the pituitary gland, the optic chiasm, and the hypothalamus. Symptoms of this brain tumor include depression of sexual function, secondary hypothyroidism, and adrenal hypofunction (amenorrhea, impotence, loss of hair, weakness, hypotension, low basal metabolism, hypoglycemia, and electrolyte disturbances).

Eosinophilic adenoma is generally a smaller and slower-growing tumor than the chromophobe tumor. The symptoms include acromegaly in adults and gigantism in children, headache, sweating disturbance, paresthesias, muscular pains, and loss of libido. Disturbances in visual fields (bitemporal hemianopsia) are rare.

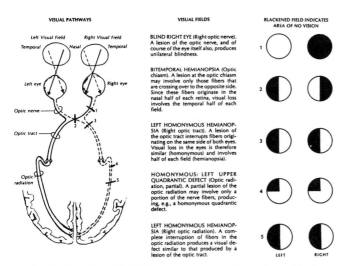

FIGURE 51-1 Visual field defects produced by selected lesions in the visual pathways. (From Programmed Practice in Anatomy and Physiology of the Nervous System, Prentice-Hall, Washington, D.C., 1972, p. 49.)

Basophil adenomas are generally small. These tumors are associated with the symptoms of Cushing's syndrome (obesity, muscle wasting, skin atrophy, osteoporosis, plethora, hypertension, salt and water retention, hypertrichosis, and diabetes mellitus).

Neurilemmoma (auditory nerve tumor)

Auditory nerve tumors comprise 3 to 10 percent of intracranial tumors. They probably arise from the Schwann cells of the nerve sheath. The nerve fibers in the eighth cranial nerve become destroyed. Bilateral auditory neurilemmoma may occur in von Recklinghausen's disease. Generally benign, these tumors occasionally undergo malignant change.

Symptoms of auditory neurilemmoma include first deafness, tinnitus, loss of caloric vestibular reactivity, and vertigo, followed by suboccipital discomfort, staggering gait, involvement of adjacent cranial nerves, and signs of increased intracranial pressure. Nystagmus is usually present, especially horizontal. Treatment consists of complete removal of the tumor, if possible, since incomplete removal is generally accompanied by recurrence of the tumor. As a result of surgery, the patient is left with facial paralysis and deafness.

Metastatic tumors

Metastatic lesions account for approximately 5 to 10 percent of brain tumors and may originate from any primary site. The most common primary tumors are from the lung and breast. But neoplasms from the genitourinary tract, gastrointestinal tract, bone, and thyroid may metastasize to the brain. The metastatic lesion may be single or multiple and may be a late stage in the metastatic process or may be the first sign of a previously unrecognized primary tumor.

Blood vessel tumors

These tumors include the angiomas, the hemangioblastoma, and the endotheliomas and make up a small percentage of brain tumors. The angiomas are congenital arteriovenous malformations, present from birth, which slowly enlarge. They may compress surrounding brain tissue and bleed intracerebrally or into the subarachnoid space. Hemangioblastomas are neoplasms composed of embryological vascular elements most commonly found in the cerebellum. The von Hippel-Lindau syndrome is a combination of cerebellar hemangioblastoma, angiomatosis of the retina, and cysts of the kidney and pancreas.

Tumors of developmental defects (congenital)

Rare congenital tumors include chordoma, which is composed of cells derived from the embryonic notochord remnants and are found at the base of the skull. They grow slowly but are highly invasive, making complete surgical removal impossible. Dermoids and teratomas may occur anywhere in the central nervous system. Teratomas frequently occur in the ventricular system and obstruct the third ventricle, the aqueduct, or the fourth ventricle. Craniopharyngiomas arise from remnants of the embryonic craniopharyngeal duct (Rathke's pouch) and are usually located posterior to the sella turcica. Symptoms for congenital tumors generally manifest themselves early in a child's life but may be silent for many years. The symptoms include defects in visual fields—generally irregular, with hypothalamic and pituitary dysfunctions.

Pinealomas (adnexal tumors)

These tumors account for a very small number of intracranial lesions seen and include tumors that originate within the pineal body (pinealoma) as well as those from the surrounding choroid plexus (choroid papilloma). Pinealomas compress the aqueduct causing obstructive hydrocephalus, as well as the hypothalamus giving rise to precocious puberty and diabetes insipidus. Choroid papilloma causes intraventricular bleeding and also obstructs the ventricular system.

Pathophysiology of brain tumors

Brain tumors give rise to progressive neurological deficit. The symptoms occur on a continuum. This underscores the importance of the history when examining the patient. Symptoms should be discussed within a time perspective. When did the symptom develop? Was it associated with anything? How long have you had this?

The neurological deficit in brain tumors is generally thought to be caused by two factors: the focal disturbances caused by the tumor and the increased intracranial pressure.

Focal disturbances occur when there is compression of brain tissue and infiltration or direct invasion of brain parenchyma with destruction of neural tissue. Dysfunction, of course, is greatest with the fastest-growing infiltrating tumors (e.g., glioblastoma multiforme).

Alteration in blood supply because of compression due to the growing tumor causes necrosis of brain tissue. Interference with arterial blood supply is usually manifested by an acute loss of function and may be confused with primary cerebrovascular disorders.

Seizures as a manifestation of altered neuronal excitability are related to the compression, invasion, and alteration in the blood supply to the brain tissue. Some tumors form cysts which also compress the surrounding brain parenchyma increasing the focal neurological deficit.

The increased intracranial pressure may be due to several factors: an increase in the mass within the skull, edema formation around the tumor, and alteration in cerebrospinal fluid circulation. The tumor's growth causes an increase in mass because it occupies space within the relatively fixed volume of the rigid compartment of the skull. Malignant tumors produce edema in the surrounding brain tissue. The mechanism is not completely understood but is thought to be due to an osmotic gradient causing an absorption of fluid by the tumor. Some tumors may cause hemorrhage. Venous obstruction and edema due to breakdown of the blood-brain barrier all cause an increase in intracranial volume and increase the intracranial pressure.

Obstruction of cerebrospinal fluid circulation from the lateral ventricles to the subarachnoid space causes hydrocephalus.

Increased intracranial pressure becomes life-threatening when rapid development of any of the previously discussed causes occur. Compensatory mechanisms require days or months to be effective and are therefore not useful when intracranial pressure develops rapidly. These compensatory mechanisms include decreased intracranial blood volume, decreased cerebrospinal fluid volume, decreased intracellular fluid contents, and decreased parenchymal cell numbers (Schwartz, 1974). Untreated increased pressure causes herniation of the uncus or the cerebellum. Uncal herniation is caused when the medial gyrus of the temporal lobe is displaced inferiorly through the tentorial notch by a mass in the cerebral hemisphere. This compresses the midbrain, causing loss of consciousness and compression of the third cranial nerve. The cerebellar tonsils are displaced downward through the foramen magnum by a posterior mass in cerebellar herniation. Compression of the medulla and respiratory arrest rapidly ensue. Other physiologic changes that occur with rapidly developing increased intracranial pressure include progressive bradycardia, systemic hypertension (widening pulse pressure), and respiratory failure (Beeson and McDermott, 1975).

Clinical manifestations

The classic triad of symptoms in brain tumor are headache, vomiting, and papilledema. But there is great variety in symptomatology depending upon the site of the lesion and rapidity of growth.

HEADACHE

Headache is perhaps the most common symptom found in patients with brain tumors. The pain may be described as deep, aching, steady, dull, and sometimes agonizingly severe. It is most severe in the morning and is aggravated by activities that normally increase intracranial pressure, such as stooping, coughing, or straining at the stool. The headache is somewhat relieved by aspirin and application of cold packs to the site.

The headache associated with brain tumor is caused by traction and displacement of pain-sensitive structures within the intracranial cavity. These pain sensitive structures include the arteries, veins, venous sinuses, and cranial nerves.

The headache has a localizing value in that one-third of headaches overlie the tumor site whereas two-thirds of headaches are near or above the tumor. Occipital headache is the first symptom in tumors of the posterior fossa. Approximately one-third of supratentorial lesions give rise to a frontal headache. A complaint of a generalized headache has little localizing value and usually indicates extensive displacement of intracranial contents with increased intracranial pressure (Beeson and McDermott, 1975).

NAUSEA AND VOMITING

Nausea and vomiting occur as a result of stimulation of the emetic center in the medulla. Vomiting occurs most frequently in children and in association with increased intracranial pressure with brainstem displacement. The vomiting may occur without preceding nausea and may be projectile.

PAPILLEDEMA

Papilledema is caused by venous stasis which leads to engorgement and swelling of the optic disc. When seen on the fundoscopic exam, it suggests increased intracranial pressure. It is often difficult to use this sign as diagnostic for brain tumor since the fundi in some individuals may not show papilledema even with very elevated intracranial pressure.

In association with the papilledema some disturbances in vision may occur. These include enlargement of the blind spot and *amaurosis fugax* (fleeting moments of dimmed vision).

LOCALIZING SYMPTOMS

Other signs and symptoms of brain tumor occur, but these tend to have a greater localizing value.

Tumors of the *frontal lobe* give symptoms of mental changes, hemiparesis, ataxia, and disturbances of speech. Mental changes are manifested by subtle changes in personality. Some patients experience periods of depression, confusion, or periods of bizarre behavior. The most common changes involve higher level reasoning and judgment skills. Hemiparesis is caused by pressure on the neighboring motor areas and pathways. If the motor area is involved, Jacksonian seizures and obvious motor weakness may occur. Tumors involving the lower end of the precentral cortex cause weakness of the face, tongue, and thumb, whereas tumors of the paracentral lobule produce weakness in the foot and lower extremity. Tumors of the frontal lobe may cause unsteadiness in the gait, often imitating cerebellar ataxia. When the left or dominate frontal lobe is affected, aphasia and apraxia may be evident.

Tumors of the *occipital lobe* may give rise to convulsive seizures preceded by an aura. With involvement of occipital cortex contralateral homonymous hemianopsia occurs (Fig. 51-1). There may be visual agnosia, difficulty in judging distances, and the tendency to get lost in familiar surroundings.

Temporal lobe tumors cause tinnitus and auditory hallucinations probably due to irritation of the temporal auditory receptive or adjacent cortex. Varying degrees of sensory aphasia beginning with difficulty in naming objects appear when the temporal lobe of the dominant hemisphere becomes involved. Mental symptoms similar to those that occur with frontal lobe tumors are not uncommon. Due to the pressure from a growing tumor on the frontal cortex, facial weakness may occur. Lesions of the anterior temporal pole cause a superior quadrantanopsia which may progress to a complete hemianopsia.

Tumors in the *parietal lobe* of the parietal sensory cortex cause loss of cortical sensory function, impairment of sensory localization, two-point discrimination, graphesthesia, position sense, and stereognosis. Visual defects from parietal or parieto-occipital tumors ordinarily involve inferior homonymous quadrants.

Cerebellar tumors cause early papilledema and frequently produce nuchal headache. Cerebellar lesions cause disorders of movement. These disorders will vary depending on the size and specific location of the tumor within the cerebellum. The most common of these are listed in Table 51-2. Less conspicuous but equally characteristic of cerebellar tumor is hypotonia, which is an absence of normal resistance to stretch, displacement of a limb from a given posture, and hyperextensibility of joints. In speech there is a tendency to decompose

TABLE 51-2
Disorders of movement seen in cerebellar tumors

DISORDER OF MOVEMENT	DESCRIPTION
Intention tremor	An oscillating tremor most marked at the end of fine movements.
Asynergia	Lack of cooperation between muscles, e.g., failure of the wrist extensors during flexion of the fingers, allowing the wrist to flex.
Decomposition of movement	The performance of actions in successive parts rather than as a whole, e.g., touching the nose by first flexing the forearm, then the arm, and lastly adjusting the wrist and forearm.
Dysmetria	Errors in the range of movement, e.g., in touching a point, stopping the action before reaching the point or moving past it.
Deviation from line of movement	E.g., carrying food to the ear instead of mouth.
Adiadochokinesis	Inability to perform alternating movements, e.g., tapping quickly and smoothly.
Nystagmus	While fixing the gaze on region and object, the eyes oscillate quickly.

words into separate syllables pronounced in a staccato rhythm—this is also called scanning speech.

Tumors of the *ventricles* and *hypothalamus* produce varied deficits. Invasive lesions of the third ventricle and the hypothalamus produce somnolence, diabetes insipidus, obesity, and disturbances of temperature regulation. A small tumor in the third ventricle, on the other hand, causes steady headache and papilledema with few localizing signs. Tumors involving the fourth ventricle give rise to rapid development of increased intracranial pressure with papilledema and cerebellar symptoms.

Diagnosis

Any patient suspected of having an intracranial lesion should undergo a complete medical evaluation with special attention to the neurological examination. Specific diagnostic studies are done after the neurological exam and proceed from the noninvasive procedures that cause the least risk to those that use more dangerous, invasive techniques.

Skull x-rays give valuable information concerning bone structure, thickening, and calcifications; the position of the calcified pineal gland; and the position of the sella turcica. The electroencephalogram gives information concerning the altered excitability of the neurons. A shift of intracerebral contents can be seen on the echoencephalogram. A radioactive brain scan will show areas of abnormal accumulation of radioactive substances. Brain tumors as well as vascular occlusion, infection, and trauma cause breakdown of the blood-brain barrier causing an abnormal accumulation of the radioactive substance.

Pneumoencephalogram and cerebral angiography are two invasive procedures which aid in the final diagnosis and aids the physician in deciding what treatment measures are to be carried out.

SPINAL CORD TUMORS

Spinal tumors are those which develop in the spine or its contents and generally produce symptoms by involvement of the spinal cord or nerve roots. Primary cord tumors are about one-sixth as common as brain tumors and have a better prognosis since about 60 percent are benign. The spinal cord suffers not only from actual tumor growth but also from compression caused by an encroaching tumor.

Spinal tumors occur in all age groups but are rarely encountered before the age of 10.

Spinal tumors are classified according to the location of the tumor in relation to the dura and the spinal cord. The major classification divides tumors into extradural

and intradural. Intradural tumors are then subdivided into extramedullary and intramedullary (see Table 51-3).

Extradural tumors generally arise from the bone of the spinal column or within the extradural space. Ninety percent of extradural tumors are malignant. The most common tumor affecting the spinal vertebral column is a metastatic carcinoma. Extradural neoplasms within the extradural space are commonly metastatic carcinomas and lymphomas.

Intradural extramedullary tumors lie between the dura mater and the spinal cord (Fig. 51-2). The most common tumors in this area are benign neurofibroma or meningioma. These tumors compress the spinal cord and can be surgically removed.

Intradural intramedullary tumors arise from within the spinal cord itself. The same tumors that affect the brain also affect the spinal cord. Ependymomas are the most common, followed by astrocytomas, gliblastomas, and oligodendrogliomas.

The spinal cord accommodates to compression that occurs slowly, as seen in meningiomas and neurofibromas, producing few signs and symptoms, especially in the early stages. An acute compression of the cord, as occurs with metastatic lesions, causes rapid, progressive neurological deficit. Resulting symptomatology depends largely upon the area affected as well as the location of the lesion within the spinal column.

Because of the anatomic organization within the cord, compression from lesions outside the cord generally produces symptoms well below the site of the lesion, the level of sensory impairment gradually ascending as the compression increases, affecting areas deeper within the cord. Lesions located deep within the cord may spare superficially arranged fibers and may give rise to sensory dissociation with loss of pain and temperature with preservation of touch. Also by disturbing position sense, cord compression may result in ataxia.

Spinal cord compression at different levels

TUMORS OF THE FORAMEN MAGNUM

Tumors of the foramen magnum are most commonly meningiomas. Symptoms of spinal cord compression at this level are due to compression of spinal cord, nerve roots, and intracranial contents. Suboccipital pain is, perhaps, the earliest symptom. This pain is aggravated by nodding the head. Nerve root compression causes sensory and motor weakness in the occipital head region (C2 dermatome) and the neck (C3 dermatome). Extension of tumors into the intracranial cavity causes increased intracranial pressure, cerebellar dysfunction,

TABLE 51-3
Spinal cord lesions

1 Extradural
2 Intradural
  a Extramedullary
  b Intramedullary

nystagmus, and compression of cranial nerve nuclei, causing trigeminal sensory loss and atrophy of the tongue.

TUMORS OF THE CERVICAL REGION

Cervical lesions produce radicularlike motor and sensory signs that involve shoulders and arms and may involve the hands. Involvement of the hands from a upper cervical lesion (i.e., above C4) is thought to be due to compression of the descending blood supply to the anterior horns via the anterior spinal artery. There is generally weakness and atrophy involving the shoulder girdle and arms. Lower cervical tumors (C5, C6, C7) may cause the loss of upper extremity tendon reflexes (biceps, brachioradialis, and triceps). Sensory loss extends along the radial border of the forearm and thumb in a C6 compression, involves the middle and index finger in lesions at C7, and C7 lesions cause sensory loss of the ring and middle fingers (see Table 51-4).

TUMORS OF THE THORACIC REGION

Lesions of the thoracic area often present with insidiously developing spastic weakness in the lower extremities with later development of paresthesia. Patients may complain of pain and a tight, binding feeling across the chest and abdomen and may be confused with pain from intrathoracic and intraabdominal disorders. In lower thoracic lesions there may be loss of lower abdominal reflexes and Beevor's sign (the umbilicus elevates when the patient, in the supine position, raises the head against resistance).

TUMORS OF THE LUMBAR-SACRAL REGION

A complex diagnostic situation exists in the case of a tumor involving the lumbar and sacral region because of the close proximity of the lower lumbar and sacral segments and the descending nerve roots from higher levels of the cord. Upper lumbar cord compression spares the abdominal reflexes, abolishes the cremasteric reflexes, and may produce weakness of hip flexion and spasticity of the lower legs. Also occurring are the loss of the knee jerk reflex with brisk ankle reflexes and bilateral Babinski signs. Pain is usually referred to the groin. Lesions involving the lower lumbar and upper sacral segments cause weakness and atrophy of perineal, calf, and foot muscles and loss of angle jerk reflex. Loss of sensation in the perianal and genital area with impairment of bowel and bladder control are characteristic signs of lesions involving the lower sacral area.

TUMORS OF THE CAUDA EQUINA

Lesions of the cauda equina cause early sphincteric symptoms and impotence. Other characteristic signs include dull, aching pain in the sacrum or perineum, sometimes radiating to the legs. Flaccid paralysis corresponds to the nerve roots involved and is sometimes asymmetrical.

Symptoms are not only produced by the anatomical location of the spinal cord but by its position within the spinal canal. The following is a discussion of the pathology of extradural and intradural tumors.

Extradural tumors

Extradural tumors are primarily metastases from a primary lesion in the breast, prostate, thyroid, lungs, kidney, and stomach. Pain is generally the first symptom, and it is described as being dull, constant, and localized over the area of the tumor, followed by pain radiating along the dermatome pattern. The localized pain is most severe at night and is aggravated by movements of the spine and bed rest. The radicular pain is intensified by coughing and straining. Pain may be present for weeks or months prior to spinal cord involvement.

The common clinical course of extradural tumors is rapid compression of the spinal cord due to encroachment of the tumor on the cord, collapse of the vertebral column, or hemorrhage from within the metastasis. Once symptoms of spinal cord compression develop, they rapidly cause total loss of spinal cord function. Spas-

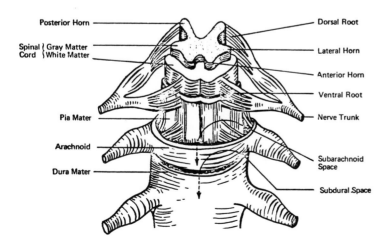

FIGURE 51-2 Structure of the spinal cord. (From Programmed Practice in Anatomy and Physiology of the Nervous System, *Prentice-Hall, Washington, D.C., 1972.*)

tic weakness and loss of vibration and joint position sense below the level of the lesion are the first signs of cord compression. Without prompt surgical decompression paresthesia and sensory loss progress quickly to irreversible paraplegia.

Diagnosis of extradural spinal cord tumors can be made by x-rays of the spine. Most patients with tumors will demonstrate osteoporosis or obvious bone destruction of the vertebral body and pedicles. Myelogram definitely localizes the tumor. Cerebrospinal fluid will show elevated protein and normal glucose levels.

Surgical decompression with laminectomy is the treatment of choice when symptoms of cord compression are present. Used as adjunctive measures are hormones, radiation, and chemotherapy.

Intradural tumors

The intradural tumors, in contrast to the extradural, are generally benign. The clinical course is much slower and may extend over a period of months to years. Intradural tumors are divided into two types—extramedullary and intramedullary.

EXTRAMEDULLARY

Approximately 65 percent of all intradural tumors are extramedullary and are basically two types, neurofibromas or meningiomas.

Neurofibromas arise from the dorsal nerve roots. They sometimes form a dumbbell or an hourglasslike growth extending into the extradural space. A small percentage of neurofibromas undergo sarcomatous changes and become invasive or metastasize.

Meningiomas are usually loosely attached to the dura, arising probably from the arachnoid membrane, and approximately 90 percent are found in the thoracic region. These tumors are more frequent in middle-aged females. The posterior-lateral aspect of the cord is the most common site on the cord for these tumors.

Extramedullary cord lesions cause compression of the spinal cord and the nerve roots at the affected segment. The Brown-Séquard syndrome may result from lateral compression of the cord. This syndrome, caused by damage to one-half of the cord, is characterized by ipsilateral signs of dysfunction of the corticospinal tract and the posterior column below the level of the lesion and contralateral reduction in pain and temperature perception below the level of the lesion. The patient complains of pain first in the back and then along the spinal roots. As with the extradural tumors, pain is aggravated by movement, coughing, sneezing, or straining and is most severe at night. The nocturnal aggravation of pain is caused by traction on the diseased nerve roots when the spine elongates with removal of the shortening effect of gravity. The sensory loss is at first vague and occurs below the level of the lesion (because of dermatome overlap). It gradually rises to below the segmented spinal cord level. Tumors of the posterior aspect may be manifested by paresthesia and later proprioceptive sensory loss adding ataxia to the weakness. Anteriorly situated tumors may cause little sensory loss with severe motor disability.

With extramedullary tumors cerebrospinal fluid protein is almost always elevated. Spine x-rays may show enlargement of a foramen and thinning of the adjacent pedicle. As with extradural tumors myelogram is essential for precise localization. Early surgical removal is essential for a complete recovery.

TABLE 51-4
Symptoms and signs of common root lesions

ROOT	LOCATION OF PAIN	SENSORY LOSS	REFLEX LOSS	WEAKNESS AND ATROPHY
C5	Lower neck, tip of shoulder, arm	Deltoid area (inconsistent)	Biceps	Shoulder abductors, biceps
C6	Lower neck, medial scapula, arm, radial side of forearm	Radial side of hand, thumb index finger	Biceps	Biceps
C7	Lower neck, medial scapula, precordium, arm, forearm	Index finger, middle finger	Triceps	Triceps
C8	Lower neck; medial arm and forearm, ulnar side of hand; fourth and fifth fingers	Ulnar side of hand, fourth and fifth fingers		Intrinsic hand muscles
L4	Low back, anterior and medial thigh	Anterior thigh	Quadriceps	Quadriceps
L5	Low back, lateral thigh, lateral leg, dorsum of foot, great toe	Great toe, medial side of dorsum of foot, lateral leg and thigh		Toe extensors, ankle dorsiflexors and evertors
S1	Low back, posterior thigh, posterior leg, lateral side of foot, heel	Lateral foot, heel, posterior leg	Achilles	Ankle dorsiflexion and plantar flexion

Source: John Simpson, and Kenneth Magee, *Clinical Evaluation of the Nervous System*, Little, Brown, Boston, 1970, p. 114.

The histological structure of intramedullary tumors is essentially that of intracranial tumors. Over 95 percent of these tumors are gliomas. In contrast to intracranial tumors they tend to be more benign histologically and have a more benign course. Approximately 50 percent of intramedullary tumors are ependymomas, 45 percent are astrocytomas, the rest are oligodendrogliomas and hemangioblastomas.

Ependymomas arise at all levels of the spinal cord but are found most commonly in the conus medullaris of the cauda equina. All other tumors occur equally frequently in all areas of the spinal cord.

These tumors grow into the central part of the spinal cord and destroy crossing fibers and neurons of the gray matter. The destruction of crossing fibers results in bilateral sensory loss of pain and temperature extending throughout the segments involved in the lesion. This causes damage to peripheral skin areas due to loss of perception of pain and temperature. The senses of touch, motion, position, and vibration are usually preserved unless the lesion is large. This loss of pain and temperature sensation with preservation of the other senses is known as *dissociated sensory loss*. Alteration in the function of muscle stretch reflexes results from damage to the anterior horn cells. Weakness, with atrophy and fasciculations, is due to involvement of the lower motor neurons.

Intramedullary tumors may extend through several segments of the spinal cord. As the lesion progresses, involvement of the corticospinal and spinothalamic tracts cause loss of pain and temperature sense, and upper motor neuron signs extend below the level of the lesion. See Table 51-5, which lists some differentiating features between upper and lower motor neuron lesions.

Other signs and symptoms include dull, aching pain localized to the level of the lesion, impotence in males, and sphincter disturbances in both sexes.

X-rays will show visible widening of the spinal canal and erosion of the pedicles. On myelogram the spinal cord appears enlarged.

Surgical removal is sometimes possible with intramedullary tumors especially ependymomas and hemangioblastomas, but recurrences are not uncommon. Again early diagnosis is imperative to ensure good prognosis.

QUESTIONS

Central nervous system tumors—Chap. 51

Directions: Answer the following questions on a separate sheet of paper.

1 Why is the diagnosis of a brain tumor so difficult to make? What are the most common general signs and symptoms?

Directions: Match the type of glioma in col. A with its characteristic in col. B.

Column A	Column B
2 ___ Glioblastoma multiforme	a Often contains calcium
	b Most malignant
3 ___ Medulloblastoma	c Commonly arises in the fourth ventricle in children
4 ___ Oligodendroglioma	d Radiosensitive posterior fossa tumor of childhood
5 ___ Ependymoma	

Directions: Match the brain tumors in col. A to the statements in col. B.

Column A	Column B
6 ___ Chromophobe adenoma	a Arises from remnants of Rathke's pouch; pre-

TABLE 51-5
Differentiation between upper and lower motor neuron weakness

	UPPER MOTOR NEURON*	LOWER MOTOR NEURON†
Type and distribution of weakness	Lesions in brain—"pyramidal distribution," i.e., distal, especially hand muscles; weaker extensors in arm and weaker flexors in legs. Lesions in cord—variable, depending on location	Depends on which lower motor neurons are involved, i.e., which segments, roots, or nerves
Tone	Spasticity—greater in flexors in arms and extensors in legs	Flaccidity
Bulk	Slight atrophy of disuse only	Atrophy—may be marked
Reflexes	Accentuated; Babinski sign present	Decreased or absent; no Babinski sign
Fasciculations	No	Yes
Clonus	Frequently present	Absent

*Synonyms: pyramidal tract (referring to fibers in the medullary pyramids), corticospinal tract, corticobulbar tract.
†Synonyms: anterior horn cell, ventral horn cell, somatic motor portions of cranial nerves, final common pathway.
Source: John Simpson, and Kenneth Magee, *Clinical Evaluation of the Nervous System*, Little, Brown, Boston, 1970, p. 60.

7 ____ Basophilic adenoma

8 ____ Eosinophilic adenoma

9 ____ Craniopharyngioma

10 ____ Neurilemmoma

11 ____ Hemangioblastoma

12 ____ Pinealoma

dominantly a tumor of childhood.

b Associated with acromegaly; does not cause chiasmal compression.

c Symptoms include tinnitus, deafness, vertigo, and caloric vestibular reactivity.

d Associated with Cushing's syndrome.

e Symptoms include those of hypopituitarism, hypothyroidism, hypoadrenalism, and often visual field defects.

f Often compresses the aqueduct, causing obstructive hydrocephalus, and the hypothalamus, causing precocious puberty and diabetes insipidus.

g Often bleeds intracerebrally or into the subarachnoid space; most common in cerebellum.

Directions: Match the following localizing symptoms of brain tumors in col. A with their probable location in col. B.

Column A

13 ____ Homonymous hemianopsia

14 ____ Impairment of sensory localization, two-point discrimination

15 ____ Superior quadrantanopsia progressing to hemianopsia

16 ____ Disturbances of judgment; Jacksonian seizures; ataxia and tremor

17 ____ Obesity and disturbance of temperature regulation

Column B

a Frontal lobe

b Temporal lobe

c Occipital lobe

d Parietal lobe

e Hypothalamus

Directions: Match the following disorders of movement seen in cerebellar tumors in col. A with its proper description in col. B.

Column A

18 ____ Nystagmus

19 ____ Dysmetria

20 ____ Asynergia

21 ____ Intention tremor

22 ____ Deviation from line of movement

23 ____ Adiadochokinesis

Column B

a Error in range of movement: carrying food to ear instead of mouth

b Inability to perform tapping movement smoothly and quickly

c Quick oscillation of eyes while fixing gaze on an object

d Lack of cooperation between muscles, e.g., failure

of wrist extensors during flexion of the fingers allowing the wrist to flex

e Oscillation tremor most marked at the end of fine movements

f Inability to arrest the movement at a given point and difficulty in performing successive movements

Directions: Circle the letter preceding each item that correctly answers each question. Only ONE answer is correct. Exceptions will be noted.

24 Each of the following statements concerning brain tumors is true *except:*
a A glioblastoma is the most malignant form of brain tumor. b Brain tumors in children occur most often in the posterior fossa. c Astrocytomas are generally nonmalignant. d Glioblastomas are generally cured by surgical excision. e Meningiomas are benign tumors of perineural tissue.

25 The two most common sources of metastasis to the brain are from the:
a Lung and colon b Colon and rectum c Lung and breast d Uterus in women and prostate in men

26 Chordomas:
a Are highly invasive, making complete surgical excision impossible b Arise at the base of the skull c Grow slowly d All of these

27 Compensatory mechanisms for increased intracranial pressure include all of the following *except:*
a A decrease in the systemic blood pressure b A decrease in intracerebral blood volume c A decrease in the volume of CSF d A decrease in the number of parenchymal cells

28 Noninvasive techniques helpful in the diagnosis of brain tumors include which of the following? (More than one answer may be correct.)
a History and neurological exam b Pneumoencephalogram c Electroencephalogram d Arteriogram e Echoencephalogram

29 The most common cause of extradural extramedullary cord compression:
a Metastatic disease b Gliomas c Astrocytomas d Ependymomas

30 The most common types of intradural extramedullary spinal tumors:
a Gliomas and angiomas b Meningiomas and neurofibromas c Sarcomas and lymphomas d Gliomas and discs

31 A spinal cord tumor which caused weakness and atrophy of the intrinsic hand muscles, sensory loss in the ulnar side of the hand, Horner's syndrome, together with a "claw hand" would most likely be:
a Intramedullary at C6 b Extramedullary at C6 c Extramedullary at C7 d Intramedullary at C8

32 One of the most important tests in the diagnosis of spinal cord compression is:
a Ultrasound b Marked electromyelographic abnormality c Spinal x-ray d Myelography

33 All of the following are characteristics of lower motor neuron lesions *except:*
a Fasciculations b Depressed reflexes below level of lesion c Spastic paralysis below level of lesion d Marked atrophy of muscle innervated below level of lesion

Directions: Answer T if the statement is true and F if it is false. Correct the false statements.

34 T F An osmotic gradient causing absorption of fluid into a malignant brain tumor is the most likely mechanism causing cerebral edema.

35 T F Hypotonia is an absence of normal resistance to stretch and is seen in cerebellar tumors.

36 T F Astrocytes function as cerebral phagocytes.

37 T F Oligodendroglia are involved in myelin formation.

38 T F Ependymomas are the most common type of intradural intramedullary spinal cord tumors.

39 T F Meningiomas of the spinal cord tend to be located in the cauda equina.

40 T F Papilledema is enlargement of the blind spot in the eye.

Directions: Match the site of spinal cord pathology in col. A with the signs and symptoms in col. B. (Letters may be used more than once.)

Column A
41 ____ Pain increased by coughing or sneezing
42 ____ Loss of vibratory and position sense
43 ____ Babinski reflex
44 ____ Fasciculations
45 ____ Spasticity
46 ____ Ataxia

Column B
a Posterior (dorsal) root
b Posterior column (major ascending tract)
c Corticospinal tract (major descending tract)
d Anterior horn cells

REFERENCES

ALPERS, B. J. and E. I. MANCALL: *Essentials of the Neurological Examination*, Davis, Philadelphia, 1971.

ALPERS, B. J., et al.: "Anatomical Studies of the Circle of Willis in Normal Brain," *Archives of Neurology and Psychiatry*, **81**: 409, 1959.

AMERICAN HEART ASSOCIATION, *Stroke*, **8:** 1, 1977.

AMERICAN SOCIETY OF HOSPITAL PHARMACISTS, *American Hospital Formulary Service*, **28**: 12, 1977.

BATES, B.: *A Guide to Physical Examination*, Philadelphia, Lippincott, 1974.

BEESON, P. B. and W. McDERMOTT (eds.): *Cecil and Loeb Textbook of Medicine*, 14th ed., Saunders, Philadelphia, 1975.

BERK, JAMES, JAMES SAMPLENER, J. SHELDON ARTZ, and BARRY VINOCUR, *Handbook of Critical Care*, Little, Brown, Boston, 1976.

BROBECK, J.: *Best and Taylor's Physiologic Basis of Medical Practice*, 9th ed., Williams & Wilkins, Baltimore, 1973, section 9.

BURCH, G. E. and N. P. DePASQUALE: "Axioms on Cerebrovascular Disease," *Hospital Medicine*, **11**(6): 8–21.

CARINI, E. and G. OWENS: *Neurological and Neurosurgical Nursing*, 6th ed., Mosby, St. Louis, 1974, p. 19.

COHEN, ALAN, RALPH FREIDAN, and MARTIN SAMUELS: *Medical Emergencies*, Little, Brown, Boston, 1977.

COHEN, S. R., B. M. HERNDON, and G. M. McKHANN: "Radioimmunoassay of Myelin Basic Protein in Spinal Fluid. . . . an Index of Active Myelinization," *New England Journal of Medicine*, **295**: 1455, 1976.

CURTIS, B., S. JACOBSON, and E. MARCUS: *An Introduction to the Neurosciences*, Saunders, Philadelphia, 1972.

DeLONG, W. B.: "Microsurgical Revascularization for Cerebrovascular Insufficiency," *Currents Concepts of Cerebrovascular Disease—Stroke*, **11**(4): 15–20, 1976.

DiPALMA, JOSEPH (ed.): *Basic Pharmacology in Medicine*, McGraw-Hill, New York, 1976, pp. 115–124.

DRACHMAN, D. B., I. KAO, and A. PESBRONK, et al.: Myasthenia Gravis as a Receptor Disorder," *Annals of the New York Academy of Sciences*, **274**: 226–234, 1976.

DUVOISIN, ROGER: "Parkinsonism," *Ciba Clinical Symposia*, **28**: 1, 1976.

EDITORIAL: *Archives of Neurology*, **33**: 395, 1976.

ELLIOTT, FRANK F.: *Clinical Neurology*, 2d ed., Saunders, Philadelphia, 1971, p. 383.

FIELDS, WILLIAM: "Aortocranial Occlusive Vascular Disease," *Ciba Clinical Symposia*, vol. 26, no. 4, 1974.

FISHER, M. "Occlusion of the Internal Carotid Artery," *Archives of Neurologic Psychiatry*, **65**: 346–377, 1951.

FROHLICH, EDWARD: *Pathophysiology*, Lippincott, Philadelphia, 1972.

GARDNER, ERNEST: *Fundamentals of Neurology*, 6th ed., Saunders, Philadelphia, 1975.

GLASER, G.: "Are the Benefits of Steroid Therapy in Myasthenia Gravis Worth the Risk?" *Modern Medicine*, May 15, 1976, pp. 61–72.

GOODMAN, L. S. and A. GILMAN: *The Pharmacological Basis of Therapeutics*, 5th ed., Macmillan, New York, 1975, pp. 201–226.

GOSS, C. M. (ed.): *Gray's Anatomy of the Human Body*, 29th ed., Lea & Febiger, 1973.

GUYTON, ARTHUR: *Textbook of Medical Physiology*, 5th ed., Saunders, Philadelphia, 1972.

HARVEY, A., R. JOHNS, A. OWENS, and R. ROSS: *The Principles and Practice of Medicine,* 19th ed., Appleton-Century-Crofts, New York, 1976.

JACKSON, F. E.: "The Pathophysiology of Head Injuries," *Ciba Clinical Symposia,* vol. 18, no. 3, 1966.

JOHNSON, R. and P. E. MILBOURN, "Main CNS Complications in Chickenpox," *Modern Medicine,* **38**: 148, 1970.

KLAWANS, H. L., et al.: "Treatment and Prognosis of Hemiballism," *New England Journal of Medicine,* **295**: 1348, 1976.

KULLER, LEWIS H.: "The Transient Ischemic Attack," *Current Concepts of Cerebrovascular Disease—Stroke,* **9**(6): 23–26, 1974.

LANGLEY, L. L., J. R. TELFORD, and J. B. CHRISTENSEN: *Dynamic Anatomy and Physiology,* 4th ed., McGraw-Hill, New York, 1974.

MANCALL, E.: "The Stroke: A Review of Current Diagnostic and Therapeutic Considerations," *Hospital Medicine,* **11**(4): 8–25, 1975.

McHENRY, L. C.: "Cerebral Blood Flow Measurement and Regulation in Man, Part II," *Current Concepts of Cerebrovascular Disease—Stroke,* **11**(2): 5–8, 1976.

McLAURIN, ROBERT: "Answers to Questions on Head Injuries," *Hospital Medicine,* **5**(1): 54–69, 1969.

Medical Notes on Parkinsonism and Pseudoparkinsonism: PI 99-14, rev. April 1972, Burroughs Wellcome Co., Research Triangle Park, North Carolina.

MOUNTCASTLE, VERNON B.: *Medical Physiology,* Mosby, St. Louis, 1968.

NIEDERMEYER, E.: *Epilepsies,* Charles C Thomas, Springfield, Ill., 1974.

Nurses' Drug Alert, **1**(7): 46, 1977.

NORMAN, R., W. BLACKWOOD, and J. CORSELLEYN: *Greenfield's Neuropathology,* 2d ed., Arnold, London, 1963.

PEERY, T. M. and F. N. MILLER, JR.: *Pathology,* 2d ed., Little, Brown, Boston, 1971, pp. 689–690.

PRIOR, JOHN and JACK SILBERSTEIN: Physical Diagnosis, Mosby, St. Louis, 1973.

Programmed Practice in the Anatomy and Physiology of the Nervous System, Prentice-Hall, Washington, D.C., 1972.

ROBBINS, S. L.: *Pathologic Basis of Disease,* Saunders, Philadelphia, 1974.

RUBIO, R. and R. BERNE: "Intrinsic Factors in the Control of the Cerebral Circulation," *Current Concepts of Cerebrovascular Disease—Stroke,* **11**(5): 21–25, 1976.

SCHWARTZ, S. I. (ed.): *Principles of Surgery,* 2d ed., McGraw-Hill, New York, 1974.

SILBERBERG, DONALD H.: "Recent Concepts of Etiology: Implications for Treatment," *Modern Treatment,* **7**(5): 879–889, 1970.

SIMPSON, J. and K. MAGEE: *Clinical Evaluation of the Nervous System,* Little, Brown, Boston, 1973.

SODEMAN, WILLIAM, JR. and WILLIAM SODEMAN: *Pathologic Physiology,* 5th ed., Saunders, Philadelphia, 1974.

SUNDT, T. METAL: "Bypass Surgery for Vascular Disease of the Carotid System," *Mayo Clinic Proceedings,* vol. 51, November, 1976.

THOMAS, J. and G. MALNER: "The Unconscious Patient," *Hospital Medicine,* **4**(11): 6, 1968.

THORN, GEORGE, et al. (eds.): *Harrison's Principles of Internal Medicine,* 8th ed., McGraw-Hill, New York, 1977, p. 1832.

VANDER, A., J. SHERMAN and D. LUCIANO, *Human Physiology—The Mechanisms of Body Function,* 2d ed., McGraw-Hill, New York, 1975.

WANG, R. and R. LAMID: "Restoring Strength in Myasthenia Gravis," *Drug Therapy,* January, 1976.

PART IX Endocrinology and Metabolism. Principles of Pathophysiology, Clinical Presentation and Management of Selected Clinical Disorders

DAVID E. SCHTEINGART

This part deals with basic concepts in endocrinology and metabolism. These concepts should help you acquire an understanding of clinical problems associated with endocrine diseases. The part examines general physiological concepts including structure and mechanism of action of hormones, principles of neurohypothalamic control of pituitary function, circadian rhythms, feedback control of endocrine function, and mechanisms which control blood glucose.

The following clinical entities have been selected for discussion: Cushing's syndrome, Addison's disease, primary and secondary aldosteronism, hirsutism, hyperparathyroidism, hypoparathyroidism, panhypopituitarism, acromegaly, diabetes mellitus, hyperthyroidism, and hypothyroidism.

OBJECTIVES

At the end of Part IX you should be able to:

1 Describe the basic functions of the endocrine system and the structure of hormones, their mechanisms of action, and the regulation of their secretion.

2 Identify the etiology, pathogenesis, and clinical expression of selected endocrine diseases.

3 Explain the rationale for the treatment of these diseases.

4 Describe the regulation of blood glucose.

5 Give a definition of diabetes mellitus and describe its prevalence, possible etiology, clinical presentation, biochemical diagnosis, treatment, and complications.

CHAPTER 52 Concepts Applied to Endocrinology and Metabolism

OBJECTIVES

At the completion of Chap. 52 you should be able to:

1 Explain the mechanism by which the central nervous system and the endocrine system are integrated.

2 Describe the five vital functions of the endocrine system.

3 Explain the three mechanisms by which hormones work on their target tissues.

4 Differentiate between the two types of hormones as to their chemical structure and sites of production. Give two examples of each type.

5 Describe the characteristics of hormone receptors including location and degree of specificity.

6 Draw a flow diagram showing how the tropic hormone angiotensin II is synthesized in the blood and stimulates a peripheral gland.

7 Identify at least two examples of diseases caused by hormonal deficit.

8 Identify examples of diseases caused by hormonal excess.

9 State the general principles of treatment of diseases caused by hormonal deficit or excess.

10 Describe the function of the hypothalamic-hypophyseal portal system.

11 Give an example of the way a feedback control mechanism regulates hormone secretion.

12 Explain a circadian rhythm by describing changes in ACTH levels (high or low) and the time of day each level occurs.

13 Describe the cyclic pattern of gonadotropin secretion.

14 Explain the way the central nervous system controls pituitary function through the hypothalamus.

15 Describe the process by which corticotropin-releasing factor (CRF) influences adrenocorticotropic hormone (ACTH).

16 Explain the feedback control of follicle-stimulating hormone (FSH) and thyroid-stimulating hormone (TSH).

17 Describe the feedback mechanism involved when plasma cortisol levels rise above normal or drop below normal.

As living organisms develop complex structure and function, integration of their various components becomes essential to their survival. This integration is effected by two systems: (1) the central nervous system and (2) the endocrine system. These two systems are related from the embryological, anatomical, and functional stand-points. For example, many of the endocrine glands originate from the neuroectoderm, an embryonic layer which also gives origin to the central nervous system. In addition, there are anatomical connections between the developed central nervous system and the endocrine system, primarily through the hypothalamus. As a consequence, stimuli which disturb the central nervous system frequently also alter the function of the endocrine system. The integrated operation of the nervous and endocrine systems helps to maximize the response of the organism to stressful stimuli.

FUNCTIONS OF THE ENDOCRINE SYSTEM

The endocrine system helps maintain and regulate vital functions such as: (1) Response to stress and injury, (2) growth and development, (3) reproduction, (4) ionic homeostasis, and (5) energy metabolism.

When injury or stress occurs, the endocrine system triggers a series of responses aimed at maintaining blood pressure and preserving life. The hypothalamic-pituitary-adrenal axis is chiefly involved in this response.

Without the endocrine system there is failure to grow and reach maturity; infertility also occurs. The hypothalamic-pituitary-gonadal axis is chiefly involved in this function.

The endocrine system is important in maintenance of ionic homeostasis. Mammalian organisms live in an external environment which changes constantly. However, tissues and cells live in an internal environment which must remain constant. The endocrine system participates in the regulation of this internal environment through maintenance of sodium, potassium, water, and acid-base balance. Aldosterone and antidiuretic hormone are responsible for this function. The calcium concentration is also controlled by endocrine function. Calcium is required for regulation of many biochemical reactions in living cells and for normal neural activation of muscle cell function. The parathyroid glands regulate calcium homeostasis.

Finally, the endocrine system acts as a regulator of energy metabolism. The basal metabolic rate is increased by thyroid hormone, and energy is made available to cells through the integrated action of gastrointestinal and pancreatic hormones.

HORMONES

The endocrine system is made up of glands which synthesize and secrete substances called *hormones*. Hormones cause the physiological and biochemical changes which mediate the types of regulation described above. Once they are released into the bloodstream, hormones are transported to target tissues where they exert their effects. These effects frequently involve the regulation of ongoing enzymatic reactions. Hormones are generally secreted in very low concentrations. For instance, hormones are present in blood at a concentration of 10^{-6} to 10^{-12} molar. In contrast, another blood component, sodium, is usually present at a concentration of 10^{-1} molar. Despite these low concentrations, hormones exert marked metabolic and biochemical effects on their target tissue. From the structural standpoint, hormones are either proteins or steroids. Some hormones are glycoproteins, a combination of a sugar moiety and a protein. Figure 52-1 illustrates the molecular structure of insulin, a protein hormone. Examples of protein hormones are thyroxine, parathormone, the tropic hormones of the pituitary gland [with the exception of thyroid-stimulating hormone (TSH) and gonadotropins], pitressin, insulin, glucagon, and the hormones of the adrenal medulla (epinephrine and norepinephrine). Examples of glycoprotein hormones are TSH and gonadotropins. Examples of steroid hormones are the adrenal cortical hormones and the hormones produced by the gonads (both male and female).

The main characteristic of steroid hormones is the presence of a multicyclic structure, the cycloperhydrophenanthrene nucleus (see Fig. 52-2). Biochemically, steroids are lipids.

Not all hormones present in the blood are produced by a specific endocrine gland. There are compounds which are hormonelike in their mechanism of action but are produced in the blood itself. An example is angiotensin II, a protein hormone which stimulates the adrenal cortex to secrete aldosterone. Angiotensin II is synthesized in the blood from renin substrate (a hepatic protein) under the catalytic effect of renin, an enzyme secreted by renal cells.

Much is known about the way hormones work on their target tissues or cells. Protein hormones act by first interacting with the cell membrane. The cell membrane contains the adenyl cyclase system. The hormone

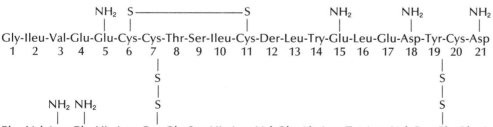

FIGURE 52-1 Molecular structure of insulin, a protein hormone. The hormone has two chains, A and B. The A chain has 21 amino acids, and the B chain has 30 amino acids. The two chains are linked to each other by disulfide linkages.

binds to specific receptors in the cell membrane and subsequently activates this system. Once activated, adenyl cyclase, an enzyme, converts adenosine triphosphate (ATP) into 3',5'-cyclic AMP, which acts as the secondary messenger. Cyclic AMP, the secondary messenger, then moves to other structures inside the cell and produces changes in the rate of protein synthesis in that cell. This sequence of events is illustrated in Fig. 52-3. In addition to cyclic AMP, another substance, prostaglandin, can act as mediator of hormone action by influencing either protein synthesis or the synthesis of other precursors inside the cell.

Steroid hormones work directly inside the cell by binding to intracellular receptor proteins and ultimately affecting the transcription of DNA. By changing messenger RNA, steroids can modify the way in which protein is synthesized (see Fig. 52-4).

In summary, there are specific receptors for each hormone in tissues which are the target of hormone action. Estrogen receptors are found in the uterus, androgen receptors in the skin, and insulin receptors in adipose, muscle, and liver cells. The physiological action of a hormone is intimately linked to its interaction with its specific receptor.

DISEASES OF THE ENDOCRINE SYSTEM

The best way to understand diseases of the endocrine system is to keep in mind that most of their symptoms can be explained by the metabolic action of the hormone(s) involved. Most endocrine diseases are related to either excessive or deficient hormone production. Thus, knowledge of the metabolic consequence of ex-

cessive or deficient hormone secretion will help identify the clinical picture emerging from these disturbances. For example, if there is excessive production of thyroxine, the thyroid hormone, one can predict an increase in the basal metabolic rate and in heat production. In effect, patients with hyperthyroidism demonstrate a high metabolic rate, increased heat sensitivity, and weight loss. Conversely, lack of thyroxine results in opposite metabolic effects such as low basal metabolic rate and increased sensitivity to cold temperature.

Treatment of endocrine diseases

The treatment of endocrine diseases is based on the change in hormone production underlying the specific disease. In simple terms, patients who have a disease caused by a deficit of hormone secretion are treated by replacement of these hormones. Consider as an example a diabetic who is not making enough insulin. Treatment for the metabolic consequence of insulin insufficiency is the administration of insulin. Similarly, a patient who is not making enough thyroid hormone and becomes hypothyroid is treated with replacement amounts of thyroxine.

The treatment of diseases of hormone excess is more complex since several therapeutic alternatives are usually available. Removal of the whole gland or part of the gland which produces the hormone in excess is one such alternative. The removal of the entire gland, however, results in total deficit of hormone, necessitating hormonal replacement to restore levels to normal. In contrast, removal of part of a gland can eliminate the hormone excess, leaving only enough hormone production to maintain normal function.

The pituitary gland provides an example of the consequence of total glandular removal. Since it is a gland with multiple functions—the anterior lobe secretes tropic hormones, and the posterior lobe antidiuretic hormone, among others—its removal leads to cessation of secretion of many hormones, or panhypopituitarism. Modern surgical techniques allow for removal of only the part of the gland that is abnormal. These techniques are used when a small tumor of the pituitary gland causes excessive hormone production. The tumor can be resected under microscopic view without removing the rest of the pituitary gland. In other cases, removal of only a part of a gland is not possible. For example, if the adrenal glands are removed, both the adrenal cortex and the adrenal medulla must be removed. Although the body can function well without the adrenal medulla, the capacity of the body to secrete catecholamines might be impaired.

Another alternative for dealing with hormone excess is the administration of drugs which interfere with hormone production by either blocking or destroying the tissue that makes the hormone. For example, a patient who has an overactive thyroid can be given radioactive iodine in large concentrations. The radioactive iodine concentrates in the thyroid gland and destroys the cells that make thyroxine, causing remission of the disease. Another example is adrenal hyperfunction in

FIGURE 52-2 A steroid nucleus. It has four rings, A, B, C, and D. The numbers designate the carbons within the molecule. Groups attached to different carbons are recognized by the respective number. For example, 17-hydroxy steroids have a hydroxyl group attached to the carbon in the 17 position.

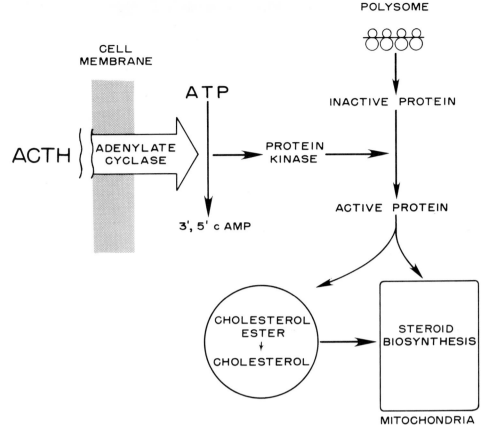

FIGURE 52-3 Mechanism of action of ACTH, a protein hormone. ACTH activates adenylate cyclase, increasing the synthesis of 3',5'-cyclic AMP. In turn, cyclic AMP stimulates a protein kinase which activates rapid turnover protein. This protein causes (1) increased release of cholesterol for use in steroid biosynthesis and (2) stimulation of conversion of cholesterol to pregnenolone in the cell mitochondria.

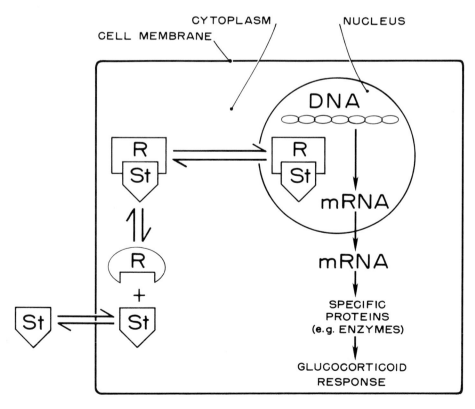

FIGURE 52-4 Mechanism of action of steroid hormones. These hormones bind to intracellular receptor proteins which subsequently carry the steroid molecule to the cell nucleus. In the nucleus the steroid modifies the formation of messenger RNA and protein synthesis.

which the glands can be blocked by drugs which interfere with the biosynthesis of adrenal cortical hormones.

Suppression of hormone production is also illustrated by oral contraceptives. Estrogens and progestogens are given to inhibit pituitary release of gonadotropins; this, in turn, suppresses normal ovarian function and ovulation.

Another method of controlling excessive hormone effects is by hormone antagonism. An excess production of female hormone can be counteracted by administering male hormone, or vice versa. Thus, the metabolic effects of a hormone are opposed by the metabolic effects of an opposite hormone, causing cancellation of the effects of the first one. A hormone can also antagonize the effect of another hormone by blocking binding of the latter to its receptors in its target cells.

In summary, endocrine diseases are those of either hormone deficit or hormone excess; the deficit state is treated by replacing the deficient hormone, while the excessive state can be treated either by surgically removing the whole gland or part of the gland that is working excessively or by giving drugs that block or destroy the tissues making the hormone.

The central nervous system is connected to the pituitary through the hypothalamus; this is the most clearly established link between the central nervous system and the endocrine system. The two systems are interrelated by both neural and vascular connections.

As demonstrated in Fig. 52-5, the pituitary is divided into an anterior, a posterior, and an intermediate lobe. Blood vessels link the hypothalamus with the cells of the anterior pituitary gland. These blood vessels end in capillaries at both ends and, for this reason, are known as a *portal system*. In this particular case, the system connects the hypothalamus with the pituitary gland (hypophysis) and is called the *hypothalamic-hypophyseal* portal system. The portal system is an important vascular channel since it allows for the movement of releasing hormones from the hypothalamus to the pituitary gland, enabling the hypothalamus to modulate pituitary function. Stimuli originating in the brain activate neurons in the hypothalamic nuclei which synthesize and secrete low molecular weight proteins. These proteins or neurohormones are known as *releasing hormones*. They are discharged into the blood vessels of the portal system through which they reach cells in the pituitary gland. The pituitary gland responds to these releasing hormones by discharging pituitary tropic hormones. In this chain of events, the hormones which are released by the

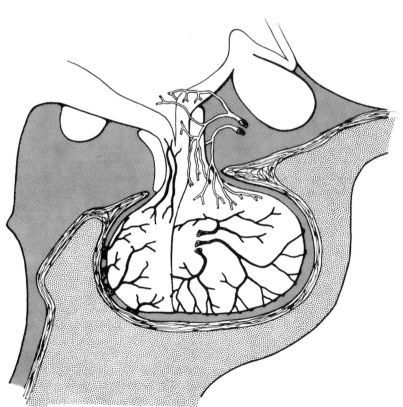

FIGURE 52-5 Schematic representation of the pituitary gland. Hypothalamic-hypophyseal portal vessels connect the hypothalamus with the anterior pituitary lobe and act as a transport channel for releasing hormones formed in the hypothalamus.

pituitary gland travel with the blood and stimulate other glands, causing the release of target gland hormones. The target gland hormones will, in turn, act upon the neuromechanism or the pituitary cells and inhibit hormone secretion (see Fig. 52-6). This type of regulation of hormone secretion is known as a *negative feedback control system.*

Another physiological characteristic of the hypothalamic-pituitary axis is the presence of rhythms. Rhythms are a common feature of the production of many hormones, and they originate in brain structures. Adrenocorticotropic hormone (ACTH) provides an excel-

lent example of rhythmic or cyclic hormone release. When ACTH and cortisol levels are measured on an hourly basis for 24 hours, the levels are seen to rise early in the day, decline later, and rise again during the night to reach a peak by the next morning (see Fig. 52-7). This type of rhythm is referred to as a *diurnal* or *circadian rhythm.* Since hormonal release by the

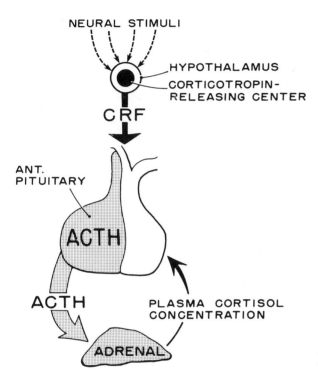

FIGURE 52-6 Feedback regulation of adrenocortical function and ACTH release.

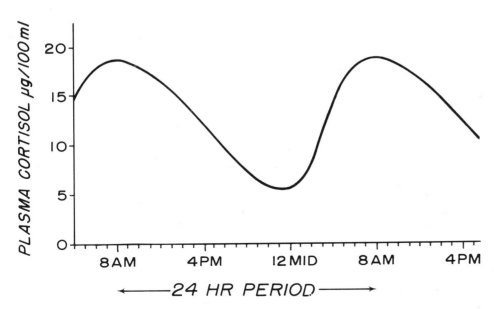

FIGURE 52-7 Circadian rhythm of cortisol secretion.

pituitary gland occurs in short spurts, it is also said that there is *episodic hormonal release*.

Gonadotropins, the tropic hormones of the pituitary gland which control gonadal function, are an example of a different kind of cycle or rhythm. In the female, the release of gonadotropins is cyclic and occurs on a monthly basis rather than on a diurnal basis (see Fig. 52-8). The presence of the normal cyclic release of gonadotropins is specific and characteristic of female reproductive endocrine function. In the male, on the other hand, the release of the same gonadotropins does

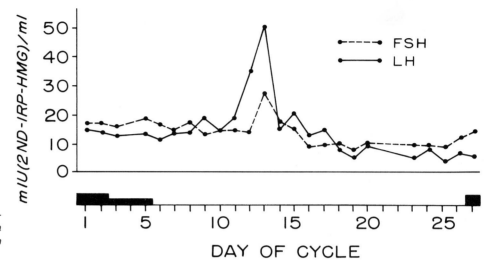

FIGURE 52-8 Monthly cyclic release of gonadotropins. There is a midcycle surge of FSH and LH in normally menstruating women.

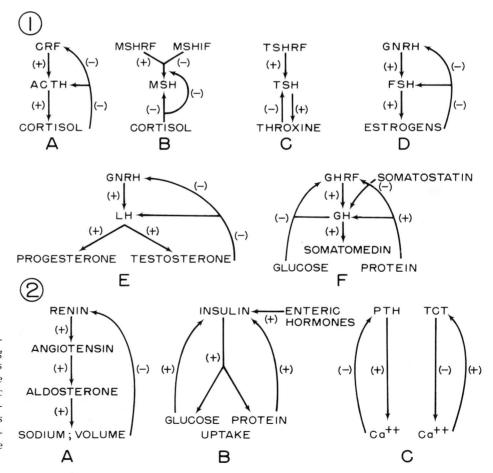

FIGURE 52-9 Diagrammatic representation of feedback regulating systems. Group 1 depicts systems where the target gland hormone feeds back on the hypothalamic pituitary release of the tropic hormone. Group 2 depicts systems where physiological or biochemical factors modulate the release of the regulating hormone.

not have this cyclic character, and it occurs at a constant rate. If the cyclic release of gonadotropins in the female is abolished, there is cessation of normal menstrual cycles, disappearance of ovulation, and infertility.

There are other hormones which are not released with a spontaneous rhythm, but are released in response to a stimulus. For example, insulin and growth hormone are released in response to food intake.

Figure 52-9 shows a number of systems which illustrate the concept of feedback control. In the case of the hypothalamic-pituitary-adrenal system, corticotropin-releasing factor (CRF) causes the pituitary to release ACTH. ACTH then stimulates the adrenal cortex to secrete cortisol. Cortisol, in turn, feeds back on the hypothalamic-pituitary axis and inhibits the production of CRF-ACTH. The system fluctuates, varying with the physiological requirements for cortisol. If the system produces too much ACTH and, therefore, too much cortisol, cortisol feeds back and inhibits the production of ACTH. This is a sensitive system, since an excessive production of cortisol or the administration of cortisol or other synthetic glucocorticoids can quickly inhibit the hypothalamic-pituitary axis and shut off the production of ACTH. The concept of feedback control has practical implications in patients on chronic corticosteroid therapy. These patients have suppressed ACTH release. If steroids are suddenly withdrawn, patients may develop adrenal insufficiency.

Another example of feedback control is the action of gonadotropin-releasing hormone (GNRH), which stimulates the pituitary to secrete follicle-stimulating hormone (FSH) and luteinizing hormone (LH). In the female, estrogens are initially produced by the ovary in small amounts; then estrogens feed back on the hypothalamus, stimulating the secretion of GNRH. This, in turn, triggers FSH and LH release, ovulation, and secretion of estrogen and progesterone. Another example shown in Fig. 52-9 is release of TSH-releasing hormone (TRH) which is secreted by the hypothalamus and causes the pituitary to secrete TSH. TSH, in turn, stimulates the thyroid to secrete thyroxine. Thyroxine then feeds back on the pituitary and inhibits the production of TSH.

There are other systems which regulate hormone production independently of the hypothalamic-pituitary axis. One example is the renin-angiotensin-aldosterone system. As illustrated in Fig. 52-10, the kidney has juxta-glomerular (JG) cells which are located in the wall of the afferent arteriole of the glomerulus. These cells secrete the enzyme renin. The production of renin is influenced by the perfusion pressure in the renal arteriole. Changes in the pressure of blood flowing through the afferent arteriole into the glomerulus are sensed by stretch receptors near the JG cells. This causes changes in the secretion of renin, which in turn activates angiotensin II. Angiotensin II stimulates the production of aldosterone by the adrenal cortex. Aldosterone promotes renal tubular reabsorption of sodium. As sodium is reabsorbed, volume is expanded, the pressure rises in the afferent arteriole, and renin production is shut off. Thus, renin, angiotensin, and aldosterone release are determined by volume and pressure changes affecting the JG cells. This is in contrast to the hypothalamic-pituitary–target gland regulation described above.

Another system which operates differently from those described involves insulin and glucose. Insulin responds to changes in the level of glucose in blood. When glucose levels increase, insulin is secreted. When glucose levels decrease, insulin is shut off. Although some of the pituitary hormones may indirectly influence insulin release, there is no clear evidence that the pituitary gland directly and specifically controls insulin secretion.

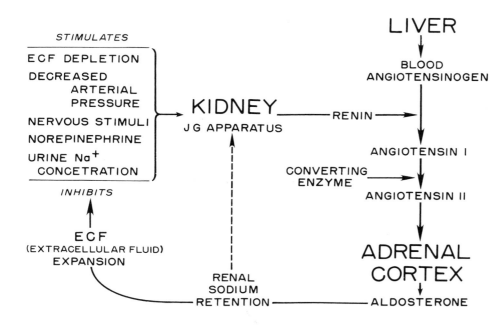

FIGURE 52-10 Regulation of aldosterone secretion by the renin-angiotensin system. ECF depletion, decreased arterial pressure, nervous stimuli, norepinephrine, and increased urinary sodium stimulate renin release, while ECF expansion inhibits renin release.

Parathormone and calcium make up another unique control system. A drop in calcium level stimulates parathormone secretion. Conversely, an increase in calcium shuts off parathormone production.

QUESTIONS

Concepts applied to endocrinology and metabolism—Chap. 52

Directions: Answer the following questions on a separate sheet of paper.

1 List in any order the five vital functions of the endocrine system.

2 List three mechanisms by which hormones can work on their target cells.

3 In Table 52-1 list the two types of hormones which are differentiated by their chemical structure. State two examples of each type and identify the location of production for each example.

TABLE 52-1
Type of hormones, location of production, and examples of each type

TYPE OF HORMONE	LOCATION OF PRODUCTION	EXAMPLES
a _____	1 _____	1 _____
	2	2
b _____	1 _____	1 _____
	2	2

4 Write a brief description and draw a flow diagram showing the way angiotension II is synthesized in the blood and stimulates a peripheral gland.

5 Identify the role played by the hypothalamus in the hypothalamic-pituitary system.

6 What is the function of the hypothalamic-hypophyseal portal system?

7 Give an example of the way the feedback control mechanism operates to regulate endocrine hormone secretion.

8 Define *circadian rhythm* by identifying the hormonal levels (high or low) of ACTH and the time of day each level occurs.

9 State the rationale for providing hormone replacement or suppresion as treatment for endocrine diseases caused by hormonal deficit or excess.

Directions: Complete the following statements by filling the blanks with the appropriate words.

10 An overproduction of thyroxine may cause a condition known as _____.

11 The system that connects the hypothalamus with the pituitary gland is called the _____.

12 Thyroid releasing hormone (TRH) secreted by the hypothalamus causes release of _____.

Directions: Circle T if the statement is true, F if the statement is false. Correct any false statements.

13   T   F   Receptors for hormone action are located in the membrane of the cell.

14   T   F   Receptors for hormone action are usually not specific for a particular hormone.

CHAPTER 53   Cushing's Syndrome and Aldosteronism

OBJECTIVES   At the completion of Chap. 53 you should be able to:

1   Describe the effects of glucocorticoid excess on the distribution of adipose tissue and on carbohydrate and protein metabolism.

2   Describe the effect of high or low plasma cortisol levels on the feedback control mechanism.

3   Differentiate between a glucocorticoid and a mineralocorticoid.

4   Explain the rationale for altering the basic chemical structure of cortisol in the manufacturing of synthetic steroid analogues.

5   Identify one consequence of glucocorticoid therapy involving large amounts for a long period of time.

6   Describe Cushing's syndrome: include at least three causes, the clinical signs and symptoms, diagnostic tests, and treatment.

7   Differentiate between primary and secondary aldosteronism as to etiology and pathophysiology.

This chapter will focus on two selected clinical entities—Cushing's syndrome and aldosteronism. The first section will concentrate on situations in which the plasma concentration of cortisol increases above normal physiologic levels and results in Cushing's syndrome. The discussion will include some aspects of the pharmacology of synthetic corticosteroids and the metabolic side effects which result from their chronic administration. Causes of spontaneously abnormal elevations of plasma cortisol will be considered. The second section will focus on another hormone of the adrenal cortex, aldosterone, and the condition known as *aldosteronism*.

The adrenal cortex synthesizes and secretes four types of adrenocortical hormones: (1) glucocorticoids, (2) mineralocorticoids, (3) androgens, and (4) estrogens. The physiological glucocorticoid secreted by the human adrenal is cortisol; the physiological mineralocorticoid is aldosterone. There are other compounds, either naturally occurring or synthetic, which may have glucocorticoid or mineralocorticoid activity.

Cushing's syndrome is a clinical condition resulting from the combined metabolic effects of persistently elevated blood levels of glucocorticoids. In order to better understand the clinical manifestations of Cushing's syndrome, it is useful to begin with a review of the metabolic consequence of glucocorticoid excess.

METABOLIC EFFECTS OF GLUCOCORTICOIDS

Effects of glucocorticoid excess alters (1) protein and carbohydrate metabolism, (2) distribution of adipose tissue, (3) electrolytes, (4) the immune system, (5) gastric secretion, (6) brain function, and (7) erythropoiesis. A most important pharmacological effect of glucocorticoids is their ability to suppress inflammation.

Glucocorticoids have catabolic and antianabolic effects on protein, causing a decrease in the ability of protein-forming cells to synthesize protein. As a consequence, there is loss of protein from tissues such as skin, muscles, blood vessels, and bone. Clinically, the skin atrophies and breaks down easily; wounds heal slowly. Rupture of elastic fibers in the skin causes purple stretch marks, or striae (see Fig. 53-1). Muscles also atrophy and become weak. Thinning of blood vessel walls and weakening of perivascular supporting tissue result in easy bruising (see Fig. 53-2). This condition can be severe enough for petechiae or even large areas of ecchymosis to appear under the cuff when the patient's blood pressure is taken. Bone is also affected. The protein matrix of bone becomes weak, causing a condition known as *osteoporosis*. This may be a serious complication of glucocorticoid excess since it causes the bone to become brittle and develop pathological fractures.

Osteoporosis occurs most frequently in the spine, causing vertebral collapse with back pain and loss of height.

Carbohydrate metabolism is also affected by abnormally high levels of glucocorticoids. Glucocorticoids stimulate gluconeogenesis and interfere with the action of insulin in peripheral cells. As a consequence, patients may develop hyperglycemia. People without diabetes are able to compensate for the effect of glucocorticoids by increasing insulin secretion and subsequently normalizing glucose tolerance. In contrast, patients with diminishing insulin-secreting capacity—prediabetics or subclinical diabetics—are unable to compensate and develop abnormal glucose tolerance tests, fasting hyperglycemia, and clinical manifestations of overt diabetes.

Excessive glucocorticoid levels also affect the distribution of adipose tissue which accumulates in the central areas of the body with development of truncal obesity, round face ("moon facies"), supraclavicular fossa fullness, and cervicodorsal hump ("buffalo hump") (see Fig. 53-3). The truncal obesity together with thinning of

the upper and lower extremities as a result of muscle atrophy gives patients the classic cushingoid appearance. This appearance is illustrated in Fig. 53-4.

Glucocorticoids have minimal effects on serum electrolytes. However, when given or produced in very large concentrations, they may cause sodium retention and potassium waste, leading to edema, hypokalemia, and metabolic alkalosis.

Glucocorticoids can inhibit the immune response. Immune responses are of two major types; one results in production of humoral antibodies by plasma cells following antigenic stimulation; the other depends on sensitized "cell-bound antibody" resulting in delayed hypersensitivity reactions. Glucocorticoids impair humoral antibody production and inhibit proliferation of germinal centers of spleen and lymphoid tissue in the primary response to antigen. Impairment of the immunological response can occur at each of the stages of this response: (1) Initial processing of antigens by cells of the reticuloendothelial system; (2) induction and proliferation of immunocompetent lymphocytes; (3) antibody production, and, (4) the inflammatory reaction. Glucocorticoids also suppress delayed hypersensitivity reactions. For example, they may convert the skin test for tuberculosis from positive to negative. In addition, the glucocorticoid-mediated inhibition of cellular immunity

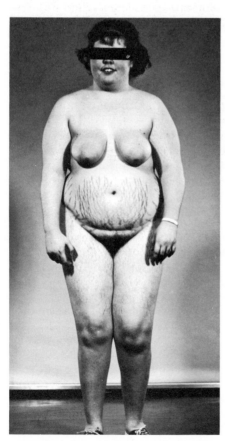

FIGURE 53-1 Abdominal striae in a patient with Cushing's syndrome produced by chronic administration of large amounts of glucocorticoids.

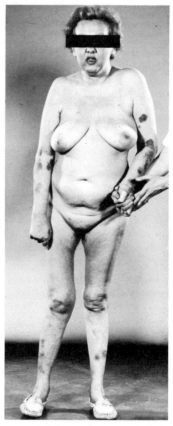

FIGURE 53-2 Marked protein catabolism in a patient with Cushing's syndrome. Muscles are markedly atrophic, and there are multiple ecchymoses in the upper and lower extremities.

is probably important in suppressing transplant rejection.

Gastric secretory activity is increased by glucocorticoids. Hydrochloric acid and pepsin secretion may be increased in certain individuals taking glucocorticoids. It has also been suggested that mucosal protective factors are altered by steroids and that this may contribute to ulcer formation.

Psychic changes are frequently seen with glucocorticoid excess. In general, it is likely that glucocorticoids have a stimulating effect on the excitability of the brain cells.

Glucocorticoids cause involution of lymphoid tissue, stimulation of neutrophil release, and enhancement of erythropoiesis.

The most important and clinically useful pharmacological effect of glucocorticoids is their ability to suppress the inflammatory response. In this regard, glucocorticoids can inhibit hyperemia, extravasation of cells, cellular migration, and cellular permeability. They also inhibit the release of vasoactive kinins from plasma proteins and suppress phagocytosis. By their effects on mast cells, glucocorticoids inhibit histamine synthesis and suppress the acute anaphylactic reaction based on antibody-mediated hypersensitivity. The anti-inflammatory properties of glucocorticoids have placed them in the foreground of therapeutic agents available for the treatment of a variety of disorders in which suppression of inflammation is desirable. There are clinical conditions in which the immune suppression and anti-inflammatory effect of glucocorticoids may be a disadvantage to the patient. With acute infection, hosts may be unable to defend themselves appropriately while receiving pharmacological doses of glucocorticoids.

Suppression of the hypothalamic-pituitary-adrenal axis

It is well known that the administration of glucocorticoids in doses which surpass the physiologic concentrations can significantly suppress the ability of the hypothalamic-pituitary axis to release ACTH. This is important since the administration of corticoids on a long-term basis may result in adrenal insufficiency (1) when steroids are withdrawn and (2) in response to stress.

CUSHING'S SYNDROME

Cushing's syndrome may result from long-term administration of pharmacologic doses of glucocorticoids (iatrogenic) or from excessive cortisol secretion caused by a disturbance in the hypothalamic-pituitary-adrenal axis (spontaneous).

Iatrogenic Cushing's syndrome is seen in patients with conditions such as rheumatoid arthritis, asthma,

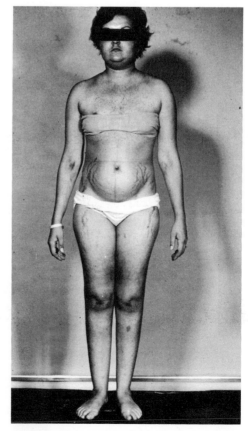

FIGURE 53-4 Patient with Cushing's syndrome with acne over the chest, striae over the abdomen and upper thighs, and relatively thin upper and lower extremities. She also has pretibial edema.

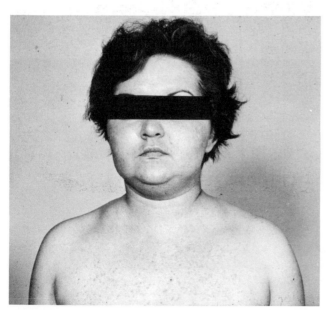

FIGURE 53-3 Typical cushingnoid facies with roundness of the face, double chin, prominent upper lip, and fullness of the supraclavicular fossae.

lymphoma, and generalized skin disorders who receive synthetic glucocorticoids as anti-inflammatory agents. In spontaneous Cushing's syndrome, adrenocortical hyperfunction develops either as a result of excessive stimulation by ACTH or as a consequence of adrenal pathology leading to abnormal production of cortisol.

Cushing's syndrome can be divided in two types: (1) ACTH dependent and (2) ACTH independent (see Fig. 53-5). Among the ACTH-dependent types, adrenocortical hyperfunction may result from abnormal and excessive secretion of ACTH by the pituitary gland. In these cases there is either a disturbance in CRF-ACTH release or an ACTH-secreting pituitary adenoma. In either case there is excessive secretion of ACTH, loss of normal circadian rhythm of ACTH release, and diminished sensitivity of the feedback control system to levels of circulating cortisol. ACTH may be secreted excessively in patients with ectopic hormone production. These are patients who have neoplasms which have acquired the capacity to synthesize and release peptides resembling ACTH both chemically and physiologically. The excessive amounts of ACTH produced under these circumstances lead to excessive stimulation of cortisol secretion by the adrenal cortex and secondarily suppression of pituitary ACTH release. Thus, the high ACTH levels in these patients come from the neoplasm and not from the patient's own pituitary gland. A large number of neoplasms can cause the ectopic secretion of ACTH. These neoplasms are usually derived from tissues originating in the neuroectodermal layer during embryonic development. Oat-cell carcinoma of the lung is the most common of these neoplasms.

Adrenocortical hyperfunction can occur independently of ACTH control. This happens in conditions where a tumor develops in the adrenal cortex with a capacity to secrete cortisol in an autonomous fashion. Adrenocortical tumors leading to Cushing's syndrome may be benign (adenomas) (see Fig. 53-6) or malignant (carcinomas) (see Fig. 53-7).

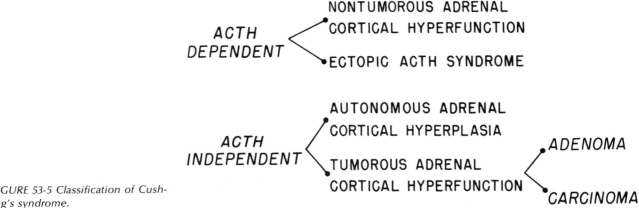

FIGURE 53-5 Classification of Cushing's syndrome.

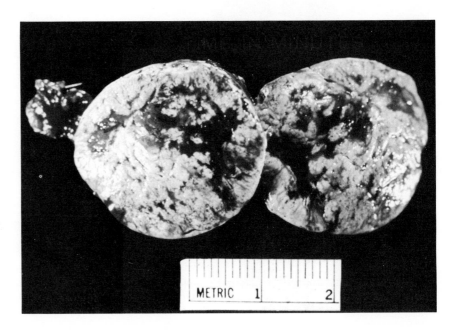

FIGURE 53-6 Benign adrenocortical adenoma.

The presence of Cushing's syndrome can be determined on the basis of the medical history and the physical findings described above. The diagnosis is usually confirmed by the measurement of abnormally high levels of cortisol in plasma and urine. There are specific tests which can be performed to determine the presence or absence of a normal circadian rhythm of cortisol release and a sensitive feedback control mechanism. Absence of circadian rhythm and diminished or absent sensitivity of the feedback control system are characteristic of Cushing's syndrome.

The types of Cushing's syndrome associated with excessive ACTH secretion—pituitary or ectopic—are frequently associated with hyperpigmentation. The pigmentation is recognized in both skin and mucous membranes.

Adrenocortical adenomas may lead to severe Cushing's syndrome, but they usually develop slowly, and symptoms may be present for several years before the diagnosis is finally made (see Fig. 53-6). In contrast, adrenocortical carcinomas develop rapidly and may lead to metastasis and early death (see Fig. 53-7).

Several diagnostic procedures can be used to establish the nature of the underlying pathology in Cushing's syndrome and to help localize a lesion amenable to surgical management.

X-ray examinations of the skull are necessary for examining the sella turcica. ACTH-secreting pituitary tumors may partly destroy the sella turcica (see Fig. 53-8). The presence of a pituitary tumor may be important not only in the diagnosis of Cushing's syndrome but also in deciding on the most appropriate modality of treatment.

Adrenal venous angiography is another radiological method which can be used to visualize the adrenal glands and possible adrenal pathology. A contrast medium is injected into the left and right adrenal veins through a catheter inserted percutaneously into the

femoral vein and inferior vena cava in order to visualize the adrenal venous system. Normal glands have a typical venous pattern (see Fig. 53-9). Distortion of this pattern suggests either adrenal hyperplasia (see Fig. 53-10) or the presence of an adrenal tumor (see Fig. 53-11).

Another technique involves the intravenous administration of radioactive cholesterol. Cholesterol labeled with ^{131}I is taken up and concentrated by the adrenal cortex. Images of the adrenal glands can be obtained by scanning techniques within 5 to 12 days after injection of the tracer (see Fig. 53-12). Patterns suggestive of normal adrenal glands, adrenal hyperplasia, or adrenal adenoma or carcinoma can be obtained with adrenal photoscanning.

Treatment of Cushing's syndrome

Treatment of ACTH-dependent Cushing's syndrome differs depending on whether the source of ACTH is pituitary or ectopic. Several approaches to therapy can be used in patients with pituitary hypersecretion of ACTH. If a pituitary tumor is recognized, a transphenoidal resection of the tumor should be attempted. If there is evidence of pituitary hyperfunction but a tumor is not clearly detected, cobalt irradiation of the pituitary gland can be used instead. This is a treatment modality which is effective, particularly in young people with Cushing's syndrome. Alternatively, cortisol excess can be controlled by a total adrenalectomy and subsequent administration of physiological doses of cortisol or by

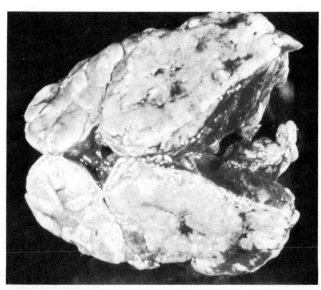

FIGURE 53-7 Malignant adrenocortical carcinoma.

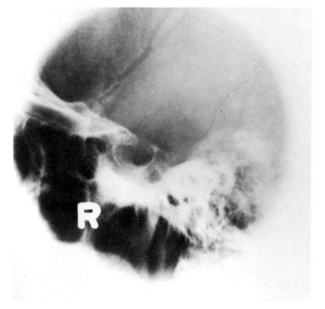

FIGURE 53-8 Enlargement and destruction of the sella turcica caused by an ACTH-secreting pituitary adenoma.

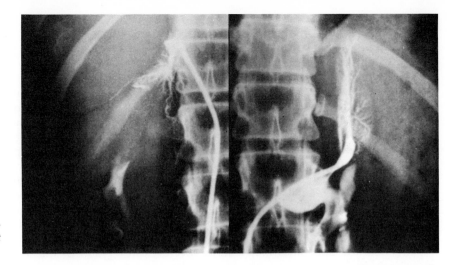

FIGURE 53-9 Right and left adrenal venous angiograms obtained in a subject with normal adrenal function.

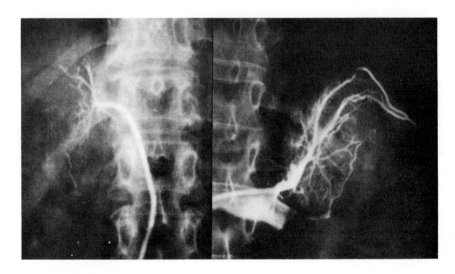

FIGURE 53-10 Right and left adrenal venous angiograms obtained in a patient with bilateral adrenocortical hyperplasia.

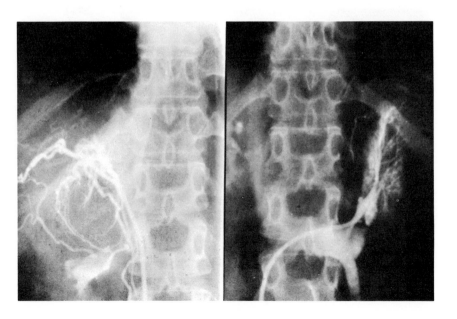

FIGURE 53-11 Right adrenal venous angiogram demonstrating a right adrenocortical tumor. In contrast, the left adrenal angiogram shows an intact adrenal gland.

chemical agents capable of blocking or destroying cortisol-secreting adrenal cortical cells. When the treatment of Cushing's syndrome is successful, remission of the clinical manifestations takes place within 6 to 12 months after institution of therapy (see Fig. 53-13).

When adrenal neoplasms are the cause of cortisol excess, removal of the neoplasm followed by chemotherapy in patients with carcinoma is the preferred mode of treatment.

Treatment of ectopic ACTH syndrome is based on (1) resection of the neoplasm secreting ACTH or (2) adrenalectomy or chemical suppression of adrenal function as prescribed for the patients with pituitary ACTH–dependent type of Cushing's syndrome.

ALDOSTERONISM

Aldosteronism is a clinical condition resulting from excessive production of aldosterone, the mineralocorticoid steroid hormone of the adrenal cortex. The metabolic effects of aldosterone relate to electrolyte and fluid balance. Aldosterone enhances proximal renal tubule reabsorption of sodium and causes potassium and hydrogen-ion excretion. The clinical consequences of aldosterone excess are sodium and water retention, expansion of the extracellular fluid volume, and hypertension. In addition, there are hypernatremia, hypokalemia, and metabolic alkalosis.

There are two types of aldosteronism: (1) primary and (2) secondary. Aldosteronism is primary when the production of aldosterone occurs as a result of a tumor (see Fig. 53-14) or hyperplasia of the adrenal cortex. The majority of the aldosterone-secreting tumors are benign and of small size—0.5 to 2 cm. Primary aldosteronism represents a form of endocrine hypertension and probably affects 1 to 2 percent of patients with hypertension. Recognition of this condition may lead to the cure of hypertension.

Secondary aldosteronism is present in conditions where there is a decrease in afferent arteriolar pressure in the renal glomerulus, leading to stimulation of the

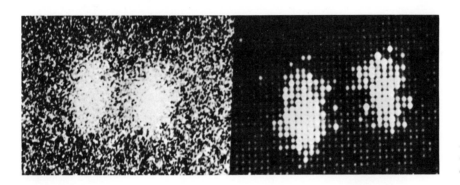

FIGURE 53-12 Image of the adrenal glands obtained by scanning with radioactive cholesterol.

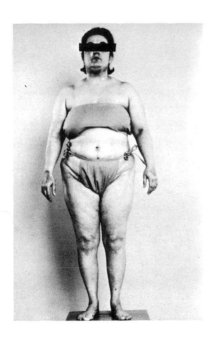
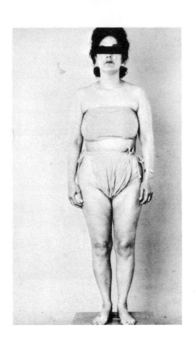

FIGURE 53-13 Response to treatment of Cushing's syndrome with o,p'-DDD and adrenal inhibitor.

renin-angiotensin system. Angiotensin stimulates aldosterone production. Secondary aldosteronism is seen in congestive heart failure, cirrhosis of the liver, and nephrotic syndrome, conditions in which edema is a prominent clinical feature. Congestive heart failure provides a good example of the way secondary aldosteronism may develop. Patients in congestive heart failure cannot pump blood normally and develop a fall in cardiac output. Perfusion pressure to the afferent arteriole of the renal glomerulus decreases. The fall in pressure is sensed by stretch receptors in the juxtaglomerular apparatus, and renin is secreted in increased amounts. Renin activates angiotensin production which in turn stimulates aldosterone secretion by an otherwise normal adrenal cortex. The increased production of aldosterone will, in turn, promote sodium and water reabsorption, expansion of the extracellular fluid compartment, and possibly an increase in afferent arteriolar pressure.

Secondary aldosteronism also develops in conditions where there is a partial occlusion of the renal artery leading to renal vascular hypertension.

The diagnosis of aldosteronism is based on the measurement of increased levels of aldosterone in plasma and urine and measurements of plasma renin. Plasma renin is low in primary aldosteronism, while it is high in secondary aldosteronism.

Adrenal angiography and photoscanning can also help detect and localize an adrenal lesion in patients with primary aldosteronism. Measurements of serum electrolytes will disclose the presence of hypokalemia and metabolic alkalosis.

Treatment of primary aldosteronism includes partial adrenalectomy, resection of an aldosterone-secreting adenoma, subtotal or total adrenalectomy in patients with adrenal hyperplasia, and the administration of aldosterone antagonists such as spironolactone.

PHARMACOLOGY AND USE OF SYNTHETIC CORTICOSTEROIDS

Synthetic analogues of cortisol with glucocorticoid and anti-inflammatory activity, are frequently employed either topically or systemically in the treatment of many

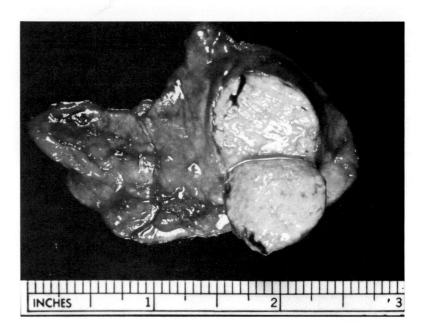

FIGURE 53-14 Aldosterone-secreting adrenocortical adenoma.

medical conditions. For example, steroids are used topically for the treatment of skin disorders. They are used systemically for treatment of conditions such as rheumatoid arthritis, asthma, and acute allergic reactions. Although therapeutically effective, steroids also have side effects. These side effects are related to the metabolic activity and action on various organ systems as described above.

By altering the basic chemical structure of cortisol, the naturally occurring glucocorticoid, the pharmacologic characteristics of this compound may be altered (see Fig. 53-15). For example, if a double bond is introduced between carbons 1 and 2 in the cortisol molecule, prednisolone is produced which has, on a milligram-per-milligram basis, less sodium-retaining and more antiinflammatory activity than the parent compound, cortisol. That is, 1 mg prednisolone is a much more potent antiinflammatory and immunosuppressive agent than 1 mg cortisol. Another possible structural alteration is the introduction of a fluorine atom in an alpha position on carbon 9 of the steroid nucleus. The resulting compound, 9-alpha-fluorocortisol, has strong sodium-retaining properties similar to aldosterone, a naturally occurring mineralocorticoid. By this substitution a compound with predominantly glucocorticoid activity becomes a mineralocorticoid.

Dozens of synthetic compounds have been created in the manner described above. In most cases, the objective has been the development of steroid compounds with strong anti-inflammatory activity and minimal undesirable metabolic side effects. Although this objective has been reached to some extent, therapy with any of the currently available synthetic corticosteroid preparations, if given long enough and in sufficiently high doses, will result in Cushing's syndrome and persistent suppression of endogenous hypothalamic-pituitary-adrenal function. In many instances, steroids are the only effective medication available for treatment of serious systemic diseases. Under those circumstances the development of Cushing's syndrome may be a necessary trade-off in the control of a serious and crippling disease.

QUESTIONS

Cushing's syndrome and aldosteronism—Chap. 53

Directions: Circle the letter preceding every correct response in each of the items below. More than one answer may be correct.

1 Glucocorticoids affect the following when present in excess:
   a Adipose tissue distribution   *b* The immune system
   c Protein metabolism   *d* Carbohydrate metabolism

FIGURE 53-15 Changes in the basic chemical structure of cortisol leading to compounds with different pharmacological characteristics than the parent compound. A, cortisol. B, prednisolone. C, 9-alpha-fluorocortisol.

2 When synthetic glucocorticoids are administered orally over a long period of time, which of the following events are likely to occur?
   a The adrenal gland continues to function normally   *b* The hypothalamic-pituitary axis is suppressed   *c* CRF and ACTH levels are increased   *d* Endogenous cortisol secretion is stimulated

3 Abrupt interruption of corticosteroid therapy may result in:
   a Hyperglycemia   *b* Severe salt depletion   *c* Nausea, vomiting, hypotension   *d* Marked hyperpigmentation

4 Which of the following pathological conditions may cause Cushing's syndrome?
   a Hypothalamic-pituitary hyperfunction   *b* Adrenal adenoma   *c* Ectopic hormone production by a neoplasm   *d* Atrophy of the adrenal glands

5 Which of the following diagnostic tests can be used to determine whether Cushing's syndrome is caused by an adrenal neoplasm or by a primary abnormality of the hypothalamic-pituitary axis?
   a Adrenal venous angiography   *b* Adrenal biopsy   *c* Adrenal photoscanning   *d* Myelogram

6 Mrs. A., 35, presents with the typical signs and symptoms of Cushing's syndrome. All the following signs and symptoms are characteristic of this condition *except:*
   a Moonface (full, round face)   *b* Hypotension   *c* Purple abdominal striae   *d* Truncal obesity   *e* Osteoporosis

7 Which of the following are characteristic metabolic effects of aldosterone?
   a Decreased potassium excretion   *b* Sodium retention   *c* Regulation of blood glucose   *d* Suppression of ACTH release

8 Primary aldosteronism occurs when the overproduction of aldosterone results from a tumor or enlargement of the:
   a Pituitary gland   *b* Adrenal cortex
   c Adrenal medulla   *d* Hypothalamus

9 Which of the following findings are characteristic of primary aldosteronism?
   a Hypokalemia   *b* Hyponatremia
   c Hypertension   *d* Nephrotic syndrome

10 The direct effect of stress is an increased secretion of corticotropin by the anterior pituitary. Corticotropin acts on the adrenal cortex to increase secretion, primarily of:
   a Glucocorticoids   *b* Mineralocorticoids
   c Epinephrine

11 Cushing's syndrome may develop when the _____

_____ _____ secretes abnormal amounts of _____ hormone.

a Adrenal cortex, aldosterone b Anterior pituitary, aldosterone c Adrenal cortex, adrenocorticotropic d Anterior pituitary, adrenocorticotropic

Directions: Answer the following questions on a separate sheet of paper.

12 Explain the statement that glucocorticoids have a catabolic effect on protein metabolism.

13 What effects do abnormally high levels of glucocorticoids have on glucose utilization?

14 The hypothalamic-pituitary axis may be activated under stress. Explain the process by which it occurs.

15 How do the basic chemical structures of 9-alpha-fluorocortisol and prednisolone differ? In relation to pharmacological effects, what is achieved by altering the basic chemical structure of cortisol?

16 List three types of treatment for pituitary ACTH–dependent Cushing's syndrome. What is the purpose of the treatment modalities?

17 What is the preferred treatment for Cushing's syndrome, secondary to an adrenal tumor?

18 Explain the way secondary aldosteronism develops in response to congestive heart failure.

Directions: Circle T if the statement is true, F if the statement is false. Correct any false statements.

19 T F CRF is secreted by the hypothalamus.

20 T F CRF stimulates the release of ACTH from the anterior pituitary.

21 T F High plasma cortisol levels exert a negative feedback effect on CRF release in the normal state.

22 T F CRF directly initiates the secretion of cortisol.

CHAPTER 54   Addison's Disease

At the completion of Chap. 54 you should be able to:

1 Identify several causes of Addison's disease.

2 Describe the possible etiologies of primary adrenal insufficiency.

3 Explain why hypoglycemia is often a manifestation of glucocorticoid insufficiency in Addison's disease.

4 State the effect of cortisol insufficiency on the production of melanocyte-stimulating hormone (MSH) and on the response to stress.

5 Identify the fluid and electrolyte disturbances which may result from a deficit in aldosterone production.

6 Define postural hypotension and tachycardia and explain the relationship between these conditions and Addison's disease.

7 Identify the effect of Addison's disease on plasma renin levels.

8 Differentiate between the signs in males and females that result from decreased production of adrenal androgens in Addison's disease.

9 Describe the most common tests used to diagnose Addison's disease.

10 Describe the treatment of Addison's disease.

Adrenocortical hormone secretion may be insufficient to maintain normal life because of: (1) primary disease or insufficiency of the adrenal cortex or (2) deficient secretion of ACTH. When the cause of adrenocortical insufficiency is a pathological process of the adrenal cortex, the condition is known as Addison's disease. With pituitary ACTH insufficiency there is secondary failure of the adrenal cortex. Patients with Addison's disease have involvement of all zones of the cortex. As a result of this involvement there is deficiency of all the adrenocortical secretions—glucocorticoids, mineralocorticoids, and androgens. Occasionally patients present with partial deficiencies of adrenocortical hormone secretion. This is seen in states of hypoaldosteronism which involves the zona glomerulosa only and its secretion of aldosterone or in the adrenogenital syndrome where an enzyme defect blocks the secretion of a specific steroid hormone.

Addison's disease occurs with an incidence of 4 per 100,000. In the past, tuberculosis was the main cause of Addison's disease. Presently, with better chemotherapy for tuberculosis, this pathological process is the cause of adrenal insufficiency in less than 50 percent of patients with this condition. Another cause of adrenal insufficiency is metastasis to the adrenal glands from a neoplasm located elsewhere. For example, carcinoma of the lung may metastasize to the adrenal glands and destroy most of the functioning adrenal cortex. In approximately 50 percent of patients with Addison's disease, destruction of the adrenal cortex occurs as a manifestation of an autoimmune process. Adrenal antibodies have been found in high titers in some patients with Addison's disease. These antibodies react with antigens in the adrenocortical tissue and cause an inflammatory reaction which eventually leads to destruction of the adrenal gland. Usually, well over 80 percent of both glands must be destroyed before signs and symptoms of insufficiency develop. Addison's disease may occur concurrently with other endocrine diseases of autoimmune origin. Among these are Hashimoto's thyroiditis, diabetes mellitus, and hypoparathyroidism. There also appears to be a familial predisposition for autoimmune endocrine disease which is probably related to abnormal reactivity of the patient's immune system.

METABOLIC CONSEQUENCES OF CORTISOL, ALDOSTERONE, AND ANDROGEN DEFICIENCIES

The clinical picture of Addison's disease results from the lack of cortisol, aldosterone, and androgens. Cortisol insufficiency has metabolic consequence in terms of maintenance of blood glucose levels. In the absence of cortisol, gluconeogenesis is diminished, liver glycogen is decreased, and there is increased sensitivity of peripheral tissues to insulin. The combination of these changes in carbohydrate metabolism may cause inability to maintain normal blood glucose levels in the fasting state. Because of the low glycogen storage, patients with adrenal insufficiency are unable to withstand food deprivation for a long period of time. Sensitivity to insulin observed in the presence of cortisol insufficiency may be a problem for insulin-requiring diabetics who also develop Addison's disease. These patients may notice that insulin doses which kept them under control in the past now cause hypoglycemia.

Another consequence of cortisol insufficiency is an increase in ACTH release. This occurs as a result of diminished feedback inhibition of the hypothalamic-pituitary axis. Melanocyte-stimulating hormone (MSH) is also suppressed by cortisol. Lack of cortisol is usually associated with an increase in MSH secretion. The clinical consequence of this hormonal response is hyperpigmentation.

Since cortisol is required for a normal stress response, patients with cortisol insufficiency are unable to withstand surgical stress, trauma, infection, etc. Under these circumstances patients may become acutely adrenal insufficient and develop evidence of vascular collapse.

Aldosterone deficiency is manifested by increased renal sodium loss and enhanced potassium reabsorption. Salt depletion is associated with water and volume depletion. The decrease in circulating plasma volume leads to hypotension. This change is most strikingly evident when the patient changes from the recumbent to the upright position. Patients with Addison's disease may record a normal blood pressure when they are lying down but marked hypotension and tachycardia when they stand up for several minutes. By definition, postural hypotension occurs when systolic and diastolic blood pressures drop by more than 20 mmHg when the patient assumes the upright posture. Postural tachycardia exists when the pulse rate increases by more than 20 beats per minute (bpm) under these circumstances. In both cases, the decrease in blood pressure and the increase in pulse rate should persist for more than 3 minutes after the change in posture. Thus, a person with Addison's disease may have a blood pressure of 120/80 mmHg in the recumbent position but of 60/40 mmHg after assuming the upright posture. Likewise, the pulse may rise from 80 to 140 bpm with a change in posture.

The plasma renin activity is also affected in Addison's disease. The decrease in plasma volume and in arteriolar pressure causes stimulation of renin release and increased production of angiotensin II. The problem in Addison's disease is that since the adrenal cortex is destroyed, angiotensin II will not be able to stimulate aldosterone production and bring the serum level back to its initial physiologic range. Therefore, high renin levels and low aldosterone secretion are characteristic of aldosterone deficiency.

Androgen deficiency may affect growth of axillary and pubic hair. This effect is masked in the male where testicular androgens exert the major androgenic metabolic effects. In the female, androgen insufficiency will cause loss of axillary and pubic hair and decrease of hair over the extremities.

Pigmentation in Addison's disease

Hyperpigmentation is an important characteristic of primary adrenocortical insufficiency. It is localized to the distal portion of the extremities and sun-exposed areas.

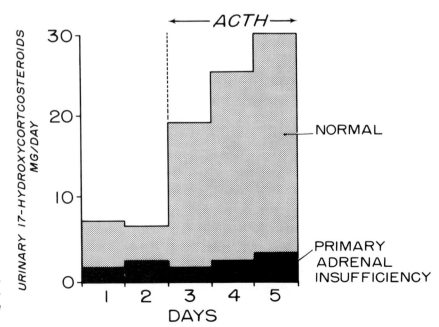

FIGURE 54-1 ACTH stimulation test. Patients with primary adrenocortical insufficiency fail to respond to the administration of ACTH.

It is also present in areas which are not normally exposed to the sun. These areas include the nipples, extensor surfaces of the extremities, genitalia, buccal mucosa, tongue, palmar creases, and knuckles. The assessment of pigmentation may be more difficult in a Negro than in a Caucasian. In these patients history of color change as ascertained by the patients or their relatives may be the only way of assessing the development of hyperpigmentation. Treatment of Addison's disease will reverse the hyperpigmentation.

Diagnosis and treatment

The diagnosis of Addison's disease is based upon the recognition of cortisol, aldosterone, and androgen deficiency. In addition, there are laboratory tests indicative of adrenocortical insufficiency. Patients have decreased excretion of the degradation products or metabolites of cortisol, the urinary 17-hydroxycorticoids. Plasma cortisol levels are low, while plasma ACTH levels are found to be elevated. If patients with Addison's disease receive an intravenous infusion with ACTH, there is a lack of rise of plasma cortisol levels in response to ACTH (see Fig. 54-1). Serum electrolytes are abnormal in patients with Addison's disease, who demonstrate hyponatremia, hyperkalemia, and metabolic acidosis.

Treatment of Addison's disease is based on replacement with cortisol—usually 20 to 30 mg per day in divided doses—and an aldosterone analogue, 9-alpha-fluorocortisol. When both cortisol and 9-alpha-fluorocortisol are employed, patients may return to a normal metabolic state and be able to live a normal life. While in the past patients used to die of Addison's disease, presently patients with this condition, if properly treated, are able to live a normal life and reach normal life expectancy.

QUESTIONS

Addison's disease—Chap. 54

Directions: Circle the letter preceding every correct response in each of the items below. More than one answer may be correct.

1 Addison's disease occurs when:
   a There is an increase in levels of aldosterone b Both glucocorticoid and mineralocorticoid deficiency develop simultaneously c Serum potassium levels decrease d There is increased sodium reabsorption by the kidney

2 Autoimmune destruction of the adrenal gland is caused by:
   a Tuberculosis or other granulomatous diseases b Malignant neoplasm of the lung which metastasizes to the adrenal gland c Adrenal tissues become antigenic, causing the production of antibodies

3 Factors contributing to hypoglycemia in Addison's disease are:
   a Decreased gluconeogenesis in the liver b In-

creased glycogen storage in the liver c Increased sensitivity of the peripheral tissues to insulin d Increased insulin secretion by the pancreas

4 Which of the following sequences best explains the postural hypotension and tachycardia associated with Addison's disease?
   a Aldosterone deficiency → increased sodium and water excretion → hypovolemia → fall in systolic and diastolic blood pressure upon standing → compensatory increase in heart rate to maintain cardiac output
   b Cortisol deficiency → decreased protein synthesis → hypoproteinemia → decreased osmotic pressure → edema → decreased intravascular plasma volume → fall in systolic and diastolic blood pressure upon standing → compensatory increase in heart rate to maintain cardiac output
   c ADH deficiency → inability of kidney to conserve water → hypovolemia → fall in systolic and diastolic blood pressure upon standing → compensatory increase in heart rate to maintain cardiac output

5 Adrenocortical insufficiency is associated with:
   a Increased plasma renin activity, decreased plasma aldosterone b Decreased plasma renin activity, increased plasma aldosterone c Hyperkalemia and hyponatremia d Hypokalemia and hypernatremia

6 The pigmentary changes observed in patients with Addison's disease are a result of:
   a Decreased production of MSH b Decreased production of ACTH by the pituitary gland with associated increased production of MSH c Decreased production of cortisol, causing an increase in ACTH and MSH secretion d Increased production of cortisol by the adrenal cortex causing increased production of MSH

7 The diagnosis of Addison's disease can be made with certainty when:
   a Plasma cortisol levels are low b Hyperkalemia, hyponatremia, and hypertension are present c 24-Hour urinary 17-hydroxycorticosteroids are less than 2 mg (normal = 2 to 8 mg/24 hours) and fail to rise after ACTH infusion d 24-Hour urinary 17-ketosteroids are less than 10 mg in an adult male (normal = 10 to 22 mg/24 hours)

8 Treatment of Addison's disease commonly includes the administration of:
   a ACTH b Cortisol c Pitressin d 9-alpha-Fluorocortisol e Pituitary extract

9 Loss of pubic and axillary hair:
   a May be a manifestation of adrenal androgen insufficiency in females but not in males b Commonly occurs in males with Addison's disease c Is uncommon in males with Addison's disease since serum testosterone levels are generally normal

CHAPTER 55 Glucose Metabolism and Diabetes Mellitus

OBJECTIVES   **At the completion of Chap. 55 you should be able to:**

1 Explain the mechanism which regulates blood glucose levels.

2 Identify a condition leading to fasting hyperglycemia.

3 Identify a condition leading to fasting hypoglycemia.

4 Explain the difference in response to a glucose load exhibited by nondiabetic and diabetic individuals.

5 Define in milligrams percent of glucose each of the following: normal blood glucose, hyperglycemia, hypoglycemia, normal renal threshold for glucose.

6 Explain the following tests of glucose tolerance in relation to administration, interpretation, sensitivity, and applicability to the diagnosis of the various stages of diabetes mellitus:
a Fasting plasma glucose   *b* 2-Hour postprandial plasma glucose *c* Glucose tolerance   *d* Cortisone glucose tolerance

7 Give a general definition of diabetes mellitus.

8 Describe the types of disturbances presently being postulated as possible etiologies of diabetes.

9 State the prevalence rate for diabetes in the United States.

10 Differentiate between the following stages of diabetes as to clinical manifestations and results of glucose tolerance tests:
a Prediabetes   *b* Subclinical   *c* Latent   *d* Overt

11 Differentiate between juvenile-onset and maturity-onset type diabetes as to age group involved, severity, symptoms, and rationale for treatment.

12 List the complications usually associated with diabetes mellitus.

13 State the principles that guide any management program for a diabetic patient.

14 Explain the purpose of the food exchange system.

15 Identify the treatment of a patient with severe insulin deficiency, and describe the rationale for that treatment.

16 Differentiate between the three types of insulin preparations as to their time action and indications for use.

17 Explain the way exercise influences blood glucose levels in both nondiabetic and diabetic patients.

18 Given a case study, identify the stage of diabetes of which the case is characteristic and the preferred treatment for that case.

19 State two examples in each of the two major categories of complications of diabetes mellitus: metabolic and peripheral vascular.

Carbohydrates are important components of the diet. They are chemical substances present in various forms, including simple sugars, or monosaccharides, and complex chemical units, disaccharides and polysaccharides. Following ingestion, carbohydrates are digested to monosaccharides and absorbed, preferentially in the duodenum and proximal jejunum. Following absorption, the blood glucose level rises temporarily and eventually returns to baseline. The physiological regulation of blood glucose levels depends to a large extent on hepatic (1) extraction of glucose, (2) synthesis of glycogen, and (3) glycogenolysis. In addition, peripheral tissues—muscles and adipocytes—utilize glucose for their energy needs. Although quantitatively in lesser magnitude than the liver, these tissues also contribute to the maintenance of normal blood glucose levels.

The hepatic uptake and output of glucose and the utilization of glucose by peripheral tissues depend on the physiologic balance of several hormones. These hormones can be classified as those which (1) lower blood glucose and (2) raise blood glucose. Insulin is the blood glucose–lowering hormone. It is produced by the beta cells of the islets of Langerhans of the pancreas. In contrast, several hormones are capable of raising blood glucose levels. These include (1) glucagon secreted by the alpha cells of the islets of Langerhans, (2) epinephrine secreted by the adrenal medulla and other chromaffin tissues, (3) glucocorticoids secreted by the adrenal cortex, and (4) growth hormone secreted by the anterior pituitary gland. Glucagon, epinephrine, glucocorticoids, and growth hormone constitute a counterregulatory mechanism which prevents a fall in blood glucose levels to hypoglycemic range under the effect of insulin.

A normal fasting plasma glucose level (autoanalyzer technique) is 80 to 110 mg%. Hyperglycemia is defined as a fasting plasma glucose level greater than 110 mg%, and hypoglycemia as a level less than 80 mg%. Glucose is filtered by the renal glomerulus and almost totally reabsorbed by the renal tubule as long as the concentration of glucose in plasma does not exceed 160 to 180 mg%. When the plasma glucose concentration rises above this level, glucose appears in the urine, a condition called *glycosuria*. A plasma glucose concentration of 160 to 180 mg% is the renal threshold for glucose.

Tests of carbohydrate tolerance

There are various methods of testing an individual's ability to regulate plasma glucose levels within the normal range. These methods test (1) the fasting plasma glucose and (2) the plasma glucose response to a glucose load.

In the fasting state when food is not being absorbed, maintenance of normal fasting plasma glucose levels depends upon a well-integrated interaction among the liver, peripheral tissues, and hormones which lower and raise plasma glucose levels. If an individual is unable to regulate plasma glucose normally, this inability will be reflected by either an increase or decrease in fasting plasma glucose. For example, a patient with an insulin-producing tumor which secretes insulin in inappropriately large amounts will develop hypoglycemia. On the other hand, a patient with insulin deficiency will be unable to maintain glucose levels at a normal range and will become hyperglycemic. Thus, the measurement of fasting plasma glucose levels can help evaluate the integrity of the mechanism regulating plasma glucose. In general, these levels become abnormal only in the advanced state of a disease. Therefore, their measurement does not provide information about early abnormalities in glucose metabolism.

A more sensitive method for uncovering abnormalities in glucose metabolism is the measurement of plasma glucose following a glucose load. A nondiabetic individual who ingests a glucose load absorbs this glucose and exhibits a temporary rise in plasma glucose levels. Mechanisms for glucose disposal are then brought into action, and the plasma glucose level returns to normal. The mechanism which mediates this response is insulin, and the main stimulus to insulin release is glucose. The tests used to make the pertinent measurements after a glucose load are the: (1) 2-hour postprandial plasma glucose, (2) glucose tolerance, and (3) cortisone-glucose tolerance tests.

The 2-hour postprandial plasma glucose test is a simple *screening test* for the ability of an individual to dispose of a glucose load. The test consists of measuring the patient's fasting plasma glucose level and then administering 100 g glucose orally. Two hours after the glucose is administered a second plasma glucose level is measured. If the plasma glucose is 80 to 110 mg% fasting and less than 110 mg% 2 hours after the ingestion of the glucose load, it can be concluded that the plasma glucose level must have returned to baseline after an initial rise, indicating that the subject has a normal mechanism for glucose disposal. In contrast, if the patient's plasma glucose level is still high after 2 hours, it can be concluded that there is a disturbance in the mechanism regulating glucose levels.

If a 2-hour postprandial plasma glucose is abnormal, an *oral glucose tolerance test* (OGTT) can provide additional and more complete information about the presence of a disturbance in carbohydrate metabolism. For a glucose tolerance test, a patient receives 100 g glucose orally within a few minutes. Plasma glucose levels are measured fasting and at half-hourly intervals for a period of 3 hours after the glucose load. In healthy, ambulatory people with normal glucose tolerance, the fasting plasma glucose is 80 to 110 mg%. After the ingestion of glucose, the plasma glucose level rises initially but returns to baseline within 2 hours. Normal values for the OGTT have been defined: plasma glucose at 1 hour <195 mg%, at 1½ hours <160 mg%, and at 2 hours <140 mg% (Fajans and Conn criteria) (see Fig. 55-1).

Criteria differing slightly from the values described above have been proposed by other investigators and health organizations. Values also vary with age. The ones described apply to individuals under age 50. Although there are no reliable universal diagnostic criteria for healthy subjects over age 50, it is likely that a progressive impairment of glucose tolerance occurs with advancing age.

The most sensitive test of carbohydrate tolerance is the cortisone glucose tolerance test (cortisone GTT). Cortisone, a glucocorticoid, increases glucose production through stimulation of gluconeogenesis and interference with the action of insulin at the cell level. When glucose levels rise under the effect of cortisone, people without diabetes secrete more insulin and bring plasma glucose levels back to normal. For example, a non-diabetic individual who is treated with large amounts of cortisone will be able to maintain normal blood glucose levels within a few days. Despite the fact that cortisone interferes with normal glucose regulation, the pancreas will secrete enough insulin to overcome this interference. Diabetic people or those with predisposition toward diabetes are unable to secrete the increased amount of insulin required to maintain normal glucose levels in the presence of excessive amounts of glucocorticoids. Their glucose tolerance test then becomes abnormal. For a cortisone GTT the patient receives corti-sone (50 to 62.5 mg) orally prior to receiving the glucose load. A GTT is then carried out as previously described. A test is positive for diabetes when plasma glucose levels are >195 mg% at 1 hour, >175 mg% at 1½ hours, and >160 mg% at 2 hours.

In summary, the cortisone GTT is the most sensitive test for detecting early abnormalities in glucose metabolism (subclinical diabetes). In contrast, the fasting plasma glucose test is the least sensitive of all available tests since the fasting plasma glucose level becomes abnormal only in the late stage of the disease (overt diabetes). The 2-hour postprandial plasma glucose test and the oral GTT are sensitive clinical tests for detection of latent diabetes.

DIABETES MELLITUS

Diabetes mellitus can be defined as a genetically determined disorder of metabolism of heterogeneous etiology which is manifested ultimately by insulin deficiency and loss of carbohydrate tolerance. In its fully developed clinical expression, diabetes is characterized by fasting hyperglycemia, atherosclerotic and microangiopathic vascular disease, and neuropathy. The clinical manifestations of hyperglycemia usually precede by many years the clinical recognition of vascular disease. Occasionally, however, there are patients with only mild abnormality of glucose tolerance who suffer the severe clinical consequences of vascular disease.

There is evidence that diabetes mellitus has heterogeneous etiology; that is, different types of lesions may

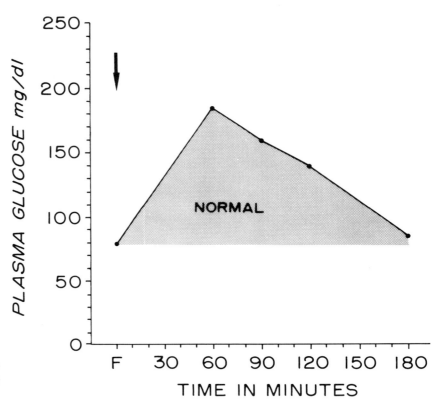

FIGURE 55-1 Normal glucose tolerance test. Values above the shaded area may be diagnostic of diabetes mellitus.

ultimately lead to insulin insufficiency. The following types of disturbances are presently being postulated as possible etiologies of diabetes:

1 A genetically determined abnormality of beta-cell function or number
2 Environmental factors altering beta-cell function and integrity
3 A defective immune system
4 Abnormality of insulin activity
5 Abnormality of glucagon secretion

While there is substantial evidence in favor of some of these proposed etiologies, the role played by others is still hypothetical.

1 A genetically determined abnormality of beta-cell function could affect the operation of the cell at various levels. It may alter the ability of the cell to:
   a Recognize the secretory stimulus
   b Propagate the secretory stimulus within the cell
   c Trigger the complex series of steps involved in the synthesis and release of insulin

Any of these alterations will cause deficient release of insulin in reference to physiological stimuli.

2 Several environmental factors can alter the integrity and function of the beta cell. These factors include:
   a Infective agents, such as Cocksackie B and mumps viruses
   b Diet—excessive intake of calories, carbohydrates, refined sugars
   c Obesity
   d Pregnancy

Most of these factors do not, by themselves, cause diabetes but may affect genetically susceptible individuals and precipitate decompensation of beta-cell function.

3 A defective immune system may be the basis for development of diabetes in certain people. It may operate by:
   a Autoimmunity with development of antipancreatic cell antibodies and eventual destruction of insulin-secreting cells
   b Increased susceptibility to beta-cell damage by viral agents
4 Insensitivity to endogenous insulin and increased secretion of glucagon are theoretically possible causes of diabetes. Insensitivity to insulin is found in patients with obesity and diabetes. The reason for this impaired sensitivity of tissues to insulin may be a decreased number of insulin receptor sites in the cell membrane of insulin-responsive cells or interference with intracellular glycolysis. Abnormalities in glucagon secretion are present in patients with diabetes, but it is unclear whether these abnormalities are primary or secondary to insulin deficiency.

In most cases of insulinopenic type of diabetes a combination of etiologic factors is likely involved. For example, environmental factors—viruses, diet—may act on genetically susceptible individuals to cause injury and destruction of beta cells and lead to insulin insufficiency and loss of ability to maintain glucose hemostasis.

Epidemiology

The prevalence rate of diabetes is high. Estimates are that there are 10 million cases of diabetes in the United States and that 600,000 new cases are diagnosed every year. Diabetes is the third leading cause of death in the United States by disease and the leading cause of blindness, through the development of diabetic retinopathy. Heart attacks occur at least 2½ times as frequently in diabetics as in nondiabetics of a comparable age. Seventy-five percent of diabetic patients eventually die of vascular disease. Heart attacks, kidney failure, strokes, and gangrene are the major complications. In addition, there is an increased rate of intrauterine neonatal death in infants of diabetic mothers.

The economic impact of diabetes is substantial. The approximate loss is $5 billion a year in medical expenses and lost wages without even including the financial consequence of many of the complications such as blindness and vascular disease.

Natural history of diabetes mellitus

Figure 55-2 depicts the natural history of diabetes mellitus. The earliest stage is known as prediabetes. In the prediabetic stage there is no detectable biochemical abnormality of glucose homeostasis. In individuals with genetic diabetes the prediabetic stage exists from the time of birth to the time when clinically apparent manifestations of glucose abnormality are first detected. Prediabetes is suspected in children born of two diabetic parents (conjugal diabetes). It is also suspected in women who give birth to babies weighing over 9 lb, women with recurrent spontaneous abortions, and patients with renal glycosuria (glucose in the urine at normal blood glucose concentrations) in the nonpregnant state.

A second stage in the natural history of diabetes is *preclinical* or *subclinical diabetes*. Patients are identified as having preclinical diabetes if they have a normal OGTT but an abnormal cortisone GTT. That is, patients are unable to compensate for the increased demands for insulin secretion caused by the administration of cortisone. The preclinical stage can persist without any further change for many years, and it ends when the standard OGTT becomes abnormal. At this point patients are said to have developed *latent* or *chemical diabetes*. The latent diabetic does not usually complain of clinical manifestations of the disease.

Overt diabetes is the final stage in the natural history of the disease. In this stage, patients develop symptoms of abnormal glucose tolerance. Not only are they unable to control the glucose load, but they are also unable to maintain normal fasting blood glucose levels. Hyperglycemia is accompanied by glycosuria if the blood glucose level exceeds the renal threshold for this sub-

matic, with the diagnosis made only following laboratory examination of the blood and performance of tests of glucose tolerance.

stance. Glycosuria leads to osmotic diuresis which causes increased urinary output—polyuria—and thirst —polydipsia. Because of the loss of glucose in the urine, patients develop a negative caloric balance and exhibit weight loss. Also, increased hunger, or polyphagia, may develop as a result of calorie loss. Patients complain of fatigue and sleepiness.

Most patients with diabetes progress from prediabetes to overt diabetes (see Fig. 55-2). Occasionally, a patient may improve his or her glucose tolerance and regress to an earlier stage of the disease.

Two clinical types of diabetes have been classically described: (1) growth-onset or juvenile-onset type and (2) maturity-onset type. Juvenile-onset type diabetes is characterized by markedly reduced islet-cell reserve, insulin insufficiency, tendency to diabetic ketoacidosis, and sensitivity to administered insulin. In contrast, maturity-onset type diabetes has, in general, milder clinical manifestations of hyperglycemia and less tendency to ketoacidosis. Islet-cell reserve is diminished but still present. Occasionally, in obese patients, insulin levels are high but inadequate to maintain normal blood glucose levels. Obese patients are insulin resistant. High-carbohydrate intake and large adipose cells appear to be responsible for the decreased sensitivity of the obese diabetic to insulin.

It was previously held that juvenile-onset type diabetes occurred only in people below age 40 and maturity-onset diabetes in individuals above that age. However, there are young people whose diabetes has the clinical characteristics described in maturity-onset diabetes (maturity-onset diabetes of the young) and older patients who exhibit the clinical characteristics of juvenile-onset diabetes.

Clinical manifestations of diabetes

Patients with juvenile-onset type diabetes generally present with rapid onset of polydipsia, polyuria, weight loss, polyphagia, fatigue, and somnolence. They may become very ill, develop ketoacidosis, and may die if treatment is not instituted promptly. In contrast, maturity-onset type diabetes may be completely asympto-

Principles of management of diabetes

The management of diabetes is based on (1) diet, (2) hypoglycemic agents, and (3) controlled physical activity.

In people without diabetes an intact capacity to secrete insulin will compensate for varying amounts of food intake and exercise. In diabetics who are unable to secrete insulin normally, this ability is lost. While normal individuals adjust to hour-to-hour changes in food intake and exercise by varying their insulin secretion, diabetic patients must maintain these factors constant in order to prevent wide fluctuations in blood glucose levels.

The diet of diabetic patients is aimed at controlling the number of calories and the amount of carbohydrates ingested daily. The recommended number of calories will vary depending on the need for maintaining, reducing, or increasing body weight. For example, if the patient is obese, a calorie-restricted diet should be prescribed until weight has dropped into the ideal range for that person. In contrast, young patients with juvenile-onset type diabetes may have lost weight during the state of decompensation. They should receive sufficient calories to help restore their best weight.

Diabetic patients should avoid intake of excessive amounts of carbohydrates in order to prevent excessive postprandial hyperglycemia and glycosuria. Usually, carbohydrates make up 40 percent of the total daily calorie allowance. This carbohydrate allowance must be distributed in such a way that the intake matches the patients' requirements throughout the day. For example, larger amounts are given at times of greater physical activity. A food exchange system has been developed to help patients manage their own diet. Food exchange lists are available which identify food choices on the basis of calorie and carbohydrate values and compare these values among various types of food.

In general, a diabetic patient is instructed on the food exchange system by a dietician. Alternatively, patients may receive standardized diets of appropriate calorie value and composition prepared by the American Diabetes Association (ADA diets).

Patients with mild diabetes may be able to maintain normal blood glucose levels by means of a diet alone.

	PREDIABETES	SUBCLINICAL DIABETES	LATENT DIABETES	OVERT DIABETES
Fasting glucose	Normal	Normal	Normal or ↑	↑
OGTT	Normal	Normal Abnormal during pregnancy, stress	Abnormal	Not necessary for diagnosis
Cortisone GTT	Normal	Abnormal	Not necessary	

FIGURE 55-2 Stages in the natural history of diabetes mellitus.

Patients with severe insulin insufficiency, however, require a hypoglycemic agent in addition to the diet. The physiologic hypoglycemic agent is insulin, which is available only in injectable form. Several insulin preparations are available for treatment of insulin-dependent diabetics (see Table 55-1). They are classified as short acting, intermediate acting, or long acting, according to the time required for maximal plasma glucose-lowering effect following their injection. Short-acting insulins produce their maximal effect within 2 to 4 hours after injection and are employed in the treatment of acute diabetic decompensation and in the management of patients with diabetic ketoacidosis. They also may be used to supplement longer-acting insulins. Intermediate-acting insulins have their peak effect within 8 to 16 hours after their administration and are usually used for day-to-day control of the diabetic patient. Long-acting insulin preparations with a peak effect within 18 to 24 hours after their administration are rarely used in the routine management of diabetic patients.

Control of the diabetic patient is usually achieved by the use of intermediate-acting insulin administered either as a single dose before breakfast or as a split dose, with the largest portion being given before breakfast and the smallest before supper. Short-acting insulin is frequently combined with intermediate-acting insulin for tighter regulation of glucose levels during postprandial periods. In any case, it is important to know the kind of insulin preparation a patient receives in order to anticipate maximal effects and possible hypoglycemic reactions.

Other hypoglycemic agents can be administered orally. They include drugs like sulfonylureas and biguanides. They should be used only in patients with mild diabetes who have some remaining islet-cell function. This *excludes* patients with juvenile-onset type diabetes who are insulinopenic and insulin dependent. Sulfonylureas stimulate beta-cell function and increase secretion of insulin. Biguanides enhance glucose utilization by stimulating anaerobic glycolysis.

There are potential side effects from the use of oral hypoglycemic drugs. Chronic use of sulfonylureas may be associated with increased incidence of cardiovascular deaths among diabetics. Biguanides may cause lactic acidosis (see Table 55-2).

Physical exercise also influences the control of blood glucose levels in patients with diabetes. Exercise appears to facilitate the transport of glucose into cells. Normally, nondiabetic individuals are able to decrease insulin release during exercise and avoid hypoglycemia. In contrast, patients who receive insulin are unable to exert this control. In these patients, exercise can potentiate the hypoglycemic action of insulin. This is particularly important when a patient engages in physical exercise at the time when the insulin dose has maximally depressed the glucose level. By appropriate timing of their physical exercise, patients may be able to improve the control of their glucose levels. For example, if patients exercise at the time when the blood glucose level is high, they might be able to lower this level with exercise alone. Conversely, if patients need to exercise when the blood glucose level is low, it is important that they receive additional carbohydrate in order to prevent hypoglycemia.

Diabetic patients can lead a relatively normal life if they are well informed about their disease and its management. Juvenile-onset type, insulin-dependent diabetics learn in time to regulate their insulin dose, administer their own insulin, and plan their diet and exercise in such a way that they will minimize hyper- or hypoglycemia. Patients with maturity-onset type dia-

TABLE 55-1
Insulin

TYPE	Description	EFFECT ON BLOOD GLUCOSE (HOURS AFTER ADMINISTRATION)		
		Onset	Peak	Termination
Short acting				
Crystalline zinc	Clear	Immediate	2	6–8
Insulin (regular)	Unmodified			
Semilente (SL)*	Cloudy: Amorphous insulin Zn suspension, no protamine	1	4–8	8–10
Intermediate acting				
NPH†	Cloudy: Crystaline Zn insulin suspension 50% sat. with protamine	2–3	8–16	32–36
Lente	Cloudy: Mixture 30% SL + 70% UL, no protamine	2–3	8–16	32–36
Long acting				
PZI†	Cloudy: Excess protamine	6	18–24	48–72
Ultralente (UL)*	Cloudy: Crystaline insulin suspension, high Zn content, no protamine	6	18–24	48–72

*Lente insulins (semi and ultra) do not contain protamine and are prepared in sodium acetate buffer. Their time action depends on their variable Zn contents and crystal sizes.
†Delayed action of NPH and PZI is controlled by their protamine content; they are prepared in sodium phosphate buffer.

betes who are obese and asymptomatic, with moderately elevated glucose levels, learn that the treatment of choice is dietary restriction and weight reduction. However, the success rate in weight reduction among these patients is low, and they may eventually require therapy with hypoglycemic agents.

Complications of diabetes mellitus

Complications of diabetes mellitus can be divided into two major categories: (1) acute metabolic complications and (2) long-term vascular complications.

The metabolic complications of diabetes are the consequence of relatively acute changes in plasma glucose concentration. The most serious metabolic complication is diabetic ketoacidosis. With severe insulin insufficiency, patients develop severe hyperglycemia and glycosuria, decreased lipogenesis, increased lipolysis, and increased oxidation of free fatty acids with production of ketone bodies (acetoacetate, hydroxybutyrate, and acetone). The increase in ketones in plasma causes ketosis. The increased production of ketones causes an increased hydrogen ion load and metabolic acidosis. Marked glycosuria and ketonuria also lead to osmotic diuresis with dehydration and loss of electrolytes. Patients may become hypotensive and develop a state of shock. Eventually, owing to decreased cerebral oxygen utilization, patients may go into coma and die. Coma and death from ketoacidosis are a rare occurrence today because patients and physicians are aware of the potential dangers of this complication and treatment of ketoacidosis can be instituted early.

The principles of therapy of diabetic ketoacidosis involve (1) reversal of the metabolic derangement caused by the lack of insulin, (2) restoration of water and electrolyte balance, and (3) treatment of conditions which might have precipitated ketoacidosis. Treatment with short-acting (regular) insulin—administered as a continuous intravenous infusion or as frequent intramuscular injections—and glucose will increase glucose utilization, decrease lipolysis and ketone body production, and restore acid-base balance. In addition, patients are treated with intravenous infusions of water, bicarbonate, and electrolytes, especially potassium. Since intercurrent infections can increase insulin requirements in diabetic patients, it is not unusual for infection to precipitate acute diabetic decompensation and ketoacidosis. Thus, treatment with antibiotics may be necessary in the management of patients with this condition.

Another frequent metabolic complication of diabetes is hypoglycemia. This is mainly a complication of insulin therapy. Insulin-dependent diabetics may, at times, receive insulin in amounts larger than needed to maintain normal glucose levels. Hypoglycemia will follow. Symptoms of hypoglycemia are caused by epinephrine release (sweating, shakiness, headache, palpitations) and by lack of glucose in the brain (bizarre behavior, dullness of sensorium, and coma). Management of hypoglycemia requires the prompt administration of

TABLE 55-2
Oral hypoglycemic agents

AGENT	ACTION	HALF-LIFE	DIVIDED DOSE	INITIAL PRIMING (NOT NECESSARY)	MAINTE-NANCE	TOXICITY	TABLET SIZE
Tolbutamide (Orinase)	Stimulates insulin release	4.5–6 h	BID or TID	2–3 g 2–4 days	0.5–2.0	Skin GI Hematology	0.5 g
Chlorpropamide (Diabinese)	Stimulates insulin release	36 h	Single	250–500 mg	100–500	Hepatic Hematology Skin GI	100 mg 250 mg
Acetohexamide (Dymelor)	Stimulates insulin release	4–6 h	Single or divided	250 mg–1.5 g	250 mg–1.5 g	Hepatic Hematology Skin GI	250 mg 500 mg
Phenethylbiguanide (DBI, Phenformin)*	Unknown Inhibits tissue oxidative enzymes, increases glucose utilization through anaerobiosis		(a) TID or QID (b) Single or BID	None, gradual increase from 100 mg None	75–150 50–200	GI	25 mg 50-mg spansule (DBI-TD)

*DBI can be used in combination with sulfonylureas if either gives only a partial response.

carbohydrate, either orally or intravenously. Occasionally, glucagon, a glycogenolytic hormone, is administered intramuscularly to raise blood glucose levels.

The long-term vascular complications of diabetes involve small vessels—microangiopathy—and middle- and large-size vessels—macroangiopathy. Microangiopathy is a specific lesion of diabetes which affects capillaries and arterioles of the retina—diabetic retinopathy—and of the muscles and skin. Histologically and by electron microscopy there is evidence of thickening of the capillary basement membrane. Histochemically, there is evidence that this thickening is accompanied by increased accumulation of glycoprotein. In addition, since all the chemical components of the basement membrane can be derived from glucose, there is an increased rate of formation of basement membrane cells with hyperglycemia. These cells do not require insulin for glucose utilization.

Histological evidence of microangiopathy is already apparent in patients with latent diabetes. However, clinical manifestations of vascular disease, retinopathy, or nephropathy usually appear 15 to 20 years after the onset of overt diabetes.

An early manifestation of retinopathy is the presence of microaneurysms (tiny sacular dilatations) of the retinal arterioles. Subsequently, hemorrhages, neovascularization, and retinal scars may lead to blindness (see Fig. 55-3).

Early manifestations of nephropathy are proteinuria and hypertension. As the loss of functioning nephrons progresses, patients develop renal insufficiency and uremia.

Other frequent complications resulting from insulin insufficiency are neuropathy and cataracts. They result from disturbances in the polyol pathway (glucose → sorbitol → fructose) caused by lack of insulin. In the lens, there is increased accumulation of sorbitol, leading to formation of cataracts and blindness. In nerve tissue, there is an increased accumulation of sorbitol and fructose and decreased concentration of myoinositol, leading to neuropathy. The biochemical alteration in nerve tissue interferes with metabolic activity of the Schwann cells and causes axonal loss. Motor conduction velocity decreases early in the course of neuropathy. Subsequently, there are pain, paresthesias, decreased vibratory and propioceptive sensations, and motor impairment with loss of deep tendon reflexes, muscle weakness, and atrophy. Neuropathy may involve peripheral nerves (mono- and polyneuropathy), cranial nerves, or the autonomic nervous system. Involvement of the autonomic nervous system may be accompanied by nocturnal diarrhea, delayed gastric emptying, postural hypotension, and impotence.

Diabetic macroangiopathy has the histopathological characteristics of atherosclerosis. A combination of biochemical disturbances caused by insulin insufficiency probably leads to this type of vascular disease. The disturbances include (1) accumulation of sorbitol in the vascular intima, (2) hyperlipoproteinemia, and (3) abnormality in blood coagulation. Diabetic macroangiopathy eventually leads to vascular occlusion. When it involves peripheral arteries, it may result in peripheral vascular insufficiency with intermittent claudication and gangrene of the extremities. When it involves the aorta and coronary arteries, it may lead to angina and myocardial infarctions.

Diabetes also interferes with pregnancy. Diabetic women are prone to spontaneous abortions, intrauterine fetal death, large fetal size, and premature infants with high incidence of respiratory distress syndrome and fetal malformations. The outcome of preg-

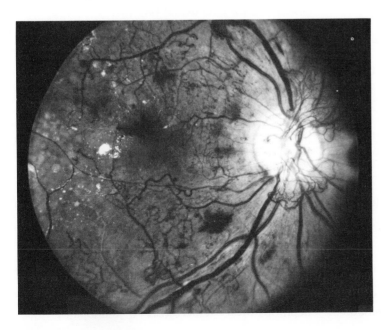

FIGURE 55-3 Diabetic retinopathy. Note the hemorrhages, exudates, neovascularization, and dilatation of veins in the fundus of a patient with diabetes mellitus. (Reproduced with permission from the Ophthalmology Department, University Hospital, University of Michigan.)

nancy in diabetic mothers has improved with tighter diabetic control during pregnancy, early delivery, and advances in the field of neonatology and in the management of complications in the newborn.

Present clinical and experimental evidence suggests that development of long-term diabetic complications relate to the chronic abnormality in metabolism caused by insufficient insulin secretion. It is possible that diabetic complications could be minimized or prevented if diabetic patients were able to completely normalize glucose metabolism with appropriate insulin therapy at all times. Unfortunately, even with the best possible control, the treatment of diabetes is not effective enough to totally normalize glucose metabolism. Persistent abnormalities in glucose metabolism are likely to lead to the vascular complications which can eventually bring death to diabetic patients.

QUESTIONS

Glucose metabolism and diabetes mellitus—Chap. 55

Directions: Circle the letter preceding every correct response in each of the items below. More than one answer may be correct.

1 Glucose is removed from the bloodstream by:
   a Conversion to glycogen by the liver *b* Peripheral glucose utilization by muscle or adipose tissue

2 Fasting hypoglycemia will usually occur when there is (are):
   a Pancreatic islet-cell tumor *b* Cirrhosis of the liver where the patient is unable to synthesize glycogen *c* Excessive production of cortisol *d* Excessive production of growth hormone

3 Which of the following test(s) is (are) the most sensitive in the diagnosis of diabetes mellitus?
   a Fasting plasma glucose *b* Cortisone glucose tolerance test *c* 2-Hour postprandial plasma glucose *d* Standard oral glucose tolerance test

4 The purpose of the cortisone GTT is to:
   a Test the insulin-secreting capacity of the islets of Langerhans under stress *b* Diagnose overt diabetes *c* Determine insulin requirements *d* Detect subclinical diabetes

5 The major defect in diabetes mellitus is a disorder of _____ secretion.
   a Epinephrine *b* Cortisol *c* Insulin *d* Growth hormone

6 Current theories of the pathogenesis of diabetes mellitus include:
   a Autoimmune destruction of beta cells *b* Viral destruction of beta cells *c* Genetically determined

defects in insulin release *d* Decreased growth hormone production

7 The prevalence rate of diabetes mellitus is calculated at a *minimum* of _____ million cases in the United States.
   a 1 *b* 3 *c* 6 *d* 10

8 Robert M., a 30-year-old male, is being treated in an out-patient clinic. His history reveals that he has a bilateral family history of diabetes mellitus. His 2-hour postprandial blood glucose test shows levels of 110 mg%. His cortisone glucose tolerance test shows 135 mg% at 2 hours. Robert would most probably be classified as a:
   a Subclinical diabetic *b* Prediabetic *c* Latent diabetic *d* Overt diabetic

9 Mrs. M., a 24-year-old female, has a bilateral family history of diabetes. Her first pregnancy resulted in a spontaneous abortion. Her second child was full-term with a birth weight of 11 lb. A glucose tolerance test was ordered, and the results were within normal limits. A cortisone GTT was ordered, and the results indicated an abnormal level. Which stage of diabetes could Mrs. M.'s case be characteristic of?
   a Prediabetes *b* Subclinical *c* Latent *d* Overt

10 Which of the following are the usual characteristics of a maturity-onset diabetic patient?
   a Relatively insensitive to insulin *b* Likely to be obese *c* Very low islet-cell reserve *d* Prone to diabetic ketoacidosis

11 The individual with juvenile-onset type diabetes usually presents with all the following except:
   a Weight gain *b* Polydipsia *c* Polyuria *d* Fatigue *e* Polyphagia

12 Jane S., a 10-year-old, was admitted to the hospital and diagnosed as having juvenile-onset type diabetes. The medical management that would most likely be prescribed for Jane would be:
   a A fixed amount of carbohydrate, fats, and protein distributed throughout the day, plus an oral hypoglycemic agent *b* A fixed amount of calories and carbohydrate, protein, and fat; insulin therapy *c* Education about diabetes and oral hypoglycemic agents

13 If a diabetic patient is given an excessive dose of lente insulin at 7 A.M., when would one expect to see a hypoglycemic reaction (if such a reaction occurs)?
   a Within one-half hour *b* 11 A.M. *c* 4 P.M. *d* 12 Midnight

14 The most common metabolic complication of insulin therapy is:
   a Hypoglycemia *b* Hyperglycemia *c* Ketoacidosis *d* Diabetic coma

15 Long-term complications of diabetes mellitus include which of the following?
   a Peripheral vascular insufficiency *b* Diabetic nephropathy *c* Ketoacidosis *d* Retinopathy

Directions: Answer the following questions on a separate sheet of paper.

16 What is the purpose of measuring the fasting blood glucose level?

17 Administration of a glucose load to a nondiabetic individual will cause a rise in blood glucose. Which is the mechanism that brings glucose back to baseline levels?

18 What is the purpose of the food exchange system?

Directions: Match the glucose level in col. B with the appropriate term in col. A.

Column A	Column B
19 _____ Hypoglycemia	a 160–180 mg%
20 _____ Normal plasma glucose	b 210 mg%
21 _____ Renal threshold for glucose	c 40 mg%
22 _____ Hyperglycemia	d 80–110 mg%

Directions: Circle T if the statement is true and F if the statement is false. Correct any false statements.

23 T F Heart attacks occur at least 2½ times as frequently in diabetics as in nondiabetics of comparable age.

24 T F Twenty-five percent of all diabetics eventually die of vascular disease, heart attacks, kidney failure, strokes, or gangrene.

25 T F Exercise tends to increase blood sugar by blocking transport of glucose into the tissues.

CHAPTER 56 Syndromes of Androgen Excess, Disorders of the Pituitary Gland, and Disorders of Calcium Balance

OBJECTIVES   At the completion of Chap. 56 you should be able to:

1 Identify factors which determine hair growth patterns in men and women.

2 Describe the typical manifestations of hirsutism and virilism in females.

3 Identify and describe the source, metabolism, and excretion of three types of androgens in men and women.

4 Compare the androgenic potency of dehydroepiandrosterone, $\Delta 4$-androstenedione, and testosterone.

5 Identify several possible causes of hirsutism in females.

6 Describe the pathogenesis of adrenal cortical hyperplasia and its consequences in congenital deficiency of C_{21}-hydroxylase.

7 Describe clinical differences among various etiologies of hirsutism.

8 Describe the treatment of androgen excess.

9 Locate the pituitary gland and describe its structure, embryologic origin, and anatomic relations with the hypothalamus.

10 Describe the origin, chemistry, control, and function of the following hormones:
a Growth hormone
b Prolactin
c Melanocyte-stimulating hormone
d Adrenocorticotropic hormone
e Follicle-stimulating hormone
f Luteinizing hormone
g Thyrotropin
h Antidiuretic hormone

11 Identify the etiology, pathogenesis, characteristic manifestations in children and adults, and treatment of panhypopituitarism.

12 Describe the etiology, characteristic manifestations in children and adults, and treatment of excessive secretion of growth hormone.

13 Describe the function of calcium in the body, normal serum values, and the role of parathormone, calcitonin, and vitamin D in its regulation.

14 Describe hypercalcemia and hypocalcemia (etiology, pathogenesis, clinical manifestations, diagnosis, and treatment).

One of the most common problems seen by the endocrinologist among young women is hirsutism. It is the simplest and earliest clinical expression of androgen excess.

It is well documented that there is a complex relationship between the growth of hair in men and women and sex hormones. For example, the growth of beard, hair in the ears, nasal tip, and upper pubic triangle, and the growth of coarse hair over the trunk and limbs are dependent upon adult male levels of circulating androgens. The growth of hair in the axilla, lower pubic region, and in part, at least, the limbs, is initiated by pubertal events in both sexes and is mediated by weaker adrenal androgens. Androgen-type hair is coarse and dark. Certain hair growth appears to be independent of sex hormones. This hair is fine and light in color and includes the lanugal hair, the eyebrows, and the eyelashes.

Hirsutism is defined as excessive growth of body hair in the female with characteristic masculine distribution over the facial, periareolar, abdominal, and sacral areas (see Fig. 56-1). It may be associated with baldness (see Fig. 56-2) or temporal recession of the hairline (see Fig. 56-3). It may be present by itself or be part of a virilizing syndrome, which is the clinical picture observed in girls and women of all ages with signs and symptoms of defeminization and masculinization. The characteristic findings in defeminization include amenorrhea, decrease in libido, atrophy of the breasts, and loss of feminine body contour. Masculinization includes hirsutism, seborrhea, acne, deepening of the voice, increased muscular development, and enlargement of the clitoris (see Fig. 56-4).

True virilism is currently recognized as a rare condition, almost always associated with adrenal or ovarian tumors or with the syndrome of congenital adrenal hyperplasia. In contrast, hirsutism often without any other signs of virilism but frequently accompanied by irregular or absent menstrual periods and acne is a common clinical entity. While it is often thought that simple hirsutism is a mild form of virilism because it has a similar etiology, no specific hormonal abnormality or etiological mechanism has been found as the sole cause of these types of hirsutism. Ethnic and genetic factors play an important role in the developmental of hair growth patterns. However, there is evidence that androgen excess is present in most cases of hirsutism.

Androgen physiology

Various types of androgens are normally secreted by both men and women. The three major types are: (1) Dehydroepiandrosterone (DHEA), (2) Δ4-androstenedione, and (3) testosterone (see Fig. 56-5).

Dehydroepiandrosterone and its metabolites, dehydroepiandrosterone sulfate and androstenediol, are generally considered to be weak androgens. The adrenal is the main source of this type of androgen, although the ovary also contributes to the level of androstenediol. These androgens can be measured in the urine as 17-ketosteroids of which dehydroepiandrosterone makes up 60 percent of the total.

Δ4-Androstenedione is a stronger androgen product than dehydroepiandrosterone but weaker than testosterone, of which it is a precursor. Like dehydroepiandrosterone, Δ4-androstenedione is also produced by the adrenal cortex and the ovary.

Testosterone is the most potent of the three androgen compounds. There are several sources of testosterone, including the adrenal cortex, the ovary, the testes, and peripheral tissues. Testosterone is metabolized to a potent androgen, dihydrotestosterone (DHT); finally, both testosterone and DHT may be converted to androstenediol in peripheral tissues and excreted as such in the urine.

Testosterone can be produced in several endocrine and peripheral tissues from precursors. It circulates in the plasma partially bound to a carrier protein (testosterone-binding protein), and it is removed through metabolic degradation in the liver and other peripheral tissues (see Fig. 56-6). Testosterone levels are therefore

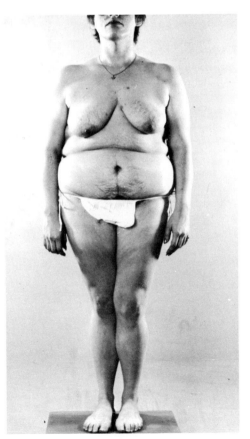

FIGURE 56-1 Hirsutism in the female. Excess of body hair over the breasts, abdomen, and extremities.

a balance between production and metabolic clearance. While a large portion of circulating androgens are bound to protein, a small fraction is present in a free state. The biological effects of circulating androgens are related to the level of free androgens in plasma. Women with hirsutism usually present with abnormalities in testosterone secretion and metabolism. For example, in normal women testosterone is extracted and metabolized almost in its entirety by the liver; in contrast, in virilized women 32 percent of secreted testosterone is extracted and metabolized by extrahepatic peripheral tissues. These tissues are then subject to greater androgenic activity than that found in normal women. Similarly, hirsute women have lower testosterone-binding, higher free-testosterone levels, and more active metabolic clearance rates than women without hirsutism.

Differential diagnosis of androgen excess

Four major categories of conditions are associated with androgen excess: (1) Adrenal cortical, (2) ovarian, (3) simple or idiopathic hirsutism, and (4) miscellaneous (see Table 56-1).

Among the adrenal cortical states associated with androgen excess is Cushing's syndrome. In Cushing's syndrome manifestations of androgen excess are superimposed on signs and symptoms of cortisol excess.

Clinically, patients demonstrate coarse, dark hair growth, balding, deepening of the voice, and occasional clitoral enlargement. Biochemically, they demonstrate high urinary 17-ketosteroids and high levels of dehydroepiandrosterone and androstenediol. Androgen excess is found most commonly among the ACTH-dependent type of Cushing's syndrome and in patients with adrenal carcinoma.

There are adrenocortical disorders associated with androgen excess only and with normal secretion of cortisol. Prenatally, such a disorder is found in patients

TABLE 56-1
Androgen excess: Differential diagnosis

I Androgen excess of adrenal cortical origin
  A Associated with cortisol excess: Cushing's syndrome
  B Androgen excess only
    1 Prenatal: congenital adrenal hyperplasia (CAH)
    2 Postnatal: prepubertal
      a Late manifestations of CAH
      b Carcinoma
    3 Pubertal or postpubertal
      a Hyperplasia, with or without polycystic ovaries
      b Carcinoma
II Androgen excess of ovarian origin
  A Neoplasms: arrhenoblastoma, adrenal rest cell, hilar cell, luteoma
  B Hilar cell or Leydig cell hyperplasia
  C Polycystic ovary syndrome
III Simple or idiopathic hirsutism
IV Miscellaneous causes
  A Endocrine
    1 Acromegaly
    2 Pregnancy
    3 Hypothyroidism
    4 Menopause
    5 Androgen therapy
    6 Inanition
  B Nonendocrine
    1 Immobilization
    2 Body cast
    3 Porphyria
    4 Congenital ectodermal dysplasia

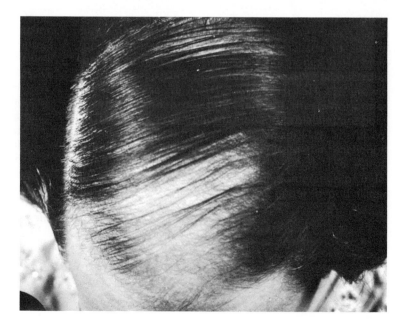

FIGURE 56-2 Baldness in a woman with androgen excess.

with congenital adrenal hyperplasia. In this condition there is an inborn defect in one of the enzymes involved in cortisol biosynthesis. The most common type is a defect in 21-hydroxylase (see Fig. 56-7). As a consequence of 21-hydroxylase deficiency the adrenal cortex has an impaired capacity to secrete cortisol. The decrease in cortisol production causes an increase in ACTH secretion in response to the negative feedback activation of pituitary function. ACTH stimulates the adrenal cortex in such a manner that the precursors of cortisol biosynthesis prior to the deficient step are shunted to the biosynthesis of androgens (see Fig. 56-8). When the fetus is exposed to increased androgen production, it undergoes changes in the development of the external genitalia. For example, a female fetus with this defect develops an enlargement of the clitoris and fusion of the labia majora. The genitalia then resemble male external genitalia. At the time of birth this ambiguity in sexual development may create difficulties in sexual identification of the newborn. The syndrome of a masculinized genetic female fetus caused by androgen excess in utero is called *female pseudohermaphroditism* (see Fig. 56-9).

Manifestations of androgen excess of adrenal origin can also develop postnatally and before puberty. Such a condition may be the result of late manifestation of congenital adrenal hyperplasia as described above or an androgen-secreting adrenal carcinoma. Finally, the clinical picture of androgen excess may develop at puberty or after puberty. It may be part of the syndrome of polycystic ovaries or secondary to an adrenal carcinoma.

Several ovarian conditions can cause androgen excess. Tumors of the ovary such as arrhenoblastomas and hilar-cell neoplasms are capable of secreting large amounts of testosterone. Other types of androgens are seen in patients with these tumors depending on the cell type involved. Manifestations of androgen excess can also be seen in patients with Leydig-cell hyperplasia. These patients usually have high plasma testosterone levels. Occasionally masculinization in association with Leydig-cell hyperplasia and Leydig-cell tumors are seen in patients with gonadal dysgenesis, a sex chromosome abnormality leading to abnormal development of the ovaries.

In polycystic ovary syndrome, hirsutism is frequently associated with infertility, amenorrhea, obesity, and enlarged ovaries. In these patients, testosterone production rates are clearly increased and are responsible for the manifestations of androgen excess. The increased production of androgens in the polycystic ovary syndrome may result from biosynthetic defects in the production of estrogens or by abnormalities in the physiological cyclic release of gonadotropins. Patients with polycystic ovary syndrome frequently present with sustained elevations of serum luteinizing hormone, or LH. These changes in gonadotropin secretion may lead to anatomical changes in the ovary and stimulation of ovarian androgen production.

Many women present with hirsutism without any other clinical manifestations of androgen excess. The

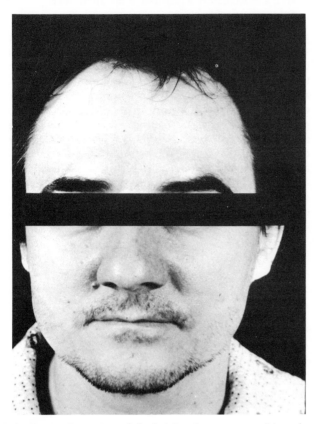

FIGURE 56-3 Recession of the hairline in a woman with androgen excess. Note the excessive facial hair growth over the upper lip, chin, and sideburn areas.

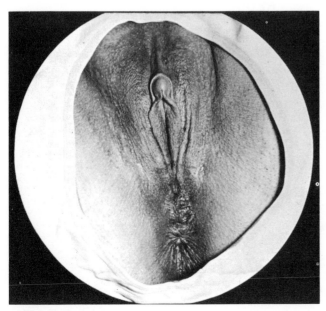

FIGURE 56-4 Clitoral enlargement in a woman with androgen excess.

problem usually begins after puberty and progresses slowly over a period of years. Patients may or may not have menstrual irregularities and may or may not present with polycystic ovaries. Urinary 17-ketosteroids are frequently slightly or moderately elevated, and testosterone production rates are increased. Free testosterone levels are also elevated. The specific biochemical defect and pathophysiology of this type of androgen excess is not well understood.

There are a number of miscellaneous causes of hirsutism. Some of them are of endrocrine origin and include the hirsutism associated with acromegaly, pregnancy, hypothyroidism, menopause, androgen therapy, and inanition. Increased hair growth may occur without hormonal stimulation. It is seen in disorders such as

porphyria and congenital ectodermal dysplasia or in areas of the body which have been either immobilized or placed in a body cast.

Clinical and laboratory evaluation of hirsute women

If a patient presents with complaints of excessive hair growth, it is necessary to determine whether the hirsutism is present by itself or accompanied by manifestations of virilization as described above. It is also important to determine whether the symptoms are those of androgen excess alone or are accompanied by symptoms of cortisol excess. A history of recent onset and rapid progression of excessive hair growth frequently suggests a malignancy as the source of excessive androgen production. In that case, one should suspect either an adrenal or ovarian tumor and perform such procedures as a pelvic examination, laparoscopy, adrenal venography, and adrenal photoscanning in order to confirm or rule out this diagnosis. In patients with simple or

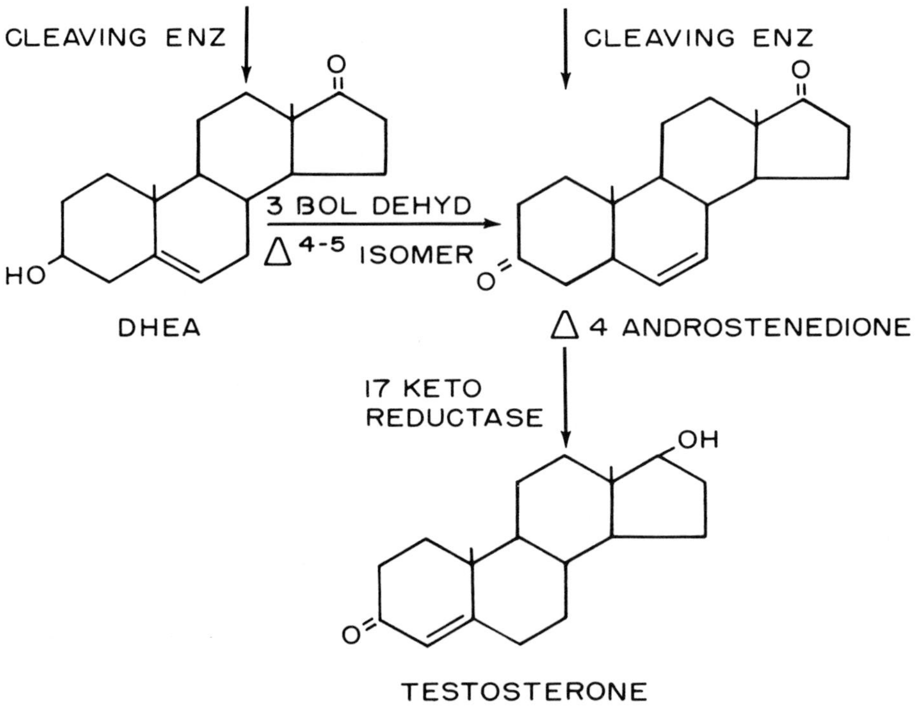

FIGURE 56-5 Three major types of androgens in the female. 17α-Hydroxypregnenolone is the immediate precursor of DHEA, while 17α-hydroxyprogesterone is the immediate precursor of Δ4-androstenedione. The transformation of the precursors to the androgen hormones is catalyzed by a cleaving enzyme. Δ4-Androstenedione can, in turn, be converted to testosterone by a step catalyzed by 17-ketoreductase.

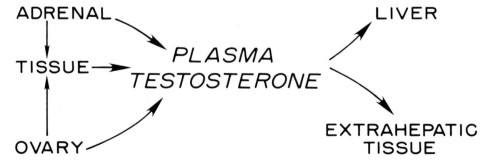

FIGURE 56-6 Metabolism of plasma testosterone. The plasma level of testosterone results from a balance between adrenal, ovarian, and peripheral tissue production of testosterone and clearance by the liver and extrahepatic tissues.

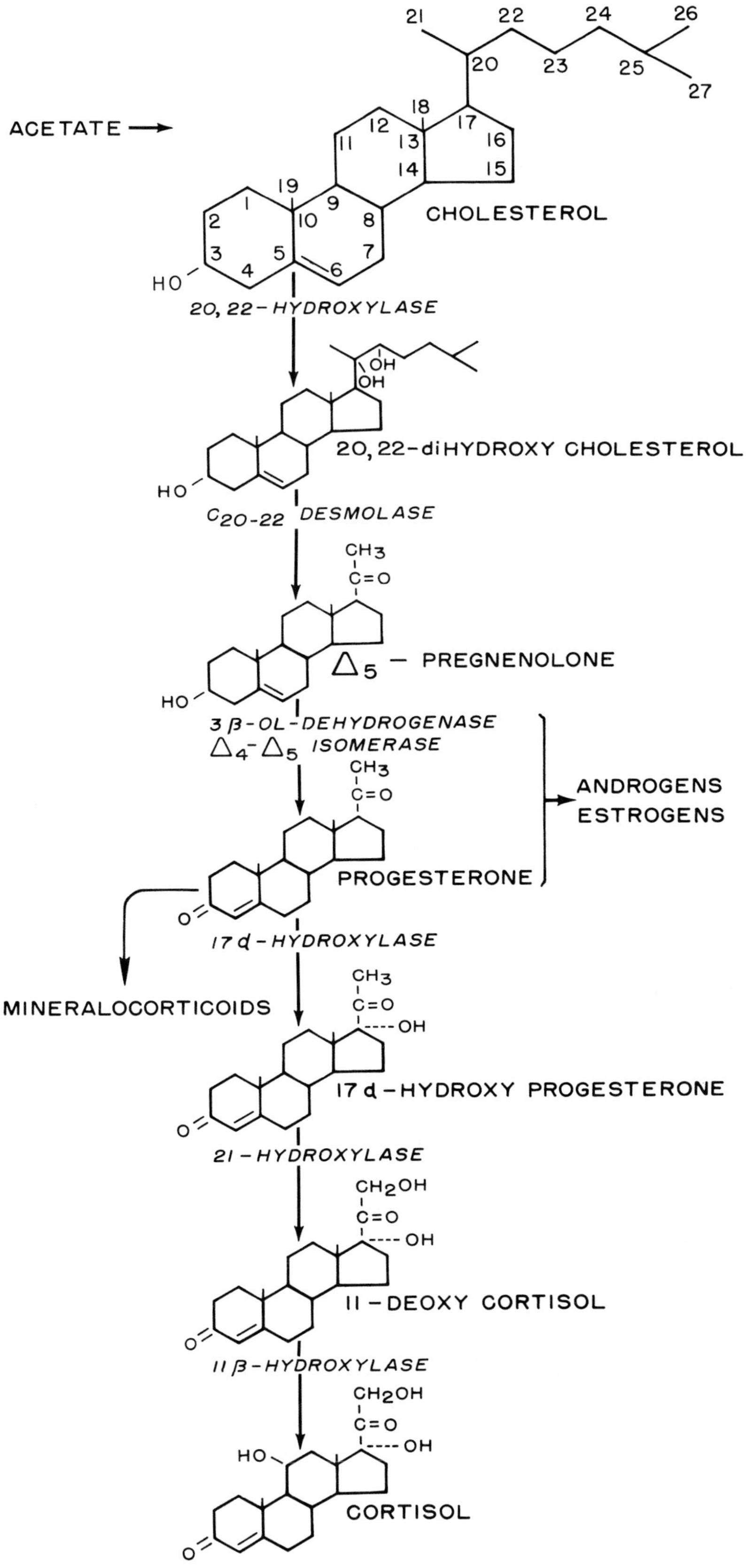

FIGURE 56-7 Pathway of cortisol biosynthesis. Δ5-Pregnenolone and progesterone are also precursors of androgens and estrogens. Progesterone is also a precursor of mineralocorticoids. The biosynthesis of cortisol takes place in the adrenal cortex. Each step is controlled by specific enzymes. A defect in 21-hydroxylase is the cause of the most common type of congenital adrenal hyperplasia.

idiopathic hirsutism, measurements of androgens in the urine and plasma will help confirm the presence of excessive androgen production. If one desires to identify the source of the androgens, suppression tests with glucocorticoids, estrogens, and progestogens as well as ovarian and adrenal-vein catheterization for measurement of regional androgen levels might help distinguish between adrenal and ovarian sources.

The treatment of states of androgen excess relates to the underlying pathology. If androgen excess is part of Cushing's syndrome, correction of Cushing's syndrome in the manner described in Chap. 53 will result in remission of the manifestations of androgen excess. Patients with congenital adrenal hyperplasia can be effectively suppressed by chronic suppressive therapy with glucocorticoid analogues. Patients with adrenal or ovarian tumors should undergo resection of these tumors. Patients with simple or idiopathic hirsutism can be treated with suppression of androgen production by means of glucocorticoid analogues (which suppress both adrenal and ovarian androgen production) as well as depilatory procedures aimed at removing excessive hair.

PITUITARY DISORDERS

General concepts

The pituitary gland is a complex structure at the base of the brain lying within the confines of a bony wall cavity, the sella turcica in the sphenoid bone at the base of the skull. It is formed early in embryonic development from the fusion of two ectodermal hollow processes. An invagination from the roof of the primitive oral region, Rathke's pouch, extends upward toward the base of the brain and is met by an outpouching of the floor of the third ventricle destined to become the neurohypophysis. The developed human pituitary gland is thus formed by a posterior lobe, or neurohypophysis, in continuity with the hypothalamus and an anterior lobe, or adenohypophysis, connected to the hypothalamus through the pituitary stalk. A vascular structure—the hypothalamic-hypophyseal portal system—also connects the hypothalamus with the anterior pituitary gland. It is through this system that releasing hormones from the hypothalamus reach the cells of the pituitary gland to promote hormone release.

The posterior lobe of the pituitary gland, or neurohypophysis, is mainly concerned with the regulation of fluid balance. Antidiuretic hormone is synthesized primarily in the supraoptic and paraventricular nuclei of the hypothalamus and stored in the neurohypophysis. The anterior pituitary gland has multiple functions, and because of its ability to regulate the function of other endocrine glands, it is also known as the *master gland*. The anterior pituitary cells are specialized to secrete specific hormones. Seven such hormones have been well identified, and their physiological metabolic roles defined. These are ACTH, MSH, TSH, FSH, LH, growth hormone, and prolactin. Some of these hormones (ACTH, MSH, growth hormone, and prolactin) are polypeptides, while others (TSH, FSH, and LH) are glycoproteins. Morphologic studies indicate that each hormone is synthesized by a specific cell type. In a sense, the anterior pituitary gland is a conglomeration of independent glands all of which are under hypothalamic control.

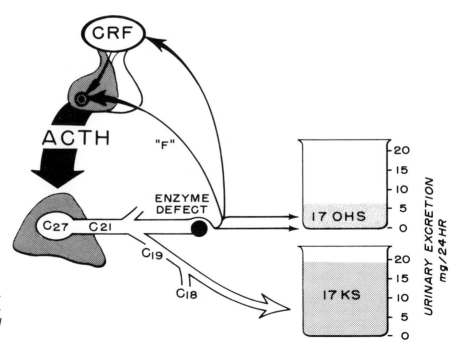

FIGURE 56-8 Biochemical and physiological consequence of enzyme deficiency in patients with congenital adrenal hyperplasia.

Growth hormone, prolactin, and MSH have direct metabolic effects on target tissues. In contrast, ACTH, TSH, FSH, and LH exert their main effect through the regulation of secretion of other endocrine glands and are therefore known as tropic hormones.

Growth hormone, or somatotropin, has major metabolic effects in both children and adults. In children, growth hormone is required for somatic growth. In adults, it may preserve normal adult organ size, and it participates in the regulation of protein synthesis and nutrient disposal. The growth-promoting effect of growth hormone appears to be mediated through the production by growth hormone of somatomedin. It is likely that without somatomedin growth hormone cannot promote growth. Secretion of growth hormone is regulated by a growth hormone–releasing hormone from the hypothalamus and by somatostatin, an inhibiting hormone. The release of growth hormone is stimulated by hypoglycemia and by amino acids such as arginine.

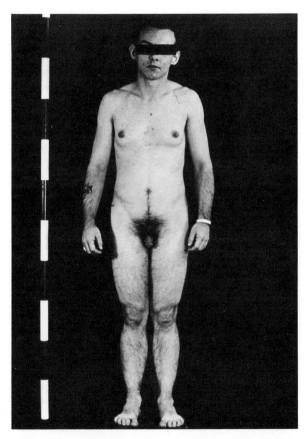

FIGURE 56-9 Female pseudohermaphroditism in a patient with congenital adrenal hyperplasia due to 21-hydroxylase deficiency. This patient had a male phenotype but was a genetic female. Note the masculine muscle development and body hair growth. On casual examination the patient appeared to have a developed penis. However, on closer examination this penis was seen to be an enlarged clitoris. The patient also had developed gynecomastia as a result of increased estrogen production accompanying the androgen excess.

Melanocyte-stimulating hormone (MSH) is similar in structure to a portion of the ACTH molecule. It appears to increase skin pigmentation by stimulating the dispersion of melanin granules in melanocytes. It is likely that its secretion is regulated by an MSH-releasing hormone and that it may be inhibited by a rise in cortisol. In fact, deficient secretion of cortisol can stimulate MSH release, while high cortisol levels suppress its secretion.

Prolactin has similarity in its molecular structure with growth hormone and some overlap with some of its biological properties. Prolactin is one of a group of hormones necessary for breast development and milk secretion. The release of prolactin is mediated mainly by the secretion of the hypothalamic inhibitory factor (PIF). In its absence prolactin secretion and lactation may occur.

ACTH regulates the growth and function of the adrenal cortex and is especially important in the control of the production and release of cortisol. By itself, ACTH does not appear to have significant extraadrenal effects.

TSH stimulates the growth and function of the thyroid gland. TSH causes thyroxine and triiodothyronine release, and these in turn regulate the secretion of TSH.

Follicle-stimulating hormone (FSH) and luteinizing hormone (LH) are also known as gonadotropins. In the male, FSH maintains and stimulates spermatogenesis, and LH the secretion of testosterone by the Leydig or interstitial cells of the testes. FSH and LH are secreted in the male in a continuous or tonic fashion. In contrast, in the female, FSH stimulates follicular development and the secretion of estrogens by the follicular cells. LH maintains and stimulates the secretion of progesterone by the corpus luteum which develops from the follicle after ovulation has occurred. The release of FSH and LH in the female follows a cylic pattern such that the levels of these two hormones rise at midcycle, triggering ovulation, and slowly decline toward the end of the cycle when menstruation occurs.

The clinical consequences of deficiencies in ACTH and TSH release are adrenal insufficiency and hypothyroidism, respectively. Absence of gonadotropin release leads to hypogonadism. Conversely, excessive secretion of ACTH leads to adrenocortical hyperfunction, or Cushing's syndrome. Syndromes of excessive TSH or gonadotropin release are more rare.

Clinical disorders of the pituitary gland

Clinical syndromes associated with abnormal function of the pituitary gland include diseases of hormone deficit and of hormone excess.

Pituitary insufficiency commonly affects all the hormones normally secreted by the anterior pituitary gland. The clinical manifestations of panhypopituitarism are, therefore, a composite of the metabolic effects caused by the deficient secretion of each one of the pituitary hormones.

Several pathological processes may result in pituitary insufficiency: (1) A pituitary tumor which destroys normal pituitary cells; (2) vascular thrombosis leading to necrosis of the normal pituitary gland; (3) infiltrative granulomatous diseases which destroy the pituitary; and (4) idiopathic or possible autoimmune destruction of pituitary cells.

The clinical syndrome resulting from panhypopituitarism differs in children and in adults. In children, there is interference with somatic growth caused by deficiency of growth hormone release. Pituitary dwarfism develops as a consequence of this deficiency. As the child reaches adolescence, there is absence of development of secondary sexual characteristics and of the external genitalia (see Fig. 56-10). In addition, patients may present with various degrees of adrenal insufficiency and hypothyroidism. They may have difficulty in school and exhibit slow intellectual development. Their skin is usually pale because of the absence of MSH.

When hypopituitarism develops in adults, loss of pituitary function frequently has the following chronol-ogy: loss of growth hormone, hypogonadism, hypothyroidism, and adrenal insufficiency. Since the adult has already completed somatic growth, adult patients with hypopituitarism are of normal height. Manifestations of growth hormone deficiency might be expressed by unusual sensitivity to insulin and fasting hypoglycemia. With the development of hypogonadism, male adults exhibit a decrease in libido, impotence, and a progressive decrease in body hair growth, beard, and muscular development (see Fig. 56-11). In women, cessation of menstral periods, or amenorrhea, is one of the early manifestations of pituitary failure. This is accompanied by atrophy of the breasts and of the external genitalia. Both men and women will show various degrees of hypothyroidism (see Chap. 57) and adrenal insufficiency (see Chap. 53). Deficiency of MSH will cause a sallow or pale appearance in these patients.

Occasionally, patients exhibit isolated pituitary hormone failure. Under these circumstances the cause of the deficiency is likely to be in the hypothalamus and involve the corresponding releasing factor.

GIANTISM AND ACROMEGALY

Giantism and acromegaly are caused by excessive secretion of growth hormone. This can result from a pituitary tumor which secretes growth hormone or from a hypothalamic abnormality involving growth hormone release.

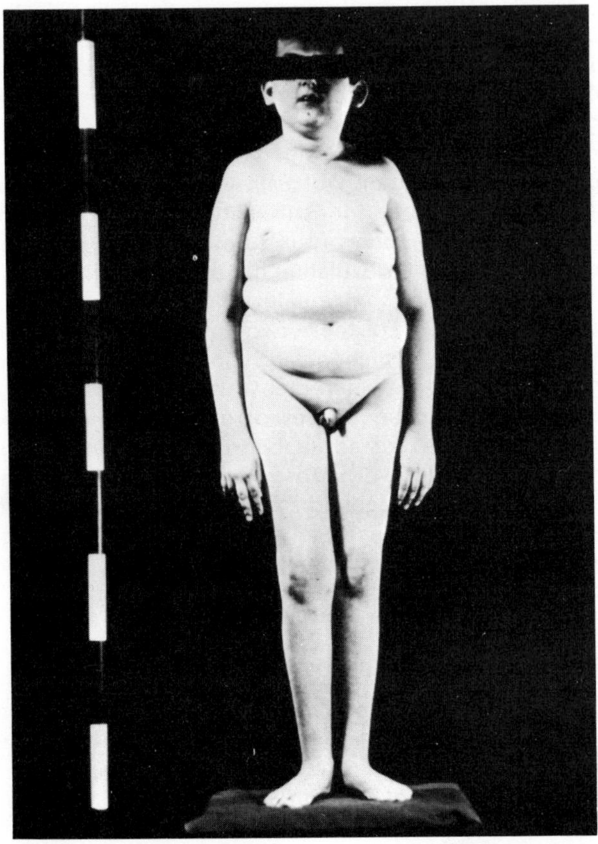

FIGURE 56-10 Short stature and absence of secondary sexual characteristics in a patient with panhypopituitarism developing during childhood.

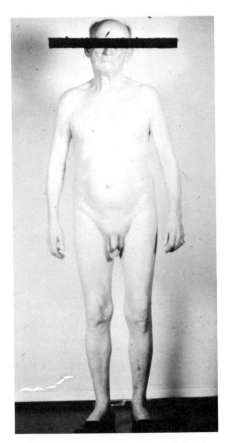

FIGURE 56-11 Panhypopituitarism in the adult. There is loss of body hair growth and pallor.

When growth hormone excess occurs during childhood and adolescence, the patient experiences rapid longitudinal growth and becomes a giant. After somatic growth is completed, growth hormone hypersecretion will not cause giantism but thickening of bones and soft tissue. This condition is termed *acromegaly,* meaning large hands and feet. Patients with acromegaly exhibit enlargement of hands and feet. Hands become not only larger but also more square (spadelike) and the fingers more round and stubby (see Fig. 56-12). Patients may relate the need for larger glove size. The feet also become larger and wider, and patients describe changes in shoe size (see Fig. 56-13). The enlargement is usually caused by growth and thickening of bones and by increased growth of soft tissue (see Fig. 56-14). In addition, there are changes in facial features which help diagnose the condition on simple observation. Facial features become coarse, and there is enlargement of the paranasal and frontal sinuses. There are frontal bossing, prominence of the supraorbital ridges, and deformity of the mandible with development of prognathism and overbite (see Fig. 56-15). Enlargement of the mandible causes the teeth to spread apart. There is enlargement of the tongue which causes difficulty with speech (see Fig. 56-16). The voice becomes deeper as a result of thickening of the vocal chords. Deformities of the spine, caused by overgrowth of bone, lead to back pain and changes in the physiological curvature of the spine. The x-ray examination of the skull in acromegaly shows typical changes with enlarge-

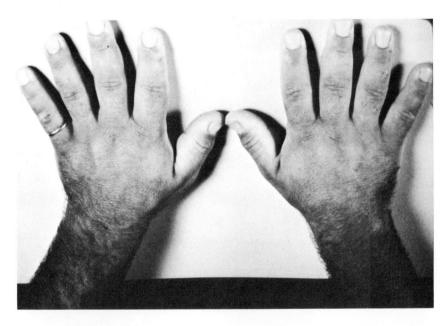

FIGURE 56-12 Hands of a patient with acromegaly.

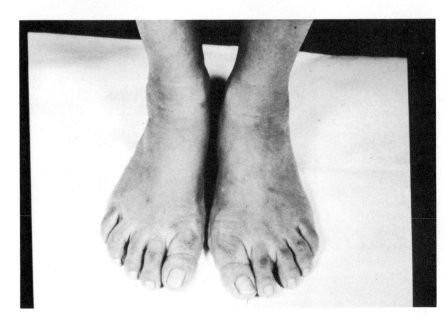

FIGURE 56-13 Feet of a patient with acromegaly.

ment of the paranasal sinuses, thickening of the calvarium, deformity of the mandible which resembles a boomerang, and, most important, enlargement and destruction of the sella turcica suggesting a pituitary tumor (see Fig. 56-17).

When acromegaly is associated with a pituitary tumor, the patients may exhibit bitemporal headaches and visual disturbance with bitemporal hemianopsia resulting from suprasellar extension of the tumor and compression of the optic chiasma.

The treatment of hypopituitarism is simple. It consists of replacement of the deficient hormones. Human growth hormone, the only one effective in humans, is available in small quantities for experimental studies. When administered to patients with pituitary dwarfism, it may cause significant increase in height. All the pituitary hormones can be administered only by injection. Thus, for long-term, daily replacement therapy, the hormones of the target glands affected by the pituitary deficiency are administered instead. For example, treatment of adrenal insufficiency caused by deficiency of ACTH secretion consists of the administration of hydrocortisone orally. Treatment of hypothyroidism caused by TSH deficiency consists of the administration of thyroxine orally. Gonadotropin deficiency can be treated by administering androgens and estrogens. However, induction of ovulation necessitates the administration of gonadotropins.

Treatment of acromegaly or giantism is rather complex. Pituitary irradiation, surgery to the pituitary gland in order to resect a pituitary tumor, or combinations of these procedures may result in amelioration or remission of the disease.

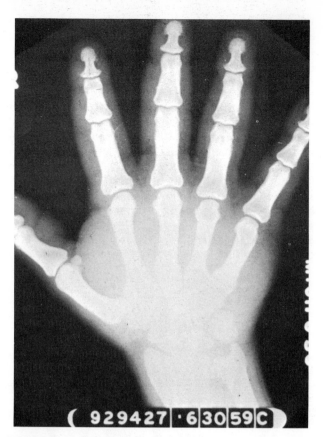

FIGURE 56-14 *Radiographic appearance of the hand of an acromegalic patient. There is increase in soft tissues and in density of the bones, squaring of the phalanges, and increased tufting of the terminal phalanges.*

DISORDERS OF CALCIUM BALANCE

General concepts

Calcium plays an important role in biological processes. It is an important constituent of biological membranes, affecting their permeability and electrical properties. For example, a lowering of the concentration of calcium outside the cell causes an increase in permeability and excitability of the cell membrane. Calcium also has an effect on neuromuscular activity. A decrease in calcium concentration increases the excitability of nerve tissue and can stimulate muscle contraction. In fact, calcium acts as a coupling factor between muscle excitation and contraction of actomyosin. Calcium is involved in the release of preformed hormones by endocrine cells and in the secretion of transmitter substances at synaptic junctions. It also participates in the mechanism of action of hormones within the cells. For example, it may be an important component in the action of cylic AMP, the secon-

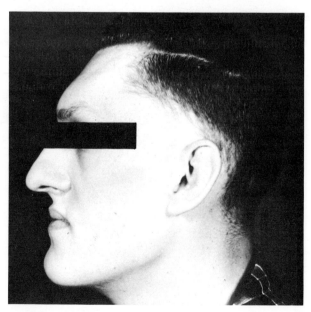

FIGURE 56-15 *Profile of a patient with acromegaly. There is prominence of the supraorbital ridges, prognathism, and coarsening of facial features.*

dary intracellular messenger. Calcium is important in the property of adhesiveness that binds cells together, in enzyme activity, and in blood coagulation.

The maintenance of normal serum calcium levels depends on the balance between calcium input and output from the bloodstream. The main sources of calcium are the diet and the skeleton with its large pool of calcium salts. The average adult intake of calcium in the North American diet is 600 to 1000 mg/day. This calcium is absorbed widely from the gastrointestinal tract. Calcium output is through the kidney and bone; 98 percent of the filtered calcium load is reabsorbed by the renal tubule by a process similar to that which regulates sodium excretion. Gastrointestinal losses, deposition of calcium into the bone mineral, and urinary clearance of calcium are the major mechanisms of calcium loss.

Several factors regulate or alter the movement of calcium in the bloodstream. Parathyroid hormone, calcitonin, and vitamin D are the three major factors concerned with this regulation.

Parathyroid hormone (PTH) is a polypeptide secreted by the parathyroid glands which are located in the neck, behind the lobes of the thyroid gland. There are four parathyroid glands, two right and two left, two superior and two inferior. Release of PTH varies with the concentration of calcium perfusing the parathyroid glands. For example, PTH release occurs in response to hypocalcemia, while secretion is suppressed by hypercalcemia. PTH acts on the gastrointestinal tract, bone, and kidney. It stimulates calcium absorption through the intestinal mucosa, it stimulates bone reabsorption by enhancing osteoclastic activity, and it increases the renal clearance of phosphorus by diminishing its tubular reabsorption. Excessive PTH secretion results in hypercalcemia and hypophosphatemia, while deficiency of PTH secretion leads to hypocalcemia and hyperphosphatemia.

Calcitonin is a hormone produced by the C cells, or parafollicular cells, of the thyroid gland. Calcitonin is released in response to hypercalcemia. It lowers serum calcium levels by inhibiting bone reabsorption. The actual physiologic role of calcitonin in the minute-to-minute regulation of calcium levels has not yet been clarified.

Vitamin D works in concert with parathyroid hormone in the regulation of calcium levels. Vitamin D_3, or cholecalciferol, is either ingested with the diet or synthesized through activation of 7-dehydrocholesterol in the skin by ultraviolet radiation from sunlight. Vitamin D_3 is absorbed in the jejunum and ileum and subsequently metabolized into an active form, first in the liver and ultimately in the kidney. The metabolism of vitamin D_3 involves sequential hydroxylations. In the liver it is converted to 25-hydroxycholecalciferol and in the kidney to 1,25-dihydroxycholecalciferol. Vitamin D_3 in its active form acts on the intestine and the bone. In the intestine it promotes absorption of calcium, while in the bone it stimulates bone reabsorption. Vitamin D_3 is an essential cofactor for PTH in both bone and kidney. In its absence, hypocalcemia and disturbances in bone mineralization may occur.

The total serum calcium concentration reflects the concentration of calcium present in several physical chemical states. As indicated in Table 56-2, slightly less than 50 percent of the circulating calcium is present in a form bound to protein. The rest is non–protein bound, of which the major portion is ionized and freely diffusible. It is this fraction which exerts biological effects and best correlates with the physiological actions of calcium in body fluids and systems perfused by them. The normal total serum calcium level is 9 to 10.5 mg%.

HYPERCALCEMIA

Hypercalcemia is defined as a calcium level above 10.5 mg%. There are many conditions which may lead to hypercalcemia, but PTH excess is by far the most common cause. Excessive production of PTH may occur as the result of primary hyperparathyroidism or secretion of

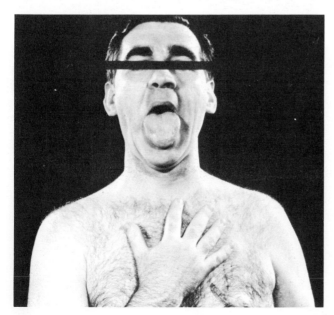

FIGURE 56-16 Enlargement of the tongue in a patient with acromegaly. Also, note a typical acromegalic hand.

TABLE 56-2
State of calcium in blood

	AMOUNT OF mg%
Total Serum Ca	9.5
Bound to protein	4.0
Not bound to protein	5.5
Ionized	4.5
Complexed (citrate, bicarbonate, phosphate)	1.0

a PTH-like peptide by nonparathyroid malignancies. In addition, hypercalcemia may be found in association with tertiary hyperparathyroidism observed in chronic uremia and after dialysis or renal transplantation. Usually, hyperparathyroidism is caused by a benign adenoma of the parathyroid glands. The excessive secretion of PTH by these adenomas is responsible for hypercalcemia, hypophosphatemia, and increased bone reabsorption. Occasionally, hyperparathyroidism may result from hyperplasia of all four parathyroid glands. In this case, all four parathyroids are the source of excessive PTH secretion. Several types of nonparathyroid neoplasms have been found to be associated with hypercalcemia. Parathormone-like peptides have been identified in patients with these neoplasms. It is postulated that the neoplasm has acquired the capacity to synthesize and release peptide hormones. Bronchial carcinomas, squamous-cell carcinomas, hypernephromas, and carcinoma of the liver are among those neoplasms associated with hypercalcemia.

There are many other types of conditions in which hypercalcemia develops independently of PTH. In fact, PTH is suppressed by the high calcium level. Included among these conditions are vitamin D intoxication, sarcoidosis, acute immobilization, hyperthyroidism, multiple myloma, and metastatic malignancy with skeletal involvement.

Symptoms and signs of hypercalcemia vary greatly depending on the rapidity of onset and the degree of elevation of serum calcium levels. In mild cases, one may find patients who are completely asymptomatic and whose hypercalcemia is discovered only through a routine laboratory investigation. On the other hand, there are severe cases where patients deteriorate rapidly and become dehydrated, confused, and lethargic. Their serum calcium levels are markedly elevated.

Symptoms of hypercalcemia involve the gastrointestinal tract, with anorexia, nausea, vomiting, weight loss, and constipation; the urinary tract, with polydipsia, polyuria, and nephrocalcinosis; the cardiovascular system, with hypertension and electrocardiographic changes, and neuropsychiatric manifestations such as lethargy, apathy, myopathy, and electromyographic abnormalities. Patients whose hypercalcemia is secondary to hyperparathyroidism have, in addition to the changes described, skeletal changes caused by the effect of parathyroid hormone on bone. Usually there is increased bone reabsorption with formation of bone cysts and erosion in the subperiosteal edges of the long bones (see Fig. 56-18). In its fully developed stage, the skeletal manifestations constitute osteitis fibrosa cystica.

The diagnosis of hyperparathyroidism is based on the demonstration of high serum calcium and low serum phosphate levels together with elevated serum PTH levels. When the hypercalcemia is caused by one of the PTH-independent conditions, the hypercalcemia may not be associated with hypophosphatemia, and the serum parathyroid hormone level is usually suppressed.

Treatment

If the condition is caused by hyperparathyroidism, treatment involves the excision of the parathyroid tumor or subtotal removal of all four parathyroid glands. In the PTH-independent types of hypercalcemia, correction depends on the treatment of the underlying disease. Since the underlying disease may be a malignancy which does not respond to therapy, it may be necessary to lower the serum calcium level by other means. These generally include effective hydration and the use of agents that enhance renal calcium excretion or drugs like calcitonin

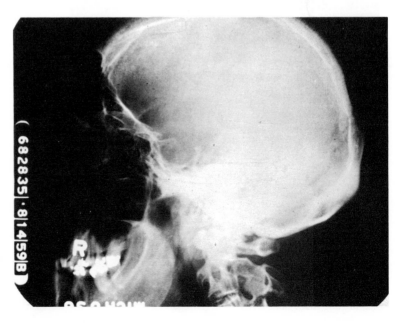

FIGURE 56-17 Radiographic appearance of the skull of a patient with acromegaly. There is marked enlargement and destruction of the sella turcica with suggestion of intrasellar calcifications. The calvarium is thick, and there is marked prominence of the frontal and paranasal sinuses. The angle of the mandible is rounded. There is also evidence of overbite.

and mithramycin which inhibit calcium reabsorption. Phosphate salts are frequently used for correction of hypercalcemia because phosphate binds calcium and precipitates it out of the bloodstream. A side effect of this treatment might be precipitation of calcium phosphate in the renal parenchyma. Thus, it should not be administered to patients with impaired renal function.

HYPOCALCEMIA

Hypocalcemia is defined as the clinical condition caused by serum calcium levels of less than 9.0 mg%. It may result from the surgical removal of all four parathyroid glands or may develop as the result of autoimmune destruction of these glands. The parathyroid glands may be removed accidentally in the course of a thyroidectomy. The condition associated with autoimmune destruction of the glands is known as *idiopathic hypoparathyroidism*.

The clinical manifestations of hypocalcemia are: tetany, seizures, mental disturbances, and ectodermal lesions. Tetany is characterized by involuntary muscle spasms. This may involve muscles of the upper and lower extremities causing carpopedal spasms, paresthesias, and occasionally laryngeal stridor. When respiratory muscles are involved, respiratory distress may be a manifestation of hypocalcemia. Usually, the increased neuro-

muscular excitability can be demonstrated by tapping over the facial nerve anterior to the ear. A unilateral contraction of the facial muscle occurs (Chvostek's sign). It can also be demonstrated by the Trousseau test, which is the carpal spasm induced by placing a blood pressure cuff on the arm and inflating it above systolic pressure. Occasionally, epileptiform seizures can occur in patients who have an underlying seizure disorder and who subsequently develop hypocalcemia. Patients with hypocalcemia usually complain of a variety of emotional disturbances, including irritability, emotional instability, impairment of memory, and confusion. Prolonged hypocalcemia, as seen in idiopathic hypoparathyroidism, may cause changes in the skin, hair, and nails as well as in the teeth and lenses. The skin may be coarse, dry, and scaly, and alopecia may develop with patchy or absent eyelashes and eyebrows. The nails become thin and brittle with transverse grooves. The teeth may erupt late and appear hypoplastic. Cataracts may develop within a few years of untreated hypocalcemia.

Treatment

Treatment of hypocalcemia is based on the administration of calcium salts and vitamin D in order to enhance intestinal absorption of calcium. Calcium salts are available as calcium gluconate, calcium lactate, or calcium choloride. Giving 10 to 15 g calcium gluconate or lactate daily is usually necessary. Vitamin D is given in doses of 50,000 to 150,000 units/day. When patients are treated with the proper combination of calcium and vitamin D, serum calcium levels can be maintained within the normal range.

QUESTIONS

Syndrome of androgen excess—Chap. 56

Directions: Circle the letter preceding every correct response in each of the items below. More than one answer may be correct.

1 A female with hirsutism may present with which of the following signs and symptoms?
a Amenorrhea, or irregular menstrual periods   b Increased breast size   c Hair growth under the chin   d Increased fertility

2 Androstenedione, a steroid precursor of testosterone, is:
a Produced in the ovary and adrenal cortex of adult females   b Produced only in the male testis   c A 17-ketosteroid   d Present in higher concentration in the plasma of hirsute and virilized females   e A less potent androgen than dehydroepiandrosterone

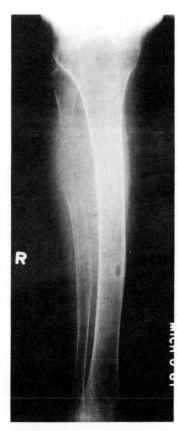

FIGURE 56-18 Lesions of osteitis fibrosa cystica in the tibia and fibula of a patient with hyperparathyroidism.

3 Congenital adrenal hyperplasia, of the 21-hydroxylase variety, is characterized by:
a A masculinized genetic female fetus b A feminized genetic male fetus c High ACTH levels d Low serum cortisol levels e Increased urine 17-keto-steroids

4 Which of the following conditions may result in excessive androgen production?
a Polycystic ovary syndrome b Arrhenoblastoma c Adrenal carcinoma d Hilus-cell tumor of the ovary

5 Manifestations of virilism include all the following except:
a Acne b Receding hairline, balding c Decreased body hair growth d Clitoral enlargement e Deepening of voice

Match the statements in col. A with the structures in col. B.

Column A
6 ___ Derived from neural cells of the developing 3d ventricle
7 ___ Derived from Rathke's pouch
8 ___ Connected to hypothalamus by the hypothalamic-hypophyseal portal system
9 ___ Confined within the sella turcica of the sphenoid bone

Column B
a Adenohypophysis
b Neurohypophysis
c Both of the above

Match the hormones in col. A with one of the functions in col. B.

Column A
10 ___ Adrenocorticotropic hormone (ACTH)
11 ___ Growth hormone (GH)
12 ___ (LH) Luteinizing hormone
13 ___ Follicle-stimulating hormone (FSH)
14 ___ Prolactin
15 ___ Thyrotropin (TSH)
16 ___ Melanocyte-stimulating hormone (MSH)
17 ___ Antidiuretic hormone (ADH)

Column B
a Stimulates spermatogenesis in the male
b Stimulates the formation and release of thyroid hormones
c Initiates milk secretion after delivery
d Stimulates the secretory activity of the adrenal cortex
e Stimulates somatomedin
f Decreases free water clearance
g Stimulates the corpus luteum to secrete progesterone and estrogens in human females
h Increases pigmentation of the skin

Directions: Circle the letter preceding every correct response in each of the items below. More than one answer may be correct.

18 The hypothalamus secretes neurohormones which:
a Facilitate the formation of a corpus luteum in the ovary b Inhibit the release of prolactin from the pituitary c Increase the synthesis of hydrocortisone by the adrenal cortex d Facilitate thyroid growth e Increase the release of parathormone by the parathyroid glands

19 Antidiuretic hormone is:
a Synthesized in the neurohypophysis b Secreted by the adenohypophysis c Secreted by the supraoptic and paraventricular nuclei in the hypothalamus d Stored and released from the neurohypophysis

20 MSH secretion is:
a Inhibited by high serum levels of cortisol b Depressed in Cushing's disease caused by pituitary ACTH excess c Greatly increased in Addison's disease d Probably controlled by a releasing hormone

21 Which of the following statements about growth hormone is false?
a It is released in response to hypoglycemia b Its release is controlled by a hypothalamic-releasing factor and somatostatin c Its release is inhibited by the administration of arginine d Its anabolic effect is mediated through somatomedin

22 Prepuberal panhypopituitarism may be manifested by:
a Acromegaly b Retardation of growth c Pale, dry skin d Precocious sexual development e Slow intellectual development

23 A 35-year-old multiparous female seeks medical help because of vague symptoms of lethargy, lack of energy, and intolerance to cold. The history reveals that her menstrual periods ceased 1 year earlier following the birth of her last child which was complicated by postpartum hemorrhage. She is concerned that she is losing her sexual attractiveness. Physical examination reveals an asthenic female with thin hair, atrophied breasts, and thin pubic hair. Blood pressure 94/60; TPR 97-54-16. Laboratory findings include: low thyroidal radioiodine uptake; normal serum cholesterol; depressed serum levels of ACTH; depressed urinary levels of 17-ketosteroids, 17-hydroxysteroids, and gonadotropins. The above data are suggestive of:
a Primary hypothyroidism b Premature menopause in an otherwise healthy female c Psychoneuroticism d Primary adrenal insufficiency e Panhypopituitarism

24 A possible explanation for this patient's condition is:
a A congenital disorder b Postpartum necrosis of the pituitary c Adrenal carcinoma d Autoimmune disease of the thyroid

25 Acromegaly results from:
a Hypersecretion of growth hormone in a child b Hypersecretion of growth hormone in an adult c Parathormone hypersecretion d Pituitary insufficiency

26 Physical signs of acromegaly include:
a Frontal bossing b Prominence of the supraorbital ridges c Broad, greatly enlarged, spadeshaped hands d Prognathism

27 Patients with acromegaly often experience:
a Slurred speech b Weight loss c Hypoglycemia d Headaches

28 Common radiologic signs in acromegaly include:
a Thickened calvarium b Enlargement of the paranasal and frontal sinuses c Increased length and thickness of the mandible d Enlargement of the sella turcica

29 Bodily processes affected by the concentration of calcium ion include:
a Contractility of cardiac and skeletal muscle b Permeability of the cell membrane to sodium and potassium c Release of neurotransmitters at synaptic junctions d Excitability of nerve tissue

30 The calcium in plasma:
a Exists only in the ionized form b Is bound to protein to the extent of about 42 percent c Normally has a total concentration of 9 to 10 mg% d Is precisely regulated at a constant level

31 The two most important factors affecting calcium homeostasis are:
a Active form of vitamin D_3 b Parathormone c Calcitonin d Thyroxine

32 Vitamin D_3 is converted to 1,25-dihydroxycholecalciferol in the:
a Skin b Intestine c Lung d Kidney

33 In primary hyperparathyroidism:
a Serum levels of PTH are always greater than in persons with hypercalcemia due to vitamin D_3 intoxication b An adenoma of one or more of the parathyroids is often the cause of the hypersecretion c Secretion of parathormone is no longer influenced by the level of serum calcium d There may be a generalized loss of bone density on x-ray examination

34 Parathormone-independent causes of hypercalcemia include:
a Vitamin D intoxication b Malignant neoplasm with osseous metastasis c Multiple myeloma d Chronic renal failure e Prolonged immobilization

35 The most common cause of hypoparathyroidism is:
a Autoimmune destruction of the parathyroid glands b Damage to the parathyroid glands during thyroid surgery or following removal of the parathyroid glands for hyperparathyroidism

36 Deficiency of parathyroid hormone results in:
a Increased renal tubular reabsorption of phosphate b Hypoplasia of developing teeth c Decreased density of bones d Increased neuromuscular irritability

Directions: Circle T if the statement is true and F if it is false. Correct any false statements.

37   T   F   Hypocalcemia may be treated by the administration of vitamin D and calcium salts.

38   T   F   A deficiency of 21-hydroxylase causes an increase in cortisol production and decrease in ACTH secretion.

39   T   F   Patients with congenital adrenal hyperplasia may be effectively treated by prednisone therapy.

40   T   F   Gonadotropin deficiency in hypopituitarism may be treated by the administration of androgens and estrogens.

41   T   F   Growth hormone for treatment of hypopituitary dwarfs is obtained by extraction of the hormone from the pituitary glands of cattle and swine.

CHAPTER 57 Diseases of the Thyroid Gland

OBJECTIVES **At the completion of Chap. 57 you should be able to:**

1 Differentiate between thyroxine (T_4) and triiodothyronine (T_3) in terms of structure, function, and potency.

2 Give a classification of thyroid diseases on the basis of disturbances in thyroid function.

3 Describe tests of thyroid function.

4 Indicate the rationale for measuring thyroid-stimulating hormone (TSH) levels in the diagnosis of hypothyroidism.

5 Define hyperthyroidism.

6 Identify the etiology and major signs and symptoms associated with Graves' disease. Describe its thyroidal and extrathyroidal manifestations.

7 Identify three types of approaches that may be used for the treatment of hyperthyroidism.

8 Differentiate between primary and secondary hypothyroidism.

9 Differentiate between cretinism, juvenile hypothyroidism, and adult hypothyroidism according to age group affected, signs and symptoms, reversible changes, and treatment.

10 Describe clinical features and diagnostic studies which may help distinguish benign from malignant thyroid nodules.

GENERAL CONSIDERATIONS

The thyroid is a gland with two lobes joined by a thin isthmus located below the cricoid cartilage in the neck. Embryologically, the thyroid gland descends from the base of the tongue into the neck; some thyroid tissue may occasionally be seen along this track. The thyroid gland normally weighs between 10 and 20 g in adults. Histologically, the gland is made up of nodules composed of tiny follicles. These follicles are separated from each other by connective tissue (see Fig. 57-1). The thyroid follicles are lined by cuboidal epithelium made up of cells which synthesize and release hormones. In addition, the follicles contain a homogeneous colloid material where thyroid hormones are stored. Another type of hormone-secreting cell, the parafollicular or C cell, is found in the basal portion of the follicle and in contact with the basal follicular membrane.

The thyroid gland secretes two types of hormones: (1) Thyroxine and triiodothyronine which are involved with iodine metabolism and the regulation of basal metabolic rates, and (2) calcitonin, a hormone which is involved in calcium metabolism. Thyroxine and triiodothyronine are produced by the follicular epithelial cells. Thyroxine contains four iodine atoms (T_4), and triiodothyronine three iodine atoms (T_3). When compared on a milligram-per-milligram basis, triiodothyronine is the most potent of the two hormones; it is also present in much lower quantities than thyroxine. Calcitonin is a hormone which lowers serum calcium levels and is produced by the parafollicular cells.

One of the principal functions of the thyroid gland is the regulation of iodine metabolism. Ingestion of iodine varies quite widely throughout the world, and some populations suffer from iodine deficiency. In modern communities most table salt has been iodized in order to provide an adequate dietary supplement of iodine. From the gastrointestinal tract, iodine enters the body and is transported in the circulation as inorganic iodide. The thyroid gland takes up between 10 and 40 percent of circulating iodide. Almost all the remainder is lost in the urine.

The biosynthesis of thyroid hormones involves a sequence of steps which are regulated by specific enzymes. These steps are (1) trapping of iodide; (2) oxidation of iodide to iodine; (3) organification of iodine into monoiodotyrosine; (4) coupling of iodinated precursors; (5) storage; and (6) release of hormones (see Fig. 57-2).

The trapping of iodide by the thyroid follicular cells is an active, energy-requiring process. The thyroid concentrates large amounts of iodide which it takes up from the circulating iodide pool. The thyroid:plasma gradient is 20:1 at a wide range of plasma inorganic iodide concentration. Iodide is converted to iodine, catalyzed by a peroxidase enzyme. Iodine is then incorporated into a tyrosine molecule, a process which is described as organification of iodine. The resulting compounds, monoiodotyrosine and diiodotyrosine, are then coupled as follows: two molecules of diiodotyrosine make thyroxine (T_4), and one molecule of diiodotyrosine and one molecule of monoiodotyrosine make triiodothyronine (T_3). The coupling step usually takes place within thyroglobulin, a protein present in the lumen of the thyroid follicle. Thyroxine and triiodothyronine are subsequently stored within the thyroglobulin. Hormone release from storage is catalyzed by proteases acting on thyroglobulin. The various steps involved in the synthesis of thyroid hormones are stimulated by thyrotropin (TSH).

Thyroid hormones circulate in plasma bound to three plasma proteins: (1) a specific glycoprotein, thyroxine-binding globulin (TBG); (2) thyroxine binding pre-albumin (TBPA), and (3) thyroxine-binding albumin

(TBA). Of the three proteins, TBG has the greatest specificity for thyroxine binding. In addition, thyroxine has much greater affinity than triiodothyronine for these binding proteins.

Thyroid hormones are chemically altered before excretion. An important alteration is deiodination. Thyroxine (T_4) may be converted into triiodothyronine (T_3) or reverse triiodothyronine (RT_3), a metabolically inactive hormone. In addition, thyroid hormones may be altered by deamination and decarboxylation or by conjugation with glucuronic acid and sulfate.

Thyroid function is controlled by the pituitary glycoprotein hormone TSH, which in turn is regulated by thyroid-releasing hormone (TRH), a hypothalamic neurohormone. In turn, thyroxine exerts negative feedback regulation of TSH secretion by a direct effect on the pituitary gland.

Actions of thyroid hormones

Both thyroxine and triiodothyronine stimulate calorigenesis, potentiate epinephrine, lower serum cholesterol, and stimulate growth. It is likely that the effects of these hormones require protein synthesis. In addition, they may stimulate oxidative processes within the mitochondria of the cells on which they act. Thyroid hormones are also involved in the normal development of the central nervous system. In their absence, mental retardation and delayed neurological maturation may be present at birth and in infancy.

Tests of thyroid function

The functional status of the thyroid gland can be ascertained by means of thyroid function tests. The following tests are frequently used in the diagnosis of thyroid disease: (1) Radioactive iodine (RAI) uptake, (2) serum thyroxine and triiodothyronine, (3) T_3 resin uptake, and (4) serum TSH levels. These tests assess the physiological steps described above. For example, the radioactive iodine (^{131}I) uptake test measures the ability of the thyroid gland to trap iodide. The measurement of the serum level of thyroxine gives a good estimation of the circulating level of this hormone, and the T_3 resin uptake test measures the saturation of plasma-binding proteins by thyroxine. When the radioactive iodine uptake test is performed, the patient receives a tracer dose of radioactive iodine (^{131}I) which the thyroid traps and concentrates over a 24-hour period. By counting the radioactivity concentrated by the thyroid, it is possible to calculate the percent of tracer which has been taken up by the thyroid over that period of time. Normally, the radioactive iodine uptake ranges from 10 to 35 percent. Values are high in hyperthyroidism and low in hypothyroidism. The serum thyroxine and triiodothyronine levels can be measured by radioligand assays. Normal levels for thyroxine

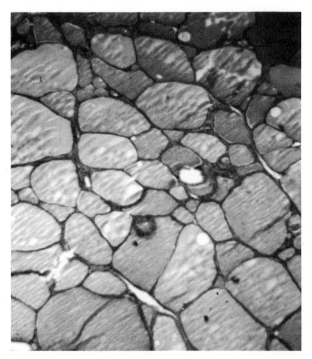

FIGURE 57-1 Histology of the thyroid gland. Note colloid of filled follicles. (Courtesy of Dr. Ronald Nishiyama, Pathology Department, University of Michigan.)

are 3.6 to 8.5 μg% and for triiodothyronine are 60 to 200 ng/ml. The T_3 resin uptake test measures the saturation of thyroxine-binding proteins by thyroxine and indirectly the level of thyroid hormone. When this test is performed, the patient's plasma is placed in a test tube together with radioactive T_3 and a resin. The radioactive T_3 will bind to both the plasma and the resin. A normal T_3 resin uptake test ranges between 86 and 110 percent. When the plasma level of thyroxine is high and the protein is completely saturated by thyroid hormone, more of the T_3 will be bound by the resin and less by the protein. Conversely, when the thyroxine level is low and the binding proteins are at a low level of saturation, more of the T_3 will bind to the protein and less to the resin. Thus, indirectly one can assess the level of thyroxine by the degree of saturation of its binding protein. Plasma TSH levels can be measured by radioimmunoassay. Normal values range from 0 to 10 μ/ml. Values are high in patients with primary hypothyroidism.

At the present time there is no single thyroid function test which will consistently provide all the answers in any given patient with thyroid disease. Therefore, combinations of tests are frequently necessary in order to diagnose the nature of a patient's thyroid problem. Hyper- and hypothyroidism are the two major functional abnormalities for which one needs to have reliable laboratory tools. Although in severe cases a clinical diagnosis may require very few supportive laboratory investigations, in milder cases the latter may become essential. Table 57-1 summarizes the changes in thyroid function tests observed in patients with hypo- and hyperthyroidism.

DISEASES OF THE THYROID GLAND

As with other endocrine diseases, those of the thyroid gland may involve: (1) Excessive thyroid hormone production—hyperthyroidism—or (2) deficient hormone production—hypothyroidism. In addition, patients may have (3) thyroid enlargement—goiters—without evidence of abnormal thyroid hormone production (see Fig. 57-3).

Hyperthyroidism

Also known as thyrotoxicosis, hyperthyroidism may be defined as the body tissue's response to excessive thyroid hormone. Graves' disease is the most common form

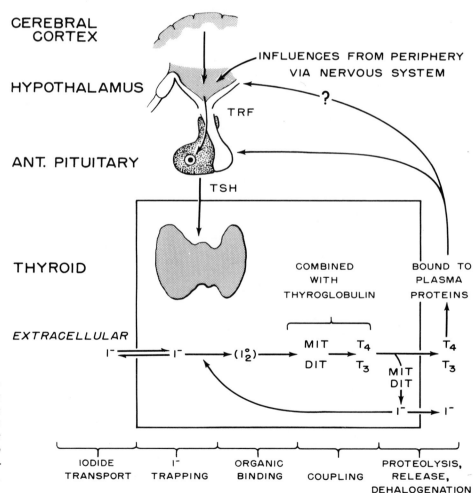

FIGURE 57-2 Synthesis and secretion of thyroid hormones. The box indicates steps which occur within the thyroid gland. Thyroid function is regulated by the hypothalamic pituitary axis. (Adapted from Ezrin et al. (eds.), Systematic Endocrinology, Harper & Row, New York, 1973 p. 58.)

of hyperthyroidism. In Graves' disease there may be two major groups of features, thyroidal and extrathyroidal, either of which may be absent. The thyroid features include a goiter, caused by diffuse hyperplasia of the thyroid gland and hyperthyroidism which results from the consequence of excessive thyroid hormone secretion. Symptoms include fatigue and tremor, heat intolerance and increased sweating with warm, moist skin, weight loss often with increased appetite, palpitations, and tachycardia. The extrathyroidal changes include opthalmopathy and localized skin infiltrations, usually occurring on the lower legs (see Fig. 57-4).

The clinical manifestations of hyperthyroidism may be less obvious in elderly patients in whom it may present as an arrhythmia and heart failure. Occasionally, severe manifestations of hyperthyroidism may lead to a thyroid crisis, or storm. In these cases there is a general worsening of the manifestations described above to the point that they become life-threatening. Fever is almost always present and may be an important clue to the onset of this serious complication. Thyroid crisis may be precipitated by minor trauma and stress. The ophthalmopathy of Graves' disease may be mild. If so, the patient presents with prominent eyes, a stare, and periorbital swelling. It is present in 50 to 80 percent of patients with Graves' disease. In less common cases, the ophthalmopathy may be severe, and vision may be threatened.

In the presence of clinical manifestations of hyperthyroidism laboratory tests will show a high thyroxine (T_4) and triiodothyronine (T_3) resin uptake.

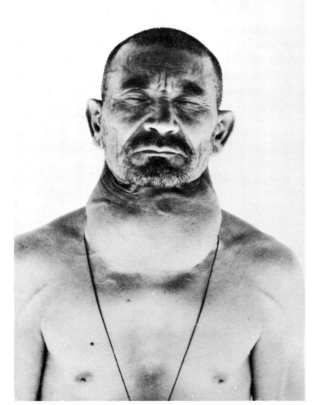

FIGURE 57-3 Large colloid goiter in a patient from an area of endemic iodine deficiency.

Management of this condition may include one or several of the following procedures:

1 Prolonged treatment with antithyroid drugs such as propylthiouracil or methimazole given for at least 1 year.
2 Surgical subtotal thyroidectomy after preoperative drug therapy with propylthiouracil.
3 Treatment with radioactive iodine.

Hypothyroidism

There are several types of hypothyroidism. In primary hypothyroidism, the disease is caused by a pathological process which destroys the thyroid gland. It may be the result of chronic thyroiditis or of therapy directed to the thyroid gland. Depending on the age of onset of the hypothyroid state, it can be classified as : (1) adult hypothyroidism or myxedema, (2) juvenile (onset after ages 1 to 2 years), or (3) congenital hypothyroidism or cretinism caused by lack of thyroid hormone before or shortly after birth. Secondary hypothyroidism may develop as a result of deficiency of TSH present as either an isolated phenomenon or as part of the clinical picture of hypopituitarism.

Clinical manifestations of hypothyroidism in the adult and juvenile forms include fatigue, hoarseness, cold intolerance and decreased sweating with a cool, dry skin, puffiness of the face, and slow movements. In the infant, hypothyroidism may be manifested by lethargy, an unusually quiet infant, constipation, umbilical hernia, feeding problems or failure to gain weight, retarded growth, respiratory problems, thick tongue, hoarse cry, bradycardia, dry skin, and hypothermia.

Among the laboratory tests used to confirm the diagnosis of hypothyroidism, serum TSH is the most sensitive available. In primary hypothyroidism serum TSH levels are high, together with low serum T_4 and T_3 resin tests. In contrast, in patients with secondary hypothyroidism all three measurements are low.

Treatment of hypothyroidism includes the administration of thyroxine which is usually instituted and gradually increased over days to weeks to a full maintenance dose of 120 mg/day.

Goiters

Diffuse colloid goiters and colloid nodular goiters are a very common disorder which affects 16 percent of

TABLE 57-1

TEST	HYPERTHYROIDISM	HYPOTHYROIDISM
RAI uptake	↑	↓
Serum thyroxine	↑	↓
T_3 resin uptake	↑	↓
Serum TSH	↓	↑

women and 4 percent of men age 20 to 60 as demonstrated in a survey of a Michigan community. Usually there are no symptoms other than cosmetic appearance, but occasional complications may occur. The thyroid may be diffusely enlarged and/or contain nodules.

The etiology of goiter includes iodine deficiency or an intrathyroidal biochemical defect caused by a variety of factors.

In order to ascertain whether the goiter is associated with hyper- or hypothyroidism, measurements of serum T_4 and T_3 resin tests may be necessary. A radioactive iodine scintiscan of the thyroid gland will show whether the nodules are "cold" or "hot." Cold nodules may represent carcinoma, while hot nodules are nearly always benign. Ultrasound scanning of the thyroid gland may be used to detect cystic changes in thyroid nodules. Cystic nodules are almost never cancerous.

Therapy of goiter involves suppression of TSH by thyroid hormone. Prolonged treatment with thyroxine will result in suppression of pituitary TSH and inhibition of thyroid function with atrophy of the thyroid gland. For complications of large goiters, surgery may be indicated aimed at removing most of the thyroid gland. In communities where goiters develop as a consequence of iodine insufficiency, the addition of iodine to table salt should be instituted.

Neoplasms of several types usually present as single nodules or masses. When present, they should be removed surgically.

Chronic thyroiditis (Hashimoto's disease) is a common pathological process of autoimmune origin. It causes destruction of the thyroid gland, giving rise to a diffuse goiter and occasionally to hypothyroidism.

QUESTIONS

Diseases of the thyroid gland—Chap. 57

Directions: Circle the letter preceding each item below that correctly answers each question. More than one answer may be correct.

1 Which of the following are characteristics of triiodothyronine (T_3) as compared with thyroxine (T_4)?
a More potent effects on body tissues in regulating general metabolic rate *b* Present in serum in greater concentrations *c* Both *a* and *b* *d* Neither *a* nor *b*

2 Which of the following levels of TSH indicate primary hypothyroidism (hypothyroidism of thyroidal origin)?
a Above normal serum TSH levels *b* Normal TSH levels *c* Undetectable TSH levels

3 Which of the following are characteristic signs and symptoms of Graves' disease?
a Weight gain *b* Diffuse hyperplasia of the thyroid gland *c* Muscle fatigue *d* Bradycardia

4 Mr. B., 40 years of age, was found to have Graves' disease. Which of the following treatment programs may be prescribed?
a Long-term administration of propylthiouracil *b* Subtotal thyroidectomy following short-term administration of antithyroid drugs and ¹³¹I treatment *c* Total thyroidectomy *d* Any one of the above

5 A nurse in the newborn nursery observes a newborn baby boy who is very lethargic, has an umbilical hernia, and dry skin. His respirations are noisy, and he has an abnormally hoarse cry. These signs suggest:
a Hyperthyroidism *b* Cretinism *c* Colloid goiter *d* Euthyroidism

6 Which of the following signs and symptoms is (are) characteristic of hypothyroidism?

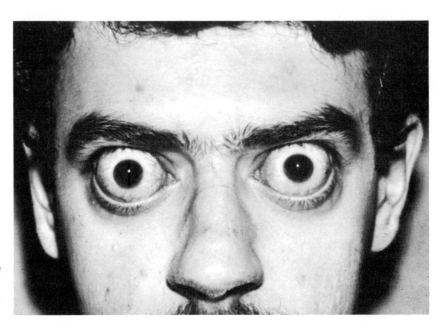

FIGURE 57-4 Exophthalmos with increased palpebral fissure and proptosis of the eyeballs. (From the Ophthalmology Department, University of Michigan.)

a Weight loss   *b* Mental, physical slowness   *c* Cold intolerance   *d* Moist skin

7 Which of the following is *not* characteristic of a malignant thyroid nodule?

a It usually presents as hot nodules   *b* It usually appears as a single, firm, fixed nodule   *c* It is functioning   *d* Prognosis following early detection and treatment is excellent

Directions: Circle T if the statement is true and F if the statement is false. Correct the false statements.

8   T   F   The T₃ resin test indicates the rate of secretion of thyroid hormone and transport.

9   T   F   The most common form of hypothyroidism is caused by a lesion in the pituitary gland.

10   T   F   Hypothyroidism of all forms is best treated with thyroxine hormone.

BIBLIOGRAPHY

Baxter, J. D. and P. H. Forsham: "Tissue Effects of Glucocorticoids," *Am J Med,* **53**: 573–589, 1972.

Catt, K. J. *An ABC of Endocrinology,* Little, Brown, Boston, 1971.

Edis, A. J., L. A. Ayala, and R. H. Egdahl: *Manual of Endocrine Surgery,* Springer-Verlag, New York, 1975.

Ezrin, C., J. E. Godden, R. Jolpe, and R. Wilson: *Systematic Endocrinology,* Harper & Row, New York, 1973.

Kirschner, M. A. and C. W. Bardin: "Androgen Production and Metabolism in Normal and Virilized Women," *Metabolism,* **21**: 7, 1972.

Williams, R. H. (ed.), *Textbook of Endocrinology,* 5th ed., Saunders, Philadelphia, 1974.

PART X Orthopedics

LARRY S. MATTHEWS

Orthopedics is concerned with prevention or corrective treatment of deformities or diseases of the musculoskeletal system including bones, muscles, joints, ligaments, tendons, and fascia of the body. This part includes a discussion of fractures (accidental injury and its initial treatment, definitions, the four "Rs" of fractures, and fracture complications) and dislocations (types, diagnosis, and treatment). Also included is a discussion of orthopedic diseases of children and a rationale for the treatment of tumors of the musculoskeletal system.

OVERALL OBJECTIVES

At the completion of Part X you should be able to:

1 Identify the characteristics of fractures and dislocations according to their classification, description, recognition, reduction, retention of reduction, complications, types of dislocations, and treatment.

2 Develop skill in identifying etiology, pathogenesis, and treatment of various orthopedic diseases of children.

3 Explain the rationale for the treatment of tumors of the musculoskeletal system.

CHAPTER 58 Fractures and Dislocations

OBJECTIVES

At the completion of Chap. 58 you should be able to:

1 State the prime objective of treatment at the scene of a serious accident.

2 Describe external cardiac massage by identifying the purpose, time to begin, and necessary duration of massage.

3 Describe the emergency treatment of any injured person who is cyanotic and in obvious respiratory distress.

4 List the characteristics of arterial bleeding.

5 Describe the sequence of steps used to stop arterial bleeding.

6 Explain the procedure used in the application of a tourniquet and the precautions that must be taken.

7 Explain the rationale for treatment of a seriously injured limb.

8 Differentiate between the emergency treatment if the fracture is located at the midportion of long bones, lower and upper extremity, or if the deformity is near a joint.

9 Describe the rationale for the procedure used in applying splints.

10 Locate and describe the function of the parts of the long bone—diaphysis (shaft), metaphysis, physis, epiphysis, periosteum, nutrient arteries.

11 Explain why the specific histology of the physis is important in understanding some specific injuries in children.

12 Define a *fracture.*

13 Differentiate between nine types of fractures (transverse, oblique, spiral, segmental, fatigue, greenstick, pathologic, compression, avulsion) in terms of radiologic appearance, location, cause, treatment, and complications.

14 Explain the significance of angulation and opposition in the description of long-bone fractures.

15 Differentiate between open and closed fractures in terms of area involved, treatment, and likely complications.

16 Explain what comminution indicates.

17 Identify the four "Rs" of fractures.

18 Name at least three considerations when dealing with recognition of fractures.

19 Define *reduction.*

20 Identify the characteristics of both closed and open reductions.

21 Identify the advantages and disadvantages of closed reduction and external immobilization of the various types of retention, and of open reduction and retention by fixation.

22 Identify the medical implications of fracture treatment.

23 Explain the purpose of and general rule for the application of casts.

24 Describe the optimal appearance of a cast and the purpose of careful molding of the soft plaster over bony prominences.

25 List the signs and treatment of neurovascular dysfunction of the exposed portions of the distal limb.

26 State the rationale for the treatment of a limb with a compromised neurovascular supply.

27 Identify the signs, symptoms, and immediate treatment if a cast has not been properly applied over bony prominences.

28 Describe traction by identifying the contribution that it makes to maintenance of limb length, position control, and observation.

29 State at least two important factors that must be considered when applying or maintaining traction.

30 List at least three advantages traction provides as the definitive early treatment of fractures.

31 Describe the potential complication associated with the use of skin tractions.

32 Identify, for Bryant's skin traction, the location of the fracture, positioning, and the rationale for age and weight requirements.

33 Describe balanced skeletal traction by identifying the type of fracture it is used with, position of skeletal pin and traction bail, and application and use of Thomas splint and Pearson attachment.

34 List the advantages of using balanced skeletal traction for the treatment of fractures.

35 Describe Russell's traction as to the type of fracture it is used with, positioning of patient, purpose of, and problems associated with this treatment.

36 Explain the purpose of the 90-90-90 traction.

37 Describe the operative procedure referred to as *open reduction and internal fixation* (ORIF).

38 List the advantages and disadvantages of operative fracture treatment.

39 Identify the characteristics of osteomyelitis in children and adults in terms of the etiology, pathogenesis, signs, and symptoms, prevention, treatment, and prognosis.

40 State the most frequently encountered reasons for using open reduction and internal fixation of fractures.

41 State the rationale for operative fracture treatment in an elderly patient with a hip fracture.

42 Identify the advantages of the telescoping hip nail and other implant devices.

43 Explain the major advantage of a femoral head replacement arthroplasty in an elderly patient.

44 State the rationale for planning for an orderly rehabilitation program from the first day of injury.

45 Differentiate between malunion, delayed union, and nonunion of a fracture and identify an example of each type.

46 Differentiate between dislocation and subluxation.

47 Describe shoulder dislocation by identifying its appearance, the age group affected, and treatment.

48 At the time of initial evaluation of a shoulder dislocation, explain the rationale for examining the neurovascular status of the limb prior to any manipulative reduction.

49 Describe the sustained anterior traction method of reduction of a dislocated shoulder.

50 Identify the characteristics of a dislocated hip according to the signs, symptoms, prognosis, and consequences of delayed reduction.

51 Explain the advantages and disadvantages of arthroplasty in the treatment of arthritis.

INITIAL TREATMENT OF ACCIDENTAL INJURY

Circulation and respiration

At the scene of a serious accident the prime objective is to preserve life and to maximize the potential for rapid and complete rehabilitation of the injured person. Death begins approximately three minutes after cardiac standstill. The time to begin external massage is *immediately* when pulselessness is discovered. External cardiac massage must be effectively continued until either the individual's own heart has resumed function or the patient is under the care of appropriate emergency personnel. Likewise, respiration must be continuous and effective, or death begins in approximately seven minutes. The most frequent cause of failure of respiration at the scene of an accident is obstruction of the nasopharynx. Debris and clotted blood must be manually removed from the mouth and throat immediately. The prone position allows continuous drainage. When any injured person is cyanotic and in obvious respiratory distress, obstructing material should immediately be removed from the nasopharynx. Success is obvious with a rapid rush of air and change in the patient's color. Another maneuver which is frequently successful is to rapidly compress the chest from behind. This raises the intrathoracic pressure and may "blow out" debris which was lodged in the trachea. Finally, if all attempts to remove the obstruction have failed, a tracheostomy must be done if the injured person is to survive. If obstruction is not the problem, or if it has been successfully eliminated and no respiratory efforts are being made by the injured individual, external respiration should be started and continued until definitive care is available.

Arterial bleeding is red, pulsatile, and voluminous. A transected femoral artery can lead to exsanguination and death in a few minutes. Such bleeding must be stopped.

If the application of a simple pressure dressing over the wound does not stop the bleeding, then digital pressure on the major artery proximal to the area of bleeding will usually be temporarily effective. A tourniquet (a belt, rope, tape, or the like) should be tightened circumferentially, proximal to the wound until the bleeding is controlled. The time of application of a tourniquet must be recorded since the limb will begin to sustain irreversible damage if reparative surgery is not initiated within approximately 1½ hours. The injured individual must be rapidly transported to a hospital where such surgery may be performed.

Splinting of limb deformities

Limb deformities and obvious skeletal instability are frequently evident. Motion of sharp fracture fragments can shear and irreparably damage the neurovascular supply to a limb. All seriously injured limbs should be splinted to prevent this unnecessary damage during transportation of the patient. If the fracture is located at the midportion of a long bone, the limb should be gently straightened to a nearly normal position and bound to an appropriate stable object. For the lower extremity, tying the injured limb to the naturally adjacent, uninjured one is frequently convenient. An upper extremity can be supported in a sling or simply bound to the chest. If the deformity is near a joint, e.g., elbow or knee, *no* attempt should be made to straighten the limb since in these locations the nerves and vessels lie close to bone and further damage may result from attempts at fracture reduction. The limb should be secured in a soft support such as a pillow in its deformed state.

The distal pulse should be checked before and after splinting to ensure that the circulation has remained intact. All splints should be extremely well padded to prevent skin ulceration. An ulceration over a bony prominence may cause more disability and require more care than the fracture itself. Open wounds should be bandaged to prevent further contamination. Any clean cloth is satisfactory if sterile bandages are not available. In many cases the time from the incident until final emergency room treatment may determine the outcome, so be sure that an ambulance is called.

ANATOMY AND HISTOLOGY OF THE LONG BONE

Figure 58-1 illustrates the location of the parts of a long bone. The *diaphysis,* or shaft, is the cylindrical midportion of the bone. It is composed of cortical bone which has great strength. The *metaphysis* is the flared region near the end of the bone. This region is largely composed of trabecular or spongy bone and contains marrow. It also supports the joint and provides appropriate areas for attachment of tendons and ligaments. The *physis* is the longitudinal growth region in children. It disappears at skeletal maturity. The *epiphysis* is directly adjacent to the joint in children. It fuses to the metaphysis at the end of the growth period. The entire bone is covered with a fibrous layer, the *periosteum,* which contains the proliferating cells that contribute to the transverse growth of a long bone. Most long bones have specific nutrient arteries. The location and patency of these vessels may determine the success of bone healing after fracture.

The specific histology of the physis, or growth plate is important in understanding some specific injuries in children (see Fig. 58-2). The uppermost layer of cells near the epiphysis is referred to as the area of resting cells. The next layer is the area of zone of proliferation. In this area active cell division is occurring, and this is where the growth of long bones begins. These cells are pushed toward the shaft into the area of hypertrophy where they swell and become metabolically inactive. These swollen cells are weak. Epiphyseal fracture separations in children commonly occur in this region with extension of the injury into the area of provisional calcification. In the zone of provisional calcification the cells first begin to become hard and resemble normal bone. Damage to the proliferating area may cause a growth arrest with either retardation of the longitudinal growth of the limb or progressive deformity in case of serious damage to only a portion of the plate.

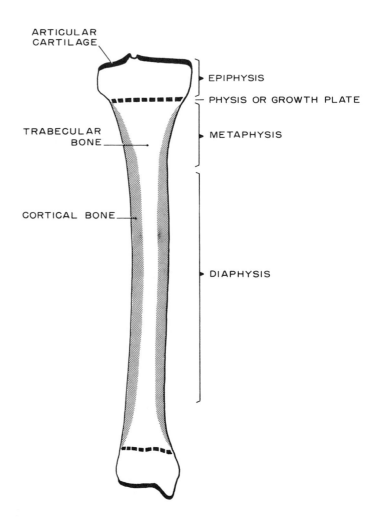

FIGURE 58-1 Anatomy of a long bone.

A fracture is a structural discontinuity in a bone. For effective communication regarding fractures, several important descriptive terms must be introduced. A *transverse* fracture is one which proceeds directly across the bone. When the broken segments of such a transversely fractured bone are repositioned, or reduced back to their original location, they are stable and usually easy to control with casts (see Fig. 58-3A). *Oblique* fractures proceed at an angle across the bone. They are unstable and difficult to control (see Fig. 58-3B). *Spiral* fractures are the result of torsion of a limb. They are typical in ski injuries where the toe of the ski may become lodged in a snowbank and the ski twists around until the bone breaks. Interestingly, this low-energy injury is associated with little soft tissue damage, and such fractures tend to heal readily with external immobilization (see Fig. 58-3C).

Segmental fractures are two adjacent fractures which isolate a central segment from its blood supply. These fractures are difficult to treat. Frequently the fracture at one or the other end of the avascular segment fails to heal and may require operative treatment (see Fig. 58-4A). *Fatigue* fractures occur in people who have recently increased their activity level—recruits in the army in basic training or people who have recently taken up jogging. With the onset of symptoms, the radiographs may not demonstrate a fracture. However, usually 2 weeks later linear radiopaque lines will appear perpendicular to the long axis of the bone. Such fractures heal well if the bone is immobilized for a few weeks. However, if they are not diagnosed, they can become displaced and will cause an increase in morbidity. Thus, any patient with severe extremity pain after a recent increase in activity may have such a lesion and should be protected by the use of crutches or an appropriate cast. After 2 weeks, radiographs should be obtained (see Fig. 58-4B). *Greenstick* fractures occur in children and are incomplete fractures. The periosteal layer is partially intact. They will heal

readily and remodel rapidly back to a normal shape and function (see Fig. 58-4C).

Pathologic fractures occur through regions of bone that have been weakened by a tumor or some other pathologic process. Frequently the adjacent bone shows decreased bone density. The most frequent cause of such fractures is a primary or metastatic tumor (see Fig. 58-5A). *Compression* fractures of the vertebral bodies are diagnosed by their radiographic appearance. Lateral views of the spine show a decrease in vertical height and a mild angulation at one or a few vertebrae. Although patients do not usually require sophisticated treatment, they should be hospitalized to care for the possible serious, indirect complications which may arise. In young people, a compression fracture may be associated with considerable retroperitoneal hemorrhage. As in pelvic fractures, the patient may rapidly develop hypovolemic shock and die if repeated accurate assessments of the pulse, blood pressure, and respiration are not obtained during the first 24 to 48 postinjury hours. Ileus and urinary retention may also result from these injuries (see Fig. 58-5B).

Avulsion fractures separate a fragment of the bone at a site of tendon or ligament insertion. Frequently no specific treatment is required. However, if joint instability or another cause of disability is expected to result from such a fracture, the displaced fragment may be operatively excised or replaced in most cases (see Fig. 58-5C).

Specific note should be made of fractures which involve a joint, particularly if the joint geometry is significantly disturbed by displacement of these fragments. Unless adequately treated, this type of injury may lead to a progressive posttraumatic degenerative arthritis of the injured joint (see Fig. 58-6).

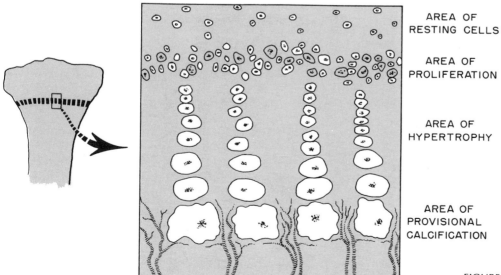

AREA OF
RESTING CELLS

AREA OF
PROLIFERATION

AREA OF
HYPERTROPHY

AREA OF
PROVISIONAL
CALCIFICATION

FIGURE 58-2 Growth of normal bone.

When a bone is fractured, the adjacent soft tissues are damaged, the periosteum is separated from the bone, and considerable bleeding takes place. A blood clot develops in the damaged area. It organizes within a few days and is invaded by new blood vessels. It then matures to become provisional callus. This early callus undergoes metaplasia to cartilage which ossifies, forming bony callus. The bony callus remodels to assume the shape of intact bone.

Description of fractures

Angulation and *opposition* are two terms frequently used in the description of long-bone fractures. The degree and direction of angulation from the normal position of a long bone may indicate the degree of fracture severity and the type of treatment program. Angulation is described by estimating the degrees of deviation of the longitudinal axis of the distal fragment from the normal longitudinal axis indicating the direction of the apex of the angle. *Opposition* refers to the extent of displacement of the fracture surfaces and is used to describe what proportion of the fractured portion of one fragment touches its mate (see Fig. 58-7).

Two other terms frequently used in fracture descriptions are *open* and *closed.* Technically, an open fracture is one in which the skin on the involved limb has been penetrated. The important concept is whether the contaminated outside environment has come into contact with the fracture site. A fracture fragment may frequently perforate the skin at the time of injury, become contaminated, and then return to near its normal position. Under these conditions operative irrigation, debridement, and administration of intravenous antibiotics may be necessary to prevent osteomyelitis. In general, open fractures should have operative irrigation and debridement within 6 hours of the time of injury for the best chance of preventing infection. *Comminution* indicates the presence of more than two fracture fragments.

A typical description of a fracture might then be: "This patient has a midshaft, open, transverse, uncomminuted fracture of the right femur. It is angulated 30°, the apex directed posteriorly. The fragments are separated widely with no opposition. The neurovascular supply to the limb is intact." Such a description would immediately indicate that the limb is apt to survive but that surgery is needed within a short time. The purpose of the surgery is to protect the patient from infection and, if necessary, to reposition the fracture fragments.

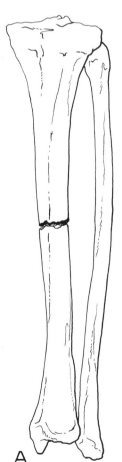 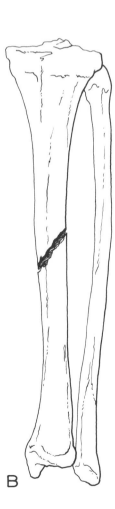 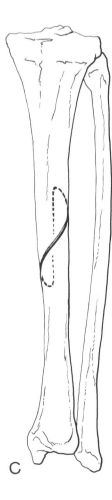

FIGURE 58-3 Classification of fractures. A, transverse. B, oblique. C, spiral.

A   B   C

Four basic concepts should be considered for fractures: *recognition, reduction, retention,* and *rehabilitation. Recognition* concerns the diagnosis at the scene of the accident and later in the hospital. *Reduction* is the repositioning of the fracture fragments as nearly as possible to their normal location. *Retention* refers to the methods which are applied to hold the fragments while they are healing. A *rehabilitation* plan should be initiated immediately and concurrently with the fracture treatment.

Recognition

The history of the accident, the severity, the force involved, and the description of the event by the patient determine the likelihood of broken bones and the need for specific examination for fractures. The pain of fractures of long bones is very specific. For example, the patient's leg will be severely painful and tender at the fracture site, but other areas such as the knee and ankle may feel nearly normal. Obvious deformities define discontinuities in the skeletal integrity. The association of localized pain and tenderness, deformity, and instability frequently leads to the presumptive diagnosis of fracture at the scene of the injury. *Crepitus,* the feeling as of two pieces of rough sandpaper rubbed together, indicates the presence of a fracture and is in fact the sensation generated by rubbing the fracture fragments together. Fracture fragments may be sharp and hard. Their relative motion after injury may sever the neurovascular supply to the limb. Therefore, upon recognition of the possibility of fracture of a long bone, the injured limb should be splinted to protect it from further damage.

Obvious soft tissue damage may also indicate the possibility of a fracture and the need for immediate splinting and further examination. This is especially true for injuries to the cervical spine where contusions and lacerations of the face and scalp indicate the need for radiographic evaluation which may demonstrate a cervical spine fracture and/or dislocation and the possible need for surgical stabilization.

Reduction

The act of manipulating broken bone fragments back as nearly as possible, to their original location is known as *reduction.* Closed fractures of long bones are frequently treated by closed reduction. This may often be effectively

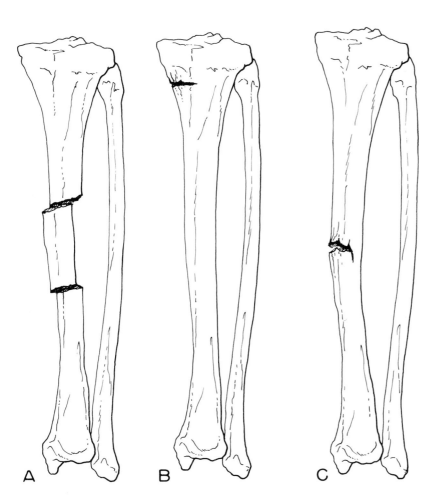

FIGURE 58-4 A, segmental. B, fatigue. C, greenstick.

carried out in the emergency room or cast room at the time of the initial evaluation. Intravenous narcotics, sedatives, or local nerve block anesthesia may be used to diminish the patient's pain during the procedure. It is very important that the patient and family recognize the extent of the injury and the need for repositioning of the fracture fragments and for immobilization. Since all forms of outpatient analgesia require several minutes for maximum effect, this allows sufficient time for reevaluating the nature of the injury. It is necessary to assess the following factors when planning the patient's treatment program: the social situation, the availability of family support, the likely effect of the injury on the patient's life during the next several months, and the expectations of the patient. During the initial treatment, the patient's family should be instructed regarding the reduction. These instructions include the possibility that reduction will not be successful, the expected consequences of the fracture, and the expected period and nature of disability. It is also very important to outline problems and complications which may possibly be associated with the injury, rather than to have to explain them after their occurrence. For example, after an elbow fracture it is rare for the patient to be able to fully extend and to "lock" the elbow. An early explanation will eliminate the necessity of exhaustive excuses for the patient's inability to regain full range of motion several weeks after the incident.

When the patient and the family are aware of the medical implications of the fracture and when analgesia is maximal, a manual effort is generally used to reposition the broken bones. It is more advantageous to use all necessary force on the first attempt, which will often rapidly accomplish a satisfactory reduction, than to be excessively gentle and make multiple skin-damaging attempts. If a closed manual reduction is not successful under outpatient analgesia, it is *mandatory* that the physician cease repeating similar efforts. Under such circumstances, the patient should be admitted to the hospital, prepared for a general anesthesia, and scheduled for a reduction under anesthesia in the operating room. In this situation a fracture table can greatly amplify the force which needs to be used and can frequently ensure control of the fragments until a cast is applied to maintain the reduction.

Retention of reduction

As a general rule, casts applied to maintain a reduction should extend past the joint above and the joint below the fracture. If adjacent joints are positioned at an angle

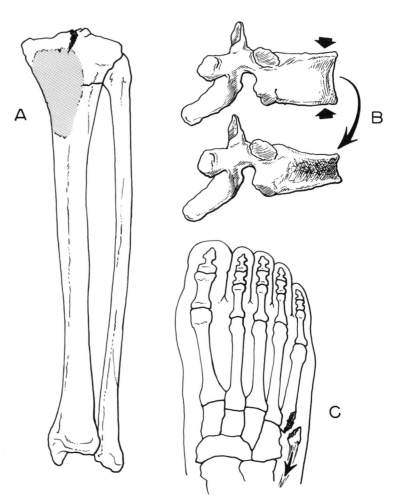

FIGURE 58-5 A, *pathologic.* B, *compression.* C, *avulsion.*

to the central longitudinal axis of the broken bone, angulation and opposition corrections may be maintained, and at the same time rotational displacements may be prevented. A cast should always be smooth, nonlaminated, and in conformity with the geometry of the limb to which it is applied. Careful molding of the soft plaster over bony prominences will generally prevent the development of pressure ulcerations and will maximize the

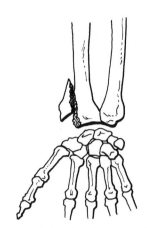

FIGURE 58-6 Fracture of the distal radius with extension into wrist joint.

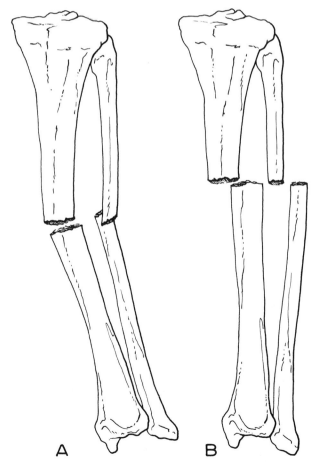

FIGURE 58-7 A, angulation. B, opposition.

ability of the cast to retain the fracture fragment positions.

Reduction and cast application are frequently completed a few hours after the injury when the maximum soft tissue swelling has not occurred. In addition, the act of reduction itself may cause further tissue edema. Consequently, because a cast is an unyielding circumferential dressing, great attention must be paid to the postreduction neurovascular supply to the limb. Therefore, the limb should be elevated, usually by a rope and sling to a fracture frame. The exposed portions of the distal limb should be repeatedly examined for the development of pain, pallor, paresthesias, and pulselessness, all of which are signs of neurovascular dysfunction. If there is any indication that the neurovascular supply to the limb is being impaired, the cast should be split from one end to the other. *All* layers should be cut, and the cast loosened until the signs and symptoms of neurovascular dysfunction have been reversed. Usually most limbs with fractures are not very painful after reduction and immobilization. All persistent patient complaints during this postreduction period must be taken seriously, and effective steps initiated to relieve the source of discomfort.

A limb with a compromised neurovascular supply may sustain irreversible pathologic changes within 1½ hours; thus an immediate effective response to these signs of danger is mandatory. During the first several hours after injury, repeated administration of narcotic medication is definitely *contraindicated*. For example, if a cast has not been molded or padded sufficiently over bony prominences—the ulnar styloid, olecranon, medial, and lateral malleoli—the patient will develop persistent burning pain at the pressure sites. This is a sign of developing skin and soft tissue necrosis. Immediate relief from the localized pressure is necessary. This excessive pressure may be relieved by cutting and reforming the cast; however, on occasion a new, properly fitted, and molded cast may be necessary to prevent costly and painful soft tissue ulceration.

Traction

Another excellent method of maintaining a satisfactory reduction of limb fractures is traction. In general, traction is achieved by weights which are attached by ropes to the patient's limb. The location of pulleys through which the ropes run is adjusted until the direction of pull is in line with the long axis of the fractured bone.

Although longitudinal traction will often maintain a satisfactory reduction, usually splints, casts, or slings are used to cradle the limb and assist in holding the fracture fragments in place. As a general rule, skeletal traction with a sterile surgical steel pin drilled through the distal fragment or a more distal bone is preferable to skin traction. When skeletal traction is used, skin necrosis and the neurovascular complications of circumferential dressings tend to be avoided. Although requiring hospitalization, traction provides many advantages as the definitive method of maintaining a reduction. Most forms of traction ensure dependable limb elevation which minimizes swelling and promotes soft tissue healing. The injured extremity may be easily observed for compromised neurovascular circulation. Wound care is facilitated. Appropriate application of traction allows convenient bed care for the patient. The patient may be quite mobile in bed if the longitudinal ropes are appropriately positioned and the splints, casts, or slings used to support the limb are properly balanced. Bedpans can be positioned and removed without discomfort, and bedclothing may be changed without fear of displacement of the fracture fragments.

Some important factors must be considered when applying or maintaining traction. The major rope, which is usually attached to a skeletal pin, should generally pull in line with the normal long axis of a fractured long bone. Both the weight of the limb and the supporting devices should be balanced by weights to ensure stable maintenance of reduction and support of the injured limb during bed care. As much as possible, pulleys and ropes should be located well above and to the side of the patient. Great care should be taken that bony prominences, i.e., the heel, malleoli, fibular head, are properly padded or otherwise protected. The traction ropes should run freely through the pulleys. The weights should be sufficiently high above the floor with the patient in a normal bed care position so that required routine repositioning does not allow a weight to rest on the floor, thereby removing the necessary tension from the attached rope. Appropriately applied and maintained traction is always comfortable.

The simplest form of traction is *Buck's skin traction.* This traction method is appropriately used in young people for short periods of time. The most frequent indication for this form of traction is the need to rest the knee joint after trauma prior to possible knee exploration and repair. Utilization of this method of traction should ideally begin with application of a thick coating of skin cement, tincture of benzoin, or elastic adherent to the patient's skin below the knee. A rolled tubular stockinette

is then applied smoothly over the distal limb below the knee. Adhesive traction strips are applied medially and laterally to the stockinette, and they are, in turn, wrapped smoothly and gently with an elastic bandage. The ends of the traction strips at the ankle are connected to a spreader bar to prevent pressure on the malleoli. A rope which is attached to the center of the spreader bar is then threaded through a pulley at the foot of the bed. Rarely should a weight greater than 5 lb be applied. Many potential complications are associated with the use of skin traction. The circumferentially wrapped elastic bandage can further compromise the circulation to the foot in a patient with prior vascular disease. Skin allergies to the adhesives may cause a problem. If great care is not taken, pressure ulceration may develop at the malleoli. Excessive traction can avulse the fragile skin of the elderly. In general, this form of traction should not be used to treat elderly patients. Even in the treatment of young adults, skeletal pin traction is preferable if such treatment will be required for more than a few days (see Fig. 58-8).

Bryant's skin traction is frequently used in the treatment of a small child with a femoral fracture or fractures. In this type of fracture the patient is positioned with the hips flexed, the knees extended, and the limbs in a vertical position slightly spread apart. Because the periosteum of children's bones is so strong, it is rarely completely separated at the time of fracture; thus this pure longitudinal form of traction almost always accomplishes an adequate reduction and maintenance of fragment position until early healing. Bryant's traction should not be applied to children over the age of *3 years* or to children weighing greater than *30 lb.* Severe damage to the skin can result from exceeding these limits. In addition, the vascular supply to the feet in older and larger children may be compromised by the considerable hydrostatic effect of vertical limb placement and by the constrictive elastic wraps. Posttraction x-rays often demonstrate bayonette apposition with approximately ½ in of overriding of the bone fragments. This is not only acceptable, but also advantageous since usually the injured limb of a child will grow faster than the normal one for several years following a fracture (see Fig. 58-9).

Balanced skeletal traction, used primarily for the treatment of femoral shaft fractures in adults, at first glance appears complex. In essence, however, a skeletal pin is positioned transversely through the distal femur or proximal tibia. A traction bail is attached, and the pri-

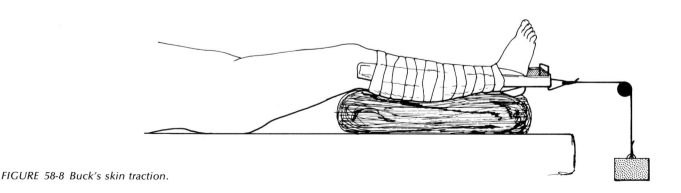

FIGURE 58-8 Buck's skin traction.

mary traction rope is attached to the bail. The patient's limb is positioned with the hip and knee in approximately 35° of flexion. The primary pulley is adjusted so that the line of tension is coaxial with the longitudinal axis of the fractured femur. Sufficient weight is attached to achieve normal femoral length.

The patient's thigh is supported by a sling or padding attached to the proximal portion of a *Thomas splint*. The distal limb is supported by the Pearson attachment to the Thomas splint. Then the Thomas splint, Pearson attachment, and the limb itself are suspended by appropriate ropes, pulleys, and weights so that the limb is freely suspended in air. Thus bed care is greatly facilitated. This form of traction is extremely valuable for the treatment of many varieties of femoral fracture. The entire splint may be adducted or abducted to correct angular deformities in the mediolateral plane. Greater or lesser degrees of hip and knee flexion allow lateral corrections. The postion and angulation of the Pearson attachment may be adjusted to correct rotational deformities.

Balanced skeletal traction demonstrates many of the major advantages of traction treatment of fractures (see Fig. 58-10). The advantages are elevation, longitudinal coaxial traction on the fractured long bone, easy access

to the injured limb for repeated examination of the neurovascular status and for local wound care, and facilitation of nursing care. As is the case with all forms of traction utilizing skeletal pins, the patient should be examined daily for signs of pin tract inflammation or infection, of loosening or sliding of the pin, and of the pin having been pulled from the bone.

While balanced skeletal traction may be used for the treatment of most fractures of the femur, better reductions of fractures of the hip may frequently be obtained by using *Russell's traction*. In this case the thigh is supported by a sling. The longitudinal traction is applied by a pin positioned through the tibia and fibula transversly above the ankle. The effect of this arrangement is to provide a traction force (derived from the vertical pull of the thigh sling combined with the horizontal pull of the two ropes at the foot) which is in alignment with the injured bone and is of appropriate magnitude. This type of traction is most frequently used to provide comfort for patients with hip fractures during the preoperative evaluation and preparation for surgery.

Although Russell's traction (see Fig. 58-11) may be used as the definitive and final treatment of hip fractures in selected patients, the elderly or debilitated patient with a fractured hip cannot usually tolerate the dangers of long-sustained bed rest, i.e., decubitus ulcers, pneumonia, and thrombophlebitis. The most common problem seen with Russell's traction is slipping of the patient toward the foot of the bed, the distal pulleys jamming together, and the weight then resting on the floor. Considerable care must be directed toward maintaining the position of the patient in bed; it may be necessary to place blocks under the foot casters of the bed to gain the assistance of gravity.

Ninety-ninety-ninety traction is particularly useful in the treatment of children from the age of 3 years through young adulthood (see Fig. 58-12). Control of fragments in a femoral shaft fracture is nearly always satisfactory with 90-90-90 traction. The patient has considerable mobility in bed.

While only lower limb traction methods have been described in detail, all the principles apply to the treatment of fractures of the upper limb.

Traction treatment of fractures is generally safe, provides considerable patient comfort and mobility in bed, allows for repeated examination of the injured limb, provides valuable elevation, and does not increase the risk of infection. However, traction treatment of fractures should be used with caution with the elderly patient since it requires continuous hospitalization with the associated danger of complications, expense, and inconvenience.

Surgical procedures

At times, the most advantageous fracture treatment method may include surgery. This method of treatment

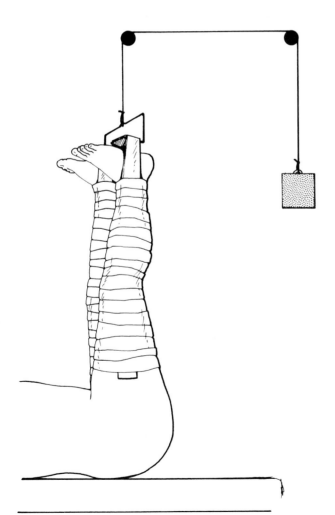

FIGURE 58-9 Bryant's skin traction.

is referred to as *open reduction and internal fixation* (ORIF). In general, an incision is made at the fracture site and carried along anatomic planes to the fracture. The fracture is observed and studied. Fracture hematoma and nonviable fragments are irrigated from the wound. The fracture is then manually repositioned to a normal position. The fracture fragments, after reduction, are stabilized by the use of appropriate orthopedic devices such as pins, screws, plates, and nails. The advantages of operative fracture treatment include accuracy in repositioning of the fracture fragments, the opportunity for inspection of the adjacent vessels and nerves, the considerable fixation stability that may be achieved, the frequent absence of a need for external casts or appliances after stabilization, a relatively short hospital course in uncomplicated cases, and the potential for maintenance of nearly normal joint function and muscular strength during fracture treatment. However, there are also potential disadvantages. Every anesthesia and operation has a possible risk of complication, even death, from the procedure itself. While closed fractures treated conservatively by casts or traction rarely become infected, operative management greatly increases the chances of infection. The use of a metallic internal stabilization device allows for the possibility of device failure. Surgery itself is additional trauma to the soft tissues, and a previously uninjured structure could accidentally be cut or damaged at operation.

It is extremely difficult to treat the deep infection that may occur. Infection of bone, osteomyelitis, is extremely resistant to successful antibiotic treatment. It is thought that this is partially due to the relative avascular nature of cortical bone. Appropriate quantities of antibiotics may never reach areas of infected tissue. The presence of implanted metal devices increases the difficulties of treating the infection. In cases of postoperative infection it is usually necessary to remove the metal device before the infection can be controlled. The decision to use open reduction and internal fixation is of critical importance because of the potential serious complications that can result from this treatment.

An individual with a femoral shaft fracture who is treated by nonoperative methods will usually spend 6 weeks in a hospital in traction. When the fracture is partially healed, a cast will be applied extending from the toes to the nipple line. The cast will be worn until the fracture demonstrates clinical and radiographic evidence of healing stability and cortical remodeling. It is rare that a person can return to work during this period which may extend from 6 to 12 months. Because employment medical benefits are generally 50 to 60 percent of regular earnings and remaining immobile at home usually causes the patient additional expenses, a simple closed fracture of the femur treated by closed techniques may be a tragedy for the family.

The nonoperative methods should be compared with treatment by open reduction and internal intramedullary fixation where, in successful cases, the patient may be discharged from the hospital 3 weeks after the injury. At the time of discharge from the hospital the patient is usually able to ambulate on crutches with partial weight

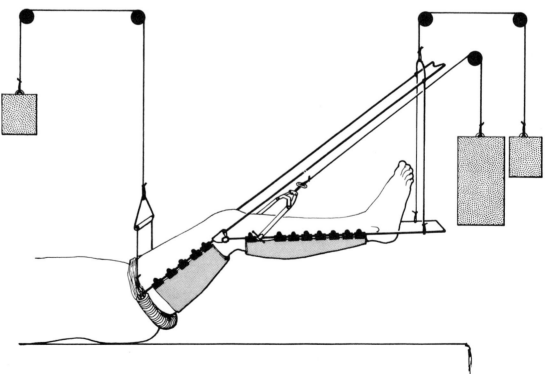

FIGURE 58-10 Balanced skeletal traction.

bearing and may frequently return to many types of employment. Self-care, shopping, and virtually any other activities that can be engaged in while using crutches can frequently be managed after the third week. Although this may seem to be the best form of therapy, the omnipresent danger of infection which occurs in 2 to 6 percent of cases must always be considered. Deep-wound infection following intramedullary fixation of a fractured femur requires long-term antibiotic therapy. It may require removal of the intramedullary rod and other operative

procedures, and it may endanger the life of the patient. Obviously the decision as to the most appropriate form of treatment is a major one and requires a major consideration of the patient, physician, and family.

One of the most frequently encountered reasons for

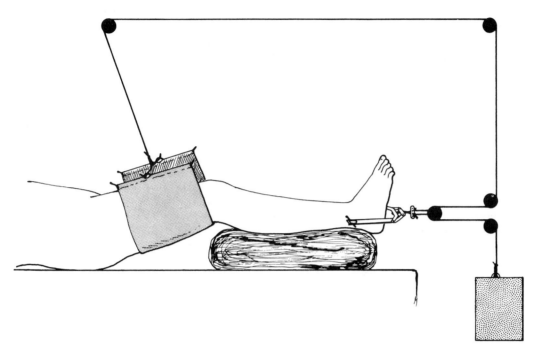

FIGURE 58-11 Russell's traction.

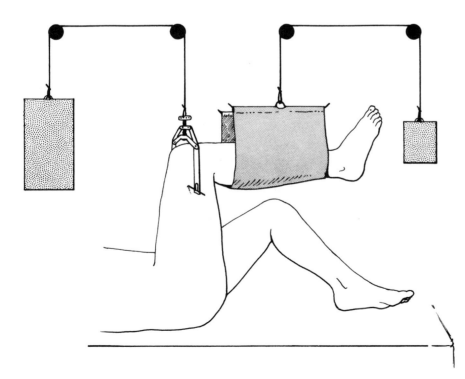

FIGURE 58-12 Ninety-ninety-ninety traction.

using open reduction and internal fixation of fractures is the inability to obtain an adequate reduction by closed means. This is a frequent occurrence in the treatment of midshaft fractures of the radius and ulna in adults. After three or four failed attempts to achieve a manual reduction, the following conditions occur: the skin becomes red, the soft tissue has sustained further damage, and there is no certainty that the reduction, if it is obtained, can be maintained in a cast for a sufficient period of time. Therefore, a decision for open reduction and internal plate or intramedullary rod fixation of the fractured bones is reasonable and prudent.

In other instances an excellent anatomic reduction is possible, but on repeated radiographic examination the reduction cannot be maintained by cast or traction. A typical example is a Piedmont or Galeazzi fracture of the radius with disassociation of the distal radioulnar joint (see Fig. 58-13). Although these fractures are often easily reduced, the reductions are unstable and may lead to malposition of the fragments a short time later. If this failure to maintain reduction is disregarded and if the radius is allowed to heal in this displaced position, the wrist is likely to develop severe arthritis with painful permanent limitation of forearm pronation and supination. Thus, failure of maintenance of adequate reduction by closed means is an excellent reason for open therapy. Another rationale for surgical treatment of fractures is the need for direct observation and possible repair of vital neurovascular structures.

In open fractures irrigation, mechanical cleansing of the wound, and debridement of necrotic tissue are essential to prevent postinjury osteomyelitis. Frequently, the contaminated wound can be converted to the equivalent of a clean, aseptic surgical wound. Under these circumstances internal fixation may be a rational treatment choice. If surgical cleansing of an open fracture is required, and adequate irrigation and debridement are accomplished, then internal fixation may be deemed advantageous and utilized immediately, although there is increased risk of infection.

In some cases open reduction and internal fixation may be the optimal form of treatment of the general condition of the patient. For example, elderly patients with hip fractures treated by traction, frequently succumb to the complications of bed rest: pressure ulceration, pneumonia, and pulmonary embolism after an extended period of painful hospitalization. Nursing care of these patients is extremely difficult. Adequate bed mobilization is nearly impossible owing to the fracture pain. The extended period of hospitalization required is expensive, and often the social isolation of the patient displaced from the normal environment leads to an emotional state which may contribute to death. Although the surgical risks and complications of open reduction and internal fixation in this patient population are serious, there is no other method of treatment that will result in a rapid recovery to a nearly pain-free, mobile, state. Thus, in many cases of fractures in the elderly patient a surgical procedure is the optimal elective form of treatment.

Recent advances in metallurgy and in the design of implant devices have made open reduction and internal fixation more attractive. The telescoping hip nail (see Fig. 58-14A) has great intrinsic strengths and allows the fracture fragments to settle toward each other as necessary during the healing process. Other devices such as the Holt nail (see Fig. 58-14B) are exceptionally strong. Implanted in a fractured human femur, the Holt nail will support loads in excess of 2000 lb, far more than the loading expected during normal unsupported walking.

Surgical open reduction and internal fixation may allow accurate reduction, increased stability of reduction, examination of neurovascular structures, a decreased need for external immobilization, rapid mobilization of joints adjacent to the fracture, shorter hospitalization, and a more rapid return to previous life-style. The risks and potential complications demand a sophisticated analysis of the patient's situation and a choice for the most satisfactory overall treatment program.

Another surgical method to treat fractures is replacement of the damaged part. Even with the most optimal combinations of device and surgical technique, the complication rates for displaced femoral-neck fractures have remained at a high level. Nonunion and aseptic necrosis of the femoral head usually result in a painful, nonfunctional outcome. Since the elderly patient with a displaced femoral-neck fracture usually cannot physiologically afford such a complication, femoral-head replacement arthroplasty has become a frequently utilized treatment method (see Fig. 58-15). Nonunion of the fracture and aseptic necrosis are impossible with this technique. Full weight bearing may be tolerated soon after the surgery. Yet, this method has its own difficulties. Postoperative dislocation of the femoral-head replacement prosthesis is possible. At times, this may be prevented by avoidance of lower-limb flexion, adduction, and internal rotation. Fol-

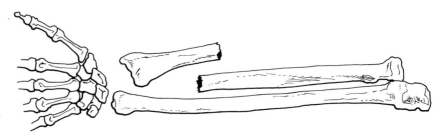

FIGURE 58-13 Galeazzi fracture with disruption of the distal radioulnar joint.

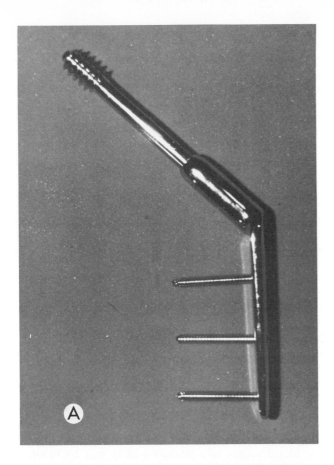

lowing femoral-head replacement, patients should not cross their legs nor should they sit in low chairs until several weeks after their surgery. Migration of the metallic femoral head through the osteoporotic bone into the pelvis has been reported. Finally, after years of satisfactory service, the prosthesis may become painfully loose within the proximal femur, and reoperation may become necessary.

Total hip arthroplasty with stable surgical replacement both of the acetabulum and proximal femur has been infrequently utilized in the past. However, the extraordinary results of this procedure in the treatment of arthritic patients may hasten its use in selected elderly patients with this fracture. The role of total hip arthroplasty as the primary treatment of femoral-neck fractures in the elderly will certainly be investigated and defined in the near future.

Rehabilitation

Recognition of a fracture, accurate reduction, and maintenance of reduction are the primary treatment modalities while a fourth major one remains sadly neglected: *rehabilitation*. The ultimate goal of fracture treatment is to return the patient as rapidly as possible to the pre-injury state.

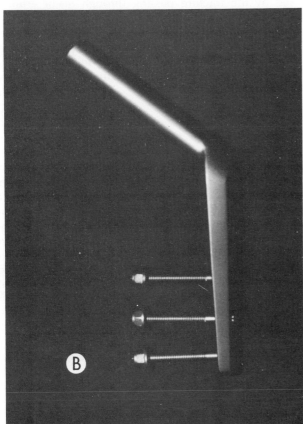

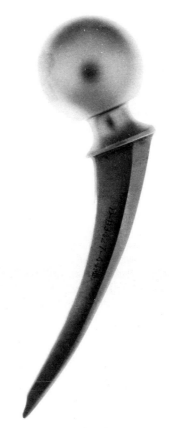

FIGURE 58-14 A, telescoping hip nail. B, Holt nail.

FIGURE 58-15 Femoral-head replacement.

Frequently the effects of the injury and the associated treatment program may unnecessarily result in imperfect or delayed recovery. Since the approximate duration of serious disability may frequently be predicted, it is important to plan for an orderly rehabilitation program from the day of injury. If social assistance is to be required for the family, the appropriate time to initiate procurement procedures is shortly after the injury. It should be anticipated that a patient with severely injured lower extremities will be required to use crutches for an extended time period. Accordingly, exercises to maintain upper extremity strength and mobility should be initiated as soon as feasible after the injury. Plans for a rational vocational rehabilitation program are best organized during the initial period of hospitalization when all the concerned individuals can conveniently meet, discuss the problem, and plan for the future. If special assistive devices will be required upon discharge from the hospital, this is the time to plan for their construction. The nurse, social worker, physical therapist, occupational therapist, vocational rehabilitation representative, and prosthetist-orthotist should during this period develop a comprehensive treatment program rather than wait until the day of discharge from the hospital to formulate a plan.

Fracture complications

Although most patients with fractures progress toward rapid healing and recovery using standard treatment techniques, there are a significant number who are disabled because of complications of the injury and the treatment program. Therefore, it is appropriate to examine some of the specific complications which relate to fracture treatment and to discuss some of the techniques which may be used to minimize their incidence and severity.

Malunion is, as the term implies, a condition in which the fracture has healed in an inappropriate, angulated, or twisted position. A typical example is that of a fractured femur treated by traction and later cast immobilization where insufficient attention was paid to the rotational alignment of the fracture fragments. The results, discovered upon removal of the final cast, are that the distal limb is either internally or externally rotated and the patient is unable to maintain it in a neutral position. These complications may be avoided by both careful analysis of the reduction and accurate maintenance of reduction during the initial healing period.

Loose casts should be changed as needed. Slippage of fracture fragments following reduction should be detected early by sequential radiographic examination. This condition should be reversed as indicated by repeat reduction and immobilization or perhaps by operative treatment.

Delayed union is a term which describes healing that is continuing to occur but at a rate slower than average.

Nonunion of a fracture may be a catastrophic complication for the patient. There are many factors which may predispose a fracture to nonunion, among them inadequate reduction with continued separation of the fracture fragments, inadequate immobilization either by open or closed means, interposition of soft tissues (usually muscle) between the fragments, severe degrees of soft tissue injury, massive bone loss, infection, and specific anatomic circulatory patterns in which the fracture may damage the blood supply to one or more of the fragments.

If postreduction radiograms demonstrate excessive separation of the fragments, the reduction must be repeated. At times, it will be necessaary to perform an open reduction to reposition the fracture fragment to an acceptable position. During surgery, a large mass of muscle may be found lying between the fragments. This mass must be displaced to achieve reduction. The quality of maintenance of reduction position and degree of immobilization should be assessed repeatedly throughout the entire treatment program. At times, it may be necessary to apply new casts successively to eliminate excessive fragment mobility when there is a progressive reduction in the size of the limb due to a loss of edema fluid and muscle atrophy. Early aggressive treatment of soft-tissue infection may prevent osteomyelitis with its associated nonunion implications.

The overwhelming majority of nonunions of fractures are related to a specific anatomic circulatory situation. The blood supply to a fractured bone may be compromised by the fracture passing through major arteries to major fragments. Fractures of the carpal navicular (scaphoid) are particularly prone to nonunion since they pass through the vascular supply to the proximal fragment (see Fig. 58-16). A similar situation holds for fractures of the femoral neck and fractures of the neck of the talus.

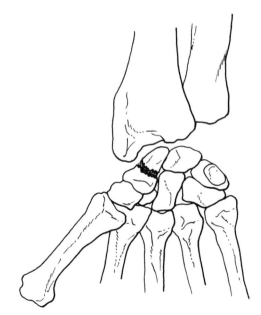

FIGURE 58-16 Fracture of carpal navicular (scaphoid).

The mating articular cartilage-bearing surfaces of normal joints fit one another with considerable accuracy. Thus, for the ball-in-socket hip joint there is little deviation from sphericity of the component parts (see Fig. 58-17). *Subluxation* refers to any deviation from the normal relationship where the articular cartilage is still touching any portion of its mating cartilage. If no portion of its articular cartilage touches the usual mate, the joint is said to be *dislocated*.

Shoulder dislocations are most common in the young and usually result from a traumatic exaggerated abduction, extension, and external rotation position of the upper extremity (see Fig. 58-18). The cocked position for throwing a ball is an example of the position which most frequently, if exaggerated, may cause dislocation. The humeral head is generally displaced anteriorly and inferiorly through a traumatic rent in the shoulder capsule. Characteristically the patient is seen in the emergency room sitting bent over, supporting the injured limb in a flexed position away from the chest or the side. The humeral head may be easily palpated in the anterior axilla. There is a palpable depression beneath the central origin of the deltoid at the acromion. This situation in addition to the patient's pain and appropriate history of the incident is sufficient to indicate the need for roentgenograms for confirmation of the diagnosis. When these films are ordered, it is important to specifically request an axillary view which documents the position of the humeral head with respect to the glenoid and clearly defines the anterior or posterior nature of the dislocation.

During the initial evaluation it is important to examine the neurovascular status of the limb by testing the sensation in the area of the insertion of the deltoid on the humerus. This area is uniquely served by the sensory fibers of the axillary nerve. Local circumscribed anesthesia indicates the likelihood of an axillary nerve injury. Similarly, the ability of the patient to minimally tense the deltoid in a voluntary attempt to initiate abduction also

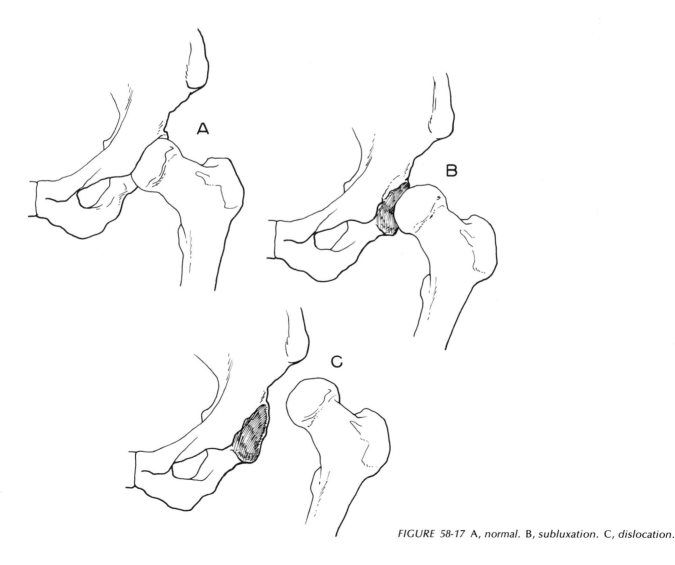

FIGURE 58-17 A, *normal.* B, *subluxation.* C, *dislocation.*

allows an estimate of the function of the axillary nerve. Axillary nerve function is necessary for shoulder abduction so that the patient is able to functionally position the arm. Since this nerve is frequently injured by the trauma of dislocation, it is imperative that the injury be recognized *prior* to any attempts at replacement of the shoulder or reduction. If this very serious axillary nerve deficit is discovered after manipulation, there is no convincing proof that the attempts to treat the patient did not cause this injury.

Ulnar nerve deficit occurs with nearly the same frequency as axillary nerve injury in shoulder dislocations. Ulnar nerve palsy has a severe effect on hand function, and it is equally imperative that the ability to actively abduct and adduct the four lateral digits be initially evaluated. It is absolutely essential that the neurovascular status of the entire extremity be *recorded* prior to any attempt at manipulative reduction lest the damage be attributed to the medical care.

Circulation, sensation, reflexes, and motor power must be examined repeatedly in all injured limbs, primarily for the patient's benefit and secondarily to ascertain the true relationship of the lesion to the trauma. This examination allows the recognition of any additional dysfunction which may have been caused by attempts at reduction.

Sustained anterior traction is the safest and most dependable method of reduction of a dislocated shoulder. With this type of traction, the patient is given an analgesic, generally a narcotic, and is in a prone position on an examination table or cart with the affected limb hanging over the side. Slow, gentle, sustained traction toward the floor is applied. In the majority of cases the reduction

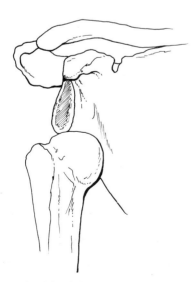

FIGURE 58-18 Shoulder dislocation.

can be felt as a "clunk." This method of reduction is extremely successful and virtually without complications. A post reduction roentgenogram should demonstrate normal anatomy.

Dislocation of the hip is one of the few orthopedic emergencies. If a dislocated hip is not reduced within 12 or at the most 24 hours of the injury, the probability of the patient developing aseptic necrosis is extremely great. Hip dislocation is recognized usually by gluteal, groin, and thigh pain in association with a rigid position of the limb in adduction, internal rotation, and flexion. With appropriate initial reduction of uncomplicated hip dislocations, the patient is frequently capable of living a normal postinjury life. However, with delay and possible aseptic necrosis the individual may be crippled for life. Thus, early recognition and early reduction of hip dislocation are the key elements to a satisfactory end result.

In general, early recognition and reduction of all dislocations are essential for a satisfactory end result. The circulation, sensation, reflexes, and motor power examination of the injured limb should be recorded immediately and repeated several times during the care of a patient with a dislocation.

ARTHRITIS

While many forms of arthritis may be well controlled by medical management, at times the progressive destruction of a major joint or joints may prematurely disable an individual. When the pain and disability are so great that the person is unable to independently carry out the basic activities of living, surgical replacement of the diseased joint may be indicated.

Over 10 years ago John Charnley in England developed the first generally successful prosthetic hip joint. His design included a prosthetic acetabular socket made of ultra–high molecular weight polyethylene mated to a prosthetic femoral head of polished metal. Significantly, the friction between the plastic socket and the metal ball is very low during normal activities, and there is little tendency for the prosthetic components to become loosened from the pelvis or femur. In addition, he discovered that very firm and lasting fixation of the prosthetic components could be accomplished by the use of self-polymerizing methylmethacrylate cement.

Now, with more than 10 years experience and after hundreds of thousands of total hip replacements, it is evident that in more than 90 percent of cases the severe disability due to hip arthritis can be virtually eliminated by total hip arthroplasty.

The same technology has also been applied to the knee, ankle, wrist, and shoulder. Because of the lack of knowledge regarding the long-term effects of implanted methylmethacrylate on the body, the possibility of the component loosening, and danger of infection, these operations have been done primarily on the elderly arthritic patient. However, outstanding rehabilitation successes have resulted from these procedures, and there is a continued interest in both the technical development of the implants and the identification of appropriate patients to maximize the value of surgical joint reconstruction.

OSTEOMYELITIS

Infection of the bone is termed *osteomyelitis*. In children infections of bone commonly develop as a complication of infection from other sites such as the pharynx (pharyngitis), ear (otitis media), and skin (impetigo). The bacteria travel via the bloodstream to the metaphysis near the growth plates where the blood flows into sinusoids. With bacterial proliferation and tissue necrosis, the localized area of inflammation is very tender and painful.

It is extremely important that osteomyelitis, especially in children, be diagnosed early so that appropriate antibiotic and surgical treatment can be administered to prevent the local spread of infection and crippling destruction of the entire bone. Any severely ill child with a painful limb should be examined with osteomyelitis as the likely diagnosis, not thrombophlebitis which is extremely rare in children. An incorrect diagnosis in children with osteomyelitis can lead to serious delay in the initiation of appropriate therapy.

In adults osteomyelitis may also be initiated by blood-borne bacteria but more frequently is the result of tissue contamination at the time of injury or surgery. Bone infections are extremely difficult to eradicate, and even the treatment of surgical drainage and debridement with appropriate antibiotic therapy is often insufficient to eliminate the disease.

QUESTIONS

Fractures and dislocations—Chap. 58

Directions: Circle the letter preceding each item below that correctly answers the question. More than one answer may be correct.

1 When treating an orthopedic emergency, the *primary* objective(s) is (are) to:
   a Reduce the fracture   *b* Preserve the life of the injured person   *c* Use a sling to cradle the limb and hold it in position   *d* Maximize the potential for rapid and complete rehabilitation of the injured person

2 External cardiac massage should be started immediately when there is a (an):
   a Weak, thready pulse   *b* Absence of a pulse   *c* Slow, shallow respiration   *d* Gurgling sound on inspiration and expiration

3 Which of the following techniques of emergency treatment should be used for an injured person who is cyanotic and in obvious respiratory distress?
   a Place in the supine position to allow for continuous drainage   *b* Manually remove debris and clotted blood from the mouth and throat   *c* From the front

position, rapidly compress the chest   *d* After all attempts to remove the obstruction have failed, a tracheostomy must be performed

4 Which of the following best describes arterial bleeding?
   a Red, pulsatile, and voluminous   *b* Continuous flow, dark red   *c* Red and scant

5 At the scene of an accident you have been unable to stop the victim's massive femoral arterial hemorrhaging by applying a series of compress pressure dressings. You decide to apply a tourniquet. A tourniquet should always be applied _____ the hemorrhaging site.
   a Distal to   *b* Proximal to   *c* At

6 The most *important* precaution, when using a tourniquet, is to note the exact time of application. Although changes are usually reversible up to 2 hours, an extremity is likely to die if a tourniquet is left in place longer than _____ hours.
   a 4   *b* 6   *c* 10   *d* 12

7 The correct emergency treatment for a limb deformity near a knee joint is to:
   a Tie the injured limb to the adjacent uninjured one
   b Straighten the limb to a near normal position and bind it to a stable appropriate object   *c* Not attempt to straighten the limb because of the close proximity to nerves and blood vessels to the fractured fragments
   d Support the limb on a soft support without attempting to straighten it

8 When splinting an injured limb, the following applies (apply):
   a No padding is necessary   *b* Check distal pulse before and after the procedure   *c* Only sterile bandages are to be applied to open wounds   *d* Ample padding is necessary

9 Which type of fracture is illustrated in the accompanying diagram? (See Fig. 58-19A on p. 724)
   a Greenstick   *b* Oblique   *c* Spiral   *d* Transverse

10 Which type of fracture is illustrated in the accompanying diagram? (See Fig. 58-19B on p. 724)
   a Pathologic   *b* Greenstick   *c* Fatigue
   d Compression

11 *Opposition* refers to the
   a Degree of fracture severity   *b* Degrees of deviation from the normal longitudinal axis and the direction of the apex of the angle   *c* Extent of displacement of the fracture surfaces   *d* Percentage of the fractured portion of one fragment that touches its mate

12 Which of the following is a definite sign of a fracture?
   a Generalized pain and tenderness   *b* Crepitus
   c Abrasions   *d* Shock

13 A cast that is applied to maintain a reduction should usually be placed:
a Past the joint above and the joint below the fracture *b* Over the fractured area only *c* Over the smallest area possible to prevent pressure and decubiti formation

14 The advantages of operative fracture treatment include:
a Increased accuracy in repositioning the fracture fragments *b* Opportunity for inspection of adjacent vessels and nerves *c* No need for external casts or appliances after stabilization *d* Potential for maintenance of nearly normal joint function and muscular strength during fracture treatment

15 The most frequent reasons for using open reduction and internal fixation of fractures are:
a To avoid deep-wound infections *b* Inability to obtain an adequate reduction by closed means *c* To avoid complications resulting from prolonged bed rest in early patients

16 Mr. M. was diagnosed with a fractured femur and was treated by traction and later cast immobilization. Upon removal of the final cast, the distal limb is either internally or externally rotated and cannot be maintained in a neutral position by the patient. This fracture complication is referred to as:
a Nonunion *b* Delayed union *c* Malunion *d* Osteomyelitis

17 Tom, a 20-year-old college student, severely injured his knee while playing soccer. At the time of admission his knee was too severely swollen, painful, and tender to make a definitive diagnosis. The most appropriate traction to use for comfort until his condition improves and a diagnosis can be made is:
a Buck's *b* Balanced skeletal *c* Russell's *d* Bryant's

18 Balanced skeletal traction is frequently used in the treatment of fractures of the:
a Patella *b* Tibia *c* Femur *d* Humerus

19 The traction illustrated in the figure below is used in the treatment of femoral fractures in children:
a Above 5 years of age and weighing over 40 lb *b* Three years of age and weighing 30 lb *c* Three years of age and weighing 40 lb *d* Six years of age and weighing 60 lb

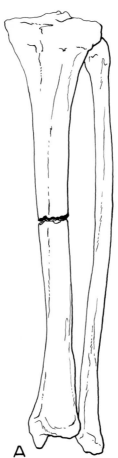
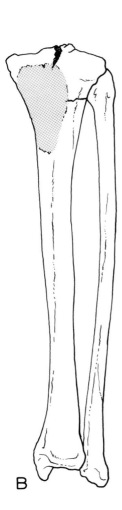
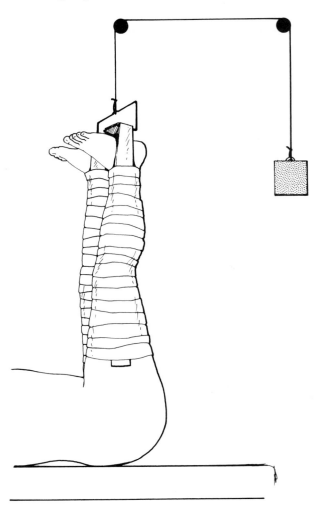

A   B

FIGURE 58-19

20 Which of the following are possible complications if the age and weight limitations are exceeded in Bryant's traction:

a The vascular supply to the feet in older and larger children may be compromised by the hydrostatic effect of vertical limb placement and constrictive elastic wraps b The osmotic pressure of the blood is decreased c Severe damage to the skin can result from exceeding these limits d The heart rate is slower

21 One complication of operative fracture treatment is osteomyelitis. Which of the following is a characteristic of osteomyelitis:

a A benign neoplasm consisting of osteoblastic connective tissue b Infection of the bone marrow and adjacent bone and cartilage c A sarcoma in bone containing foci of neoplastic cartilage

22 Subluxation:

a Occurs when no portion of a cartilaginous surface is in contact with its mating cartilage b Refers to the angle of fracture in the femur c Occurs when parts of articular cartilage are partially separated d Is a method of reducing a fractured limb

23 All the following are signs and symptoms indicative of a shoulder dislocation except:

a The patient supports the injured limb in a flexed position away from the chest or the side b The humeral head can be palpated in the anterior axilla c There is localized pain in the area of the injury d There is a definite sensation of crepitus

24 Before attempting to reduce a dislocated shoulder, one must observe and record which of the following:

a The amount and duration of pain the victim is experiencing b The presence of tactile sensation within a small designated area over the deltoid muscle c Blood pressure and pulse rate d Ability of the patient to minimally elevate the injured limb away from the body

25 The important structure that is necessary for shoulder abduction and is most frequently injured as a complication of a shoulder dislocation is the:

a Radial nerve b Brachial artery c Axillary nerve d Radial artery

26 Mr. S., 35 years old, was brought to the emergency room after falling down his basement stairs. He is experiencing pain in his left groin and in the gluteal region. His right leg is flexed at the hip, adducted, and internally rotated. Mr. S.'s most likely diagnosis is a:

a Fractured acetubulum b Dislocated hip c Fractured femoral head d Fractured femur

27 Label the parts of the long bone—diaphysis, epiphysis, physis, periosteum—in the accompanying diagram.

Directions: Circle T if the statement is true and F if it is false. Correct any false statements.

28   T   F   A closed fracture is one where the skin on the involved limb has been penetrated.

29   T   F   The most frequent method of reduction is by manual manipulation.

30   T   F   Comminution involves more than two fracture fragments.

31   T   F   Closed reduction of a fracture involves detailed and precise surgical approximation of the bone ends.

Directions: Match the type of fracture in col. A with its characteristic in col. B. Each letter may be used more than once.

Column A	Column B
32 ____ Spiral	a Heals rapidly; occurs in children
33 ____ Oblique	b Results from torsion of a limb
34 ____ Greenstick	c Occurs in people who have recently increased their activity level
35 ____ Pathologic	d Typical in ski injuries
36 ____ Fatigue	e Primary or metastatic tumors are most frequent cause
	f Proceeds at an angle across bone

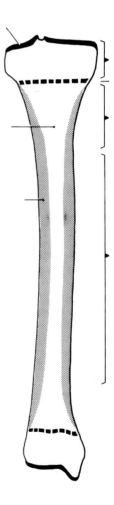

Directions: Answer the following questions on a separate sheet of paper.

37 List all the signs of neurovascular dysfunction.

38 Why is it important to immediately treat a limb with a compromised neurovascular supply by splitting all layers of the cast from one end to the other?

39 Describe the type of pain, what this usually indicates, and the treatment when a cast has not been molded or padded sufficiently over bony prominences.

40 Why is skeletal traction generally preferable to skin traction?

41 What are the principles used in traction to maintain a satisfactory reduction of limb fractures?

42 List the advantages of traction as a method of reduction of a limb.

43 List the advantages of implant devices such as the telescoping hip nail.

44 What is the ultimate goal of fracture treatment and how is this achieved?

CHAPTER 59   Orthopedic Diseases of Children

HEALING POTENTIAL OF CHILDREN'S FRACTURES

Children's fractures heal rapidly and well. The active periosteal sleeve around the tubular bones in children is very strong. Since this area is rarely completely ruptured, fracture fragments tend to be maintained in acceptable position after fracture. Children's bones have great potential for corrective remodeling. Thus, a considerable postreduction angular deformity may be accepted with confidence that the mature bone will be straight without evidence of injury. In addition, there is a tendency of the injured limb to grow faster than normal. *Bayonette apposition* is often preferable to an end-on-end reduction in order to achieve equal adult limb lengths (see Fig. 59-1). While angular deformities do rapidly correct, there is no similar tendency for rotational deformities to spontaneously resolve. Thus it is of utmost importance to maintain a normal rotational position during healing.

Most fractures in children are appropriately treated by closed reduction and external immobilization with casts or traction. Only a few very specific children's fractures are optimally treated surgically. An example is a fracture of the lateral condyle of the humerus which extends into the joint and which may also involve an injury to the

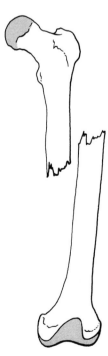

FIGURE 59-1 Bayonette apposition.

epiphyseal growth plate. Failure to accurately reduce the fragment back to its normal anatomic position may lead to a reduction of elbow function and growth arrest of the limb, which may result in gross deformity developing with increasing maturity. Fractures of the head of the radius and of the hip in children also frequently demand surgical treatment. In general, fractures which extend into joints or which pass across or through growth plates require surgery more often than do other fractures.

SPECIFIC DISEASES

Congenital dislocation of the hip is a condition in which the femoral head is not positioned normally in the acetabulum at birth (see Fig. 59-2). In addition, there is usually a delay in the maturity, size, and development of both the femoral head and the socket itself. The femoral head is small and frequently located superiorly and laterally out of the acetabulum.

Normal congruous development of the hip requires a normal congruent relation between the femoral head and the acetabulum. Long-term dissociation (separation) leads to inadequate development of both the femoral head and acetabulum and will result in ultimate *crippling* of the individual. *All* newborn children should be examined for congenital hip dislocation within a few days of birth. This neonatal examination should specifically test for the ability to manually dislocate and then reduce the abnormal hip. The baby is placed in a supine position

with both hips flexed. A gentle pressure is applied at the knees toward the examining table and the knees and the thighs are manually abducted. At the same time an upward and medial pressure is applied to the proximal thighs. This initial downward knee pressure causes complete dislocation of the affected hip. When the thighs are abducted as described above, the hip can be felt to spontaneously reduce with a "clunk." Then with adduction the hip can be felt to dislocate. The hip instability demonstrated by this provocation test is diagnostic of congenital hip disease and is known as a *positive Ortolani's sign* (see Fig. 59-3).

An inability to fully *abduct* one or both hips is frequently seen in a congenital dislocated hip (see Fig. 59-4). Additional signs include the Addis test where obvious pathologic shortening of the thigh is noted (see Fig. 59-5). Asymmetric skin folds, extra gluteal folds, or inguinal creases are less definitive signs, but they do identify the need for further careful examination.

The most important radiographic view is an anterior posterior projection of the pelvis and hips with the hips extended, the thighs together, and the lower limbs in neutral rotation. This position ensures maximal separation of the femoral head and acetabulum. If the femoral head does not lie in the lower inner quadrant as defined by Hilgenringer's line (drawn horizontially through the triradiate cartilage connecting the bones of the pelvis) and Perkin's line (drawn vertically downward from the superior lateral margin), congenital dislocation of the hip is the most likely diagnosis (see Fig. 59-6). The femoral head of the affected side is usually smaller than normal. The acetabular angle is greater than normal. However, of greater diagnostic significance is absence of the normal cupping depression of the acetabulum.

If congenital hip disease is diagnosed in the newborn infant, the appropriate treatment is reduction or relocation of the femoral head within the socket. This reduction must be maintained until the mutual relationship between the ball and the socket have stimulated a normal development and resolution of the disease. Gentle manipulation will generally allow seating of the femoral head in the acetabulum. Immobilization to maintain reduction must not be in an extreme position. Forceful reduction and extreme positions often lead to rapid development of aseptic necrosis of the femoral head which may be a situation *more disabling* than the congenital hip dislocation itself. Many orthopedists rely on casts applied during anesthesia to maintain the first reduction for a period of a few months and continue the treatment with splints or braces until the radiograms demonstrate symmetric and normal hip development.

While braces may be used from the outset, it is possible for the hip to become dislocated during the infant's diaper changes. When the brace or splint is reapplied, the femoral head may be forced against the pelvic wall in a dislocated position. It is more advantageous to maintain the limb in a reduced position in a carefully applied cast until a relative degree of stability is achieved.

Nearly all patients with congenital dislocation of the hip who are diagnosed in the neonatal period and treated as described above will develop hips which function nor-

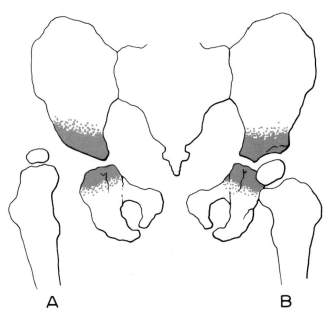

A   B

FIGURE 59-2 A, Congenital dislocation of the hip. B, Normal hip.

mally throughout their lives. The success of this treatment in the neonatal period emphasizes the need for early diagnosis of *all* cases. If the diagnosis is not made until the child is 1 or 2 years of age, the chances for success are greatly compromised. Although closed reduction and immobilization may be a successful mode of treatment, operative care is often necessary. Many operative procedures have been described for the late treatment of congenital dislocation of the hips; this wide variety of treatment indicates the lack of predictable success for any specific procedure.

Talipes equinovarus (clubfoot) is another childhood disease which is optimally treated by early diagnosis and conservative management. In this condition the newborn foot is abnormally directed downward and turned in (see Fig. 59-7). It cannot be passively corrected to a normal position. While some spontaneous normalization may occur with time, the optimal immediate treatment to achieve maximal correction is the application of a small, short leg cast in the position of correction. This treatment is repeated on a daily or alternate-day basis. The newborn has an amazing potential for a plastic response to corrective forces which are applied early. Most clubfoot deformities can be corrected in a few weeks, and the correction need be maintained only until the foot is stable in the new, more normal position. With this treatment program the need for operative repositioning is decreased enormously. Prior treatment programs involved manipulation and cast application on an every-other-week basis. This procedure is to be condemned since it

fails to take maximal advantage of the great flexibility and rapid corrective response characteristic of the neonatal period.

Calvé-Legg-Perthes' disease is a condition affecting the hip joint of children, the majority of whom are 5 to 7 years of age. Although frequently classified as an osteochondritis, the etiology is unknown. The specific pathophysiology remains uncertain. Frequently a healthy child will begin to complain of groin or knee pain on an intermittent but increasingly frequent basis. The knee is often examined. The negative examination and normal knee roentgenograms delay the important process of hip evaluation. The fact that the pain usually originates in the hip region and radiates directly to the knee tends to delay the diagnosis. Finally, the continued pain and limp eventually lead to an examination of the hip. The hip is painful during a forced range of motion examination. Roentgenograms usually demonstrate an increase in the apparent joint space and a slight lateral displacement of the femoral head owing to the presence of moderately tense effusion. At times, the joint capsule may be seen bulging. The femoral epiphysis appears somewhat flat (see Fig. 59-8B). In this early stage the epiphysis is probably relatively avascular and somewhat soft.

With time cystic changes (see Fig. 59-8C) appear, and

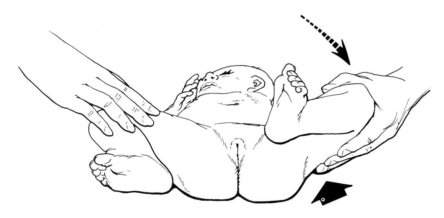

FIGURE 59-3 Ortolani's sign.

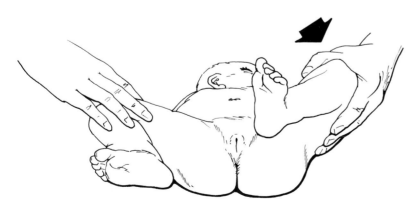

FIGURE 59-4 Limitation of abduction.

frequently the epiphysis appears to fragment (see Fig. 59-8D). After many months revascularization (see Fig. 59-8E) occurs, and the epiphysis regains its blood supply and strength.

Historically, treatment has relied on methods which can minimize the deforming forces on the affected epiphysis such as crutches with a leather sling to support

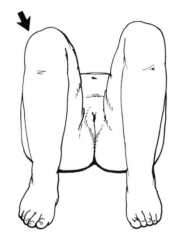

FIGURE 59-5 Addis test.

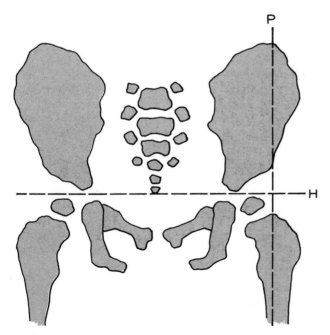

FIGURE 59-6 X-ray changes in congenital dislocation of the hip. (Modified from Smith, Badgley, Orwig, and Harper, "Correlation of Postreduction Roentgenograms and Thirty-one Year Follow-up in Congenital Dislocation of the Hip," J. Bone Joint Surg., 50-A: 6, 1968.)

the distal limb and discourage weight bearing, non–weight-bearing crutch walking, or bed rest. After a few weeks, the child usually becomes symptom-free and discontinues the treatment program before reconstitution has progressed. With unprotected ambulation the femoral head becomes increasingly deformed, and a permanent crippling deformity results.

For many years long-limb suspension ischial weight-bearing braces were used to attempt to accomplish the goal of sustained protection of the hip. Frankel recently proved that the voluntary acceleration of the brace and limb during normal gate required muscular activity about the hip which imposed loads on the involved epiphysis. These loads were at least as great in magnitude and deformation potential as those experienced during normal unprotected gait. This type of brace is therefore ill advised.

Another more recent treatment method depends upon the normal spherical anatomy of the uninvolved acetabulum. This concept is that if the capital femoral epiphysis can be positioned and maintained within the spherical acetabulum, it will be protected from significant deformation during the natural course of the disease. Thus, abduction braces and casts have been used to accomplish this goal. Although theoretically correct, the treatment method is cumbersome, and the brace is often discarded before the final safe stage of the disease.

In Scandinavia, bed rest or bed rest with traction (Mose) imposed throughout the course of the disease has been demonstrated to produce the best results, as documented by repeated roentgenograms. However, the required period of inactivity is approximately 18 months. There is considerable disagreement whether the disease has such serious or disabling consequences as to warrant this extreme treatment.

In summary, the essence of treatment would appear to be minimization of muscular and weight forces on the femoral head until reconstitution has occurred. Contain-

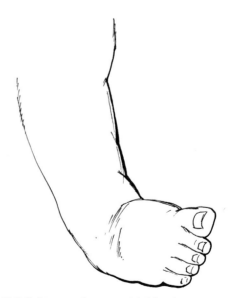

FIGURE 59-7 Talipes equinovarus (clubfoot).

ment of the soft femoral head in the acetabulum may be of some value. Surgical reshaping or repositioning of the acetabulum to increase the coverage or protection of the femoral head has recently been attempted. Until the end results have been documented, it is too soon to adequately judge this new treatment method.

Slipped capital femoral epiphysis is another fairly common disease of children. These children are usually in their early teens and have no associated disease. They are usually obese but may also be notably thin. The incidence is greater in males.

In this condition the epiphyseal plate of the proximal femur has insufficient sheer strength to prevent deformation, and slippage of the femoral epiphysis occurs from its normal position directly on the end of the femoral neck. It may progressively slip medially (into varus) and posteriorly relative to the femoral neck (see Fig. 59-9).

These patients also complain of pain on a forced end range of motion examination. When hip flexion is attempted, the limb automatically assumes a position of external rotation. Internal rotation in a flexed position is markedly limited. The knee on the same side feels painful and again excessive medical interest in the knee may misdirect the diagnosis away from the diseased hip joint. Children, as well as adults, with complaints of knee pain should have an examination of the hips. In this condition an accurate early diagnosis may make a great difference in the patient's subsequent course. If the disease is diagnosed early, when minimal slippage and deformity has occurred, a simple internal pin fixation may stabilize the epiphysis, and nearly normal function frequently may be expected. However, if the individual continues untreated with unrestricted activity, increased deformity with the associated loss of normal range of motion may result. The incidence of aseptic necrosis and resultant crippling hip disease parallels delay in treatment. When a teen-ager is examined for suspicious knee, groin, or hip pain, an x-ray is indicated. A positive result for slipped capital femoral epiphysis indicates the immediate need for crutches at least, and possibly for early or immediate hospitalization and treatment (see Fig. 59-10A, B).

While multiple pin stabilization is frequently satisfactory treatment for mild slips, those with more deformity may require extensive surgery to identify the diseased epiphyseal plate. The growth plate is then wholly or partially removed. An iliac bone graft is impacted across the plate region into the epiphysis. This procedure ensures immediate mechanical stability and early solid union of the epiphysis to the shaft. It is important to note that full unprotected activity is not completely safe until this union has taken place. Since forceable attempts at reduction of the epiphysis to its normal position are strongly related to head necrosis, it is generally best to accept even a moderate degree of deformity and to attempt union in this postion. Since the bulge of the lateral proximal femoral neck may restrict abduction and internal rotation, this protrusion is surgically removed during the operation (see Fig. 59-10C).

Scoliosis means curvature of the spine as observed by an anteroposterior x-ray. Although there are many recognized causes of scoliosis, the most frequent type is re-

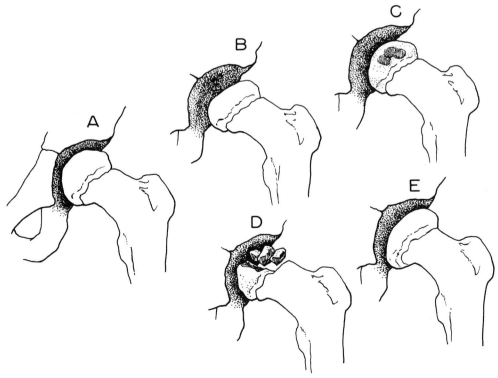

FIGURE 59-8 Stages of Calvé-Legg-Perthes' disease. A, normal. B, flattening. C, cystic changes. D, fragmentation. E, reconstitution.

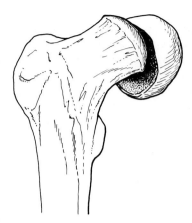

FIGURE 59-9 Slipped capital femoral epiphysis.

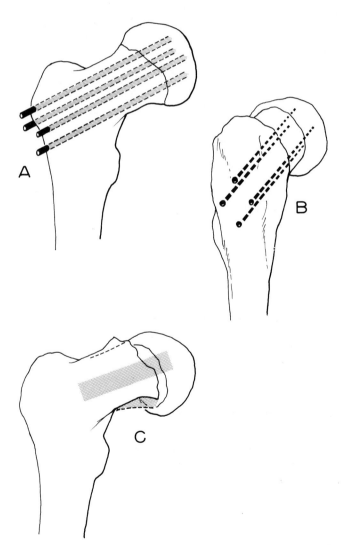

FIGURE 59-10 Surgical treatment for slipped capital femoral epiphysis.

ferred to as *idiopathic scoliosis*. A typical example of this condition would be an 11- or 12-year-old girl noted to have a protrusion of the right posterior chest with the right scapula appearing high and prominent. Her clothing would drape poorly, and there would be an apparent difference in the lengths of the lower limbs. Initially although mildly deforming, with adolescent prematuration rapid growth the curvature may very quickly become much more severe. As the curvature increases, a rotation of the spine develops, and the deformity of the thorax becomes very offensive (see Fig. 59-11).

If an early diagnosis of idiopathic scoliosis is made, the youngster may usually be effectively treated with a Milwaukee brace. This sophisticated device not only tends to hold the spine straight in tension, but, of greater importance, it encourages the patient to use his or her own muscles to maintain the correction. With further growth in the corrected position, progression of the deformity is halted and at times reversed. The brace must be worn 23 hours daily, and a series of breathing, straightening, and strengthening exercises must be carried out. The brace must be worn until there is definite objective evidence of skeletal maturity with cessation of further spinal growth. The iliac apophysis must have appeared and progressed toward the sacrum (Risser sign), and the vertebral ring apophysis must have fused to the central mass of the vertebral bodies (see Fig. 59-12). A regular menstrual cycle, secondary sex characteristics, i.e., development of axillary and pubic hair and of breasts,

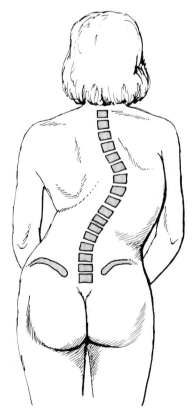

FIGURE 59-11 Scoliosis.

should be established before brace treatment may be safely discontinued. Although the deformity documented at diagnosis can rarely be reversed by brace treatment, further progression is usually prevented. After skeletal maturity, a slight progression of the deformity is anticipated, but the patient can be expected to lead a nearly normal life.

In the case of a late diagnosis or failure of brace treatment, surgical straightening of the spine and spinal fusion in the corrected position may be the best treatment. Special surgical implants such as Harrington rods may be used to straighten the spine at fusion. A skeletal brace traction, the Halo pelvic brace, may be required in severe cases. Spinal fusions are massive operations with a significant complication rate. Therefore, the best expected end result is a stiff spine in a partially corrected position. It is very important that the diagnosis be made early and the Milwaukee brace therapy be initiated before the deformity becomes excessive or the spine too stiff.

QUESTIONS

Orthopedic diseases of children—Chapter. 59

Directions: Circle the letter preceding each item below that correctly answers the question. More than one answer may be correct.

1 All newborn babies in the nursery should be examined for the presence of the following signs of congenital hip dislocation:

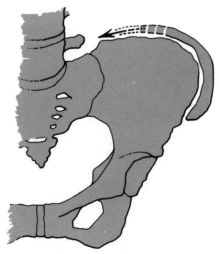

FIGURE 59-12 Risser sign. (Modified from Hugo Keim, "Scoliosis," Clinical Symposia, **24:** 1, Ciba-Geigy Corp., Summit, N.J., 1972.)

a Limitation of abduction in initial flexion *b* Impaction of the two bone ends *c* A positive Ortolani's sign (palpable click on adduction and abduction) *d* Limitation of adduction

2 The treatment (early after birth) of a congenital dislocated hip is:
a To place the proximal head of the ischium into the acetabulum and hold until stable in position *b* Open reduction to establish a new acetabulum and to reposition the head of the femur in that *c* To place the proximal head of the femur into the acromion process and hold in a cast until stable *d* To relocate the femoral head within the socket and to maintain this reduction in a cast in abduction with the femoral head reduced in position

3 Talipes equinovarus is best treated by:
a Use of multiple casts *b* Surgical procedure to shorten the calcaneal tendon *c* Bryant's traction *d* Buck's traction

4 The condition characterized by flattening, cystic changes, breakup, and reconstitution of the femoral head is:
a Slipped capital femoral epiphysis *b* Calvé-Legg-Perthes disease *c* Osteoarthritis of the femoral head *d* Osteogenic sarcoma

5 John, an overweight 13-year-old, presents with moderate groin and knee pain in his left leg. While flexing his hip, John's leg abducts and externally rotates. The most likely diagnosis of John's condition is:
a Congenital dislocation of the hip *b* Slipped capital femoral epiphysis *c* Calvé-Legg-Perthes disease *d* Fracture of the femoral head

6 Optimum treatment for idiopathic scoliosis depends primarily upon:
a Surgery after the curvature is of significant magnitude and fixed *b* Brace treatment for 2 years *c* Early examination and diagnosis at a stage of relative skeletal immaturity *d* Use of casts prior to surgery

Directions: Answer the following questions on a separate sheet of paper.

7 Explain why children's fractures usually heal rapidly and well.

8 Why is bayonette apposition often preferable in reduction of children's fractures?

CHAPTER 60   Tumors of the Musculoskeletal System

OBJECTIVES

At the completion of Chap. 60 you should be able to:

1 List the signs and symptoms associated with tumors of the musculoskeletal system.

2 Explain the rationale for treatment of a lesion that is benign and self-limiting as opposed to a lesion that is less certainly benign. State an example of each type of lesion.

3 List the complications that may result in the use of a cannulated needle to obtain a tissue biopsy.

4 State the advantages and disadvantages of performing an open excisional biopsy to obtain a tissue specimen.

5 For osteogenic sarcoma identify the age group affected, sites of occurrence, appearance, treatment, and prognosis.

6 List the clinical signs and symptoms that increase concern for malignant tumor potential.

7 Identify the radiographic appearance and the cause for the "onion-skin" appearance of Ewing's sarcoma.

8 Describe the specific radiologic signs that may be associated with a chondroblastoma, a benign unicameral cyst, giant-cell tumor, osteogenic sarcoma, Ewing's sarcoma, and osteoid osteoma.

9 State the etiology of the major type of bone tumor in adults.

PRESENTING SIGNS AND SYMPTOMS AND DIAGNOSTIC MEASURES

A complete presentation of the diagnosis, characterization, pathophysiology, and treatment of tumors of the musculoskeletal system is beyond the scope of this chapter. Therefore, it is more appropriate to focus the discussion on information pertaining to these lesions as they confront the medical team. The emphasis of this chapter will be on the rationale for an appropriate medical care plan.

The patient frequently presents with a painful, enlarging mass. Characteristically the pain is minimal, related to activity, and frequently more intense at night. There is usually no previous history of specific serious trauma. Occasionally the tumor will have weakened the bone to such an extent that a pathologic fracture has occurred. The tumor may have been discovered by x-ray examination that was done for unrelated reasons. No matter how the patient presents, the immediate concern is whether the mass should be biopsied.

Some tumors or lesions may be directly identified by a consideration of the characteristics of the patient, the family history, the course of the condition, and the radiographic appearance of the lesion. In cases where the condition is definitively diagnosed as benign and self-limiting, e.g., a bone island or degenerative cyst, no further diagnostic studies are needed and no further medical care is usually necessary. In other cases the lesion may be diagnosed as benign with a lesser degree of certainty, e.g., osteochondroma or unicameral bone cyst. When uncertainty exists about the lesion, it may be reasonable to reexamine the patient at intervals and to repeat the radiograms. The dimension of time and the rate of change used in this treatment regimen may eliminate the need for a surgical procedure. When this method of treatment is used, an assessment must be made as to whether the patient and the family are responsible and will return for repeat examinations. If a series of examinations over several months reveals no change in the lesion or in the condition of the patient, follow-up visits may be discontinued. The patient should be instructed to return for a further examination should any changes become evident. Many lesions may not be easily identified and may leave doubts as to the possibility of malignancy. Under these circumstances and especially if the patient is not likely to return for repeated examinations, a biopsy is necessary for a definitive diagnosis.

When obtaining a sample of tissue from the lesion, use of a cannulated needle is convenient and often successful. However, several problems are associated with this technique. The needle may macerate the tissue and thus destroy its important architecture. There is no certainty as to the exact location sampled, and so the tumor cells may not be included in the examined material. There is also the potential of injury to vascular or vital structures which may be recognized as a late complication.

Although inconvenient for the patient and usually requiring hospitalization, open excisional biopsy may be the procedure of choice. This procedure is most appropriate for a patient who has a small, circumscribed lesion of uncertain identity. For example, in osteoid osteoma the lesion may be totally removed, positively identified, and the treatment completed with an excisional biopsy, or such a biopsy may identify a tumor with considerably greater malignant potential which may require more extensive definitive treatment.

TYPES OF TUMORS

A characteristic feature of a *giant-cell tumor* is the vascular and cellular stroma which is made up of oval-shaped cells containing small, elongated, darkly staining nuclei. The giant cell is a large cell with pink-staining cytoplasm; it contains numerous nuclei which are vesicular and appear similar to stromal cells. Although this tumor is usually considered to be benign, there are varying degrees of malignancy, depending upon the sarcomatous nature of the stroma. In the malignant types, the tumor becomes anaplastic with areas of necrosis and hemorrhage. Such tumors occur chiefly in young adults. The common sites are the ends of the long bones, especially at the knee and the lower end of the radius. This type of tumor usually requires a definitive gross local excision after biopsy identification. Removal of a safe border of normal tissue is in this case necessary. Characteristics of this tumor are that it tends to be locally recurrent and of increasingly malignant character after incomplete excision. With prior biopsy, diagnosis, and gross local removal, an immediate

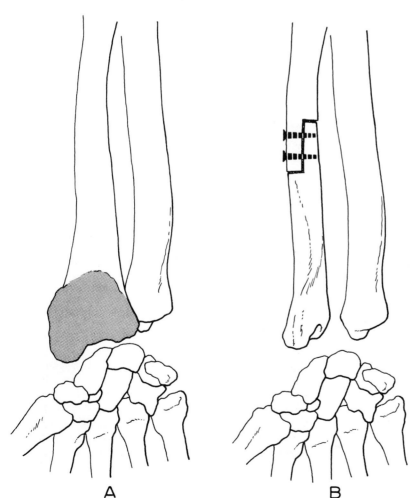

A   B

FIGURE 60-1 A, giant-cell tumor of the distal radius. B, use of a bone transplant to reconstruct the limb after total excision of a giant-cell tumor.

reconstruction of the area may be possible. In the case of a large giant-cell tumor of the distal radius (see Fig. 60-1A) the patient's proximal fibula can be substituted to reconstruct the forearm (see Fig. 60-1B).

Osteogenic sarcoma, or osteosarcoma, is a very malignant primary neoplasm of bone. The tumor arises in the metaphysis of the bone. The most common sites are at the ends of the long bones, especially at the knee. The incidence of osteogenic sarcoma is greatest in adolescents and young adults, but it may also affect people, usually over 50 years of age, who have Paget's disease.

The gross appearance of osteogenic sarcoma is variable. It may be (1) osteolytic where the bone is destroyed and the soft tissue invaded by the lesion, or (2) osteoblastic as a result of the formation of new sclerotic bone. Periosteal new bone may be deposited adjacent to the lesion itself appearing as a triangle on x-rays (see Fig. 60-2). Although this is seen with many malignancies of bone, it is characteristic of osteogenic sarcoma; the tumor itself may produce a somewhat abortive form of bone. The radiographic appearance of such a lesion is referred to as a "sunburst," as depicted in Fig. 60-3.

Some primary tumors such as osteogenic sarcoma may be best treated by amputation or radical ablative surgery. While chemotherapy and immunotherapy appear to have some potential benefits, complete surgical removal of the tumor and all surrounding tissue is usually necessary. The most satisfactory operative procedure is amputation.

Ewing's sarcoma is another very malignant bone tumor. This tumor is most often seen in preteen-age children. The common site is the shaft of long bones. The gross appearance is a soft, gray tumor arising in the bone marrow which erodes bone cortex from within. Under the periosteum, layers of new bone are deposited parallel to the shaft producing an "onion skin" effect (see Fig. 60-4). The typical signs and symptoms are pain, tender swelling, fever, and leukocytosis. Treatment consists of radiation therapy and surgical removal of the tumor. A poor prognosis is associated with this tumor. Recent reports indicate that new techniques of chemotherapy may significantly increase the survival rate.

SIGNS AND SYMPTOMS ASSOCIATED WITH MALIGNANT TUMORS

What are the clinical signs and symptoms that may indicate a malignant tumor potential? The rate of increase in the size of the mass is important. Benign lesions grow

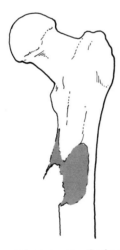

FIGURE 60-2 Osteogenic sarcoma—Codman's triangle.

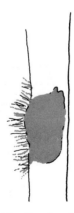

FIGURE 60-3 Radiographic "sunburst" appearance seen in osteogenic sarcoma.

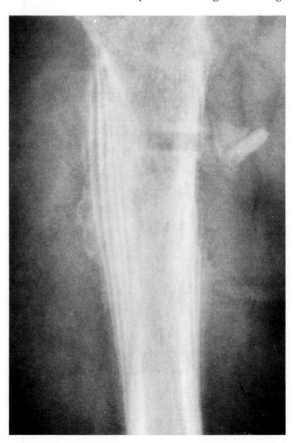

FIGURE 60-4 Radiographic "onion skin" appearance seen in Ewing's sarcoma. Courtesy of Dr. William Martel.

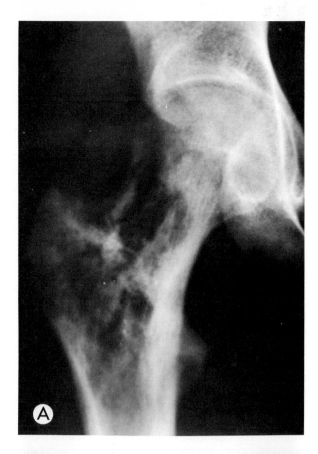

very slowly or not at all, while a very malignant tumor may double in size within a month. Increasing night pain and sleeplessness that are associated with weight loss in a healthy individual are important indications. Fatigability in a young person is a very significant sign. A persistent fever and localized temperature increase in the region of the tumor indicate an increase in cellular activity. Finally, a physiologic dysfunction such as obstruction of the ureters, an obstruction of a major vessel, or neurologic dysfunction is frequently seen in malignant tumors.

DIAGNOSTIC STUDIES

As a general rule the radiographic appearance of a specific lesion may be very helpful in determining its relative malignancy. For example, a lesion with discrete rounded margins tends to be benign. Such a lesion fre-

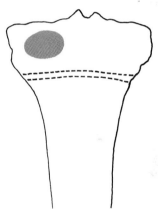

FIGURE 60-6 Chondroblastoma.

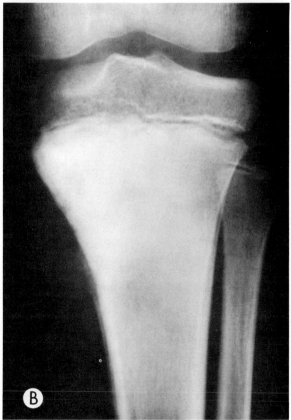

FIGURE 60-5 Radiographic appearance of a malignant tumor. A, femur. B, tibia. Courtesy of Dr. William Martel.

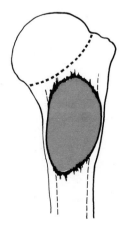

FIGURE 60-7 Unicameral bone cyst.

quently has a sclerotic margin, indicating that the bone has had the time and ability to respond to the mass. The lack of a definable margin indicates invasion of the tumor into adjacent bone (see Fig. 60-5A). This lesion is growing rapidly and the bone has not had sufficient time or a defense response to react against it. Extension of the lesion

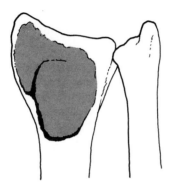

FIGURE 60-8 Radiographic appearance typical of a giant-cell tumor.

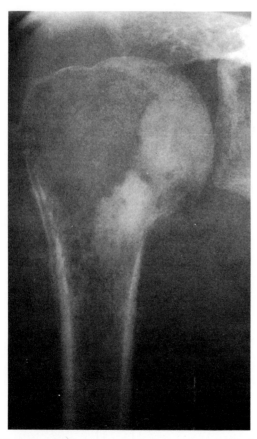

FIGURE 60-9 Radiolucent cortical lesion typical of Ewing's sarcoma. Courtesy of Dr. William Martel.

through the cortex of the bone is typical of a malignancy. When the tumor penetrates the cortex, the periosteum may be lifted off. It may respond by depositing a thin layer of reactive bone, then be lifted off, and the periosteal reaction begins again. As mentioned previously, this produces an "onion skin" effect typical of Ewing's sarcoma (see Fig. 60-5B).

While the previous radiographic signs indicate the degree of malignancy of a lesion, there are other specific x-ray signs that lead to a more definitive diagnosis. For example, a radiolucent lesion located within the epiphysis of a growing bone is apt to be a chondroblastoma (see Fig. 60-6). A sclerotic marginated cystic lesion in the metaphysis of a long bone near an active growth plate is likely to be a benign unicameral bone cyst (see Fig. 60-7). A lucent lesion in an adult in the metaphysis near the old growth plate is likely to be a giant-cell tumor (see Fig. 60-8).

A large, destructive lesion penetrating the cortex of the metaphysis of a long bone of an adolescent or young adult is very indicative of osteogenic sarcoma. A reticulate, spotty, and extensive radiolucent cortical lesion in a child is very likely to be Ewing's sarcoma (see Fig. 60-9). A "target" or "bullseye" lesion, sclerotic bone around a radiolucent area surrounding a central dense nucleus, in an individual with night pain which responds to salicylates is nearly always an osteoid osteoma.

The age of the patient offers significant diagnostic information. For example, children are often affected by a unicameral cyst, eosinophilic granuloma, or Ewing's sarcoma, while slightly later chondroblastoma becomes relatively more prevalent. As mentioned previously, adolescents and young adults are the usual victims of osteogenic sarcoma, which also affects people in the late middle years who have Paget's disease.

The major type of bone tumor in adults is metastasis from other primary sites such as the lungs, breasts, thyroid, kidneys, and the prostate. Multiple myeloma is the most common primary tumor of bone in adults.

QUESTIONS

Tumors of the musculoskeletal system—Chap. 60

Directions: Circle T if the statement is true and F if the statement is false. Correct any false statements.

1 T F Osteochondroma occurs frequently near joints and has a potential for malignant change.

2 T F Pathologic fractures usually do not result from metastasis of malignant tumor to bone.

3 T F Benign giant-cell bone tumors have a tendency to become aggressive and spread locally if there is incomplete surgical removal and/or unsuccessful radiation therapy.

4   T   F   The major type of bone tumor found in children results from metastasis from the primary tumor site to bone.

Directions: Circle the letter preceding each item below that correctly answers each question.

5 The onion skin pattern of subperiosteal new-bone formation would be most likely in which of the following tumors involving long bones?
a Ewing's sarcoma   b Osteosarcoma
c Chondroblastoma   d Reticulum cell sarcoma

6 John B., age 18, was admitted to the hospital with an enlarging primary mass in the right distal femur at the knee. Microscopic studies revealed numerous abnormal bone forming cells with great variation in size and shape. Radiologic studies revealed extension of tumor into adjacent soft tissue—cortical breakthrough. Which one of the following diagnoses would you suspect?
a Ewing's sarcoma   b Osteogenic sarcoma
c Osteoid osteoma   d Giant-cell tumor
e Osteoporosis

7 The most likely malignant tumor to arise from pre-existing Paget's disease is:
a Giant-cell tumor   b Osteochrondroma
c Osteosarcoma (osteogenic sarcoma)   d Ewing's sarcoma

8 All the following signs and symptoms are associated with tumors of the musculoskeletal system *except:*
a Painful, enlarging mass   b History of specific serious trauma   c Nocturnal pain is frequently more intense   d Pathologic fractures

BIBLIOGRAPHY

BLOUNT, WALTER: *Fractures in Children*, Williams & Wilkins, Baltimore, 1955.

BRUNNER, LILLIAN and D. SUDDARTH: *Textbook of Medical-Surgical Nursing*, 3d ed., Lippincott, Philadelphia, 1975, pp. 962–1021.

COZEN, LEWIS: *An Atlas of Orthopedic Surgery*, Lea & Febiger, Philadelphia, 1966.

DUTHIE, ROBERT and A. B. FERGUSON: *Mercer's Orthopaedic Surgery*, 7th ed., Williams & Wilkins, Baltimore, 1973.

KEIM, HUGO: "Scoliosis," *Clinical Symposia*, **24**: 1, Ciba-Geigy Corp., Summit, N.J., 1972.

LANGLEY, L. L. and I. TELFORD: *Dynamic Anatomy and Physiology*, McGraw-Hill, New York, 1974.

LARSON, CAROLL and M. GOULD: *Orthopedic Nursing*, 5th ed., Mosby, St. Louis, 1974.

MACAUSLAND, WILLIAM and R. MAYO: *Orthopedics*, Little, Brown, Boston, 1965.

MUSTARD, WILLIAM et al. (eds.): *Pediatric Surgery*, 2d ed., Year Book, Chicago, 1969.

ROCKWOOD, CHARLES and D. GREEN (eds.): *Fractures*, Vols. 1 and 2, Lippincott, Philadelphia, 1975.

RUBIN, PHILIP: *Dynamic Classification of Bone Dysplasia*, Year Book, Chicago, 1964.

SALTER, BRUCE: *Textbook of Disorders and Injuries of the Musculoskeletal System*, Williams & Wilkins, Baltimore, 1970.

SMITH, WILLIAM et al.: "Correlation of Postreduction Roentgenograms and Thirty-one Year Follow-up in Congenital Dislocation of the Hip," *J Bone Joint Surg*, **50-A**: 6, 1081–1098, September 1968.

PART XI Rheumatic Disorders

CATHY M. IDEMA

Rheumatology is the study of arthritis and allied conditions, including connective tissue disease and other inflammatory, degenerative, and metabolic disorders of the musculoskeletal system. Inflammation of connective tissue, frequently manifesting itself as arthritis, is characteristic of several of these disorders.

As an area of interest for health care professionals, rheumatology has grown dramatically. Research has proved successful by providing both methods for earlier diagnosis and more effective modes of therapy. In order to provide high-quality health care to patients with rheumatic disease, health care professionals must have an understanding of the pathophysiology of rheumatic diseases as well as the usual therapeutic regimes.

The demand for the care of these patients is growing because of the large number of people afflicted. Earlier detection of some of the rheumatic diseases has had an influence on the apparent increase in the number of patients. A national health survey conducted by the US Department of Health, Education, and Welfare in 1960 estimated that nearly 11 million adults were suffering with arthritis or rheumatism.[1] Current estimates approximate 20 million cases. Many of those adults afflicted are also disabled. Days lost from work and unemployment due to disability have tremendous impact on our economic system. The social and economic implications of rheumatic disease are further affected by the chronicity of the disease process. The rheumatic diseases kill relatively few; however, the disability affects millions for a lifetime.

This section is devoted to the study of some of the major rheumatic diseases, their pathophysiology, and their treatment, however, one must first understand that arthritis itself is a *symptom,* not a disease. That is, arthritis, or inflammation of a joint, may be a manifestation of many diseases, but it is not itself a disease.

OVERALL OBJECTIVES

At the completion of Part XI you should be able to:

1 Identify arthritis as a symptom, not a disease.

2 List the common clinical manifestations and basic medical treatments for each of the major rheumatic diseases discussed.

3 Identify the role of health care professionals in patient care.

CHAPTER 61 Anatomy and Physiology of the Joints

OBJECTIVES **At the completion of Chap. 61 you should be able to:**

1 List the three major categories for classifying connective tissue according to their cell composition.

2 State the major function(s) of connective tissue.

3 Describe the three types of connective tissue.

4 Differentiate between the three types of joints as to the degree of movement and location. Give an example of each type.

5 Describe the way selected rheumatic diseases affect synovial fluid.

6 List the four basic kinds of angular movement of the joint.

7 Describe the inflammatory process seen in the autoimmune diseases.

Tendons, ligaments, cartilage, bone, periosteum, the outer wall of blood vessels, and the dermis of the skin all contain specialized forms of connective tissue. All the different forms of connective tissue can be classified into three major categories, on the basis of their cellular component. The three categories are (1) fibrous connective tissue, (2) cartilage, and (3) bone.[2]

The major function of connective tissue is to provide support and protection for the body and internal organs. In addition, connective tissue has a major role in (1) the transmission of nutrients and waste products and (2) the inflammatory and reparative processes that occur in injured tissues.

Elastin, reticulin, and collagen are three types of fibrillar proteins found in connective tissue, with collagen being the most abundant. These three differ on the basis of their physical properties, chemical composition, and occurrence in various types of connective tissue throughout the body.

Cartilage is a dense form of connective tissue which may be found in or around joints (called *articular* cartilage), the external ear, the larynx, and the nose. Articular cartilage is the type most affected in rheumatic diseases. There are usually no blood vessels or nerves in articular cartilage. The cartilage receives nourishment from the joint fluid bathing it, or from vessels feeding the end plate of the bone. The articular cartilage covering the ends of the bone functions to cushion the movement of one bone on another.

The place where bones meet is referred to as a *joint* or *articulation* (see Fig. 61-1). Bones are held together by various means: capsules, fibrous bands, ligaments, tendons, fascia, or muscle. There are basically three types of joints. Synarthrodial, or fibrous, joints allow little or no movement because of the binding substance between the bones. Skull sutures are a form of synarthrodial joints.

The second type of joint is the cartilaginous joint, in which the bones are joined by cartilage. The symphysis pubis and the intervertebral disks are examples of the cartilaginous joint.

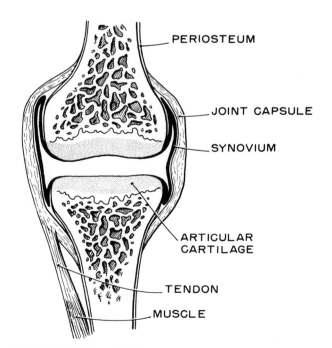

FIGURE 61-1 Normal joint.

PERIOSTEUM

JOINT CAPSULE

SYNOVIUM

ARTICULAR CARTILAGE

TENDON

MUSCLE

The third type of joint is the diarthrodial, or synovial, joint which allows for freer movement. These joints are the ones most frequently affected by rheumatic disease. The joined bones are enveloped by a joint capsule which is lined by synovial tissue. The synovial tissue, or synovium, is a specialized form of connective tissue which covers the inner surface of the joint capsule and forms a sac. The synovium produces synovial fluid, a clear non-clotting thick fluid which contains complex polysaccharide substances. It moistens and lubricates the joint and is a source of nutrition for the articular cartilage. Friction caused by joint movement is reduced by lubrication from synovial fluid.

Normal synovial fluid is a clear, thick, straw-colored fluid. Relatively small amounts (1 to 3 ml) are found in normal joints. The white blood cell count of the fluid is less than 200 cells/mm³. Hyaluronic acid, a constituent of synovial fluid, is responsible for its viscosity.

The synovial fluid may be affected differently by each of the rheumatic diseases (see Table 61-1). Synovial fluid in osteoarthritis, for example, may very nearly approximate normal fluid, with a slight elevation of the white blood cell count. The fluid of systemic lupus erythematosis (SLE) may demonstrate LE cells. Synovial fluids of rheumatoid arthritis and gout are very inflammatory with white blood cell counts in excess of 10,000 to 15,000 cells/mm³. Urate crystals are seen in the synovial fluid of gout. The most inflammatory synovial fluid, however, is that which is infected; white blood cell counts usually are above 50,000 cells/mm³. Bacteria can be cultured from such synovial fluid.

The mucin clot test, a laboratory test, is performed by adding acetic acid to the synovial fluid which then forms a precipitate by interaction with hyaluronic acid. The mucin clot is poorer with the more inflammatory fluids because the hyaluronic acid has been broken down by lysosomal enzymes and therefore does not precipitate when treated with the acetic acid. The clarity of normal synovial fluid is diminished by an increase in the cells and protein in pathlogical conditions.

The blood supply of the synovial joint arises from the subchondral bone (beneath the cartilage). The blood vessels divide into very small vessels that provide a rich blood supply to portions of the synovium.

Nerves, both autonomic and sensory, are widely distributed in the ligaments, joint capsule, and synovium. The nerve innervations account for the sensitivity of these structures to position and movement. Free nerve endings in the capsule, ligaments, and adventitia of blood vessels are particularly sensitive to stretching or twisting. Pain arising from the joint capsule or synovium, however, tends to be diffuse rather than localized. Hip pain, for example, may be perceived as knee pain.[3]

There are four basic kinds of angular movement of the joint: (1) *Flexion,* which decreases the angle between bones, or brings the bones together, (2) *extension,* which increases the angle or separates the bones, (3) *abduction,* which is movement away from the body, and (4) *adduction,* which is movement toward the body.[4]

Connective tissue is affected in a variety of ways by the rheumatic diseases. The cartilage may wear down, and bony changes may occur with aging as in osteoarthritis. Joint inflammation may occur, resulting in overproduction of synovial fluid, or be induced by precipitation of an irritating crystal (such as uric acid in gouty arthritis). The connective tissues of the lungs, blood vessels, or kidney may be damaged as a result of the inflammatory process in the rheumatic disease called systemic lupus erythematosus.

The terminology used in referring to the joints of the hand is illustrated in Fig. 61-2. Note that with the excep-

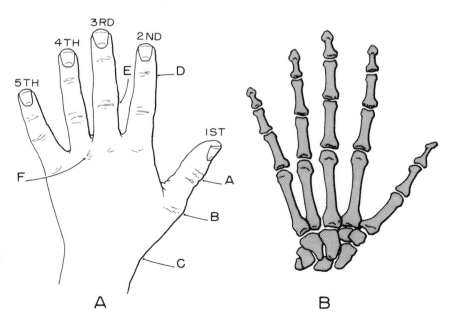

FIGURE 61-2 A, *first IP (first interphalangeal joint).* B, *first MCP (first metacarpophalangeal joint).* C, *first CMCP (first carpalmetacarpophalangeal joint).* D, *second DIP (second distal interphalangeal joint).* E, *third DIP (third peripheral interphalangeal joint).* F, *fourth MCP (fourth metacarpophalangeal joint).*

tion of the thumb, the same term is used for each of the three joint levels, with the number of the finger preceding the joint term.

INFLAMMATORY PROCESS

In order to understand the rheumatic diseases, one needs a basic understanding of the inflammatory process. First, there is an arousal of the inflammatory process by an injurious stimulus (physical, chemical, foreign proteins, or antigen). However, in autoimmune diseases such as rheumatoid arthritis, systemic lupus erythematosus, polymyositis, and scleroderma, the body's immune system no longer accepts certain body proteins and reacts as if they were foreign; this leads to the production of antibodies. The antigen reacts with an antibody to form an immune complex, which then reacts with complement. Complement is a series of proteins which help to stimulate the inflammatory reaction. After the immune complex is formed and deposited in vessel walls, the complement system is activated. This causes the release of cell-damaging enzymes which ordinarily work to rid the body of the foreign substance. The result of this enzyme release is tissue damage.

The signs of inflammation are rubor (redness), calor (heat), dolor (pain), and tumor (swelling). These signs occur because of the increased vascular supply and vascular permeability at the site of the inflammatory reaction. Heat and redness are brought about by the increased blood supply. Swelling occurs because of the increased permeability which allows the escape of fluid into the surrounding tissues. The pressure of the swelling may then cause pain.

Different body reactions may occur depending on the site of origin of the inflammatory process. The lungs may produce fluid resulting in chest pain and/or difficulty in breathing as a result of the inflammatory process.

Kidney function may be impaired and lead to the release of red blood cells and/or protein into the urine. An increase in blood pressure may occur as a consequence of the impaired renal function. The synovial lining of joints may increase production of synovial fluid and become swollen, red, and hot as a result of the inflammatory reaction. Another result of the inflammatory process (particularly with a perpetuating chronic inflammatory process) is permanent tissue damage and/or tissue scarring.

QUESTIONS

Anatomy and physiology of the joint—Chap. 61

Directions: Answer the following questions on a separate sheet of paper.

1 List the three major types of connective tissue based on their cellular component.

2 What is (are) the major function(s) of connective tissue?

Directions: Circle the letter preceding each item below that correctly answers the question. More than one answer may be correct.

3 Of the three types of connective tissue, which is the most abundant?
   a Reticulin *b* Elastin *c* Collagen

TABLE 61-1
Synovial fluid

	NORMAL	DEGENERA-TIVE JOINT DISEASE	SYSTEMIC LUPUS ERYTHE-MATOSUS*	GOUT†	RHEUMA-TOID ARTHRITIS	REITER'S SYNDROME	INFECTIOUS ARTHRITIS‡
Color and clarity	Straw colored; clear	Straw colored; clear	Straw colored; clear	Straw colored or white; cloudy	Straw colored or light yellow; cloudy	Opaque	Gray, purulent; cloudy
Mucin clot	Good	Usually good	Fair to good	Poor	Poor	Poor	Poor
White blood cell count (average)	<200/mm³	1000/mm³	5000/mm³	10,000–20,000/mm³	15,000–20,000/mm³	20,000/mm³	50,000–75,000/mm³

*LE cells may be present.
†Uric acid crystals present.
‡Bacteria can be cultured.

4 Which of the following best describes a freely movable joint?
   a Diarthrodial (synovial) b Synarthrodial (fibrous)
   c Cartilaginous

5 An example of a cartilaginous joint is:
   a Skull sutures b Symphysis pubis c Synovium
   d Intervertral joints

6 Synovial fluid with white blood cell counts in excess of 10,000 to 15,000 cells/mm³ may be observed in:
   a Systemic lupus erythematous b Rheumatoid arthritis c Gout d Degenerative joint disease

7 In autoimmune disease the body immune system:
   a Does recognize all proteins and releases antibodies. b Links antigen to an antibody which is joined by complement. c Seldom activates complement system. d Does not accept certain proteins and reacts by producing antibodies.

CHAPTER 62 Rheumatoid Arthritis

OBJECTIVES At the completion of Chap. 62 you should be able to:

1 Identify the major characteristics of rheumatoid arthritis.

2 List four of the eight clinical features of rheumatoid arthritis.

3 Identify the most commonly involved joints in rheumatoid arthritis.

4 List two of the systemic organ involvements which may be seen in rheumatoid arthritis.

5 Name two laboratory tests which can be helpful in diagnosis of rheumatoid arthritis.

6 State the three goals of treatment for rheumatoid arthritis.

7 List the five basic components of the treatment program for rheumatoid arthritis.

8 List at least one therapeutic use and one side effect for each of the following medications: salicylates, gold salts, phenylbutazone (Butazolidin), indomethacin (Indocin), and corticosteroids (Prednisone).

9 Identify the drug of choice in treating rheumatoid arthritis.

10 Identify at least three ways in which a health care professional can help a patient with rheumatoid arthritis develop a home care plan.

RHEUMATOID ARTHRITIS

Rheumatoid arthritis is a chronic systemic disease characterized by inflammation of connective tissue. The most common manifestation of this disease is joint involvement which is generally persistent and progressive, initially involving the small joints of the hands and feet. Joint deformity and disability, accompanied by pain, often result. Rheumatoid arthritis is characterized by spontaneous flares and remissions (see Fig. 62-1). Although it may occur at any age, affecting either sex, it occurs most frequently in women (the female/male ratio is 3:1) during the childbearing years. Rheumatoid arthritis occurs with a frequency of approximately 500 cases per year per 1 million population.[5]

The onset of rheumatoid arthritis is usually insidious. Constitutional symptoms such as fatigue, fever, loss of appetite, and weight loss frequently are the primary presenting symptoms. The small joints of the hands and feet may be painful and stiff. However, the initial disease presentation is highly variable. The onset may be insidious or may be acute and fulminate, involving many joints.

Clinical features

The common clinical features of rheumatoid arthritis are the following:

1 *Constitutional symptoms,* such as fatigue, anorexia, weight loss, and fever are present.

2 *Symmetrical polyarthritis* of the peripheral joints most frequently involves the small joints of the hands and feet, and the wrists, although larger joints may also be involved.

3 *Morning stiffness* is common. This may be generalized stiffness but primarily involves the joints. The stiffness generally lasts more than 30 minutes and may last for many hours into the day. This differs from the stiffness of osteoarthritis, which occurs in the later part of the day after use of the joints.

4 *Erosive arthritis* is a radiologic characteristic of this disease. The chronic inflammation of the joints results in erosions at the marginal aspects of the bones which can be demonstrated on x-ray (see Fig. 62-2).

5 *Deformity* can result from this chronic disease. Ulnar drift, or deviation of the fingers, subluxation of the metacarpophalangeal (MCP) joints, boutonniere and

swan neck deformities (see Fig. 62-3) are some of the common deformities involving the hands. The larger joints may also be involved with a decrease in extension and/or flexion. Joints also may become alkylosed with complete loss of motion.

6 *Rheumatoid nodules* are subcutaneous masses occurring in approximately one-third of adult rheumatoid arthritis patients. They occur commonly in the olecranon bursa (elbow) or along the extensor surface of the forearm, but can occur elsewhere. They are firm, nontender, round, or oval masses which are usually movable but may be fixed to the periosteum of bone. The presence of these nodules is usually associated with active or more severe disease[6] (see Fig. 62-4).

7 *Chronicity* is an important characteristic of rheumatoid arthritis. When the diagnosis is made, objective joint inflammation should be present for at least 3 months. The disease is characterized, however, by remissions and flares; hence joint inflammation may not be constant.

8 *Extraarticular manifestations.* Rheumatoid arthritis is a systemic disease which may include organ involvement other than joints. The heart (pericarditis), lungs (pleuritis), eyes (scleritis), and vessels (vaculitis) can be inflamed as a result of the disease (see Fig. 62-5). See Table 62-1 for further delineation of extraarticular manifestations.

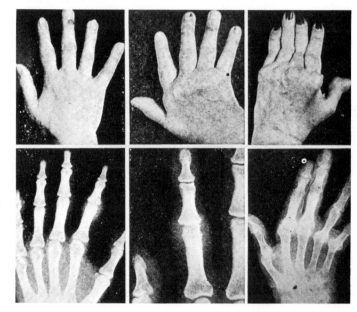

FIGURE 62-1 *Early, moderate, and advanced rheumatoid arthritis: Hands. Note the swelling of the second PIP joint as part of the early changes. In the moderate stage there is swelling of the MCP joints. The advanced stage shows subluxation of the MCP joints. (Reproduced with permission from Dwight C. Ensign, "Osteoarthritis and Rheumatoid arthritis,"* Modern Medicine, *March 1, 1955, p. 128, copyright 1955 by Harcourt Brace Jovanovich.)*

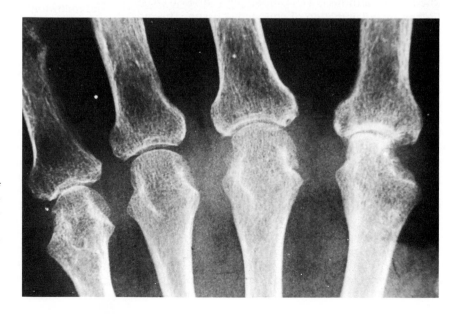

FIGURE 62-2 *X-ray of rheumatoid hand. Note the joint space narrowing, erosion of the second metacarpal head with early erosion of the third metacarpal head. The cortex of the fourth metacarpal head remains indistinct. Compare this with the nice, well-defined cortex of the fifth metacarpal head. (Reproduced with permission from the Canadian Arthritis and Rheumatism Society, Dr. J. B. Houpt, Editor.)*

Several laboratory findings may be helpful in diagnosing rheumatoid arthritis. Approximately 85 percent of patients with rheumatoid arthritis have the autoantibody known as the *rheumatoid factor* in their serum. This factor is an anti–gamma globulin factor. Higher titers of rheumatoid factor do not always reflect disease activity; however, they are usually associated with rheumatoid nodules, severe disease, vasculitis, and a poor prognosis. Although the rheumatoid factor test is helpful diagnostically, it is not specific for rheumatoid arthritis. Rheumatoid factor is seen in other connective tissue disease (e.g., systemic lupus erythematosus, scleroderma, dermatomyositis), as well as in a small percentage (3 to 5

percent) of the normal population. In the normal population, the seropositivity increases with aging, with as many as 15 to 20 percent of people over 60 having a positive rheumatoid factor in low titer.

The blood may also be tested for an elevated erythrocyte sedimentation rate (ESR); this is a nonspecific index of inflammation which can be elevated with any inflammatory process. Anemia may also be present in patients with rheumatoid arthritis.

Normal synovial fluid is a clear, light-yellow fluid with

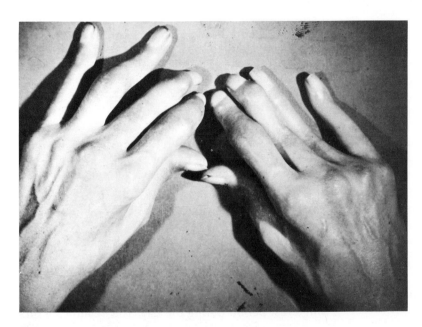

FIGURE 62-3 Rheumatoid hand: Boutonniere and Swan neck deformity. Polyarthritis of the joints of the hands. Among the advanced deforming changes is the muscle wasting in the anatomical snuff box (between thumb and forefinger). Boutonniere deformity of the left fourth digit. Swan neck deformity involving the right third and fourth digits. (Reproduced with permission from the Arthritis Division, University Hospital, University of Michigan.)

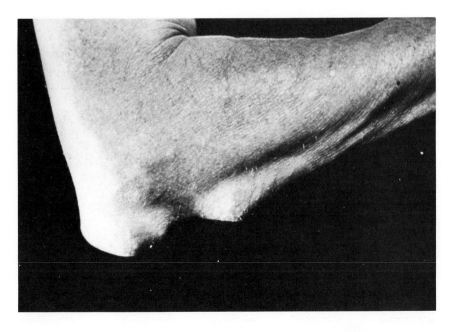

FIGURE 62-4 Rheumatoid nodules, elbow. Two large subcutaneous nodules are located about the elbow. One is in the olecranon bursa and the other on the extensor surface of the forearm. Nodules may be fixed or movable and are usually nontender. They occur most commonly at the elbow, but may also be found elsewhere, as on the feet, fingers, occiput, heels, and buttocks. Nodules occur in about 20 percent of patients with rheumatoid arthritis, may fluctuate in size, and are usually associated with high titers of rheumatoid factor. (Reproduced with permission from The Arthritis Foundation, New York, copyright 1972.)

a white blood cell count of less than 200 cells/mm³. Because of the inflammatory process occurring in the joints in rheumatoid arthritis, the synovial fluid loses its viscosity and the leukocyte count increases to 5000 to 50,000 cells/mm³, which makes the fluid turbid.

Radiologic features

Narrowing of the joint space is one of the characteristic radiologic findings. Damage to articular cartilage results from this uniform narrowing. Bone erosions, occurring at the marginal aspects of the bones, are another radiologic feature of rheumatoid arthritis. Neither narrowing of the joints nor bone erosion is reversible.

Diagnostic criteria

The diagnosis of rheumatoid arthritis does not rest on any single feature of the disease, but rather is based on careful clinical evaluation of all available evidence. It is convenient to consider such evidence within the framework of the diagnostic criteria for rheumatoid arthritis adopted by the American Rheumatism Association in 1956 (revised in 1958) which follows:

1 Morning stiffness
2 Pain on motion, or tenderness in at least one joint
3 Swelling (not bony) in at least one joint
4 Swelling of at least one other joint within a 3-month period
5 Symmetrical joint swelling
6 Subcutaneous nodules
7 X-ray changes typical of rheumatoid arthritis
8 Positive serologic test for rheumatoid factor
9 Poor mucin precipitate from synovial fluid
10 Characteristic histologic change in nodule
11 Characteristic histologic change in synovial tissue

To be diagnosed as having *classic* rheumatoid arthritis, the patient must exhibit at least *seven* of the above criteria. *Definite* rheumatoid arthritis is diagnosed when at least *five* of the above criteria are met, while *probable* rheumatoid arthritis exists when *three* of the above criteria are exhibited. These criteria are employed in conjunction with a list of exclusions, which serve to rule out the other rheumatic diseases.[8,9]

Treatment

The fluctuating course of rheumatoid arthritis makes therapeutic efforts difficult to evaluate. Since the disease is characterized by remissions and flares, it is difficult to determine whether a particular therapeutic effort has resulted in a remission or whether the remission is a natural occurrence. The goal of treatment is to achieve and maintain a remission, or, failing that, to suppress, insofar as possible, the activity of the disease.

The main goals of the therapeutic program are:

1 Relief of pain and inflammation
2 Maintenance of joint function and maximum functional capacity of the patient
3 Prevention and/or correction of deformities

The basic therapeutic program consists of the following five components which aid in achieving these goals.

1 Rest

Since fatigue accompanies this disease, patients must be helped to regulate their activities of daily living in such a way that severe fatigue does not occur. Optimally, the patient must get adequate rest at night (8 to 10 hours) with a rest period during the day. The health care pro-

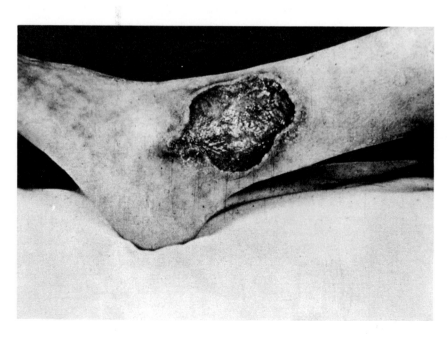

FIGURE 62-5 Rheumatoid arthritis: Vasculitis, leg ulcer. A large, painful, sharply demarcated ulcer can be seen on the lateral side of the ankle. This type of ulcer is caused by vasculitis of small vessels and is commonly associated with peripheral neuropathy and a high titer of rheumatoid factor. (Reproduced with permission from The Arthritis Foundation, New York, copyright 1972.)

fessional can assist patients in pacing their activities, thus providing for alternation of heavier duties with light tasks and short periods of rest in between.

2 Exercises

Specific exercises are useful in maintenance of maximal joint function. Overuse of such exercises, however, can result in pain which discourages the patient from continuing the program. The use of medication and heat prior to exercises provides a time of minimized discomfort and may result in greater willingness on the part of the patient to carry out the exercise program. Significant pain after exercising indicates a need to modify the program.

TABLE 62-1
Extraarticular manifestations of rheumatoid arthritis[7]

1 Subcutaneous and subperiosteal (rheumatoid granulomas)
2 Organ Involvement:

Heart	Pericarditis: only occasionally symptomatic and only rarely progressing to chronic constricting disease
	Valvular lesions: chiefly aortic due to rheumatoid granulomas (rare)
Lung	Pleurisy: with or without effusion
	Multiple pulmonary (rheumatoid) nodules
	Rheumatoid pneumoconiosis (Caplan's syndrome)
	Progressive interstitial fibrosis, with formation of honeycomb lung
Eye	Scleritis
	Iridocyclitis (in *juvenile* rheumatoid arthritis)
Nervous system	Peripheral neuropathy (associated with vasculitis)
	Peripheral compression syndromes, including carpal tunnel syndrome (median nerve neuropathy), ulnar nerve neuropathy, peroneal palsy, and cervical spine abnormalities

3 Systemic complications:
Anemia (common)
Generalized osteoporosis
Felty's syndrome (in 10% of cases of rheumatoid arthritis)
Sjögren's syndrome (keratoconjunctivitis sicca)
Amyloidosis (rare)
4 Features associated with vasculitis:
Fever
Digital arteritis (focal ischemic areas in nail fold, nail edge, or digital pulp; gangrene, rare)
Raynaud's phenomenon
Skin lesions (rash and gangrene)
Chronic leg ulcers
Peripheral neuropathy (mononeuritis multiplex)
Erosions in mucosa of gastrointestinal tract with hemorrhage
Necrotizing arteritis involving mesenteric, coronary, renal vessels

Source: Modified from Committee of the American Rheumatism Association, 1973.

3 Heat

There are many types of heat application, any of which can provide relief of pain. A wide variety of moist heating techniques can be used: Hubbard tanks (available in physical therapy departments), bathtubs, even simple bath towels soaked in warm water and applied locally to a painful joint can be helpful. Using dry heat such as heat lamps or heating pads can also be helpful. Each patient may have a preference for a particular type of heat but should be cautioned against investing money in expensive gadgets since simple home methods are usually just as effective.

4 Medications

Several medications may be employed in the treatment of rheumatoid arthritis. The objective is to relieve pain and inflammation with the safest medications possible and to reserve the more potent agents for use after reasonable trials of the safer agents have failed.

Aspirin is the primary drug of choice in treating rheumatoid arthritis because it is relatively safe, inexpensive, and effective. Aspirin is an analgesic as well as an anti-inflammatory medication. It can, however, be irritating to the stomach, and therefore should be taken with meals or antacids. Ringing in the ears and muffled hearing are signs of aspirin toxicity. These symptoms will usually disappear when the dosage is decreased. The dose may range anywhere from 8 to an excess of 20 tablets per day, depending on the need as well as the tolerance of the patient.

Antimalarials (hydroxychloroquin, chloroquin) have been used for over 20 years in the treatment of rheumatoid arthritis, although their primary use is in the treatment of malaria. They are effective in treating the joint complaints, as well as the cutaneous manifestations of systemic lupus erythematosus. In the treatment of SLE, antimalarials are sometimes used for their steroid-sparing effect; that is, use of these drugs may result in lower requirements of steroids. Usual dosage of the antimalarials ranges from 200 to 600 mg daily. Side effects may include headache, dizziness, and gastrointestinal complaints. Long-term effects may include corneal damage and possible retinal damage resulting in loss of vision. In order to prevent these side effects, the patient should have a detailed ophthalmologic examination every 3 to 6 months.

Indomethacin (Indocin) is a relatively potent (nonsteroidal) anti-inflammatory agent used in treating rheumatoid arthritis. The dose may range from 50 to 200 mg/day. Toxic side effects may include headaches, dizziness, nausea, diarrhea, skin rash, and, rarely, hallucinations. It may also cause gastrointestinal bleeding, ulceration, or perforation.

Phenylbutazone (Butazolidin), another anti-inflammatory agent, is similar in potency to indomethacin. Doses usually range from 200 to 400 mg/day. Side effects include nausea, vomiting, diarrhea, salt and water retention, vertigo, and gastritis. This drug may cause bone marrow suppression, and therefore the patient is advised to have a complete blood count every 2 to 4 weeks. This drug is only moderately effective in the treatment of chronic rheumatoid arthritis.

Several newly released nonsteroidal anti-inflammatory agents are available for the treatment of rheumatoid arthritis. They seem, in general, to be tolerated as well as or better than aspirin, cause less gastrointestinal distress, and are at least one-half as effective, but usually more expensive, than aspirin.

Gold salts [aurothioglucose (Solganal) and gold sodium thiomalate (Myochrysine)] are also prescribed as treatment for rheumatoid arthritis. There are many theories as to the mode of action of gold salts, none of them universally accepted. Gold salts are employed *only* in the treatment of rheumatoid arthritis and are given intramuscularly with initial test doses of 10 mg followed by 25 mg in 1 week. Generally, patients remain at 50 mg at weekly intervals until 800 to 1000 mg have been given. At this time the effectiveness of treatment should be evaluated. If improvement has occurred, the gold may be continued, with the interval between injections being slowly increased. Side effects from treatment with gold salts include stomatitis, pruritus, rash, blood dyscrasias, and nephritis (proteinuria, red blood cells). A complete blood count and urinalysis should be done prior to each gold injection, as well as an examination for other possible side effects. If the patient is carefully watched and the gold is discontinued at the first sign of toxicity, the adverse reactions are reversible.

Corticosteroids are a hormone produced daily in small amounts by the adrenal glands. When hydrocortisone or a synthetic corticosteroid (e.g., prednisone) is given orally in larger doses, the drug is useful as an anti-inflammatory and immunosuppressive agent. It is important to remember that the body's own secretion of corticosteroids is suppressed when oral dosages of corticosteroids are being administered. When the oral dose is reduced, the patient must be slowly tapered off so as to allow the adrenals to reactivate and thus begin to produce this vital hormone again. Because steroids have the potential to produce severe complications, they are reserved for patients who have not responded to more conservative measures. In treating rheumatoid arthritis, steroids are usually given in relatively small doses, and patients are tapered off the drug if possible. There are many side effects, some of which are fullness of face ("moon face"), easy bruisability, gastrointestinal disturbances, salt and water retention, increased appetite, mood changes, adrenal suppression, osteoporosis, increased susceptibility to infection, decreased healing ability, and cataracts. Because of the extensive side effects, especially those affecting body image, patients are often reluctant to be treated with corticosteroids. For this reason, patients must be taught about this drug treatment: the reason for its use, the importance of consistent doses, and, especially, the importance of not discontinuing the drug on their own.

Immunosuppressive agents (cyclophosphamide, azathioprine) have some use in the treatment of certain rheumatic diseases. These are very potent drugs with potentially severe side effects. They are not commonly employed but may be used for the special patient whose disease is resistant to other therapeutic measures, or the patient who is experiencing such severe side effects from steroids that they must be discontinued.

5 Nutrition

There is no special diet which will affect or cure rheumatoid arthritis. It is important, however, that patients with rheumatoid arthritis follow nutritionally adequate diets. Patients who are overweight are placing an additional source of stress on the joints and should be encouraged to lose unnecessary weight.

Patient care implications

Health care professionals have the responsibility to provide patients with knowledge of the disease and the treatment program so that they can better cope with this chronic illness. Generally, patients are less interested in the technicalities of the disease itself and are more concerned with the way it will affect their daily lives. For this reason, each aspect of the treatment program should be discussed with the patient in detail.

The following points regarding daily activities should be stressed. Patients should be advised to get adequate rest and should be helped to plan their days in such a way that there is a balance of heavier and lighter tasks, with adequate rest periods between. An occupational therapist can be very helpful in teaching the techniques of pacing and joint protection. Two examples are (1) planning housework so that one finishes all chores on one floor before going to the next, thus avoiding running up and down stairs, and (2) sitting while gardening, and gardening in a square area around oneself, instead of bending over to garden in rows, in order to protect the back and knees.

The physical therapist will also be involved in helping the patient with exercise. The nurse can reinforce the efforts of the physical therapist by reviewing the schedule of exercises with the patient before discharge in order to determine the level of patient understanding. It is important that the patient understand that the exercises being taught cannot be replaced by the exercise one gets in the course of a busy day.

The nurse can also help by reviewing methods of heat treatment with the patient. Patients who choose methods of dry heat should especially be cautioned against burning themselves by leaving heating pads on all night, by setting heating pads on "high," or by coming too close to a heat lamp.

The patient should be made aware of all the medications that there have been prescribed, their use, and their side effects. Many of the medications can be irritating to the gastric mucosa. The patient may need to be reminded that this irritation can be relieved by taking the medications with meals or antacids. Patients should be taught what to do if they experience side effects. It may also be helpful to patients who are taking many medications or are somewhat forgetful to assist them in making up a chart as a daily reminder of when to take their medications. These patients can also be advised that they may request their pharmacist not to use the child protector caps on their medication bottles; these caps are very difficult to open by anyone whose hands are painful and weak.

The health care professional can also review the four basic food groups and caution patients about the many advertisements they will encounter regarding diet cures for arthritis. Most of these diets are not helpful, and some can be expensive as well as nutritionally inadequate. Referral to a dietician is of benefit for those patients needing specific diet instruction.

Patients should be cautioned against the expensive and sometimes harmful devices often advertised as a cure for arthritis. People with arthritic diseases are frequent targets of quackery. When in doubt about an advertised product, they should check with their physician, their nurse, or the local chapter of the Arthritis Foundation.

QUESTIONS

Rheumatoid arthritis—Chap. 62

Directions: Circle the letter next to each item that correctly answers the question.

1   Rheumatoid arthritis affects which segment(s) of the population?

a Females only   *b* Females more than males (3:1)   *c* Males more than females (3:1)   *d* Both sexes equally

2   The joints most commonly affected by rheumatoid arthritis are the:
    a Small joints of the hands, feet, and the wrists   *b* Knees and hips   *c* Ankles

Directions: Answer the following questions on a separate sheet of paper.

3   What are the three main goals of the treatment program for rheumatoid arthritis?

4   What is the main drug of choice in treating rheumatoid arthritis? (Consider effectiveness, safety, and cost.)

5   Identify two types of heat used for treating rheumatoid arthritis. Name two examples of each type of heat.

6   List at least four of the clinical features of rheumatoid arthritis.

CHAPTER 63 Psoriatic Arthritis, Ankylosing Spondylitis, and Reiter's Syndrome

OBJECTIVES

At the completion of Chap. 63 you should be able to:

1 Identify the characteristics of psoriatic arthritis.

2 Differentiate between psoriatic and rheumatoid arthritis in terms of joint manifestations.

3 Identify one medication which is used for the treatment of psoriatic arthritis.

4 Identify the characteristics of ankylosing spondylitis including age at onset and sex predilection.

5 State two treatment measures commonly employed for ankylosing spondylitis.

6 State the three main conditions that can be identified as Reiter's syndrome.

7 Identify the clinical characteristics of Reiter's syndrome.

8 State two components of the treatment program for Reiter's syndrome.

PSORIATIC ARTHRITIS

Psoriatic arthritis is now recognized as a distinct clinical entity.[10] Usually the arthritis of psoriatic arthritis occurs after the appearance of the psoriasis but can occur before or simultaneously with it.

Clinical features

The articular manifestations of psoriatic arthritis most commonly occur in the form of asymmetric inflammation involving only a few peripheral joints at a time. The joints of the feet and interphalangeal joints of the hands are commonly involved with a striking predilection for the distal interphalangeal joints (see Fig. 63-1). There is a tendency for the activity of the arthritis to vary with the psoriasis, particularly the nail involvement of psoriasis (see Fig. 63-2).

The joint involvement (other than the distal interphalangeal joints) does not differ greatly from rheumatoid arthritis, except that rheumatoid arthritis tends to be symmetrical. Some question the possibility of rheumatoid arthritis occurring simultaneously with psoriasis, particularly in those cases where there are subcutaneous nodules and a positive rheumatoid factor. Psoriatic arthritis tends in most cases to be less debilitating than rheumatoid arthritis, even though it can cause joint damage.

Laboratory and radiologic findings

There are no specific laboratory tests for psoriatic arthritis, though the rheumatoid factor test is usually negative and the sedimentation rate may be elevated. X-ray changes characteristic of psoriatic arthritis can also be detected.

Treatment

Aspirin is the treatment of choice for psoriatic arthritis, although other anti-inflammatory drugs may be used. Corticosteroids are generally not used because of the large doses needed, even though they may improve both skin and joints. Intraarticular injection of cortisone may provide temporary relief without the consequence of side effects produced by oral administration of cortisone. Since there is a tendency for the arthritis to flare with increased activity in the skin disease, a special effort is made to control the psoriasis with drug and topical therapy.

Ankylosing spondylitis is a chronic, progressive inflammatory disease primarily involving the sacroiliac joints and spinal articulations. The costovertebral articulations and paravertebral soft tissue may also be affected as the disease progresses up the spine.

It was once thought that ankylosing spondylitis was a spinal version of rheumatoid arthritis. Several differences, such as absence of rheumatoid nodules, low incidence of rheumatoid factor, and dissimilarities in sex predilection, have proved this not to be the case. Ossification, bony bridging (syndesmophytes), and ankylosis of the spinal articulations, which differ from rheumatoid arthritis, may result in the fused "poker-spine."

The disease has been described from skeletons dating back to as early as 2900 B.C. Marie Strümpell, by whose name the disease used to be known, described the clinical picture of several cases in the late 1800s.

Although the etiology is still unknown, hereditary factors are thought to play an important role. Recently a high incidence (>95 percent of cases) of histocompatibility antigen HLA-B27 has been found in this disease. The disease demonstrates a predilection for males with a ratio of 8 or 9:1. Onset commonly occurs in men between 20 and 40 years of age and is uncommon after 50 years of age.[11]

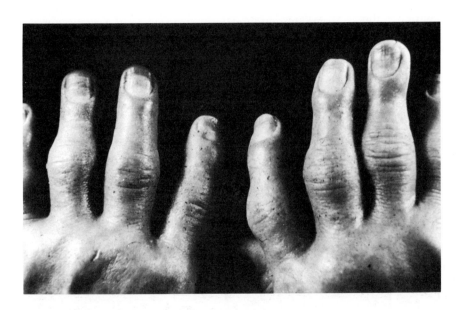

FIGURE 63-1 Psoriatic arthritis: Hands. Somewhat diffuse swelling involving many joints of the hands. Note the slight sausage shape of the fingers. (Reproduced with permission from the Arthritis Division, University Hospital, University of Michigan.)

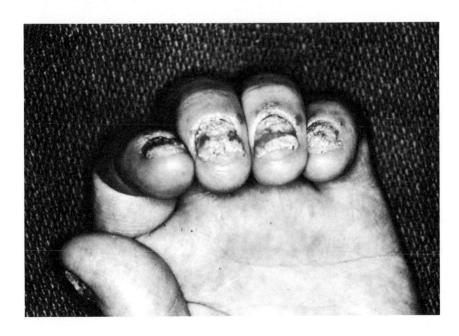

FIGURE 63-2 Psoriatic arthritis: Nails. Psoriasis with extensive nail involvement. (Reproduced with permission from the Canadian Arthritis and Rheumatism Society, Dr. J. B. Houpt, Editor.)

Clinical features

The onset of ankylosing spondylitis is usually insidious. Complaints of fatigue, weight loss, and intermittent low-back pain are common. Morning stiffness which is relieved by mild activity may occur. Although pain over the sacroiliac joints is the most common initial complaint, peripheral joints may be involved with pain and swelling. Hips, shoulders, and knees are the most commonly involved peripheral joints. Except for the hips and shoulders, peripheral joint involvement is usually transient and benign.

Initial physical examination may reveal a healthy patient except for pain over the sacroiliac joints and a guarded spinal motion. As the disease progresses, the lumbar and dorsal spine are affected. Costovertebral involvement at the thoracic level may compromise chest expansion, resulting in chest pain and breathing difficulties. Fusion of the spine, at late stages of the disease, usually results in hip flexion contractures and flexed knees in order for the patient to maintain an erect position (see Fig. 63-3). Pain is usually diminished after ankylosis occurs.

Laboratory findings

The erythrocyte sedimentation rate is usually elevated at the onset and during active phases of the disease. The rheumatoid factor is usually negative. Tests for the histocompatibility antigen HLA-B27 are positive in 95 percent of patients.

Radiologic findings

There are characteristic x-ray changes which occur in ankylosing spondylitis. Joint space narrowing and erosions occur at the sacroiliac joints. There is eventual fusion of these joints. Ultimately there is a squaring of the vertebral bodies. Syndesmophytes, or vertical bony growths, can be demonstrated bridging the gaps between the vertebral bodies (see Fig. 63-4). Calcification of the intevertebral disks may be followed by calcification and ossification of paravertebral ligaments later in the disease.

Treatment

Consistent, regular doses of aspirin may be of benefit in ankylosing spondylitis. However, phenylbutazone or indomethacin, stronger anti-inflammatory agents, are

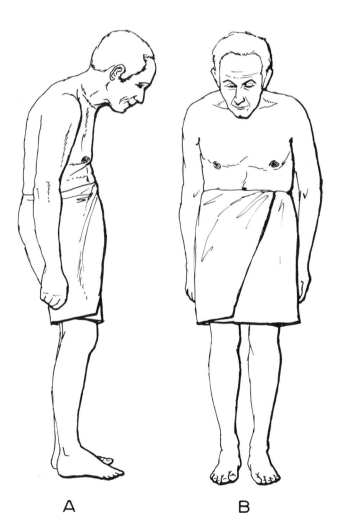

A   B

FIGURE 63-3 Ankylosing spondylitis: Posture changes.

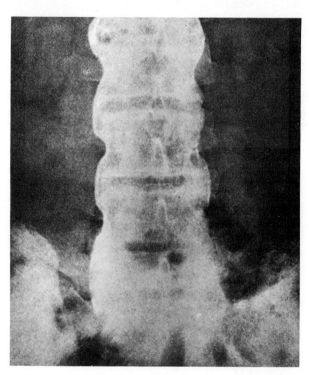

FIGURE 63-4 Ankylosing spondylitis: Spine x-ray. Advanced ankylosing spondylitis of the lumbar spine. There is generalized symmetrical osseous bridging between the vertebrae (syndesmophytes). The apophyseal and sacroiliac joints are fused. (Reproduced with permission from J. L. Hollander (ed.), Arthritis and Allied Conditions, A Textbook of Rheumatology, *8th ed., Lea & Febinger, Philadelphia, 1972.)*

sometimes more effective than salicylates. Corticosteroids are rarely used and only in the most severe cases.

A patient education program, including physical therapy, is vital in preventing long-term deformities. A flexed position is frequently assumed by the patient because this position may reduce the pain; however, fusion in this position must be prevented. It is critical that the patient be taught proper positioning for rest. The patient's mattress should be firm (a bed board may be indicated), and the patient should sleep flat, without a pillow, in order to prevent flexion deformity as the spine fuses. Proper breathing exercises are useful to increase the breathing capacity, especially in view of decreased chest expansion. The patient's height should be recorded at regular intervals in order to detect spine flexion.

REITER'S SYNDROME

Although Hans Reiter in the early 1900s was not the first to describe the clinical picture of nongonoccocal urethritis, arthritis, and conjunctivitis, the disease carries his name. Reiter's syndrome rarely occurs in women, but

rather affects men, often after sexual exposure. Cases, however, involving both men and women have been reported after a dysentery outbreak.

The triad of symptoms—urethritis, arthritis, and conjunctivitis—have become the cardinal signs of Reiter's syndrome. However, oral muccocutaneous lesions and keratodermia blennorrhagicum (a characteristic dermatitis) are also common clinical features.

The etiology of Reiter's syndrome is still unknown, yet sexual exposure seems to occur just prior to onset in many cases. There is some thought that Reiter's syndrome and psoriatic arthritis are nearly the same disease, since the dermatitis and nail changes may be indistinguishable between the two diseases.

Clinical features

Constitutional symptoms, weight loss, and fever may occur at the onset of Reiter's syndrome. Urethritis, purulent or watery, frequently is the motivating factor for the patient to seek health care. There is usually a history of recent sexual exposure.

Articular manifestations involve the larger joints in an asymmetric fashion. Heel pain is common. The sacroiliac joints may also be involved, resulting in low-back pain.

Ocular involvement is usually manifested by conjunctivitis with a mild burning sensation.

Painless oral and penile ulcerations are common. Other skin manifestations include pustular lesions which become keratotic (see Fig. 63-5). Nails may be separated from the beds owing to keratotic lesions.

Diarrhea may occur a few weeks prior to any of the other symptoms. The diarrhea may be bloody.

All these symptoms will usually resolve on their own, without residual effects. However, the rate of recurrence is high. Severe joint involvement may leave residual damage, and the sacroiliac involvement may continue for long periods of time.

Laboratory and radiologic findings

The synovial fluid is inflammatory, with 15,000 to 20,000 white blood cells/mm³.

Osteoporosis and bony erosions may occur as a result of chronic severe disease. X-ray findings can simulate those found in psoriatic arthritis.

Treatment

Therapeutic doses of salicylates or other anti-inflammatory agents are of benefit in the treatment of Reiter's syndrome. Intraarticular steroids may provide relief of joint pain. A balanced physical therapy program of rest and exercise may deter joint deformities.

Some authors have written of the benefit of antibiotic therapy for aborting or preventing the attacks. Although

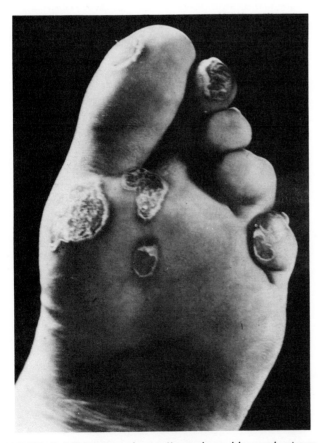

FIGURE 63-5 Reiter's syndrome: Keratoderma blennorrhagicum, foot. Discrete, circinate, scaly, and plaquelike lesions on the foot are due to Reiter's syndrome and resemble secondary syphilis and psoriasis. Note two small lesions in an early phase of keratoderma. (Reproduced with permission from The Arthritis Foundation, New York, copyright 1972.)

this therapy is not universally accepted, penicillin is, however, indicated for those patients who may simultaneously have gonoccocal urethritis.

QUESTIONS

Psoriatic arthritis—Chap. 63

Directions: Circle T if the statement is true and F if it is false. Correct any false statements.

1 T F The psoriasis usually precedes the arthritis in psoriatic arthritis.

2 T F Psoriatic arthritis is usually much more destructive to the joints than rheumatoid arthritis.

3 T F Tetracycline is the treatment of choice for Reiter's syndrome.

4 T F Corticosteroids are generally not used in the treatment of psoriatic arthritis.

Directions: Answer the following questions on a separate sheet of paper.

5 Name the three major symptoms of Reiter's syndrome (triad).

6 In which sex is Reiter's syndrome most commonly found?

7 Name at least two medications which are particularly helpful in treating ankylosing spondylitis.

8 List two therapeutic measures for ankylosing spondylitis.

Directions: Circle the letter preceding each item below that correctly answers the question.

9 The joints which are most commonly involved in Reiter's syndrome are:
a Weight-bearing joints (knees, ankles, feet)
b Upper extremity joints (shoulders, wrists, hands)
c Hips and neck joints

Directions: Complete the following statements by filling in the blanks.

10 The male/female ratio for occurrence of ankylosing spondylitis is ___:___.

11 The most common initial complaint in ankylosing spondylitis is _____.

CHAPTER 64 Polymyositis, Dermatomyositis, and Progressive Systemic Sclerosis (Scleroderma)

At the completion of Chap. 64 you should be able to:

1 Define *polymyositis* in a sentence or two.

2 Define *dermatomyositis* in a sentence or two.

3 Identify the clinical features of polymyositis and dermatomyositis.

4 Name the muscles which are usually involved in the onset of polymyositis and dermatomyositis.

5 List two components of the treatment program for polymyositis.

6 State the common characteristics of progressive systemic sclerosis (PSS or scleroderma).

7 Describe the appearance of the skin in patients with scleroderma.

8 Identify at least two clinical features of scleroderma.

POLYMYOSITIS AND DERMATOMYOSITIS

The first case of polymyositis was described in the middle to late 1800s, and yet there is still much to be learned about this disease. Both polymyositis and dermatomyositis are inflammatory diseases affecting the striated muscle groups, usually in a symmetrical fashion. They can affect any age group; however, dermatomyositis more often occurs in children or in persons over 40 years of age, sometimes in association with a malignancy. Females are affected twice as often as males except in the presence of a malignant tumor, when a more equal distribution is demonstrated. Malignancies are associated with these diseases approximately five times more frequently than in the general population. Prognosis is brighter for children and young adults and also better for those without a malignancy.

Clinical features

The onset generally presents a gradual weakening of the proximal muscles. Severe constitutional symptoms such as weight loss, fever, and fatigue may also be present. Many patients experience arthralgias or arthritis, particularly involving the small joints of the hands, the wrists, and the knees.

Muscle weakness generally affects the proximal muscles of the lower extremities first. This may be perceived by the patient as difficulty climbing stairs. Upper extremity involvement of the proximal muscles may present the patient with difficulty in caring for the hair. Neck musculature can also be affected, although facial muscles are rarely involved. Dysphagia (difficulty swallowing) may result from inflammation of the voluntary muscles of the pharynx. Hypomotility of the lower esophagus, such as is found in scleroderma, may occur. Pain and tenderness of the affected muscles seem to be directly related to the acuity of the disease process.

Pulmonary function may be impaired owing to inflamed intercostal muscles. The patient may also develop pulmonary fibrosis or aspiration pneumonitis.

Involvement of distal muscles may occur in severe or chronic disease. Long-term complications may include muscle atrophy and contractures. Calcinosis may result from severe muscle inflammation and is seen more frequently in children or adolescents than in adults.

The dermal involvement of dermatomyositis includes the appearance of dark red patches which are slightly scaly (see Fig. 64-1). These eruptions often appear over the peripheral interphalangeal and metacarpophalangeal joints, as well as over elbows and knees. A butterfly malar rash may appear as in systemic lupus erythematosus. A dusky erythematous rash on the eyelids is referred to as a *heliotrope* rash and is considered pathognomonic.

The occurrence of malignancy in conjunction with these disorders is demonstrated at a higher frequency rate than the occurrence of malignancies alone. Malignancies can be demonstrated approximately five times more frequently in people 40 years or older who have either polymyositis or dermatomyositis. However, these findings are presently being refuted. The lungs, breasts, ovaries, uterus, and prostate are the most common sites for the malignancy. Generally, the myositis presents itself 1 to 2 years prior to the discovery of the malignancy. The successful treatment of the malignancy may also resolve the myositis.

Laboratory findings

The erythrocyte sedimentation rate is often elevated. Positive rheumatoid factors may also be demonstrated in the patient's serum. The most helpful laboratory tests, however, for both diagnosis and regulation of therapy are the serum muscle enzymes (creatine phosphokinase, aldolase, and transaminases). These enzymes, which are normally found in the muscle tissue, are released from damaged tissue into the serum. Measurement of the elevated serum enzymes is therefore an indication of muscle injury. Electromyography and muscle biopsy are also useful in establishing the correct diagnosis.

Treatment

The first principle of therapy is rest, particularly during the acute and active phase of the disease. Corticosteroids, usually in the range of 40 to 60 mg/day in divided doses, should be promptly instituted. Steroid doses in this range will generally suppress the disease activity, although patients with malignancies are often steroid-resistant.

As the muscle strength improves and the serum muscle enzymes approach normal, the steroid dose may be gradually tapered. Too-rapid reduction may result in a flare of the disease. Some patients may require long-term low-dose steroid therapy. Those patients who are resistant to steroid therapy may need to be considered for immunosuppressive medications.

The diagnostician must always look for the possible presence of a malignancy (especially in patients over 40 years of age).

Patient care implications

It is the responsibility of the nurse and the family to provide an atmosphere at home in which the patient can get the amount of rest needed. Community agencies may be useful in providing help in achieving these goals in the home. The nurse can help the family reorganize schedules so that the chores for which the patient was responsible are redistributed among family members or community agency helpers.

Since these patients are frequently taking high doses of prednisone for a period of weeks, months, or longer, they can expect to experience many of the side effects ("moon face" and other side effects) common to patients on long-term steroid therapy. The nurse can inform the patient and family of these side effects and the reasons for taking this medication.

Because of the extreme weakness which can occur, precautions should be taken as with any immobilized patient. Passive range of motion exercises may be indicated in order to prevent muscle contractures, without placing undue strain on the inflamed muscles.

PROGRESSIVE SYSTEMIC SCLEROSIS

Progressive systemic sclerosis (PSS) is often referred to as *scleroderma*. It is, as the name indicates, a progressive and generalized disorder. Connective tissues, both cutaneous and visceral, undergo inflammatory and sclerotic changes.[12] The cause is as yet unknown.

All races can be affected, and progressive systemic sclerosis generally involves women twice as frequently as men. Onset is usually in the third to fifth decades and the disease only rarely affects children.

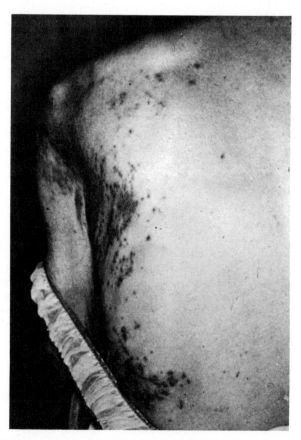

FIGURE 64-1 Dermatomyositis: Skin rash. Dermatomyositis with pruritic eruption over the back and upper arm. (Reproduced with permission from the Canadian Arthritis and Rheumatism Society, Dr. J. B. Houpt, Editor.)

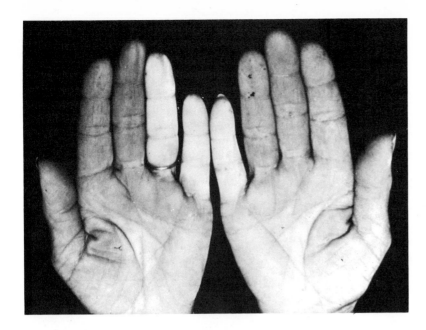

FIGURE 64-2 Scleroderma: Raynaud's phenomenon. The marked pallor of the fourth and fifth digits of the left hand and of the fifth digit of the right hand is characteristic of Raynaud's phenomenon. Vasospastic changes are common in systemic sclerosis. (Reproduced with permission from the Arthritis Foundation, New York, copyright 1972.)

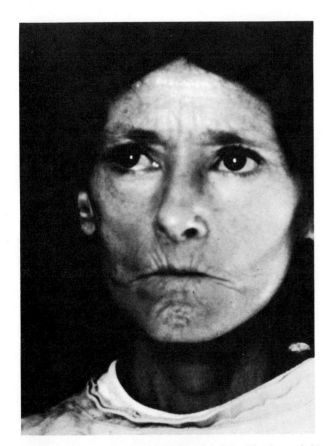

FIGURE 64-3 Scleroderma: Skin changes, face. The face of this young woman demonstrates many features of systemic sclerosis including drawn pursed lips, shiny skin over the cheeks and forehead, and atrophy of muscles of the temple, face, and neck. These changes in the face are known as "Mauskopf" (mousehead). (Reproduced with permission from the Arthritis Foundation, New York, copyright 1972.)

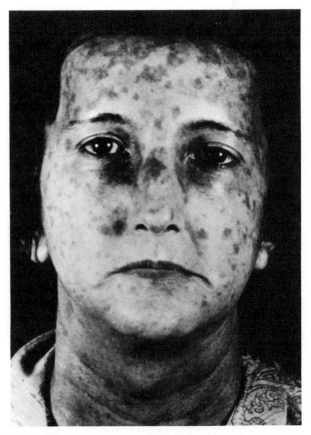

FIGURE 64-4 Scleroderma: Telangiectasias. Multiple telangiectases are present on the face. They blanch with pressure. Telangiectasia occurs frequently in this disorder, at times leading to confusion in differentiation from hereditary hemorrhagic telangiectasia. (Reproduced with permission from the Arthritis Foundation, New York, copyright 1972.)

PSS, as do many other connective tissue disorders, may remit and flare, progressing slowly and allowing for a reasonably long life. However, when vital organs are involved and damaged, PSS may be rapidly progressive and lead to an early death. Renal failure is the leading cause of death in patients with PSS.

Clinical features

Raynaud's phenomenon (see Fig. 64-2), a paroxysmal vasospastic disorder, is a presenting symptom in at least one-half of the cases of PSS. This abnormal spasm of the vessels, usually in response to cold or extreme emotions, cause the digits to become white, then red, then blue. Raynaud's phenomenon usually affects the fingers and, less often, the toes. Nearly all patients with PSS experience Raynaud's phenomenon at some time during the course of the disease. Some patients experience mild Raynaud's, which may result in small pitted scars, while others may experience more severe Raynaud's, resulting in gangrene of the digits.

Another initial complaint is the swelling of the fingers, which have a sausagelike appearance. The skin slowly thickens and becomes very taut, shiny, and bound-down. This process progresses proximally involving the arms, chest, and face. The face becomes very taut (see Fig. 64-3), the oral orifice becomes wrinkled, and the opening of the orifice is restricted. The forehead loses its normal wrinkles.

Contractures of the extremities may result from the thickened hide-bound skin. Telangiectasias (see Fig.

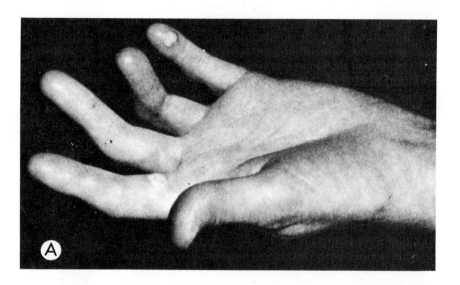

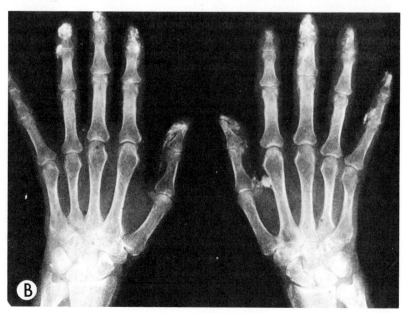

Figure 64-5 Scleroderma: Subcutaneous calcification. A, hand of adolescent girl with progressive systemic sclerosis. Note the circumscribed lesions of calcinosis in the skin of the volar surface of the proximal portion of the second and distal portion of the fifth digit. B, x-ray of the hands of a woman with progressive systemic sclerosis as depicted by the extensive subcutaneous calcinosis in the fingers and near the joint of the right hand. (Reproduced with permission from J. R. Hollander (ed.), Arthritis and Allied Conditions, A Textbook of Rheumatology, 8th ed., Lea & Febinger, Philadelphia, 1972.)

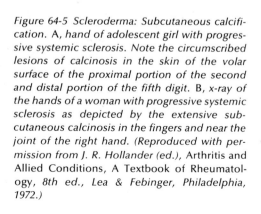

64-4), small spots consisting of tiny dilated blood vessels, are common on the face and hands. In the later stages of the disease, subcutaneous calcifications may develop on the fingers. The skin may ulcerate, discharging a white chalky substance from the deposits.

Arthralgias and arthritis may affect some patients, especially at the onset of PSS. Pain and stiffness usually affect the fingers, knees, and wrists; however, joints are not usually swollen or hot.

As PSS progresses, many organ systems may become involved. The majority of patients develop some dysfunction of the neuromusculature of the esophagus, leading to dysphagia. This may, in turn, lead to weight loss or aspiration pneumonitis. Hypomotility or strictures of the lower esophagus may also develop.

The colon may be affected, resulting in diarrhea or constipation, cramping, malabsorption, and, in a few cases, perforation.

Exertional dyspnea is usually the first sign of pulmonary involvement. Pulmonary function studies may show alteration in the gas exchange, that is, decrease in breathing capacity and an increase in the residual air. Pericarditis, arrythmias, and/or electrocardiogram changes may occur with cardiac involvement.

Renal involvement manifested as proteinuria, microscopic hematuria, and hypertension may rapidly progress to renal failure. Renal disease is the leading cause of death in patients with progressive systemic sclerosis. Any vital organ involvement, especially when rapidly progressive, indicates a poorer prognosis for the patient.

Laboratory and x-ray findings

The erythrocyte sedimentation rate may be elevated. A small group of the patients may demonstrate rheumatoid factor in their serum. Many of the patients with PSS have a positive antinuclear antibody, and hypergammaglobulinemia may be demonstrated. Skin biopsies are the most specific way of making the diagnosis.

Radiologic examination may demonstrate subcutaneous calcifications of the digits of the hand (see Fig. 64-5). Esophageal and intestinal abnormalities may also be detected.

Treatment

These patients must protect themselves from the cold in order to decrease the frequency of attacks of Raynaud's phenomenon. Vasodilators are sometimes of benefit in the treatment of Raynaud's phenomenon.

Low doses of corticosteroids may relieve joint complaints but are usually not of great benefit for treatment of PSS.

Antibiotics have been used with some success in the treatment of small-bowel involvement. The theory is that the hypomotility allows for an overgrowth of microorganisms which interferes with absorption. Treatment with antibiotics reduces the overgrowth and allows for a more regular absorption.

Para-aminobenzoic acid (PABA) has been used in the treatment of scleroderma with variable results. Immunosuppressive drugs and alkylating agents have been used to treat some patients.

Physical therapy is of benefit for decreasing or preventing contractures.

QUESTIONS

Polymyositis, dermatomyositis, and progressive systemic sclerosis (scleroderma)—Chap. 64

Directions: Complete the following statements by filling in the correct word in the blank.

1 The treatment of choice for polymyositis is _____.

2 In polymyositis (and dermatomyositis) the proximal pelvic girdle and the proximal muscles of the _____ extremities are usually initially involved.

3 Scleroderma is also known as _____.

4 Involvement of the esophagus in cases of scleroderma can produce _____.

Directions: Answer the following questions on a separate sheet of paper.

5 In which sex does polymyositis occur more commonly?

6 In the 30 to 50 year age group, which sex does PSS most commonly affect?

7 Describe the skin changes which occur in patients with PSS.

8 Name two systems which may be involved in PSS.

9 Describe a potential problem which may occur in a patient with polymyositis when the *intercostal* muscles are involved.

Directions: Circle T if the statement is true and F if it is false. Correct the statement if it is false.

10 T   F   In polymyositis, children and young adults usually have a better prognosis.

CHAPTER 65   Systemic Lupus Erythematosus (SLE)

OBJECTIVES   **At the completion of Chapter. 65 you should be able to:**

1 Define *systemic lupus erythematosus* (SLE) with regard to its main characteristics.

2 Define *autoimmunity.*

3 Differentiate between the arthritis associated with SLE and the arthritis associated with rheumatoid arthritis.

4 Define *antinuclear* antibody (ANA).

5 List two laboratory tests which may be helpful in diagnosing SLE.

6 Name at least four of the clinical features of SLE.

7 List two medications useful in treating SLE and identify the range of doses appropriate for treating SLE.

8 Identify at least two health care professional implications for patients with SLE.

9 Identify symptoms that the SLE patient should recognize as critical to report to the attending physician.

SYSTEMIC LUPUS ERYTHEMATOSUS

Systemic lupus erythematosus (SLE) is a multisystem, chronic, autoimmune disease. It involves immunologic reactions which attack the "self" as if it were foreign, resulting in a chronic inflammatory process. Although SLE can affect either sex from infancy to old age, it mainly involves women in their childbearing years (the female/male ratio is 7:1). It is characterized by episodic flares and remissions. The flares can be characterized by a recurrence of symptoms experienced in the past or by totally new symptoms.

SLE originally was described as a skin disorder (in the 1800s) and given the name *lupus* because of the characteristic "butterfly rash" across the bridge of the nose and cheeks that resembles the coloring of a wolf (*lupus* is the Latin word for wolf). Discoid lupus is the name now given to the disorder when it is limited to cutaneous involvement.

In the late 1800s, the systemic involvement of SLE was noted, and it was recognized as a progressive or fatal disease. Since the advent of laboratory tests for earlier diagnosis and the use of steroids for treatment (1940s and 1950s), SLE patients now have a much better prognosis. Today a spectrum of mild to severe diseases is recognized.

Clinical features

Constitutional symptoms such as fever, fatigue, weakness, and weight loss generally occur early in the disease process but may recur throughout the course of the disease.

Skin manifestations include an erythematous rash which may appear on the face (in which case it is referred to as the "butterfly-rash") (see Fig. 65-1), the neck, the extremities, or the trunk. Sun exposure may aggravate this rash. The patient may also experience alopecia (hair loss); however, even if the loss is severe, the hair generally grows back. Small ulcerations of the oral or nasopharyngeal mucous membranes are another clinical feature of SLE.

Polyarthritis or arthralgias are evident in 90 percent of the patients, often as an initial manifestation. The polyarthritis of SLE differs from that of rheumatoid arthritis in that it is nondeforming. Subcutaneous nodules are rarely seen in SLE.

Pleurisy (chest pain) may occur as a result of the chronic inflammatory process of lupus; however, bacterial infection may be the causative factor of the chest pain, and so one must make a careful diagnosis. Carditis is another clinical manifestation of systemic lupus erythematosus. The myocardium, endocardium, or pericardium may become involved.

Raynaud's phenomenon has been noted to occur in up to 15 to 20 percent of SLE patients.[13] Some cases may be so severe as to result in gangrene of the digits. Arteries and veins, both small and large, may be affected by vasculitis.

Lupus nephritis occurs as the antinuclear antibody (anti-DNA) attaches to its antigen (deoxyribonucleic acid) and is deposited in the renal glomerulus. DNA is not usually antigenic in humans, but, because of the effects of SLE on the immune system, it acts as an antigen. Complement, a series of proteins in the serum, is fixed to this immune complex, and the inflammatory process begins. Inflammation, tissue damage, and/or scarring may result.

Lupus nephritis is a frequent, as well as serious, feature of SLE. It is the most frequent cause of death. It may be clinically recognized by protein, red blood cells, and/or casts in the urine, although the urine may be negative. It can be diagnosed by kidney biopsy.

Central nervous system disease causing behavioral changes (depression, psychosis), convulsions, cranial nerve disorders, and peripheral neuropathies can also occur with SLE. These disorders are usually associated with severe disease and poor prognosis.

Not every patient experiences all these clinical fea-

tures; some patients have mild disease and may experience only the rash and arthritis. Some patients, on the other hand, experience very severe disease involving several major organ systems.

Diagnosis

The American Rheumatism Association has developed criteria for the diagnosis of systemic lupus erythematosus. The presence of *four* of these criteria with a positive ANA yields a definite diagnosis (90 percent confidence).

1 Facial erythema
2 Oral or nasopharyngeal ulcerations
3 Alopecia
4 Photosensitivity
5 Discoid lupus (a form of lupus affecting only the skin)
6 Pleuritis or pericarditis
7 Raynaud's phenomenon
8 Arthritis without deformity
9 Central nervous system disease
10 Cytopenia (hemolytic anemia, leukopenia, or thrombocytopenia)
11 Positive LE cell test
12 Chronic false positive serologic test for syphilis
13 Profuse proteinuria (3.5 g/day)
14 Cellular casts[14]

Laboratory findings

The ANA (antinuclear antibody) test should be positive in 95 to 100 percent of SLE patients. This test indicates whether there are antibodies capable of destroying the nucleus of one's own body cells. This test also has a positive result in other autoimmune diseases and in a small percentage of the normal population as well (increases with aging). Therefore, the ANA test is not specific for SLE. Anemia, leukopenia, and occasionally a thrombocytopenia are present.

The LE (lupus erythematosus) factor is demonstrated in a test that shows a white blood cell that has ingested other nuclear material after incubation in a simple test system (see Fig. 65-2). This factor can usually be demonstrated at some time in the course of the disease. Al-

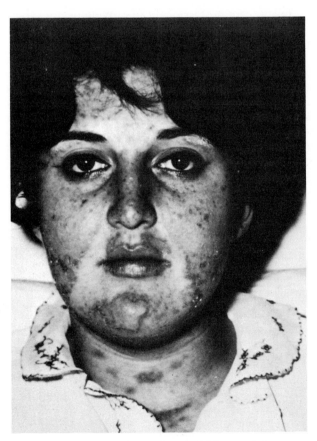

FIGURE 65-1 SLE: Rash, face and neck. Widespread discrete and confluent erythematous lesions are present on the face and neck. Typical peeling is noted on the chin and cheeks. (Reproduced with permission from The Arthritis Foundation, New York, copyright 1972.)

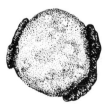

FIGURE 65-2 SLE: LE cell. A neutrophil within which is contained homogeneous material, the LE body. The nucleus is pushed to one side and flattened around the mass.

though it can be seen in other autoimmune diseases, it is strongly suggestive of SLE, particularly in the presence of clinical symptoms.

The most specific test for SLE is the anti-DNA test because it rarely is positive in any other situation, while it is positive in the majority of patients with SLE. Positivity generally correlates with active disease and renal involvement and, hence, may be useful in guiding therapy. The hemolytic complement test is also useful in following inflammatory activity in patients with SLE. In the immune reaction, the complement is fixed to the antibody-antigen complex, and the level of free complement in the serum is thus decreased, indicating an increase in the activity of the disease.

Urinalysis, including examination for protein, white blood cells, red blood cells, and casts, may be of help in both the diagnosis and the management of the renal disease.

Treatment

PROPHYLAXIS

Patients should be advised to take certain precautions. They should avoid the sun, particularly direct exposure at the time of day when the sun is strongest. Exposure of a photosensitive patient to the sun can induce a flare.

Patients should avoid certain drugs, such as diphenylhydantoin (Dilantin), contraceptives, sulfas, isoniazid, and procainamide, all of which may aggravate SLE. Unnecessary transfusions should also be avoided because of the possibility of transfusion reactions.[15]

Fatigue is a constantly recurring problem for patients with systemic lupus erythematosus; thus, patients should avoid fatigue as much as possible by getting adequate amounts of rest and by pacing their daily activities.

Pregnancy may cause a flare in the disease and can be dangerous, particularly for patients with renal disease. Also, patients who are taking cytotoxic drugs should be informed of the potential ill effects on the fetus. Birth control methods should be discussed with these patients. Contraception methods *other* than the birth control pill should be used since the pill may aggrevate SLE. The intrauterine device also is a relative contraindication for patients on prednisone because of the potential for infection.

HEAT

Heat can be very helpful for symptomatic relief of articular manifestations of SLE. Refer to Rheumatoid Arthritis chapter for a review of the appropriate types of heat.

MEDICATIONS

Salicylates can be useful in treating the arthritis associated with SLE. Hydroxychloroquine (Plaquenil) is used for treating the rash and the joint manifestations. As is the case with rheumatoid arthritis, precautions should be taken to prevent eye toxicity from the drug.

Corticosteroids (prednisone) are very useful and important agents in the treatment of SLE; they are the mainstay of therapy. The lowest dose possible to achieve results is used because of the many side effects associated with long-term use of this drug. Doses used in treating SLE range widely and depend on the activity of the disease and the organ system involved. Doses in excess of 80 mg/day have been used for short periods of time to treat life-threatening central nervous system disease. As the disease becomes inactive, the dose of prednisone is tapered to as low a dose as possible. Because of the immunosuppressive nature of steroids, infection is always a hazard.

Immunosuppressive therapy (cyclophosphamide or azathioprine) can be used in an effort to suppress the autoimmune activity of SLE. Such therapy is generally prescribed under the following circumstances: (1) Well-established diagnosis, (2) severe, life-threatening disease, (3) failure of other therapeutic measures (e.g., failure to respond to steroids or the need for reduction of steroids because of side effects), and (4) absence of infection, pregnancy, and neoplasm.

Patient care implications

The health care professional can provide useful service in helping the patients and interested family members to understand the effect of SLE on their lives.

SLE involves long-term medical management, and informed patients are better equipped to care for themselves. It is essential for patients to understand protective measures which can be taken, such as avoidance of the sun and avoidance of fatigue. It is also important that patients and their families understand the reasons for taking the medications and the importance of taking them consistently. An explanation of the effect prednisone has upon suppressing the body's adrenal production of cortisone is essential. Patients must understand that if they were to stop taking prednisone, the force suppressing the disease would be removed. In addition, the body would be left without any of this essential hormone since the body's production of it has been suppressed.

It is critical that patients know which problems they should report to their physician. Any recurrence of symptoms experienced in past flares (fever, severe fatigue, arthritis, chest pain) or any new symptoms should be reported. Severe side effects from drugs such as black, tarry stools, which may indicate gastrointestinal bleeding, should also be reported. The patient should make an active attempt to avoid exposure to infections and should inform the health care provider if exposures or infections occur. Vomiting, making it impossible to keep down medications (especially prednisone), must be reported immediately. The patient may have to be admitted for parenteral administration of the prednisone.

As with any chronic disease, the health care professional can help the patient in adjusting to this new illness. The professional may be able to direct the patient and family to a variety of community agencies. For example, homemakers may need to be directed to agencies that provide assistance with household duties. Financial aid agencies may help to deal with loss of income, as well as financial stress due to the cost of medications, of medical care, and of transportation. Counseling agencies may aid the patient and family in coping with the major change in life-style required by this disease.

As the health care professional becomes involved in teaching the patient about SLE, its treatment, and the side effects of medications, the patient may become more comfortable and want to confide in that person. Personal thoughts about having a chronic disease and feelings about the reaction of the family may all be shared. These actions generally indicate an acceptance of the health care professional by the patient. This is an opportune time for the professional to offer professional skills in helping the patient cope with SLE. Health care professionals can provide assistance to the patient in many ways, but should refer the patient to a counseling professional or agency for patient needs which they cannot meet. If referral is necessary, the reasons for the referral should be discussed with the patient.

QUESTIONS

Systemic lupus erythematosus (SLE)—Chap. 65

Directions: Answer the following questions on a separate sheet of paper.

1 Define *autoimmunity*.

2 List three clinical features of SLE.

3 Differentiate between the arthritis of SLE and rheumatoid arthritis.

Directions: Complete the following question by filling in the blank with the appropriate response.

4 The _____ test should be positive in order to make the diagnosis of SLE.

Directions: Circle T if the statement is true and F if it is false. Correct any false statements.

5　T　F　Prednisone is always used in doses above 60 mg/day in the treatment of SLE.

6　T　F　Infection is always a potential hazard in a patient taking large doses of prednisone.

Directions: You are a public health nurse visiting a patient with SLE. She is taking 20 mg prednisone per day for arthritis as well as for control of her renal disease. For which of the following symptoms would you encourage her to promptly contact her physician? State your rationale for your choices.

7 Severe chest pain which increases with deep breathing

8 Mild fatigue

9 Increase in appetite

10 Black tarry stools

11 Missed menstrual period

12 Rounded face ("moon face")

13 Fever of 101° and a swollen knee

CHAPTER 66 Gout

OBJECTIVES **At the completion of Chap. 66 you should be able to:**

1 Define the clinical characteristics of gout.

2 Differentiate between acute and chronic gout in terms of clinical features.

3 List two criteria for diagnosing gout.

4 List two drugs useful for treating an acute attack and one drug used for maintenance therapy of gout.

GOUT

Gout is a metabolic disease which was described by Hippocrates in ancient Greece. It was then thought to be a disease of the social elite caused by an overindulgence in food, wine, and sex. Since then, many etiologic and therapeutic theories have been proposed. Today, gout is probably one of the best understood of all the rheumatic diseases and has the highest rate of success derived from therapeutic efforts.

The classic picture of the acute severe arthritis of gout is directly associated with hyperuricemia (high serum uric acid). Gout may be primary or secondary. Primary gout is the direct result of the body's overproduction or decreased excretion of uric acid. Secondary gout occurs when the body's overproduction or reduced excretion of uric acid is a result of another disease process or of medication.

Urate deposits in the joints as well as in the urinary tract result from the low solubility of the uric acid and its salts. The excess uric acid and salts precipitate out of the serum and urine and are deposited in the joints and urinary tract, respectively.

Clinical features

Acute gout generally occurs after puberty in males and after menopause in females with peak incidence being in the fifth and sixth decades. Gout occurs much more frequently in males, with almost 95 percent of patients with gout being males. The serum urate of the normal female population is around 1 mg/100 ml less than that of males until after menopause, when the difference becomes

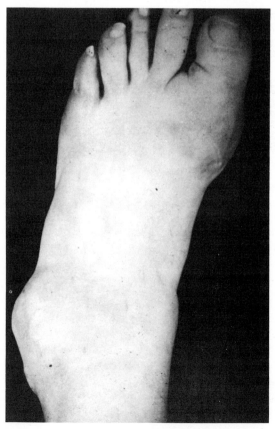

FIGURE 66-1 Gout: Great toe. Typical inflammatory response of gout involving the great toe. This is the most common site of acute gout. (Reproduced with permission from the Arthritis Division, University Hospital, University of Michigan.)

less marked. In males, hyperuricemia does not usually appear until adolescence.

Acute gout is usually monoarticular and sudden in onset. Severe pain and signs of local inflammation are common signs of the onset of a gout attack. The patient may also experience fever and an elevated white blood cell count. Surgery, local trauma, drugs, alcohol, and emotional stress may precipitate acute attacks. Although involvement of the great toe (metatarsophalangeal joint) is most common initially (see Fig. 66-1), other joints may become involved. Finger joints, knees, wrists, and elbows may be sites for a gout attack as the disease progresses. An acute attack of gout is usually self-limited; most of the symptoms of the acute attack may subside within 10 to 14 days, even without treatment.

The development of the acute attack of gout generally follows a set sequence of events. First there is a supersaturation of urate in the plasma and body fluids. This is followed by a precipitation of urate crystals out of the body fluids and deposition into and around the joints. The mechanism of the crystalization of urates out of the serum is not clearly understood; however, gout attacks frequently follow local trauma or the rupture of tophi (deposits of sodium urate), which would account for a rapid increase in local concentrations of uric acid. The body may not be able to appropriately handle this increase, resulting in the precipitation of uric acid out of the serum. Crystalization and deposition of the uric acid then triggers the gout attack. These uric acid crystals trigger a phagocytic response by leukocytes, and, as the leukocytes ingest the urate crystals, the responses of other inflammatory mechanisms are triggered. The inflammatory response may be influenced by the site and magnitude of uric acid crystal deposition. The inflammatory reaction may become self-propagating and self-enhancing owing to the deposition of additional crystals from the serum.

The period between acute attacks of gout is referred to as *intercritical gout*. The patient at this time is free from clinical symptoms.

Chronic gout develops over a period of years and is characterized by pain, aching, and stiffness. Chronic inflammation results from the presence of urate crystals, the joint swelling of chronic gout often being large and nodular. Acute attacks of gout may occur simultaneously with the symptoms of chronic gout. Tophi develop in chronic gout because of the relative insolubility of urates (Fig. 66-2). The onset and the size of tophi may be proportionally related to the level of serum urate. The olecranon bursa, Achilles tendon, extensor surface of the forearm, infrapatellar bursa, and helix of the ear (see Fig. 66-3) are common sites for tophi. These tophi may be virtually impossible to distinguish clinically from rheumatoid nodules. On occasion, the tophi may ulcerate and drain and may also limit the motion of a joint. Renal disease may result from chronic hyperuricemia but can be prevented with adequate management of gout.

Diagnostic criteria

Gout should be a consideration in any patient with a history and physical findings compatible with those described above, particularly the classic clinical picture. An elevated serum uric acid is very helpful in making the diagnosis. It should be kept in mind, however, that many drugs have an effect on the serum uric acid levels and also that there are many asymptomatic individuals in the normal population with an elevated uric acid.

Another diagnostic test for supporting the diagnosis of gout is determining the response of the joint symptoms to colchicine. Colchicine is a medication which provides a dramatic relief of symptoms of an acute attack of gout. Characteristic radiologic changes can be very helpful in making a diagnosis of gout, but striking changes are usually not present at the onset of the disease.

Once a diagnosis of gout is suspected, it can be confirmed by two methods: (1) Demonstration of urate crystals in the synovial fluid (Fig. 66-4), and (2) demonstration of urate in tophaceous deposits.

Contributing factors

Certain factors may contribute to hyperuricemia. A diet high in purines may be one contributing factor since uric acid is formed from the purines, adenine and guanine. Starvation and excessive ethyl alcohol intake

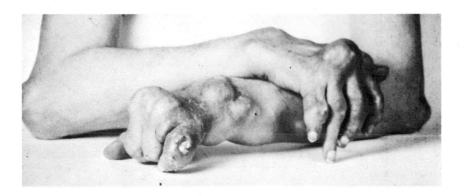

FIGURE 66-2 Gout: Tophi, hands and olecranon bursa. Many tophi are present on the hands. One asymmetrically shaped tophus on the little finger has ulcerated. The characteristic whitish to yellowish color of urate deposits can be seen. Tophi are also present in both olecranon bursae; these are common sites for tophi. Swelling of some joints due to synovitis is also present. (Reproduced with permission from The Arthritis Foundation, New York, copyright 1972.)

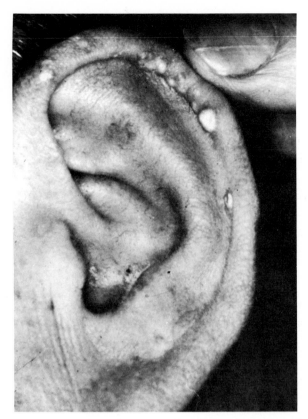

FIGURE 66-3 Gout: Tophi, ear. Small tophi can be seen on the helix of the ear having a typical whitish appearance as a result of urate deposition. Small cartilaginous nodules are commonly present in the ears of normal individuals and can be mistaken for tophi. A tophus will characteristically stand out as a discrete white nodule when pressed by the examiner's fingers; in contrast, the cartilaginous nodule will blanch out and blend with the rest of the ear. Transillumination reveals an opaque center in the tophus but not in the cartilaginous nodule. (Reproduced with permission from The Arthritis Foundation, New York, copyright 1972.)

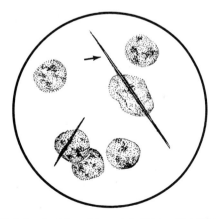

FIGURE 66-4 Gout: Uric acid crystal. One uric acid crystal in a white blood cell in synovial fluid.

may cause hyperuricemia. An increase in keto acid levels results from prolonged fasting, and these keto acids interfere with the renal excretion of uric acid. Blood lactate levels increase as a by-product of the normal metabolism of alcohol, and these increased levels also interfere with renal excretion of uric acid. Salicylates in low doses (less than 2 to 3 g/day) and certain diuretic antihypertensive medications (chlorthiazide, ethacrynic acid) contribute to a rise in the serum uric acid.

Treatment

Colchicine, an anti-inflammatory agent, has traditionally been employed as a treatment for acute gout attacks, as well as to prevent future acute gouty attacks. It is also used as a diagnostic aid. The usual treatment for an acute attack is one 0.5 mg tablet every hour until a relief of symptoms has occurred or there is evidence of gastrointestinal side effects. A maximum dose is 4 to 8 mg, depending on the weight of the patient. Some patients experience severe nausea, vomiting, and diarrhea and must discontinue use at that time. Relief of symptoms occurs within about 10 to 24 hours for the majority of patients. Colchicine in doses of 0.5 to 2 mg/day has shown to be effective in complete or near complete prevention of further gout attacks. Daily doses of colchicine also tend to reduce the severity of gouty episodes when they do occur. Long-term use of colchicine has not been shown to produce severe side effects.

Phenylbutazone, a potent anti-inflammatory agent, may also be useful in treating acute gouty arthritis. However, because of the side effects of phenylbutazone, colchicine is used for preventive therapy.

Three other medications are useful in maintenance or preventive therapy. Allopurinol decreases the formation of uric acid. A daily dose of 200 to 400 mg reduces the levels of serum uric acid. Probenecid and sulfinpyrazine are uricosuric agents, which means that they block reabsorption of urate by the renal tubule and thus increase the excretion of uric acid. Checking levels of serum uric acid is useful to determine the effectiveness of therapy.

Avoidance of foods high in purines may be indicated. Among these foods are organ meats such as liver, kidneys, sweetbreads, and brains. Sardines and anchovies would also be restricted.

Surgery is advised for the removal of bulky draining tophi, particularly if the tophi are impeding joint motion.

QUESTIONS

Gout—Chap. 66

Directions: Complete the following statements by filling in the blanks with the correct response.

1 The clinical manifestations of gout are directly caused by _____.

2 A medication used for both acute attacks and mainte-

nance therapy is _____. (It often is used as a diagnostic test because of the dramatic response from gout patients.)

Directions: Answer the following question on a separate sheet of paper.

3 Name one of the long-term manifestations of hyper-uricemia.

Directions: Circle T if the statement is true and F if it is false. Correct any false statements.

4   T   F   Gout affects males more than females.

5   T   F   An acute attack of gout is usually self-limiting even without treatment.

6   T   F   Demonstration of urate crystals in the joint fluid yields a definite diagnosis of gout.

CHAPTER 67 Infectious Arthritis and Degenerative Joint Disease (Osteoarthritis)

OBJECTIVES

At the completion of Chap. 67 you should be able to:

1 Define *infectious arthritis.*

2 State the procedure used in diagnosing infectious arthritis.

3 State the general treatment for infectious arthritis.

4 List two of the common organisms that invade joints.

5 State two predisposing factors to infectious arthritis.

6 Identify the characteristics of osteoarthritis in relation to age, sex, and predisposing factors.

7 List two of the clinical features of osteoarthritis.

8 Describe at least two therapeutic measures which may be employed in treatment of osteoarthritis.

INFECTIOUS ARTHRITIS

Invasion of a joint space by an infectious agent is known as infectious arthritis. This condition is also referred to as suppurative, pyogenic, or septic arthritis.

Common organisms which may invade the joint are *Staphylococcus aureus, Diplococcus pneumoniae, Streptococcus pyogenes,* and *Neisseria gonorrhea.*

Some factors which may predispose the patient to a joint infection include other systemic diseases (e.g., malignancies), treatment with cytotoxic drugs or corticosteroids (which depress the patient's immune reaction), joint trauma or a preexisting inflammatory joint process, a septic area elsewhere in the body, or an invasive procedure such as a joint aspiration.

The production and accumulation of pus in the joint cavity, which may result from the severe inflammatory response, can cause rapid destruction of the cartilage and subchondral bone. Therefore prompt diagnosis and treatment are of utmost importance.

Clinical features

Severe pain, swelling, and erythema involving one joint is often the initial presenting symptom. However, more than one joint may be involved, and the inflammatory response may be less severe. When the presentation is mild, infectious arthritis may become very difficult to

diagnose in a patient who has an already existing joint disease such as rheumatoid arthritis.

Infectious arthritis generally affects the larger joints such as the hips, knees, elbows, and wrists; however, any joint may be involved. As with many septic processes, a fever may be present.

Laboratory and radiologic findings

Diagnosis of infectious arthritis can be made by culturing joint fluid obtained by joint aspiration. Blood cultures may also be helpful in diagnosis. Demonstration of the invading organism is the only way to make a definite diagnosis.

The joint fluid in septic arthritis is a very inflammatory fluid with a cell count usually in excess of $50,000/mm^3$. The fluid is usually watery, losing its normal viscosity, and is usually turbid (not clear).

Characteristic x-ray changes occur much more rapidly in infectious arthritis than in other joint disorders. Changes in the joint space (cartilage damage) and bony changes may occur as soon as 1 or 2 weeks after the infectious process begins.[16]

Treatment

The patient should be treated promptly with the appropriate antibiotic drug(s), that is, the antibiotic drug(s) indicated by sensitivity tests of the invading organism. It is also important to remove purulent fluid from the joint as it accumulates, so as to reduce chances of articular damage. Removal may involve daily aspirations of the purulent exudate.

Parenteral antibiotics readily gain access to the joint cavity, and there is thus no indication for intraarticular injection of antibiotic (especially since it may cause a local inflammatory reaction).

The duration of antibiotic therapy is dependent on the invading organism but may extend anywhere from 2 to 6 weeks. Joint fluid cultures and cell counts are helpful in evaluating therapy.

Splinting of a painful joint may be helpful during the initial stages of the disease, but gradual passive range of motion exercises leading up to active range of motion exercises will aid in preventing loss of motion.

Tuberculosis arthritis

Tuberculosis may also involve a joint. Symptoms of such involvement usually have a more insidious onset. Diagnosis can be made by joint fluid cultures, synovial biopsy, positive history of tuberculosis, and radiologic changes. Antituberculosis therapy is employed for treatment.

DEGENERATIVE JOINT DISEASE (OSTEOARTHRITIS)

Degenerative joint disease is a chronic, slowly progressive, and noninflammatory disorder which seems to be a natural element of the process of aging. There is a deterioration or degeneration of the joint cartilage and growth of new bone at the marginal aspects of the joint (bony spurs).

The degeneration is caused by a breakdown of chondrocytes, which are an essential element of articular cartilage. This breakdown is thought to be initiated by biomechanical stresses. A release of lysosomal enzymes leads to the breakdown of protein polysaccharides, which form the matrix surrounding the chondrocytes, thus resulting in damaged cartilage. The most commonly affected joints are the weight-bearing joints: the hips, the knees, and the vertebral column. The distal interphalangeal joints and the proximal interphalangeal joints are also frequently involved.

There are several synonyms for osteoarthritis, among them degenerative joint disease (DJD), hypertrophic arthritis, and "wear and tear" arthritis. Degenerative joint disease is presently the more accurate, and hence preferred, name.

Although the disease process may begin as early as the second decade, it most commonly affects the elderly. Osteoarthritis affects men and women, blacks and whites. However, apparently more women suffer from moderate to severe disease than do men. Radiologic evidence of osteoarthritis may, however, be demonstrated on as many as 85 percent of those persons over the age of 75, although clinical signs of pain and stiffness may not be present.

Secondary osteoarthritis involves degenerative changes which result from events such as joint injury, joint infection, congenital deformities, and other inflammatory joint diseases including rheumatoid arthritis. This process may affect younger persons more than those affected by primary osteoarthritis.

Clinical features

Joint pain is the primary feature of osteoarthritis. The patient may induce or aggravate pain with moderate to vigorous exercise. The characteristic aching pain is generally not induced or present when the patient is at rest. Periods of rest may, however, result in joint stiffness which is another characteristic manifestation of osteoarthritis. The stiffness of osteoarthritis is not as severe as that of rheumatoid arthritis. Mild activity will usually dissipate the stiffness.

Degenerative joint disease may in some cases cause limitation of motion. This may be intentional because of pain or may result from joint space narrowing or from lack of use of the joint.

Characteristic changes may occur in the hands. Heberden's nodes or bony enlargements of the distal interphalangeal joints are a common feature of degenerative joint disease. Less commonly seen are Bouchard's nodes (see Fig. 67-1), which are bony enlargements of the proximal interphalangeal joints. Pain, stiffness, and sometimes a reduction of motion may affect the knees and hips. Although degenerative joint disease is noninflammatory, effusions may be detected in involved joints (especially the knees).

The vertebral column may be affected by pain, stiffness, and limited range of motion. Bony overgrowths or spurs may irritate the nerve roots as they pass through the vertebrae, resulting in neuromuscular changes such as numbness and tingling. Degeneration of the vertebral disks, which may also be attributed to the aging process, can contribute to nerve root irritation or nerve root compression.

The etiology of degenerative joint disease is as yet unknown; however, certain factors may contribute to its development. The aging process, as has been mentioned, is a contributing factor. Excessive use of a joint or trauma may predispose an individual to osteoarthritis. Obesity may influence the age of onset as well as the severity of the disease. The weight-bearing joints are the ones most greatly affected by obesity.

Laboratory findings

There are usually no serum abnormalities unless their presence is related to another disease process. The rheumatoid factor test is generally negative. If the rheumatoid factor is found in the serum of older patients, its presence may be unrelated to the arthritis since false positivity of rheumatoid factor increases with age in the normal population.

Synovial fluid is usually noninflammatory, that is, clear and viscous, with a total cell count of less than 1000/mm³.

Radiologic findings

Narrowing of the joint space, moderate malalignment, and osteophytes (spurs) at the marginal aspects of the joints may be demonstrated radiographically (see Fig. 67-2).

Treatment

The use of heat over involved joints may provide temporary relief of pain. Certain range of motion exercises may be useful in maintaining full range of motion of involved joints. When joints are particularly painful, the health care professional or a member of the patient's family may assist the patient by putting the joints through

their range of motion. This is done passively, that is, without active involvement of the patient.

Cervical collars may provide relief of pain when there is severe osteoarthritis of the cervical spine. These collars provide mild traction which may relieve the nerve root irritation by the bony overgrowths at the edge of the vertebrae.

There are many techniques for joint protection and work simplification which can be learned by the patient. These are energy-saving techniques employed in order to minimize joint trauma and overuse. For examples refer to chapter 62.

Since osteoarthritis usually involves the weight-bearing joints (the hips and knees), it is very important that the patient maintains an optimal weight. There are no special foods which cause or cure osteoarthritis, but proper nutrition is vital, and weight reduction is mandatory for overweight individuals.

Aspirin is usually the drug of choice, but when it is not well-tolerated or effective, other medications may be used. Indomethacin (Indocin) may provide relief of the symptoms of osteoarthritis, but it usually is reserved until the effectiveness of aspirin has been tested. Propoxyphene hydrochloride (Darvon) is a medication which is often used to supplement aspirin therapy, particularly during times of increased pain. New non-

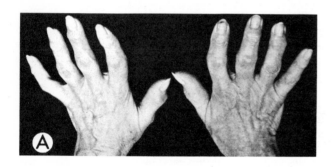

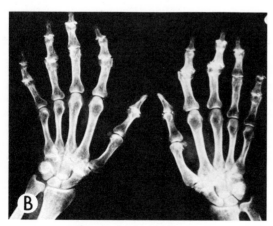

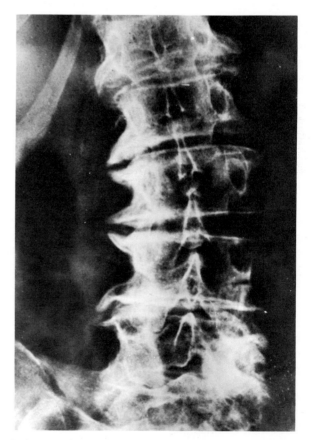

FIGURE 67-1 Degenerative joint disease. A, primary osteoarthritis of the hands with marked proximal interphalangeal involvement (Bouchard's nodes) along with distal interphalangeal joint involvement. B, x-ray of the same hands. (Reproduced from J. L. Hollander (ed.), Arthritis and Allied Conditions, A Textbook of Rheumatology, 8th ed., Lea & Febinger, Philadelphia, 1972.)

FIGURE 67-2 Denerative joint disease: Spine x-ray. This antero-posterior projection of the lumbar spine shows scoliosis and narrowing of the intervertebral spaces on the concave side where extensive osteophyte formation is present. The osteophytes are not continuous as seen in ankylosing spondylitis. Adjacent bony margins are sclerosed. (Reproduced with permission from The Arthritis Foundation, New York, copyright 1972.)

steroidal anti-inflammatory agents are now available, and these can be useful when aspirin is not well-tolerated. Oral steroids and phenylbutazone should be avoided because of their potential toxicity. Intraarticular steroids may provide relief for an inflamed painful joint (usually the knee).

Canes or crutches can provide stability and relief of strain on weight-bearing joints. Patients usually resist using these walking aids because they fear dependency on them, but patients can be helped to realize that canes and crutches are only an *aid* in walking.

For patients with severe pain which is not being relieved by medication, or patients with severe joint limitation, orthopedic surgery may be indicated. There has been increasing success with total knee and hip replacements.

Patient care implications

As with all the rheumatic diseases, the patient must adjust to a new life-style. The health care professional can be helpful in assisting older patients to make adjustments in their lives so that they can live effectively within their limitations. It is particularly important that the professional recognize how difficult it is for people to change life-styles suddenly. Frequently, arthritis complaints take a back seat to the more life-threatening chronic ailments afflicting the geriatric population; yet osteoarthritis can be a disabling disorder forcing the patient to limit or give up many of the activities which have made life enjoyable. The health care professional must employ all professional skills as well as common sense in order to assist the patient to adapt to limitations in a reasonable and acceptable fashion. The goal is to allow patients to partake in the activities they enjoy without inducing severe joint pain and stiffness.

QUESTIONS

Infectious arthritis and degenerative joint disease (osteoarthritis)—Chap. 67

Directions: Answer the following questions on a separate sheet of paper.

1 Name one common invading organism of infectious arthritis.

2 Name one predisposing factor to infectious arthritis.

3 List the three clinical features of osteoarthritis.

4 Name two predisposing factors contributing to the development of osteoarthritis.

5 Name two medications which may be used in the treatment of osteoarthritis.

Directions: Complete the following statement by filling in the blank.

6 _____ should be cultured in order to isolate the causative organism in infectious arthritis.

Directions: Circle T if the statement is true and F if it is false. Correct any false statements.

7 T F Steroids are used to treat septic arthritis.

8 T F The joint fluid in septic arthritis is an inflammatory fluid with a cell count that ranges around 50,000/mm³.

9 T F There are no specific laboratory tests for diagnosing osteoarthritis.

10 T F Although patients have x-ray changes of osteoarthritis, they may not experience any symptoms of pain and stiffness.

11 T F Osteoarthritis can occur in any age group.

REFERENCES

[1] *Health Statistics, Series B, No. 20,* U.S. Department of Health, Education, and Welfare, Washington, 1960.

[2] Committee of the American Rheumatism Association, Section of the Arthritis Foundation, 7th ed., *Primer on the Rheumatic Diseases,* reprint ed., JAMA, **224**: 51, suppl., 7–15, April 30, 1973.

[3] *Ibid.,* pp. 14–15.

[4] ESTHER M. GREISHEIMER, *Physiology and Anatomy,* Lippincott, Philadelphia, 1963, pp. 123–124.

[5] Committee of the American Rheumatism Association, p. 18.

[6] Committee of the American Rheumatism Association, p. 31.

[7] Committee of the American Rheumatism Association, p. 34.

[8] M. W. ROPES et al., "1958 Revision of Diagnostic Criteria for Rheumatoid Arthritis," *Bull Rheum Dis,* **9**: 175, 1958.

[9] B. BLUMBERG et al., "ARA Nomenclature and Classification of Arthritis and Rheumatism (tentative)", *Arthritis Rheum,* **7**: 93–97, 1964.

[10] G. G. BOLE, "Collagen and Rheumatic Disease," in Frederick A. Mausolf (ed.), *The Eye and Systemic Diseases,* Mosby, St. Louis, 1975.

[11] *Ibid.,* p. 87.

[12] *Ibid.,* p. 94.

[13] *Ibid.,* p. 92.

[14] A. S. COHEN et al., "Preliminary Criteria for the Classification of Systemic Lupus Erythematosus," *Bull Rheum Dis,* **21**: 643–648, 1971.

[15] JAMES T. CASSIDY, "Systemic Lupus Erythematosces," in *Tice's Practice of Medicine,* Vol. V, Chap. 30, Harper & Row, Hagerstown, Md., 1970.

[16] Committee of the American Rheumatism Association, p. 91.

Answers

ANSWERS

General concepts of disease—health vs. disease—Chap. 1

1 Pathology is the science or study of disease. It includes study of the pathogenesis of disease and the structural and functional alterations which result from disease. Pathology is literally abnormal biology, the study of sick or disordered life.

2 Anatomic pathology is the study of morphology of cells, organs, and tissues in disease. Clinical pathology refers to the application of many other laboratory techniques to the study of disease. Examples of anatomic pathology include surgical pathology, exfoliative cytology, autopsy pathology. Examples of clinical pathology include clinical chemistry, microbiology, hematology, immunology, and immunohematology.

3 Etiology refers to the causal agent(s) of disease. Pathogenesis is the way disease unfolds, the mechanism of development.

4 The concept of normalcy is a very complex one and difficult to define succinctly. Selecting any parameter which might be applied to an individual or group of individuals, the concept of "normal" involves some average value for that parameter. For example, average values for height and weight are derived from observations on many individuals. Implicitly a certain amount of variation from the average is accepted as being permissible or normal. The usual concept of normalcy involves both an average value and some range of variation either above or below that value.

5 b

6 d

ANSWERS

Heredity, environment, and disease interaction of heredity and environment—Chap. 2

1 (a) DNA may instruct a cell to produce a specific chemical product. (b) Other kinds of DNA can instruct cells to develop certain kinds of structures. (c) Portions of the DNA thus determine the limits of the individual's stature, facial features, etc. (d) DNA molecules can instruct the cell to make exact duplicates of themselves when the cell is about to divide.

2 During the process of cell division DNA is duplicated, and there is splitting of each chromosome and then a separation of the newly formed structures so that identically endowed daughter cells are formed. Beginning with the fertilized ovum at the moment of conception, identical genetic information is passed to every cell of the developing body.

3 One way for a chromosomal abnormality to develop is for one or more chromosomes to break and have the broken ends stick inappropriately to other chromosomes forming a fused, abnormal chromosome. Another type of abnormality involves failure of separation of the two chromosomes of a given pair during the special reduction division which normally leads to 23 chromosomes. A germ cell would be formed with a pair of chromosomes in a particular location instead of a single one, which would result in 24 instead of 23 chromosomes.

4 The prevention of genetic disorders requires the identification of couples that are capable of producing defective genotypes. The task of human genetics is also one of identifying subjects at unusual risk on a genetic basis and minimizing that risk by some environmental manipulation. The genetic counselor must render as accurate a diagnosis as possible. When parental genotypes are determined, the genetic prognosis is usually presented in terms of probability that a given couple will produce an affected offspring. The counselor must make certain that the couple understands the meaning of these absolute figures and the variability in clinical expression. The counselor must possess the ability to explain to the parents, humanely but understandably, the nature and prognosis of the disease and its impact on affected individuals, the mode of available treatment, and the means of preventing the occurrence of the disease.

5 a, d

6 c

7 b

8 b, c

9 a, c d

10 c

11 False; these abnormalities cannot be identified by microscopic examination since the karyotype of the affected individual is normal.

12 True

13 True

14 True

Cellular injury and death—Chap. 3

1 d
2 b
3 d
4 e
5 b
6 c
7 b
8 d
9 a
10 d
11 Biochemical, functional, anatomic
12 Dystrophic, metastatic, stone formation
13 Rigor mortis
14 d
15 c
16 b
17 e
18 a

ANSWERS

Response of the body to injury—Chap. 4

1 d
2 c
3 a, b, c
4 a, c, e
5 b, d
6 a, c
7 a, b, c
8 a, c
9 b
10 a, c, d
11 a, d
12 a, b, d
13 d
14 e
15 d
16 a
17 a, b, d
18 a, c
19 All are correct.
20 b, c, e
21 All are correct.
22 b, d, e
23 a, c
24 a, b, c
25 b, d, e
26 All are correct.
27 a, b, c
28 True
29 False; the host is capable of forming and liberating endogenous substances with a chemotactic effect.
30 True
31 True

32 True
33 True
34 False; it is called a macrophage.
35 True
36 True
37 True
38 True
39 False; they are formed by fusion of macrophages.
40 False; this is characteristic of chronic inflammation. Subacute inflammation involves only *early* repair.
41 False; it is caused by abnormal production or remodeling of collagen in the healing wound.
42 b
43 e
44 a
45 d
46 c
47 Abscess
48 Ulcer
49 Empyema
50 Sinus
51 Fistula
52 -itis
53 Margination
54 Emigration
55 Resolution
56 Repair
57 Lymphadenitis
58 a, b, e, d, c

ANSWERS

The response of the body to immunologic challenge—Chap. 5

1 The offending foreign material is neutralized, destroyed, or eliminated from the host more rapidly than would otherwise occur, i.e., in the absence of immunity.
2 Antigens are of relatively high molecular weight. Most antigens are proteins, but particularly polysaccharides, polypeptides, or nucleic acids of large sizes may also function antigenically. Antigens may be chemically pure proteins, or they may be incorporated in complex form as part of the structure of a bacterium, a virus, or a living tissue. In provoking an immunologic response, only certain active portions of the molecule (determinant groups) are essential to the specificity of the reaction. Certain molecules too small to behave as antigens by themselves are able to join chemically with larger molecules within the host creating molecules which may behave as an antigen.
3 (a) Humoral immunity, in which immunoglobulin antibodies are formed, or (b) cellular immunity, in which a population of specifically sensitized lymphocytes is

developed; the result in either case is enhanced elimination of the antigen.

4 (a) Self-recognition—these reactions will be mounted only against materials which are sensed as being foreign and will not ordinarily be mounted against constituents of the host's own body. (b) Memory—immunologic reactions proceed more rapidly with repeated introduction of the antigen. (c) Specificity—antibodies whose formation is elicited by a particular antigen react uniquely with that antigen.

5 Some stimulated lymphocytes are capable of secreting lymphokines. Other types of lymphocytes modulate their structure, acquire the cytoplasmic "machinery" of protein synthesis, and produce immunoglobulin antibody. Other lymphocytes undergo "blast formation," that is, they become dividing lymphoblasts, giving rise to expanding numbers of cells having the same properties.

6 When the antigen enters the body, phagocytosis of the antigen by macrophages occurs. The macrophages present the antigen to the B-lymphocytes, which have surface receptors to which the antigen binds. The stimulated B-lymphocytes differentiate into plasma cells and secrete an antibody which is specific for the original antigen. In the case of most antigens a population of T-lymphocytes function as helper cells, influencing B-lymphocyte activities. Thus, the induction of antibody response generally involves the collaboration of B-cells, T-cells, and macrophages.

7 False; they are filled with blood.

8 True

9 False; the spleen is a major locus of antibody production.

10 False; it is active not passive immunization that is described.

11 True

12 False; this is an antibody-mediated not a cell-mediated response.

13 True

14 c

15 a

16 e

17 c

18 d

19 a, c

20 d

21 c

22 c

23 d

24 b

25 b

26 d

27 d, e

28 c

29 a

30 a

31 b

32 a

33 a

34 a

35 a

36 b

ANSWERS

The response of the body to infectious agents—Chap. 6

1 Infection can be said to be present if some microbial agent has been able to adhere to the body surface, or to colonize and invade the tissues of the host, and then grow and multiply. The presence of infection, however, only indicates the relationship of the parasite to the host and does not necessarily indicate disease. Infectious disease is usually manifested by clinical illness. Infection may be totally asymptomatic.

2 *Skin* (especially if traumatized): Ordinarily the multilayered epithelium, dry keratin layer, and shedding of cells provide a mechanical barrier to infection. The chemical properties of sweat and sebaceous secretions have a mild bactericidal effect, and the normal flora provides a biological barrier.

Mouth, pharynx, gastrointestinal tract: The entire alimentary canal is lined with mucous membrane which, along with the protective layer of mucus, provides a mechanical barrier to invasion by microbes. The flow of saliva washes away many microbes mechanically. Rapid peristalsis in the stomach and especially in the small intestine provides another mechanical barrier. The high acidity of the stomach provides an excellent chemical barrier. Finally, the normal flora of the mouth, throat, and especially the large intestine provides a biological barrier to microbial proliferation and invasion. The gastrointestinal mucus contains antibody which provides immunologic defense.

Respiratory tract: A mechanical barrier is provided by a layer of mucus covering the surface and the constant action of the cilia which move the secretions toward the exterior of the body. Antibody is present in respiratory secretions, and motile macrophages in the alveoli engulf and destroy microbes.

Urinary tract: Defense is provided by the multilayered epithelium and the flushing action of urine flow.

Eyes: The flow of tears is a defense; antibody also is present in tears.

The general nature of the defenses of the body surfaces against microbial invasion are mechanical, chemical, biological (normal flora of each surface area), and immunological.

3 The microorganisms may spread locally along fascial planes or tubular structures such as a bronchus or ureter. The organisms may be passively carried by the fluid currents of the body. They may spread via lymphatics, ultimately to infect lymph nodes, or may be transferred to another location by a phagocyte if it does not kill the ingested organism. The next step is

systemic spread of the microorganisms via the circulating blood. Organisms may even enter blood vessels directly in the local area of initial invasion.

4 If an infectious agent is not contained locally by the inflammatory response or the regional lymph nodes, the microorganisms may enter the systemic blood (bacteremia) and possibly disseminate throughout the body. The phagocytic cells of the reticuloendothelial system, chiefly in the liver and spleen, cleanse the blood of the microorganisms.

5 An infectious disease in a debilitated host produced by an organism ordinarily harmless to a healthy individual with intact defenses.

6 (a) Antimicrobial therapy, which would suppress part of the normal flora and allow a normal resident organism to overgrow or might cause the treated person to become very susceptible to an exogenous invader. (b) Adrenocorticosteroids, which would be affecting inflammatory and immunologic mechanisms, might allow overgrowth of bacteria which would ordinarily be held in check. (c) Radiation therapy and cancer chemotherapy, which might depress the bone marrow and lymphoid tissue, possibly resulting in severe infection. (d) Immunosuppressive therapy (used to prevent rejection of a transplanted organ) causes a depression of immune defenses against microbes. (e) Unavoidable situations in hospitalized patients—anesthesia, shock, burns which lower many defenses. (f) Primary disease conditions—for example, virus infection of upper respiratory tract, which may be followed by bacterial pneumonia. (g) Environmental factors—overcrowding, famine, weather, etc.

7 Bacterial flora modifies the surface on which it grows and by competitive or direct inhibition prevents other potentially more pathogenic microorganisms from establishing residence.

8 Some pathogenic organisms may damage tissue by immunologic means, producing cellular hypersensitivity (tuberculosis), or may produce circulating antigen-antibody complexes (poststreptococcal glomerulonephritis). Others may produce exotoxins or endotoxins. Viruses act as intracellular parasites, altering cellular metabolism and synthetic activity.

9 d
10 c
11 b, d
12 c
13 b
14 a
15 d
16 b
17 a
18 c

ANSWERS

Disturbances of circulation—Chap. 7

1 In active congestion more blood than usual is actively flowing into the area. This increase in local blood flow is accomplished by dilatation of arterioles which be-

have as valves governing the flow into the local microcirculation. In passive congestion there is some impairment of drainage of blood from the area. Anything which compresses the venules and veins draining a tissue or otherwise hinders flow may produce passive congestion.

2 When the heart fails in its pumping action, impaired venous drainage results. For example, if the left side of the heart fails in its pumping action, the flow of blood returning to the heart from the lung will be impaired. The blood will be dammed back into the lung producing passive congestion of the pulmonary vasculature.

3 If the passive congestion is short-lived, there are no effects on the involved tissue. However, in chronic passive congestion there may be permanent effects on the tissue. This is due to the fact that in a passively congested area if the change in blood flow is severe enough, there is an element of tissue hypoxia which may lead to shrinkage or loss of cells of the involved tissue. Also, in many areas there is evidence of local breakdown of red blood cells which results in the deposition of certain pigments within the tissues. Fibrosis may also ensue.

4 Edema is an accumulation of excess fluid between the cells of the body or within the various body cavities.

5 c
6 c
7 a, d
8 c
9 a, c
10 a, b, c
11 c
12 a, c
13 b

14 The commonest cause of hemorrhage is loss of integrity of vascular walls, permitting the escape of blood. This is most often due to external trauma such as with injuries accompanied by bruising.

15 (a) Blood platelet system. With a small hole in the blood vessel, the blood platelets may aggregate over the hole and simply plug it up. (b) Blood clotting system. A fibrin clot is formed due to the activation of a series of clotting factors in the blood.

16 The local effects of hemorrhage are related to the presence of extravasated blood in the tissues and can range from trivial to lethal. The most trivial local effect is perhaps a bruise, which may be of only cosmetic importance, whereas a small volume of hemorrhage in a vital area of the brain can produce death. Systemic effects depend on two factors: (a) rate of loss and (b) volume of blood extravasated. If a rapid loss of blood occurs, the patient may actually die or may go into a state of hemorrhagic shock. With survival and the passage of time, the patient may develop blood-loss anemia.

17 (a) Thrombosis may result in obstruction of an artery

or vein, with possible ischemia or congestion, respectively. (b) It provides a source of possible emboli.

18 (a) Thrombus in an artery, (b) narrowing of an atherosclerotic artery, (c) embolus in an artery, (d) tumor pressing on a vessel.

19 (a) Functional disturbance (pain, such as angina), (b) atrophy of ischemic tissue, (c) infarction of ischemic tissue.

20 c
21 a
22 a
23 c
24 a, c
25 a, b
26 d
27 b
28 a
29 b
30 False; Monckeberg's sclerosis is not clinically significant; the lining of the involved vessel is not roughened nor is the lumen narrowed.
31 True
32 True
33 False; atherosclerosis is a multifactorial disease.
34 True
35 True
36 False; infarct is used to denote tissue necrosis *due to* a circulatory abnormality.

ANSWERS

Disturbances of growth, cellular proliferation, and differentiation—Chap. 8

1 c
2 d
3 h
4 e
5 a
6 g
7 b
8 b, c
9 b
10 a
.11 b
12 b
13 a, c
14 c
15 d
16 c
17 d
18 True
19 False; the current state of knowledge about the existence of immunologic defenses against the neoplasm does not permit the routine widespread use of immunotherapeutic measures.

20 False; this tumor is sometimes referred to as scirrhous.
21 True
22 False; this smear may be made of any of a variety of body fluids such as gastric aspirates or sputum specimens as well as uterine cervical scrapings.
23 Some causes of atrophy are ischemia, advancing age related to decreasing hormone production (e.g., breast tissue), and disuse (e.g., leg in a cast).
24 (a) The ability to invade normal tissue, (b) the ability to form metastases.
25 (a) Via lymphatic channels, (a) via direct "transplantation," as across serosal cavities (or, in fact, into incisions via surgical instruments), (c) via the bloodstream.
26 Neoplasms can produce a variety of local-mechanical symptoms by impinging upon normal structures, producing obstruction of passages, destroying vital functions, etc. They may ulcerate, may become secondarily infected, or may give rise to hemorrhages. Neoplasms may have endocrine function and produce signs and symptoms on that basis. Advanced malignancies may produce a state of cachexia.
27 The criteria used include the appearance of individual cells, their level of differentiation, their arrangement, and the presence or absence of certain cell products. Also included is the cell type of origin of the neoplasm and the organ of origin of the neoplasm.
28 This concept is not completely understood at the present time. It is thought that the behavior of cancer cells is "antisocial" with regard to normal cells of the body. Malignant cells disobey the usual territorial rules and grow in inappropriate locations. Evidence is beginning to accumulate which indicates that the important abnormalities of cancer cells seem to lie within the cell membrane. On the cell membrane homeostatic signals are received from other cells and from other points in the body and are transmitted to the interior of the cell. Abnormalities in this membrane may result in abnormal reception of control signals or abnormal responses to them. Evidence also indicates that events at the cell membrane are important in controlling cellular proliferation. The antigenic structure of cell membranes is important with regard to the immunologic interactions of the cell with its surroundings.
29 (a) A classical notion is that of somatic mutation which suggests that the basic cancerigenic event involves a chemical change in the DNA of a cell, that is a mutation. This type of mutation would involve a nongerm cell or somatic cell. This theory of mutation would explain the fact that once a cell is transformed into a neoplastic cell its characteristics breed true giving rise to an expanding clone of cells with similar properties, determined by the mutated DNA. (b) Another explanation for the expression of malignant behavior is the "addition" of genetic information to the cell by viral infection, with the "new" genetic information being expressed as abnormal cellular behavior. (c) Finally, there is some evidence that malignancy may

be a matter of abnormal differentiation, i.e., abnormal and inappropriate expression of genetic information always present in each cell of the body but usually kept repressed except, for instance, in embryonic life.

30 In most instances of human neoplasia the causes are as yet unknown. However, circumstantial and experimental evidence seems to indicate that the environment is the source of most tumorigenic agents. Many chemical substances within the environment are carcinogenic. This is evident from animal experimentation, from the incidence of certain tumors in industrial workers, and from the devastating incidence of lung cancer in cigarette smokers. The role of viruses of various types in tumorogenesis has been elucidated in many species of animals. Genetic factors do seem to be important in neoplasia. Generally there is not inheritance of an overall susceptibility to cancer of various kinds but of an inherited increased likelihood of developing one particular type of tumor or another.

31 The criteria used include the precise type and the extent of a neoplasm, the presence or absence of metastases, etc., as determined by combinations of radiologic, pathological, and endoscopic means.

ANSWERS

Familiar allergic disorders: anaphylaxis and the atopic diseases—Chap. 9

1 c
2 d
3 a, d
4 a, c
5 d
6 b
7 c
8 a, b, c
9 d
10 b, c, d
11 c
12 a, c, d
13 b
14 d
15 d
16 a
17 a
18 c
19 Evidence suggests that clinical anaphylaxis in both animal and humans involves a sudden multifocal reaction of allergen with mast cell–bound, specific IgE followed by widespread tissue response to the mediator substances (e.g., histamine, SRS-A) released; other factors appear to be of secondary importance.
20 This seems to reflect differences in both the distribution of mast cells and relative responsiveness of tissues to mediator substances.
21 This generally requires the injection of potent allergens, although certain gastrointestinal and respiratory parasites also elicit prominent IgE responses. Many

persons also make specific IgE responses to mucosal contact with innocuous materials including foods, pollens, and animal emanations (danders).

22 1 Efforts to reduce allergen (and irritant) exposure.
2 Suppressive medications to mitigate symptom severity nonspecifically.
3 Specific hyposensitization to reduce responsiveness to unavoidable allergen challenge.

23 True
24 True
25 False. Strongly positive reactions indicate only the immunologic "apparatus" for response and provide no assurance that symptoms arise from exposure to the allergens in question.
26 False. Aqueous extracts are used, and testing by pricking through the skin is *usually* done first; negative reactors are considered for intracutaneous (IC) tests. However, where IC tests are done exclusively, very dilute materials must be used.
27 True

ANSWERS

Bronchial asthma—allergic and otherwise—Chap. 10

1 A clinically defined condition marked by recurrent, discrete episodes of reversible bronchial narrowing, separated by periods in which ventilation approaches normal. Asthma is an abnormal pattern of response rather than a discrete disease.

2 These changes are confined to bronchial airways and include smooth muscle spasm, mucosal edema, and hypersecretion of viscid mucus. Mobilization of lumenal secretion is compromised by airway narrowing and by the shedding of ciliated bronchial epithelial cells.

3 Bronchial narrowing produces an increased resistance to airflow which underlies an inability to achieve normal rates of flow during respiration (especially expiration). This results in uneven lung aeration and a loss of the normal spatial matching of ventilation and pulmonary blood flow. These defects may produce no symptoms or merely a sense of tracheal irritation; alternatively, respiratory distress may be intolerable.

4 Although atopy is implicated in many instances of bronchial asthma, there are a substantial number of asthmatics who lack demonstrable allergic factors even after exhaustive study. These individuals are often said to have "intrinsic" asthma, although their problem is more properly idiopathic. In addition, many allergic (atopic) asthmatics also respond adversely to nonallergic factors.

5 Asthmatic airways behave as if their beta-adrenergic innervation were incompetent, and, at least function-

ally, partial "beta blockage" seems to exist. Without adequate bronchodilator tone, bronchoconstrictor influences, known to be mediated normally by parasympathetic (cholinergic) and alpha-adrenergic pathways, would tend to predominate. In clinical practice, the bronchial lability of asthmatics may be confirmed by demonstrating their brisk airway obstructive responses to extremely *low* concentrations of inhaled histamine and methacholine.

6 Since invading organisms frequently destroy ciliated epithelium and localize agents of inflammation in labile bronchi, their adverse effect on asthma is predictable. In addition, animal studies have suggested that microbial substances may further weaken beta-adrenergic activity.

7 The effectiveness of these agents is thought to reflect *direct* stimulation of an enzyme, adenyl cyclase, which promotes the synthesis of 3′,5′-cyclic AMP. Cyclic AMP–induced effects (i.e., relaxation of bronchial smooth muscle and inhibition of mediator release from mast cells and basophils) are, therefore, shared by beta-adrenergic agents with theophylline, and additive effects of these two groups of drugs often result.

8 When atopic factors are evident, efforts to reduce exposure and immunotherapy for selected inhalant allergens have established merit. Avoidance of irritants—especially tobacco smoke—as well as prompt treatment of unresolved bacterial respiratory infections are of major benefit to asthmatics. Perfumes, aerosol cleaners and cosmetics, solvents, and paint fumes also pose potentially avoidable risks that must be appreciated. Cold air is a bronchoconstrictor that may be mitigated by wearing a scarf or gauze mask over the nose and mouth. Adding moisture to dry indoor air is desirable. Programs of regular medication also can effectively reduce bronchial lability and thereby raise the threshold for obstructive airway responses.

9 b, d, e
10 b
11 e
12 b, d
13 c
14 b
15 e
16 a, b, c
17 b
18 a
19 a
20 False. EIA is most commonly evident in children and characteristically appears in subjects who are symptom-free before beginning exertion.
21 False. Other conditions may lead to diffuse wheezing simulating asthma such as the impaction of a foreign body or growth of a localized tumor in the bronchi, as well as pulmonary emphysema.

ANSWERS

Atopic dermatitis—urticaria—Chap. 11

1 a
2 b
3 a, b, d
4 a, d
5 b
6 c
7 a, b, c
8 a
9 b, d
10 a
11 c, d
12 b, d
13 False. These factors probably act by direct contact with an abraded epidermis but are implicated rarely.
14 True
15 False. These drugs should be employed for their anti-inflammatory properties.
16 True
17 False. Tars are rarely used today to reduce lichenification and cracking; urea-containing ointments are more cosmetically acceptable agents to promote healing and restoration of skin texture, and topical corticosteroids are quite helpful for this purpose.
18 False. Organic solvents that defat even normal skin must be avoided.
19 True
20 False. The resemblance of urticarial wheal to IgE-mediated skin reactions has promoted this false inference.
21 True
22 True
23 a Ingestants such as egg, fish, shellfish, and nuts including peanuts.
  b Drugs and drug metabolites capable of stable bonding to proteins (e.g., penicillins) or are themselves complete antigens.
  c Many drugs also appear to cause urticara by mechanisms exclusive of IgE (e.g., aspirin), though not typical anaphylaxis.
24 Since bouts of hives generally are self-limited and vary in duration as well as severity, the value of treatment measures for affected individuals often is difficult to discern. Epinephrine has demonstrated effectiveness in speeding this resolution. Agents such as diphenhydramine and hydroxyzine also are acknowledged to have value in this condition. Adrenal corticosteroids have been beneficial in severe acute hives. Hydroxyzine often is the single most valuable agent in *chronic* urticaria.

Autoimmune and immune complex-induced diseases—Chap. 12

1 The appearance of autoantibodies (antibodies reactive with autologous tissue components) denotes a failure of diverse safeguards which normally prevent their emergence. The responsible factors are rarely demonstrable. These autoantibodies have potential for causing tissue damage and are implicated in various illnesses. In addition, they may serve as diagnostic markers of conditions such as lupus erythematosus.

2 In certain instances the inciting antigens are normally sequestered and may remain "foreign" even to mature tissue. These responses could arise following subtle injury incident to microbial invasion. The possibility that infecting bacteria and viruses may produce limited changes in host tissue components rendering them "foreign" to immune surveillance has been proposed. Antibodies (or sensitized lymphocytes) resulting from this process might have specificities broad enough to permit reaction with native as well as modified tissue determinants. Autoimmune phenomena could arise if an invading organism and host tissues shared an antigen or closely similar antigenic groups as a result of parallel evolution. "Mutant" forbidden clones of immunocompetent cells could be involved, as well.

3 Circulating antibodies, reactive with glomerular and alveolar basement membranes, are usually present and, along with complement components, form linear deposits at these sites in vivo. The associated tissue damage is thought to reflect complement-mediated cytotoxicity and local effects of recruited neutrophils.

4 Chills, fever, and low-back pain occasionally preceded by urticaria or flushing, uneasiness, and mild air hunger. When cell lysis is massive, the resulting debris may trigger widespread intravascular clotting with depletion of coagulation factors and bleeding from wounds and venipuncture sites.

5 a Identifying the source and proper recipient of blood products.

b Continual surveillance of persons receiving blood—especially of those whose mobility or awareness is impaired.

c Any serious question of an incipient reaction should prompt discontinuance of the questioned unit, maintenance of intravenous access, and careful clinical observation.

d A carefully drawn venous sample from the recipient should be checked for serum hemoglobin and the compatibility of donor and recipient reconfirmed.

e *All* materials used for transfusion should be saved to facilitate serological and microbiological testing.

f Special precautions to monitor urine output are essential, and examination of serial centrifuged specimens for hemoglobin may be instructive.

g Maintenance of adequate hydration and urine flow are important considerations in all survivors, and osmotic diuresis with cautiously administered IV mannitol may help in achieving this goal.

h Safe fluid therapy demands precise and regular evaluation of cardiopulmonary and renal function. Measures to combat shock, pulmonary edema, acute renal failure, and/or defibrination (i.e., consumptive coagulopathy) may be required.

6 a Recipients of leukoagglutinins have developed fever, cough, shortness of breath, and lung shadows on chest x-ray; several days have been required for full resolution. Persons deficient in IgA also may suffer severe reactions from transfused IgA in plasma as a result of antibodies formed to this immunoglobulin. These episodes often resemble anaphylaxis with dyspnea, flushing, abdominal cramps and diarrhea, fever, and chills.

b The latter reactions may be averted by using IgA-deficient donors or thoroughly washed red blood cells.

7 False. Platelets and red blood cells are attacked predominantly.

8 True

9 a, d

10 c

11 a, c

12 c

13 c

14 b

15 c

16 a, c

17 e

18 b, c

19 b

20 d

ANSWERS

Adverse reactions to drugs and related substances—Chap. 13

1 a, c, d

2 a, c

3 c

4 a, b

5 b

6 c, d

7 a, b

8 False. Since this response is to be expected to injected antigens in most persons, it is not confined to the atopic population.

9 True

10 True

11 a, c

12 b, c, d

13 e

14 b, d

15 c

16 Initially, complexes of host IgG or IgM and drug (or drug protein conjugate) become attached to one or more blood cell types. Complement components are localized to the cell surface, and their interaction results in discrete membrane lesions, the formed elements being injured as "innocent bystanders" rather than direct participants. Following fixation of complement factors, the immune complexes often dissociate from affected membranes.

17 a Syncope, hypotension, cardiac rhythm disturbances, and, at times, convulsions.

b These reactions are probably a direct toxic effect of large doses required for local infiltration.

18 a An effective approach to the prevention of adverse drug reactions requires knowledge of the potential complications of medication and a willingness to consider adverse drug reactions as a possible cause of *any* unexpected clinical event.

b Since untoward responses usually are repetitive, no drug should be given without first assessing the individual's past experience with that agent. The clinical data base requires no less than a comprehensive assessment of past drug reactivity. Health care personnel must also be prepared to accept, on face value, reports of past problems arising from medication until these have been disproved conclusively.

c Close surveillance can reveal the earliest stigmata of drug reactions, facilitating prompt withdrawal of the offender and, often, abbreviating morbidity. Once recognized, adverse reactivity must be clearly indicated in the clinical record, and, if possible, the sensitivity identified for the patient or responsible family members. Documentation is aided if the patient carries a card, bracelet, or medallion indicating medication(s) to be avoided. Exhaustive instruction is necessary where a risk of reaction from related agents exists or when the offender has many readily available, poorly identified sources.

ANSWERS

Approaches to immune deficiency states—Chap. 14

1 d

2 c, d

3 c

4 a, b, c

5 True

6 False. Selective deficit of IgA.

7 True

8 False. T cell defects are generally more evident.

9 False. Relatively complete absence of T cell function occurs selectively when the thymus fails to develop.

10 True

11 a Determination of naturally occurring (IgM) antibodies to ABO blood group substances absent from the subject's red cells. Normal persons consistently demonstrate such "isohemagglutins" by the age of 1 year.

b Schick-testing of persons previously immunized with diphtheria toxoid. If adequate levels of (IgG) specific antibody have been produced, tissue breakdown at the site of toxin injection is prevented.

c Determination of antibody titers before and after nonviable immunizing materials such as tetanus toxoid and typhoid vaccine.

12 Intradermal injections are performed with 0.1-ml portions of substances that elicit DTH and to which a previous sensitizing exposure may be assumed; commonly used materials include: PPD (of the tubercle bacillus); streptokinase and streptodornase, enzymes of beta-hemolytic streptococci, etc. Test sites are observed and palpated after 48 hours, and an indurated area with a diameter of 10 mm or larger generally is regarded as a positive reaction. Using a battery of such materials, at least one positive test should be evident in the vast majority of normal individuals (excluding infants). For nonreactors, a more stringent test of cellular competence is provided by attempting contact sensitization with dinitrochlorobenzene (DNCB).

13 a Response of lymphocytes in short-term tissue culture to antigens and nonspecific agents that stimulate cell division and associated nucleic acid synthesis. An increase in the incorporation of thymidine tagged with tritium is observed normally in response to these agents.

b Peripheral aggregation of sheep red blood cells around human peripheral (T) lymphocytes when the two are mixed and incubated. Normally, over 60 percent of lymphocytes demonstrated rosetting, although a teleological basis for the sheep cell receptor is unknown.

c Assays of lymphokines produced in response to appropriate antigens added to lymphocyte preparations. To date, most studies have focused on the macrophage inhibiting factor (MIF), and defects at several stages prior to its release have been described.

ANSWERS

The composition of the blood and lymphoreticular system—Chap. 15

1 The study of blood, its nature, function, and disease.

2 a Red blood cells (RBCs) *b* White blood cells (WBCs) *c* Platelets

3 c

4 d

5 a

6 g

7 b

8 e
9 i
10 c
11 f
12 h
13 False. Men, 4.7–6.1
14 True
15 True
16 False. 4000–10,000
17 False. 200,000–400,000.
18 True

ANSWERS

The red blood cell—Chap. 16

1 *a* Oxygen is transported from the lungs to the tissues in the RBC in combination with the hemoglobin. (The hemoglobin, not the RBC, is what carries the oxygen.)
b Carbon dioxide is carried from the tissues to the lungs in the RBC, chiefly as sodium bicarbonate.
2 In many instances there is not a lack of blood. A more accurate definition is a reduction below normal of red blood cells, the concentration of hemoglobin, and the volume of packed cells per 100 ml blood.
3 *a* Pallor (skin, mucous membranes, skin folds, nail beds) *b* Shortness of breath *c* Headache, vertigo, faintness (snycope), easy fatigability
4 *a* Removal of RBCs from the circulation
hemorrhage—blood loss
—acute-peptic ulcer
—chronic-menstrual blood loss
hemolysis —hereditary—sickle cell
b Inadequate production of red blood cells.
Deficiencies of essential substances (B_{12} or folic acid) for RBC production
Deficiencies occurring primarily in the marrow resulting in deficient RBC production
5 *a* Determine the exact cause of the anemia. *b* If possible, correct the underlying cause. *c* Start specific treatment only if indicated.
6 Uncontrolled proliferation of red blood cells in the circulating blood which results in increased whole-blood viscosity and increased blood volume.
7 It may be classified as primary and secondary.
a Primary polycythemia: Polycythemia vera is due to a primary bone marrow defect in the regulation of the production of RBCs.
b Secondary polycythemia: Secondary to some underlying medical problem such as lung disease.
8 Compare your drawing with Fig. 16-1.
9 Normocytic, normochromic
10 a, c
11 b
12 c
13 a, d
14 True. This condition is usually not a hematologic disorder but a disturbance in the regulation of plasma volume. Through the loss of plasma, the concentra-

tion of red corpuscles increases above normal in the circulating blood.
15 True. It is the opposite of relative polycythemia which has a normal red blood cell mass.

ANSWERS

The white blood cell—Chap. 17

1 d, e
2 f
3 f, g
4 a, e
5 c
6 b
7 False. Plasma cells do not normally circulate and are found in small numbers in the bone marrow.
8 False. Viral infection is the most frequent cause of neutropenia; the amount of neutrophils is below normal.
9 True
10 Leukocytosis
11 Reed-Sternberg cells
12 Leukopenia
13 Neutrophils (neutrophilia), Eosinophils (eosinophilia), Basophils (basophilia)
14 a, b, d
15 d
16 a, b, c
17 b
18 b
19 a, b, c, d
20 A group of neoplastic diseases characterized by an uncontrollable proliferation of one of the types of white blood cells: granulocytes, lymphocytes, or monocytes.
21 *a* Type of cell involved in the malignant process.
b Clinical course of the patient depends on the maturity of the white blood cell.
22 b, d
23 a
24 e, f
25 c, b

ANSWERS

Coagulation—Chap. 18

1 False. Platelets function to maintain capillary integrity, initiate and retract clots.
2 True
3 True
4 a
5 c
6 Formation of the platelet plug, release of platelet factor III, clot retraction.

7 Factors V and X

8 It is thought that once the platelet level reaches a certain peak level, spontaneous aggregates of platelets occur. In the large vessels this has little effect, but the platelets do plug off the tiny capillaries. In the process, the capillary wall is damaged, and bleeding occurs into the tissues.

9 b, d

10 a

11 d

12 b

13 a

14 b, d

ANSWERS

The esophagus—Chap. 19

1 Transportation of ingested material from the pharynx to the stomach.

2 Lower esophageal closure strength has not developed fully in the infant. In adults, regurgitation reflects both lower esophageal sphincter incompetence and failure of the upper esophageal sphincter to serve as a regurgitation barrier.

3 Varicose veins of the esophagus (enlarged tortuous veins). Esophageal varices develop in cases of hepatic cirrhosis and portal hypertension because of the communication between the portal and esophageal veins providing a bypass of the liver to the vena cava. Esophageal varices may rupture, causing a fatal hemorrhage because they are unable to withstand the high-pressure flow.

4 An esophagomyotomy is an operation on the lower esophagus to enlarge the opening into the stomach. A pyloroplasty is an operation to repair the pylorus, especially to enlarge the gastric outlet. These procedures are often used to treat achalasia and are often combined because incompetence of the LES and reflux esophagitis may follow the myotomy. Enlarging the gastric outlet helps to prevent gastric reflux into the esophagus.

5 Avoid hot, cold, or spicy foods; eat bland foods
Eat slowly and chew food well before swallowing
Sleep with head of bed elevated
Take antacids
Avoid eating just before going to bed
Avoid tight clothes
Lose weight, if overweight
Avoid stooping, bending
Avoid straining to have a bowel movement (stool softeners may be necessary)
Eat in a quiet, relaxed environment
Avoid alcohol and tobacco

6 Check your drawing with Fig. 19-5.
The most important mechanism preventing reflux is the zone of high pressure between the esophagus and stomach (physiologic lower esophageal sphincter).

The acute gastroesophageal angle produces a flap-valve effect. The phrenoesophageal ligament produces a pinchcock valve effect.

7 Chronic reflux esophagitis causes esophageal inflammation, ulcer formation, bleeding, and eventually scarring and stricture.

8 Because these patients often aspirate esophageal or gastric contents into the lungs, especially during sleep.

9 The symptom of pyrosis, or heartburn, is poorly correlated with the presence or absence of esophagitis. Some patients with heartburn do not have evidence of esophagitis and some patients with esophagitis due to reflux may not have symptoms until the condition is advanced. The acid perfusion test is the best method of identifying esophagitis.

10 d

11 c

12 b

13 c

14 a

15 b

16 a

17 a, c

18 a

19 a

20 a

21 a, c, d

22 b

23 b

24 d

25 c

26 a, c

27 a

28 b

29 b, c

30 c

31 e

32 d

33 a

34 b

35 b

36 c, e

37 a, d

38 True

39 True

40 False

41 True

42 False

43 True

44 True

ANSWERS

Stomach and duodenum—Chap. 20

1 Refer to Fig. 20-1.

2 The outer layer of the stomach consists of peritoneum which is reflected off the lesser curvature as the lesser omentum and off the greater curvature as the greater omentum.

3 Mucosal folds which allow for expansion of the stomach.

4 Pepsinogen is converted to pepsin in the presence of a low pH. Pepsin digests proteins.

5 The extrinsic nerve supply of the stomach is entirely from the autonomic nervous system. Parasympathetic fibers travel via the vagus nerve and control gastric motor and secretory activity. Sympathetic fibers travel via the greater splanchnic nerves. Sympathetic stimulation inhibits gastric secretion and motility, which is opposite to the effect of vagal stimulation. Auerbach's and Meissner's nerve plexuses are involved in local reflexes and help to coordinate peristalsis. These plexuses comprise the intrinsic gastric innervation.

6 Celiac artery comes off the aorta; right and left gastric arteries and gastroepiploic supply most of the stomach.

7 Because posterior wall duodenal ulcers frequently erode into the gastroduodenal and pancreaticoduodenal arteries located just behind the duodenum.

8 Reservoir function, mixing function, and emptying function.

9 Approximately 1 to 2 liters; there is a receptive relaxation of the smooth muscle as food and liquids are ingested.

10 Intrinsic factor combines with vitamin B_{12} and is necessary for its absorption in the ileum. Vitamin B_{12} is necessary for the normal maturation of red blood cells.

11 There is a basic intrinsic rhythm to the peristaltic activity of the stomach which is modified by nervous and hormonal factors. Gastrin stimulates gastric motility as does parasympathetic stimulation, while sympathetic stimulation inhibits motility. Gastric emptying is also controlled by nervous and hormonal factors which are elicited by distention of the duodenum and the physical and chemical state of the chyme as it enters the duodenum.

12 The gastric mucus forms a protective coat for the gastric mucosa against mechanical and chemical injury (Hollander). The mucus in the columnar epithelial cells and the tight junctions between the epithelial cells prevent back diffusion of hydrogen ion (Davenport). Aspirin, alcohol, and bile salts are the most common substances causing disruption of the gastric mucosal barrier. The result is increased back diffusion of H^+, mucosal injury, and ulceration due to the action of gastric acid and pepsin.

The duodenum is protected by secretion of a highly alkaline, viscid mucus which neutralizes the acid chyme from the stomach. It is produced by Brunner's glands in the duodenum.

13 Increases closure strength of the lower esophageal sphincter, thus preventing gastric reflux into the esophagus during gastric mixing; increases pyloric sphincter tone, thus preventing gastric emptying until mixing is completed; stimulates the secretion of acid and pepsin in the stomach so that protein digestion may begin; promotes receptive relaxation of the stomach so that filling can occur without an increase in intragastric pressure; stimulates gastric and intestinal motility so that mixing and propulsion of chyme is promoted; stimulates secretion of insulin, bile, and pancreatic juice.

14 Superficial inflammation of the gastric mucosa. If you have ever had "food poisoning" or "intestinal flu" with nausea, vomiting, or diarrhea, you no doubt have had acute superficial gastritis.

15 Cephalic phase—sight, smell, or thought of food mediated through parasympathetic fibers of the vagus nerve which stimulates gastric acid secretion.

Gastric phase—antral distention is the prime stimulus to release of the hormone gastrin which stimulates gastric acid secretion.

Intestinal phase—of little importance in stimulating gastric acid secretion. Influence is mainly inhibitory.

16 d
17 a, b, c, d
18 a, c, d
19 a, b, e
20 b
21 a, c, d
22 c
23 a
24 c, d
25 c
26 d
27 a, c, d
28 c
29 a, c
30 d
31 b
32 a, b, d, e
33 e
34 a
35 c
36 b
37 a, d
38 a, b, e, f
39 False, pepsinogen
40 True
41 True
42 True

ANSWERS

Small intestine—Chap. 21

1 Cytotoxic drugs interfere with the metabolism of all rapidly proliferating cells (cancer and leukemic cells). Since hair cells and the epithelial cells of the gastrointestinal mucosa are the most rapidly proliferating cells in the body, they are especially vulnerable to the effects of these drugs. Cell division is inhibited, resulting in atrophy of both the villi and crypts of Lieberkuhn and sometimes there is ulceration and bleeding of the mucosa.

2 Bile salts act as detergents solubilizing fatty acids, glycerides, and fat-soluble vitamins by the formation of micelles. These substances are thus held in solution until absorption takes place.

3 Maldigestion means that digestion of a particular nu-

trient did not take place somewhere in the stepwise process of food breakdown into the most simple products which can be absorbed. Maldigestion could be caused from general lack of a secretion containing enzymes (pancreatic insufficiency) or lack of a specific enzyme (lactase insufficiency). Other causes of maldigestion are lack of mechanical breakdown of food particles, so that digestive enzymes cannot reach all of the food substances, or a transit time through the intestine which is too rapid to allow time for hydrolysis by enzymes. Of course, maldigestion always results in malabsorption, since nutrients cannot be absorbed until they have been hydrolized into the most simple substances.

Malabsorption refers to lack of transport of a substance across the intestinal mucosa.

4 The stool is pale, large in volume, greasy, frothy, and tends to float. It tends to stick to the side of the toilet and is difficult to flush away.

5 The lesion is granulomatous and similar to the lesion of tuberculosis except that cavitation does not occur. Since the tubercular lesion represents a hypersensitivity reaction (cellular immune mechanism), medical scientists have looked for an infectious agent and autoantibodies but have not been successful in identifying either.

6 Valvulae conniventes, villi, and microvilli

7 (1) Inadequate digestion due to rapid emptying of stomach and poor mixing

(2) Insufficient stimulation of CCK-PZ release (which stimulates pancreatic secretion) due to bypass of duodenum in Billroth II gastrectomy

(3) Deconjugation of bile salts by abnormal bacterial proliferation in blind loop after Billroth II

(4) Loss of reservoir function resulting in dumping of stomach contents into small bowel with rapid transit time

8 When the small bowel is obstructed either mechanically or functionally, it loses its absorptive and forward propulsive capacity so that gastrointestinal secretions pool within the lumen. The resulting ischemia of the intestinal wall from the distention further compromises the absorptive and motile function of the bowel so that a vicious cycle of degeneration develops. The pooling of fluids in the gut depletes the ECF volume, resulting in hypovolemic shock. Bacterial proliferation occurs in the pooled fluids, and increased permeability of the ischemic mucosa allows absorption of bacteria and its toxins into the circulation, causing septicemia and toxemia.

9 Superior mesenteric

10 Pyloric; ileocecal

11 Mesentery

12 Greater omentum; infection

13 Ligament of Treitz

14 Valvulae conniventes

15 Villi

16 Crypts of Lieberkuhn

17 Lacteal

18 umbilicus; iliac; appendix

19 d, f

20 c, g

21 a, h

22 b, e

23 b

24 d

25 c

26 b

27 c

28 d

29 a

30 c

31 b

32 d, e

33 f

34 g

35 c, h

36 a, f

37 b

38 d

39 g, e

40 b

41 c

42 a

43 c

44 d

45 b

46 a, b, d

47 b

48 c

49 c

50 d

51 a, b, c, d

52 c

53 a, b, c, d, e

54 c

55 c, d, e

56 a, b, d

57 a, b, c, d

58 True

59 False

60 True

61 True

62 True

ANSWERS

Large intestine—Chap. 22

1 Check your drawing with Fig. 22-1.

2 The absorption of water and elimination of the wastes of digestion.

3 Compared to the small intestine, the large intestine is more than twice as long. It has a diameter more than twice that of the small intestine. The external anal

sphincter is under voluntary control, while the sphincters at each end of the small intestine are under autonomic control. The large intestine has no villi, its longitudinal muscle layer is incomplete throughout most of its length, and the mucosa contains more goblet cells compared to the small intestine. These structural differences between the small and large intestine are in keeping with their primary functions. The villi, large volume of secretions, and very active motility pattern of the small intestine serve well its primary function of digestion and absorption. In contrast, the motility pattern of the large intestine is much slower, and although one of its main functions is absorption of water, it only absorbs about 1/13 the amount of the small intestine. The slower motility pattern allows more time for absorption since its ability to absorb is less as a result of a lack of villi. One of the functions of the large intestine is to act as a reservoir until elimination can take place. The increased number of goblet cells and increased mucus secretion is important, since the feces is semisolid in the large intestine and lubrication is more necessary for propulsion of the fecal mass.

4 Haustral churning are back and forth pendular movements, especially prominent in the transverse colon caused by annular contractions of short segments of the bowel, especially of the circular muscles. These movements allow time for the absorption of water. Mass peristalsis is a contraction involving a long segment of the large intestine which serves to propel a large amount of fecal material forward. Feces is frequently moved into the rectum by mass peristalsis and the defecation reflex is initiated.

5 Hemorrhoids, constipation, cancer of the rectum, anorectal abscesses, fissures, and fistulae

6 Palpation of the abdomen: presence of mass, tenderness

Rectal digital exam: palpation of tumors, hemorrhoids

Proctosigmoidoscopic exam: direct visualization of tumors, internal hemorrhoids, ulcerated or hyperemic mucosa; biopsy or cell washings may also be obtained for histologic study (lower 25 cm of bowel observed)

Colonoscopy: direct visualization of entire large bowel with same information obtained as above

Barium enema x-ray: neoplasms, strictures, diverticula, and polyps may all be visualized

Stool exam: blood, parasites, shape, size, etc. may give clues to many disorders of the GI tract

7 Only a very small percentage of the patients with diverticulitis require surgery. Surgery is indicated when there is severe and extensive disease or complications such as perforation. During an attack of acute diverticulitis, the medical treatment usually consists of bed rest, liquid diet, stool softeners, and antibiotics.

8 Ulcerative colitis of more than 10 years duration; certain types of colonic polyps; eating a diet low in fiber and high in refined carbohydrates

9 Burkitt proposed that slow transit with low-fiber diets permits bacterial action on bile acids or other normal bowel constituents to produce carcinogens, which then act on the colonic mucosa.

10 Since the superior hemorrhoidal vein is connected to the portal system, increased portal pressure may cause backflow into these veins and hemorrhoids.

11 A fissure in ano is a persistent crack in the perianal skin. A fistula in ano is an abnormal granulation-lined tract connecting two epithelial surfaces—in this region running between the anal canal and the skin of the perianal area. It is the consequence of anorectal abscess which has been inadequately treated. Any of these conditions may be a complication of hemorrhoids. Crohn's disease of the colon is especially likely to be associated with anorectal fistulae.

12 a
13 a
14 e
15 a
16 a, b, c, d
17 a, b, c
18 e
19 e
20 c
21 b
22 a, c, d, e
23 e
24 a
25 b, c, d
26 c
27 e
28 a, c, e
29 d
30 a, b, c, e
31 b
32 All of these
33 b, d, e
34 b
35 c
36 a
37 d
38 b
39 a, c, d
40 a, b, d, e
41 a, b, c
42 a
43 diverticulosis; diverticulitis
44 pedunculated; juvenile; villous; familial polyposis
45 annular; polypoid
46 direct extension to adjacent structure; lymph nodes; blood stream
47 Superior; middle; inside; inferior
48 Bleeding, thrombosis, strangulation
49 d
50 a
51 c
52 a

53 a
54 b
55 b
56 b
57 b
58 a
59 c
60 a
61 a-2; b-1; c-3
62 True
63 False; it is under voluntary control
64 False; only a few severe or complicated cases
65 False; vitamin K and some of B group
66 True
67 True
68 False; they are inside both sphincters
69 True
70 False; 35 percent
71 True
72 True
73 True
74 True

ANSWERS

Liver, biliary tract, and pancreas—Chap. 23

1 Blood circulation through the liver is unusual because a mixture of portal venous blood and arterial blood flows through the liver sinusoids. The portal blood contains many nutrients absorbed from the intestines which are metabolized in the liver.

2 The gallbladder is a pear-shaped hollow muscular bag having a capacity of about 45 ml. Its primary function is to concentrate hepatic bile which is transported to the gallbladder via the cystic duct. Bile is stored in the gallbladder and released as needed for digestion of fats in the intestine. Cholecystokinin–pancreozymin stimulates the gallbladder to contract and release bile.

The pancreas is about 6 in long and 1½ in wide and resembles a bunch of grapes. The main pancreatic duct runs through the entire length of the organ and opens into the duodenum. An accessory pancreatic duct (duct of Santorini) may also open into the duodenum at a different point. The pancreas has an exocrine secretion, pancreatic juice from the acini, and endocrine secretions, glucagon and insulin, produced by the alpha and beta cells in the islands of Langerhans. The release of pancreatic juice is controlled by CCK-PZ and secretin.

3 Formation and excretion of bile; carbohydrate metabolism including synthesis, storage, and release of glucose to maintain proper blood level; protein metabolism including synthesis of most proteins, urea formation, and storage of amino acids; fat metabolism including cholesterol synthesis and fat storage; storage of many vitamins and minerals; metabolism of steroid hormones; detoxification of both endogenous and exogenous substances potentially harmful; acts as flood chamber and filter.

The liver is called an organ of defense because of its large concentration of phagocytic Kupffer cells lining the sinusoids. These cells are actually part of the reticuloendothelial defense system.

The liver detoxifies drugs and other potentially harmful chemicals by oxidation, reduction, hydrolysis, or conjugation so that they become physiologically inactive. Conjugation with glucuronic acid, for example, makes the substance water-soluble so that it may be excreted in the urine.

The liver is capable of holding a liter or more of blood and holds a strategic position between the intestinal and general circulation. It can serve as a reservoir (flood chamber) when blood backs up as in right heart failure. Sudden release of the blood from this reservoir could cause circulatory overload and pulmonary congestion.

The liver is the central chemical laboratory for the metabolism of carbohydrates, fats and proteins, and this role alone makes the liver essential for life. It plays a major role in the regulation of blood glucose, serum lipids, serum proteins, and coagulation factors.

4 Excess production of bilirubin exceeding the processing ability of the liver; impaired uptake of unconjugated bilirubin; impaired conjugation; and impaired excretion of bilirubin.

5 Kernicterus is the deposition of bilirubin in lipid-rich brain, especially the basal ganglia, causing damage to the cells by its toxic action. Kernicterus occurs when there are high levels of unconjugated bilirubin (lipid-soluble) in the blood.

6 The jaundice is physiologic because the immaturity of the liver leads to relative deficiency of the glucuronyl transferase which conjugates free bilirubin with glucuronic acid. The accepter proteins may also be inadequate, so that uptake by the hepatocyte is also deficient.

7 No, it is only useful in helping to prevent hepatitis in exposed individuals, especially hepatitis A.

8 Community: Safe and inspected water supply and sewage disposal; inspection of all wells and septic tanks; restaurant inspection; inspection of public swimming pools and beaches for safety of water

   Home: Good general sanitary habits—handwashing, separate drinking glasses and eating utensils, adequate dish washing and sterilization

   Clinical unit: Use of disposable syringes, needles, catheters; screening of blood for hepatitis B antigen; careful disposal of urine and feces from infected individuals; handwashing; avoidance of needle puncture; isolation of infected individuals in a private room with separate bathroom facilities, disposable dishes, and gowns and gloves worn by those attending patient.

9 About 90 percent removal or destruction of the liver is compatible with life. Complete removal results in death in about 10 hours.

10 Triangular, 1500, right upper, kidney, gallbladder, stomach, pancreas; falciform; Glisson

11 Bile, hepatic; hepatic; cystic, bile; pancreatic, Oddi

12 Hepatic, portal, hepatic, vena cava; portal, hepatic; spleen, esophageal, rectal

13 Lobule, sinusoids, Kupffer; canaliculi

14 b

15 d

16 a, b, c, d

17 d (bile is catabolized in the intestine)

18 a, b, c, d, e

19 c

20 c

21 c

22 a

23 c

24 c

25 d

26 a

27 a, b, d

28 d

29 b

30 d

31 d

32 a

33 d

34 a, c, d, e

35 c, b, a, b, a, b, d, b, a, b, a

36 d, b, c, i, a, g, e, f, h

37 Alcoholic hepatitis is a lesion characterized by hepatocellular necrosis and infiltration with inflammatory cells. It is associated with alcohol ingestion and is believed to be the critical lesion in the development of Laennec's cirrhosis.

38 Because cirrhosis is generally silent until far advanced when major signs and symptoms appear. Early symptoms are vague and nonspecific so that patients do not seek medical help.

39 Portal hypertension is a sustained elevation of the portal venous pressure above the normal 6 to 12 cm water. The primary mechanism causing portal hypertension is increased resistance to blood flow through the liver. This could occur in cirrhosis, congestive heart failure (backup of blood from right atrium), and from hepatic vein thrombosis. Increased inflow through the splanchnic arteries in cirrhosis also contributes to portal hypertension.

40 Compression of varices by esophageal and gastric balloons (Sengstaken-Blakemore tube); vasopressin infusion. It is important to remove the blood from the gastrointestinal tract because large amounts of ammonia may be produced from the action of gut bacteria on the blood protein. The ammonia may reach the systemic circulation, causing hepatic encephalopathy by interfering with cerebral metabolism. Recurrent bleeding from esophageal varices may be prevented by reducing the pressure and blood flow through the varices by creating a surgical shunt between the portal and systemic circulation. Flow through the esophageal veins is reduced, but ammonia and other protein metabolites may pass directly into the systemic circulation, causing hepatic encephalopathy.

41 Hepatic encephalopathy is a form of cerebral intoxication caused by ammonia and/or other protein metabolites. It is manifested clinically by a neuropsychiatric syndrome characterized by mental clouding and neuromuscular dysfunction progressing to coma.

It occurs when more ammonia is presented to the liver than the failing cells can synthesize into urea or when the ammonia bypasses the liver through shunts and enters the systemic circulation.

It is important to detect hepatic encephalopathy during the early stages because prompt treatment may be successful in reversing the process. The mortality is very high if it progresses to an advanced stage.

42 Asterixis is a peripheral manifestation of impaired cerebral metabolism characterized by a peculiar flapping tremor of the wrists and metacarpophylangeal joints. It is tested by having the patient extend both arms out with fingers spread.

43 Constructional apraxia is the inability to construct simple diagrams or to write legibly in the absence of paralysis or motor weakness. Deterioration in the ability to perform purposeful, skilled constructions or to write reflects the progress of the encephalopathy and a serial record can be kept in the patient's records.

44 Stage I   Slowness of mentation and affect, untidiness, slurred speech, personality change, inappropriate behavior, disordered sleep rhythm

Stage II   Accentuation of Stage I, inappropriate behavior, lethargy, asterixis, muscle tremor

Stage III   Sleeps most of time but can be aroused, marked confusion, may be abusive and violent, abnormal EEG pattern

Stage IV   Comatose, positive Babinski, hyperactive reflexes, abnormal EEG, hepatic fetor sometimes detected

45 In acute cholecystitis the patient has a sudden onset of severe pain in the right upper quadrant which may last for several hours. It is often associated with the passage of a gallstone through the cystic or common bile duct. There may be tenderness over the gallbladder. Chronic cholecystitis is characterized by symptoms which are much milder. There may be episodes of mild pain in the right upper quadrant and a long history of dyspepsia, flatulence, heartburn, and fat intolerance.

46 Because the liver acts as a filter with about one-third of the cardiac output traversing it each minute. Malignant cells transported from the intestines, stomach or pancreas through the portal vein are readily trapped in the liver capillary bed.

47 a, b, c, d

48 c

49 d
50 a
51 d
52 a, c, d
53 a, c
54 b
55 a, b, d
56 c
57 d
58 e
59 d
60 c
61 b
62 c, d
63 d
64 b
65 c
66 a, b, c, d, e
67 a
68 d
69 a, b, d
70 a, b, c
71 False; it is within the peritoneal cavity
72 True
73 True
74 False; more common in females; history of alcoholism more common in males
75 True
76 True
77 False; pure bilirubin stones
78 False; a pseudocyst forms outside the pancreas, often within lesser omental sac
79 False; they are uncommon in the United States and are usually diagnosed late when they are beyond hope; early symptoms are insidious
80 True
81 True
82 True
83 False; it is a cholecystectomy
84 f, c, a, b, e, d

ANSWERS

Anatomy of the cardiovascular system—Chap. 24

1 Venae cavae → right atrium → pulmonary artery → lung capillaries → pulmonary veins → left atrium → left ventricle → aorta → systemic arteries → arterioles → capillaries → venules → systemic veins.

2 The AV node delays the wave of electrical excitation to allow time for ventricular filling during atrial contraction prior to ventricular contraction. It also prevents an excessive number of electrical impulses from reaching the ventricles.

3 The thickness of the right ventricle is only one-third that of the left ventricle. These differences in muscular size reflect their respective pumping functions in the circulatory system. The right ventricle pumps blood through the low pressure, low resistance pulmonary circuit. The work load of the left ventricle is much greater than that of the right, since it must generate pressure about five times as high in order to overcome the high resistance of the systemic circulation.

4 To support the atrioventricular valves during ventricular contraction and prevent leaflet eversion into the atria.

5 Three; aortic valve; sinuses of Valsalva; to protect the coronary orifices from occlusion by the aortic valve cusps during ventricular ejection.

6 The visceral and parietal pericardium. This small space contains a small amount of lubricating fluid which functions as protection against friction.

7 Lymph is propelled by muscle compression of the lymph vessels. Flow is aided by lymphatic peristalsis.

8 Sympathetic stimulation of the alpha receptors causes vasoconstriction while stimulation of beta receptors causes vasodilation.

9 d
10 c
11 c
12 b
13 b
14 c
15 d
16 c
17 d
18 b
19 a, b, c
20 a, c, d
21 e
22 c, d
23 a, b
24 c, e, f, a, d, b
25 c
26 a
27 e
28 d
29 b
30 f
31 Automaticity; excitability; conductivity; rhythmicity
32 Valves
33 Collateral
34 Right coronary; left anterior descending
35 60 to 100; 40 to 60; 20 to 30

ANSWERS

Physiology of the cardiovascular system—Chap. 25

1 Systole and diastole represents the *mechanical activity* of the heart. Systole is the period when the heart muscle contracts. Diastole indicates the resting period of

the heart when the muscles relax. The terms systole and diastole are commonly used in referring to ventricular activity. The ECG represents a body surface recording of the summated *electrical* activity of *all* the myocardial cells. An action potential is an intracellular recording of the electrical activity of a *single* cell. Electrical activity stimulates mechanical activity.

2 Starling's law states that the force of contraction is a function of the length of the muscle fiber. However, the ventricular function curve shows that stroke volume can only increase up to a point (cardiac reserve) and then stroke volume decreases (cardiac failure) when end-diastolic volume increases.

3 Poiseuille's law stated in terms of the circulation says that the volume of blood circulated per minute is directly related to the systemic blood pressure gradient and inversely related to the resistance ($F = \Delta P/R$). The systemic blood pressure gradient is calculated by subtracting pressures at the arterial and venous end of the circulation (i.e., mean arterial pressure − central venous pressure).

4 SV = EDV − ESV = 100 ml − 30 ml = 70 ml (This is in the normal range). CI = CO/body surface area = 4.5 liters/min · 1.5 m²) = 3.0 (this is also in the normal range). EF = SV/EDV = 70/100 = 0.70 (the ejection fraction should be 2/3 or 0.67, so it is normal).

5 a
6 c
7 a, b, c, d
8 c
9 a, c
10 a
11 a
12 a, b, c
13 a, c
14 b
15 b
16 b
17 a
18 All of these
19 d
20 c
21 a
22 e
23 b
24 f
25 a, h, d, f, g, c, i, b, e
26 Absolute refractory; relative refractory
27 Negatively; potassium; sodium
28 Open; closed
29 Closed; open
30 AV node

ANSWERS

Diagnostic procedures—Chap. 26

1 Class III
2 The left carotid may be partially occluded possibly because of an atherosclerotic plaque. Her mean arterial pressure is about 126 mmHg. MAP = diastolic BP + pulse pressure/3 = 100 + 78/3 = 126

3 The hepatojugular test is performed by manually applying pressure over the right upper quadrant of the abdomen for 30 to 60 seconds and simultaneously observing the jugular veins. A rise in the level of the venous pressure head in the neck veins indicates a positive test. A positive test signifies that the right heart was not able to accept the increased venous return (main source from venous reservoir in the liver which is being compressed) which could result from right ventricular failure.

4 The hexaxial reference system is a representation of all the limb leads of the electrocardiogram. It is formed by moving the bipolar limb leads centrally so that these lines intersect. The position of the heart may be pictured at the center of this electrical reference system. When the unipolar limb leads are added to the reference system, the hexaxial reference system is produced. Using this reference system, the summation vector or electrical axis for the P, QRS, and T waves can be derived. An analysis of deviations of the electrical axis from the various leads assists in diagnosing conditions such as conduction abnormalities and chamber enlargement.

5 Pressures in the various cardiac chambers and great vessels may be recorded and the waveforms of the pressure tracings analyzed to detect valvular stenosis and regurgitation. The injection of radiopaque material into the various cardiac chambers allows visualization of chamber size and visualization of wall movement so that deviations from normal may be detected. Cardiac output may also be detected. Sampling of oxygen content in the right and left sides of the heart allows detection of right-to-left shunts such as from a ruptured septum. Selective coronary artery angiography allows detection of lesions in these vessels.

6 Indications for coronary arteriography: (1) to determine the feasibility of coronary bypass surgery; (2) to evaluate atypical angina; (3) to evaluate the results of coronary revascularization surgery. Characteristics of a bypassable coronary artery lesion: the lesion must be located proximally, reveal greater than 75 percent obstruction of the lumen and there must be a patent artery distal to the lesion which can be anastomosed to the bypass graft.

7 d
8 c
9 a, c
10 b
11 d
12 d
13 a
14 b
15 d
16 All of these

17 d
18 a
19 b, c
20 c
21 c
22 c
23 c
24 b
25 b
26 a
27 b
28 d
29 b
30 c
31 a
32 d
33 a
34 c
35 d
36 c
37 b
38 c
39 c
40 d
41 b
42 f
43 a
44 e
45 c
46 b
47 a
48 a
49 d
50 c
51 c
52 c
53 d
54 b
55 a
56 b
57 c
58 a
59 b
60 c
61 a
62 b
63 d
64 e
65 b
66 c
67 a
68 f
69 f
70 a
71 b
72 e

73 c
74 g
75 h
76 d
77 False; it is on top of the foot.
78 True
79 True
80 False; the CVP increases during inspiration
81 True
82 False; it is normal
83 True
84 False; they are caused by turbulent blood flow through the partially occluded artery during the recording of blood pressure in an extremity.
85 True
86 Regurgitation
87 5; aortic stenosis
88 Turbulent

ANSWERS

Coronary atherosclerotic disease—Chap. 27

1 Oxygen demand is greater for the left ventricle than for the right because of its greater work load and larger muscle mass. Oxygen supply is more restricted because very little coronary perfusion of the left ventricle occurs during systole. The firm compression of blood vessels by the thick muscular wall limits perfusion during systole. On the other hand, the thinner-walled right ventricle continues to have some perfusion during systole.

2 Atherosclerotic lesions tend to occur in the epicardial proximal segments of the right and left coronary arteries and at points of abrupt curvature such as where the left coronary artery branches into the left anterior descending.

3 Size and location of the infarct; function of the uninvolved myocardium; collateral circulation; cardiovascular compensatory mechanisms.

4 It is a reflex parasympathetic response resulting from pain or stimulation of parasympathetic ganglia in the myocardium. The effect is to slow the heart rate and reduce the blood pressure and cardiac output. Thus the response has an adverse effect in myocardial infarction since sympathetic support of the compromised circulation is needed.

5 Severe, prolonged chest pain; elevated serum cardiac enzymes; ECG changes in leads overlying the area of necrosis (deep Q waves, S-T segment elevation, and inverted T waves).

6 Since cardiac output is a function of heart rate and stroke volume, a slow heart rate can reduce the total volume ejected in a given time by lowering the frequency of ejection. On the other hand, a rapid rate reduces ventricular filling time so that less blood is ejected per beat. Tachycardia also reduces the length of diastole so that perfusion time of the myocardium is limited. Thus oxygen supply is reduced at the same time that demand is increased because of the increased cardiac work.

7 Heart rate, force of contraction, and arterial pressure (a determinant of wall tension).

8 Because the diseased coronary blood vessels have a limited ability to dilate and thus increase perfusion and oxygen delivery to the myocardium. Total coronary perfusion is not increased by nitroglycerin, although there is some improvement of flow to ischemic areas by dilation of collaterals.

9 To allow healing of the infarcted tissue, decrease the incidence of complications, and to salvage the ischemic zone surrounding the infarct.

10 In congestive heart failure, digitalis, diuretics, and restriction of fluid and salt intake are utilized to improve cardiac function and prevent the development of pulmonary edema.

The first priority in the treatment of severe pulmonary edema is to reduce the increased intravascular volume and pressure in the pulmonary vessels and thus reduce transudation of fluid. This may be achieved quickly by the use of rotating tourniquets, phlebotomy, and by elevating the trunk with the legs dependent. Additional treatment includes the use of morphine which causes peripheral dilatation and helps to pool blood in the extremities. Aminophylline relieves bronchospasm and increases the contractility of the heart. Oxygen therapy helps to correct the hypoxemia and positive pressure breathing may reduce transudation by opposing the increased pulmonary hydrostatic pressure.

Cardiogenic shock is treated utilizing vasopressor drugs (and sometimes vasodilators) and sometimes circulatory assistance devices to reduce the cardiac workload. Sodium bicarbonate is utilized to correct acidosis.

11 The intra-aortic balloon is a device placed in the descending thoracic aorta. Inflation of the balloon during systole improves coronary perfusion and systemic perfusion. Balloon deflation during systole increases cardiac output and decreases cardiac work and oxygen demand. An external counterpulsation device assists circulation by the application of positive pressure to the lower extremities during diastole and negative pressure during systole, effecting similar physiologic changes. Left heart assist devices reduce the work of the left ventricle by shunting blood from the left atrium to the systemic circulation.

12 The patient needs individualized guidance and teaching to achieve maximum functional ability. Both psychological and physical variables are involved.

13 b
14 b
15 c
16 All of these
17 c
18 b
19 b
20 b
21 a
22 a
23 b
24 c

25 d
26 c
27 All of these
28 a, b, d, e
29 c
30 c
31 b
32 d
33 e
34 All of these
35 d
36 c
37 d
38 a, d, e
39 d
40 All of these
41 b
42 c
43 a
44 b
45 a, c
46 d
47 a
48 b
49 True
50 True
51 False; this is a complication of saphenous vein bypass graft.
52 False; it increases muscle mass and oxygen demand.
53 False; they are a protective response to sinus node failure.
54 Ischemia
55 Increases
56 b, d, a, c
57 a
58 b
59 b
60 a
61 b
62 a
63 a
64 a
65 b
66 b
67 c
68 d
69 a
70 d
71 a
72 c
73 b
74 c
75 a
76 b
77 e
78 d

ANSWERS

Valvular heart disease—Chap. 28

1 Recurrent attacks of rheumatic fever—most common cause

Subacute bacterial endocarditis—most infections occur in patients with rheumatic or congenital heart deformities

Papillary muscle dysfunction or rupture—may be a complication of myocardial infarction

Congenital malformations

Inborn defects of connective tissue

2 It is regurgitation secondary to chamber enlargement. As a result of ventricular chamber enlargement the papillary muscles and chordae tendenae are unable to anchor the valve leaflets securely. The valvular annulus may also enlarge.

3 Prophylactic antibiotics are necessary in order to reduce the risk of bacterial endocarditis in susceptible patients. These patients include those with a history of rheumatic carditis or those with cardiac deformities. Even minor procedures such as dental work and catheterization may cause a transient bacteremia and the implantation of organisms on the endocardial surface.

4 Pulmonary congestion—diuretics to decrease blood volume; digitalis to increase heart contractility

Atrial fibrillation—antiarrhythmic drugs

Systemic emboli—anticoagulant drugs

5 Splitting of fused valvular commissures by the surgical introduction of an instrument to dilate them by blunt pressure

6 It is a device consisting of an oxygenator, pump, and viaducts which performs the basic functions of the heart and lungs as the circulation to these organs is bypassed during open heart surgery.

7 a

8 c, b, d, a

9 a

10 c

11 d

12 b

13 c

14 c

15 b

·16 b

17 b

18 c

19 All of these

20 b

21 c

22 d

23 c

24 a

25 b

26 c

27 e

28 c

29 a

30 All of these

31 c

32 b

33 b

34 c or *d*

35 c

36 c

37 b, d

38 c

39 c

40 a, c

41 c

42 a, b, d

43 a, c, e

44 b, d, f

45 Venae cavae; oxygenator; aortic arch or femoral artery

ANSWERS

Peripheral vascular disease—Chap. 29

1 Atherosclerosis; thromboangiitis obliterans

2 The site of the lesion; severity of the lesion; metabolic demand of the tissue beyond the lesion; the extent of collateral circulation. For example, occlusion by a large atherosclerotic plaque of the main renal artery (an end artery) would have more serious consequences than occlusion of the radial artery since the ulnar artery may provide adequate perfusion to the hand.

3 Atherosclerotic plaques commonly form at points of arterial branching and abrupt curvature—bifurcation of the abdominal aorta, common iliac, or common femoral, popliteal. Other sites include the renal, superior mesenteric, celiac, subclavian and other aortic arterial branches. Plaque formation is more common in the lower extremities.

4 Varicose veins are dilated, tortuous veins generally seen in the lower extremities. Pathogenetic factors include inflammatory destruction of valves, weak vein walls, and increased venous pressure (as in pregnancy) all causing varying degrees of valvular incompetence and regurgitation. The two major complications of varicosities are thrombosis and venous ulcer. Both of these complications are a result of venous stasis. A varicosity differs from an aneurysm in that the vessel is affected throughout a significant segment of its length whereas an aneurysm generally involves a short segment of a blood vessel.

5 Deep venous thrombosis, because it may be asymptomatic or difficult to detect and more often leads to pulmonary embolism.

Superficial veins may dilate to compensate for deep venous thrombosis providing a route for venous return to the heart. There are many communicating veins between the deep and superficial veins.

6 Early ambulation following surgery; avoid prolonged bed rest; leg exercises in patients confined to bed; elastic hose; avoiding prolonged sitting, garters, crossing knees. In some high-risk patients, anticoagulants may be indicated to prevent recurrent thrombosis.

7 An aneurysm is a dilated area of artery which may be saccular or fusiform in shape. Aneurysms form due to weakening of the elastic layer of the artery walls by atherosclerosis, infection such as syphilis, or occasionally trauma. The dangers of an aneurysm are progressive enlargement, rupture, or thrombosis and embolism. A dissecting aneurysm occurs when blood penetrates between the media and intima so that an increasing area of intima is dissected off the arterial wall. This forms a sac which blocks the arterial lumen causing severe pain and inadequate circulation below the dissection and often results in sudden death.

8 The color change results from the extrasavation of red cells from the capillaries to the extravascular space. Breakdown of the red cells causes release of hemoglobin and deposition of hemosiderin with consequent pigmentation of the skin in the region of the ankle and lower leg.

9 Atherosclerotic plaque, aneurysm, myocardial infarction, atrial fibrillation, mitral stenosis.

10 e

11 a

12 b

13 c

14 d

15 d

16 c

17 b, c

18 d

19 b, c, d (generally the temperature is not elevated to this extent)

20 a, d, e

21 b, c, d

22 b

23 b

24 b

25 c

26 a

27 d

28 d

29 b

30 c

31 a

32 Thrombophlebitis; phlebothrombosis

33 Thromboangiitis obliterans

34 False; it increases oxygen demand and the ischemic tissue may easily be burned

35 True

36 False; it is called an embolectomy

37 False; they should be slightly dependent

38 True

ANSWERS

Normal respiratory function—Chap. 30

1 Infections, malignancies, and chronic bronchitis and emphysema

2 Respiration is the combined activity of the various

mechanisms which supply oxygen to the body cells and remove carbon dioxide.

3 See inset of Fig. 30-1 if you have forgotten the structure of the mucosal lining of the airways.

The blanket of mucus serves to trap dust and bacteria which is then moved by ciliary action to the pharynx where it is swallowed or expectorated. Inspired air is also humidified and warmed by the mucus blanket and underlying vascular network.

4 The right mainstem bronchus is larger and runs a more vertical course from the trachea than the left.

5 The lung would collapse (atelectasis).

6 Review Fig. 30-4 if you have forgotten the functional position of the lungs in the circulation. Did you remember to include the bronchial circulation?

The lung has a dual blood supply—the bronchial and pulmonary circulation. The pulmonary circulation is a low-pressure, low-resistance system (the mean pulmonary artery pressure at 15 mmHg is only about one-sixth of that of the systemic circulation at about 90 mmHg).

7 Yes, there is a net pressure of 10 mmHg in the direction of the alveolus.

8 larnyx or glottis

9 surfactant; surface tension

10 ventilation; respiratory bellows; diaphragm; external intercostal

11 Hering-Breuer

12 pons and medulla

13 c

14 c

15 c

16 e

17 a

18 b

19 e

20 d

21 c

22 c

23 a-6, b-3, c-1, d-5, e-7, f-8, g-9, h-4, i-10, j-2, k-12, l-11

24 a-4, b-5, c-2, d-1, e-7, f-6, g-3

25 Because of dilution with water vapor and other gases in the anatomic dead space

26 The volume of anatomic dead space is equal to 1 ml/lb of body weight; if you weigh 120 lb, your anatomic dead space is about 120 ml.

27 Diffusion; the driving force is the pressure gradient between the partial pressure of the gas in the alveolus and in the pulmonary capillary.

28 No; perfusion increases going from the apex to the base of the lungs due to the effect of gravity in the low-pressure, low-resistance pulmonary circulation. The overall ventilation/perfusion ratio is 0.8, which is less than unity.

29 $\dot{V}/\dot{Q} = 3$ liters/minute $\div$ 6 liters/minute $= 0.5$. This value would represent wasted perfusion and would be present in a shunt-producing disease.

30 More oxygen could be transported to the tissues in

physical solution, which might make the critical difference in cases where there is very little hemoglobin available to transport oxygen to the tissue cells.

31 No; increasing the concentration of oxygen in the inspired air will be wasted because the blood is already 97 to 98 percent saturated when it leaves the lungs, and the oxygen content is normal. An examination of the oxyhemoglobin dissociation curve (flat upper portion) shows that very little if any advantage could be gained.

32 The S shape of the oxyhemoglobin dissociation curve indicates that under normal environmental conditions large changes of the PO_2 of the inspired air causes only small changes in oxyhemoglobin saturation. Even at a PO_2 of 50 mmHg in the alveoli, hemoglobin is 80 to 85 percent saturated with oxygen which is sufficient to meet tissue demands for oxygen under most conditions.

33 The Bohr effect is the slight shift to the right of the oxyhemoglobin dissociation curve caused by the increase in acidity due to the effect of carbon dioxide being released from the tissues. The rightward shift in the curve causes oxygen to be more easily released from its association with hemoglobin and thus facilitates tissue uptake of oxygen.

34 Although alveolar oxygen tension may be increased slightly by hyperventilation, this does not significantly increase the oxygen content of the arterial blood because of the sigmoid shape of the oxygen dissociation curve and because blood leaving normally ventilated alveoli is already almost fully saturated with oxygen. The carbon dioxide dissociation curve, however, is linear in shape indicating that the CO_2 content of the blood is directly related to the alveolar PCO_2. When CO_2 is "washed out" of the lungs during hyperventilation, the carbon dioxide content of the blood is likewise reduced.

35 If diffusion were impaired enough to affect CO_2 transport, the patient would be dead. Carbon dioxide diffuses more readily than oxygen at the same pressure gradient. Even a minute pressure gradient (less than 1 mmHg) is enough to ensure elimination of all the CO_2 produced at rest.

36 No; knowledge of the blood gases does not give information about how well the tissues are being perfused, how much oxygen is being delivered to the tissues, and the PO_2 in the tissue cells. One must have data on hemoglobin concentration and adequacy of cardiac function and make other clinical observations to assess whether respiratory function is adequate. All data must be correlated and the final judgment is a clinical one.

37 All of the following are examples of altered mechanisms or conditions which may interfere with normal respiration.

(1) low PO_2 of inspired air—high altitudes

(2) depression of respiratory center—barbiturate overdose

(3) alveolar hypoventilation due to inadequate bellows function—obesity, deformed chest cage, weak respiratory muscles

(4) impaired diffusion of gases at the alveolar-capillary membrane—pulmonary edema or fibrosis

(5) ventilation/perfusion imbalance—pneumonia or pulmonary embolism

(6) impaired transport of blood gases by systemic circulation—anemia, carbon monoxide poisoning, inadequate cardiac output or shunting by tissues as in shock

(7) impairment of gas diffusion at tissue level—edema

38 Stage 1 is ventilation—flow of air into and out of the lungs effected by the respiratory bellows.

Stage 2 is transportation—includes the diffusion of gases between the alveolus and the pulmonary blood and between the tissue cells and the systemic blood. Transportation also includes the distribution of the pulmonary and systemic blood and the distribution of air in the lungs.

Stage 3 is cell respiration—oxidation of cell metabolites with the production of energy, water, and carbon dioxide.

39 The diaphragm and external intercostals are used in quiet inspiration. The scalene and sternocleidomastoid muscles are additional accessory muscles of respiration which are involved in maximum inspiration.

40 201 ml/minute = (12 gm/100 ml × 1.34 ml/gm × 5000 ml/minute × 0.25)

41 Mixed venous blood containing reduced hemoglobin from the bronchial circulation is mixed with oxygenated pulmonary blood leaving the lungs thus accounting for the slight reduction in hemoglobin saturation.

42 Decreases; increases (alkalosis); shifts to the left so that hemoblobin is reluctant to release oxygen to the tissues

43 42 mmHg = [(247 − 47) × 0.21]; no, a PO_2 of 42 would barely be able to supply tissue oxygen requirements at rest. The climber might be expected to pass out unless he uses cylinder oxygen supply.

44 a

45 a, b, c

46 b

47 increase, decrease, less, into

48 ascends, decreasing

49 increase, more, out of

50 normal, low, low

51 decrease, increase, alkalosis

ANSWERS

Diagnostic procedures in respiratory disease—Chap. 31

1 Routine chest film, fluoroscopy, bronchography, angiography, and lung scans.

2 (a) Status of the thoracic cage including the ribs,

pleura, the contour of the diaphragm and of the upper airway as it centers the chest

(b) The size, contour, and position of the mediastinum and hilus of the lung including the heart, aorta, lymph nodes, and root of the bronchial tree

(c) The texture and degree of aeration of the lung parenchyma

(d) The size, shape, number, and location of pulmonary lesions including cavitation, fibrous markings, and zones of consolidation

3 c
4 c
5 a
6 b
7 f
8 d
9 e
10 g
11 d
12 e
13 a, f, g
14 c
15 b
16 f

17 The chief value of ventilatory function tests is that quantitative data is provided to assess the degree of pulmonary disability, to follow the progress of the disability, and assess response to treatment. Ventilatory function test data is not generally specifically diagnostic, although patterns of disordered pulmonary function may be discriminated. Blood gas measurements, like ventilatory function tests, provide quantitative data to assess the degree of respiratory insufficiency and are particularly helpful in guiding oxygen therapy, but these data do not provide all the information necessary to assess total respiratory function.

18 Alveolar ventilation takes into account the amount of air wasted in ventilating the deadspace.

19 Measurements of the change in volume at different degrees of lung inflation and the change in alveolar or intrapleural pressure measured by means of an esophageal balloon are made simultaneously. Compliance is then calculated by the following formula:

$$\text{Compliance} = \frac{\Delta \text{ Volume}}{\Delta \text{ Pressure}}$$

20 Causes of decreased lung compliance include pulmonary fibrosis, pulmonary edema, pneumonia, and deficiency of surfactant.

Causes of decreased thoracic cage compliance include obesity, abdominal distention, and skeletal deformities of the chest cage.

21 The emphysema patient whose main problem is increased airways resistance due to premature collapse of the airways during expiration adopts a slow, deep pattern of respiration to minimize the work of breathing. Airflow is less turbulent with slow, deep respirations.

22 The chief problem for a patient with very stiff lungs is an increase in the elastic resistance. The work of breathing is minimized by a rapid, shallow pattern of respiration.

23 The radial artery is usually chosen for the arterial puncture because of its easy access. The wrist is extended (positioned over a rolled towel), the artery is stabilized with two fingers of one hand while the arterial puncture is made with the other hand using a heparinized syringe. Air is displaced from the blood specimen. Finally, the specimen is placed on ice and taken to the blood gas laboratory.

24 Hyperventilation can occur as a result of anxiety, brain injury, and pneumonia. It may also result secondarily to metabolic acidosis as a compensation. Causes of hypoventilation include narcotic or barbiturate overdose, and increased physiologic deadspace. It may also occur as a compensation for metabolic alkalosis.

25 Hypoxemia is caused by: ventilation–perfusion imbalance, alveolar hypoventilation, impaired diffusion, and intrapulmonary anatomic shunts. Hypoxemia caused by intrapulmonary anatomic shunting is not corrected by oxygen administration because the blood bypasses the pulmonary unit.

26 False; the reason is incorrect. In this case, less effective ventilation results because the total amount of air wasted as deadspace ventilation is greater.

27 True
28 False; $V_A = (200 - 120) \times 30 = 2.4$ liters/minute
29 True
30 True
31 True
32 True
33 a
34 b
35 c
36 c
37 b
38 d
39 a, b
40 a, c
41 f
42 c
43 d
44 e
45 b
46 a
47 Check your answer by referring to Table 31-5.

ANSWERS

Cardinal signs and symptoms of respiratory disease—Chap. 32

1 c
2 f
3 g

4 *b*

5 *a*

6 *e*

7 *d*

8 True

9 False; a P_aO_2 of less than 85 mmHg may or may not be associated with hypoxia. One can be fairly certain, however, that there is associated hypoxia if the P_aO_2 is persistently below 50 mmHg.

10 False; the detection of cyanosis is difficult, the cause is highly variable, and it may be absent in the presence of severe hypoxia or present when there is no hypoxia.

11 True

12 False; anemic persons (e.g., Hb = 7 g%) may never develop cyanosis even though they have severe hypoxia because it would be difficult to have 5 out of 7 g% reduced hemoglobin at any one time. Even in patients with normal hemoglobin concentration, cyanosis generally is an advanced sign of respiratory insufficiency.

13 True

14 True

15 False; alveolar hyperventilation is the cause of hypocapnia.

16 True

17 Digital clubbing refers to a loss of the base angle of the nail so that this angle is greater than the normal 160°; bulbous changes in the digital tips are also indicative of clubbing. Loss of the base angle is the earliest sign of digital clubbing, while the bulbous change is a late sign. Digital clubbing is important to detect because it is frequently associated with pulmonary disease (especially bronchogenic carcinoma), cardiovascular disease, and gastrointestinal disease.

18 Inspection of the buccal mucosa, especially under the tongue, is the most reliable method of detecting central cyanosis in both black and white patients. The lighting must be good, preferably daylight.

ANSWERS

Obstructive patterns of respiratory disease—Chap. 33

1 An increased resistance to airflow

2 All three diseases may exist in the pure form, although it is more common for patients to manifest aspects of all these diseases. It is especially common for patients to have features of chronic bronchitis and emphysema at the same time. This overlap and difficulty in separating the diseases is the reason for the label COPD.

3 An asthmatic attack is characterized by orthopnea (having to sit up to breathe), dyspnea, fear of suffocation, prolonged wheezing expirations, and later, cough and sputum production. Treatment consists of bronchodilator drugs and oxygen if the blood gases

are abnormal. Corticosteroid drugs are used occasionally for severe attacks. Long-term therapy consists of desensitization and avoidance of known allergens. Status asthmaticus is a prolonged, severe attack of asthma which may cause ventilatory insufficiency so severe that death results.

4

Feature	CLE	PLE
1. Sex prevalence	More common in males	Equal sex distribution
2. Etiology	Associated with smoking	Possible genetic factor
3. Pathologic anatomy	Respiratory bronchioles primarily affected	Entire acinus affected
4. Part of lung affected	Uneven distribution; upper lobes may be more severely affected	Uniform in distribution; basal lung more severely affected
5. Type of COPD associated with	Chronic bronchitis	Primary emphysema; chronic bronchitis; aging

5 Measures to relieve obstruction of the small airways; cessation of smoking; avoidance of air pollutants; prompt treatment of infection; cautious oxygen administration

6 Excessive production of mucus, chronic cough; 3 months per year and 2 consecutive years

7 Abnormal enlargement of the alveoli and the alveolar ducts, and destruction of the alveolar walls

8 Blebs; ruptured alveoli

9 Bullae; check valve obstruction of the bronchiole

10 In asthma there is hypersensitivity of the tracheobronchial tree to various stimuli, manifested by periodic, reversible airway narrowing due to bronchospasm.

11 Chronic inflammation causes weakening of the bronchial walls so that they become dilated. The dilated areas may be cylindrical or saccular in shape. The dilated areas serve as a reservoir for the collection of sputum. The stagnant sputum collection, in turn, may lead to chronic reinfection so that there is progressive destruction and persistence of the process. Precipitating factors include whooping cough, measles, pneumonia, aspiration of a foreign body, and bronchial obstruction due to a tumor.

12 Chronic loose cough, expectoration of a large amount of (up to 200 ml/day) of foul-smelling sputum, malnutrition, digital clubbing, cor pulmonale, and right heart failure.

13 Daily bronchial hygiene with postural drainage, antibiotics

14 Removal of the obstructing bronchial secretions

15 *b, a, c*

16 *a, c, d*

17 *b, d*

18 *c*

19 *b*

20 a, b, c
21 d
22 True
23 True
24 False; cystic fibrosis is more common in Caucasians
25 True
26 True
27 True
28 False; the prognosis is poor and few patients live beyond adolescence
29 a
30 b
31 a
32 b
33 a
34 b
35 b
36 b
37 a
38 b
39 b, e
40 a, c
41 d, e

ANSWERS

Restrictive patterns of respiratory disease—Chap. 34

1 f
2 e
3 a
4 b
5 d
6 c
7 True
8 False; pectus excavatum is a congenital deformity in which the lower end of the sternum is attached to the thoracic spine by fibromuscular bands, giving the lower end of the anterior chest a "caved-in" appearance.
9 True
10 False; the deformity is symmetrical
11 c
12 a
13 d
14 b
15 Alveolar hypoventilation, and an inability to maintain normal blood gas tensions
16 Traumatic—penetrating wound to the chest (knife or gunshot wound)
   Therapeutic—induced pneumothorax which was a common treatment for tuberculosis until about 1960
   Spontaneous—rupture of blebs and bullae in emphysema, pneumonia, neoplasm
17 Airtight seal is placed over the wound immediately.
18 Air gains access to the pleural cavity through the defect.
19 A large pneumothorax (greater than 20 percent lung collapse) is treated by closed (water-sealed) chest tube drainage. A large pleural effusion may be removed by thoracentesis. If a pleural effusion is an exudate it is treated by closed chest tube drainage to prevent fibrothorax.
20 Pleural effusion
21 Pulmonary venous pressure
22 An exudate
23 A transudate
24 (1) Invasion by bacteria, viruses, fungi, malignant cells—infection and destruction of lung tissue
   (2) Inhalation of irritating dusts—inflammation and pulmonary fibrosis
   (3) Inhalation of irritating gases—inflammation, and pulmonary fibrosis
   (4) Damage to the alveolar capillary endothelium—edema
   (5) Deficiency of pulmonary surfactant—atelectasis

25	*Absorption atelectasis*	*Compression atelectasis*
Common cause	Intrinsic obstruction of airway due to mucus plug	Extrinsic pressure on lung due to pleural effusion, hemothorax, pyothorax, or pneumothorax
Mechanism	Obstruction prevents air from entering alveoli distal to the obstruction. Air in alveoli is gradually absorbed into bloodstream and alveoli collapse	External pressure due to the fluid or air causes compression collapse of the alveoli

26 These small pores (between the alveoli) provide a path for collateral ventilation between alveoli and whole segments of the lung in case the normal airway is obstructed. Deep inspiration is effective in opening up the pores and providing ventilation to adjacent obstructed alveoli. Collapse due to absorption of gases into the bloodstream is thus prevented. (Once collapse occurs, reexpansion is much more difficult.) During expiration the pores close and pressure builds up, aiding in the explusion of the mucus plug.
27 (1) Engorgement (4 to 12 hours)—serous exudate from leaking blood vessels pour into alveoli
   (2) Red hepatization (next 48 hours)—lung, red and granular in appearance (RBCs, PMNs, and fibrin fill alveoli)
   (3) Gray hepatization (3 to 8 days)—lung has grayish appearance (leukocytes and fibrin consolidate in alveoli)
   (4) Resolution (7 to 11 days)—lysis and resorption of exudate by macrophages and restoration of tissue to normal

28 Administration of antibiotic effective against the specific infecting organism, oxygen therapy for hypoxemia, and treatment of complications

29 (1) Size of dust particle—those 1 to 5 μm can easily reach alveoli

(2) Concentration and length of exposure—high concentration and long exposure generally needed to produce adverse affects

(3) Nature of the dusts—some organic dusts produce an allergic alveolitis; the chemical nature of inorganic dust is important; some are harmless and inert, while others harm macrophages by which they are phagocytized and form fibrotic nodules

30 Infant—deficiency of surfactant

Adult—loss of surfactant secondary to damage to alveolar-capillary membrane

31 Since the condition results from a number of diverse insults, treatment is aimed at correcting the shock, acidosis, and hypoxemia. Positive end expiratory pressure (PEEP) is used to reexpand atelectic areas of lung and prevent further collapse of alveoli.

32 Histoplasmosis, coccidioidomycosis, and blastomycosis

33 Decreased lung compliance; interference with the gas diffusion pathway

34 Restrictive lung disease

35 interstitial

36 parenchyma; lung abscess, empyema; poor

37 atelectasis, pulmonary edema, congestion; hyaline

38 True

39 True

40 False; the prognosis is generally good

41 False; erythromycin is effective against mycoplasmal pneumonia. Antibiotics are not effective against viral infections.

42 True

43 False; this statement describes hypostatic pneumonia

44 True

45 True

46 c

47 a

48 b

49 c, g, and j

50 d, h, and i

51 a and f

52 b and e

53 c, f, h, and i

54 a, b, and g

55 d and e

56 c and h

57 c

58 f and g

59 d

60 a and e

61 b

62 h

63 b, c, d, e
64 b, e, f
65 a
66 a, c, e, g
67 d
68 a
69 b
70 e
71 c
72 d
73 b
74 c

ANSWERS

Respiratory insufficiency and respiratory failure—Chap. 35

1 Respiratory insufficiency refers to an impairment of the normal ability to oxygenate arterial blood and eliminate carbon dioxide so that there is an inability to maintain normal arterial blood gas levels under conditions of increased demand such as increased activity or exercise.

2 Chronic obstructive pulmonary disease

3 Hypoxemia without hypercapnia (hypoxemic respiratory failure or oxygenation failure); hypoxemia with hypercapnia (hypercapnic respiratory failure or ventilatory failure)

4 High concentrations of oxygen will reduce the hypoxic drive for breathing (which these patients depend on) and may aggravate hypoventilation and carbon dioxide retention.

5 P_aO_2 about 40 mmHg; P_aCO_2 60 to 70 mmHg

6 Liquefy and remove secretions by adequate hydration and administration of expectorants, aerosols; supervised coughing of patient; suctioning, percussion, vibration, postural drainage; treat respiratory infection with the appropriate antibiotic

7 Ensure that hypoxemia, acidosis, and hypercapnia do not reach hazardous levels

8 False, the point when respiratory insufficiency has progressed to failure is hard to detect in these patients since they have adapted somewhat to the abnormal blood gas tensions.

9 False, it is highly unreliable. If you missed this question, go back and read the section on cyanosis in Chap. 32.

10 True

11 True

12 False, hyperventilation causes this

13 True

14 True

15 True

16 d

17 b, c

18 a

19 b, c

20 a, b, c, d

Cardiovascular disease and the lung—Chap. 36

1 Local injury to the vascular wall; stasis of blood flow; hypercoaguability

2 Chronic obstructive pulmonary disease

3 Increased hydrostatic pressure within the pulmonary capillaries

Decrease in the colloid osmotic pressure (as in nephritis)

Damage to the capillary walls (as when noxious gases are inhaled)

Left ventricular heart failure

4 It is the name given to attacks of dyspnea caused by pulmonary edema at night. The increased hydrostatic pressure in the lungs is due to the horizontal position in patients with chronic passive congestion of the lungs resulting from left ventricular failure.

5 It is the condition in which hypertrophy and dilatation of the right ventricle develops due to disease affecting the structure and function of the lung. (Congenital and left heart disease are not included.)

6 When the left ventricle fails while the right ventricle continues to pump blood, the pulmonary hydrostatic pressure rises until pulmonary edema results. Yes

7 Prevent the recurrence of pulmonary embolism; relieve symptoms resulting from the embolism; surgical removal of a massive embolus

8 To improve the underlying pulmonary disorder and correct the hypoxemia

9 Two mechanisms leading to increased pulmonary vascular resistance are (1) anatomic alterations in the pulmonary blood vessels leading to a reduction of the pulmonary vascular bed and (2) pulmonary functional disorders caused by alveolar hypoventilation or $\dot{V}/\dot{Q}$ imbalances which cause hypoxemia, hypercapnia, and acidosis (blood gas abnormalities); the blood gas abnormalities then cause pulmonary arteriolar vasoconstriction.

10 a, b, c, e; d is associated with a massive pulmonary embolism

11 c

12 a, b, d

13 c

14 b, c, d, e

15 c

16 a, c

17 c

18 a

19 a, b, c, d

20 Congestive heart failure is first in importance and the postoperative bedridden condition is second.

21 True

22 True

23 True

24 False

25 embolism

26 5

27 pulmonary hypertension

ANSWERS

Pulmonary malignant neoplasms—Chap. 37

1 The carcinoid syndrome is a symptom complex characterized by attacks of anxiety, tremulousness, hypotension, flushing, dyspnea, and cyanosis due to bronchoconstriction. It is caused by the elaboration of serotonin and other biologically active substances secreted by a carcinoid type of bronchial adenoma.

2 Cough, chest pain, sputum expectoration, mild dyspnea, digital clubbing and hemoptysis are common, but symptoms may be minimal. Diagnosis on the basis of symptoms is difficult since the onset may be insidious and the symptoms are not specific. Lung cancer may imitate a number of other lung disorders.

3 Radiology—"coin lesion" on x-ray

Bronchoscopy—direct visualization of tumor and biopsy identification of malignant cells

Cytology—examination of sputum, bronchial washings, or pleural fluid for malignant cells

4 b, c, h, j

5 d, h, j, m, n, o

6 e, i, k, l

7 a, f, g, i, k, l

8 True

9 False; there is a positive relationship. The greater the number of cigarettes smoked, the greater the risk.

10 False; it is asbestos.

11 False; secondary metastases are more common.

12 True

13 True

14 a, c

15 d

16 a, c, and d

ANSWERS

Pulmonary tuberculosis—Chap. 38

1 b, c

2 c

3 a

4 c

5 c

6 d

7 b

8 b

9 d

10 d

11 c

12 b, c, d

13 c

14 a, d

15 True

16 False; the risk of hepatitis is very low in persons under 20 years of age and reaches a peak among persons over 50 years of age.

17 False; the classification system is based on the broad host–parasite relationships as described by exposure history, infection, and disease.

18 True

19 These risk factors are: (1) risk of acquiring the infection and (2) developing clinical disease after the infection has occurred. The risk of acquiring the infection and developing the disease is dependent on the following: infection in the population, crowding, socially disadvantaged populations, and inadequacy of medical care.

20 The primary public health measures for prevention and control of tuberculosis in the United States are early detection of cases and sources of infection. Preventive therapy with antimicrobial drugs is an effective tool in the control of the disease.

ANSWERS

Normal renal function—Chap. 39

a. *1* 1 Left kidney; 2 right kidney; 3 ureter; 4 bladder; 5 urethra; 6 urinary meatus.

b. *2* 1 Eleventh rib; 2 twelfth rib; 3 transversus abdominus muscle; 4 psoas major muscle.

c. *3* 1 Fibrous capsule; 2 cortex; 3 medulla; 4 column of Bertin; 5 papilla; 6 pyramid; 7 minor calyx; 8 major calyx; 9 renal pelvis; 10 ureter.

d. *4* 1 Proximal convoluted tubule; 2 glomerular capillary tuft; 3 Bowman's capsule; 4 efferent arteriole; 5 juxtaglomerular cells; 6 afferent arteriole; 7 macula densa; 8 loop of Henle; 9 distal convoluted tubule; 10 collecting duct.

5 Check your drawing with Fig. 39-1. The hilus of each kidney should be at about the level of the second lumbar vertebra. The superior pole of the left kidney is at about the level of the lower border of the eleventh rib, while the right is at about the level of the twelfth rib.

6 (a) Bowman's capsule; (b) proximal convoluted tubule; (c) distal convoluted tubule; (d) collecting ducts; (e) papillary ducts of Bellini; (f) minor calyces; (g) major calyces; (h) renal pelvis; (i) ureter; (j) bladder.

7 (a) Abdominal aorta; (b) renal artery; (c) interlobar arteries; (d) arcuate arteries; (e) interlobular arterioles; (f) afferent arterioles; (g) glomerular capillaries; (h) efferent arterioles; (i) peritubular capillaries; (j) interlobular veins; (k) arcuate veins; (l) interlobar veins; (m) renal vein; (n) inferior vena cava.

8 More than 25 percent of the population has more than one renal artery supplying a kidney, which may cause technical difficulties for the surgeon. Some difficulties presented by aberrant blood vessels may be insurmountable.

9 A decrease in the hydrostatic pressure of the blood flowing through the afferent arteriole sensed by the JG cells or a decrease in sodium concentration in the distal tubule filtrate sensed by the macula densa cells causes the release of renin from the JG cells. This results in the conversion of angiotensinogen to angiotensin I and finally to the active form, angiotensin II. Angiotensin II increases arterial blood pressure by causing peripheral vasoconstriction and stimulates the secretion of aldosterone. Increased aldosterone levels cause increased sodium reabsorption in the distal tubule. More water is then reabsorbed, resulting in an increase in plasma volume. Both vasoconstriction and increased plasma volume help to elevate blood pressure. An increase in the blood pressure in the afferent arteriole or an increase in the sodium concentration of the distal tubular filtrate has the opposite effect.

10 A severe blunt impact over the back, flank, or even the abdomen can cause trauma to the kidney. This situation is common following traffic accidents. The most common trauma in such cases results from the kidney being pushed against a transverse process or being punctured by a fractured twelfth rib. The resulting injury can vary from a simple bruise to a shattering of the renal parenchyma. Complete transection of a kidney by the twelfth rib is not uncommon in severe cases.

11 d

12 f

13 b

14 e

15 c

16 a

17 d

18 a

19 c

20 b

21 d

22 c

23 c

24 a

25 e

26 It is called ultrafiltration because the glomerular filtrate has the same composition as plasma with the absence of proteins—almost everything is filtered through and at a very high flow rate.

27 The differences in the pressures in the glomerulus and in Bowman's capsule tend to force fluid into the capsule. Net filtration pressure = intracapillary hyrostatic pressure − colloid osmotic pressure of the blood − intracapsular hydrostatic pressure.

28 The GFR is the rate of the appearance of glomerular filtrate from filtration of the blood at the glomerulus. The average GFR in men is 125 ml/minute and in women, 110 ml/minute.

29 To measure the GFR a substance must be used which is freely filtered by the glomerulus but is neither secreted nor reabsorbed along the tubules. A substance which was cleared by both filtration and secre-

tion along the tubule would cause the apparent GFR to be higher than the true GFR. A substance which was both filtered and reabsorbed would cause the apparent GFR to be lower than the true GFR.

30 $GFR = \dfrac{UV}{P} = \dfrac{(500 \text{ mg}/100 \text{ ml})(2 \text{ ml/minute})}{25 \text{ mg}/100 \text{ ml}}$

= 40 ml/minute.

A GFR of 40 ml/minute indicates that this patient has moderately severe impairment of renal function. The calculated value is normally corrected for body surface area by means of a normogram. The standard body surface area is 1.73 m² (the body surface area of an average man). The final result is then reported in milliliters/minute/1.73 meters squared.

31 Regulation of water and acid-base balance. Water is reabsorbed in the presence of ADH. Acid-base balance is regulated by regeneration of bicarbonate and hydrogen-ion excretion in combination with phosphates and ammonia.

32 The lungs control the excretion of carbon dioxide, and the kidneys control the reabsorption of bicarbonate, both important components of the bicarbonate–carbonic acid buffer system in the blood. The ratio of these two components is important in maintaining a normal blood pH. This subject may be explored in greater detail in many fine texts dealing with fluid and electrolyte homeostasis.

33 H^+ is excreted in the urine by combining with HPO_4^{2-} to form $H_2PO_4^-$ and by combining with NH_3 to form NH_4^+.

34 (a) Maintain water balance to keep plasma osmolality at 285 mosmol, (b) maintain electrolyte balance, (c) maintain acid-base balance, (d) excrete nitrogenous end products of protein metabolism, (e) produce renin for regulation of blood pressure, (f) produce erythropoietin important in RBC formation, (g) activate vitamin D.

35 (a) Vapor pressure is lowered. (b) Boiling point is elevated. (c) Freezing point is lowered. (d) Osmotic pressure is increased. Osmotic pressure refers to the external pressure which would have to be applied to a solution with the greater number of particles to prevent water from diffusing across a semipermeable membrane from a solution with a lesser number of particles. It is a measure of water concentration, and there are no real physical pressures present in the solutions—it is only the pressure used to characterize the system. Adding particles to water lowers its chemical potential (molar free energy), and water always flows from an area of higher potential (more dilute) to an area of lower potential (more concentrated). The attainment of equilibrium by the application of pressure to the more concentrated solution is due to raising its chemical potential so that it is equal to the water in the more dilute solution on the other side of the membrane. The application of pressure prevents an increase in volume in the more concentrated solution due to water diffusion.

36 The osmometer is an apparatus for measuring the freezing point of a solution. The freezing point depression below that of pure water can then be used

to very accurately calculate the osmotic concentration of the solution since it depends only on the number of particles in solution. The urinometer actually measures the density or specific gravity of a solution and does not measure true concentration which depends on the number of particles in solution. Therefore, the osmometer is more accurate in estimating the concentration of a solution.

37 $Osmolality = \dfrac{\Delta T}{K_f} = \dfrac{-0.53}{-1.86} \times 1000 = 285 \text{ mOsm}$

The result is multiplied by 1000 to convert to milliosmols.

38 Check your drawing with Fig. 39-15. Cortical glomeruli should be located high in the cortex with relatively short loops of Henle which extend slightly into the medullary area. Juxtamedullary glomeruli should be located deep in the cortex next to the medulla, and the loops of Henle should be relatively long, extending deep into the medulla.

39 The vasa recta are medullary blood vessels which form hairpin loops beside the juxtaglomerular loop of Henle. They help maintain the concentration gradient of the medullary interstitial fluid.

40 The purpose of the countercurrent mechanism is the conservation of water (or the concentration of urine) by the kidney. The two basic processes involved are the loop of Henle acting as a countercurrent multiplier of concentration to build up the concentration gradient in the medulla and the vasa recta acting as a countercurrent exchanger to prevent washing out the hyperosmolality built up by the loop of Henle.

41 d
42 a
43 b
44 c
45 c
46 d
47 c
48 d
49 d
50 b; it is hyperosmotic even during diuresis.
51 d; increase in medullary blood flow washes out medullary hypertonicity.
52 b, c
53 a, d; reabsorption in the proximal tubule is obligatory.
54 b; maximum concentration is about 1400 mOsm; plasma concentration is 285 mOsm.
55 a
56 b
57 a
58 c
59 b
60 d; hypoosmotic during diuresis due to Na^+ reabsorption and water cannot passively follow; isosmotic when water is reabsorbed with Na^+ during antidiuresis.

61 a, b, or *c*

62 c

63 b

64 All except *f, l.*

65 e, g

66 c, d

67 i, j, p

68 i

69 h, j, n; actually ammonia is also a nitrogenous substance synthesized from amino acids, especially glutamine, and secreted along the tubule.

70 a, b

71 b, o

72 m

73 k

74 a

75 b

76 c

77 c

78 c

79 a

ANSWERS

Diagnostic procedures in renal disease—Chap. 40

1 A normal healthy adult may excrete up to 150 mg of protein in the urine per day. Amounts in excess of 150 mg/day are considered pathologic and occur most frequently in renal disease, particularly glomerulonephritis. Patients with the nephrotic syndrome excrete more than 3.5 g of protein per day and may excrete as much as 20 to 30 g.

2 The direct cause of proteinuria is always an increase in glomerular permeability.

3 When urine stands for a period of time, urea breaks down to ammonia and the urine becomes more alkaline.

4 Uric acid is derived principally from the catabolism of nucleoproteins in the cells. Cytotoxic drugs cause increased degradation of the rapidly proliferating cells, and thus uric acid production is increased. Two-thirds of the uric acid is normally excreted by the kidneys. The uric acid may crystallize and obstruct the tubules under conditions of acid urine.

5 (a) Infection with urea-splitting organisms producing alkaline urine; (b) hypercalciuria due to prolonged immobilization; (c) urinary stasis due to low fluid intake. All three of these conditions are often present in patients with chronic illness who are confined to a bed, thus favoring the formation of urinary calculi which form in alkaline urine. Calcium salts are mobilized from bone, and precipitation is favored by highly concentrated, alkaline urine.

6 High fluid intake

7 (a) The accuracy of the urinometer; (b) a uniform solution; (c) avoid errors of surface tension; (d) read the calibrated units from top to bottom at eye level; and (e) correct for temperature.

8 Creatinine is a nitrogenous end product of muscle metabolism. The normal plasma level is 0.7 to 1.5 mg%. The plasma level is constant in the healthy person and depends on muscle mass.

9 A substance which is filtered by the glomerulus and is neither secreted nor reabsorbed by the tubules is required for a true measurement of GFR. Creatinine is secreted by the tubules, and there is an error inherent in the laboratory method of measuring the plasma level. These two large errors nearly cancel each other out so that creatinine clearance approximately equals GFR.

10 GFR decreases with increasing age. After age 30 it decreases at the rate of about 1 ml/minute/year.

11 The PAH excretion test is the most accurate test of effective renal plasma flow.

12 The plasma creatinine level, because its production rate in the body is constant. It depends on muscle mass, which changes very little. Urea production varies with dietary protein intake and catabolism of body protein. Azotemia means that there is an increase in nitrogenous substances in the blood. This occurs when the kidneys are not able to excrete these substances as rapidly as they are produced.

13 (a) The correct interpretation of a "trace" reading must take into account the concentration of the urine specimen and the time of the day it is collected. A trace reading in an early morning concentrated specimen is probably within normal limits. If the urine is collected later in the day and is dilute, a trace response might indicate excessive proteinuria. (b) Contamination by vaginal secretions in the female (contain protein).

14 Albumin; Tamm-Horsfall

15 6

16 a; alkaline

17 b, c, nocturnal acid

18 285

19 1.001, 1.040; to maintain the osmolality of the ECF at a constant value.

20 28 percent; this is the minimum for normal renal function; average excretion is 35 percent.

21 1.025, 1.003

22 Urine acidification or ammonium chloride; 5.3

23 Sodium conservation; *a*

24 c

25 c

26 a, c

27 c. $C_{cr} = \dfrac{U_{cr}V}{P_{cr}} = \dfrac{50 \text{ mg/100 ml} \times 1 \text{ ml/minute}}{2 \text{ mg/100 ml}}$
$= 25$ ml/minute.

It is necessary to convert the 24-hour urine volume to milliliters per minute to calculate the problem: 1400 ml/24 hours × 24 hours/1440 minutes = 1 ml/minute.

28 b; decrease is at the rate of 1 ml/minute/year after

the age of 30. A decrease of 60 ml/minute is expected in this 90-year-old man, which is about a 50 percent decrease of the normal GFR in the young, healthy male.

29 Red blood cells, white blood cells, casts, bacteria

30 A bacterial count of 10^5 (100,000) organisms per milliliter urine is considered significant and is an indication of urinary tract infection (more than three or four WBCs per high-power field during microscopic examination of the urine sediment suggests significant bacteriuria and indicates that a bacterial count should be done). However, the urine must not have been contaminated by bacteria from other sources such as from the container or from the genitalia. Therefore the genitalia must be cleansed with soap and water before voiding into the sterile specimen bottle and care must be taken to avoid contamination of the urine by the labia or vaginal secretions in the female ("sterile-voided"). Catheterization gives greater insurance that the specimen is "sterile." The urine must be examined immediately or a preservative should be added and the specimen refrigerated to avoid bacterial growth.

31 An IVP is accomplished by injecting into a vein x-ray contrast medium which is then excreted by the kidneys, while in the retrograde pyelogram a catheter is passed up a ureter, and contrast medium is injected directly into the renal pelvis.

The purpose of an IVP is to visualize the cortex, calyces, renal pelvis, ureters, and bladder. The adequacy of filling of the calyces and renal pelvis may also be determined. The purpose of the retrograde pyelogram is to obtain better visualization when the IVP is not clear and to investigate a nonfunctioning kidney.

32 (a) Hypertension—may be due to renal artery stenosis or other obstruction, (b) possible neoplasm—blood vessels of tumor can be visualized, (c) transplant—to visualize the precise vascular supply prior to surgery, (d) to visualize the blood supply to the cortex—may have patchy appearance indicating ischemia.

33 The GFR is probably very low and the dye will not be excreted well; the pyelogram will be difficult to visualize.

34 The entry site should be checked periodically for signs of hematoma or inflammation. Vital signs are checked every 15 minutes until stable and then every 4 hours for 24 hours. Peripheral pulses (in the leg when the femoral artery is used as the entry site) should be checked for diminished strength at the same time intervals as above in order to detect occlusion of blood flow due to thrombus or embolus formation. Color and skin temperature are other signs which should be observed to detect occlusion.

35 The patient should lie prone with a sandbag under the abdomen for 30 minutes after a renal biopsy. Firm pressure with 4 × 4 sponges is applied over the biopsy site for 10 minutes followed by application of a pressure dressing. The patient should be kept in bed and as quiet as possible for 24 hours. Vital signs are checked and the abdomen observed for swelling during this period. The urine should also be observed for gross and occult blood.

36 Microscopic; bacteriologic; radiology; biopsy

37 Tamm-Horsfall; distal

38 Cylindruria, protein

39 Culture and sensitivity

40 Clubbing (also may be seen in some other forms of chronic renal disease).

41 b

42 a

43 c

44 a; death occurs in only 0.17 percent of the cases

45 c

46 d

47 a

48 b

ANSWERS

Chronic renal failure—Chap. 41

1 The time period of development of the disease condition; chronic renal failure is a progressive, slow process over a period of years, whereas acute renal failure develops over a period of a few days to weeks. In both cases the kidneys lose their ability to keep the internal environment of the body normal.

2 (a) Chronic glomerulonephritis with primary glomerular involvement; (b) chronic pyelonephritis with primary involvement of renal tubules and interstitium; (c) polycystic disease with primary involvement of renal tubules; (d) hypertensive nephrosclerosis with primary involvement of renal vasculature.

3 Stage I = decreased renal reserve—up to 75 percent of nephron mass destroyed. Stage II = renal insufficiency—75 to 90 percent nephron mass destroyed. Stage III = uremia or end-stage renal failure—90 percent or more of the nephron mass destroyed.

4 First stage—BUN and plasma creatinine levels both normal; second stage—BUN and plasma creatinine levels rising just above normal, unstable; third stage—BUN and plasma creatinine levels both rising very sharply with each decrement of GFR.

5 The creatinine clearance progresses towards zero as nephrons are progressively destroyed by the renal disease process (creatinine clearance rate gives a fairly good estimate of the true GFR in the middle range but is much less accurate at either high or low filtration rates).

6 Polyuria means an increase in the *volume* of urine whereas oliguria is just the opposite—urine output is decreased below the normal range. (Do not confuse polyuria and frequency, a common mistake made by students. Frequency means an increase in the *number*

of voidings, but there is not necessarily an increase in the volume. With moderate polyuria, there is not necessarily an increase in frequency.) Nocturia means that a person has to get up more than once to void during normal sleeping hours or output is 700 ml or more during the night.

7 Polyuria and nocturia occur because of the solute diuresis and inability to concentrate the urine. Both symptoms occur early in the course of progressive renal failure and are compensatory. When most of the nephrons are destroyed, the patient becomes oliguric because total net filtration rate is low (because there are few nephrons) even though the GFR for each individual intact nephron may be high (decompensation stage). Primary lesions of the medulla might interfere with the chloride pump, the countercurrent mechanism, and tubular secretion and reabsorption, while lesions of the glomerulus might prevent glomerular filtration from occurring or cause the loss of protein and formed elements into the urine.

8 An increased solute load may be induced in a normal person by the ingestion of a very high protein diet or by giving mannitol intravenously. The usual solute load of the kidneys is thus extended many times. Each normal nephron is undergoing an osmotic diuresis which results in an obligatory loss of water. The kidney loses its flexibility to either concentrate or dilute the urine from the plasma osmolality of 285 mOsm under the stress of water deprivation or overload. Identical principles are involved in progressive renal failure, and both conditions are explained by the intact nephron hypothesis.

9 The remaining intact nephrons compensate by hypertrophying. Filtration rate, solute load, and tubular reabsorption per nephron are all increased, and glomerular-tubular balance is maintained until most of the renal nephrons are destroyed.

10 The renal disease may not be diagnosed until it is far advanced when functional and morphological characteristics may be similar for a number of chronic renal diseases.

11 Bacteriuria (10^5 bacteria per ml urine) means that there is an infection in the urinary tract, whether symptomatic or asymptomatic so that there is an increased risk of developing an acute, symptomatic pyelonephritis or perhaps an asymptomatic chronic pyelonephritis.

12 The patient may have a persistent or recurrent asymptomatic bacteriuria, indicating urinary tract infection which is perhaps in the kidney or, if located in the lower urinary tract, can ascend to the kidney.

13 Symptoms may be very mild and not revealed by the patient, or the patient may be entirely asymptomatic until end-stage renal disease. Thus the patient may not seek help.

14 Arguments for bacterial etiology of chronic pyelone-

phritis: (1) at least half of the patients have a history of urinary tract infections including acute pyelonephritis, while the remainder of patients may have had subclinical infections; (2) the hypertonic medulla is especially susceptible to infection since bacteria can thrive there in the form of protoplasts which can be converted to active bacteria from time to time causing recurrent or chronic infection; (3) bacteria and leukocyte casts may only be discharged into the urine periodically and consequently may be difficult to detect.

Arguments against bacterial etiology of chronic pyelonephritis: (1) many patients have no recallable history of urinary tract infection; (2) sex incidence of chronic pyelonephritis is about equal although the female/male ratio of urinary tract infection and acute pyelonephritis is about 10:1; (3) urinary tract infection is a frequent complication of other renal disease; (4) lesions similar to chronic pyelonephritis are caused by nonbacterial factors such as phenacetin.

15 Acute pyelonephritis: the kidney is swollen with multiple abscesses on the surface and within the parenchyma; hydronephrosis and blunting of the calyces may be present. Chronic pyelonephritis: the kidney is contracted, has a coarsely granular surface with U-shaped depressions, irregular outline with scarring and distortion of the pelvis and calyces.

16 b

17 c, d

18 d

19 b, c

20 a

21 a, b; poor blood supply is probably not important since most infecting bacteria are not anaerobic; high glucose content is not normally present.

22 c

23 e

24 a; because it is a result of bacterial infection of the urinary tract which then infects the kidney. Public efforts are needed to detect urinary tract infections (significant bacteriuria) in the population, especially those at high risk. Those infections detected then need to be treated and adequately followed. There is also a need for public health education with respect to prevention measures and information on the signs and symptoms of urinary tract infection or renal disease. Chronic glomerulonephritis might be reduced a small amount by prompt treatment of all streptococcal infections. However, 90 percent of chronic glomerulonephritis has an insidious onset and is not associated with streptococcal infections and cannot be cured. Health education or mass screening programs to ensure early detection of renal disease might be helpful so that conservative medical management could begin and thus prolong renal function.

25 True

26 False; it may be intermittent and so easily missed.

27 True

28 PMNs; tubules; lymphocytes; plasma

29 a, Atrophied tubule containing cast; b, normal

tubule; *c*, area of interstitial fibrosis; *d*, hypertrophied tubule with atrophy of epithelial cells; *e*, inflammatory cells (PMNs)

30 The original meaning of the term glomerulonephritis was to describe a primary renal disease which involved an inflammatory lesion of the glomerulus and whose chief manifestations were hematuria and proteinuria. This term was also applied to many renal diseases which were poorly understood. Today the term is often used to describe any inflammatory lesion of the glomerulus even if secondary to a systemic disease.

31 Confusion exists because of the many emerging categories based on histologic findings which do not always correlate with the clinical features of glomerulonephritis. Glomerulonephritis is much more complex than originally believed, and the exact etiology is unknown in most cases.

32 Acute glomerulonephritis: In the classic poststreptococcal GN, about 90 percent of the children have a complete recovery, but the prognosis is not as good for adults. About 10 percent develop CGN. Acute GN can occur following bacterial endocarditis and during the course of many other renal diseases.

Subacute or rapidly progressive glomerulonephritis: Rapid progression to end-stage renal failure within 2 years; 4 percent of the cases follow APSGN, but in most cases the cause is unknown.

Chronic glomerulonephritis: Slowly progressing GN leading to end-stage renal failure over a period varying from 2 to 40 years; 90 percent of the cases have an insidious onset, or the precipitating cause is unknown.

33 Classic case of acute poststreptococcal GN: most prevalent in children aged 3 to 7 years; common nephrotogenic organism is group A β-hemolytic streptococcus, Types 12 and 4 most common; follows strep sore throat or skin infection in about 10 days; common signs and symptoms: anorexia, fatigue, fever, headache, nausea and vomiting, hypertension, edema (especially of face), hematuria; major physiologic disturbances: glomerular damage resulting in hematuria, albuminuria, and urinary casts; decreased GFR from glomerular damage resulting in oliguria, azotemia, salt and water retention. Salt and water retention contributes both to the edema and the development of hypertension. Vasospasm may also play a role in the development of hypertension. Usual treatment is penicillin to eradicate any streptococcal infection, salt restriction, antihypertensive drugs.

34 The nephrotic syndrome is a clinical condition characterized by the loss of large amounts of protein in the urine (more than 3.5 g/day), hyperlipidemia, hypoalbuminemia, and edema. Massive edema is common when there is massive loss of protein (rate of loss greater than rate of production by the liver). The resulting hypoalbuminemia reduces the colloid osmotic pressure in the blood vessels so that fluid tends to move from the intravascular to the interstitial spaces. The edema is further aggravated by the resulting hypovolemia which causes a decrease in the renal blood flow and GFR, and an increase in aldosterone and salt and water retention. More than 75 percent of the cases are associated with the various types of primary glomerulonephritis. About 50 percent of patients with chronic GN have the nephrotic syndrome at some time during the course of the disease. Other diseases commonly associated with the nephrotic syndrome are SLE, diabetes mellitus, amyloidosis. Principles of treatment include corticosteroid and immunosuppressive drugs directed against the primary disease when appropriate, high protein, salt-restricted diet, diuretics, and protection against infection.

35 Early diagnosis of renal artery obstruction is important because surgical correction of hypertension may be possible. If left uncorrected, the affected kidney will undergo ischemic atrophy, and the contralateral kidney will develop nephrosclerosis from the systemic hypertension which is mediated through the renin-angiotensin system of the originally affected kidney.

36 (a) High renal blood flow, (b) hyperosmotic interstitium, (c) excretory route for most drugs and chemicals.

37 *c*

38 *b*

39 *a*

40 *b, c, g*

41 *a, d, e, f, h*

42 *c, d*

43 *b, e*

44 *a, e*

45 *b, f*

46 *b, g*

47 *b, d, i, j*

48 *b, c, d, i*

49 *a, b*

50 *b, h*

51 *d*

52 *e*

53 *c*

54 *d*

55 *c*

56 *b*

57 *a*

58 *a*

59 *c*

60 *b*

61 *c*

62 *d*

63 *b, c*

64 *c*

65 False; not if the contralateral kidney has developed nephrosclerosis. The ischemic kidney may have better function than the contralateral kidney, so that the latter should be removed.

66 False; about two-thirds or more.

67 True

68 True

69 False; the loss of protein is usually not sufficient to cause hypoproteinemia.

70 False; it is often very small with a granular surface due to ischemia.

71 True

72 True

73 False; it signifies rapid or an advanced state of destruction; prognosis is very poor.

74 True

ANSWERS

The uremic syndrome—Chap. 42

1 The uremic syndrome refers to a symptom complex that results from or is associated with retention of nitrogenous metabolites related to renal failure.

2 The first group of symptoms relates to deranged regulatory and excretory functions (i.e., fluid and electrolyte disturbances, acid-base imbalances). The second group of symptoms refers to cardiovascular, neuromuscular, gastrointestinal, and other system abnormalities.

3 Because the total number of nephrons is decreased, and not because of a tubular transport problem.

4 H^+ is probably being buffered by calcium carbonate from the bones. No doubt, this process contributes to the dissolution of bone though it is not as important as the increased parathormone levels.

5 Because of the increased solute load of each intact nephron. The osmotic diuresis results in obligatory salt losses.

6 Milk of magnesia and magnesium citrate

7 A fixed urine specific gravity of 1.010 means that the patient has severe renal failure with no ability to either concentrate or dilute the urine. Consequently, there is little ability to regulate the fluid balance in the body, and fluid intake must be carefully prescribed.

8 When the GFR falls to about 5 ml/minute in terminal renal failure, both males and females lose their libido and are generally sterile. The male is generally impotent, and the female ceases to menstruate.

9 Poor nutrition, overhydration, indwelling catheters and cannulas, immunosuppressive drugs.

10 Caucasian—waxy yellow (bronze) cast to the skin; brown-skinned person—yellowish brown coloration; black-skinned person—ashen-gray with yellow tones. All of these skin color changes are due to the anemia and retention of urochrome pigments in the uremic patient. Skin color changes in the dark-skinned per-

sons are due to a loss of the red undertones which gives the dark skin a "look-alive" appearance. Yellow tones are more evident in the conjunctiva, and on the palms and soles.

11 GI bleeding → hypotension → decreased renal
⌐→ perfusion → ↓ GFR
└→ digestion of blood protein → ↑ BUN

Vomiting → dehydration → hypovolemia
⌐→ → ↓ renal perfusion → ↓ GFR
Diarrhea → loss of HCO_3^- → aggravation of acidosis

12 You might expect the patient to complain of tiring easily, not able to work very long without resting, to be unable to sleep at night or lethargic during the day. You might observe that the patient's affect seemed flat, and there was difficulty in following a complex train of thought. Muscular weakness and muscular twitching might be complaints. The untreated patient in terminal renal failure will eventually become confused and comatose and may have convulsions, especially if severely hypertensive.

13 Stage I: nerve conduction test reveals decreased velocity of nerve conduction. Patient may complain of needing to walk or move the legs (restless leg syndrome). Stage II: sensory nerve changes. Patient complains of burning sensation on the soles of the feet; numbness or prickling sensation moving up legs in stockinglike fashion; may have paresthesias of the hands. Stage III: motor nerve involvement. Loss of motor function usually is first observed as foot drop and may progress to paraplegia.

14 Check your illustration with the hand x-ray in Fig. 42-2. The radial aspect of the bone is eroded and has a jagged appearance.

15 See Fig. 42-3 if you have forgotten this sequence of events. Bone disorders associated with secondary hyperparathyroidism might include "honeycombing" demineralization of the bone, especially notable on skull x-ray, subperiosteal bone resorption, giving the phylanges a ragged border. Pathological fractures of the long bones and ribs may result. Calcium salts may be deposited in the soft tissues of the body, around joints, in the arteries, and in the eyes.

16 This patient has a calcium-phosphate cross product of $8 \times 10 = 80$, which exceeds the solubility product of calcium and phosphate by a large margin. Soft tissue deposition of calcium phosphate would certainly be expected.

17 Check your illustration with Fig. 42-4. Irritation from the calcium salts deposited in the eye may cause conjunctivitis called "uremic red eye" due to its appearance.

18 b

19 c

20 a

21 c

22 b

23 a

24 c

25 b, c, d

26 c

27 a, b, c, d

28 *a, c, e* (It is possible to have iron deficiency, especially if the patient is not eating well. The factors related to uremia are those listed.)

29 *a, c*

30 *d*

31 True

32 False (If you missed this question, review the description in this chapter.)

33 True

34 False; it has no effect on the GFR.

35 True

36 False; certain amino acids are elevated while others are depressed.

37 False; uremic patients are often hyperglycemic.

38 True

39 True

40 Urea, ammonia, infection

41 (a) Osteitis fibrosa; (b) osteomalacia (rickets); (c) osteosclerosis

42 *c*

43 *a, d*

44 *b, e*

45 *b*

46 *f*

47 *d*

48 *e*

49 *c*

50 *a*

ANSWERS

The treatment of chronic renal failure—Chap. 43

1 When the patient becomes azotemic. The physician searches out and treats any reversible factors, such as hypertension, urinary tract obstruction or infection. The principles of conservative measures are based on regulating individual solutes and fluids in order to achieve as normal an internal milieu as possible in view of the kidney's decreased ability to adapt to a variable intake.

2 Death in terminal renal failure, dialysis, or renal transplantation. Unfortunately, only about one-half of the patients who could benefit from renal transplantation or chronic dialysis are actually being treated. The main reason is because of lack of referral to a treatment center. Lack of skilled health care personnel, facilities, and financial support are not as important limiting factors as they were in the 1960s.

3 Some nephrologists restrict protein to 40 g when the GFR is 10 ml/minute; 25 to 30 g with a GFR of 5 ml/minute; and 20 g with a GFR of 3 ml/minute or less. Allowance is much more liberal after dialysis is begun. Protein foods must be restricted somewhat to avoid a high intake of potassium, phosphate, and acid production. Care is taken to provide an adequate carbohydrate intake in order to provide calories and prevent catabolism of body protein. It is usually necessary to restrict dietary potassium even after the patient

is being dialyzed regularly. Sodium intake must be adjusted carefully to avoid fluid overload or a negative sodium balance which might lead to dehydration and deterioration of renal function.

4 About 500 ml + 500 ml = 1000 ml

5 Chronic intermittent dialysis and renal transplantation. Dialysis may be used for long-term maintenance of the end-stage renal failure patient. Even if the patient chooses renal transplantation as the mode of therapy, dialysis will undoubtedly play a role in treatment. Dialysis can be used to restore and maintain the uremic patient in an optimal physical state before the transplant kidney is available and as a backup treatment modality should the transplanted kidney fail. The patient who has chosen maintenance home or satellite-center dialysis may also opt for a transplant at a later date.

6 Dialysis is the process by which water and small-molecular-weight solutes pass through a semipermeable membrane from one fluid compartment to another and achieve equilibrium.

7 The two common methods are the creation of an internal AV fistula by anastomosing an artery and a nearby vein in an extremity, and the creation of an external AV shunt, or cannula system, by placing cannula tips in an artery and nearby vein and directing flow from artery to vein through a silicone rubber tubing. In both cases blood is shunted from an artery to a vein, but in one case the shunt is internal, and in the other case it is external.

8 *a, b, d, i*

9 *g*

10 *e, k*

11 *h*

12 *f*

13 *j*

14 *c*

15 *c*

16 *a*

17 *b*

18 *b, c, d;* a BUN of 60 mg% is not by itself an indication for dialysis.

19 *c*

20 *c*

21 *c*

22 *a;* not entirely true—some albumin does pass through the pores in the semipermeable membrane. The amount of albumin lost from the blood is generally insignificant during hemodialysis but is quite substantial during peritoneal dialysis.

23 *b*

24 *d*

25 *b;* to provide a high blood-flow rate adequate for hemodialysis. The enlarged vein also allows large-bore needles to be easily inserted.

26 *b*

27 c
28 a, d, e
29 a, b
30 b
31 a

ANSWERS

Acute renal failure—Chap. 44

1 Because inhalation of fumes of CCl₄ (and other organic solvents) and the ingested ethyl alcohol react chemically in the body to produce a very potent nephrotoxin which may produce acute tubular necrosis.
2 Nephrotoxic injury and renal ischemia
3 Acute renal failure is superimposed on persons with chronic renal insufficiency due to intrinsic renal disease. Precipitating causes include nausea, vomiting, and infections.
4 There are two basic types of lesions involved in ATN, though in some cases there may be a mixture of both. The less serious lesion results in necrosis of the tubular epithelium only. This lesion commonly results from mild doses of CCL₄ or HgCl₂. When only epithelial damage takes place, complete healing of the lesion commonly occurs in 3 to 4 weeks. In the second type of lesion there is necrosis of the epithelium and also the basement membrane. This is commonly associated with severe renal ischemia. The prognosis of this type of lesion depends on the extent of damage. When the basement membrane is disrupted, epithelial regeneration occurs in a haphazard manner frequently leading to obstruction of the nephron at the site of necrosis.
5 Acute cortical necrosis means that the entire nephron is infarcted. It is commonly associated with pregnancy complications such postpartum hemorrhage, premature separation of the placenta, eclampsia, and septic abortion. The prognosis is generally poor. If the patient survives the acute phase of illness, calcification and permanent renal damage often occur in the area of cortical necrosis. Glycol (antifreeze) poisoning may also cause this lesion.
6 Infection
7 c
8 b
9 a, b, d, f
10 e
11 b, c, d
12 b
13 c
14 a
15 a
16 a
17 a
18 b

The nervous system—Chap. 45

1 True
2 True
3 False; toward the cell body.
4 True
5 True
6 False; except olfactory.
7 False; brain and spinal cord.
8 False; gray matter.
9 False; lateral white matter.
10 False; nerve fibers are classified according to the direction in which they conduct impulses; they cannot be reversed.
11 b
12 c
13 d
14 d
15 a
16 b
17 a
18 c
19 d
20 b
21 e
22 a, c
23 b, c, d
24 d
25 a
26 a, c, d
27 c
28 b

ANSWERS

The neurologic examination: evaluation of the neurologic patient—Chap. 46

1 Neurologic illness is usually well defined, and a clear history will provide clues that will assist in an accurate assessment of the patient's condition.
2 Examination of the motor system (i.e., testing the gait, voluntary muscle strength, muscle tone)
Sensory examination (i.e., pain, temperature, vibration sense, examination of the reflexes)
Coordination of arms and legs
Examination of mental status and speech
Examination of cranial nerves
Examination of the reflex status
3 False; the parietal cortex.
4 True
5 False; the left hemisphere is dominant.
6 True
7 e
8 h
9 d
10 g
11 a
12 f
13 b

14 c
15 d
16 i
17 f
18 g
19 j
20 b
21 e
22 h
23 a
24 b
25 e
26 b
27 c
28 c
29 b
30 a
31 b
32 c
33 b
34 b
35 c
36 a
37 d

38 (a) Superficial tactile sensation, (b) proproceptive (motion or position sense), (c) vibratory sense, (d) cortical sensory function.

ANSWERS

Cerebrovascular disease—Chap. 47

1 b
2 b, d
3 c
4 b, d
5 The internal carotid enters the skull through the carotid canal, where it gives rise to the ophthalmic artery. The internal carotid then divides into the anterior and middle cerebral arteries. The anterior cerebral artery supplies the medial surface of the cerebrum and anastomoses with the anterior communicating artery. The middle cerebral artery supplies the lateral surfaces of the cerebral cortex. This branch joins, via the posterior communicating artery, the posterior cerebral branch of the basilar artery. The cerebral arteries and their communicating branches to the basilar artery form the circle of Willis. The basilar artery supplies the cerebellum and the brainstem. It terminates in two posterior cerebral arteries, which supply the inferior surfaces of temporal and occipital lobes. They communicate with the middle cerebral artery via the posterior communicating artery to complete the circle of Willis.
6 Extrinsic factors: (a) Systemic blood pressure: If the BP drops below 60 mmHg, the autoregulatory mechanism of the brain becomes less effective. If the BP continues to drop until CBF is decreased to 30 ml/100 g of tissue per minute, signs of cerebral ischemia will appear. (b) Cardiovascular function: If cardiac output is decreased by more than one-third, there is

likely to be a fall in CBF. (c) Blood viscosity: CBF may increase by as much as 30 percent with anemia; in polycythemia it may decrease by 50 percent.

Intrinsic factors: (a) Cerebral autoregulatory mechanism is related to cerebral perfusion pressure (difference between the cerebral artery and veins). When systemic BP decreases, there is a compensatory increase in cerebral vascular pressure, whereas, when BP increases the opposite occurs. (b) Cerebral blood vessels: These vessels are considered the most important factor relating to cerebrovascular resistance. A myogenic response proposes that parenchymal tissue of arterioles releases a vasodilatory metabolite in response to their oxygen needs on arterial smooth-muscle tone. (c) Intracranial pressure (ICP): An increase in the ICP will increase cerebrovascular resistance. However, CBF does not decrease until ICP has increased to 450 mm water.
7 200,000; 2 million
8 (a) Transient ischemic attacks (TIAs): Focal neurological deficits that develop suddenly and disappear within a few minutes to hours. (b) Progressive (stroke in evolution): Evolution of stroke is gradual though acute. (c) Completed stroke: Deficits are maximal at onset with little improvement.
9 c, d
10 a, b, c, d
11 e
12 True
13 True
14 False; cerebral tissue necrosis is not associated with TIA
15 True
16 a
17 d
18 a
19 b
20 d
21 c
22 c
23 c
24 a, b, c
25 c
26 b
27 b
28 a, b, c
29 These factors are (a) stabilization of vital signs—maintaining a patent airway and blood pressure control on an individualized basis, (b) detection and correction of cardiac arrhythmias, (c) bladder care, (d) proper positioning stressed immediately (frequent turning, ROM).
30 (a) Vasodilators have increased CBF experimentally but have not proved beneficial in human strokes. It should be noted that the use of vasodilators may exert an adverse effect on CBF by lowering systemic BP and thereby decreasing intracerebral anastomotic flow. (b) Anticoagulants exert no beneficial effect with

established strokes or those in active evolution. In TIAs they appear to decrease the frequency and severity of attacks. (c) Platelet antiaggregants have not had long-term clinical trials as yet.

31 The primary goal of surgical intervention is to improve the cerebral blood flow.

32 (a) A revascularization technique where a superficial temporal artery is anastomosed to a superficial cortical artery, or a segment of the saphenous vein is anastomosed to the subclavian artery and the proximal end of the internal carotid. (b) A carotid endarterectomy where the neck of the carotid artery is exposed. The vessel is incised at the site of stenosis, and the clot and plaque material are removed.

33 To prevent recurrent hemorrhage.

34 (a) Decrease in salt intake—especially with the elderly, extreme care to maintain blood pressure during surgical procedures; (b) avoid oversedation and prolonged bed rest; (c) Increased activity; (d) weight control, especially if obese; (e) stop cigarette smoking.

ANSWERS

Epilepsy—Chap. 48

1 A paroxysmal disorder of the nervous system characterized by recurrent attacks of loss or alteration of consciousness with or without motor convulsive phenomena. This is usually caused by excessive, uncontrolled, local discharges of a group of cerebral neurons, usually in the cortex.

2 (a) 1:200; (b) 1:20 or 10 times as frequent.

3 Cerebral vascular disease, cerebral atrophy, meningitis, diabetic acidosis, acute alcoholism

4 Midbrain, thalamus, cerebral cortex

5 Current theory refers to the possibility of "epileptic neurons" that have lower thresholds for firing abnormal discharges. A deafferented neuron has been identified in some focal lesions. These neurons are hypersensitive and in a chronic state of depolarization. The cytoplasmic membranes exhibit increased permeability making them susceptible to activation by various factors (hypoxia, hyperthermia) and circumstances (repeated sensory stimuli).

6 Metabolic needs are increased during convulsions; the electrical discharges of motor nerve cells may be increased to 1000 per second. Cerebral blood flow is increased, along with some increase in respiration and glycolysis. Acetylcholine appears in CSF during and following seizures. Glutamic acid may be depleted during seizure activity.

7 Status epilepticus refers to a state in which there is a succession (two or more) of generalized seizures with no recovery of consciousness between them.

8 a, b, c, d
9 a, b
10 c
11 d
12 b, d
13 a, c, d
14 b
15 c
16 a
17 e
18 f
19 d

ANSWERS

Degenerative diseases of the nervous system—Chap. 49

1 Caudate nucleus }
Lenticular { putamen } Corpus striatum (some authors include part of adjacent internal capsule)
nucleus { globus pallidus }
Amygdaloid nucleus
Claustrum
Red nucleus
Substantia nigra }
Subthalamic nucleus { structures closely associated with basal ganglia
(corpus Luysii)

The basal ganglia function in some way to prevent oscillation and afterdischarge in motor systems, probably by direct action on the midbrain centers and in part as inhibitory-feedback to the motor cortex. They are also involved in the control of stretch reflexes and in the generation of mannerisms and automatic activity.

2 Basal ganglia. Slow degeneration of nerve cells. Below the Cortex (subcortical).

3 Extrapyramidal motor nerve tract; it regulates semi-automatic movements, such as coordination of hand movements and swallowing.

4 It is a chronic disorder of the central nervous system characterized by a specific group of symptoms which get progressively worse (until the patient is unable to perform the activities of daily living and becomes bedridden).

Idiopathic, postencephalitic, and drug-induced Parkinsonism (the latter is a type of pseudoparkinsonism).

5 Dopamine. In the basal ganglia there is a deficiency of this substance, which is a neurotransmitter.

6 (a) Resting tremor—fine or course rhythmic alternating contraction of opposing muscle groups. Occurs at rest in disease of the basal ganglia and decreases with voluntary motion.

(b) Choreiform movement—Rapid, irregular, jerky, purposeless contractions of random muscle groups followed by prompt relaxation.

(c) Athetoid movement—continuous, slow writhing movements that may be tonic avoiding or grasping reactions.

(d) Dystonia—slow, powerful movements, like bending a lead pipe.

(e) Hemiballism—flailing, intense, violent movements involving one side of the body.

7 Phenothiazine, *Rauwolfia*

8 Hyperactive glabellar reflex; palmomental reflex; resting tremor (pill-rolling); expressionless face; festinating gait; micrographia; monotone voice; plastic or cogwheel rigidity to movements

9 Acute disseminated encephalomyelitis, in which patchy areas of demyelinization occur in the brain and spinal cord. Preventive measures include regular vaccination for measles in children and avoiding routine smallpox vaccination. The newer, killed-duck-embryo rabies vaccine should be given when it is necessary to give this drug.

10 There are widespread patches of myelin destruction and gliosis in the central nervous system. If the patient reported to you a *temporary* condition of blurring of vision in one eye, blindness, or an episode of weakness or tingling in an extremity, this would be grounds for suspicion.

11 c
12 b
13 a
14 a, c
15 c
16 b
17 b
18 d
19 c
20 c
21 c
22 d
23 c
24 d
25 c

ANSWERS

Central nervous system injury—Chap. 50

1 Normal intracranial pressure (ICP) is about 4 to 15 mmHg. The basic cause of increased ICP is an expanding mass within the rigid, bony cranium which allows very little room for expansion (about 5 cm³) before pressure starts to increase. Normally the cranial contents consist of tissue, blood, and cerebrospinal fluid (CSF). An increase in ICP can be caused by increased tissue as from a growing tumor, blood (hematoma secondary to rupture of a blood vessel), blockage of the flow of CSF and its accumulation, and cerebral edema (commonly associated with cerebral trauma). Increased ICP is dangerous because it causes cerebral ischemia, hypoxia, compression of the cortex and herniation of the brainstem through the foramen magnum. The latter causes cessation of function of the vital regulatory centers within the brainstem and death.

2 Compression of cortex: hemiparesis is due to compression of motor cortex; seizures may be due to local cortical disruption; mental dysfunction because cortex is concerned with higher thought processes.

Displacement of brainstem down into foramen magnum causing its compression: reticular formation in brainstem is concerned with level of consciousness; systolic blood pressure increases so that it will be higher than ICP and cerebral circulation will be maintained; this also causes decerebrate rigidity due to removal of normal influence of higher centers on muscle tone.

Compression of the oculomotor nerve by herniated uncus causes ipsilateral dilated pupil.

3 (a) Local tissue damage due to direct force (penetration or compression by missiles, bone fragments, or damage due to displacement of cranial contents in rapid acceleration or deceleration). (b) Cerebral ischemia due to lack of autoregulation secondary to increasing intracranial pressure.

4 Forceful thrusting of the brain contents against the inner surface of the skull on the side opposite the impact. The areas most likely to be damaged in a decelerating automobile accident are the anterior portion of the frontal and temporal lobes and the upper section of the midbrain.

5 The most common sites are where a relatively mobile portion of the vertebral column meets a relatively fixed segment. These are between the lower cervical and upper thoracic spine, between the lower thoracic and upper lumbar spine, and between the lower lumbar spine and the sacrum.

6 Stabilize the spinal column to prevent contusion, laceration, and further damage to the spinal cord from bony fragments and foreign bodies.

7 Epidural hematomas usually result from a tear in the middle meningeal artery. The bleeding occurs between the dura mater and the skull, usually in the temporal area. The development of clinical symptoms and the course is rapid and proceeds to completion within a few hours since the bleeding is arterial. On the other hand, subdural hematomas usually result from the tearing of veins which pass from the surface of the brain to one of the major dural sinuses. Blood escapes between the dura and the arachnoid. Since bleeding is under venous low pressure, the accumulation of blood may be much more prolonged, and the clinical course much more protracted.

8 a
9 All of these
10 d
11 b, c
12 c
13 b
14 a, b, c
15 b, d

16 c

17 a

18 c; loss of vibration due to destruction of dorsal (uncrossed ascending) columns and increased touch threshold due to destruction of ventral spinothalamic tract (crossed ascending axons).

19 c, d

20 c, e

21 a, d

22 b

23 False; it is between the dura and skull.

24 False; this causes quadriplegia.

25 True

26 True

27 True

28 False; surgical decompression is controversial; all agree that it should be done if there is progressive neurological deficit.

29 True

30 True

ANSWERS

Central nervous system tumors—Chap. 51

1 Because the symptoms are very diverse and depend on the location and size of the growth. However, the symptoms tend to progress. The most common general symptoms are headache, vomiting, and papilledema, all a result of increased intracranial pressure from the expanding mass.

2 b

3 d

4 a

5 c

6 e

7 d

8 b

9 a

10 c

11 g

12 f

13 c

14 d

15 b

16 a

17 e

18 c

19 f

20 d

21 e

22 a

23 b

24 d

25 c

26 d

27 a

28 a, c, e

29 a

30 b

31 d

32 d

33 c

34 True

35 True

36 False; microglia function as phagocytes.

37 True

38 True

39 False; most commonly in thoracic region.

40 False; this is amaurosis fugax. Papilledema involves engorgement and swelling of the optic disc.

41 a

42 b

43 c

44 d

45 c

46 b

ANSWERS

Concepts applied to endocrinology and metabolism—Chap. 52

1 a Response to stress and injury

b Growth and development

c Reproduction

d Maintenance of ionic homeostasis

e Control of energy metabolism

2 a One mechanism by which hormones work on cells is the adenyl cyclase system. In this case, the protein hormone interacts with its cell receptor and activates the system. Adenyl cyclase then converts adenosine triphosphate (ATP) into cyclic AMP, a secondary messenger, which enters structures of the cell to regulate the rate of protein synthesis in the cell.

b Some hormones interact with the target-cell membrane and activate prostaglandins, fatty acids which serve as intracellular messengers. It is thought that prostaglandins influence either protein synthesis or synthesis of other precursors inside the cell.

c A third mechanism by which hormones work on target cells is exemplified by steroid hormones which appear to work directly inside the cell to change the transcription of messenger RNA (and also to affect protein synthesis).

3 See Table 52-2

4 A decrease in the pressure of the blood flowing through the afferent arteriole of the renal glomerulus is sensed by JG cells causing release of renin. This results in the following sequence of events:

Renin → Renin substrate
      ↓
   Angiotensin I
      ↓
   Angiotensin II
          └────────→ Adrenal cortex
                          ↓
                      Aldosterone

TABLE 52-2

TYPE OF HORMONE	LOCATION OF PRODUCTION	EXAMPLES
a Proteins (polypeptides, glycoproteins)	Posterior pituitary gland	Pitressin
	Beta cells of islets of Langerhans	Insulin
	Adrenal medulla	Epinephrine Norepinephrine
	Thyroid gland	Thyroxine
	Parathyroid gland	Parathyroid hormone
	Anterior pituitary	Tropic hormones
b Steroids (lipids)	Adrenal cortex	Cortisol
	Gonads	Estrogen Progesterone

5 The hypothalamus possesses a variety of nuclei which are made up of neurons having a secretory function. These neurons manufacture proteins called releasing hormones which are secreted through axons into blood vessels. The hypothalamus receives fibers from other areas of the brain which influence hypothalamic neuronal function.

6 This anatomical mechanism permits the movement of neurostimuli from the hypothalamus to the pituitary gland; this is the mechanism by which the CNS influences the pituitary gland.

7 Any neurostimuli reaching the CR center causes release of CRF into the portal system. CRF causes release of ACTH by cells in the anterior pituitary gland. ACTH stimulates the adrenal cortex to produce cortisol, which affects the rate and amount of CRF-ACTH secreted by the hypothalamic pituitary axis.

8 ACTH production typically exhibits a cyclic pattern throughout the 24-hour period. The levels usually go up early in the day, go down later in the day, and go up again during the night to reach a peak level by the next morning.

9 If a disease arises from excessive production of a hormone, the problem may be treated surgically by removing the gland or part of the gland that produces the hormone. This is followed by replacement with normal amounts of the hormone. If a disease is caused by hormone deficit, the treatment is replacement of the hormones which are not being produced.

10 Hyperthyroidism
11 Hypothalamic-hypophyseal portal system
12 Thyroid-stimulating hormone (TSH)
13 True
14 False. They are specific.

ANSWERS

Cushing's syndrome and aldosteronism—Chap. 53

1 a, b, c, d
2 b
3 c
4 a, b, c
5 a, c
6 b
7 b
8 b
9 a, c
10 a
11 d
12 The catabolic effect of glucocorticoid excess causes a decrease in the ability of protein-forming cells to synthesize protein from amino acids.
13 Interferes with the action of insulin in the peripheral cells which results in the impairment of the ability of the receptor cells to metabolize glucose.
14 Stress causes the CNS to activate the corticotropin-releasing center, causing CRF and ACTH to be released. Increased ACTH leads to an increase in cortisol release. The important concept is that stress causes an increased secretion of cortisol by the adrenal gland.
15 9-Alpha-fluorocortisol has a fluorine group in the 9-alpha position of the cortisol molecule. Prednisolone has a double bond between carbons 1 and 2 of this molecule. These compounds have different metabolic effects than the parent compound. For example, prednisolone, as compared with cortisol, has less sodium-retaining activity and more anti-inflammatory activity on a per-milligram basis. 9-Alpha-fluorocortisol has much greater sodium-retaining activity than cortisol.
16 Pituitary irradiation, removal of a pituitary tumor, and adrenalectomy. The excess cortisol is eliminated if the procedure is successful.
17 Surgical removal of the neoplasm.
18 In congestive heart failure, patients are unable to pump blood normally, and cardiac output decreases. The renal afferent arteriole experiences a change in perfusion pressure causing increased production of renin which activates synthesis of angiotensin. This will stimulate aldosterone production, causing reabsorption of Na and water and volume expansion.
19 True
20 True
21 True
22 False. CRF directly initiates the secretion of ACTH.

ANSWERS

Addison's disease—Chap. 54

1 b
2 c
3 a, c
4 a
5 a, c
6 c
7 c
8 b, d
9 a, c

ANSWERS

Glucose metabolism and diabetes mellitus—Chap. 55

1 a, b
2 a, b
3 b
4 a, d
5 c
6 a, b, c
7 d
8 b
9 b
10 a, b
11 a
12 b
13 c
14 a
15 a, b, c, d
16 Fasting plasma glucose is measured in order to check the function of the regulating mechanisms which control carbohydrate metabolism. It should be noted that this method is a relatively insensitive way of checking carbohydrate metabolism.
17 Insulin. In people without diabetes, a rise in blood glucose stimulates release of insulin which triggers disposal of excess glucose.
18 This system assists diabetics in managing their own diets. The food exchange lists help patients identify food alternatives.
19 c
20 d
21 a
22 b
23 True
24 False. Seventy-five percent of diabetics die from these complications of diabetes.
25 False. Exercise appears to facilitate the transport of glucose into cells.

ANSWERS

Syndrome of androgen excess—Chap. 56

1 a, c
2 a, c, d
3 a, c, d, e
4 a, b, c, d
5 c
6 b
7 a
8 a
9 c
10 d
11 e

12 g
13 a
14 c
15 b
16 h
17 f
18 a, b, c, d
19 c, d
20 a, c, d
21 c
22 b, c, e
23 e
24 b
25 b
26 a, b, c, d
27 a, d
28 a, b, c, d
29 a, b, c, d
30 b, c, d
31 a, b
32 d
33 a, b, d
34 a, b, c, e
35 b
36 a, b, d
37 True
38 False. A 21-hydroxylase deficiency causes a decrease in cortisol and an increase in ACTH secretion.
39 True
40 True
41 False. Human growth hormone is the only one effective in humans and is used in experimental study for the treatment of hypopituitary dwarfism.

ANSWERS

Diseases of the thyroid gland—Chap. 57

1 a
2 a
3 b, c
4 d
5 b
6 b, c
7 a
8 False. This test relates the binding of thyroxine to serum proteins and the concentration of serum thyroxine.
9 False. Thyroid gland.
10 True

ANSWERS

Fractures and dislocations—Chap. 58

1 b, d
2 b
3 b, d

4 *a*
5 *b*
6 *b*
7 *c, d*
8 *b, d*
9 *d*
10 *a*
11 *c, d*
12 *b*
13 *a*
14 *a, b, d*
15 *b, c*
16 *c*
17 *a*
18 *c*
19 *b*
20 *a, c*
21 *b*
22 *c*
23 *d*
24 *b, d*
25 *c*
26 *b*
27 Refer to Fig. 58-1 below

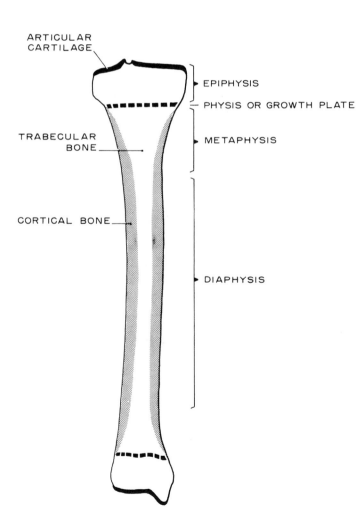

ARTICULAR CARTILAGE

EPIPHYSIS

PHYSIS OR GROWTH PLATE

TRABECULAR BONE

METAPHYSIS

CORTICAL BONE

DIAPHYSIS

FIGURE 58-1

28 False. Penetration of the skin occurs in open fractures.
29 True
30 True
31 False. In many cases, closed reduction is the act of manipulating fragments of broken bone back to their original location without surgical incision.
32 *b, d*
33 *f*
34 *a*
35 *e*
36 *c*
37 Pain, pallor, pulselessness, paresthesias
38 The limb may sustain irreversible pathologic changes within 1½ hours.
39 Persistent burning pain at the pressure sites indicates developing skin and soft-tissue necrosis; pressure may be relieved by cutting and reforming the cast.
40 Skin necrosis and neurovascular complications of circumferential dressing are avoided when skeletal traction is used.
41 Weights are attached by ropes to the patient's limb. The location of pulleys through which the ropes run is adjusted until the direction of pull is in line with the long axis of the fractured bone.
42 Traction (a) provides for limb elevation (reduces swelling) in a dependable way; (b) promotes soft-tissue healing; (c) provides for easy observation for neurovascular dysfunction; and (d) allows convenient bed care for the patient.
43 Implant devices have great intrinsic strengths and allow the fracture fragments to settle toward each other as is necessary during the healing process.
44 The goal is to return the patient as rapidly as possible to the preinjury state. The approximate duration of serious disability is often predictable, and therefore it is important to plan for rehabilitation from the day of the injury.

ANSWERS

Orthopedic diseases of children—Chap. 59

1 *a, c*
2 *d*
3 *a*
4 *b*
5 *b*
6 *c*
7 In children, the periosteal sleeve around the tubular bones is *strong and active,* allowing for rapid healing.
8 Children's limbs grow very quickly; bayonette apposition is often used to achieve equal length by adulthood.

f Rheumatoid nodules
g Chronicity
h Extraarticular manifestations

ANSWERS

Tumors of the musculoskeletal system—Chap. 60

1 True
2 False. Pathologic fractures are generally the result of metastasis of malignant tumor to bone.
3 True
4 False. Metastasis from a primary site to bone is frequently found in adults, not children.
5 a
6 b
7 c
8 b

ANSWERS

Anatomy and physiology of the joints—Chap. 61

1 The three categories are:
  a Fibrous connective tissue b Cartilage c Bone
2 The major function of connective tissue is to provide support and protection for the body and internal organs. Connective tissue also has a major role in the transmission of nutrients and waste products, and in the inflammatory and reparative processes that occur in injured tissue.
3 c
4 a
5 b, d
6 b, c
7 b, d

ANSWERS

Rheumatoid arthritis—Chap. 62

1 b
2 a
3 a Relief of pain and inflammation b Maintenance of joint function and maximum functional capacity of the patient c Prevention and/or correction of deformities
4 Aspirin
5 a Moist heat: bath, wet towels
  b Dry heat: lamp, heating pad
6 a Constitutional symptoms: fatigue, anorexia, weight loss, fever
  b Symmetrical polyarthritis
  c Morning stiffness
  d Erosive arthritis
  e Deformity

ANSWERS

Psoriatic arthritis, ankylosing spondylitis, and Reiter's syndrome—Chap. 63

1 True
2 False. Psoriatic arthritis is usually not as destructive to the joints as rheumatoid arthritis.
3 False. Therapeutic doses of salicylates or other anti-inflammatory agents are used to treat Reiter's syndrome.
4 True
5 Urethritis, conjunctivitis, and arthritis (may include mucocutaneous lesions and keratodermia blennorrhagicum)
6 Male
7 Aspirin, indomethacin (Indocin), and phenylbutazone (Butazolidin)
8 Firm mattress, sleeping flat without a pillow; breathing exercises in order to increase breathing capacity as chest expansion decreases.
9 a
10 9:1
11 Low-back pain

ANSWERS

Polymyositis, dermatomyositis, and progressive systemic sclerosis (scleroderma)—Chap. 64

1 Prednisone (steroids, corticosteroids)
2 Upper
3 Progressive systemic sclerosis (PSS)
4 Dysphagia, or difficulty in swallowing
5 Female
6 Female
7 Early edematous changes progressing to thickening and tightening of skin; finally, the skin appears taut and shiny ("hide bound") (further description: telangiectasis, subcutaneous calcifications).
8 Possible answers are: Gastrointestinal, cardiac, pulmonary, renal, skin, and musculoskeletal.
9 Respiratory infections (e.g., pneumonia, aspiration pneumonitis) or difficulty in breathing (dyspnea)
10 True

ANSWERS

Systemic lupus erythematosus (SLE)—Chap. 65

1 Autoimmunity is a condition in which a patient's antibodies attempt to destroy the patient's own tissue or cells as if they were foreign.

2 Match your answer against the clinical features listed in this section.

3 The arthritis in SLE is a nondeforming arthritis as opposed to the erosive, destructive, and deforming type in rheumatoid arthritis.

4 Antinuclear antibody, or ANA

5 False. The lowest dose possible is used to treat SLE because of the side effects of long-term use of this drug.

6 True

Should contact her physician:

7 May be pleuritis, a reactivation of her lupus; she may need a brief boost in prednisone dose.

10 May indicate gastrointestinal bleeding as a side effect of the prednisone.

13 May indicate a flare of lupus; especially since arthritis is a problem for this patient, there is also the possibility that this is an infection which must be promptly treated.

Not necessary to contact physician:

8 Mild fatigue is a common part of this disease, and unless it increases and becomes severe, it is not indicative of a flare.

9 Increase in appetite is an expected side effect of prednisone which is important only to the patient who should not gain weight.

11 A missed period need not be promptly reported since prednisone can cause menstrual disorders. It is important, however, if the patient thinks she is pregnant to follow up this possibility with a pregnancy test.

12 It is an expected side effect from prednisone.

ANSWERS

Gout—Chap. 66

1 Hyperuricemia, or high serum uric acid
2 Colchicine
3 Chronic gouty arthritis, tophaceous deposits (urate deposits) in tissue, or urinary calculi
4 True
5 True
6 True

ANSWERS

Infectious arthritis and degenerative joint disease (osteoarthritis)—Chap. 67

1 *Staphylococcus aureus, Diplococcus pneumonia, Streptococcus pyogenes,* or *Neisseria gonorrhea*
2 Any of the following:
   a Other systemic disease b Treatment with immunosuppressives c Joint injury or inflammatory process d Septic area elsewhere in body e Invasive procedure (source of infection)
3 Pain, stiffness, and deformity
4 Any two of the following:
   a Sex b Excessive use c Trauma
   d Genetic influence
5 Aspirin, Indocin, Darvon
6 Joint fluid
7 False. Steroids would lower the patient's ability to fight the infection. Antibiotics are used as therapy.
8 True
9 True
10 True
11 False. Although the disease process may begin as early as the second decade, it most commonly affects the elderly.

Index